ASTHMA IN THE WORKPLACE

THIRD EDITION

ASTHMA IN THE WORKPLACE

And Related Conditions

THIRD EDITION

edited by

I. Leonard Bernstein
University of Cincinnati
Cincinnati, Ohio, U.S.A.

Moira Chan-Yeung
University of British Columbia
Vancouver, British Columbia, Canada

Jean-Luc Malo
Université de Montréal
Montreal, Quebec, Canada

David I. Bernstein
University of Cincinnati
Cincinnati, Ohio, U.S.A.

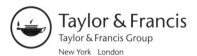

Taylor & Francis
Taylor & Francis Group
New York   London

Published in 2006 by
Taylor & Francis Group
270 Madison Avenue
New York, NY 10016

Library of Congress Cataloging-in-Publication Data

Catalog record is available from the Library of Congress

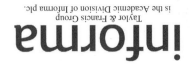

informa

Taylor & Francis Group
is the Academic Division of Informa plc.

Visit the Taylor & Francis Web site at
http://www.taylorandfrancis.com

Preface

Interest in occupationally induced lung diseases has been focused chiefly on dust-induced disorders since the earliest description of miners' lung disease by both Agricola and Paracelsus in the middle of the 16th century. It is therefore not surprising that contemporary textbooks of occupational lung disease have emphasized ailments that, until recently, were very common in industrialized countries and could be detected by progressive radiological changes, permanent loss of pulmonary function, and unique structural histological characteristics. In industrialized countries, the "picture" has changed in recent years with the significant reduction in dust-induced lung diseases (e.g., silicosis, asbestosis) because of efficient environmental control. However, the effect of asbestos exposure can still be seen from the steady increase in mesothelioma and bronchial carcinoma. On the other hand, the frequency of occupational asthma has increased with a recent plateau and is now the most prevalent occupational lung disease in these countries (see Chapter 14). Although occupational asthma was recognized as early as the 18th century by Ramazzini, its importance as a significant hazard in the workplace was not widely appreciated until the spurt in industrial technology after World War II. The literature concerning workplace asthma has steadily increased since the great impetus given by Professor Jack Pepys, who can be considered the father of occupational asthma and to whom this book is dedicated. Specialists have recognized that asthma may now be one of the most common work-related respiratory diseases. Recent journal reviews, book chapters, monographs, and Web sites also document the proliferation in the number of specific causes of occupational asthma.

Asthma in the workplace is a complex entity that is not equivalent to new onset occupational asthma as defined in the first chapter of the book. The chapter on definitions (Chapter 1) has been revised to account for the fact that approximately 10% of asthmatic subjects note that the workplace worsens their asthma symptoms. A proportion develop new onset occupational asthma, defined as "asthma caused by the workplace," whereas many others are affected by work-exacerbated asthma. The diagnosis of occupational asthma is often difficult because of multiple causality in many occupational environments, the variability of symptoms and patterns of late-phase asthmatic reactions, the requirements for special diagnostic procedures, and the unpredictability of onset and persistence of symptoms. Outbreaks of occupational asthma in specific work settings are ideal, mini-epidemiological paradigms of nonoccupational asthma. Such outbreaks provide excellent opportunities for investigating the source, the characteristics of the emission–dispersion cycles, and the health impact of inciting agents. Environmental sampling for monitoring the concentration of both chemicals and proteins is available in many occupational situations where work-related asthma has occurred (see Chapters 11–13). The ready access to such integrated data in a defined milieu provides an ideal setting for further advancement of knowledge about the pathophysiological pathways and natural history of asthma.

These expanded opportunities have attracted the collaborative interests of allergists, immunologists, pulmonologists, immunotoxicologists, occupational health specialists, aerosol scientists, hygienists, and epidemiologists. In addition, the economic and social hardships imposed on workers who have refractory symptoms associated with occupational asthma require consultation with medicolegal experts. These interactions have clearly established that the features of occupational asthma are unique and often at odds with medical dogma derived from the surveillance, diagnosis, and prevention of mineral dust–induced lung disorders. Combined with the recent upsurge of scientific interest and literature in the pathophysiology of asthma in the general population, these considerations convinced us that a textbook dealing with occupational asthma was overdue. The enthusiastic response to publication of the first and second editions and the number of literature citations attributed to it have more than justified preparation of a third edition.

As is the case with most new fields of health-related expertise, discovery and research in workplace-related asthma have continued at a rapid pace and have served as the impetus for this updated and revised edition. In addition, coverage of several specific areas of interest that had not yet clearly evolved prior to publication of the first and second editions has been either added or expanded.

Because new advances in workplace-related asthma are international in scope, the coalition of editors and individual contributors in this book is a reflection of this orientation. The common goal of this cooperative effort was to prepare an authoritative, educational resource for primary care physicians, occupational health specialists, allergists, and pulmonologists. A reference book of this type was considered particularly germane for primary care providers because current mandates for early detection and reporting of occupational asthma require that these physicians develop skills that lead to early recognition of this disease. To this end, special emphasis has been given to an algorithm of clinical diagnosis, immunological evaluation, and physiological methods of evaluation (see Chapters 7–10) as a practical guide for primary care physicians. Special chapters on medicolegal aspects, compensation, assessment of disability, prevention, and surveillance (Chapters 14 and 15) address the social outcomes of workers disabled by asthma and should serve as useful reference sources for occupational health physicians, workers' compensation administrators, private insurers, attorneys, adjudicators, and legislators. The chapters concerning epidemiology and disease entities have been prepared to provide sufficient in-depth information for occupational health and other medical subspecialists primarily concerned with asthma in the workplace. Although occupational asthma represents the core of this book, this third edition includes new chapters on asthma exacerbated at work and asthma-like syndromes, with all conditions being grouped under the general theme of "asthma in the workplace." Conditions that share clinical, functional, or immunological features to workplace asthma (chronic obstructive pulmonary disease due to occupational exposure, hypersensitivity pneumonitis, building-related illnesses) are covered in specific chapters (Chapters 28–30). The relationship of conditions frequently associated with workplace asthma is reviewed in Chapters 31 and 32 ("Upper Airways Involvement" and "Occupational Urticaria").

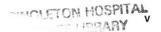
This book is organized into four main sections:

Part I, "General Considerations," contains chapters on definitions, historical background, epidemiology, genetics, pathophysiology, and animal models.

Part II, "Assessment and Management," includes chapters that delineate the basic guidelines for clinical and objective evaluation, environmental monitoring, and prevention of occupational asthma. Medicolegal aspects and surveillance strategies are also discussed in this section.

Part III, "Specific Agents Causing Occupational Asthma with a Latency Period," provides detailed information about specific agents (including a variety of high- and low-molecular-weight agents) that induce asthma or asthma-like diseases.

Part IV, "Specific Disease Entities and Variants," covers other types of work-related asthma conditions, e.g., irritant-induced asthma, asthma exacerbated at work and asthma-like syndromes. Chronic airflow obstruction due to occupational exposure, hypersensitivity pneumonitis, and building-related illnesses are also covered in this part of the book.

The book also contains a compendium, in particular a table that lists the major protein and chemical inducers of occupational asthma, the type of workplaces or occupations in which these occur, pertinent immunological and physiological evidence, and key literature references.

In a sense, the preparation of individual chapters by multiple authors and the endeavor that the authors have put forth in this third edition is similar to meta-analyses that compare different published health-related data pertaining to a given research question. As often occurs with meta-analyses, agreement at times is incomplete. Above all, the authors and editors have attempted to balance opposing views as objectively as possible. In most cases, this balancing process was successful in arriving at editorial consensus. Where this was not possible, the data appear with the caveat that a controversy exists and resolution is not possible, because definitive data are either not yet available or under investigation. These critical assessments have been rewarding educational experiences for the editors and authors. We hope that this joint effort will not only provide pragmatic information for current clinical applications, but also serve as a foundation for significant new research information that will most assuredly advance the discipline during this new millennium.

I. Leonard Bernstein
Moira Chan-Yeung
Jean-Luc Malo
David I. Bernstein

Contents

PART I: GENERAL CONSIDERATIONS

Contents

Contents

PART IV: SPECIFIC DISEASE ENTITIES AND VARIANTS

25. Reactive Airways Dysfunction Syndrome and Irritant-Induced Asthma · 581
Denyse Gautrin, I. Leonard Bernstein, Stuart M. Brooks, and Paul K. Henneberger

26. Asthma Exacerbated at Work · · · · · · · · · · · · · · · · 631
Gregory R. Wagner and Paul K. Henneberger

Contributors

Xaver Baur Department of Occupational Medicine, Ordinariat und Zentral Institut für Arbeitsmedizin Hamburg, Institute of Occupational Medicine, University of Hamburg, Hamburg, Germany

Margaret R. Becklake Respiratory Epidemiology and Clinical Research Unit, Departments of Medicine and Epidemiology, Biostatistics, and Occupational Health, McGill University, Montreal, Quebec, Canada

Donald Beezhold Analytical Services Branch, NIOSH, Morgantown, West Virginia, U.S.A.

David I. Bernstein Division of Allergy–Immunology, Department of Internal Medicine, College of Medicine, University of Cincinnati, Cincinnati, Ohio, U.S.A.

I. Leonard Bernstein Division of Allergy–Immunology, Department of Internal Medicine, College of Medicine, University of Cincinnati, Cincinnati, Ohio, U.S.A.

Jonathan A. Bernstein Division of Allergy–Immunology, Department of Internal Medicine, College of Medicine, University of Cincinnati, Cincinnati, Ohio, U.S.A.

Raymond E. Biagini Biomonitoring and Health Assessment Branch, Robert A. Taft Laboratories, NIOSH/CDC, Cincinnati, Ohio, U.S.A.

Paul D. Blanc Division of Occupational and Environmental Medicine, Department of Medicine, University of California–San Francisco, San Francisco, California, U.S.A.

Stuart M. Brooks College of Public Health, University of South Florida, Tampa, Florida, U.S.A.

P. Sherwood Burge Occupational Lung Disease Unit, Birmingham Heartlands Hospital, Birmingham, U.K.

Robert K. Bush Allergy Section, William S. Middle Veterans Affairs Hospital, Madison, Wisconsin, U.S.A.

Paloma Campo   Division of Allergy–Immunology, Department of Internal Medicine, College of Medicine, University of Cincinnati, Cincinnati, Ohio, U.S.A.

André Cartier   Department of Chest Medicine, Université de Montréal and Sacré-Cœur Hospital, Montreal, Quebec, Canada

Moira Chan-Yeung   Occupational and Environmental Lung Disease Unit, Respiratory Division, Department of Medicine, University of British Columbia and Vancouver General Hospital, Vancouver, British Columbia, Canada

David C. Christiani   Department of Environmental Health, Harvard School of Public Health, and Department of Medicine, Massachusetts General Hospital/Harvard Medical School, Boston, Massachusetts, U.S.A.

Yvon Cormier   Institut Universitaire de Cardiologie et de Pneumologie, Laval University and Hospital, Laval, Quebec, Canada

Leonardo M. Fabbri   Section of Respiratory Diseases, Department of Oncology and Hematology, University of Modena, Modena, Italy

Denyse Gautrin   Université de Montréal, Montreal, Quebec, Canada

Susan Gordon   Institute of Occupational Medicine, Riccarton, Edinburgh, Scotland, U.K.

Dick Heederik   Division of Environmental and Occupational Health, Institute for Risk Assessment Sciences, University of Utrecht, Utrecht, The Netherlands

Paul K. Henneberger   Division of Respiratory Disease Studies, NIOSH/CDC, Morgantown, West Virginia, U.S.A.

Eva Hnizdo   Division of Respiratory Disease Studies, NIOSH, Morgantown, West Virginia, U.S.A.

Anthony Johnson   Research and Education Unit, Workers' Compensation (Dust Diseases) Board, Sydney, New South Wales, Australia

Victor J. Johnson   Toxicology and Molecular Biology Branch, Health Effects Laboratory Division, NIOSH/CDC, Morgantown, West Virginia, U.S.A.

Susan M. Kennedy   School of Occupational and Environmental Hygiene, University of British Columbia, Vancouver, British Columbia, Canada

Helena Keskinen   Finnish Institute of Occupational Health, Helsinki, Finland

Kathleen Kreiss   Division of Respiratory Disease Studies, NIOSH Field Studies Branch, NIOSH, Morgantown, West Virginia, U.S.A.

Catherine Lemiere   Department of Chest Medicine, Sacré-Cœur Hospital, Montreal, Quebec, Canada

Jacques Lesage   Laboratory Services and Expertise, Institut de Recherche Robert-Sauvé en Santé et en Sécurité du Travail, Montreal, Quebec, Canada

Gary M. Liss   Gage Occupational and Environmental Health Unit, Department of Public Health Sciences, University of Toronto, and Occupational Health and Safety Branch, Ontario Ministry of Labour, Toronto, Ontario, Canada

Boris D. Lushniak   Office of Counterterrorism Policy and Planning, U.S. Food and Drug Administration, Rockville, Maryland, U.S.A.

Michael I. Luster   Toxicology and Molecular Biology Branch, Health Effects Laboratory Division, NIOSH/CDC, Morgantown, West Virginia, U.S.A.

Piero Maestrelli   Department of Environmental Medicine and Public Health, University of Padova, Padova, Italy

Jean-Luc Malo   Department of Chest Medicine, Université de Montréal and Sacré-Cœur Hospital, Montreal, Quebec, Canada

Cristina E. Mapp   Section of Hygiene and Occupational Medicine, Department of Clinical and Experimental Medicine, University of Ferrara, Ferrara, Italy

C. G. Toby Mathias   Departments of Environmental Health and Dermatology, University of Cincinnati Medical Center and Group Health Associates, Cincinnati, Ohio, U.S.A.

Dick Menzies   Respiratory Epidemiology Unit, Department of Medicine and Epidemiology and Biostatistics, Montreal Chest Institute, McGill University, Montreal, Quebec, Canada

Rolf Merget   Research Institute for Occupational Medicine of the Institutions for Statutory Accident Insurance and Prevention (BGFA), Ruhr-University, Bochum, Germany

Gianna Moscato   Allergy and Immunology Unit, Fondazione Salvatore Maugeri, IRCCS, Scientific Institute of Pavia, Pavia, Italy

Anthony J. Newman-Taylor   Department of Occupational and Environmental Medicine, National Heart and Lung Institute, Royal Brompton and Harefield NHS Trust, London, U.K.

Mark Nieuwenhuijsen   Division of Primary Care and Population Health Sciences, Department of Epidemiology and Public Health, Imperial College London, London, U.K.

Henrik Nordman Department of Occupational Medicine, Finnish Institute of Occupational Health, Helsinki, Finland

Hae-Sim Park Department of Allergy and Rheumatology, Ajou University School of Medicine, Youngtongku, Suwon, South Korea

Jack Pepys[†] Royal Postgraduate Medical School, London, U.K.

Guy Perrault Consultation en R and D et Expertise en SST, Laval, Quebec, Canada

Santiago Quirce Department of Allergy, Fundación Jiménez Díaz, Madrid, Spain

Carrie A. Redlich Department of Internal Medicine, Yale University, New Haven, Connecticut, U.S.A.

Katherine Sarlo Central Product Safety Organization, Miami Valley Laboratories, The Procter and Gamble Company, Cincinnati, Ohio, U.S.A.

Mark Schuyler Department of Internal Medicine, University of New Mexico School of Medicine, Albuquerque, New Mexico, U.S.A.

David A. Schwartz Duke University Medical Center and Durham Department of Veterans Affairs Medical Center, Durham, North Carolina, U.S.A.

Jaspal Singh Department of Medicine, Duke University Medical Center, Durham, North Carolina, U.S.A.

Andrea Siracusa Department of Clinical and Experimental Medicine, University of Perugia, Perugia, Italy

Mark C. Swanson Mayo Foundation, Rochester, Minnesota, U.S.A.

Susan M. Tarlo Gage Occupational and Environmental Health Unit, Departments of Medicine and Public Health Sciences, University of Toronto, and The Asthma Centre, Toronto Western Hospital, University Health Network, Toronto, Ontario, Canada

Kjell Toren Departments of Occupational and Environmental Medicine and Allergology, Sahlgrenska University Hospital, Sahlgrenska Academy at Göteborg University, Göteborg, Sweden

Olivier Vandenplas Department of Chest Medicine, Mont-Godinne Hospital, Catholic University of Louvain, Yvoir, Belgium

---

[†]Deceased.

Susanna Von Essen   Pulmonary and Critical Care Medicine Section, Department of Internal Medicine, University of Nebraska Medical Center, Omaha, Nebraska, U.S.A.

Gregory R. Wagner   Department of Environmental Health, Harvard School of Public Health, Boston, Massachusetts, and NIOSH, Washington, D.C., U.S.A.

Adam V. Wisnewski   Department of Internal Medicine, Yale University, New Haven, Connecticut, U.S.A.

Berran Yucesoy   Toxicology and Molecular Biology Branch, Health Effects Laboratory Division, NIOSH/CDC, Morgantown, West Virginia, U.S.A.

C. Raymond Zeiss   Allergy/Immunology Division, Northwestern/Feinberg School of Medicine, Chicago, Illinois, U.S.A.

Introduction

Asthma has long been recognized as a disease associated with reversible airway obstruction. However, it was only in the latter half of the twentieth century that mechanisms of asthma pathogenesis began to be explored and effective therapies evolved. During this time, the important role of occupational exposure in the pathogenesis of asthma began to be described; occupational asthma is now recognized to be one of the most common work-related diseases.

The textbook *Asthma in the Workplace* was created to provide a comprehensive and fully documented book that provides both the scientific basis and the treatment of asthma associated with the workplace. Each subsequent edition has added new insights. The text has encouraged collaborations among multiple disciplines. Advances in the field are international in scope, and this is reflected in the list of authors. The strategy of the text has been to relate scientific principles to the diagnosis and care of asthma in the workplace. To this end, the book begins with a section describing underlying scientific principles, followed by sections on assessment and management, specific agents, and specific diseases. Future research needs are also addressed in many chapters.

During the years since the last edition, there has been growth in both the basic and clinical understanding of occupational asthma, and the third edition attempts to provide this information to the reader. For example, more attention has been given to chronic obstructive lung diseases in relation to occupational impact. The chapters on animal models, genetics, and medicolegal aspects have been expanded. The editors have brought new contributors and new issues into the text.

Finding the answers to occupational asthma continues to be similar to a "who done it" detective novel, but in this case the discoveries can save real lives. Hats off to the authors who share their expertise, provide educational opportunities to the reader, and thus improve the care of patients.

Jay A. Nadel, M.D.
University of California–San Francisco
San Francisco, California, U.S.A.

1

Definition and Classification of Asthma in the Workplace

I. Leonard Bernstein and David I. Bernstein
Division of Allergy–Immunology, Department of Internal Medicine, College of Medicine, University of Cincinnati, Cincinnati, Ohio, U.S.A.

Moira Chan-Yeung
Occupational and Environmental Lung Disease Unit, Respiratory Division, Department of Medicine, University of British Columbia and Vancouver General Hospital, Vancouver, British Columbia, Canada

Jean-Luc Malo
Department of Chest Medicine, Université de Montréal and Sacré-Cœur Hospital, Montreal, Quebec, Canada

INTRODUCTION

Definitions vary with time according to the current status of evidence and changing diagnostic means. Definitions also vary according to purposes for which they are used as in epidemiology, surveillance programs, clinical diagnosis, and medicolegal jurisdiction. Because the consensus definition of asthma has improved its recognition and management in recent years, precise and workable definitions of occupational asthma (OA) are required to improve its investigation and management.

CLASSIFICATION OF ASTHMA IN THE WORKPLACE

The workplace can trigger or induce asthma (Fig. 1). In the broad spectrum of asthma conditions related to the workplace, some nosological entities can be identified based on the strength of the causal relationship, clinical and objective features, and/or physiopathological mechanisms (Table 1) (1).

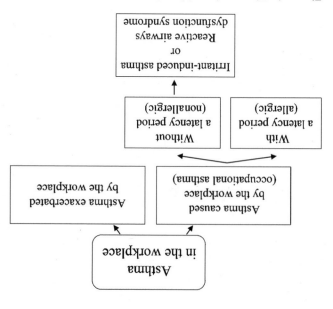

Figure 1 Phenotypic entities of occupational asthma.

DEFINITIONS

Occupational Asthma

To avoid ambiguity in defining OA in this book, an editorial basis for consensus was sought by analyzing the essential content of prior definitions of OA:

1. A broad definition that describes asthma caused by any agent specific to the workplace. Several definitions have included this feature. Those by Brooks, Sheppard, Parkes, Newman-Taylor, as well as by Chan-Yeung and Malo specify that the causal agent should be specific to the workplace.

   a. "Occupational asthma is a disorder in which there is generalized obstruction of the airways, usually reversible, caused by inhalation of a substance or a material that a worker manufactures or uses directly or is incidentally present at the worksite" (2).

   b. "Although the term 'occupational asthma' usually refers to new onset asthma caused by workplace exposure, exacerbations of preexisting asthma are an equally important cause of workplace morbidity.... extreme sensitivity of airways to chemical, physical and pharmacological stimuli is a characteristic feature of asthma. Thus many agents encountered in the workplace that have little or no effect on non-asthmatic workers can cause pronounced symptomatic broncho-constriction in workers with asthma" (3).

   c. "Occupational asthma, therefore, is caused by some specific agent or agents in the form of dust, fumes or vapors in an industrial environment" (4).

   d. "Occupational asthma is variable airways narrowing causally related to exposure in the working environment to airborne dust, gases, vapors, or fumes" (5).

Table 1 A Nosological Classification of Asthma in the Workplace

	OA		Work-aggravated asthma
	Allergic	Nonallergic (acute irritant-induced asthma)	
Causes	All high- and some low-molecular-weight agents	Exposure to agents present at high concentrations	Agents with irritant properties
Mechanisms	IgE medicated for all high- and some low-molecular-weight agents; cellular immunity?	Acute irritant injury to bronchi	Probably related to airway hyperresponsiveness caused by nonwork-related conditions
Essential features	Latency period of exposure and sensitization prior to onset of symptoms	Sudden onset No latency period	Work-related asthma symptoms
Evidence of causal relationship	Demonstration of specific IgE by skin testing or in vitro assays	Temporal relationship between exposure to agents present in high concentrations and the rapid onset of nasal and/or lower respiratory symptoms	Exclusion of OA
Objective diagnosis means used	Assessment of airway caliber, responsiveness, and inflammation at work and away from work Serial PEFR Specific inhalation challenges	Assessment of airway caliber and responsiveness after the inhalational accident(s)	Assessment of airway, caliber, responsiveness, and inflammation at work and away from work
Outcome	Improvement on removal from exposure; often with persistent airway hyperresponsiveness	Improvement on removal from exposure; often with persistent airway hyperresponsiveness	Unknown

Abbreviations: IgE, immunoglobin E; OA, occupational asthma; PEFR, peak expiratory flow rate.

e. "Occupational asthma will be defined as asthma caused by specific agents in the workplace. This will exclude bronchoconstriction induced by irritants at work, exercise and cold air." (6). The word "specific" used in these definitions can easily be understood if it is contrasted to "nonspecific" stimuli to which all asthmatic subjects react (irritants, fumes, exercise, and cold air). Therefore, "specific" used in this context refers to any agent or exposure that is present in the workplace that directly results in OA.

2. Narrower definitions can be used to describe OA caused by sensitizing agents specific to the workplace. These definitions specifically apply to agents that are present in the workplace and exert their effects through "sensitization" mechanisms. Such definitions have been proposed by Cotes and Steel as well as by Burge.

a. "Occupational asthma is caused by exposure at a place of work to a sensitizing bronchoconstrictor agent" (7).

b. "Occupational asthma is asthma which is due in whole or in part to agents met at work. Once occupational sensitization has occurred ..." (8).

In these definitions, the nature of the "sensitizing" mechanism is not alluded to, although it can be assumed as originating from a classical allergic process.

The key element common to all of the aforementioned definitions is the presence of a causal relationship between workplace exposure and the development of work-related asthma. It therefore seems logical to limit the definition of OA to those conditions in which the asthma is induced or caused by occupation, as originally proposed by professor Jack Pepys: "Having made a diagnosis of asthma ("widespread airways obstruction reversible over short periods of time, either spontaneously or as a result of treatment"), it is then necessary in occupational asthma to establish a relationship to the work as recommended by Ramazzini in 1713" (9).

Agents causing OA can be referred to as inducers. Inducers cause airway obstruction, hyperresponsiveness and inflammation but inciters do not (10). All asthmatic subjects react to inciters but only a minority to inducers.

Editorial Consensus Definition of OA

After deliberating on the diversity of opinion represented in the above references, the editors adopted the following definition, which allows sufficient latitude to include both allergic and nonallergic causes of OA:

Occupational asthma is a disease characterized by variable airflow limitation and/or hyperresponsiveness and/or inflammation due to causes and conditions attributable to a particular occupational environment and not to stimuli encountered outside the workplace.

Two types of OA are distinguished based on their appearance after a latency period.

1. After a latency period (allergic).
This category is characterized by work-related asthma appearing after a latency period and encompasses (i) OA caused by most high- and certain low-molecular-weight agents for which an allergic [immunoglobulin E

(IgE)–mediated] mechanism has been proven, and (*ii*) OA induced by specific occupational agents (e.g., western red cedar) but the allergic mechanisms responsible have not yet been fully characterized.

2. Without a latency period (nonallergic).
   This category includes irritant-induced asthma or reactive airways dysfunction syndrome (RADS), which may occur after single or multiple exposures to nonspecific irritants at high concentrations. Activation of preexistent asthma or airway hyperresponsiveness by nontoxic irritants or physical stimuli in the workplace ordinarily is excluded by this definition. (See definition of "work-exacerbated asthma.")

Work-Exacerbated Asthma

The term work-exacerbated asthma is used to describe the worsening of preexisting or coincident (adult new-onset) asthma because of workplace environmental exposure (Chapter 26) (11). Aggravation of asthma in the workplace can manifest as an increase in frequency or severity of asthma symptoms and/or increase in medication required to control symptoms on working days. These clinical features are similar to those encountered in OA; on the contrary, several studies have shown that subjects who experience exacerbation of asthma symptoms at work fail to demonstrate significant objective evidence of the asthma worsening when they are exposed to the suspected agent and monitored either in their workplace or in the laboratory (12,13). Work-exacerbated asthma and OA are not mutually exclusive, and rarely, both could coexist in certain workers.

The prevalence of work-exacerbated asthma is not known, although it is likely to be a common condition. It has been estimated that approximately 10% to 15% of all adult-onset asthma can be attributable to the workplace (14). This percentage includes both OA and work-exacerbated asthma. As the economic burden of work-exacerbated asthma to the individuals and to the society is similar to OA, we need a great deal of research on its physiopathology, optimal management, and long-term consequences.

NOSOLOGICAL WORKING DEFINITIONS FOR DIAGNOSTIC AND EPIDEMIOLOGICAL PURPOSES

The strength and the nature of the causal relationship between exposure and onset of symptoms or disease vary according to the purposes. The practicing physician has to examine if a subject referred as "asthma in the workplace" has OA. For diagnosing OA, the physician therefore needs a more stringent association and will use more time-consuming, expensive, and invasive diagnostic procedures. The epidemiologist who conducts field studies is interested in identifying cases of "asthma in the workplace"; the epidemiologist's intention is not to diagnose OA but to identify disease susceptibility factors. For the occupational physician who runs a medical surveillance program, when early detection of disease is desirable, the requirement will again be different.

It is therefore convenient to have working definitions for asthma in the workplace as for other conditions such as cardiovascular diseases (15). Such schemes for ascertaining asthma in the workplace have been proposed for clinical purposes previously (see the consensus panel of experts from the American College of Chest Physicians, Table 2) (11) and for epidemiological or surveillance surveys (see proposal

Table 2 Criteria for Defining Occupational Asthma Proposed by the American College of Chest Physicians

A   Diagnosis of asthma
B   Onset of symptoms after entering the workplace
C   Association between symptoms of asthma and work
D   One or more of the following criteria:
    1   Workplace exposure to an agent or process known to give rise to occupational asthma
    2   Significant work-related changes in FEV_1 or peak expiratory flow rate
    3   Significant work-related changes in nonspecific airway responsiveness
    4   Positive response to specific inhalation challenge tests with an agent to which the patient is exposed at work
    5   Onset of asthma with a clear association with a symptomatic exposure to an irritant agent in the workplace RADS

Requirements
  Occupational asthma:
    Surveillance case definition: A + B + C + D1 or D2 or D3 or D4 or D5
    Medical case definition: A + B + C + D2 or D3 or D4 or D5
    Likely occupational asthma: A + B + C + D1
  Work-aggravated asthma: A + C (i.e., the subject was symptomatic or required medication before and had an increase in symptoms or medication requirement after entering a new occupational exposure setting)

Abbreviations: RADS, reactive airways dysfunction syndrome; FEV_1, forced expiratory volume in one second.
Source: From Ref. 11.

by the National Institute for Occupational Safety and Health (Table 3) (17). These definitions incorporate different levels of evidence that result in various positive and negative predictive values for recognizing the link between exposure and the defined condition.

Table 3 Surveillance Case Definition of Occupational Asthma Proposed by the SENSOR

Health care professional's diagnosis of asthma
An association between symptoms of asthma and work
One or more of the following criteria:
  Increased asthma symptoms or increased use of asthma medication (upon entering an occupational exposure setting) experienced by a person with preexisting asthma who was symptomatic or treated with asthma medication within the 2 years prior to entering that new occupational setting (work-aggravated asthma)
  New asthma symptoms that develop within 24 hours after a one-time high-level inhalation exposure (at work) to an irritant gas, fume, smoke, or vapor and that persist for at least 3 months (reactive airways dysfunction syndrome)
  Workplace exposure to an agent or process previously associated with occupational asthma
  Work-related changes in serially measured FEV_1 or peak expiratory flow rate
  Work-related changes in bronchial responsiveness as measured by serial nonspecific inhalation challenge testing
  Positive response to specific inhalation challenge testing with an agent to which the patient has been exposed at work

Abbreviations: SENSOR, Sentinel Event Notification Systems for Occupational Risks; FEV_1, forced expiratory volume in one second.
Source: From Ref. 16.

Asthma-Like Disorders and Variants

Asthma-like disorders typically present with asthma-like symptoms associated with one or more objective asthmatic features, i.e., a significant cross-shift change in forced exipiratory volume (FEV), "medium-range" or partial degree of reversibility in airway obstruction, bronchial hyperresponsiveness, and airway inflammation (eosinophilic and/or neutrophilic). A cross-shift decrease in FEV_1 may predict later development of chronic airflow limitation as in byssinosis, a textile dust disease, which affects the airways of workers exposed to cotton, flax, hemp, jute, or sisal (Chapter 27). Symptoms and functional evidence of partially reversible obstructive airflow limitation occur after exposure to grain dusts or in workers of aluminum potrooms (Chapter 23). There is also evidence that exposure to inorganic dusts such as silica and silicon carbide causes airway obstruction with some reversibility and bronchial hyperresponsiveness (Chapter 28) (18,19). In another condition, eosinophilic bronchitis, there is evidence of eosinophilic airway inflammation but without evidence of reversible airway obstruction or bronchial hyperresponsiveness, which may represent a preasthmatic state.

CONCLUSION

This book aims at presenting the whole spectrum of asthma in the workplace. OA represents a condition in which the disease is asthma and the causal relationship of the disease with exposure is a key element. Therefore, this condition constitutes the principal part of the presentation. Because OA is often associated with involvement of other target organs (nose, eyes, and skin), these conditions are also addressed. Work-exacerbated asthma is relatively more common compared to OA and is frequently responsible for loss of earnings. It represents a situation in which the causal relationship between the disease and the occupational environment is uncertain, borderline, not well-characterized, or open to debate. Therefore, further research is needed as proposed in Chapter 26. Finally, asthma-like conditions and variants, which partially share one or more features of asthma, are presented in separate chapters and less extensively than OA.

ACKNOWLEDGMENTS

The authors are grateful to colleagues and contributors to this book for their most appreciated input and helpful suggestions.

REFERENCES

1. Vandenplas O, Malo JL. Definitions and types of work-related asthma: a nosological approach. Eur Respir J 2003; 21:706–712.
2. Brooks SM. Occupational asthma. In: Weiss EB, Segal MS, Stein M, eds. Bronchial Asthma. Boston: Little, Brown, 1985:461–469.
3. Sheppard D. Occupational asthma and byssinosis. In: Murray JF, Nadel JA, eds. Textbook of Respiratory Medicine. Philadelphia: WB Saunders, 1988:1593–1605.
4. Parkes WR. Occupational Lung Disorders. London: Butterworths, 1982:415–453.
5. Newman Taylor AJ. Occupational asthma. Thorax 1980; 35:241–245.

6. Chan-Yeung M, Malo JL. Occupational asthma. Chest 1987; 81:130S–136S.

7. Cotes JE, Steal J. Work-related lung disorders. Oxford: Blackwell Scientific Publ, 1987:345–372.

8. Burge PS. Occupational asthma. In: Barnes P, Rodger IW, Thomson NC, eds. Asthma: Basic Mechanisms and Clinical Management. London: Academic Press, 1988:465–482.

9. Pepys J. Occupational asthma: review of present clinical and immunologic status. J Allergy Clin Immunol 1980; 66:179–185.

10. Dolovich J, Hargreave FE. The asthma syndrome: inciters, inducers, and host character-istics. Thorax 1981; 36:641–644.

11. Chan-Yeung M. Assessment of asthma in the workplace. ACCP consensus statement. American College of Chest Physicians. Chest 1995; 108:1084–1117.

12. Malo JL, Ghezzo H, L'Archevêque J, Lagier F, Perrin C, Cartier A. Is the clinical history a satisfactory means of diagnosing occupational asthma? Am Rev Respir 1991; 143:528–532.

13. Tarlo SM, Leung K, Broder I, Silverman F, Holness DL. Asthmatic subjects symptoma-tically worse at work: prevalence and characterization among a general asthma clinic population. Chest 2000; 118:1309–1314.

14. Blanc PD, Toren K. How much asthma can be attributed to occupational factors? Am J Med 1999; 107:580–587.

15. Hurst JW, Morris DC, Alexander RW. The use of the New York Heart Association's classification of cardiovascular disease as part of the patient's complete problem list. Clin Cardiol 1999; 22:385–390.

16. Jajosky RAR, Harrison R, Reinisch F, et al. Surveillance of work-related asthma in selected U.S. states using surveillance guidelines for state health departments-California, Massachusetts, Michigan and New Jersy, MMWR 1999; 48(SS3):1–20.

17. Matte TD, Hoffman RE, Rosenman KD, Stanbury M. Surveillance of work-related asthma in selected U.S. states using surveillance guidelines for state health departments, California, Massachusetts, Michigan, and New Jersey, 1993–1995. Mor Mortal Wkly Rep CDC Surveil Summ 1999; 48:1–20.

18. Hnizdo E, Vallyathan V. Chronic obstructive pulmonary disease due to occupational exposure to silica dust: a review of epidemiological and pathological evidence. Occup Environ Med 2003; 60:237–243.

19. Petran M, Cocarla A, Baiescu M. Association between bronchial hyper-reactivity and exposure to silicon carbide. Occup Med 2000; 50:103–106.

2
Historical Aspects of Occupational Asthma

Jack Pepys[†]
Royal Postgraduate Medical School, London, U.K.

I. Leonard Bernstein
*Division of Allergy–Immunology, Department of Internal Medicine, College of
Medicine, University of Cincinnati, Cincinnati, Ohio, U.S.A.*

Editors' Note: In the first and second editions of Asthma in the Workplace, *this
chapter was coauthored by Drs. Jack Pepys and I. Leonard Bernstein. Dr. Pepys'
contribution was the "Introduction" through the section entitled "Simulated Occupational Provocation Tests," which the editors decided to retain in toto for this issue.
This section includes a review of some of Dr. Pepys' key contributions to occupational asthma and therefore reinforces the dedication of this book to him. The
remaining sections of the chapter, beginning with the section "Current Status of
Occupational Asthma," have been revised by I. Leonard Bernstein.*

INTRODUCTION

The recognition and acceptance of occupational asthma (OA) as an important and
distinct entity has depended upon clarification of the term "asthma" and upon means
of establishing its occupational relationship. Asthma translated literally means "pant-
ing," i.e., a symptom rather than a clinical disorder. Hippocrates (460–370 B.C.) cited
its presence in metal workers, fullers, tailors, horsemen, farmhands, and fishermen.
The use of the term asthma to describe a clinical disorder is attributed to Aretaeus
in the first century A.D. Maimonides, known as Rambam, discussed the disorder in
a "Treatise on Asthma" in 1190. The paroxysmal nature of the disorder interspersed
with periods of freedom was described by van Helmont in 1662 and by Floyer in 1698.

Observation of relationships of diseases to occupations has been influenced by
socioeconomic factors, according to Sigerist (1). In antiquity, industry was small
scale, employed ancient technology, and was frequently conducted outdoors. Early
examples of occupational respiratory problems can be seen in a citation from an
ancient Egyptian papyrus (Papyrus Sallier) describing "the weaver engaged in home

---

[†] Deceased.

work (who) is worse off in the house than the women: doubled up with his knees drawn up to his stomach, he cannot breathe," and in Roman times in a report by Pliny stating that "persons employed in the manufactories in preparing minimum (native cinnabar, red lead) protect the face with masks of loose bladder skin, to avoid inhaling the dust, which is highly pernicious: the covering being at the same time sufficiently transparent to admit of being seen through." There was little development in reports on occupational diseases in the Middle Ages.

With the development of trade and the need for precious and other metals in the 15th century, occupational diseases became of medical interest and were mainly concerned with mining and traumatic injuries and termed *morbi metallici*. Ellenbog in 1473 wrote a short pamphlet entitled, "On the Poisonous and Wicked Fumes and Smokes" encountered by goldsmiths and others. Paracelsus (1493–1541) wrote the first monograph on occupational diseases arising from his interest in chemistry, and this was devoted mainly to mining.

Occupational disease in general came of age when Bernardino Ramazzini published in 1713 his great classic landmark in occupational diseases, *De morbis artificum diatriba* (2). This contained important contributions to occupational respiratory disease affecting bakers, handlers of old clothes, and workers with flax, hemp, and silk, and in a section on "Diseases of sifters and measurers of grain" the description corresponds with the features of farmer's lung, the classical example of extrinsic allergic alveolitis (bronchioloalveolitis). Such subjects may also have an asthmatic component of their illness, and some may be mainly or solely asthmatic. Whereas Ramazzini was referred to as the historical source of information on farmer's lung when the main cause, *Micromonospora faeni*, was being identified (3), it was of interest to learn of a much earlier comparable description by Olaus Magnus in 1555 of respiratory disease due to threshing of grain (Fig. 1).

Ramazzini, in addition to his incisive and always topical description of diseases due to various occupations, made another great contribution. He wrote "The Divine Hippocrates informs us, that when a Physician visits a Patient, he ought to inquire into many things, by putting questions to the Patient and Bystanders" and added "To which I would presume to add one interrogation more: namely, what Trade is he of?", thus providing an indispensable dictum for occupational disease. This should, of course, include "What other occupations have you had?"

The next step in occupational diseases and priority in their description arose with the Industrial Revolution in the United Kingdom in the 1800s. Charles Turner Thackrah published in 1832 a fine book on the effects of arts, trades, and professional and civic status and habits of living on health and longevity (4). A review of this book at that time in the *Edinburgh Medical and Surgical Journal* concluded that "English literature has until now been destitute of a single general treatise on the diseases of trades and professions." Thackrah used the term asthma only twice, with reference to maltsters and coffee roasters and to hatters and hairdressers. These were thought to have chronic bronchitis, "the chronic pulmonary catarrh of Laennec." He also mentions the production of respiratory symptoms in pharmacists grinding to powder ipecacuanha, the Brazilian shrub used as an expectorant from early in 1648. The affected persons had to stay out of buildings where this was being done. Thomas Dover used ipecacuanha together with opium to form Dover's powder, widely used, even recently, for coughs and colds.

Thackrah was concerned with respiratory problems in flax mills and, like Patissier in France, described mill fever on the initial exposure followed by trouble-some cough and observed "that the respiratory symptoms evinced a great and easily

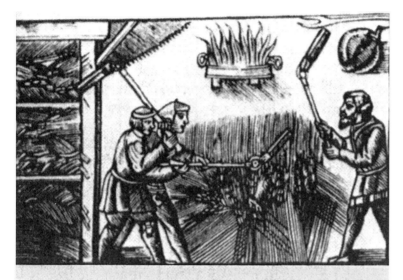

Når man skiljer agnarna från kornen tager man sorg-
fälligt i akt den tid då man kan få lämplig vind som sopar
undan sädesdammet att det icke må lända de tröskande
karlarnas lifsorgan till skada.
På grund av sin fina art tränger detta stoft nästan omärk-
ligt in i munnen och hopar sig i svalget. Om man då icke
tyr sig till snar bot och dricker färskt öl lärer man aldrig
mera eller och blott en kort tid få äta hvad man tröskat.

Olaus Magnus (1555)

Figure 1 "When sifting the chaff from the wheat, one must carefully consider the time when a suitable wind is available that sweeps away the harmful dust. This fine-grained material readily makes its way into the mouth, congests in the throat, and threatens the life organs of the threshing men. If one does not seek instant remedy by drinking one's beer, one may never more, or only for a short time, be able to enjoy what one has threshed."—Olaus Magnus, 1555.

excited irritability." The noises of flax mills made auscultation of the workers difficult, and Thackrah describes the usefulness of the "pulmometer" in diseases of the lungs. This consisted of "a large graduated glass jar, inverted over, and filled with water. The person blows through a tube, the lower end of which is under the jar, making however but one expiration at each trial. The air bubbling up displaces of course the water at the upper part of the vessel, and as this is marked from above downward, the subsidence of the water indicates the quantity of air expired." The spirometer was developed in 1836.

Just as Ramazzini instructed that questions about occupation should be put, so Thackrah stated dogmatically, "If any object, that the cure not the causes or prevention of disease, is the business of the medical practitioner, I would reply that the scientific treatment of a malady requires a knowledge of its nature, and the nature is imperfectly understood without knowledge of the cause." In other words, precise etiologic diagnosis is required, most pertinent to OA, and to be discussed further.

Major contributions to the recognition of extrinsic causes of asthma in general were made, among others, by Bostock in 1819 (5), Blackley in 1873 (6), and Salter in 1860 (7). Literature on occupational diseases in the United States began in 1837, instigated by the New York Medical Society. The first chairs in industrial hygiene were created in 1910 in New York and in Milan.

Occupational Causes of Asthma—Early 1900s to 1960s

The limited examples of asthma related to specific occupational causes are those due to both high- (mainly protein) and low-molecular-weight (mainly chemical) allergens. In chronological order, the first comprises castor bean dust (8), western red cedar (9), endemic asthma due to castor bean dust (10), atopy to acacia (gum arabic) (11), may-fly (Ephemerida) (12), asthma due to gum acacia (13), tragacanth (14), wood dust (15), and locust (16). Among low-molecular-weight chemical allergens are platinum halide salts (17), platinum salts (18), chromium (19), chromates (20), phthalic anhydride (21), sulfonechloramides (22), platinum salts (23,24), toluene diisocyanate (TDI) (25), chrome, nickel, and aniline (26), and rubber, lacquer, and shellac (27).

The reason for the above arbitrary limited selection of references is to show the great increase in reports on OA and its causes, in particular, low-molecular-weight chemicals, from about 1960 onward. For example, in 1980, more than 200 causes had been identified, and more than 2000 new substances were being synthesized each year (28). The comprehensive discussion on OA by Brooks (9) has 347 references, and the other chapters in this volume will increase these numbers.

Developments in Diagnosis

Ramazzini initiated the clinical diagnosis of the occupational nature of asthma by asking, "What is your occupation?" Support for this may be obtained by pulmonary function tests in reaction to work, as suggested by Thackrah using the pulmometer, and in etiological terms by skin and other immunological tests. The gold standard for identifying a particular occupational agent as the probable cause of asthma is the response to exposure under controlled and appropriate conditions, and most attention will be paid to its development. The use of bronchial provocation tests with common protein allergens was pioneered by Colldahl (29). A new era in which such tests are made with low-molecular-weight chemical compounds was opened by Gelfand (27). He investigated respiratory allergy due to chemical compounds encountered in the rubber, lacquer, shellac, and beauty culture industries. Almost all of his subjects were atopic with evidence of sensitivity to common allergens. He elicited immediate skin and bronchial reactions to solutions of ethylenediamine, monoethanolamine, ammonium thioglycolate, and hexamethylenetetramine. These were administered as a fine mist, and Gelfand states that "in many instances, spraying the material into the air near the patient would result in immediate symptoms." The duration of the inhalation tests was not stated. In the case of a granular product, hexamethylenetetramine, unsuitable for an aerosol test, the lacquer and hair spray product as used by the public was tested. The reactions elicited, lasting one-half to two hours, were an "uncontrollable paroxysmal cough, blocking, or running of the nose as well as precipitation of asthmatic breathing." The latter required injection of adrenaline. The sera of two patients who gave positive reactions to ethylene-diamine gave passive transfer test. Gelfand's description of the severity of reactions is not encouraging for similar tests, though the results had useful etiological diagnostic value. As for isocyanates, he states, "This chemical is too toxic for either skin or provocative inhalation testing."

In 1964, Gandevia reported on "respiratory symptoms and ventilatory capacity in men exposed to isocyanate vapour" (30). He found, as did Gelfand, that work exposure to TDI caused more cough than wheeze, suggestive of bronchitis, and that subjects regularly had nocturnal symptoms, now recognized to be a feature of OA. None had a past history of allergy. In 1967, Gandevia and Milne (31) investigated asthma in workers handling western red cedar. Bronchial provocation with an aqueous solution of an extract elicited asthmatic reactions occurring after four to six hours, again at night, and recurring on successive nights thereafter, with normal findings during the daytime. Such subjects would not notice improvement when off work over weekends, which can otherwise be so useful in diagnosing OA. This sequence of reactions corresponded with the clinical histories of affected workers of rhinitis and cough at the end of the day's work or early at night followed by later nocturnal asthma.

The next study of this sort was made in 1969 by Popa et al. (32) who investigated "bronchial asthma and asthmatic bronchitis determined by simple chemicals" using skin, serological, and bronchial provocation tests. The low-molecular-weight substances were tested as aerosols inhaled for five minutes except for a test with the fume from a heated urea formaldehyde resin. A decrease in the FEV_1 of 10% was taken as positive, in contrast to the 20% decrease required at present. Two patterns of asthmatic reaction were elicited. In one group of subjects an immediate reaction was associated with immediate intradermal and passive transfer reactions to ethylenediamine, sulfathiazole, and chloramine. These correspond with the clinical history. In another group, the inhalation test reactions came on after 2 to 12 hours. Skin tests, intradermal and patch, gave delayed 24- to 48-hour reactions, but no immediate reactions, leading to the hypothesis of a delayed hypersensitivity mechanism, as yet still subject to confirmation, a topic of much interest. The provocation test reactions corresponded to the clinical histories of dyspnea at the end of the shift persisting for one to two hours, only to recur during the night as a "classic nocturnal asthma." An explanation is needed for their finding of negative bronchial reactions to common environmental allergens to which most of the subjects had given positive intradermal tests.

Occupational-Type Bronchial Provocation Tests

The above findings raised challenging questions about low-molecular-weight chemicals as causes of OA but left open the urgent need for safe, acceptable, and reproducible procedures for definitive and analytical bronchial tests. Faced with the problems of the unsuitability of many agents for use as aerosols and the possibilities of irritant, toxic, highly potent allergenicity, and other adverse effects, Pepys et al. (33) developed a pragmatic, simulated occupational type of test. This was suggested by a patient with severe OA who was occupied in varnishing boats for the Oxford–Cambridge boat race using a two-part varnish consisting of polyurethane resin to which TDI was added prior to use. He was tested as shown in Figure 2 by painting on a surface with the polyurethane resin, which gave no reaction. This was followed the next day by painting with the mixture of polyurethane and TDI, which elicited an unequivocal and reproducible nonimmediate reaction.

This form of test avoids artificiality in the nature of the exposure, the duration of which may be as little as a few breaths with certain substances and in all cases far

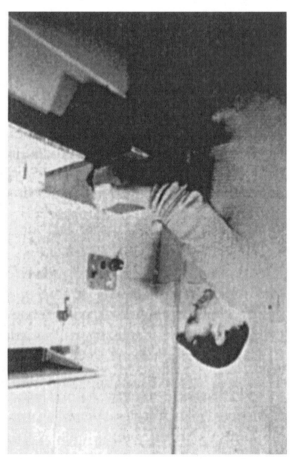

Figure 2 Occupational-type test for TDI (gaseous emanations) sensitivity. Repeated application of polyurethane varnish with and without TDI activator in proportions as used. Atmospheric concentration in test cubicle was 0.00173–0.0018 ppm. *Abbreviation:* TDI, toluene diisocyanate. *Source:* From Ref. 33.

less than the ordinary work exposure, usually of many hours each day. It is, in essence, a small piece of real life and is fully acceptable, when made with care under controlled conditions, on ethical grounds and for clinical, etiological diagnosis. Indeed, failure to establish a precise cause and leave the subject to continued exposure are undesirable. The testing is time consuming but potentially precise in identifying causes in complex exposures. The simulated occupational type of test was a landmark in future studies. Examples will be given of the various patterns of reaction, immunochemical, and other findings in response to dusts, powders, fumes, gaseous emanations, and aerosols (34).

Patterns of Asthmatic Reaction

The various patterns reported by Gelfand (27), Gandevia (30) and Milne (31), and Popa et al. (32) were observed in more detail. They consisted of (*i*) an immediate reaction starting in minutes and lasting 1.5 to 2 hours, and of nonimmediate reactions, (*ii*) an uncommon reaction starting after about one hour and lasting four to five hours, (*iii*) the common late reaction starting after several hours and lasting 12 hours or more, and (*iv*) a nocturnal reaction without any further challenge and with decreasing intensity at the same time each night for several or many nights. Isolated single reactions or late reactions or combined reactions were found. Care was needed regarding late reactions, which could develop after negative immediate reactions even to very limited challenges. Furthermore, as Gandevia (30) noted, recurrent reactions can result in persistence of asthma when off work over weekends or longer, thus giving an impression of nonoccupational asthma. Such findings showed that it is also necessary to ensure that any recurrent reactions due to previous work exposure shall have ceased before starting the tests, as otherwise a false-positive result may be elicited. In the course of these tests it was shown that sodium cromoglycate could inhibit both immediate and dual reactions, whereas corticosteroid inhalation had no effect on the immediate reaction but was very effective in inhibiting the late reaction (34,35).

These patterns are identical to those elicited by common protein environmental allergens, and they correspond to the common clinical histories of OA often starting with respiratory symptoms at the end of the day or elicited by exercise, followed later by asthmatic attacks at the end of the day and at night and in some cases later by immediate attacks on work exposure.

Simulated Occupational Provocation Tests

A number of reports have been published on the results of occupational-type tests with a variety of different exposures to gaseous emanations, fumes, and dusts of natural organic origin and of inorganic and organic chemical origin, mainly of low molecular weight. Other methods of testing aimed at quantitative aspects and many other identified causes appear in subsequent chapters. It is noteworthy that the pragmatic occupational-type exposures are capable of giving very reproducible reactions and can suffice for clinical etiological purposes (Figs. 3 and 4). Points of special interest will be cited. The test for sensitivity to TDI as made by Pepys et al. (33) is an example of its versatility. Of the subjects concerned, two were employed in soldering television wires. They were tested as if at work by soldering the relevant wire coated or uncoated with a polyurethane film and the resin flux for 10 minutes. The coated wire liberated TDI fumes, and a late asthmatic reaction was elicited. The specific sensitivity was confirmed by a painting test for 30 minutes with polyurethane varnish mixed with the TDI activator (Fig. 2).

The environmental effect of reactive chemicals was shown by the production of asthma in workers in a storeroom in East London (36). In the absence of possible causes, questions were asked about neighboring enterprises. It transpired that an adjacent factory making polyurethane foam was exhausting its products near the ventilation system of the storeroom. TDI was found in the ventilation filters, the portal of entry into the storeroom. Provocation tests by painting with polyurethane resin plus TDI established TDI as the cause. These workers were subsequently compensated by the neighboring factory. The initial presenting patient was so sensitive that he had only to approach the area to develop severe asthma that day.

In the case of amino-ethyl ethanolamine (37), a flux component for aluminum wire soldering was identified as the cause in a test consisting of three to four inhalations of the fumes, confirming the findings of Sterling (38).

In testing with dusty or powdered agents, the material was mixed with well-dried lactose, starting with a low concentration and increasing for daily tests until a reacting concentration was found. This was tipped from one receiver to another, simulating the inhalation exposure at work (Fig. 3). In two subjects working with piperazine, late reactions were inhibited by sodium cromoglycate when it was inhaled before and four hours after the challenge and before the late reaction had begun to present (39).

Tests for sensitivity to wood dusts were made by the tipping method using the wood dusts themselves and gave specific late reactions (40). Chan-Yeung et al. (41) studying the sensitivity to western red cedar, have shown that a low-molecular-weight organic acid in western red cedar, plicatic acid, is an allergen.

The acceptability of this form of occupational-type test is shown by its use in tests for sensitivity to platinum halide salts, which are of extremely high allergenicity. Starting with microgram amounts in 250 g of lactose (Fig. 3), the concentration was increased gradually, one test per day, up to 40 mg/kg, which elicited reactions to the dust after carefully monitored exposures of 4 to 30 minutes. This elicited immediate, dual, and isolated late asthmatic reactions. Skin testing was approached with caution in view of severe reactions to scratch and intradermal tests (18,42,43). Skin prick tests starting with a 10^{-6} concentration up to 10^{-3} are effective for demonstrating sensitivity (44), and subsequently specific IgE antibodies were shown in the majority

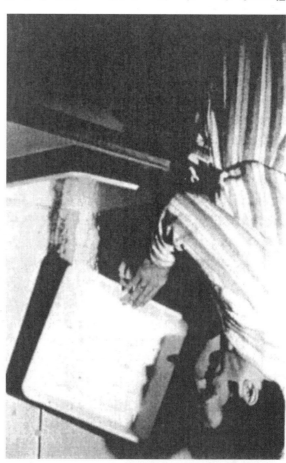

Figure 3 Occupational-type test for sensitivity to dust/powder agents mixed with lactose or unmixed, e.g., for wood dusts. Repeated tipping under controlled conditions and with increasing concentrations. Stippled areas in Figures 4, 5, 6, and 7 show duration of challenges.

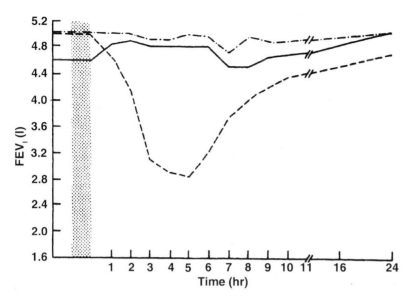

Figure 4 Occupation-type test as in Figure 3 with mixture of 1 g of 6APA in 250 g lactose. (–), Lactose control test; (– –), lactose plus commercial 6APA; (–·–), lactose plus purified 6APA. *Note*: Late asthmatic reaction to commercial and unpurified 6APA, i.e., die to a contaminant. *Source*: From Ref. 60.

by RAST (45). A number of points of basic serological and immunochemical interest (46) were present in the findings on platinum salt allergy. Passive transfer tests in humans and monkeys showed the presence in unheated serum of long-term specific IgE antibodies and also in heated serum of short-term heat-stable antibodies, presumably IgG-STS, capable of giving immediate reactions to the platinum halide salt itself and without any need for conjugation with a carrier protein for the making of the test (47). A possible role for heat-stable, short-term sensitizing antibody to low-molecular-weight chemicals merits examination.

The capacity of low-molecular-weight chemicals in themselves to elicit immediate reactions and react with specific IgE antibodies or in PK tests has been shown for a number of other occupational allergens, such as chlorhexidine (48), the anhydrides (49,50), azo and anthraquinone dyes (51), sulfonechloramides (22), and ethylenediamine and paraphenylenediamine (32).

An important area of future research on the allergenic effects of reactive low-molecular-weight chemicals is shown by the capacity of the platinum halide salts to create in affected subjects neoantigens in human serum albumin, against specific IgE antibody that is formed. This antibody can react with neoantigens in serum albumin resulting from combination with other unrelated chemical haptens. Thus in platinum salt-sensitive workers, 4 out of 38 gave positive RASTs to human serum albumin compared with 3 out of 116 nonsensitive subjects. Tests with dinitrophenyl-HSA gave positive RASTs with 8 out of 38 sera and with 4 of the 116 nonsensitive subjects (52).

Similar findings have been made in a patient allergic to nickel sulfate (53,54) and in patients allergic to phthalic anhydrides (55), trimellitic acid anhydride (TMA) (56), and diisocyanates (57). This phenomenon has been described as autoantibodies induced by extrinsic, low-molecular-weight chemical allergens, i.e., extrinsically determined autoallergy (EDAA) (58). Evidence for a possible active role of such IgE antibodies to neoantigens in human serum albumin in biological reactions is the elicitation of an immediate reaction to a skin prick test with human serum albumin in a subject sensitive to trimellitic acid who had IgE antibodies to HSA (A. Newman-Taylor, personal communication). Similar findings have been shown in guinea pigs sensitized to TDI in which reaginic antibodies were induced against both the TDI and the guinea pig serum albumin neoantigens. Skin tests with guinea pig serum albumin elicited immediate reactions (59).

A great advantage of low-molecular-weight chemicals is their known chemical structure. This can provide basic immunochemical information. For example, skin prick tests with a wide range of platinum salts (46) showed that allergenicity in eliciting reactions was related to the number of chlorine molecules in the test material. Chlorine is a leaving ligand and is loosely bound to the platinum. By contrast, palladium encountered in the refining of platinum is poorly, if at all, allergenic, and in this case the chlorine molecules are firmly bound. Investigations of this sort would be very useful with other agents containing chlorine, such as ammonium chloride, capable of eliciting immediate skin test reactions and for the identification of other possibly relevant ligands. In the context of chlorine itself it is remarkable that chlorhexidine becomes potently allergenic for inducing sensitivity and eliciting reactions by simple dilution in chlorinated water (48).

An investigation of asthma in four workers from the same firm manufacturing ampicillin and exposed also to benzyl-penicillin and 6-amino-penicillanic acid showed differences in their sensitivities (60). Tests by dust inhalation (Fig. 4) of mixtures with lactose elicited characteristic and reproducible late asthmatic reactions. In one case the reactions were elicited by commercial preparations of 6-amino-penicillanic acid and ampicillin but not by purified preparations, showing sensitivity to an unidentified impurity present in both products (Figs. 4 and 5). In another subject typical late reactions coming on after three to four hours and lasting

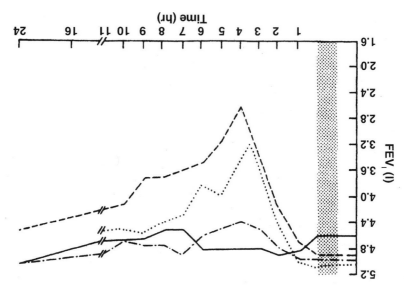

Figure 5 Occupation-type test as in Figure 3 with mixture of 1 g ampicillins in 250 g lactose as patient in Figure 4. (—), Lactose control; (– –), lactose plus commercial unpurified ampicillin; (·····), lactose plus another unpurified ampicillin; (—·—), lactose plus purified ampicillin. *Note:* Late asthmatic reaction to contaminant in unpurified ampicillin as with 6APA in Figure 4. *Source:* From Ref. 60.

more than 16 hours were elicited by both commercial and purified ampicillin (Fig. 6). Both commercial and purified preparations of 6-amino-penicillanic acid elicited quite different reactions to the ampicillin, coming on after 10 hours and maximal at 16 hours (Fig. 7). The difference between the two materials is the addition of phenylglycine acid chloride as a side chain to the 6-amino-pencillanic acid to make ampicillin. Identical asthmatic reactions were given after oral administration of a dose of the relevant antibiotic (Fig. 8). Immediate-type reactions to phenylglycine being made in large amounts have also been reported (61). Figures 4 and 5 show the reproducibility of the reactions in the occupational-type test.

Two female asthmatic hairdressers were tested as if at work by mixing in a mortar a hair-bleaching agent with hydrogen peroxide (62). One gave an acute immediate reaction and the other a late reaction. The cause in a mixture of 11 unnamed ingredients provided by the maker was identified as potassium persulfate. The immediate reactor also gave an immediate skin reaction to application of a drop of solution to unbroken skin, an example of contact urticaria. The late reactor to the bleach was also sensitive to henna, which on testing in the same way gave an immediate nasal and conjunctival reaction and a positive immediate skin prick test reaction.

A worker who developed asthma while making salbutamol noticed an association with an intermediate product termed "glycol compound" [(2-N-benzyl-N-tert-butyl-amino)-4'-hydroxy-3'-hydroxymethyl acetophenone diacetate]. Provocation tests with the powder and the lactose mixture (Fig. 3) elicited a late asthmatic reaction to the glycl compound and less so to a benzyl compound. Salbutamol itself, the final product, caused no reaction on challenge and was effective when used for relief of symptoms (63).

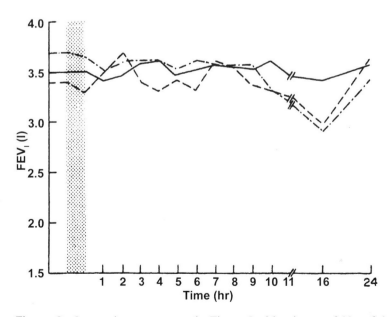

Figure 6 Occupation-type test as in Figure 5 with mixture of 10 g of 6-amino-penicillanic acid (6APA), commercial and purified in 250 g lactose. (–), lactose control; (—·—), lactose plus purified 6APA; (– –), lactose plus commercial 6APA. *Note*: Late, reproducible, 16-hour reactions to both purified and unpurified 6APA molecule. *Source*: From Ref. 60.

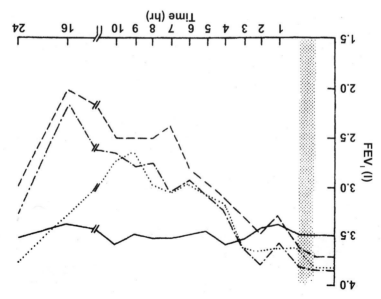

Figure 7 Occupational-type test in Figure 5 with mixture of 10 g of purified commercial ampicillins in 250 g lactose in same patients as Figure 3. (–), lactose control; (– –), lactose plus commercial unpurified ampicillin; (–·–), lactose plus purified ampicillin; (·····), lactose plus another purified ampicillin. *Note:* Late, reproducible three- to four-hour onset asthmatic reactions to purified and unpurified ampicillins, more severe than 6APA reactions (Fig. 3) and attributable to addition of phenyl-glycine to 6APA nucleus to form ampicillin. *Source:* From Ref. 60.

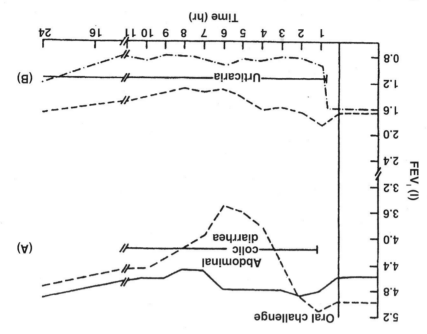

Figure 8 Oral challenge with capsule of (**A**) commercial ampicillin (2×500 mg) in patient (Figs. 3 and 4) and (**B**) benzyl penicillin (2×500 g) in another subject. *Note:* Reproducible late asthmatic reactions to ampicillin, plus gastrointestinal reactions to ingested allergen in (**A**) and to benzyl penicillin in (**B**) plus urticaria. Similar reactions were observed to oral challenges in subjects giving late reactions to tests with other inhaled and possibly ingested dusts. *Source:* From Ref. 68.

A major role in the chemical cause of OA is played by the development of synthetic resins to take the place of colophony and its derivatives, mainly acrylics, epoxy resins, and polyurethanes. The first polyurethane foams were made during World War II by I. G. Farben in Germany, using TDI as an activator. It has been calculated that 2.2 million tons are likely to be used in the United States in the next 10 years involving many thousands of workers. Occupational-type tests were made with epoxy resin systems containing phthalic acid anhydride, TMA, and triethylene tetramine (64). Their sensitivity could be shown by the test consisting of as little as a single breath of fume from heated materials. Their diagnostic value was shown in a patient thought to have asthma due to TDI to which he, however, gave a negative reaction; an acute immediate reaction was given to a heated cured resin containing phthalic acid anhydride. In another subject, painting with a liquid bisphenol A resin to which triethylene tetramine was added gave a late asthmatic reaction to the mixture but not to the resin alone. Sensitivity to TMA was demonstrated in yet another by one breath of the invisible fume from heated epoxy paint, which elicited a dual asthmatic reaction. TMA is remarkable in that it causes three different syndromes with different immunological findings (65). Immediate reactions are present with positive skin tests and IgE and other antibodies to TM-human serum albumin. Late respiratory reactions coming on 4 to 12 hours after exposure occurred in patients with negative skin tests and high total antibody levels but not IgE antibody to TM-human serum albumin. In the third pulmonary disease/anemia syndrome, very high levels of antibody to TM-human serum albumin are present but no IgE antibody.

Asthma due to the fumes from the soldering of Multicore—a tin–lead alloy containing cores of wood resin flux—has been shown to result from colophony, a pine resin widely used for soft soldering in the electronics industry and for other purposes (66). The active material in the resin is mainly abietic acid. Immediate asthmatic reactions, late, and dual, were elicited by one breath to three-minute exposure in tests made on separate days of the fumes from heating of the Multicore or the colophony resin. Up to 20% of the workers were sensitized (67), and many showed the value of frequent monitoring of the peak flow rate to show occupational effects. Affected subjects may develop symptoms in the neighborhood of pine trees that emanate resins into the air, and they can react to unheated colophony (68).

There is as yet no explanation in general for isolated late reactions or the recurrent nocturnal reaction, in contrast to immediate and many dual reactions where specific IgE antibody is present as shown by skin and serological tests. The above list of agents and reactions to occupational-type tests will be expanded considerably in the chapters to follow, as will discussions and results of tests with other methods of exposure, because of their importance in establishing etiological diagnosis in OA.

CURRENT STATUS OF OA

Greater recognition of OA is leading to improved environmental control and avoidance of the use of potent causal agents. Points of importance include greater understanding of the immunochemical properties of such agents, on the one hand, and of factors predisposing to sensitization of exposed subjects on the other. Examples of the former are the role of halide molecules, notably chlorine, behaving as leaving ligands, in bestowing sensitizing and eliciting capacity. This is shown by platinum halide salts in humans (46) and in experimental animals (69) and by the striking effect of chlorine on allergenicity of chlorhexidine (48). The well-defined structure of low-molecular-weight chemical allergens offers many opportunities for establishing more basic information like this.

Of the factors predisposing to sensitization, atopy and the induction of specific IgE have been of prime importance, supported by clinical observations with common environmental protein allergens and by investigations showing that atopics are more readily sensitized than nonatopics to allergen aerosol (70). Atopy in immunological terms can be defined as the predisposition to sensitization to common allergens as shown by immediate skin prick test reactions (71). Thirty to 40% of apparently asymptomatic subjects belong to the atopic group so defined and present a problem in deciding whether occupational exposure to potential allergens should be permitted. Recent findings, however, emphasize the importance of cigarette smoking in its own right and as an additive factor to atopy in favoring IgE sensitization to a variety of occupational agents (72). Zetterstrom et al. (73) found that cigarette smokers had raised serum levels of IgE and a higher rate of sensitization to ispaghula. Similar sensitizations are reported to tetrachlorophthalic anhydride (74), platinum halide salt (75), and *Bacillus subtilis* enzymes (76). This effect of smoking may be attributable to increased permeability of the bronchial epithelium (77) and to immunological effects. A striking contrast is the finding, in extrinsic allergic alveolitis occurring mainly in nonatopic subjects, farmer's lung, bird fancier's lung, and seasonal disease in Japan, that nonsmokers are more likely to develop precipitating antibodies and clinical disease (78–81). Uncertainty about the relationships between atopy and work is discussed by Nordman (82).

ACTIONS OF REGULATORY BODIES

In 1956 the U.S. Department of Labor noted 100 occupations apparently associated with the development of asthma. Later, on-site plant inspections under the United States National Exposure Survey (NOES) confirmed this overall prevalence. For example, significant exposure to polyisocyanates was found in 30 different occupational settings (83). The problem was to recognize this by law with rights of compensation. France in 1960 was the first country to do so and related it to the manufacturing and handling of penicillin. Additions were made in 1967 of tropical woods, followed in 1972 by low-molecular-weight chemicals, paraphenylenediamine and ethanolamine, and in 1973 by isocyanates and biological enzymes, and further agents have been added since then. In Germany a law was passed in 1961 accepting "bronchial asthma enforcing the cessation of the professional occupation or any other paid employment," with special emphasis on flour and TDI.

The United Kingdom bowed much later to the pressures of the clinical and etiological diagnoses being made from the findings with isocyanates and platinum salts. The contents of the report on OA under the Social Security Act of 1975 illustrate the approach to the problems of recognition for medicolegal purposes. The question examined was "whether there is any condition resulting from exposure to industrial asthma-inducing agents which should be prescribed under the Act." The main problem, it was stated, was that of separating asthmatics whose asthma is unrelated to their occupation from those whose asthma has been initiated by a sensitizing agent encountered at work. The first and most important step was the detailed clinical and occupational history, and the four key diagnostic points were (*i*) a sensitizing agent is present at work, (*ii*) the patient has been exposed for some time before the asthma develops, (*iii*) the symptoms improve when away from work, and (*iv*) exposure to a much smaller dose than the work exposure causes the symptoms to recur.

The last two points are relevant to the foregoing discussion. Symptoms can persist for some time after cessation of exposure in the form of recurrent nocturnal asthma and also in response to ordinary environmental exposure to the causal agents (30,84–86). For example, a patient sensitive to ampicillin developed asthma at night after visiting the town where the factory was located; a TDI-sensitive patient had the same problem in the neighborhood of the factory, and colophony-sensitive patients can react to pine trees and even to unheated colophony and turpentine (68). The acceptance of responses to minimal re-exposure emphasizes the importance of provocation studies to provide definitive evidence, especially in relation to new substances or where the cause is in doubt, so that the established knowledge cannot, for practical purposes, be assumed to suffice for the diagnosis.

The report concluded with a list of seven causal agents regarded as the most clearly established causes of OA (87). These were platinum salts, isocyanates, acid anhydride and amine hardening agents, fumes from the use of resin as a soldering flux, proteolytic enzymes, animals and insects in laboratories, and dusts arising from milling and handling flour and from harvesting, drying, transporting, and storing grains. A further seven additions made in 1986 were antibiotics, cimetidine, wood dusts, ispaghula, castor bean dust, ipecacuanha (a hark back to Thackrah and Dover's powder), and azodicarbonamide. The last nine additions in 1990 were glutaraldehyde, persulfate salts or henna arising from their use in the hairdressing trade, crustaceans or fish or products arising from these in the food-processing industry, reactive dyes, soybeans, tea dust, green coffee bean dust, fumes from stainless steel welding, and, finally, a catchall addition to the list consisting of "any other sensitizing agent inhaled at work."

In the United States adoption of a national etiologic list of OA was not possible because of the administrative heterogeneity with which individual states recognized OA. This may, in fact, have been advantageous to workers inasmuch as the number of newly discovered causal agents continues to increase.

Regulatory bodies urge that more emphasis should be given to surveillance and prevention in view of the frequency of industrial spills and other unforeseen exposures (88). In this regard, development of rapid throughput, self-reading personal monitors would prevent undue prolongation of harmful exposures. Whether prevention of work-exacerbated asthma (WEA) in workers with preexisting asthma can be accomplished is problematic. However, under certain work conditions where workers are exposed to high concentrations of nonsensitizing pollutants (e.g., ozone, sulfur dioxide, volatile organic compounds), the use of high efficiency charcoal filtration should be explored (89–91). Finally, the increased incidence of asthma in public administration workers, teachers, and other white collar workers has focused attention on better building design and proper installation of heating, ventilation, and air conditioning systems (83,92).

KEY ADVANCES FROM 1993 TO 2005

The third edition of *Asthma in the Workplace* appears 12 years after the first edition. Unfortunately, Dr. Jack Pepys can no longer personally witness the rapid evolution of the discipline he helped to pioneer, but it would have been a great source of satisfaction to him that some of his predictions about the future of OA either have already transpired or are beginning to emerge in the relatively short period of time since the original publication of this book. This remarkable upsurge in OA and the ensuing medical interest it has engendered has culminated in two major occupational symposia [the first (93) and the second Jack Pepys Occupational Symposia, Montreal and Toronto, Canada, respectively] since publication of the second edition. A significant number of attendees of these meetings are contributors to this edition, and many of the questions posed at these conferences are also addressed in this edition. In the past 12 years the recognition curve of OA has assumed a much steeper slope, as evidenced by at least a 100% increase in literature citations reviewed in this text. These were selected from a relatively greater array of relevant articles which have appeared since publication of the second edition. For example, in a recent review of all PubMed listings of "Occupational Asthma" ($n = 4691$), about 35% of these ($n = 1285$) appeared since the beginning of the new millennium. Prospective surveillance programs continue to demonstrate that OA is by far the most common disorder among all occupationally induced lung diseases (88). Commensurate with this upward trend, there also appears to be an increased awareness among adjudication officials that disability and compensation must be evaluated apart from classical fibrogenic and restrictive lung diseases (94). Longitudinal surveillance of several worksites confirms that early detection and removal from exposure are the optimal means of preventing long-term disability. When specific causal relationships can be established, employers may be able to alter the manufacturing process itself, which, in some cases, may attenuate or abolish the risks of high exposure (95). However, exhaustive environmental control measures to eliminate human exposure may not suffice to completely prevent OA due to agents such as diisocyanates even in an optimally engineered plant (95).

As morbidity and mortality statistics of asthma continue to rise in the world's developed nations, the perception that occupational allergens, nonspecific triggers, and irritants are important contributory factors has been noted in several evidentiary-based guideline documents on the diagnosis and management of asthma (96,97). Technological progress in the identification of high- and low-molecular-weight agents in the workplace environment has expanded; these developments are discussed in detail in Chapters 12 and 13. The role of nonspecific irritants in the induction of nonimmunological OA has been explored more extensively since the first edition of this book was published. First described by Brooks et al. (98) in 1985, many case reports, case series, and several epidemiological studies of reactive airways dysfunction syndrome (RADS) have appeared in the recent literature and are reviewed in the current edition (99,100). Some new cases have been described after multiple exposures to both high and low levels of workplace irritants (Chapter 25) (101). Of particular interest is additional information derived from bronchoalveolar lavage and biopsy investigation about the histopathological features of RADS. Although the overall microscopic anatomical changes of RADS are identical to asthma, immunologically unique differences between RADS, induced OA, and naturally occurring asthma have been identified (99,102). Epithelial desquamation is a common feature but is more intense in the acute phase of RADS and is often accompanied by a higher percentage of bronchoalveolar neutrophils. Some investigators have not observed many bronchoalveolar eosinophils in chronic stages of RADS. Subepithelial fibrosis is more prominent in RADS than in other forms of occupational or nonoccupational asthma. These findings, coupled with the chronic persistence of airway hyperresponsiveness, have firmly established RADS as a prototype of nonimmunological asthma. Future research in the various clinical stages of RADS and their corresponding pathophysiological mechanisms will undoubtedly expand the continued increase in incidence of asthma in industrial urban centers.

Better understanding of risk factors has evolved over the past 12 years. In the case of protein allergens, the extent and the distribution of exposure are foremost among risk assessment (103). The significance of these risk factors is illustrated by the rapid appearance of respiratory sensitization among 5% to 10% of health workers soon after universal barrier control management of AIDS patients mandated the usage of latex gloves (104,105). Determination of "safe" exposure thresholds for HMW allergens causing OA has been undertaken for laboratory urinary proteins and wheat flour (106,107). Although the risk for sensitization in all workers was associated with greater allergen exposure, considerably smaller amounts of allergen were required in atopics. Moreover, the relationship between exposure and asthma also depended on the specific processing industry (108). In wheat plants, the probability of sensitization increased with exposure up to $2.7 \, \mathrm{mg/m^3}$ inhalable dust but the risk decreased at higher exposures. It was concluded that exposure–response relationships may be non-linear and differ between industries (108). Thus far it has not been possible to develop a no-effect level standard, but further research in this area will certainly proceed.

In his historical review, Dr. Jack Pepys emphasized the role of halides in confer-ring allergenicity to certain chemicals such as platinum salts and chlorhexidine. This concept has been extended to other reactive organic chemicals and their analogs. As a result there has been renewed interest in predictive animal models based on struc-ture–activity relationships of haptenic allergenicity. For example, systemic immunolo-gical investigations of acid anhydride chemicals have demonstrated that ring structure, position of double bonds, and methyl group substitution may be critical determinants of IgE-mediated sensitization (109). A computer-assisted analysis of respiratory sensitization based on chemical structure has also been developed as a means of predicting human allergenicity (110). Pre-existent atopy also continues to be an important determinant of IgE-mediated asthma induced by workplace high-molecular-weight allergens (111,112). In some instances, new workers who are atopic may already be presensitized to occupational protein allergens (e.g., laboratory animals) prior to entering the workplace. Moreover, apprentices in this work environment have a high incidence of occupational rhinoconjunctivitis which either precedes or markedly increases their risks of OA (113). Interestingly, Brooks et al. (114) recently proposed that atopy is also a risk factor in the "not so sudden" form of RADS. Except for platinum salts, atopy does not appear to be a prerequisite for sensitization to many low-molecular-weight chemicals. Nevertheless, genetic susceptibility has been explored further and may predispose individuals to sensiti-zation by specific low-molecular-weight chemicals such as TDI and trimellitic anhydride, both of which demonstrate associations between specific HLA class II genes (115,116). Both susceptibility and protective specific class II genes have been reported in the case of TDI asthma (117). An increase in specific nucleotide poly-morphisms (e.g., glutathione S-transferase, IL-4Rα), certain gene/gene interactions and haploid prevalences have been observed in diisocyanate workers (118,119). Smok-ing is a well-established risk factor for IgE-mediated OA induced by high-molecular-weight substances and a few chemicals such as platinum salts and tetrachlorophthalic acid anhydride (120,121). Occupational exposure to environmental tobacco smoke also presents a substantial risk to workers (122). However, a susceptibility role of smoking has not been proven in workers who develop asthma after exposure to low-molecular-weight agents (e.g., TDI, western red cedar), for which immunological mechanisms do not entirely account for all the pathophysiological consequences induced by these chemicals (121).

The risk for upregulation of IgE sensitization to both HMW and LMW occupational allergens is greater with coexposure to diesel fumes (123). Increased ozone concentrations in the workplace may enhance the development of either immunologic or nonimmunologic asthma (89).

A number of recent epidemiologic reviews have called attention to the frequent occurrence of work exacerbated asthma (WEA) (124,125). In a descriptive analysis of SENSOR data, it was determined that about 20% of all reported work-related asthma was ascertained to be WEA due to irritant exposures in workers with pre-existing asthma (125). Agents that have been responsible for WEA were dusts, indoor pollutants, chemicals, cleaning agents, paints, and smoke. A retrospective survey of approved work-related asthma compensation claims revealed that 19% of these claims occurred after accidental high exposure to respiratory irritants (126). Among these workers, 75% had pre-existing asthma, as compared to 24% with irritant-induced asthma (IIA) or RADS. In workers with preexisting asthma, the main agents were dust, paints, and fumes. These combined studies suggested that there might be selective occupational or industrial differences between WEA and new onset OA. For example, the prevalence of WEA is high among workers exposed to fumes from cleaning agents. These recent epidemiologic data have necessitated a new chapter on WEA (Chapter 26).

The pathogenesis of the inflammatory milieu of immunological OA is in many respects similar to that of nonoccupational asthma, especially in those instances where TH2 cytokines, IgE antibodies, and immediate hypersensitivity mediator pathways are involved (127). However, T cells and their proinflammatory secretions are also prominent in non-IgE–mediated polyisocyanate asthma in which specific T-cell proliferation, activated T cells, and increased ratios of CD8+ T cells and T-cell–derived proinflammatory cytokines and chemokines have all been recently demonstrated (128–130). Whether innate immune responses through toll-like receptors are involved has not yet been explored. The unique aerobiological components (source, release, dispersion, and impact) of OA have stimulated design of many new rodent models that more accurately simulate the human paradigm (109,131–134). These have been designed to investigate many important components of OA (i) deposition of antigens (132); (ii) structure–function relationships (109); (iii) prediction of human sensitization (131); (iv) contrasting effects of IgE sensitizing and IgG antibodies (133); dermal sensitization (134,135) and (v) the role of cytokines, chemokines, and mediators in the inflammatory response (136,137). Advances in small animal respiratory physiological technology also enable the assessment of airway obstruction and nonspecific bronchial responsiveness in nonanesthetized animals (137).

The diagnosis of OA requires a combination of: (i) recognition of the source and dispersion of the causative agent; (ii) characteristic symptoms; and (iii) specific and nonspecific functional abnormalities related to the worksite. In the case of high-molecular-weight allergens, skin prick tests are the preferred diagnostic correlates of IgE sensitization (138). In some situations in vitro assays of specific IgE are complementary. At the IgE effector level, the role of basophil activation is being investigated as a diagnostic adjunct (139). The role of IgG antibodies is more problematic, but some investigators suggest that they could be used as biomarkers of exposure (140). What would have been especially gratifying to Dr. Pepys is that controlled, specific bronchial provocation remains the "gold standard" of diagnosis, although in many instances this can only be accomplished as a workplace challenge. Of particular interest to him would have been recent reports about the role of cytokine and chemokine networks in the pathogenesis of late or dual-phase bronchial challenge responses (127,128). He also would have been impressed that OA has evolved into an excellent model of human asthma because it affords a unique opportunity of examining pathophysiological processes during the initial phases of exposure, subsequent elicitation of symptoms after reexposure, and sequential changes on a prospective basis (141).

Several possible surrogates for specific challenge may be emerging. These are noninvasive techniques which measure inflammatory components responsible for OA. Induced sputum showing predominant numbers of either eosinophils or neutrophils is being reported with increased frequency (142,143). Recently, there are a number of reports of eosinophilic bronchitis without evidence of asthma (142,144,145). This syndrome is discussed in Chapter 28 as well as other bronchial obstructive presentations which can be confused with OA (e.g., bronchiolitis obliterans). The diagnostic potential of airways nitric oxide is being vigorously explored as a possible predictive index of active or classic OA disease (146). This is discussed in more detail in Chapter 25. Finally, examination of breath condensates, presently an experimental procedure for detecting proinflammatory cytokines in children, may have a potential for further usefulness in OA (147).

Several promising new imaging techniques may prove to be useful adjuncts in the diagnosis of OA both in workers who continue their exposure at work and in those who are removed from further exposure. These include hyperpolarized helium-3 magnetic resonance, synchrotron radiation microtomography (ultra high resolution CT), oxygen-enhanced MRI using dynamically acquired T1 parameter maps, and high-magnification bronchovideoscopy (148–151). These methods may enable non-invasive evaluation of bronchial wall thickening and other remodeled tissues. Oxygen-enhanced MRI may also be useful in assessing pulmonary function (150).

Early recognition and removal from sources of exposure are the preventive hallmarks of OA. Unfortunately, this is not always feasible in all occupations, and some workers refuse this advice because of economic hardship (152). The possibility that specific immunotherapy for HMW allergens could be an alternative strategy in such cases was investigated in latex-allergic workers. Two independent, small, double-blind, placebo-controlled studies revealed promising efficacy for cutaneous manifestations but not for asthma (153,154). Mild but treatable systemic reactions occurred in both trials during the build-up period. There may be a special niche for development of therapeutic rush immunotherapy in IgE-mediated OA due to protein allergens under protective cover of anti-IgE. Theoretically, the latter should prevent systemic reactions during the immunotherapy regimen.

FUTURE RESEARCH TRENDS

Future research in work-related asthma can be expected to focus on:

- essential differences and the status of compensatory awards between work-exacerbated and new onset OA;
- the utility of a broader definition of OA for public health purposes;
- long-term observation of atopic children when they reach employment age;
- the role of candidate genes in susceptibility, surveillance, and diagnosis;

- close surveillance and management of affected workers who continue to be exposed as well as those who are removed from exposure;
- a search for biologic markers of massive and low dose irritant effects in exposed workers;
- new diagnostic approaches to irritant-induced asthma which presents for the first time after a long absence from the alleged exposure;
- further refinements in preparation and utility of low-molecular-weight sensitizer skin and in vitro reagents (e.g., polyisocyanates, persulfate salts);
- more attention to the induction and propagation of nonasthmatic obstructive syndromes after workplace exposures (e.g., eosinophilic, neutrophilic bronchitis, bronchiolitis, and various forms of COPD);
- the inflammatory components of OA including those produced by innate immunity;
- more quality of life prospective studies;
- development of reliable exposure–response models for both high- and low-molecular-weight allergens;
- continued attention to the role of pollutants (e.g., endotoxin, ozone, and diesel fumes);
- OA as a model of environment–gene interactions;
- progress in the application of novel noninvasive techniques for estimating pathology and remodeling effects;
- the feasibility of immunotherapy for high-molecular-weight allergens under certain circumstances;
- the advantages of specialized centers offering expertise in OA for both workers and employers.

REFERENCES

1. Siegrist HE. Historical background of industrial and occupational diseases. Bull NY Acad Med 1936; 12:597–609.
2. Ramazzini B. De morbis artificum diatriba. Chicago: University of Chicago Press, 1940 (translated by WC Wright).
3. Pepys J, Jenkins PA, Festenstein GH, Gregory PJ, Lacey ME, Skinner FA. Thermophilic actinomycetes as a source of "farmer's lung hay" antigens. Lancet 1963; 2:607–611.
4. Thackrah CT (1832). The Effects of the Principal Arts, Trades and Professions, and of Civic States and Habits of Living on Health and Longevity, with Suggestions for the Removal of Many of the Agents Which Produce Disease and Shorten the Duration of Life. Reprint. Edinburgh: Livingstone, 1957.
5. Bostock J. Case of a periodical affection (?) of the eyes and chest. Med Chir Trans 1819; 10:161.
6. Blackley CH. Experimental Researches on the Causes and Nature of Catarrhus Aestivas (Hay Fever or Hay Asthma). London: Bailliere, Tindall & Cox, 1873.
7. Salter HH. On Asthma, Its Pathology and Treatment. London: Churchill, 1860.
8. Bernton HS. On occupational sensitization to the castor bean. Am J Med Sci 1923; 165:196–202.
9. Brooks SM. Occupational asthma. In: Weiss EB, Segal MS, Stein M, eds. Bronchial Asthma, Mechanisms and Therapeutics. 2nd ed. Boston: Little, Brown, 1985:461–493.
10. Figley KD, Elrod RM. Endemic asthma due to castor bean dust. JAMA 1928; 90:79–82.
11. Spielman AD, Baldwin HS. Atopy to acacia (gum arabic). JAMA 1933; 101:444–445.
12. Figley KD. Mayfly (Ephemerida) hypersensitivity. J Allergy 1940; 11:376–387.

13. Sprague PH. Bronchial asthma due to sensitivity to gum acacia. Can Med Assoc J 1942; 47:253.
14. Gelfand HH. The allergenic properties of vegetable gums. A case of asthma due to tragacanth. J Allergy 1943; 14:203–219.
15. Ordman D. Bronchial asthma caused by inhalation of wood dust. Ann Allergy 1949; 7:492–496.
16. Frankland AW. Locust sensitivity. Ann Allergy 1953; 11:445–453.
17. Karasek ST, Karasek M. The use of platinum paper. Report of Illinois State Commission of Occupational Disease, 1911:97.
18. Vallery-Radot P, Blamoutier R. Sensibilisation au chloroplatinite de potassium: accidents graves de choc survenus a la suite d'une cutireaction avec ce cel. Bull Soc Med Hop Paris 1929:222–230.
19. Joules H. Asthma from sensitisation to chromium. Lancet 1932; 2:182–183.
20. Card WI. A case of asthma sensitivity to chromates. Lancet 1935; 2:1348.
21. Kern RA. Asthma and allergic rhinitis due to sensitisation to phthalic anhydride. Report of a case. J Allergy 1939; 10:164–165.
22. Feinberg SM, Watrous BM. Atopy to simple chemical compounds, sulphonechloramides. J Allergy 1945; 16:209–220.
23. Hunter D, Milton R, Perry KMA. Asthma caused by the complex salts of platinum. Br J Ind Med 1945; 2:92–98.
24. Roberts AE. Platinosis: 5 year study of effects of soluble platinum salts on employees in platinum laboratory and refinery. Arch Ind Hyg 1951; 4:549–559.
25. Woodbury JW. Asthmatic syndrome following exposure to toluylene di-isocyanate. Ind Med Surg 1956; 25:540–543.
26. Tolot F, Broudeur P, Meulat G. Troubles pulmonaries asthmatiformes chez des ouvriers, exposes a l'inhalation de chrome, nickel, aniline. Arch Mol Prof 1957; 18: 291–293.
27. Gelfand HH. Respiratory allergy due to chemical compounds encountered in the rubber, lacquer, shellac and beauty culture industries. J Allergy 1963; 34:374–381.
28. Newman Taylor AJ. Occupational asthma. Thorax 1980; 35:241–245.
29. Colldahl H. Study of provocation tests on patients with bronchial asthma. Acta Allergol 1952; 5:133–142, 154–162.
30. Gandevia B. Respiratory symptoms and ventilatory capacity in men exposed to isocyanate vapour. Aust Ann Med 1964; 13:157–166.
31. Gandevia B, Milne J. Occupational asthma and rhinitis due to western red cedar (*Thuja plicaa*), with special reference to bronchial reactivity. Br J Ind Med 1970; 27:235–244.
32. Popa V, Teculescu D, Stanescu D, Gavrilescu N. Bronchial asthma and asthmatic bronchitis determined by simple chemicals. Dis Chest 1969; 56:395–404.
33. Pepys J, Pickering CAC, Bresin ABX, Terry DJ. Asthma due to inhaled chemical agents—toluylene di-isocyanate. Clin Allergy 1972; 2:225–236.
34. Pepys J, Hutchcroft BJ. Bronchial provocation tests in etiologic diagnosis and analysis of asthma. Am Rev Respir Dis 1975; 112:829–859.
35. Pepys J, Davies RJ, Breslin ABX, Hendrick DJ, Hutchcroft B. The effects of inhaled beclomethasone dipropionate (Becotide) and sodium cromoglycate on asthmatic reactions to provocation tests. Clin Allergy 1974; 4:13–24.
36. Carroll KB, Secombe CJP, Pepys J. Asthma due to nonoccupational exposure to toluene (tolylene) di-isocyanate. Clin Allergy 1976; 6:99–104.
37. Pepys J, Pickering CAC. Asthma due to inhaled chemical fumes—amino-ethyl-ethanolamine n aluminum soldering flux. Clin Allergy 1972; 2:197–204.
38. Sterling GM. Asthma due to aluminum soldering flux. Thorax 1967; 22:533–537.
39. Pepys J, Pickering CAC, Loudon HWG. Asthma due to inhaled chemical agents—piperazine hydrochloride. Clin Allergy 1972; 2:189–196.
40. Pickering CAC, Batten JC, Pepys J. Asthma due to inhaled wood dusts—western red cedar and Iroko. Clin Allergy 1972; 2:213 218.

41. Chan-Yeung M, Giclas PC, Henson PM. Activation of complement responsible for asthma due to western red cedar (*Thuja plicata*). J Allergy Clin Immunol 1980; 65:331–337.

42. Freedman SO, Krupey J. Respiratory allergy caused by platinum salts. J Allergy 1968; 42:233–237.

43. Levene GM, Calnan GD. Platinum sensitivity and treatment by specific hyposensitisation. Clin Allergy 1971; 1:75–82.

44. Pepys J, Pickering CAC, Hughes EG. Asthma due to inhaled chemical agents—complex salts of platinum. Clin Allergy 1972; 2:391–396.

45. Cromwell O, Pepys J, Parish WE, Hughes EG. Specific IgE antibodies to platinum salts in sensitised workers. Clin Allergy 1979; 9:109–118.

46. Cleare MJ, Hughes EJ, Jacoby B, Pepys J. Immediate (type I) allergic responses to platinum compounds. Clin Allergy 1976; 6:183–195.

47. Pepys J, Parish WE, Cromwell O, Hughes EG. Passive transfer in man and the monkey of type I allergy due to heat labile and heat stable antibody to complex salts of platinum. Clin Allergy 1979; 9:99–108.

48. Layton GT, Stanworth DR, Amos HE. Factor influencing the immunogenicity of the hapten drug chlorhexidine in mice. II. The role of the carrier and adjuvants in the induction of IgE and IgG anti-hapten responses. Immunology 1986; 59:459–465.

49. Maccia CA, Bernstein IL, Emmett REA, Brooks SM. In vitro demonstration of specific IgE in phthalic anhydride hypersensitivity. Am Rev Respir Dis 1976; 113:701–704.

50. Howe W, Venaables K, Topping MD, et al. Tetrachlorophthalic acid anhydride asthma: evidence for specific IgE antibody. J Allergy Clin Immunol 1983; 71:5–11.

51. Alanko K, Keskinen H, Bjorksten F, Ojanin S. Immediate type hypersensitivity to reactive dyes. Clin Allergy 1978; 8:25–31.

52. Murdoch RD, Pepys J, Hughes EG. IgE antibody responses to platinum group metals: a large scale refinery survey. Br J Ind Med 1986; 43:37–43.

53. Malo J-L, Cartier A, Doepner M, Nieboer E, Evans S, Dolovich J. Occupational asthma caused by nickel sulphate. J Allergy Clin Immunol 1982; 69:55–59.

54. Dolovich J, Evans SL, Nieboer E. Occupational asthma from nickel sensitivity. I. Human serum albumin in the antigenic determinant. Br J Ind Med 1984; 41:51–55.

55. Bernstein DI, Gallagher JS, D'Souza L, Bernstein IL. Heterogeneity of specific IgE responses in workers sensitized to acid anhydride compounds. J Allergy Clin Immunol 1984; 74:794–801.

56. Zeiss CR, Levitz D, Pruzansky JJ, Patterson R. Antibody to haptenized human serum albumin and human secretory IgA in workers exposed to trimellitic anhydride (TMA). J Allergy Clin Immunol 1982; 69:123 (abstract).

57. Butcher BT, Mapp C, Reed MA, O'Neill CE, Salvaggio JL. Evidence for carrier specificity of IgE antibodies detected in sera of isocyanate exposed workers. J Allergy Clin Immunol 1982; 69:123 (abstract).

58. Pepys J. Autoantibodies induced by extrinsic, low molecular weight chemical allergens. Proc XII Int Cong Allerg Clin Immunol. CV Mosby/St Louis1986:204–208.

59. Sarlo K. Inhalation sensitization of guinea pigs to toluene di-isocyanate: generation of antibodies that recognize toluene di-isocyanate and guinea pig serum albumin. Toxicology 1989; 9:72 (abstract).

60. Davies RJ, Hendrick DJ, Pepys J. Asthma due to inhaled chemical agents: ampicillin, benzyl penicillin, 6-amino-penicillanic acid and related substances. Clin Allergy 1974; 4:227–247.

61. Kammermeyer JK, Matthews KP. Hypersensitivity to phenyl-glycine acid chloride. J Allergy Clin Immunol 1973; 52:73–84.

62. Pepys J, Hutchcroft BJ, Breslin ABX. Asthma due to inhaled chemical agent—persulfate salts and henna in hairdressers. Clin Allergy 1976; 6:399–404.

63. Fawcett IW, Pepys J, Erooga MA. Asthma due to ''glycl compound'' powder—an intermediate in production of salbutamol. Clin Allergy 1976; 6:405–409.

64. Fawcett IW, Newman Taylor AJ, Pepys J. Asthma due to inhaled chemical agents—epoxy resin systems containing phthalic acid anhydride, trimellitic acid anhydride and triethylenetetramine. Clin Allergy 1977; 7:1–14.

65. Zeiss CR, Wolkonsky P, Chacon R, et al. Syndromes in workers exposed to trimellitic anhydride: a longitudinal clinical and immunologic study. Ann Intern Med 1983; 98:8–12.

66. Fawcett IW, Newman Taylor AJ, Pepys J. Asthma due to inhaled chemical agents—fumes from "Multicore" soldering flux and colophony resin. Clin Allergy 1976; 6:577–585.

67. Burge PS. Occupational asthma, rhinitis and alveolitis due to colophony. In: Pepys J, ed. Clinics in Immunology. Vol. 4. Occupational Respiratory Allergy. London: WB Saunders, 1984:55–81.

68. Burge PS, Wieland A, Robertson AS, Weir D. Occupational asthma due to unheated colophony. Br J Ind Med 1986; 43:559–560.

69. Murdoch RD, Pepys J. Immunological responses to complex salts of platinum. II. Enhanced IgE antibody responses to ovalbumin with concurrent administration of platinum salts in the rat. Clin Exp Immunol 1985; 58:478–485.

70. Salvaggio JE, Kayman H, Leskowitz S. Immunologic responses of atopic and normal individuals to aerosolized dextran. J Allergy 1966; 38:31–40.

71. Pepys J. Atopy. In: Gell PGH, Coombs RRA, Lachmann PJ, eds. Clinical Aspects of Immunology. 3rd ed. Oxford: Blackwell Scientific Publications, 1975:877–902.

72. Editorial. Smoking, occupation, and allergic lung disease. Lancet 1985; 1:965.

73. Zetterstrom O, Osterman K, Machads L, Johanson SGO. Another smoking hazard: raised serum IgE concentration and increased risk of occupational allergy. Br Med J 1981; 283:1215–1217.

74. Venables KM, Topping MD, Howe W, Luczynska CM, Hawkins R, Newman Taylor AJ. Interactions of smoking and atopy in producing specific IgE antibody. Br Med J 1985; 290:201–204.

75. Venables KM, Dally MB, Nunn AJ, et al. Smoking and occupational allergy in workers in a platinum refinery. Br Med J 1989; 299:939–941.

76. Greenberg M, Milne JE, Watt A. A survey of workers exposed to dusts containing derivatives of *Bacillus subtilis*. Br Med J 1970; 11:629–633.

77. Hulbert WC, Walker DC, Jackson A, Hogg JC. Airway permeability to horseradish peroxidase in guinea pigs: the repair phase after injury by cigarette smoke. Am Rev Respir Dis 1981; 123:320–326.

78. Morgan DC, Smyth JT, Lister RW, Pethybridge RJ. Chest symptoms and farmers' lung: a community survey. Br J Ind Med 1973; 30:259–265.

79. Morgan DC, Smyth JT, Lister RW, et al. Chest symptoms in farming communities with special reference to farmers' lung. Br J Ind Med 1975; 32:228–234.

80. Warren CPW. Extrinsic allergic alveolitis: a disease commoner in non-smokers. Thorax 1977; 32:567–569.

81. Arima K, Ando M, Yoshida K, et al. Suppressive effects of cigarette smoking on the prevalence of summer-type hypersensitivity pneumonitis caused by *Trichosporon cutaneum* and specific antibody response to the antigen. Am Rev Respir Dis 1990; 141:A316 (abstract).

82. Nordman H. Atopy and work. Scand J Work Environ Health 1984; 10:481–485.

83. De la Hoz R, Young R, Pedersen D. Exposure to potential occupational asthmagens; prevalence data from the National Occupational Exposure Survey. Am J Ind Med 1997; 31:195–201.

84. Davies RJ, Green M, Schofield NM. Recurrent nocturnal asthma after exposure to grain dust. Am Rev Respir Dis 1976; 114:1011–1019.

85. Newman Taylor AJ, Davies RJ, Hendrick DJ, Pepys J. Recurrent nocturnal asthmatic reactions to bronchial provocation tests. Clin Allergy 1979; 9:213–219.

86. Henrick DJ, Lane DJ. Occupational formalin asthma. Br J Ind Med 1977; 34:11–18.

87. Occupational asthma. Department of Health and Social Security (Social Security Act, 1975). Her Majesty's Stationery Office, 1981, Cmnd 8121.

88. Sallie B, Ross D, Meredith S, McDonald JC. SWORD '93: surveillance of work-related and occupational respiratory disease in the UK. Occup Med (London) 1994; 44(4): 172–182.

89. Olin AC, Andersson E, Granung G, Hagberg S, Toren K. Prevalence of asthma and exhaled nitric oxide are increased in bleachery workers exposed to ozone. Eur Respir J 2004; 23(1):87–92.

90. Hoppin JA, Umbach DM, London SJ, Alavanja MC, Sandler DP. Diesel exhaust, solvents and other occupational exposures as rising factors for wheeze among farmers. Am J Respir Crit Care Med 2004; 169(12):1308–1313.

91. Flodin U, Jonsson P. Non-sensitising air pollution at workplaces and adult onset asthma. Int Arch Occup Environ Health 2004; 77(1):17–22.

92. Dangman KH, Bracker AL, Storey E. Work-related asthma in teachers in Connecticut: association with chronic water damage and fungal growth in schools. Conn Med 2005; 69(1):9–17.

93. Proceedings of the First Jack Pepys Occupational Asthma Symposium. Am J Respir Crit Care Med 2003; 167:450–471.

94. Dewitte JD, Chan-Yeung M, Malo J-L. Medicolegal and compensation aspects of occupational asthma. Eur Resir J 1994; 7:969–980.

95. Bernstein DI, Korbee L, Stauder T, et al. The low prevalence of occupational asthma and antibody-dependent sensitization to diphenylmethane diisocyanate in a plant engineered for minimal exposure to diisocyanates. J Allergy Clin Immunol 1993; 92: 387–396.

96. Spector SL, Nicklas RA, eds. Practice parameters for the diagnosis and treatment of asthma. J Allergy Clin Immunol 1995; 96(suppl):707–870.

97. National Heart, Lung, and Blood Institute, National Asthma Education and Prevention Program. Expert Panel Report 2: Guidelines for the Diagnosis and Management of Asthma, pub. No. 97-4051. Bethesda, MD: National Institutes of Health, 1997.

98. Brooks SM, Weiss MA, Bernstein IL. Reactive airways dysfunction syndrome (RADS): persistent asthma syndrome after high level irritant exposure. Chest 1985; 88:376–384.

99. Gautrin D, Boulet LP, Boutet M, et al. Is reactive airways dysfunction syndrome (RADS) a variant of occupational asthma? J Allergy Clin Immunol 1994; 93:12–22.

100. Gautrin D, Leroyer C, Malo J-L. Longitudinal assessment of workers at risk of chlorine exposure. Am J Respir Crit Care Med 1996; 153:A-185.

101. Sallie B, McDonald C. Inhalation accidents reported to the SWORD surveillance project 1990–1993. Ann Occup Hyg 1996; 40:211–221.

102. Lemiere C, Malo J-L, Boutet M. Reactive airways dysfunction syndrome due to chlorine: sequential bronchial biopsies and functional assessment. Eur Respir J 1997; 10:241–244.

103. Houba R, Heederik D, Doekes G, van Run P. Exposure-sensitization relationship for α-amylase allergens in the baking industry. Am J Respir Crit Care Med 1996; 154:130–136.

104. Sussman G, Tarlo S, Dolovich. The spectrum of IgE-mediated responses to latex. JAMA 1991; 265:2844.

105. Heilman DL, Jones RT, Swanson MC, Yunginger JW. A prospective, controlled study showing that rubber gloves are the major contributor to latex aeroallergen levels in the operating room. J Allergy Clin Immunol 1996; 98:325–330.

106. Heederik D, Venables K, Malmberg P, et al. Exposure response relationships for occupational respiratory sensitizers: results from a European study in laboratory animal workers. J Allergy Clin Immunol 1999; 103:678–684.

107. Heederik D, Houba R. An exploratory quantitative risk assessment for high molecular weight sensitizers: wheat flour. Am Occup Hyg 2001; 45:175–185.

108. Peretz C, de Pater N, de Monchy J, Oostenbrink J, Heederik D. Assessment of expo sure to wheat flour and the shape of its relationship with specific sensitization. Scand J Work Environ Health 2005; 31(1):65–74.

109. Zhang XD, Lotvall JL, Skerfving S, Welinder H. Antibody specificity to the chemical structures of organic acid anhydrides studied by in vitro and in vivo methods. Toxicology 1997; 118:223–232.
110. Karol MH, Graham C, Gealy R, Macina OT, Sussman N, Rosenkranz HS. Structure activity relationships and computer-assisted analysis of respiratory sensitization potential. Toxicol Lett 1996; 86:187–191.
111. Botham PA, Lamb CT, Teasdale EL, Bonner SM, Tomenson JA. Allergy to laboratory animals: a follow-up study of its incidence and of the influence of atopy and pre-existing sensitization on its development. Occup Environ Med 1995; 52:129–133.
112. Bernstein JA, Kraut A, Bernstein DI, et al. Occupational asthma induced by inhaled egg lysozyme. Chest 1993; 103:532–535.
113. Rodier F, Gautrin D, Ghezzo H, Malo J-L. Incidence of occupational rhinoconjunctivitis and risk factors in animal-health apprentices. J Allergy Clin Immunol 2003; 112(6):1105–1111.
114. Brooks SM, Hammad Y, Richards I, Giovinco-Barbas J, Jenkins K. The spectrum of irritant-induced asthma: sudden and not-so-sudden onset and the role of allergy. Chest 1998; 113:42–49.
115. Balboni A, Baricordi OR, Fabbri LM, Gandini E, Ciaccia A, Mapp CE. Association between toluene diisocyanate-induced asthma and DQB1 markers: a positive role for aspartic acid at position 57. Eur Respir J 1996; 9:207–210.
116. Young RP, Barker RD, Pile KD, Cookson WOCM, Newman Taylor AJ. The association of HLA-DR3 with specific IgE to inhaled acid anhydrides. Am J Respir Crit Care Med 1995; 151:219–221.
117. Mapp CE, Beghe B, Balboni A, et al. Association between HLA genes and susceptibility to toluene diisocyanate-induced asthma. Clin Exp Allergy 2000; 30(5):651–656.
118. Mapp CE, Fryer AA, De Marzo N, et al. Glutathione S-transferase GSTP1 is a susceptibility gene for occupational asthma induced by isocyanates. J Allergy Clin Immunol 2002; 109(5):867–872.
119. Bernstein DI, Cartier A, Wanner M, et al. Haplotypes of IL-4 receptor and CD14 genetic polymorphisms are markers of susceptibility for diisocyanate asthma. AJRCCM 2003; 167:A580 (abstract).
120. Baker DB, Gann PH, Brooks SM, Gallagher J, Bernstein IL. Cross-sectional study of platinum salts sensitization among precious metals refinery workers. Am J Ind Med 1990; 18:653–664.
121. Venables KM, Chan-Yeung M. Occupational asthma. Lancet 1997; 349:1465–1469.
122. Hammond SK, Sorensen G, Youngstrom R, Ockene JK. Occupational exposure to environmental tobacco smoke. JAMA 1995; 274:956–960.
123. Mastrangelo G, Clonfero E, Pavanello S, et al. Exposure to diesel exhaust enhances total IgE in non-atopic dockers. Int Arch Occup Environ Health 2003; 76(1):63–68.
124. Saarinen K, Karjalainen A, Martikainen R, et al. Prevalence of work-aggravated symptoms in clinically established asthma. Eur Respir J 2003; 22(2):305–309.
125. Goe SK, Henneberger PK, Reilly MJ, et al. A descriptive study of work aggravated asthma. Occup Environ Med 2004; 61(6):512–517.
126. Tarlo SM, Liss G, Corey P, Broder I. A workers' compensation claim population for occupational asthma. Comparison of subgroups. Chest 1995; 107:634–641.
127. Beasley R, Roche WR, Roberts JA, Holgate ST. Cellular events in the bronchi in asthma and after bronchial provocation. Am Rev Respir Dis 1989; 139:806–817.
128. Bentley AM, Maestrelli P, Saetta M, et al. Activated T-lymphocytes and eosinophils in the bronchial mucosa in isocyanate-induced asthma. J Allergy Clin Immunol 1992; 89:821–829.
129. Maestrelli P, Del Prete GF, De Carli M, et al. CD8 T-cell clones producing interleukin-5 and interferon-gamma in bronchial mucosa of patients with asthma induced by toluene diisocyanate. Scand J Work Environ Health 1994; 20:376–381.
130. Lummus ZL, Alam R, Bernstein JA, Bernstein DI. Characterization of histamine releasing factors in diisocyanate-induced occupational asthma. Toxicology 1996; 111:191–206.

131. Sarlo K, Fletcher ER, Gaines WG, Ritz HL. Respiratory allergenicity of detergent enzymes in the guinea pig intratracheal test: association with sensitization of occupationally exposed individuals. Fund Appl Toxicol 1997; 38:44–52.

132. Karol MH, Jin RZ, Lantz RC. Immunochemical detection of TDI adducts in pulmonary tissue of guinea pigs following inhalation exposure. Inhal Toxicol 1997; 9:63–83.

133. Mapp CE, Lapa E, Silva JR, et al. Inflammatory events in the blood and airways of guinea pigs immunized to TDI. Am J Respir Crit Care Med 1996; 154:201–208.

134. Dearman RJ, Moussavi A, Kemeny DM, Kimber I. Contribution of CD4+ and CD8+ T lymphocyte subsets to the cytokine secretion patterns induced in mice during sensitization to contact and respiratory chemical allergens. Immunology 1996; 89:502–510.

135. Kimber I. The role of the skin in the development of chemical respiratory hypersensitivity. Toxicol Lett 1996; 86(2):89–92.

136. Faccione S, deSiqueira ALP, Jancar S, Russo M, Barbuto JAM, Mariano M. A novel murine model of late-phase reaction of immediate hypersensitivity. Media Inflamm 1997; 6:127–133.

137. Hamelmann E, Vella AT, Oshiba A, Kappler JW, Marrack P, Gelfand EW. Allergic airway sensitization induces T cell activation but not airway hyperresponsiveness in B cell-deficient mice. Proc Natl Acad Sci USA 1997; 94:1350–1355.

138. Bernstein DI, Bernstein IL, Gaines WG Jr, Stauder T, Wilson ER. Characterization of skin prick testing responses for detecting sensitization to detergent enzymes at extreme dilutions: inability of the RAST to detect lightly sensitized individuals. J Allergy Clin Immunol 1994; 49:498–507.

139. Buhring HJ, Streble A, Valent P. The basophil-specific ectoenzyme E-NPP3 (CD203c) as a marker for cell activation and allergy diagnosis. Int Arch Allergy Immunol 2004; 133(4):317–329.

140. Chan-Yeung M. Assessment of asthma in the workplace. Chest 1995; 108:1084–1117.

141. Gautrin D, Infante-Rivard C, Malo J-L. Specific IgE-dependent sensitization and change in bronchial responsiveness in a cohort of apprentices exposed to high-molecular-weight agents. Am J Respir Dis 1998; 155:A855.

142. Lemiere C, Efthimiadis A, Hargreave FE. Occupational eosinophilic bronchitis without asthma: an unknown occupational airway disease. J Allergy Clin Immunol 1997; 100:852–853.

143. Leigh R, Hargreave FE. Occupational neutrophilic asthma. Can Respir J 1999; 6(2):194–196.

144. Tanaka H, Saikaia T, Sugawara H, et al. Workplace-related chronic cough on a mushroom farm. Chest 2002; 122(3):1080–1085.

145. Birring SS, Berry M, Brightling CE, Pavord ID. Eosinophilic bronchitis: clinical features, management and pathogenesis. Am J Respir Med 2003; 2(2):169–173.

146. Piipari R, Piirila P, Keskinen H, Tuppurainen M, Sovijarvi A, Nordman H. Exhaled nitric oxide in specific challenge tests to assess occupational asthma. Eur Respir J 2002; 20(6):1532–1537.

147. Hunt J. Exhaled breath condensate: an evolving tool for noninvasive evaluation of lung disease. J Allergy Clin Immunol 2002; 110:28–34.

148. Samee S, Altes T, Powers P, de Lange EE, et al. Imaging the lungs in asthmatic patients by using hyperpolarized helium-3 magnetic resonance: assessment of response to methacholine and exercise challenge. J Allergy Clin Immunol 2003; 111(6):1201–1202.

149. Ikura H, Shimizu K, Ikezoe J, Nagareda T, Yagi N. In vitro evaluation of normal and abnormal lungs with ultra-high resolution CT. J Thorac Imaging 2004; 19(1):8–15.

150. Arnold JF, Fidler F, Wang T, Pracht ED, Schmidt M, Jakob PM. Imaging lung function using rapid dynamic acquisition of T1-maps during oxygen enhancement. MAGMA 2004; 16(5):246–253.

151. Shibuya K, Hoshino H, Chiyo M, et al. High magnification bronchovideoscopy combined with narrow band imaging could detect capillary loops of angiogenic squamous dysplasia in heavy smokers at high risk for lung cancer. Thorax 2003; 58:989–995.

152. Marabini A, Siracusa A, Stopponi R, Tacconi C, Abbritti G. Outcome of occupational asthma in patients with continuous exposure. A 3-year longitudinal study during pharmacologic treatment. Chest 2003; 124:2372–2376.
153. Leynadier F, Hermana D, Vervloet D, Andre C. Specific immunotherapy with a standardized latex extract versus placebo in allergic healthcare workers. J Allergy Clin Immunol 2000; 106(3):585–590.
154. Sastre J, Fernandez-Nieto M, Rico P, et al. Specific immunotherapy with a standardized latex extract in allergic workers: a double-blind, placebo-controlled study. J Allergy Clin Immunol 2003; 111(5):985–994.

3
Epidemiological Approaches in Occupational Asthma

Margaret R. Becklake
Respiratory Epidemiology and Clinical Research Unit, Departments of Medicine and Epidemiology, Biostatistics, and Occupational Health, McGill University, Montreal, Quebec, Canada

Jean-Luc Malo
Department of Chest Medicine, Université de Montréal and Sacré-Cœur Hospital, Montreal, Quebec, Canada

Moira Chan-Yeung
Occupational and Environmental Lung Disease Unit, Respiratory Division, Department of Medicine, University of British Columbia and Vancouver General Hospital, Vancouver, British Columbia, Canada

INTRODUCTION—THE ROLE OF EPIDEMIOLOGY

The Discipline of Epidemiology

Epidemiology has been described as a discipline and not as a science (1). As a discipline, epidemiology comprises a set of principles and approaches that, in their application to the study of human ill health, focus on the distribution and determinants of health-related states and disease in populations (2). The determinants of disease are usually considered under two broad headings—environmental and host factors. In the context of occupational asthma (OA), the environmental factors that are of interest are those encountered in the workplace and include all exposures, whether gaseous or airborne particulates, physical stress (heat and/or cold), or factors related to workplace organization. A determinant has been defined as "any physical, biological, social, cultural, or behavioral factor that influence the study outcome (in the present context, OA)" (2). It may be causal or not, and can increase or decrease risk; risk factors may be primary (i.e., they increase incidence) or secondary (i.e., they increase severity and/or trigger symptoms) (3).

Historical Perspective

The principles of epidemiology have been applied to the study of causes of work-related illness at least since the days of Ramazzini, a physician to the trade and craft workers of Padua, Italy, in the late 1600s and early 1700s (4). By recognizing

37

similarities in patterns of illness in those engaged in similar occupations, he was able to identify certain conditions as work related, for example, the "asthmatic troubles" in those who sifted and measured grain. With the social upheaval of the 1800s that accompanied the Industrial Revolution, and the concentration of labor into factories, the focus shifted from those with common occupations to those in similar workplaces. This period also saw the recognition of diseases such as "byssinosis" (a term introduced in 1887 to describe an asthma-like condition widespread in the cotton mills of North England) and pneumoconiosis (introduced to describe the harmful effects of mineral dusts on the lungs). At the end of the 20th century, the focus had again shifted both in terms of the disease outcomes and the exposures of concern. Thus, pneumoconiosis had yielded to stricter environmental controls (at least in the larger industries in countries with enforcement capability), so that the work-related diseases now of concern were airway disease (5,6) (asthma and chronic obstructive pulmonary disease) as well as lung and pleural cancer (7), all conditions that occur in the general population, but may also be caused by work-related exposures. By the 1990s, national surveys had shown that OA accounted for a substantial proportion of work-related lung disease recognized by workmen's compensation boards, ranging from 28% in the United Kingdom (8) through 38% in the United States (9) to as high as 52% and 63%, respectively, in the Canadian provinces of British Columbia (10) and Quebec (11). Not only smoking, but also the occupational environment contributes a substantial burden to chronic obstructive lung diseases (12,13). The total pollutant burden of dusts, dusts previously considered as nuisance dusts, and fumes, gases, and vapors even at quite low levels (10) as well as weather and temperature conditions in the general and occupational environments has also been examined with regard to their role in determining the outcome of airway function in the general population.

When the links between illness and work are obvious, the epidemiologic approach is similar to that used in infectious disease epidemiology; thus, the study of the sentinel case of OA (14) has much in common with the study of the index case in an outbreak of, for example, typhoid or cholera. When the link to work is less obvious, for instance, for late asthmatic reactions occurring away from work, including at night (15), then the epidemiologic approach may be closer to that used in the chronic disease epidemiology (6). Community epidemics of asthma due to environmental exposures have also been studied using the approaches of infectious disease epidemiology (16).

The increase in the frequency of OA among work-related lung diseases recognized by workmen's compensation boards in Europe and North America occurred over a period (1970 to 1990) when the prevalence, and probably the incidence, of asthma in the general population, particularly in children, had also been increasing. While environmental factors, particularly those associated with a "westernized" lifestyle, have been implicated (17), support continues to grow for the view that societies are also becoming more susceptible (18). If so, this may also have contributed to the increasing rates of OA among work-related lung diseases in these societies.

Work-Relatedness of Airway Disease Including Asthma

Because the work-relatedness of a disease differs for different disease conditions, the International Labor Office (7) suggested the use of the following categories to describe these relationships: (i) conditions caused only by agent-specific exposures; (ii) conditions of multifactorial etiology in which work exposures may be the primary or one of the several etiological factors; (iii) conditions to which an individual is

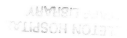

susceptible and in which the expression of disease is precipitated by a work-related exposure; and (*iv*) preexisting conditions aggravated by a work-related exposure. Conditions falling into category "i" were designated as *occupational diseases*, and those in categories "ii," "iii," and "iv" as *work-related diseases*, although this terminology is not universal. Asthma occurring at work could be considered in any one of these categories, depending on how it is defined (19), the particular agent under consideration, and the features of the asthma and/or asthma like reaction it evokes. As a consequence, definitions of OA vary, not only between clinicians in terms of the clinical diagnosis of OA (19–23), but also between jurisdictions in terms of attributability for medicolegal purposes (10,24). From the point of view of the individual suffering from work-related asthma, disability is the same, whatever the category of work-relatedness of the condition.

Determinants of OA

The classic approach to the study of occupational lung disease focuses on the environmental determinants with careful documentation of exposure levels by objective measurement (25). Objectives include characterizing the exposure–response relationships for the purposes of (*i*) establishing a causal relation between a contaminant and the respiratory effect under study, and/or (*ii*) providing the scientific basis for establishing workplace control levels (25). The epidemiologic approach to the study of OA is hampered by the nature of the condition itself for several reasons. First, asthma is usually a nonpermanent condition, and its markers may be absent during the epidemiologic survey. Second, once sensitized to an asthmogenic agent or agents in the workplace, the individual reacts to a lower level of exposure, often because of the development and persistence of nonspecific bronchial hyperresponsiveness (NSBH).

    As a result, certain prevalence studies, and even incidence studies, may fail to identify levels responsible for provoking the onset of the condition (even if the affected individual has not quit the workplace location). Furthermore, this level is likely to differ according to the mechanism triggering the hyperresponsiveness [allergic and immunoglobin (Ig) E–mediated, or irritative through stimulation of irritant receptors, or pharmacologic]. Theoretically, therefore, the slope and intercept of the exposure–response relationship might differ between individuals in the same workplace according to the mechanism of disease provocation (and therefore host factors).

    A 1988 editorial with the provocative title "Why study the epidemiology of asthma?" concluded that research into the causes of asthma should focus on its environmental determinants on the grounds that, despite extensive research on mechanisms, there is only one known host factor implicated in the development of asthma, namely atopy (both asthma and atopy may be genetically determined), in contrast to the considerable body of evidence indicating that asthma is in large measure an environmental condition (26).

METHODOLOGICAL ISSUES

Definitions of OA

Primary Definition vs. Diagnostic Criteria

As discussed above, the definition of a disease or condition varies according to the purpose for which information based on the definition is to be used. The editors of this book propose a definition of OA (Chapter 1) but recognize that other and different definitions may be desirable, depending on the circumstances. A distinction is also usually made between the primary definition of a medical term and its use as a diagnostic term to describe a particular case with certain clinical and/or laboratory features. Thus, for the clinical diagnosis of OA, these usually include the clinical and/or laboratory information necessary to establish the presence of (*i*) variable air-flow limitation and its relationship to work, (*ii*) immunologic status including atopy, (*iii*) NSBH, and (*iv*) the presence of sensitization to a specific agent (19). Clearly, also the features considered necessary to establish a clinical diagnosis of OA are more demanding and restrictive if the diagnosis is to be used for confirming the clinical diagnosis, than, for example, a screening examination in workers in a particular workplace under suspicion for causing OA. In the latter case, the findings might trigger an industrial hygiene survey (19,27), but not necessarily a clinical diagnosis or mandatory withdrawal from the workplace.

Definitions in Epidemiologic Studies

Epidemiologic studies of OA, like clinical examinations, are conducted with different objectives in mind; thus, the definition of asthma used will vary according to study question, study design, and study population. Thus, while epidemiologists accept the need for flexibility in the definition of outcome variables, they are nevertheless insistent that once a precise definition is formulated for a particular study, it must be meticulously respected. However, clinicians tend to be reluctant to accept information generated by studies using definitions that do not conform to what is necessary to describe clinical situations. To minimize clinical skepticism, the term "asthma-like" has been used (28). Nevertheless, clinical texts on asthma often start with a statement to the effect that there is no general consensus definition of asthma (29), let alone OA (Chapter 1).

Study Approaches and Design

In this section, study approaches and design are addressed both in general terms (Fig. 1) (30) and in specific terms, including their strengths and weaknesses as they apply to the investigation of the epidemiology of OA (Table 1) . Potential sources of bias are considered later.

The key to the scientific method is the experiment, a study design in which the researcher has control over all aspects of the study (Fig. 1) (Table 1) (25). This includes identification and characterization of the entire population eligible for study (or an appropriately selected sample) prior to randomization for the intervention, as well as a complete follow-up. Study inferences depend on comparing the exposed with the nonexposed, or comparing subjects receiving with those not receiving the intervention. In studies of human populations, the experimental design is exemplified in the randomized controlled trial (RCT), though even in this study design, random sampling of the entire eligible population is not usually achieved. In most other circumstances, a less than complete experimental design must be accepted as the only practical option. Such studies are classified as observational, because the key issue of allocation to exposure or not (and the issue that provides the comparisons on the basis of which study inferences are drawn) depends on circumstances beyond the control of the researcher. For instance, there is good evidence that entry into many contaminated workplaces is not a random event, but subject to selection factors, imposed either by others (for instance, by the preemployment examination) or

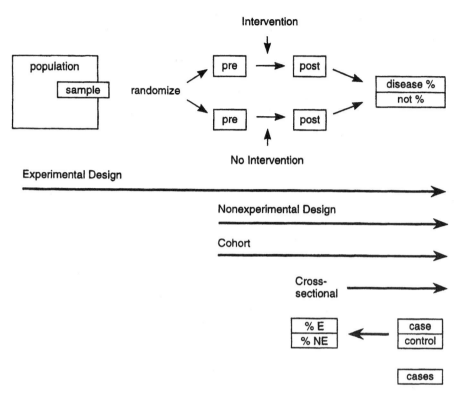

Figure 1 Design of epidemiological studies. *Source*: From Ref. 30.

by the individual, based on economic, social (31) or, more usually, health constraints, also called the "healthy hire" effect. The "healthy hire" and survivor effects are part of the healthy worker effect (32). Subjects with OA have been included in RCTs of asthma management and treatments, but the study population in such studies is seldom confined to cases of OA. A rare example of a RCT examined the effect of inhaled steroids on recovery from OA after removal from exposure (33).

 Longitudinal (cohort) studies are used to estimate incidence, i.e., the development of new cases in a specified time frame (Table 1). If the population is also stratified according to the exposure level, the relationship of incidence to exposure (exposure–response) can also be studied. Observational studies, longitudinal or cross-sectional, can be strengthened by parallel observations in a nonexposed group. However, even cohort studies, unless they account for those who leave a workplace (i.e., avoid survivor bias), may underestimate rates for OA. A study cohort can also be constituted retrospectively from data obtained in a cross-sectional study. For instance, subjects in a community-based study can be stratified into those whose asthma started prior to or after age 16 years (or prior to or after starting a given job). This would allow exposures which aggravate or induce asthma to be studied (34).

 Case–control (case-referent) studies are used to identify and amplify information about risk factors within a population. In this approach, which is closer to the clinical approach than prevalence or cohort studies, cases are identified and compared with noncases to provide additional information about environmental and/or host factors. In the investigation of OA, the case control design is greatly strengthened

Table 1 Designs Used in Epidemiological Studies: Features, Strengths, and Weaknesses

Design	Information provided	Strengths	Limitations	Comments on use
RCT	Evaluation (in terms of efficacy or effectiveness) of treatments, usually drugs, or other interventions; treatment trials may also test hypotheses about mechanisms underlying OA	All aspects of the study are under the researcher's control	Cases suitable for randomization often not representative of all cases	The design is strengthened if both observer and subject are blinded as to the nature of the intervention. Cases of OA be included in drug trails or be the target of a treatment trials to test a hypothesis
Longitudinal (cohort)	Incidence (number of new cases), determinants (host and exposure) of new cases over time; natural history of OA (studies usually workforce based and should include retirees)	Only source of direct evidence on host and exposure factors as determinants of OA; may be possible to determine the exposure dose that induces asthma, if exposure is measured in sufficient detail, e.g., in cohort of recruits	Subject to both selection and survivor bias, collectively the "healthy" worker effect; if follow-up is complete, survivor bias is minimized; loss from cohort likely due to the condition under study, i.e., asthma	Cohort studies in workforces at risk for OA are resource demanding and are less frequently undertaken than prevalence surveys; attention has more often been focused on host factors than on exposure; follow-up can be facilitated by linkage to workplace medical records or services; cohort studies should include retirees
Case-control	Additional information on host and/or environmental	Inexpensive of resources; allows detailed study of selected subjects to	Representativeness of controls not always easy to achieve except in nested	To date, infrequently used in the study of OA despite their strength in exploring

Design				
	determinants; if nested in a cohort or prevalence study, may provide information on risk factors and dose–response	facilitate contrasts, which will test hypotheses e.g., matching for exposure to focus on host factors, or vice-versa	case–control studies	causal factors, host and/or environmental
Cross-sectional (prevalence)	Prevalence (number of current cases) and potential determinants (host and exposure) at the time of study; usually workforces based	Practical: the "workhorse" of occupation epidemiology; can provide the definition of a cohort to be followed; source of evidence on exposure-response	Usually unable to establish time and cause and effect relationships; particularly subject to selection and survivor bias because of workplace turnover due to OA	The most commonly used design in occupational epidemiology; unable to establish whether atopy and/or bronchial hyperresponsiveness measured cross-sectionally preceded or followed the first clinical manifestations of asthma
Case series and case reports	Captures clinical experience (usual and unusual); able to generate hypotheses to explain cases which do not fit current clinical dogma	Provide material for laboratory study of mechanisms, e.g., inhalation challenge; may generate hypotheses from cases which do not fit current clinical dogma	Unable to provide information on rates or on workplace exposures implicated	Case reports from much of the published scientific literature on OA

Abbreviations: OA, occupational asthma; RCT, randomized, controlled trial.

if nested in a cohort or prevalence study (1). This permits cases to be matched with controls of similar exposure (if the study objective is to identify pertinent host factors), or matched with controls with comparable host factors, such as age (if the study objective is to identify pertinent exposure factors).

Cross-sectional (prevalence) studies, in which the study population is defined and described at the time of the study, give information on case rates at a given point in time (point prevalence) or on case rates up to the time of study (cumulative prevalence). In the case of OA, prevalence studies are particularly liable to underestimate rates because of the survivor bias referred to under longitudinal studies.

The term "survey" is often used. A survey is defined as "an investigation in which information is systematically collected but in which the experimental method is not used" (2). The term usually refers to prevalence studies. In the context of OA, the term invariably describes a field study in which data is gathered in a defined workplace or community. Tables 2 and 3 illustrate the type of information on the distribution and determinants of OA provided by epidemiologic studies of defined workforces or workplaces.

Clinical case studies and case reports summarize clinical experience, and will always remain a useful source of information, often providing the impetus for a planned investigation. They obviously do not provide information suitable for testing hypotheses concerning risk factors, in particular exposure, or establishing rates. In a book entitled *The Epidemiology of Work-Related Diseases*, which he edited, McDonald contributes an excellent section on study design to which the reader is referred (31). He emphasizes the concept of design for a purpose, the purpose being to answer the study question (having regard for the present state of knowledge) and this, in turn, drives the selection of the most appropriate and efficient design (i.e., a design that works), given the appropriate resources and opportunities available. In other words, the choice of design is a compromise between the feasible and the ideal, tempered by the availability of a suitable population and appropriate methods to measure the study outcome and the exposure. To capsulize his advice, McDonald cites Voltaire's admonition "*le mieux est l'ennemi du bien*," with a caution that while "perfectionism can hinder progress, the wrong answer can certainly do so." Study questions should be clear, unambiguous and, given the current state of knowledge, relevant to all parties, including the subjects, their medical advisors and the jurisdictions under which their cases are handled. They must obviously also be ethical, feasible in real time, and useful in fields beyond their own. Answers to study questions may be in the form of yes/no; i.e., a hypothesis was tested (e.g., does the administration of inhaled steroids improve the asthmatic condition of subjects with OA once they have left the workplace?) (33), or a number derived [e.g., what is the prevalence of asthma symptoms among adult Canadians (59)?] or both [e.g., what are the recent trends in physician-diagnosed asthma in Manitoba, Canada, and can they be explained by diagnostic exchange (28)?].

Target Populations

The term "target population" usually refers to the population a study seeks to describe and/or to which the results are to be generalized. The term has also been used to describe the collection of individuals about whom the study will make inferences (1). For a population at risk for OA with high employment turnover, and/or job change or rearrangement, particularly in the short term, the *survivor* effect is likely to be strong, and this has led to questions being raised as to what is

(*Text continues on page 49*)

Table 2 Workers Exposed to High-Molecular-Weight Agents: Results of Selected Cross-Sectional (Prevalence) Studies

First author, year, country, exposures/industry/occupation	No. studied	Exposure prior to diagnosis (months)	Prevalence			Determinants of the distribution of asthma symptoms in exposed workforces[c]	References
			Asthma[a] (%)	Smoking (%)	Atopy[b] (%)		
Mitchell, 1971, Australia, enzymes/detergent	98	Intermittent	50	52	64	Exposure level, not smoking or atopy	(35)
Desjardins, 1995, Québec, Canada, clam/shrimp processors	57	Intermittent	26(8)	49	21	Exposure, atopy	(36)
Malo, 1990, Québec, Canada, guar gum/carpet	162	Up to 108	23(2)	42	24	Exposure, not atopy	(37)
Cartier, 1984, Québec, Canada, snow-crab processors	303	Months	21(16)	67	11	Exposure, to a lesser extent smoking, not atopy	(38)
Burge, 1980, United Kingdom, locust research workers	109	Under 40	11	39	43	Exposure, atopy, not smoking	(39)
Slovak, 1981, United Kingdom, lab animal workers	141	36	10	n/a	24	Exposure, atopy	(40)
Gross, 1980, United States, lab animal workers	399	42	8	n/a	22	Exposure defined by job, atopy	(29)
Cullinan, 1994, United Kingdom, lab animal workers	238	26	7	30	40	Exposure intensity (dust or aeroallergens) at time of onset of symptoms; not smoking	(41)

(Continued)

Table 2 Workers Exposed to High-Molecular-Weight Agents: Results of Selected Cross-Sectional (Prevalence) Studies (*Continued*)

First author, year, country, exposures/industry/occupation	No. studied	Exposure prior to diagnosis (months)	Prevalence			Determinants of the distribution of asthma symptoms in exposed workforces[c]	References
			Asthma[a] (%)	Smoking (%)	Atopy[b] (%)		
Cullinan, 1994, United Kingdom, Bakery workers	264	12	6	57	34	Exposure intensity at time of survey, especially to flour allergens	(42)
Vandenplas, 1995, Belgium, latex, hospital workers	289	120	2(3)	24	25	Skin reactivity to latex	(43)

Note: Studies listed in decreasing order of prevalence of work-related asthma.

[a]Based on work-related chest symptoms, e.g., wheeze and/or difficulty with breathing; figures in parentheses are based on the algorithm for case identification (Fig. 2).

[b]Defined on the basis of a personal history of allergy or skin test reactivity to one or more allergens including the occupational agent(s) under investigation.

[c]Exposure usually defined by job and/or industrial hygiene measurement of airborne allergen levels (36,38,41).

Abbreviation: n/a, not applicable.

Table 3 Workers Exposed to Low-Molecular-Weight Agents: Results of Selected Cross-Sectional (Prevalence) Studies

Author, year, country, industry, occupation, (agent)	No. studied	Exposure prior to diagnosis (months)	Work-related asthma[a] (%)	Prevalence Smoking (%)	Atopy[b] (%)	Determinants of the distribution of asthma symptoms in exposed workforces[c]	References
Venables, 1989, United Kingdom, platinum refinery	91	12–24	54	63	33	Smoking, not atopy	(44)
Burge, 1979, United Kingdom, colophony electronics plant	924	24	22	47	n/a	Exposure, atopy, smoking (minimal)	(45)
Séguin, 1987, Québec, various isocyanates in secondary industry	51	54	20 (12)[d]	52	n/a	Exposure	(46)
Slovak, 1981, United Kingdom, plastics blowing (azodicarbamide)	151	n/a	19	43	48	Exposure, not smoking, not atopy	(47)
Wernfors, 1986, Sweden, phthalic anhydride	118	1–192	18	75	29	Exposure, atopy (weakly)	(48)
Burge, 1981, United Kingdom, factory making solder containing colophony	45	n/a	11	73	18	Exposure	(49)
Venables, 1985, United Kingdom toluene diisocyanate in secondary industry	241	Within 36 months in most cases	9.5	51	35	Exposure, probably not atopy	(50)
Malo, 1988, Québec, Canada, pharmaceutical company (spiramycin)	51	n/a	9 (8)	48	39	Exposure	(51)
Butcher, 1970, United States, TDI production	112	Not given	8.3	Not given	23	Exposure, not atopy	(52)
Vedal, 1986, BC, Canada, red cedar saw mills (plicatic acid)	334	120	8.0	35	n/a	Exposure level	(53)

(*Continued*)

Table 3 Workers Exposed to Low-Molecular-Weight Agents: Results of Selected Cross-Sectional (Prevalence) Studies (*Continued*)

Author, year, country, industry, occupation, (agent)	No. studied	Exposure prior to diagnosis (months)	Prevalence Work-related asthma[a] (%)	Smoking (%)	Atopy[b] (%)	Determinants of the distribution of asthma symptoms in exposed workforces[c]	References
Malo, 1994, Québec, Canada, white cedar saw mills (plicatic acid)	42[d]	13	7[d]	71	n/a	Exposure	(54)
Chan-Yeung, 1984, BC, Canada, red cedar workers (plicatic acid)	652	n/a	4	38	19	Exposure, not atopy	(55)
Ishizaki, 1973, Japan, furniture makers using red cedar (plicatic acid)	1320	12–24	3.4	n/a	n/a	Exposure, atopy	(56)

Note: Studies listed in decreasing order of prevalence of work-related asthma.

[a]Based on various reported work-related symptoms, e.g., wheeze, difficulty with breathing, chest tightness, shortness of breath upon hurrying in the level, etc. (see individual references), not present before employment started and/or improved on weekends. Figures in parentheses based on the algorithm for case definition (Fig. 2).

[b]Variously defined on the basis of a history of previous allergies or positive skin tests to one or more antigens including the occupational agent(s) under investigation.

[c]Exposure was most often defined by job, in some studies by duration, and in a few by measurement of airborne allergen levels (47, 51, 57, 58).

[d]Refers to subjects considered to have OA.

Abbreviations: n/a, not applicable; TDI, toluene diisocyanate; OA, occupational asthma.

the appropriate denominator (or target population) for prevalence and/or incidence studies (those ever exposed, those currently exposed, or the average workforce over a given period of time?) and what is the appropriate time frame for data collection (months, years, or decades?) (59,60). Obviously, results will vary with each definition of the denominator and/or time frame, and the choice will depend on the precise objective of the study. For instance, if the objective is to describe the prevalence of OA in a workforce exposed to high-molecular-weight allergens, a shorter time frame, but at least two years, should be used, given that about 40% of the subjects develop asthma within two years of exposure, and only 20% after 10 years of exposure (61). Results will also vary according to each definition of the denominator and/or the time frame, and the choice will depend on the precise objective of the study. For instance, if the data is being collected to compare with published data on similar workforces, the choice will be made to maximize comparability of the data sets. If, on the other hand, the study objective is to assess the burden of OA in the general population, then a suitable choice for the rate denominator would be those exposed and followed up in the long term, at least for years, and preferably for decades. Such studies should also be community-rather than workforce-based to include those with short exposures and thus take into account high turnover rates.

Principles of Measurement in Epidemiological Studies

Inference in science depends on comparisons of measurements made in appropriately selected material. In the case of epidemiological studies of OA, *inference depends on comparison of population groups*, which exhibit differences in health characteristics or have been subject to different exposures. Thus the measurements and the measurement tools, whether of health outcome or exposure, must be equally sensitive and/or specific for individuals in the two groups. In other words, every precaution must be taken to minimize measurement differential across the comparison groups because *imprecision in outcome or exposure measurements* can only lead to *attenuation of exposure–response* relationships, and so diminish the chances of showing a relationship between asthma and workplace contaminants. In addition, whatever outcome measurements are used must be repeatable within the same subject, and valid (i.e., measure what they purport to measure). Estimates of within-subject variation (repeatability) are also necessary for calculations of sample size and/or study power. Thus, in any epidemiological study, but particularly in epidemiologic studies of OA, no effort should be spared to assure the quality of the data in terms of reproducibility and validity of the measurements of outcome and response. This is why as eminent a biostatistician as Rothman (62) expresses the view that "an epidemiologic study is properly viewed as an exercise in measurement with accuracy as the goal."

For epidemiologic studies, *the tools used to measure health outcomes* are derived from the tools used in clinical medicine, but adapted and standardized so that the information they furnish is equally repeatable and equally valid in the comparison groups on which the study inferences will be based. Thus, the respiratory symptom questionnaire, a surrogate for the clinical history, is a means to assure that the"interview" with each study subject is conducted in a standardized fashion, rather than the process being open ended and personalized as is usual in the clinical setting. Likewise, if lung function tests are to be used, the procedure for administering them must be standardized so that each study subject is given the same instructions and the opportunity to perform the same number of trials, rather than this being left to the technician's judgement as would be the case for a clinical test (63). In the case of allergy skin tests, the wheal can be traced onto transparent tape for possible remeasurement of the wheal size at a later date.

The tools used to measure exposure in epidemiologic studies of OA vary considerably, depending on the nature of the study, its objectives, the study site(s) and resources available. All of the following have been used with success: (i) self-reported exposure by the subject (5,19,64); (ii) available industrial hygiene data on the work place, either current and collected for the purpose of the study or gathered from past company, or from other records (65); and (iii) industrial hygiene evaluation of the subject's work place exposures based on a job/industry history, often using a job exposure matrix or occupational title–based system (66). In some studies (i) has been shown to be complementary to (ii) and (iii), because it provides information not contained in (ii) and (iii) (64).

Outcome Measurements

Questionnaires

In contrast to clinical case identification, which calls for standardization, case definition and the choice of outcome measurement in epidemiological studies of OA can be expected to vary according to the purpose of the study, the study question, design and other features that include innocuousness, and easiness and cost of the investigative means. For instance, many population- and workplace-based studies have used only questionnaires to assess the frequency of OA. Indeed, the first study of OA in grain workers carried out in the early 1700s in Italy by Ramazzini was based on questionnaire information (4,67). The first report of diisocyanate-induced asthma, the most common cause of OA in developed countries, also exclusively utilized a questionnaire (68). Questionnaires have an obvious advantage of being noninvasive and easy to administer and are appropriate for population studies of prevalence and attributable risk (69). However, they have several limitations. First, although questionnaires for epidemiologic studies of chronic obstructive lung diseases developed in the 1960s by the Medical Research Council of Great Britain and by the American Thoracic Society did provide useful information on the epidemiology of OA, a standardized questionnaire for the investigation of asthma has been only recently developed and validated in international comparisons (70). Second, several but not all studies (71,72) show poor correlation between responses to questions on asthma symptoms and the presence or absence of NSBH originally regarded as the hallmark of asthma. Third, bronchial hyperresponsiveness can exist without symptoms (73). Fourth, some asymptomatic subjects with bronchial hyperresponsiveness can develop symptoms in subsequent years (73,74). Fifth, questionnaires administered by trained physicians have variable sensitivity and specificity in predicting asthma or OA (75–77). Finally, subjects may overreport or underreport their symptoms depending on the circumstances in which the questionnaire is being administered. From Table 2, it can be seen that the proportion of workers proven to be suffering from OA by specific challenge tests or by peak flow rate recording varies in different studies, ranging from 2% to 16% of workers who were considered to have OA using the questionnaire. Thus, the questionnaire is a sensitive tool but not a specific one, and while invaluable in analytical (etiological) epidemiological studies in populations at risk for OA, it is inadequate on its own for clinical case identification.

Immunological Assessment

Assessment of the atopic status of subjects is often included in epidemiologic studies of asthma and OA because atopy is the most important risk factor in asthma. Allergy skin tests using the prick method with common inhalant allergens such as house dust, house dust mite, cat epidermal antigen, and some local pollens have been found to be invaluable in field studies to assess the atopic status of subjects. They are easy to perform and do not give systemic or serious local reactions (78). Personal and family history of allergy does not correlate well with the tendency of individuals to produce IgE antibodies (79).

Many occupational agents cause asthma by sensitization with the production of specific IgE antibodies. These include mostly high-molecular-weight proteins which are complete antigens and some low-molecular-weight agents, such as phthalic anhydride, which act as haptens (80). When appropriate antigens are available, skin tests can be performed and blood samples can be taken for the determination of specific IgE antibodies at the time of the survey. These tests provide objective evidence of sensitization. They are useful in surveillance programs of at-risk subjects because they are considered as early markers of an IgE-mediated process whose history starts with immunological sensitization and proceeds toward symptomatology, either simultaneously or thereafter.

At present, immunologic assessment has little role in the clinical diagnosis or case identification in epidemiologic studies of workplaces with exposures to the majority of low-molecular-weight agents. There is a great need to develop and make available commercially standardized antigens for these investigations.

Functional Assessment

Measurement of Lung Function.   Measurement of lung function is important in assessing respiratory hazards due to various airborne pollutants. It may be necessary to perform lung function tests at the plant site and this presents special problems not usually encountered in hospitals or clinic laboratories (63). It is important to have trained technicians to calibrate the equipment and be able to deal with problems with instrumentation. The technicians should also be trained to recognize poor subject performance (81). Poor performance, in particular poor reproducibility, may also be a marker of airway dysfunction (82).

There is an array of available pulmonary function tests. Several factors need to be considered in choosing the lung function tests: the cost of equipment, the testing time, the simplicity of the test, and analysis of results, reproducibility, acceptability and the degree of standardization of the instrument and test procedures. Measurements of peak expiratory flows (PEF), forced expiratory volume in one second (FEV_1), forced vital capacity (FVC), and maximum mid-expiratory flow rate (FEF, 25–75%) by spirometry fulfill all the criteria mentioned above. However, for epidemiologic studies, measurements of PEF, FEV_1, FVC, and FEV_1/FVC are probably adequate. Although FEF 25% to 75% is considered a more sensitive test, it is more variable compared with FEV_1 and FVC. Instrument requirement, calibration techniques, test procedures, measurement of test results, and data interpretation should conform to the ATS or ERS guidelines (83).

Pre- and Postshift Spirometric Measurement.   Assessment of pre- and postshift (cross-shift) FEV_1 has been used to confirm the work-relatedness of asthma. Initial reports were to the effect that this test was neither a specific nor a sensitive method for case identification, probably due to a combination of factors such as diurnal variation (levels are lowest in the early hours of the morning, highest in the early hours of the afternoon), measurement or technical errors, and intermittent rather than daily exposure to the sensitizing agent (84). On the other hand, measurement of cross-shift change in lung function has proved a very useful way of detecting acute nonallergic airway response to exposure to occupational agents such as cotton dust and grain dust. The cross-shift change in lung function is directly proportional to the level of exposure.

Serial Measurements of PEF. Although serial measurements of PEF rate have proven to be a valuable tool in assessment of patients with OA in a clinical setting (85) and show a reasonable correlation with the results of specific challenge testing, their role in the assessment of OA in prevalence surveys is questionable. Serial PEF monitoring has been used successfully in several epidemiological surveys (38,51,77,86). To date, no study has explored the validity of PEF monitoring in comparison with specific inhalation challenges for screening of subjects with OA in a large number of subjects in the workplace. There is also the practical problem of subject compliance because the subjects are usually asked to monitor their PEF at least four times a day at work and at home for a period of three to four weeks, a commitment that many find hard to keep. More time will be needed in the field study to explain and instruct the subjects how to measure and register their own PEF properly. Moreover, there might be falsifications in the way subjects record and register the readings (38). The between-observer reproducibility of the interpretation of peak flow rate recordings obtained from surveys is, however, good (87) and comparable to the interpretation carried out in a clinical setting (88).

Nonspecific Challenge Tests. Measurement of nonspecific bronchial responsiveness has been used by a number of investigators in epidemiologic surveys of general populations (89,90) and workplace populations (91-94). These studies have shown that methacholine, histamine, and hyperventilation of unconditioned air challenge tests can be carried out in epidemiologic settings safely without the presence of physicians. As discussed in Chapter 9, measurement of nonspecific bronchial responsiveness is not specific enough to be used alone in identifying subjects who would attract a clinical diagnosis of asthma. However, when combined with questionnaire information and immunologic tests (when feasible), this test is very useful for identifying subjects with possible OA in the workplace (94).

Specific Challenge Tests. The methodology of specific challenge tests is discussed separately in Chapter 10. Specific challenge tests with the suspected offending agent have been used successfully in the clinical setting to confirm the diagnosis of OA. It is not practical to include specific challenge testing in field studies. However, these tests can be used to confirm the diagnosis in subjects suspected of OA identified through surveillance means.

Algorithm for Case Identification (Decision Tree) in Epidemiologic Studies of OA. A stepwise approach (Fig. 2) proposed elsewhere has been used successfully in several field studies (10). The first two steps have usually been carried out during field studies.

Subjects who require further investigation for the confirmation of the diagnosis of OA include those who have questionnaire responses compatible with work-related asthma, evidence of immunologic sensitization, and/or nonspecific bronchial responsiveness. Serial monitoring of PEF and specific challenge tests should also be conducted on these subjects. It is highly unlikely that subjects without evidence of nonspecific bronchial responsiveness and immunologic sensitization will react on specific challenge testing to the offending agent.

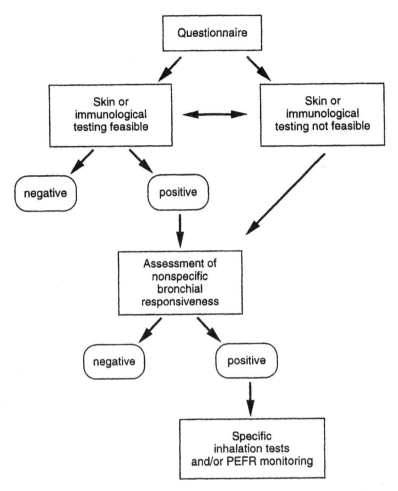

Figure 2 Epidemiological investigation of occupational asthma. *Abbreviation*: PEFR, peak expiratory flow rate.

Assessment of Risk Factors

Exposure Assessment

In occupational epidemiology studies, the strongest evidence of causality is provided by exposure–response relationships. For the pneumoconioses, the key environmental determinant of chronic respiratory effects has been shown to be the cumulative exposure to inorganic dust, measured as the product of the level and the duration of exposure, exposure–response relationships being stronger for this measurement than for either of its components. Assessment of exposure in epidemiological studies of OA is essential to determine exposure–response relationship with the ultimate aim of determining the exposure limit of asthma-inducing agents for prevention of disease. A variety of exposure-limit values have been developed to protect workers from the toxicological effects of uncontrolled exposure to chemical contaminants. Most of these thresholds are supported by or extrapolated from animal or in vitro toxicological data. These exposure limits are inadequate for the prevention of OA where individual susceptibility may play a role in the sensitization process. In OA, little work has been carried out on quantifying exposure until the last two decades. This is due to the perceived importance of individual sensitivity rather than to the dose. Moreover, as the agents responsible are often proteinaceous and exist as dry or wet aerosols, different methods of collection, measurement, and analysis are required, most of which have only been developed in the last two decades.

Several studies have shown that there is a dose–response relationship between the level of exposure and the prevalence of sensitization or asthma due to occupational agents. They include exposure to western red cedar (53,95), flour (42,96), laboratory animals (41), colophony (97), and acid anhydride (50). Some of these are HMW sensitizers such as flour and laboratory animal proteins. Most of these agents contain several allergens. In most epidemiological studies, exposure to these substances has been assessed by total dust concentration, for example, for flour, wheat dust, protein content for latex allergen, and enzyme activities for enzyme exposure. These approaches were not sensitive or specific. The introduction of specific and highly sensitive immunoassays to measure the allergen content of dust samples has permitted much more accurate assessment of exposure for determination of threshold limits.

Immunochemical methods use antibodies, which are specifically directed against the antigens or allergens to be measured. The methods are very sensitive and can detect a tiny amount of allergen present in dust samples. Antibodies in the immunoassays are specific IgE or IgG4 antibodies from sensitized workers, polyclonal antibodies from serum of animals, or monoclonal antibodies produced by hybridomas of immunized animals. Details of these assays can be found in Chapter 8. It is necessary to validate and standardize the antibodies and purify the allergen standards for epidemiological studies of exposure–response relationship in order to determine threshold limit values.

Using standardized methods for sampling and determination of allergens in dust samples, comparisons could be made between different studies and populations. A European collaborative project was carried out using data from three independent studies of 1062 laboratory animal workers with measurement of airborne allergen using immunochemical methods (98). The results showed that average exposure multiplied by the number of hours worked a week with rats was more strongly associated with sensitization than mean exposure or the number of hours worked with rats. Interestingly, atopic workers had a much higher risk of sensitization at very low levels of exposure than nonatopic workers, but the risk did not increase further with higher exposure. In nonatopic workers, the higher the exposure, the higher was the risk of sensitization. It is therefore necessary to know the slope of the exposure–response curve to determine threshold limit values. The authors also showed that there is a wide range in sensitization potency between various allergens. For example, sensitization to rat urinary proteins occurs in the pg/m^3 range, to pig and cow allergen in $\mu g/m^3$ range and in $\mu g/m^3$ range for fungal alpha-amylase.

Traditional industrial hygiene techniques are available for measuring several low-molecular-weight chemicals capable of causing asthma, such as diisocyanates. Direct reading monitors are also now available for measurement of chemicals such as formaldehyde, amines, and diisocyanates. However, these methods may not be sensitive enough for detecting low but sensitizing levels.

In acute challenges with occupational agents in the laboratory, the total dose of the agent (i.e., concentration $\times$ duration of exposure) is the most important determinant of the severity of reaction (99). It is therefore tempting to extrapolate these findings to the actual work situation, i.e., total dose of exposure rather than the concentration is probably more relevant in causing sensitization.

It has been suggested that exposure to high concentrations of diisocyanates (spills) can induce asthma (100). Intermittent exposure to levels higher than the permissible concentration (but not levels encountered in a spill) of an agent may be more important in causing OA than continuous exposure to low levels of the same agent (100). In this context, a continuous monitoring device with direct readout would be much more useful in assessing exposure than the measurement of eight-hour average, which is often the practice. Further extensive research is required in this area.

Once an individual is sensitized to an agent, a minute dose below the permissible exposure limits can bring on an attack of asthma. Concomitant environmental exposures such as to low levels of irritants and cigarette smoke may enhance sensitization to some occupational agents.

Sampling Methods. Personal sampling gives a better estimate of individual exposure than area sampling. Personal sampling of aeroallergens in the general breathing zone has become more common in occupational studies in the past 10 years (20,101) to quantitate individual exposure to biologic substances in the workplace using immunochemical methods. These new sampling devices have greatly improved the methodology for collecting high-molecular-weight aeroallergens (102).

Nasal sampling has been described for measurement of the actual inhaled amount and particle sizes of inhaled aeroallergens. This will improve our understanding of exposure–response relationships of occupational respiratory allergens relevant to their site of action (upper or lower airway) (103). The potential advantage of nasal sampling is to determine the true personal inhaled allergen exposure, provided the worker is not mouth-breathing and that the relatively short sampling time captures the appropriate work activities and exposure. Further studies are required to assess the usefulness of this new device.

Host Determinants of OA

While exposure is the single most important determinant in OA (104,105), not all subjects develop OA given the same degree of exposure. Various host markers (genetically determined) and factors (acquired) have been incriminated. Atopy has been shown to be associated with sensitization to high-molecular-weight agents. In a prospective study of apprentices of animal facilities, atopy, respiratory symptoms during the pollen season, and exposure to rodents for more then 52 hours were found to be significant determinants for specific sensitization (106). Atopy was also found to be a significant determinant for sensitization to latex in a prospective study of apprentices in dental hygiene (107) as well as in bakers (108,109). However, the positive predictive value of atopy in OA is low, 34% in laboratory animal workers (40), 8% in workers exposed to guar gum (37), and 7% in those exposed to psyllium (110). Atopy was only marginally associated with the development of probable OA in laboratory animals in a prospective study (94). These findings do not justify routine screening of atopy in high-risk workplaces. Atopic individuals who wish to enter certain high-risk workplaces should be advised of this potential risk in advance. If they do enter the workplace, regular follow up examinations for early detection of sensitization and development of NSBH (i.e., surveillance for case identification) should be carried out. Atopy is not associated with OA due to low-molecular-weight agents (54,55).

The effect of smoking on OA appears to be dependent on the type of occupational agent. When the agent induces asthma by producing specific IgE antibodies, cigarette smoking enhances sensitization. Venables et al. found an interaction between smoking and atopy in workers exposed to laboratory animals (111) and tetrachlorophthalic anhydride (50): atopic smokers had the highest and the nonatopic nonsmokers the lowest prevalence of sensitization. Among platinum refinery workers, smoking, not atopy, is the most important risk factor for sensitization (112). Cigarette smoking, however, was not associated with increased work-related asthmatic symptoms in workers exposed to detergent enzymes (35). When the agent induces asthma independent of IgE antibodies, nonsmokers may be more frequently affected than smokers as in diisocyanate-induced asthma (113), colophony (45), and red cedar asthma (114).

The role of NSBH as a host marker in OA requires more study. In most studies, NSBH appears to be an acquired phenomenon rather than a predisposition. This conclusion is based on the demonstration of improvement in NSBH in some subjects who withdraw from exposure and worsening of bronchial hyperresponsiveness on reexposure to the offending agent. In a prospective study of western red cedar sawmill workers, none of the four workers who developed red cedar asthma had NSBH before development of symptoms (115). However, in the prospective study of apprentices exposed to laboratory animals, nonallergic bronchial hyperresponsiveness and baseline skin test reactivity to pets were significant determinants of probable OA (94).

Other genetic markers may be important in OA. Recently, HLA class II genetic markers were studied in subjects with different types of OA (Chapter 4). Most of these studies involved a relatively small number of patients and in many instances, control subjects were from population samples rather than exposed subjects without asthma. Studies of genetic markers may help us to understand the pathogenic mechanism of OA.

Upper airway symptoms such as rhinitis and conjunctivitis often precede the occurrence of lower airway symptoms. They can be used as an early marker of OA. Malo et al. have shown that rhinitis and conjunctivitis often occurred before the development of asthma in patients exposed to both high- and low-molecular-weight agents (57). Gautrin et al. (116) have also shown that rhinoconjunctivitis may precede the development of OA although the predictive value is only around 30%. Finally, it was recently suggested that metal fume fever may be associated with the development of probable OA in an apprentice welders (117).

Sources of Bias in Epidemiologic Studies of OA

All observational studies, and to a much lesser extent experimental studies (RCTs), are potentially subject to bias, and the validity of study inferences depends to the extent that these sources of bias are minimized. Bias is defined as "deviation of results or inferences from the truth," or processes leading to that deviation" and the definition is further elaborated to include "any trend in the collection, analysis, interpretation, publication, or review of data that can lead to conclusions that are systematically different from the truth" (2).

The most important sources of bias are: (i) *selection bias* (the study population is not representative of the target population in terms of health or exposure characteristics); (ii) *information bias* (bias in the health and exposure information gathered, usually *recall bias* due to those who report symptoms and attribute their symptoms to work exposure, being more likely to recall any workplace exposures compared to those who report no symptoms); and (iii) *confounding bias*. A confounder is defined as "a variable that can cause or prevent the outcome of interest, is not an intermediate variable" (i.e., a step in the process of disease development) "and is associated with the factor under investigation" (2). This usually refers to the fact that the variable is unevenly distributed across the comparison groups and unless it is possible to take it into account in analysis, its effects cannot be distinguished from those of the factor under study. For instance, in a study of OA in which lung function is to be compared in groups exposed to high and low levels of a work place asthmagen, smoking (also associated with reduced lung function level) would be a confounder if smoking rates were higher (or lower) in one group compared with the other. As a result, it would not be possible to separate the independent effect of the asthmagen unless the information on smoking was available and was taken into account in analysis.

In epidemiological studies of OA, selection bias is probably the most important, due to the "healthy worker" effect, either because susceptible individuals rarely enter jobs at risk or they quit after such short periods and are never recorded as workers (the "healthy hire" effect), or because, at the time of a workplace survey, those most affected have either already left the workplace, or rearranged their jobs to minimize exposure, or changed jobs, and do not therefore appear on the company lists as holding an at-risk job (the "survivor" effect) (32). Examples of the "healthy hire" effect are to be found in studies of laboratory animal workers (100) those exposed to isocyanates at work (46), those who handle spiramycin (51), in grain workers (118), and in foundry workers (119). Examples of the "survivor" effect are also to be found in studies of grain workers and in laboratory animal workers (100,120). By contrast, community-based studies, because they minimize selection bias, have been consistent in showing associations between asthma outcomes and occupational exposures (see page 61). They have, however, the disadvantage that exposure is of necessity self-reported and therefore subject to information bias.

Practical Issues Associated with Occupational Surveys

The key to a successful occupational survey is to obtain cooperation from both the management and the labor. It should ideally be preceded by discussions with the local occupational health and safety committees (joint management and labor) about local concerns and issues to be addressed by the study. From the onset, the investigator should emphasize the necessity for confidentiality of individual medical results and that no medical information regarding an individual will be released without signed consent. Once the protocol has been agreed upon, it is usually a good idea for the investigator to meet with the workers and explain to them the purpose of the study, test procedures, possible side effects, and the rationale for each test.

Ideally, environmental monitoring should be carried out at the time of the survey to study the effects of current exposure. It is also important to obtain results of previous measurements from the management. If measurements of personal sampling were available in the past and were found to be accurate, one can construct cumulative exposure indices for effects of chronic exposure. To study the effects of acute exposure, personal sampling can also be carried out together with cross-shift measurements of lung function.

Tests in the field may not be conducted under optimal conditions. For example, there may be wide temperature fluctuation during the day if the temperature of the room cannot be regulated. It is, therefore, very important to have test procedures standardized as much as possible. The temperature and pressure should be noted at different times of the day. Calibration of lung function equipment should be done at the worksite daily before testing or twice daily, if a large number of workers are to be tested.

Confidentiality of information should be emphasized to workers to allay their fears. It should be noted that methods used in surveys can only screen for individuals with possible asthma. Further tests are necessary for confirming the diagnosis of OA. Individuals identified as having possible OA should be given the opportunity of having confirmatory tests (if those are offered) without losing their jobs. Furthermore, when the diagnosis is confirmed, every effort should be made to help the individual to obtain a transfer or to find other employment. Without such guarantee ahead of time, it will not be possible to have accurate case identification.

It is also important to have the survey conducted at the worksite and the tests performed in an organized and efficient manner to minimize the time lost from productivity. A well-organized schedule should be made to avoid individuals waiting between tests. At the end of the study, it is a good practice to send individual results directly to the worker and offer to give further explanation if necessary. Advice to the worker and an offer for further testing can be given at the same time. It is also advisable to present the group results to the local occupational health committee for further input before the preparation of the final report.

DISTRIBUTION AND DETERMINANTS OF OA

Workforce-Based Studies

There is a rich literature of workforce-based surveys, some initiated by the identification of clusters of cases, through physician referral or sentinel programs, and others seeking a priori to examine risk factors associated with particular asthmagenic exposures. Tables 2, 3, and 4 summarize the findings from selected studies, cross sectional and longitudinal, of workplaces contaminated by high- and low-molecular-weight asthmagens. All the studies listed were epidemiological in concept, i.e., population (workforce) based; all estimated the prevalence or incidence by identifying the number of cases as well as the number of subjects at risk, and in all, an analysis was made of the distribution and determinants of OA. Environmental factors examined were exposure level and duration and/or occupation (as a measure of exposure). Host factors examined included a history of atopy and skin test positivity. Note also that the tables are not comprehensive but rather illustrative of the information available to guide both clinical and public health practice. In all three tables, the studies are listed in decreasing order of prevalence of questionnaire markers of OA. In several studies in Tables 2 and 3, the algorithm for clinical case identification (see page 53) was followed, and the rate of cases so identified is included in the tables in parentheses in column 4, illustrating the differences in the rates between the two definitions, the first essentially for epidemiological (public health) purposes and the second for clinical use (36,43,86,122).

From Table 2, describing workforces exposed to HMW asthmagens, it is evident that the estimates of prevalence vary considerably, from rates as high as 50% described in workers in an Australian plant manufacturing enzyme detergents, when the process was first introduced (35), prior to the introduction of process reformulation to control exposure, to as low as 2% in hospital workers exposed to latex (43). While these between-workforce differences are no doubt due in part methodological, such as differences in the questions used to define OA, differences in the intensity of the exposures of the different workforces and in the asthmogenic potential of the different agents involved may also have played a role. By contrast, because the

Table 4 Determinants of Occupational Asthma in Workers Exposed to High and Low Molecular-Weight Agents: Results of Selected Longitudinal (Cohort)[i] and Nested Case–Control[j] Studies

First author, year, country, exposure, industry, occupation	No. studied (years of study)	Exposure prior to diagnosis (months)	Smoking (%)	Atopy[a] (%)	Occupational asthma		References
					Incidence	Determinants at baseline (RR[i] or OR[j], CI)	
Brisman, 2004, United Kingdom[i], bakers and millers	300 (up to 7 yrs)	40 (1–91)	n/a	n/a	12%[b] (36/300)	Exposure–response relationships of new chest symptoms with airborne alpha-amylase exposure	(105)
El-Zein, 2005[i], Québec, Canada, apprentice welders	286 (203 studied)	Average 15	65 (ever smokers)	47.3	13.8[c] (32/232 subjects)	Metal fume fever[d] was a risk factor for OA OR 7.4 (1.97–27.45)	(117)
De Zotti, 2000[i], Trieste, Italy, trainee bakers	125 (1992–1993)	Up to 30	24	13	9.0%[c] (47/125 subjects)	Work-related respiratory symptoms significantly related to personal history of allergic disease OR 5.8 (1.8–18.2) and to skin sensitization to flour or amylase OR 4.3 (1.2–14.9)	(121)
Brisman, 2003[j], Sweden, former bakery students	717 M (1961–1989)	n/a	n/a	51	5.9%[b] (26/44 subjects)	Given OA, OR for atopy: 5.8 (1.1–32.0)	(109)
Archambault, 2001[i], Québec, Canada, Dental hygiene, apprentices	110 (1993–1995)	3–32	9.8	43	4.5%[f] (5/282 person yrs)	All were atopic and all showed specific sensitization to latex (skin test)	(107)

(Continued)

Table 4 Determinants of Occupational Asthma in Workers Exposed to High and Low Molecular-Weight Agents: Results of Selected Longitudinal (Cohort)[i] and Nested Case–Control[j] Studies (*Continued*)

First author, year, country, exposure, industry, occupation	No. studied (years of study)	Exposure prior to diagnosis (months)	Smoking (%)	Atopy[a] (%)	Occupational asthma		
					Incidence	Determinants at baseline (RR[i] or OR[j], CI)	References
Cullinan, 2001[j], United Kingdom, bakery and flour mill workers[g]	300 new employees (1990–1993)	40 (1–91)	n/a	Cases: 38 Controls: 35	4.18 per 100 person-yrs	Chest symptoms in relation to flour allergen exposure OR 7.7 (1.8–33.0) to total dust OR 5.2 (1.3–21.0)	(104)
Gautrin, 2001[i], Québec, Canada, laboratory animal apprentices	373	8–44	11.8	40.0	2.7%[b] (28/1043 person yrs)	RR for atopy: 4.1 (1.6, 10.8) RR for PC20 < 32 mg/mL: 2.5 (1.0, 5.8) RR for lower FEV$_1$ (protective): 0.58 (0.43, 0.78)	(94)

[a] Defined as a positive skin test to at least one common allergen.
[b] Asthma defined as reporting occasions of shortness or wheeze and normal breathing in-between and/or a physician's diagnosis of asthma or hospitalized for asthma.
[c] Cumulative incidence at 30 months.
[d] Defined fever as a prerequisite with at least two of the following symptoms (cough, wheezing, and chest tightness) on exposure to welding fumes, adjusted for years of employment, pack years, and the presence of physician diagnosed asthma.
[e] Defined as asthma diagnosed by a doctor.
[f] Defined as subjects who had experienced skin sensitization to one extract of latex and a significant decrease in bronchial hyperresponsiveness (PC 20%) to methacholine since recruitment.
[g] Cases and controls (two per case) were matched for duration of employment. Cases were defined as those who developed chest related symptoms during follow-up, controls those who did not. Exposure–response relationships were seen with increasing categories of exposure (low, medium, and high) for flour allergen and total dust.
[h] Defined as skin reactivity to occupational allergens associated with the onset or increase in responsiveness to methacholine since recruitment.
Abbreviations: FEV$_1$, forced expiratory volume in one second; OA, occupational asthma.
[i] Longitudinal (cohort) studies.
[j] Case–control studies.

definition of asthma within studies was constant, the role of the determinants in the distribution of asthma within a workforce is unlikely to have been affected by this source of bias. It is therefore of interest that in all the studies listed in Table 2, the within-workforce distribution of the questionnaire markers of asthma was related to exposure, and usually, though not in all studies, to atopy or other markers of an allergic diathesis, and to smoking in some studies (38) but not in others (39). The consistency with which exposure relationships are demonstrable is surprising, given the inaccuracy of the exposure measurements used in most studies. Reasons for the less-consistent relationships with atopy and smoking may be in part methodological, but may also be due in part to different mechanisms operating to produce asthma and asthma-like symptoms in different workers, and/or differences in other features of their workplaces, such as coexposures to environmental tobacco smoke, dust, heat, and other workplace contaminants.

From Table 3, describing workforces exposed to HMW asthmagens, it is evident that estimates of prevalence also vary over much the same range as those shown in Table 2. As in Table 2, in all the studies cited in Table 3 in which exposure was examined, level and/or duration (usually defined by job and/or work area) was a determinant of the distribution within a workplace, whereas atopy was either not related to (44,47,52,55) or only weakly related (50) with exceptions (45,48,123). Despite the fact that, in all studies, exposure level was a determinant of the distribution of asthma within a workforce, and though some studies reported specific bronchial challenge tests using the agent concerned, objective measurements of levels of airborne contaminants have been infrequently reported (53).

Table 4 shows the distribution and determinants of asthma in selected longitudinal (cohort) and nested case–control studies in workers exposed to high- or low-molecular-weight agents, all of which were carried out between 2000 and 2004, i.e., since the 2nd edition of the book was published. These studies were carried out in a more limited number of workplaces/occupations (bakers and millers; dental hygienists, welding and laboratory animal apprentices), in contrast to the wide variety of occupations and exposures (mainly to chemicals) reviewed in Tables 2 and 3 in which only one study of bakers was included (41). Four of the seven studies listed in Table 4 were carried out in bakers and millers. Adjusted estimates of incidence ranged from 12% (36/300) in a 2004 U.K. study of 300 bakers and millers (105) to 4.1 per 100 person years in a 2001 U.K. case–control study of 300 new employees in three large, modern bakeries, two flour mills and a flour packing station (104), compared to 6% in the one 1994 cross-sectional study listed in Table 2 (42), which was carried out on 264 U.K. bakery workers (see Table 2).

Community-Based Studies

Community-based studies have proved surprisingly powerful in bringing to attention associations between occupational exposures and wheezing complaints despite the fact that, in such studies, the potential for misclassification, both for exposure and outcomes (which are of necessity self-reported), is considerable (Table 5) (125,127–129,133,134). The strength of community-based studies derives from the fact that they reach all individuals ever exposed in workplaces at risk, as distinct from only those currently exposed or only those exposed long enough to be registered in any workforce census. The consistency with which relationships between occupational exposures and wheezing complaints can be demonstrated in community-based

Table 5 Asthma Symptoms in Community-Based Studies: Their Relationship to Work Exposures and Population Attributable Proportion (Etiologic Fraction) in Selected Cross-Sectional (Prevalence) and Longitudinal (Cohort) Studies

First author, year, city, country	Subjects: number, age	Exposure (%) Cig.	Exposure (%) Work	Wheezing %	Wheezing OR[a] or RR	PAR[b] (%)	Exposures implicated	Definitions	References
Ng, 1994, Singapore[e]	2375 M and W 20–54 yrs	42	~59	—	1.7	33	Exposed vs. not	Asthma recorded in the case notes	(124)
Viegi, 1991, Po Valley, Italy[e]	1027 M	60	31	3	2.4	29	Any vs. none	Breathless with wheeze or reported asthma	(125)
Becklake, 1996, 4 cities, Canada[e]	602 W 18–64 yrs	38	16	4	2.9	27			(126)
	12380 M and W 20–44 yrs	31	49	10	1.9	23	Dust or gas vs. none	Doctor diagnosed asthma in the last year	
Johnson, 2000[e] 6 communities cities, Canada	2974 M and W 20–44 yrs	36	n/a	36[c] (31–41)	1.5	18	Service (nursing), manufacturing, primary industry	Asthma diagnosed by a doctor[c]	(59)
Krzyzanowski, 1988, 7 cities, France[e]	8692 M	73	34	17	1.6	17	Any vs. none		(127)
	7772 W 25–59 yrs	28	23	12	1.7	13	Any vs. none	Wheezing any time	

Study	Population				OR/RR	PAR%	Exposure	Outcome	Ref
Bakke, 1991, Bergen Co, Norway[e]	4469 M and W 15–70 yrs	43	29	29	1.9	16	Dust or gas vs. none	Occasional wheeze	(128)
Korn, 1987, 6 cities, United States[e]	8515 M and W 25–74 yrs	58	31	6	1.5	14	Dust vs. none	Persistent wheeze	(129)
					1.2		Fumes vs. none		
					1.6		Both vs. none		
Tomas, 2002, Bergen, Norway[f]	2819 M and W 26–81 yrs	39	28	31	2.1^{d} (1.3, 3.2)	14	Dust or fumes vs. none	Hospitalized or treated for asthma by a physician	(130)
Kogevinas, 1996, 5 regions, Spain[e]	2646 M and W 20–44 yrs	51	24	24	1.9	3	High vs. low risk at the time of diagnosis	Asthma symptoms or treatment	(131)
Fishwick, 1997, New Zealand[e]	1609 M and W 20–44 yrs	21	~5	41	1.6	3	High vs. low risk	Wheezing	(132)

Note: Listed in descending order of PAR%.

[a] OR (RR) were all adjusted for age and smoking and for gender when data on men and women were combined; additional adjustments were made in some studies for education, socio-economic status and air pollution (127), atopy and race (132) and city or area of residence (128,131), and educational level (130).

[b] PAR% (or etiologic fraction) for work-related asthma symptoms.

[c] OA defined as doctor-diagnosed asthma, first attack aged 15 or over, while working in an industry/occupation at high risk for OA (probable) or exposed to a sensitizing agent or irritant, not in a high risk industry (possible).

[d] RR for cumulative incidence over 11 years, adjusted for sex, age, educational level, and smoking.

[e] Cross-sectional (prevalence) study.

[f] Longitudinal (cohort) study.

Abbreviations: PAR, population attributable risk; OA, occupational asthma.

studies is thus an eloquent testimony to health-selection effects resulting from workers with such complaints leaving the workplace responsible for inducing their symptoms.

Table 5 shows the results of selected community-based studies listed in decreasing order of population attributable risk percentage. No study was performed with the objective to investigate these relationships, and yet in all but two studies (128,131), statistically significant relationships were demonstrated for wheezing in relation to occupational exposures, either to dusts alone or to dusts with fumes and/or gases. The prevalence of wheezing ranged from 3% in Italy (125) to 14% in Norway (130) and 41% in New Zealand (132). By contrast, estimates of population attributable risk (or etiological fractions) (PAR%) were low, approximately 3%, in the studies from Spain and New Zealand compared with 23% in a Canadian study (126), and were even higher, 33% in a case-control study carried out in Singapore (124) though this study design does not allow calculation of the prevalence of wheezing complaints in the general population (135). The fact that relationships between exposures and wheezing complaints are demonstrable in different populations in different countries by different researchers, using similar, but not identical study methods, lends strength to the causal hypothesis, i.e., that the wheezing complaints analyzed are the consequence of the occupational exposure (5,25). While wheezing complaints do not constitute a clinical diagnosis of OA, nevertheless it is among these individuals that one expects to find those who currently have, or will develop the clinical features necessary to attract a diagnosis of OA.

Estimates of Incidence of OA from National and Regional Statistics

Estimates of incidence of OA, important for both public health practice and policy, have been made using registers based on mandated or voluntary physician reporting, self-reporting by individuals, medicolegal statistics, and other national disease or disability registers (Table 6).

The Sentinel Event Notification System for Occupational Risks (SENSOR), introduced in several states in the United States in the 1980s (14), was based on man-datory and/or voluntary reporting of suspected work-related disease, and linked physicians who identify occupational disease with public health officials responsible for investigating workplaces thought to be at risk. Though confirmation of OA cases was labor intensive, the system was felt to be successful in increasing health provider awareness. As with infectious disease notification, underreporting was a persistent problem. In the United Kingdom, a sentinel type system, modeled on the informal reports of communicable diseases submitted by its Public Health Laboratory Service, was introduced in 1989 (136) and was based on voluntary reporting by selected physicians across the country. Systems based on this model have since been introduced on a trial basis elsewhere, for instance in Canada, in the Provinces of Quebec (138) and British Columbia (137), in France (144), and in South Africa (142). Other estimates of incidence of OA have been derived from national registers of self-reported asthma in Sweden (140), and of registers of persistent OA in Finland (139).

As Table 6 shows, there are considerable between-country differences in the estimated incidence of OA, ranging from approximately 20 per million per year (range 10–14) in the United Kingdom to 187 per million per year in Finland in 1993 (139). These are due in part to methodological difference, and in part to differences in the profile of local industries and employment opportunities, differences which assist public health authorities in directing their preventive interventions.

Table 6 Estimates of Annual Incidence of OA[a] or of Occupational Lung Disease[b] from National and Regional Statistics

First author, year, country	Sources of information	No. of cases (yrs)	Reference population (million)	Annual incidence per million (range)	Comments	References
Lagier, 1990, Québec, Canada	Workmen's compensation	~50–70/yr	n/a	~15–20	97/213 claims accepted in 1987	(11)
Meredith, 1991, United Kingdom	Voluntary by physicians	554[a] (1989)	Labor force	22 (10–114)	282/554 due to agents receiving WCB benefits	(136)
Countreras, 1994, British Columbia, Canada	Voluntary by physicians	124[a]	Labor force (1.05 M)	92	82% workers covered; not all cases proven	(137)
Provencher, 1997, Québec, Canada	Voluntary reporting by physicians	287[a] (1992–1993)	121	48% workers covered	WCB recognized one-third of cases reported	(138)
Reijula, 1994, Finland	Occupational disease register	352[b] (1981–1989)	Labor force (2.25 M)	~156	Twofold increase in registered cases	(139)
Toren, 1996, Sweden	Registers (self report)	101[a] (1990–1992)	Census 4.2 M	80[c] (22–844)[a]	Useful in surveillance and identifying at-risk work	(140)
Reijula, 1996, Finland	Registers of persistent and OA	8056, 386 (1993)	Labor force (2.026 M)	~187 ~4.8% of all new asthma cases are occupational	Since 1986 prevalences of persistent asthma and OA have increased by 21% and 70%, respectively	(141)
Hnizdo, 2000, South Africa	Voluntary reporting by doctors and nurses	225[a]	Employed people	13.1 (aver) (37.6/M in W Cape)	Isocyanates, platinum salts, and low-molecular agents accounted for ~60% of cases	(142)

(Continued)

Table 6 Estimates of Annual Incidence of OA[a] or of Occupational Lung Disease[b] from National and Regional Statistics (*Continued*)

First author, year, country	Sources of information	No. of cases (yrs)	Reference population (million)	Annual incidence per million (range)	Comments	References
McDonald, 2000, United Kingdom	Voluntary reporting by doctors	7387[a] 25,674[b] (1989–97)	Labor force	7 (5–9)[a, d], to 1464[e] (968– 2173)[a]	33% of suspected agents were organic, 33% chemical, 6% metallic and 34% mixed, or unknown	(143)
Ameille, 2003, France	Voluntary reporting by doctors	2178[a] (1996–1999)	Working population (23.06 M)	24.0 (22–25)[f]	Agents implicated: flour (20.3%), isocyanates (14.1%), latex (7.2%), aldehyde (5.9%), persulphate salts (5.8%), and wood dusts (3.7%)	(144)

Note: Listed by date of published report.
[a] Asthma.
[b] Occupational respiratory disease.
[c] For Swedish men across occupational groups.
[d] Professionals, clerical and service workers (lowest risk group).
[e] Coaches and other spray workers (highest risk group).
[f] Highest risk occupations were bakers and pastry makers (683/M), car painters (326/M), hairdressers (308/M), and wood workers (218/M).
Abbreviations: OA, occupational asthma; WCB, Workers' Compensation Board.

Whatever the reservations concerning the validity of between-country differences in the estimates of prevalence and/or incidence, within-country differences are less threatened and can be reasonably accepted as a valid reflection of time trends, providing one of the few sources of such information. An increase in prevalence and/or incidence over time, in particular the 1980s, suggested by several studies, is in keeping with general population studies (139,141,145–148) of the time also suggesting an increase in the prevalence and/or incidence of asthma (3). Another interesting aspect of these estimates lies in the analysis of causal agents. In the 1990s, the number of cases of OA diminished because latex was identified as an important agent causing OA in this period and its use was subsequently decreased (143). Surveillance programs in at-risk industries may also cause increases in rates, for instance in Ontario, Canada (149), in the case of diisocyanates. Overall, the potential weaknesses of this type of estimate are both underestimation (not all cases are reported or seen by targeted physicians) and overestimation (not all cases will conform to the criteria required for a diagnosis of OA). Moreover, it is difficult to maintain the collaboration of the systems that depend on voluntary physician reporting over time.

Most of the agents prescribed for disability benefits in the United Kingdom (flour/grain, wood and other plant dusts, etc.) are also among the most frequently implicated agents in other jurisdictions represented in Table 6. Also important is the fact that, in the SWORD reporting system in the United Kingdom, approximately half the cases reported by physicians as OA had been exposed to agents not prescribed for benefits. In Quebec, a similar percentage of cases was not confirmed for benefits, and the British Columbia report also indicated that a number of cases were not confirmed for benefits.

Cases evaluated for medicolegal benefits are another source used to estimate the incidence of OA (see also Table 5). Again the variability from country to country depends on several factors, including (*i*) the means used to confirm the diagnosis, (*ii*) the interest presented by readaptation programs, and (*iii*) real differences in the incidence (150).

Epidemic and Endemic Asthma

The term "environmental asthma" has been used to describe epidemics of asthma affecting communities and attributable to episodes of unusually high pollution by various airborne contaminants (151). Epidemics of this sort are not new. For instance, a 1928 report implicated castor bean dust residue from a plant in Toledo, Ohio, expressing plant oils (152). Post–World War II epidemics include: (*i*) Tokyo–Yokohama asthma, described in the 1950s in American military personnel in Japan but not in the Japanese, and attributed to high levels of common urban air pollutants (153); (*ii*) New Orleans asthma, described in the 1960s and attributed to simultaneously high levels of several organic pollutants in that city including coffee, grain, and bagasse emitted from local sources (154); (*iii*) Yokkaidu asthma, described in the 1980s and attributed to sulfuric acid mists emitted from a titanium manufacturing plant (155), and (*iv*) Barcelona asthma, attributable to soybean dust released over that city during unloading of ships in the harbor (156).

In Barcelona, the first outbreak was identified in 1981 in the emergency room of a city hospital clinic, and the subsequent investigations provide a model for the epidemiologic investigation of such episodes. The first step in this detective story was taken in 1983, when a retrospective investigation of six prior outbreaks and a comparison with 12 random hospital days was carried out. Features in all outbreaks were that most of those affected presented within a period of hours, shortly after the development of symptoms, and in many, the attacks were severe, requiring assisted ventilation. No etiologic hypothesis could be developed from review of existing community pollution data (smoke and sulfur dioxide). In 1984, after a seventh outbreak during a period of high NO_2 pollution, a Collaborative Asthma Group of epidemiologists and clinicians was established. On their advice, a population-based monitoring and data collection system was set in place, encompassing the city. As a result, in the eighth outbreak (November, 1984), a complete description of the episode was possible, covering the 43 adults and 22 children who sought emergency room treatment. The most affected neighborhoods were those close to the harbor and near an industrial area. In the period 1985 to 1986, six more outbreaks were confirmed by epidemiologic investigation. The time clustering of cases was confirmed, and 23 additional unusual asthma days not identified by clinicians were documented for the period 1985 to 1986. In addition, geographic clustering became evident, and the Collaborative Asthma Group postulated a point source in the harbor or a nearby industrial area and turned their strategy to focus on a specific etiologic hypothesis in several well-designed studies. Among these were (i) time–ecologic studies to link the asthma episodes with unloading soybean in the harbor, and (ii) a case–control study that showed measurable specific IgE levels to soybean in 74% of asthma cases seen during the epidemic episodes compared with 4% of asthma cases seen on nonepidemic days. At this point, the evidence was considered conclusive for a causal relationship and community air pollution by soybean dust recognized as the agent responsible for the Barcelona asthma. Outbreaks of a similar nature were subsequently described in another Spanish port, and after investigation using a similar epidemiologic approach, soybean dust was again incriminated as the responsible agent (157).

Asthma episodes less dramatic than the Barcelona epidemic and not fully explained are the peak incidences of asthma and asthma-like episodes presenting at emergency rooms that have been noted in urban centers in the fall, i.e., September–November in the northern hemisphere and in April and May in the southern hemisphere (158), attributed to the rising levels of indoor pollution that accompany the cooler weather as home dwellers close and seal their windows for the winter. Implicated could be any, several, or all of the following in varying combinations: mites and fungi, volatile organic compounds, chemical agents, smoke, and cooking fuels (159). The relationship of these episodes to increased levels of the common urban pollutants and/or to acid aerosols is also attracting increasing attention (160,161).

NATURAL HISTORY

The natural history of asthma and OA is illustrated in Figure 3. Possible determinants are shown at each step of the time course. Because workers in high-risk work-places can be examined at the time they start exposure, during exposure, and after they are removed from exposure if they develop the disease, OA offers a unique opportunity to study the natural history of allergic sensitization, rhinoconjunctivitis, and asthmatic symptoms, a situation that does not exist for common asthma because it is not generally possible to examine asthmatic subjects before they start being exposed to common allergens.

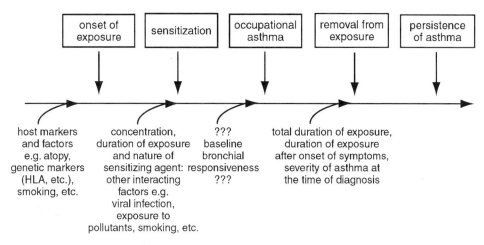

Figure 3 Natural history of occupational asthma.

Onset of Sensitization, Upper and Lower Respiratory Tract Symptoms

The latent period between onset of exposure and events such as allergic sensitization and the development of either rhinoconjunctivitis or lower respiratory symptoms vary according to the type of agent. Maximum sensitization occurs within the first two years in the case of laboratory animals (41,116). Rhinoconjunctivitis symptoms generally develop before lower respiratory tract symptoms in the case of high- but not low-molecular-weight agents, rhinoconjunctivitis symptoms being anyhow less frequent in the latter instance (57,116). A retrospective study has shown that the onset of asthmatic symptoms due to low-molecular-weight agents (diisocyanates and western red cedar) generally required a shorter interval than for high-molecular-weight compounds (Fig. 4) (61). Approximately 40% of patients exposed to low-molecular-weight agents developed symptoms within the first year after exposure started, while only 18% of patients exposed to high-molecular-weight agents developed asthma during this period (61). A small proportion of patients develop asthma after 10 years of exposure (10%). It is not known what factors initiate the onset of symptoms in these patients.

Outcome of Workers with OA Who Are Removed from Exposure

Patients with pneumoconioses such as asbestosis and silicosis often develop irreversible damage to their lungs. The fact that OA can lead to permanent disability remained unsuspected until the late 1970s. It has been taken for granted for a long time that removing patients with OA from exposure to the offending agent would lead to a cure. Chan-Yeung was the first to refute this dogma by showing that subjects with OA remain with asthmatic symptoms and physiological abnormalities even after stopping exposure (162). Thirty-eight subjects with OA caused by western red cedar were studied for at least six months after they left exposure. Although the majority (71%) became asymptomatic and had normal airway caliber at the follow-up visit, every subject was left with bronchial hyperresponsiveness. These findings were confirmed in a subsequent study carried out on a larger number of subjects and followed for a longer period, three-and-a-half years (114). The same group also found that those who remained in the same job experienced a worsening in their asthma symptoms and an increase in nonspecific bronchial responsiveness (163). Several factors of prognostic significance were identified: age, total duration of exposure, and duration of exposure after onset of symptoms. The investigators concluded that early diagnosis and removal from exposure were essential in ensuring recovery.

Several retrospective studies, summarized in Table 2, have later all confirmed that the majority of subjects with OA fail to recover years after removal from exposure. These findings have altered our perspective on the natural history of asthma. Using this analogy, one can postulate that patients who develop nonoccupational allergic asthma may have permanent asthma even though the sensitizing agent has been eliminated.

Malo et al. (58) were able to show that the improvement of bronchial caliber and responsiveness reached a plateau approximately one year and two years after leaving exposure, respectively, in the case of workers exposed to snow crab (Fig. 5). Levels of specific IgE to crab antigens (meat and boiling water) decreased progressively without reaching a plateau, confirming earlier reports that the half-life for disappearance of specific IgE antibodies could be prolonged as in the case of other occupational agents, phthalic anhydride (164), and flour (165). In the latter study, Lemiere et al. (165) showed that the level of specific IgE that remained was associated with the persistence of airway reaction on reexposure to the causal agent. More recent studies in subjects with OA due to various agents (not to snow-crab) show that there may be continuation in improvement even after the first two years of cessation of exposure, although this occurs at a slower pace (166,167).

The duration of exposure and the duration of symptoms are important prognostic factors. Thus, early diagnosis and removal from exposure are recommended. There is a physiopathological basis to the persistence of symptoms and NSBH in patients with OA. Patients who failed to recover from western red cedar asthma

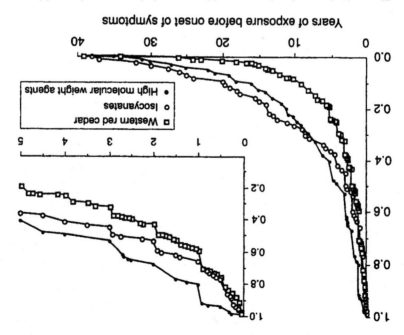

Figure 4 Occupational agents and latency period among patients with occupational asthma.

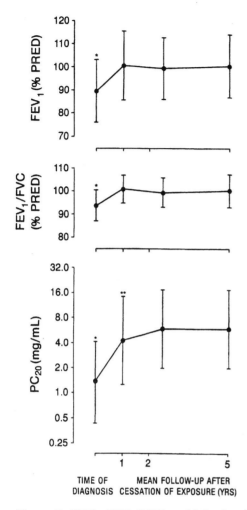

Figure 5 FEV_1, FEV_1/FVC, and PC_{20} (mg/mL) and duration after removal from exposure in patients with snow crab–induced asthma, showing more rapid improvement in FEV_1 and FEV_1/FVC and a slower improvement in PC_{20}. *Abbreviations*: FEV, forced expiratory volume; FVC, forced vital capacity.

had higher total cell count and eosinophils in bronchoalveolar lavage fluid than those who recovered completely after removal from exposure (168). Saetta et al. (169) have documented improvement in bronchial inflammation (diminution of mast cells and lymphocytes) and airway-wall remodeling (reduction in the thickness of subepithelial fibrosis and the number of subepithelial fibroblasts) in patients with TDI-induced asthma after the cessation of exposure. Although there is reduction in airway inflammation, induced sputum still shows abnormalities with regard to the percentages of eosinophils and neutrophils as well as levels of cytokines long after removal from exposure (mean duration of 10 years) in apparently cured subjects (asymptomatic subjects with normal airway caliber and responsiveness) (170).

The reasons for the persistence of NSBH after removal from exposure are not known. The persistence of NSBH could be the result of airway remodeling with subepithelial fibrosis (169) and from chronic airway inflammation (170). These persisting abnormalities may be due to a number of possibilities: (*i*) continuous exposure to the responsible agent in the environment even though the subject is not at work, for example, there is cross-reactivity between the latex antigen and a number of foods such as kiwi, avocado (171), and banana (172) and this may be responsible for symptoms in health care workers with latex-induced asthma; (ii) the development of an "autoimmune" process when agents such as diisocyanates may combine with a body protein and remain in the airways or the persistence of a protein adduct (173); (iii) genetic susceptibility that predisposes the individuals to the development and the persistence of asthma; and (iv) sensitization to other environmental allergens as a result of development of asthma, although, in the latter instance, this seems unlikely as subjects with OA do not become sensitized to common allergens after removal from exposure to the occupational agent (174).

There have been two clinical trials exploring the possibility of "curing" subjects with OA with inhaled steroids after removal from the workplace. Maestrelli et al. (175) documented a fourfold improvement in PC_{20} in the treated group after five months. Malo et al. (33) also showed improvement in various clinical and functional parameters. Although no case of cure from asthma was documented in the latter study (33), results indicated that early initiation of inhaled steroids yielded greater improvement than later initiation (one year after the cessation of exposure).

Outcome of Workers with OA Who Continue to Be Exposed

There have been case reports of subjects with OA who died while working and being exposed to the same agent as reviewed (176). Most studies have shown that subjects with OA deteriorate if they continue in the same job (113,163,177). In a study by Côté et al. (163) 48 subjects with western red cedar asthma confirmed by specific challenge testing were reassessed from 1 to 13 (mean 6.5) years after the initial examination. Using criteria based on four parameters (PC_{20}, FEV_1, asthma symptom score, and antiasthma medication requirement), the investigators found that only 10% of subjects improved, 62.5% remained stable, and 37.5% deteriorated. None of the subjects recovered. Measures to reduce dust exposure including change from daily to intermittent exposure or job relocation to a less dusty area, or use of respiratory protective devices (paper mask, twin-cartridge respirator, and air-purifying respirator) did not influence the outcome with the exception of the use of a twin-cartridge respirator.

There is no data on the use of immunotherapy with extracts of high-molecular-weight occupational allergens to allow the subject to continue to work. Such a modality seems unlikely to be helpful because continuous exposure has not led to the development of immunity and improvement of symptoms. The efficacy of inhaled steroids in the treatment of subjects with OA who opt to remain in the same job for financial reasons is not known. As fatality has been reported, every effort should be made to remove such subjects from further exposure.

OA as a Model to Study the Natural History of Asthma

Some prospective studies have been carried out to study the natural history of sensitization to occupational agents and of OA. Convincing evidence originates from studies carried out in apprentices starting exposure to at-risk agents (179). An example of the natural history of nonspecific bronchial responsiveness due to sensitization to snow-crab is illustrated in Figure 6. In this subject, increased bronchial responsiveness occurred after only eight days of exposure but took one year to return to normal.

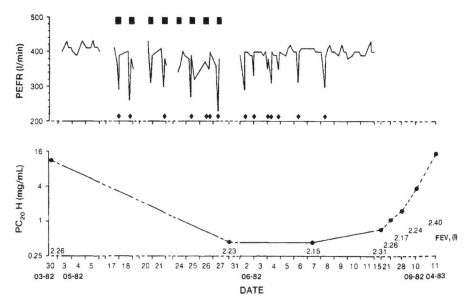

Figure 6 Change in PEF and PC_{20} in a patient with snow crab–induced asthma, showing a rapid development of NSBH after a short period of exposure and a much slower improvement in NSBH after cessation of exposure. *Abbreviations*: PEF, peak expiratory flow; NSBH, nonspecific bronchial hyperresponsiveness.

In two prospective surveys conducted in workers exposed to laboratory animals and flour, respectively, Cullinan et al. (41,42) have demonstrated that atopy and exposure intensity are significant determinants of specific sensitization. However, the subjects in these two studies had been exposed to these specific agents before the surveys. Gautrin et al. (179) have conducted a prospective study on 769 apprentices entering study programs as animal health technicians, dental hygienists, and bakers. They found that 14%, 5%, and 0.8% of the apprentices had immediate skin reactivity to animal-derived allergens, flour, and latex, respectively, before entering the programs (Table 3) (179). The incidence of sensitization was much higher in the cohort of apprentices exposed to laboratory animals than in students exposed to flour and latex (116). Specific sensitization to a program-related allergen was associated with atopic status, work-related symptoms, and NSBH (106).

Because there is no difference between occupational high-molecular-weight allergens and common inhalant allergens in inducing host response, studies of the natural history of OA due to high-molecular-weight allergens will likely reflect the origin and progression of nonoccupational allergic asthma. Studies of the natural history of OA due to low-molecular-weight compounds and/or irritant-induced asthma will be very useful in our understanding of adult-onset or intrinsic asthma.

SCREENING AND SURVEILLANCE

The terms "screening" and "surveillance," often used interchangeably, describe different activities with different objectives, and should be clearly distinguished (180). Thus, screening is directed toward the individual (has a clinical focus), whereas surveillance is directed toward the population from which the individual comes (has a public health focus).

Screening has been defined as ''the presumptive identification of unrecognized disease or defect by the application of tests, which can be applied rapidly.'' This defini-tion also points out that ''a screening test is not intended to be diagnostic'' (2). Thus screening aims to detect disease before an individual seeks medical advice, i.e., at a pre-clinical stage. The goal of screening is thus secondary prevention, i.e., to detect organ dysfunction and/or disease at a stage when intervention would be beneficial. In the case of OA, affected individuals have often themselves rearranged or adjusted their jobs to minimize exposure. In addition, for most exposures, the chances of improve-ment after exposure becomes less the longer exposure continues after the onset of asthma symptoms. For not a few individuals detected by screening, this may mean the directive or recommendation to quit their current job and/or workplace, daunting for the young person in the shrinking job market, and for the older individual in a metier that he has pursued for all his working life, and who lacks the skills to adapt to new technologies in the changing workplace. The detection of an index case or cases in a workplace may also trigger public health action in the form of an industrial hygiene investigation of the workplace implicated. A feature of the SENSOR program in the United States was to link clinicians who identify work-related disease such as asthma with public health officials who can investigate and intervene at specific work-places and alert physicians to local settings and/or workplaces at risk (14).

By contrast, surveillance is defined as ''continued watchfulness over the distri-bution and trends of disease through the systematic collection, consolidation, and evaluation of morbidity and mortality reports and other relevant data,'' and perhaps even more important, the timely distribution of data '' to all who need to know'' (180). Identifying who ''needs to know'' is clearly important because, by definition, surveillance should trigger public health action. Those who generate the surveillance data are often also responsible for public health action (140), but not always (136). National surveys are useful in identifying at-risk work and providing estimates of incidence beyond what is provided by the usually smaller workforce- or occupa-tion-based survey and in providing surveillance of time trends, again in workforces or from analysis of national databases, and perhaps even more important, in deter-mining the time trends in national data (Table 6). Examples of the use of national databases in the form of disease registers are the reports from Sweden (140), and Finland (139,141), which showed increases in the rates of OA over the 1980s. Despite the potential for bias toward both under- and overestimation, the Swedish self-reported system for registering OA was considered useful (140). Ideally, the public health action that findings of this sort might trigger include hygiene surveys in workplaces or occupations identified or suspected as at-risk (but not yet surveyed), and, perhaps even more important, follow-up on previous surveys to determine the effect of any previously implemented preventive interventions.

USES, USEFULNESS, AND APPLICATIONS

Information of the epidemiology (distribution and determinants) of asthma asso-ciated with occupational exposures is used for several purposes (25,27). These include:

1. Establishing prevalence and/or incidence data for public health purposes and as a guide to the need for preventive services and/or surveillance in any industry at risk.

2. Addressing etiologic questions relating to exposures and personal risk factors.
3. Establishing exposure–response relationships to provide the scientific basis for setting environmental control levels.
4. Evaluating preventive services or control measures.

Although none of this information can be furnished by clinical case studies, all of it informs each step in the clinical evaluation of a case of OA, namely establishing the diagnosis, setting prognosis, planning and evaluating management, and taking the appropriate steps in notification.

In the application of epidemiology to the study of OA, the importance of selecting the design most appropriate for answering the particular study question cannot be overemphasized (Table 1) (Fig. 1). Equally important is to identify the appropriate definition of the study outcome (usually asthma or some surrogate of asthma), and of careful selection of the study population to minimize underestimation of the exposure–response effect due to selection bias from the "healthy worker" effect, whether due to "healthy hire" or "survivor" effects. Tables 2 through 7 illustrate the application of epidemiology to the study of OA. Tables 2 and 3 show the prevalence of OA in relation to workplace exposure to high-and low-molecular-weight agents, respectively. This information serves as a guide to public health as well as a guide in the clinical management of OA. Table 4 shows the incidence of asthma derived from longitudinal studies published since the last edition of this book. These studies provide information on the determinants of OA, including exposure factors and, in some studies, exposure–response relationships. This represents a step toward realization of the potential of environmental measurements for evaluating workplace exposures and practices as well as environmental controls (27). The reader is also referred to this excellent document for further discussion on guidelines and approaches to the epidemiologic investigation of OA.

Table 6 shows estimates of incidence of OA in the several industrialized countries; rates range from as low as 22 per million for the year 1989 in the United Kingdom, based on voluntary physician reporting (136), to approximately 187 per million for the year 1993 for Sweden, based on self-reporting. Table 7 shows estimates of the percentage of adult asthma due to occupation range from 3% to 29%. Study rates in two U.S. panel studies ranged from 3.0% to 25.5% and from 8.8% to 14.1%, respectively, while rates based on two National Statistics U.S. studies were 3.7% for the period 1988 to 1994 and 15.4% for the period 1976 to 1978. By contrast, a lower estimate of 6% was made based on patients attending an asthma clinic in a developing country, Zambia (181). While methodological differences may account for a substantial proportion of the between-country differences in estimated rates, the increases in rates over time within countries, e.g., Finland, are likely to be valid reflections of what is happening at a time when by and large workplaces are being better maintained and environmental standards better respected. This lends credence to the view that the increase in adult asthma over the past decades may also reflect an increase in the susceptibility of today's populations (18).

RESEARCH NEEDS

The important questions to be addressed by research should include the following:

- What are the host markers for OA, rhinitis, and conjunctivitis in various susceptible populations?

Table 7 Percentage of Adult Asthma Attributable to Work Exposure Based on National Statistics and Panel Studies of Prevalence

First author, year, country	Population number, source, year of study	No. of cases (age, yrs)	Work-related asthma			Information source(s) and comment	References
			%	CI	Exposure		
Blanc, 1987, United States	6063 HIS and SSDS[a] (1976, 1978)	478	15.4	n/a	Job, employer	Questionnaire	(145)
Timmer, 1993, MI, United States	Hospital discharge patients (1990)	94 (20–65)	3.0[b] 20.2 25.5	n/a	Recognized agents; work–symptoms self-attributed	Interviewed for exposure, chart review for asthma	(146)
Blanc, 1996, CA, United States	Patient panel study	601 (18–54)	8.8 13.1 14.1	6.5–11.1 10.4–15.8 11.3–16.9	Sensitizers and irritants; high-risk job; sensitizer and high-risk job	Telephone interview for job and work exposure: 3% (8/255) have WCB benefits	(147)
Rejula, 1996, Finland, 1993	2.02 M National Register[c]	386 (15–64)	4.8	n/a	Medicolegal criteria	Since 1986 increases in persistent (21%) and OA (71%)	(141)
Arif, 2002, United States	5022 M and W (NHANES III)[d] (1988–1994)	188 (20)	3.7	2.88–4.52	Recognized	PAR[e] for work related asthma was 36.5%	(148)

Note: Listed by date of published report.
[a] 1976 Health Interview Survey and 1978 Social Security Administration Disability Survey.
[b] Based on NIOSH criteria for probable (3.0%), possible or probable (20.2%) OA and self-reported work-relatedness.
[c] National register information on persistent and OA.
[d] National Health and Nutrition Examination Survey (NHANES).
Abbreviations: OA, occupational asthma; PAR, population attributable risk %.

- What are the genetic susceptibility factors in OA, rhinitis, and conjunctivitis?
- What are the permissible exposure limits for various agents responsible for OA, rhinitis, and conjunctivitis?
- Are the permissible exposure limits to prevent sensitization to occupational agents the same as for OA?
- Are there interactions between host susceptibility factors and environmental exposure?
- What are the roles of exposure to low levels of irritants in the pathogenesis of OA?
- What are the reasons and pathogenic mechanisms for persistence of asthma in patients with OA who left exposure?
- What is the true population attributable risk of work exposure to adult-onset asthma?
- What is the prevalence of irritant-induced asthma?

SUMMARY

All of the information in this chapter has been presented with a view to underlining the role of epidemiology in the public health and clinical evaluation of OA. Studies with a public health focus include those in which sentinel cases can be identified, as well as those based on national and regional statistics. Studies of this type are currently being carried out in several industrialized countries and can monitor trends as well as trigger prompt industrial hygiene investigations of the workplaces implicated. Many of the agents involved have already been identified as causes of OA and are common to many industrialized countries; others are sufficiently under suspicion to warrant further study, and yet others remain to be identified. In addition, several cohort studies, including some in which the target population is young apprentices (94,106,107,121), reported risk factors in a number of industries that could be translated into early secondary prevention. Clinical studies are still (and are likely to remain so for a long time) the commonest source for the identification of agents not previously identified as associated with OA, as well as of workplaces and/or occupations not previously thought to be at risk.

REFERENCES

1. Miettinen OS. Theoretical Epidemiology: Principles of Occurrence Research in Medicine. New York: John Wiley and Sons, 1985:317–344.
2. Last JM. A Dictionary of Epidemiology. 4th ed. Oxford University Press, 2001:1–180.
3. Becklake MR, Ernst P. Environmental factors. Lancet 1997; 350(suppl II):10–13.
4. Ramazzini B. De Morbis Artificium Diatribas (WC Wright, trans. 1940 1713). Chicago: University of Chicago Press, 1940.
5. Becklake MR. Occupational exposures: evidence of a causal association with chronic obstructive pulmonary disease. Am Rev Respir Dis 1989; 140:S85–S91.
6. Organization World Health. Tenth report of the Joint ILO/WHO Committee on Occupational Health. Epidemiology of Work-Related Diseases and Accidents 1989; WHO, Geneva, Technical report series 777:1–23.
7. Cancer International Agency for Research on IARC monographs on the evaluation of the carcinogenic risk of chemicals to humans: chemicals, industrial processes and industries associated with cancer in humans. IARC 1982; (suppl 4):1–29.

8. Meredith SK, McDonald JC. Work related respiratory disease in the United Kingdom, 1989-1992: report on the SWORD project. Occup Med 1994; 44:183-189.

9. US Department of Health and Human Services. Work-related lung disease surveillance report 1994, NIOSH 1994; (94):120.

10. Chan-Yeung M, Malo JL. Occupational asthma. N Engl J Med 1995; 333:107-112.

11. Lagier F, Cartier A, Malo JL. Statistiques médico-légales sur l'asthme professionnel au Québec de 1986 à 1988. Médico-legal statistics on occupational asthma in Québec between 1986 and 1988. Rev Mal Respir 1990; 7:337-341.

12. Trupin L, Earnest G, SanPedro M, Balmes JR, Eisner MD, Yelin E, Katz PP, Blanc PD. The occupational burden of chronic obstructive pulmonary disease. Eur Respir J 2003; 22:462-469.

13. Balmes J, Becklake M, Blanc P, et al. Environmental and Occupational Health Assembly, American Thoracic Society. American Thoracic Society Statement: Occupational contribution to the burden of airway disease. Am J Respir Crit Care Med 2003; 167:787-797.

14. Matte TD, Hoffman RE, Rosenman KD, Stanbury M. Surveillance of occupational asthma under the SENSOR model. Chest 1990; 98:173S-178S.

15. Chan-Yeung M. Occupational asthma. Chest 1990; 98:148S-161S.

16. Anto JM, Sunyer J. Epidemiologic studies of asthma epidemics in Barcelona. Chest 1990; 98(suppl 5):185S-190S.

17. Platts-Mills TAE, Carter MC. Asthma and indoor exposure to allergens. N Engl J Med 1997; 336:1382-1384.

18. Seaton A, Godden DJ, Brown K. Increase in asthma: a more toxic environment of a more susceptible population? Thorax 1994; 49:171-174.

19. Becklake MR. Occupational asthma: Epidemiology and surveillance. Chest 1990; 98(suppl 5):165S-172S.

20. Taylor AN. Asthma. In: Mcdonald JC, ed. Epidemiology of Work Related Disease. London: BMJ Publishing Group, 1995:117-142.

21. Fish JE. Occupational asthma: a spectrum of acute respiratory disorders. J Occup Med 1982; 24:379-386.

22. Brooks SM. Bronchial asthma of occupational origin: a review. Scand J Work Environ Health 1982; 3:53-72.

23. Venables KM. Epidemiology and the prevention of occupational asthma (editorial). Br J Ind Med 1987; 44:73-75.

24. Cotes JE, Steel J. Occupational asthma. Work-Related Lung Disorders. Oxford: Blackwell Science Publications, 1987:345-372.

25. Becklake MR. Population studies in risk assessment: strengths and weaknesess. In: Mohr U, ed. Inhalational Toxicology. The Design and Interpretation of Inhalational Studies and Their Use in Risk Assessment. New York: Springer-Verlag, 1988:263-272.

26. Burney P. Why study the epidemiology of asthma? Thorax 1988; 43:425-428.

27. Smith AB, Castellan RM, Lewis D, Matte T. Guidelines for the epidemiologic assessment of occupational asthma. Report of the subcommittee on the epidemiologic assessment of occupational asthma, occupational lung disease committee. J Allergy Clin Immunol 1989; 84:794-805.

28. Manfreda J, Becker AB, Wang PZ, Roos LL, Anthonisen NR. Trends in physician-diagnosed asthma prevalence in Manitoba between 1980 and 1990. Chest 1993; 103:151-157.

29. Gross NJ. Allergy to laboratory animals: epidemiologic, clinical, and physiologic aspects, and a trial of cromolyn in its management. J Allergy Clin Immunol 1980; 66:158-165.

30. McDonald JC. Epidemiology. In: Weill H, Turner-Warwick M, eds. Occupational Lung Diseases. New York: Marcel Dekker Inc, 1981:373-403.

31. McDonald JC. Methodology. Study design. In: McDonald JC, ed. Epidemiology of Work Related Diseases. BMJ, 1995:325-351.

32. Eisen EA. Healthy worker effect in morbidity studies. Med Lav 1995; 86:125–138.
33. Malo JL, Cartier A, Côté J, et al. Influence of inhaled steroids on the recovery of occupational asthma after cessation of exposure: an 18-month double-blind cross-over study. Am J Crit Care Respir Med 1996; 153:953–960.
34. Manfreda J, Becklake MR, Sears MR, et al. Prevalence of asthma symptoms among adults aged 20–44 years in Canada. CMAJ 2001; 164:995–1001.
35. Mitchell CA, Gandevia B. Respiratory symptoms and skin reactivity in workers exposed to proteolytic enzymes in the detergent industry. Am Rev Respir Dis 1971; 104:1–12.
36. Desjardins A, Malo JL, L'Archevêque J, Cartier A, McCants M, Lehrer SB. Occupational IgE-mediated sensitization and asthma due to clam and shrimp. J Allergy Clin Immunol 1995; 96:608–617.
37. Malo JL, Cartier A, L'Archevêque J, et al. Prevalence of occupational asthma and immunologic sensitization to guar gum among employees at a carpet-manufacturing plant. J Allergy Clin Immunol 1990; 86:562–569.
38. Cartier A, Malo JL, Forest F, et al. Occupational asthma in snow crab-processing workers. J Allergy Clin Immunol 1984; 74:261–269.
39. Burge PS, Edge G, O'Brien IM, Harries MG, Hawkins R, Pepys J. Occupational asthma in a research centre breeding locusts. Clin Allergy 1980; 10:355–363.
40. Slovak AJ, Hill RN. Laboratory animal allergy: a clinical survey of an exposed population. Br J Ind Med 1981; 38:38–41.
41. Cullinan P, Lowson D, Nieuwenhuijsen MJ, et al. Work related symptoms, sensitisation, and estimated exposure in workers not previously exposed to laboratory rats. Occup Environ Med 1994; 51:589–592.
42. Cullinan P, Lowson D, Nieuwenshuijsen MJ, et al. Work related symptoms, sensitisation, and estimated exposure in workers not previously exposed to flour. Occup Environ Med 1994; 51:579–583.
43. Vandenplas O, Delwich JP, Evrard G, et al. Prevalence of occupational asthma due to latex among hospital personnel. Am J Respir Crit Care Med 1995; 151:54–60.
44. Venables KM, Dally MB, Nunn AJ, et al. Smoking and occupational allergy in workers in a platinum refinery. Br Med J 1989; 299:939–942.
45. Burge PS, Perks WH, O'Brien IM, et al. Occupational asthma in an electronics factory: a case control study to evaluate aetiological factors. Thorax 1979; 34:300–307.
46. Séguin P, Allard A, Cartier A, Malo JL. Prevalence of occupational asthma in spray painters exposed to several types of isocyanates, including polymethylene polyphenylisocyanates. JOM 1987; 29:340–344.
47. Slovak AJM. Occupational asthma caused by a plastics blowing agent, azodicarbonamide. Thorax 1981; 36:906–909.
48. Wernfors M, Nielsen J, Schutz A, Skerfving S. Phthalic anhydride-induced occupational asthma. Int Arch Allergy Appl Immunol 1986; 79:77–82.
49. Burge S, Edge G, Hawkins R, et al. Occupational asthma in a factory making flux-cured solder containing colophony. Thorax 1981; 36:828–834.
50. Venables KM. Low molecular weight chemicals, hypersensitivity, and direct toxicity: the acid anhydrides. Br J Ind Med 1989; 46:222–232.
51. Malo J-L, Cartier A. Occupational asthma in workers of a pharmaceutical company processing spiramycin. Thorax 1988; 43:371–377.
52. Butcher BT, Salvaggio JE, Weill H, Ziskind MM. Toluene diisocyanate (TDI) pulmonary disease: Immunologic and inhalation challenge studies. J Allergy Clin Immunol 1970; 58:89–100.
53. Vedal S, Chan-Yeung M, Enarson D, et al. Symptoms and pulmonary function in western red cedar workers related to duration of employment and dust exposure. Arch Environ Health 1986; 41:179–183.
54. Malo JL, Cartier A, L'Archevêque J, Trudeau C, Courteau JP, Bhérer L. Prevalence of occupational asthma among workers exposed to eastern white cedar. Am J Respir Crit Care Med 1994; 150:1697–1701.

55. Chan-Yeung M, Vedal S, Kus J, Maclean L, Enarson D, Tse KS. Symptoms, pulmonary function, and bronchial hyperreactivity in Western Red Cedar workers compared with those in office workers. Am Rev Respir Dis 1984; 130:1038–1041.

56. Ishizaki T, Sluda T, Miyamoto T, Matsumara Y, Mizuno K, Tomaru M. Occupational asthma from Western red cedar dust (*Thuja plicata*) in furniture factory workers. JOM 1973; 15:580–585.

57. Malo JL, Lemière C, Desjardins A, Cartier A. Prevalence and intensity of rhinoconjunctivitis in subjects with occupational asthma. Eur Respir J 1997; 10:1513–1515.

58. Malo JL, Cartier A, Ghezzo H, Lafrance M, Mccants M, Lehrer SB. Patterns of improvement of spirometry, bronchial hyperresponsiveness, and specific IgE antibody levels after cessation of exposure in occupational asthma caused by snow-crab processing. Am Rev Respir Dis 1988; 138:807–812.

59. Johnson AR, Dimich-Ward HD, Manfreda J, et al. Occupational asthma in adults in six Canadian communities. Am J Respir Crit Care Med 2000; 162:2058–2062.

60. Diller WF. Facts and fallacies involved in the epidemiology of isocyanate asthma. Bull Eur Physiopathol Respir 1988; 23:551–553.

61. Malo JL, Ghezzo H, D'Aquino C, L'Archevêque J, Cartier A, Chan-Yeung M. Natural history of occupational asthma: relevance of type of agent and other factors in the rate of development of symptoms in affected subjects. J Allergy Clin Immunol 1992; 90:937–944.

62. Rothman KJ. Modern Epidemiology. Boston: Little Brown and Company, 1985.

63. Becklake MR, White N. Sources of variation in spirometric measurements: identifying the signal and dealing with noise. Occup Med: State of the Art Series 1993; 8:241–264.

64. Fonn S, Groeneveld HT, deBeer M, Becklake MR. Relationship of respiratory health status to grain dust in a Witwatersrand grain mill: comparison of workers' exposure assessments with industrial hygiene survey findings. Am J Ind Med 1993; 24:401–411.

65. Fonn S, Becklake MR. Documentation of ill-health effects of occupational exposure to grain dust through sequential, coherent epidemiologic investigation. Scand J Work Environ Health 1994; 20:13–21.

66. deCrosbois S. Occupational exposures and airway disease: a study to develop a questionnaire for community based studies. PhD thesis. McGill University, Montreal, 1998.

67. Raffle PAB, Lee WR, McCallum RI, Murray R. Hunter's Diseases of Occupations. Little Brown and Company, 1987:34–38.

68. Fuchs S, Valade P. Étude clinique et expérimentale sur quelques cas d'intoxication par le Desmodur T (diisocyanate de toluylene 1-2-4 et 1-2-6). Arch Mal Prof 1951; 12:191–196.

69. Stewart PA, Stewart WF, Siemiatycki J, Heineman EF, Dosemeci M. Questionnaires for collecting detailed occupational information for community-based case control studies. Am Ind Hyg Assoc J 1998; 58:39–44.

70. Burney PGJ, Laitinen LA, Perdrizet S, et al. Validity and repeatability of the IUATLD (1984) bronchial symptoms questionnaire: an international comparison. Eur Respir J 1989; 2:940–945.

71. Enarson DA, Vedal S, Schulzer M, Dybuncio A, Chan-Yeung M. Asthma, asthma-like symptoms, chronic bronchitis, and the degree of bronchial hyperresponsiveness in epidemiologic surveys. Am Rev Respir Dis 1987; 136:613–617.

72. Dales RE, Nunes F, Partyka D, Ernst P. Clinical prediction of airways hyperresponsiveness. Chest 1988; 93:984–986.

73. Jansen DF, Timens W, Kraan J, Rijcken B, Postma DS. (A)symptomatic bronchial hyper-responsiveness asthma. Respir Med 1997; 91:121–134.

74. Laprise C, Boulet LP. Asymptomatic airway hyperresponsiveness: a three-year follow-up. Am J Respir Crit Care Med 1997; 156:403–409.

75. Adelroth E, Hargreave FE, Ramsdale EH. Do physicians need objective measurements to diagnose asthma? Am Rev Respir Dis 1986; 134:704–707.

76. Malo JL, Ghezzo H, L'Archevêque J, Lagier F, Perrin B, Cartier A. Is the clinical history a satisfactory means of diagnosing occupational asthma? Am Rev Respir Dis 1991; 143:528–532.

77. Smith A Blair, Bernstein DI, London MA, et al. Evaluation of occupational asthma from airborne egg protein exposure in multiple settings. Chest 1990; 98:398–404.

78. Barbee RA, Lebowitz MD, Thompson HC, Burrows B. Immediate skin-test reactivity in a general population sample. Ann Intern Med 1976; 84:129–133.

79. Vedal S, Chan-Yeung M, Ashley MJ, Enarson D, Lam S. Does a family history or personal history of allergy predict immediate skin test reactivity? Can Med Assoc J 1985; 132:34–37.

80. Maccia CA, Bernstein IL, Emmett EA, Brooks SM. In vitro demonstration of specific IgE in phthalic anhydride hypersensitivity. Am Rev Resp Dis 1976; 113:701–704.

81. Chan-Yeung M, Lam S, Enarson D. Pulmonary function measurement in the industrial setting. Chest 1985; 88:270–275.

82. Becklake MR. Epidemiology of spirometric test failure. Br J Ind Med 1990; 47:73–74.

83. Society American Thoracic. Standardization of spirometry. Am J Respir Crit Care Med 1995; 152:1107–1136.

84. Burge PS. Single and serial measurements of lung function in the diagnosis of occupational asthma. Eur J Respir Dis 1982; 63(suppl 123):47–59.

85. Moscato G, Godnic-Cvar J, Maestrelli P, Malo JL, Burge PS, Coifman R. Statement on self-monitoring of peak expiratory flows in the investigation of occupational asthma. J Allergy Clin Immunol 1995; 96:295–301.

86. Bardy JD, Malo JL, Séguin P, et al. Occupational asthma and IgE sensitization in a pharmaceutical company processing psyllium. Am Rev Respir Dis 1987; 135:1033–1038.

87. Venables KM, Burge P Sherwood, Davison AG, Taylor AJ Newman. Peak flow rate records in surveys: reproducibility of observers' reports. Thorax 1984; 39:828–832.

88. Malo JL, Cartier A, Ghezzo H, Chan-Yeung M. Compliance with peak expiratory flow readings affects the within- and between-reader reproducibility of interpretation of graphs in subjects investigated for occupational asthma. J Allergy Clin Immunol 1996; 98:1132–1134.

89. Burney PGJ, Britton JR, Chinn S, et al. Descriptive epidemiology of bronchial reactivity in an adult population: results from a community study. Thorax 1987; 42:38–44.

90. Woolcock AJ, Peat JK, Salome CM, et al. Prevalence of bronchial hyperresponsiveness and asthma in a rural adult population. Thorax 1987; 42:361–368.

91. Hendrick DJ. Epidemiological measurement of bronchial responsiveness in polyurethane workers. Bull Eur Physiopathol Respir 1988; 23:555–559.

92. Pham QT, Mur JM, Chau N, Gabiano M, Henquel JC, Teculescu D. Prognostic value of acetylcholine challenge test: a prospective study. Br J Ind Med 1984; 41:267–271.

93. Vedal S, Enarson DA, Chan H, Ochnio J, Tse KS, Chan-Yeung M. A longitudinal study of the occurrence of bronchial hyperresponsiveness in western red cedar workers. Am Rev Respir Dis 1988; 137:651–655.

94. Gautrin D, Infante-Rivard C, Ghezzo H, Malo JL. Incidence and host determinants of probable occupational asthma in apprentices exposed to laboratory animals. Am J Respir Crit Care Med 2001; 163:899–904.

95. Brooks SM, Edwards JJ, Apol A, Edwards FH. An epidemiologic study of workers exposed to western red cedar and other wood dust. Chest 1981; 80(suppl):30–32.

96. Musk AW, Venables KM, Crook B, et al. Respiratory symptoms, lung function, and sensitisation to flour in a British bakery. Br J Ind Med 1989; 46:636–642.

97. Burge PS, Edge G, Hawkins R, White V, Taylor AN. Occupational asthma in a factory making flux-cored solder containing colophony. Thorax 1981; 36:828–834.

98. Heederik D, Doekes G, Nieuwenhuijsen MJ. Exposure assessment of high molecular weight sensitisers: contribution to occupational epidemiology and disease prevention. Occup Environ Med 1999; 56:735–741.

99. Vandenplas O, Cartier A, Ghezzo H, Cloutier Y, Malo JL. Response to isocyanates: effect of concentration, duration of exposure, and dose. Am Rev Respir Dis 1993; 147:1287–1290.

100. Butcher BT, Jones RN, O'Neil CE, et al. Longitudinal study of workers employed in the manufacture of toluene-diisocyanate. Am Rev Respir Dis 1977; 116:411–421.

101. Newman-Taylor A. Non-malignant diseases. Asthma. In: McDonald JC, ed. Epidemiology of Work Related Diseases. London: BMJ Publishing Group, 1995:117–142 (chap 6).

102. Reed CE, Swanson MC, Agarwal MK, Yunginger JW. Allergens that cause asthma. identification and quantification Chest 1985; 87:40S–44S.

103. Poulos LM, O'Meara TJ, Hamilton RG, Tovey ER. Inhaled latex allergen (Hev b 1). J Allergy Clin Immunol 2002; 109:701–706.

104. Cullinan P, Cook A, Nieuwenhuijsen MJ, et al. Allergen and dust exposure as determinants of work-related symptoms and sensitization in a cohort of flour-exposed workers: a case-control analysis. Ann Occup Hyg 2001; 45:97–103.

105. Brisman J, Nieuwenhuijsen MJ, Venables KM, et al. Exposure-response relations for work related respiratory symptoms and sensitisation in a cohort exposed to alpha-amylase. Occup Environ Med 2004; 61:551–553.

106. Gautrin D, Ghezzo H, Infante-Rivard C, Malo J-L. Incidence and determinants of IgE-mediated sensitization in apprentices: a prospective study. Am J Respir Crit Care Med 2000; 162:1222–1228.

107. Archambault S, Malo JL, Infante-Rivard C, Ghezzo H, Gautrin D. Incidence of sensitization, symptoms and probable occupational rhinoconjunctivitis and asthma in apprentices starting exposure to latex. J Allergy Clin Immunol 2001; 107:921–923.

108. Gautrin D, Ghezzo H, Infante-Rivard C, Malo JL. Incidence and host determinants of work-related rhinoconjunctivitis in apprentice pastry-makers. Allergy 2002; 57:913–918.

109. Brisman J, Lillienberg L, Belin L, Ahman M, Jarvholm B. Sensitization to occupational allergens in bakers' asthma and rhinitis: a case-referent study. Int Arch Occup Environ Health 2003; 76:167–170.

110. Malo JL, Cartier A, L'Archevêque J, et al. Prevalence of occupational asthma and immunologic sensitization to psyllium among health personnel in chronic care hospitals. Am Rev Respir Dis 1990; 142:1359–1366.

111. Venables KM, Upton JL, Hawkins ER, Tee RD, Longbottom JL, Newman-Taylor AJ. Smoking, atopy and laboratory animal allergy. Br J Ind Med 1988; 45:667–671.

112. Calverley AE, Rees D, Dowdeswell RJ, Linnett PJ, Kielkowski D. Platinum salt sensitivity in refinery workers: incidence and effects of smoking and exposure. Occup Environ Med 1995; 52:661–666.

113. Paggiaro PL, Loi AM, Rossi O, et al. Follow-up study of patients with respiratory disease due to toluene diisocyanate (TDI). Clin Allergy 1984; 14:463–469.

114. Chan-Yeung M, Lam S, Koerner S. Clinical features and natural history of occupational asthma due to western red cedar (Thuja plicata). Am J Med 1982; 72:411–415.

115. Chan-Yeung M, Kennedy S, Vedal S. A longitudinal study of red cedar sawmill workers. Am Rev Respir Dis 1990; 139:A81.

116. Gautrin D, Ghezzo H, Infante-Rivard C, Malo JL. Natural history of sensitization, symptoms and diseases in apprentices exposed to laboratory animals. Eur Respir J 2001; 17:904–908.

117. El-Zein M, Infante-Rivard C, Malo JL, Gautrin D. Is metal fume fever a determinant of welding related respiratory symptoms and/or increased bronchial responsiveness? A longitudinal study. Occup Environ Med 2005; 62:688–694.

118. Zejda JE, Pahwa P, Dosman JA. Decline in spirometric variables in grain workers from start of employment: differential effect of duration of follow up. Br J Ind Med 1992; 49:576–580.

119. Zammit-Tabona M, Sherkin M, Kijek K, Chan H, Chan-Yeung M. Asthma caused by diphenylmethane diisocyanate in foundry workers. Clinical, bronchial provocation, and immunologic studies. Am Rev Respir Dis 1983; 128:226–230.

120. Chan-Yeung M, Ward H Dimich, Enarson DA, Kennedy SM. Five cross-sectional studies of grain elevator workers. Am J Epidemiol 1992; 136:1269–1279.

121. DeZotti R, Bovenzi M. Prospective study of work related respiratory symptoms in trainee bakers. Occup Environ Med 2000; 57:58–61.

122. Malo JL, Cartier A, L'Archevêque J, et al. Prevalence of occupational asthma and immunological sensitization to guar gum among employees at a carpet-manufacturing plant. J Allergy Clin Immunol 1990; 86:562–569.

123. Burge PS, Perks W, O'Brien IM, Hawkins R, Green M. Occupational asthma in an electronics factory. Thorax 1979; 34:13–18.

124. Ng TP, Hong CY, Goh LG, Wong ML, Koh KTC, Ling SL. Risks of asthma associated with occupations in a community-based case-control study. Am J Ind Med 1994; 25:709–718.

125. Viegi G, Prediletto R, Paoletti P, et al. Respiratory effects of occupational exposures in a general population sample in north Italy. Am Rev Respir Dis 1991; 143:510–515.

126. Becklake M, Ernst P, Chan-Yeung M, et al. The burden of asthma attributable to work exposures in Canada. Am J Respir Crit Care Med 1996; 153:A433.

127. Kryzanowski M, Kauffman F. The relation of respiratory symptoms and ventilatory function to moderate occupational exposure in a general population: Results from the French PAARC study of 16000 adults. Int J Epidemiol 1988; 17:397–406.

128. Bakke P, Eide GE, Hanoa R, Gulsvik A. Occupational dust or gas exposure and prevalences of respiratory symptoms and asthma in a general population. Eur Respir J 1991; 4:273–278.

129. Korn RJ, Dockery DW, Speizer FE, Ware JH, Ferris BG. Occupational exposures and chronic respiratory symptoms: a population based study. Am Rev Respir Dis 1987; 130:298–304.

130. Tomas M, Eagan L, Gulsvik A, Eide GE, Bakke Per S. Occupational airborne exposure and the incidence of respiratory symptoms and asthma. Am J Respir Crit Care Med 2002; 166:933–938.

131. Kogevinas M, Anto JM, Soriano JB, Tobias A, Burney P. The risk of asthma attributable to occupational exposures. Am J Respir Crit Care Med 1996; 154:137–143.

132. Fishwick D, Pearce N, D'Souza W, et al. Occupational asthma in New Zealanders: a population based study. Occup Environ Med 1997; 54:301–306.

133. Lebowitz MD. Occupational exposures in relation to symptomatology and lung function in a community population. Environ Res 1977; 14:59–67.

134. Heederik D, Kromhout H, Burema J, Biersteker K, Kromhout D. Occupational exposure and 25-year incidence rate of non-specific lung disease: The Zutphen study. Int J Epidemiol 1990; 19:945–952.

135. Burney PGJ, Luczynska C, Chinn S, Jarvis D. The European Community Respiratory Health Survey. Eur Respir J 1994; 7:954–960.

136. Meredith SK, Taylor VM, McDonald JC. Occupational respiratory disease in the United Kingdom 1989: a report to the British Thoracic Society and the Society of Occupational Medicine by the SWORD project group. Br J Ind Med 1991; 48:292–298.

137. Contreras GR, Rousseau R, Chan-Yeung M. Occupational respiratory diseases in British Columbia, Canada in 1991. Occup Environ Med 1994; 51:710–712.

138. Provencher S, Labrèche FP, Guire L De. Physician based surveillance system for occupational respiratory diseases: the experience of PROPULSE, Québec, Canada. Occup Environ Med 1997; 54:272–276.

139. Reijula K, Patterson R. Occupational allergies in Finland in 1981–91. Allergy Proc 1994; 15:163–168.

140. Toren L. Self reported rate of occupational asthma in Sweden 1990–1992. Occup Environ Med 1996; 53:757–761.

141. Reijula K, Haahtela T, Klaukka T, Rantanen J, et al. Incidence of occupational asthma and persistent asthma in young adults has increased in Finland. Chest 1996; 110: 58–61.

142. Hnizdo E, Esterhuizen TM, Rees D, Lalloo UG. Occupational asthma as identified by the surveillance of work-related and occupational respiratory diseases programme in South Africa. Clin Exp Allergy 2001; 31:32–39.

143. McDonald JC, Keynes HL, Meredith SK. Reported incidence of occupational asthma in the United Kingdom, 1989–97. Occup Environ Med 2000; 57:823–829.

144. Ameille J, Pauli G, Calastreng-Crinquand A, et al. ONAP and the corresponding members of the Reported incidence of occupational asthma in France, 1996–99. Occup Environ Med 2003; 60:136–142.

145. Blanc P. Occupational asthma in a national disability survey. Chest 1987; 92:613–617.

146. Timmer S, Rosenman K. Occurrence of occupational asthma. Chest 1993; 104:816–820.

147. Blanc PD, Cisternas M, Smith S, Yelin E. Occupational asthma in a community-based survey of adult asthma. Chest 1996; 109:56S–57S.

148. Arif AA, Whitehead LW, Delclos GL, Tortolero SR, Lee ES. Prevalence and risk factors of work related asthma by industry among United States workers: data from the third national health and nutrition examination survey (1988–1994). Occup Environ Med 2002; 59:505–511.

149. Kraw M, Tarlo SM. Isocyanate medical surveillance: Respiratory referrals from a foam manufacturing plant over a five-year period. Am J Ind Med 1999; 35:87–91.

150. Dewitte JD, Chan-Yeung M, Malo JL. Medicolegal and compensation aspects of occupational asthma. Eur Respir J 1994; 7:969–980.

151. Merchant JA. Workshop on environmental and occupational asthma: Opening remarks. Chest 1990; 98(suppl 5):145S–146S.

152. Figley KD, Elrod RH. Endemic asthma due to castor bean dust. JAMA 1928; 90:79–82.

153. Phelps HW, Koike S. Tokyo-Yokohama asthma: the rapid development of respiratory distress presumably due to air pollution. Am Rev Respir Dis 1962; 88:55–63.

154. Carroll RR. Epidemiology of New Orleans asthma. Am J Public Health 1968; 58:1677–1683.

155. Kitagawa T. Cause analysis for the Yokkaidu asthma episode. J Air Pollut Control Assoc 1984; 34:743–746.

156. Anto JM, Sunyer J, Rodriguez-Roisin R, Suarez-Cervera M, Vazquez L. Community outbreaks of asthma associated with inhalation of soybean dust. N Engl J Med 1989; 320:1097–1102.

157. Alvarez-Dardet C, Belda J, Pena M, Nolasaco A. Outbreak of asthma associated with soybean dust (letter). N Engl J Med 1989; 321:1127–1128.

158. Lee DK, ed. Environmental Factors in Respiratory Disease. New York: Academic Press, 1972:1–252.

159. Samet JM, Marbury MC, Spengler JD. Health effects and sources of indoor pollution. Part 1. Am Rev Respir Dis 1987; 136:1486–1508.

160. Bates DV, Sizto R. Relationship between air pollution levels and hospital admissions in Southern Ontario. Can J Public Health 1983; 74:117–122.

161. Bates DV, Baker-Anderson M, Sizto R. Asthma attack periodicity: A study of hospital emergency visits in Vancouver. Environ Res 1990; 51:51–70.

162. Chan-Yeung M. Fate of occupational asthma. A follow-up study of patients with occupational asthma due to western red cedar (Thuja plicata). Am Rev Respir Dis 1977; 116:1023–1029.

163. Côté J, Kennedy S, Chan-Yeung M. Outcome of patients with cedar asthma with continuous exposure. Am Rev Respir Dis 1990; 141:373–376.

164. Venables KM, Topping MD, Nunn AJ, Howe W, Newman-Taylor AJ. Immunologic and functional consequences of chemical (tetrachlorophthalic anhydride)-induced asthma after four years of avoidance of exposure. J Allergy Clin Immunol 1987; 80:212–218.

165. Lemière C, Cartier A, Malo JL, Lehrer SB. Persistent specific bronchial reactivity to occupational agents in workers with normal nonspecific bronchial reactivity. Am J Respir Crit Care Med 2000; 162:976–980.

166. Perfetti L, Cartier A, Ghezzo H, Gautrin D, Malo JL. Follow-up of occupational asthma after removal from or diminution of exposure to the responsible agent: relevance of the length of the interval from cessation of exposure. Chest 1998; 114:398–403.

167. Malo JL, Ghezzo H. Recovery of methacholine responsiveness after end of exposure in occupational asthma. Am J Respir Crit Care Med 2004; 169:1304–1307.

168. Chan-Yeung M, Leriche J, Maclean L, Lam S. Comparison of cellular and protein changes in bronchial lavage fluid of symptomatic and asymptomatic patients with red cedar asthma on follow-up examination. Clin Allergy 1988; 18:359–365.

169. Saetta M, Maestrelli P, Turato G, et al. Airway wall remodeling after cessation of exposure to isocyanates in sensitized asthmatic subjects. Am J Respir Crit Care Med 1995; 151:489–494.

170. Maghni K, Lemière C, Ghezzo H, Yuquan W, Malo JL. Airway inflammation after cessation of exposure to agents causing occupational asthma. Am J Respir Crit Care Med 2004; 169:367–372.

171. Ahlroth M, Alenius H, Turjanmaa K, Makinen-Kiljunen S, Reunala T, Palosuo T. Cross-reacting allergens in natural rubber latex and avocado. J Allergy Clin Immunol 1995; 96:167–173.

172. Alenius H, Makinen-Kiljunen S, Ahlroth M, Turjanmaa K, Reunala T, Palosuo T. Crossreactivity between allergens in natural rubber latex and banana studied by immunoblot inhibition. Clin Exp Allergy 1996; 26:341–348.

173. Jin R, Day BW, Karol MH. Toluene diisocyanate protein adducts in the bronchoalveolar lavage of guinea pigs exposed to vapors of the chemical. Chem Res Toxicol 1993; 6:906–912.

174. Perfetti L, Hébert J, Lapalme Y, Ghezzo H, Gautrin D, Malo JL. Changes in IgE-mediated allergy to ubiquitous inhalants after removal from or diminution of exposure to the agent causing occupational asthma. Clin Exp Allergy 1998; 28:66–73.

175. Maestrelli P, Marzo De N, Saetta M, Boscaro M, Fabbri LM, Mapp CE. Effects of inhaled beclomethasone on airway responsiveness in occupational asthma. Am Rev Respir Dis 1993; 148:407–412.

176. Ortega HG, Kreiss K, Schill DP, Weissman DN. Fatal asthma from powdering shark cartilage and review of fatal occupational asthma literature. Am J Ind Med 2002; 42:50–54.

177. Moscato G, Dellabianca A, Perfetti L, et al. Occupational asthma. A longitudinal study on the clinical and socioeconomic outcome after diagnosis. Chest 1999; 115:249–256.

178. Malo JL, Chan Yeung M. Occupational asthma. J Allergy Clin Immunol 2001; 108:317–328.

179. Gautrin D, Infante-Rivard C, Dao TV, Magnan-Larose M, Desjardins D, Malo JL. Specific IgE-dependent sensitization, atopy and bronchial hyperresponsiveness in apprentices starting exposure to protein-derived agents. Am J Respir Crit Care Med 1997; 155:1841–1847.

180. Wagner GR. Screening and Surveillance of Workers Exposed to Mineral Dusts. Geneva: World Health Organisation, 1996:68.

181. Sybbalo N. Occupational asthma in a developing country (letter). Chest 1991; 99:528.

4

Genetics and Occupational Asthma

Anthony J. Newman-Taylor
Department of Occupational and Environmental Medicine, National Heart and Lung Institute, Royal Brompton and Harefield NHS Trust, London, U.K.

Berran Yucesoy
Toxicology and Molecular Biology Branch, Health Effects Laboratory Division, NIOSH/CDC, Morgantown, West Virginia, U.S.A.

INTRODUCTION

Common diseases such as asthma and diabetes mellitus tend to cluster in families. The risk of developing the disease if a first-degree relative is affected is 5% to 10% greater than the prevalence of the disease in the population, but less than the 25% risk for a recessive and 50% risk for a dominant single gene disorder. The familial clustering is due not to a single gene defect, but is the outcome of multiple genes (polygenic) and their interaction with the environment.

Genetic variation between individuals, such as differences in blood groups, occurs frequently in the population. Such variants, whose frequency is stable between generations, are known as "polymorphisms." Polymorphisms are the basis of diversity within human populations and contribute not only to differences in characteristics such as height and blood pressure but also to variation in the ability to resist infection and handle environmental challenges. Such challenges include the response to agents inhaled at work, both inorganic and organic. Differences between individuals in their responses are likely to be determined, at least in part, by the functional consequences of polymorphisms of relevant genes, and their interactions with each other.

Molecular genetic studies have provided the opportunity to identify the relevant genetic polymorphisms. However, it is important to appreciate that in a multifactorial disease such as occupational asthma (OA), a single polymorphism, although increasing susceptibility to the development of asthma in those exposed to a particular agent, is unlikely to be sufficient alone, and may even not be necessary, to cause the disease. Polymorphic genes may increase susceptibility or resistance to disease but do not determine it. The identification of a single polymorphic gene alone is therefore unlikely to provide the basis for a screening test for susceptibility to OA. Knowledge of the genes involved, the function of their protein products, and of their interaction with the relevant environmental influences does however have the potential to illuminate disease mechanisms at the molecular level and provide new opportunities to treat and prevent it.

THE IMPORTANCE OF WELL-DEFINED PHENOTYPES IN GENETIC STUDIES

The genetic constitution of an organism is its genotype; the physical expression of the genotype (either as an observable characteristic or protein product) is its phenotype. Mendel inferred the patterns of inheritance in sweet peas, by studying the transmission of pairs of clearly contrasted physical characteristics (phenotypes) such as tallness versus shortness of the plant and, green versus yellow, and round versus wrinkled seeds. Similar patterns of inheritance can be inferred for human diseases such as cystic fibrosis. In such Mendelian disorders, genotype and phenotype correspond (one gene, one protein). In common diseases, such as asthma, diabetes, and hypertension, how-ever, the correspondence is not observed because the same phenotype (e.g., asthma) is associated with different genotypes (genetic heterogeneity) or vice versa because of interaction with other genes, with environmental factors, or both.

Genetic studies of disease in man require an unequivocal definition of pheno-type. This implies diagnostic criteria which are comprehensive (i.e., high sensitivity with few false negatives) and exclusive (high specificity with few false positives) to minimize misclassification bias. Genetic studies of atopy and asthma have been con-siderably impeded by the lack of widely accepted diagnostic criteria. Asthma is usually defined as reversible airway narrowing, whose characteristic symptoms are episodic wheeze and breathlessness. However, all that wheezes is not asthma and not all asthma wheezes; furthermore, cases of asthma may not have demonstrable reversibility at the time of testing. Another defining characteristic of asthma is air-way hyperresponsiveness—an increased responsiveness of the airways to nonspecific provocative stimuli such as exercise, inhaled cold air, or histamine. Airway hyperre-sponsiveness, although sensitive, is not a specific characteristic of asthma, being found in some 15% of the population. These problems make a comprehensive and exclusive definition of asthma difficult. Similarly, atopy—which was defined by Pepys as the propensity to make immunoglobulin E (IgE) antibody in response to allergens encountered in everyday life—has been identified by different investigators as one or more immediate skin test responses to common inhalant allergens, an ele-vated total IgE in serum, or the presence of specific IgE antibody in serum to one or more common inhalant allergens. Cookson and Hopkin (1) in their genetic studies decided on a comprehensive case definition, which included one or more of any of these three; in contrast, others have focused on the inheritance of total IgE.

These difficulties and differences in case definition have made genetic studies of asthma and atopy difficult to undertake and to compare the findings of different studies.

GENETIC BASIS OF ASTHMA

Asthma and atopy show clear indications of genetic susceptibility; the frequency of disease in family members of cases is greater than in the population as a whole, and is greater in identical monozygotic (MZ) twins than in nonidentical dizygotic (DZ) twins.

Family Studies

Genetic susceptibility is suggested if a disease occurs in greater frequency in the family members of a case than in the general population. The relative risk (λ_R) is the risk of a disease for the relative of an affected individual divided by the risk (prevalence) of the disease in the general population. λ_o and λ_s are the ratios for offspring and sibs to the population prevalence. The size of λ_R is taken to indicate the degree of concordant inheritance of genetic factors in affected relative pairs.

First-degree relatives—parents, brothers, sisters, and children—have half their genes in common with the index case (or proband). Second-degree relatives—grandparents, aunts, uncles, nephews, and nieces—have one-quarter of their genes in common. The most commonly reported value is for λ_s but usually sibs also share a common childhood environment and $\lambda_s > 1$ may reflect a shared environment as well as a shared inheritance. An increased frequency of disease in second-degree relatives may therefore be a more reliable indication of genetic influences. The value of λ_s for cystic fibrosis is about 500, for insulin-dependent diabetes 15, and for schizophrenia 8.5. The value for asthma probably lies between two and five.

Several family studies have provided evidence that asthma and associated atopic disease, eczema and hayfever, are more frequent in the relatives of asthmatics than in the relatives of matched controls. Sibbald (2) estimated that the population frequency of asthma was between 5% and 10%. The probability of a child of an atopic asthmatic parent having asthma varied from 14% when one parent was affected to 29% when both parents were affected. The risk for the child of a nonatopic asthmatic parent to have asthma was a little greater than the risk in the general population. Atopy increased the risk of a child developing asthma to about threefold. Similarly, Jenkins et al. (3) found that the risk of asthma and associated atopic diseases in seven-year-old Tasmanian children was greater when one or both parents were asthmatic than when neither was affected. The risk of having asthma was increased to about 2.5 times when either parent had asthma and 6.7 times when both parents had asthma.

Twin Studies

Twin studies, which compare the concordance of disease in identical (MZ) twins, who are genetically identical, and nonidentical (DZ) twins who like other sibs share half their genes, can better differentiate genetic from environmental influences than family studies. Assuming that the effect of a shared familial environment is the same for MZ and DZ twins, the frequency of a disease with no genetic component will be similar in them. A disease influenced by genetic factors will be more frequent in MZ twins than in DZ twins; the larger the difference, the more likely that genetic factors are important in the development of the disease. The results of twin studies of multifactorial diseases can be expressed as "hereditability"—the proportion of the total variation of the phenotype due to genetic factors.

Twin studies have consistently shown the concordance of asthma to be higher in MZ twins than in DZ twins. In a study of 7000 Swedish twin pairs, Edfors-Lub (4) found that the concordance of asthma between MZ twins was 19% and between DZ twins was 4.8%, giving an estimated hereditability of some 15%. More recent twin studies have reported higher estimates for the hereditability of asthma. Hopper et al. (5) estimated a hereditability of 50% in a study of 3808 Australian twins. Harris et al. (6) in a study of 5684 Norwegian twins found that the risk of developing asthma in twins whose co-twin had a history of asthma (as compared to those whose co-twin did not) was increased 18 fold in MZ twins and 2.3-fold in DZ twins.

Hanson et al. (7) studied MZ and DZ twins reared together and apart; they found in either situations, a greater concordance for asthma and specific IgE [estimated by skin test and radio-allergosorbent allergy testing (RAST)] in MZ twins than in DZ twins. Although the number of twins in this study was relatively small, the implications of its findings are considerable, suggesting a substantial genetic influence on the development of specific IgE and asthma, with little contribution from familial environment shared in childhood.

Twin studies indicate that asthma has an inherited component, but do not identify its mode of inheritance. This is usually addressed by segregation analysis in family studies, in which the occurrence of asthma is determined in terms of the degree of genetic relatedness to the index case (or proband). Families studied may be nuclear (which include only first degree relatives of the probands) or extended (which include more distant relatives and usually encompass three or more generations).

The results of such studies have been conflicting. Some have suggested that asthma is inherited as an autosomal dominant characteristic with incomplete penetrance, i.e., a single gene is responsible for asthma but not all who inherit it develop asthma (8,9). Cookson and Hopkin (1) found that 90% of atopic asthmatics had an atopic parent and suggested a dominant mode of inheritance for atopy.

Others have suggested that the inheritance of asthma is polygenic (10), implying asthma to be the outcome of an interaction between several genes. In part, these apparently striking different findings reflect differences in methods of ascertainment and phenotype definition, but probably also reflect considerable heterogeneity in the inheritance of atopy and asthma.

MOLECULAR GENETICS

Modern molecular techniques have provided the opportunity to disentangle the difficulties in genetic analysis of complex traits caused by factors such as genetic heterogeneity and polygenic inheritance. These studies allow for identification of the genes that contribute to the development of multifactorial diseases such as asthma. The ultimate purpose of these investigations is to determine the protein products of the relevant genes, their functions, and how these differ from those not at increased risk of disease. Understanding the biochemical basis of diseases such as diabetes, schizophrenia, and asthma could offer insights of therapeutic and preventative value.

Two complementary approaches have been taken: genetic linkage and investigation of candidate genes.

Genetic Linkage

The opportunity for human genetic linkage studies has been provided by recognition of the naturally occurring variation in human DNA sequences (on average, individuals differ every 200 to 500 base pairs) and the identification of a large number of polymorphic markers spaced at short intervals along human chromosomes.

Genetic linkage is based on the simple principle that the closer the marker polymorphism is to the gene of interest, the less likely is separation at meiosis and the more likely that they are coinherited (linked). The genetic locus of a particular disease can be identified by the frequency of the coinheritance of the disease with a marker of known chromosomal location. If the genetic marker and the disease are unlinked (on a separate chromosome or far apart on the same chromosome) they are as likely to cosegregate as not, and the recombination fraction will be

50% or 0.5. When the marker and disease locus are on the same chromosome, the shorter the distance between them, the less likely is crossing over during meiosis, the more likely that they are inherited together, and the fewer the recombinants. The recombination fraction will fall from 50% (reflecting independent assortment) toward zero (reflecting tight linkage).

Initial linkage studies are undertaken in families with the disease, looking for cosegregation of a marker of known chromosomal location with the gene involved in the disease. Because of the large number of markers examined in a genome screen, any suggestive linkage needs to be replicated with more refined linkage mapping to identify a "candidate gene." DNA sequencing of the candidate gene allows identification of variations in the coding sequence (polymorphisms). Finally, population studies, which investigate the association between the polymorphism and the disease of interest, allows estimation of the prevalence of the polymorphism and its contribution to the disease frequency and severity.

This was the approach taken by the Oxford group in their investigation of the genetic basis of atopy. Having observed that 90% of atopic asthmatics had an atopic parent, a result they interpreted as indicating dominant inheritance, they undertook a linkage analysis within nuclear and extended families. They found significant linkage between a marker on chromosome 11q and atopy (11) (broadly defined as one or more skin-prick test reactions, specific IgE to common inhalant allergens, or an elevated serum total IgE), which they confirmed in a subsequent study of other Oxford families (12). Linkage was found to be primarily through maternal chromosomes (13). Because of its known location on chromosome 11q and plausible relevance to atopy, they postulated the β chain of the high affinity IgE receptor (Fc εR 1-β) as the candidate gene (14). Subsequent sequence analysis identified two separate polymorphisms, Leu 181 and 183, present either separately or together (15).

They subsequently studied a random population sample from the town of Busselton, in Western Australia and found that the prevalence of the Leu 181/183 polymorphism was some 4.5%. All 13 children who had inherited the polymorphism from their mothers were atopic and all but one had hay fever, asthma, or both. In contrast, none of the eight children who inherited the gene from their fathers was atopic, confirming maternal transmission of gene expression (16). A number of other studies failed to replicate these results (17,18), which in some cases may reflect the small number of families studied, but probably primarily reflects the genetic heterogenicity of atopy and asthma.

Chromosome 5q has also been extensively investigated because it contains several candidate genes relevant to asthma and atopy. These include the interleukin-4 gene cluster, which contains IL-3, -4, -5, -9, -13, and GM-CSF, the β$_2$ adrenoceptor gene, and the corticosteroid receptor gene. Marsh et al. (19) studied 170 individuals from 11 Amish families in the United States and found significant linkage with total IgE for five markers within the 5q 31.1 region but not for the three markers (lying just) outside this region. Postma et al. (20) studied the children and grandchildren of 84 Dutch probands with asthma. They found coinheritance of increased levels of total IgE with airway hyperresponsiveness and linkage of airway hyperresponsiveness with several markers on chromosome 5q.

These studies indicate that polymorphisms of candidate genes on chromosome 5q are probably contributing to the development of asthma and atopy, but in the absence of defined polymorphisms, it is not possible to determine their prevalence or the size of their contribution to the development or severity of disease.

Candidate Genes

The second parallel approach, applicable when the biochemical basis of the disease is understood, is to seek polymorphisms of the genes encoding potentially relevant proteins. The considerable knowledge of the cellular and molecular mechanisms of asthma, both the TH2 lymphocyte response and associated eosinophilic bronchitis, provides a remarkable array of plausible candidate genes. Investigations reported to date, particularly those relevant to OA, have investigated the association of asthma and specific IgE antibody with the highly polymorphic genes encoding the major histocompatibility complex (MHC) proteins, also known as human leukocyte antigens (HLAs) in man, which play a central role in the immune recognition of foreign proteins.

MHC molecules are expressed as heterodimeric proteins on the cell surface. Foreign peptides, derived from within the cell by the degradation of endogenous or exogenous proteins, are bound in the groove of the MHC molecule and are expressed as an MHC peptide complex which is recognized in a very specific way by the T cell receptor (TCR) on the surface of T lymphocytes. This trimolecular complex [MHC protein, foreign peptide (epitope), and TCR] is at the center of immune recognition and response. MHC proteins are divided into two classes: MHC-1 and -2. MHC Class 1 proteins (HLA-A, -B, and -C antigens in man) are expressed on the surface of all cells; MHC Class 2 (HLA-DR, -DP, and -DQ antigens in man) proteins are expressed on the surface of antigen presenting cells such as dendritic cells, B lymphocytes, macrophages, and some epithelial cells. MHC Class 1 proteins present endogenous peptides which are mostly recognized by CD8+ (cytotoxic) T lymphocytes; MHC Class 2 proteins present exogenous peptides which are recognized by CD4+ (helper) T lymphocytes, although there are exceptions, where Class 1 peptide complexes are recognized by CD4+ cells and Class 2 peptides by CD8+ cells.

MHC proteins are encoded on the short arm of chromosome 6. HLA-A, -B, and -C each have one gene on each chromosome. HLA-DR has up to four genes and HLA-DP and -DQ each have two genes encoding α and β chains, a total of 12 genes on each chromosome allowing a potential 24 different HLA types in any individual. HLA genes are also highly polymorphic with more than 200 variants of these 12 genes, which are numbered in sequence (e.g., HLA-A1, -A2, -A3, etc.) providing billions of potential combinations of the 200 genes that are unique to each individual (other than identical twins who share the same HLA type). MHC proteins have evolved as a mechanism of self-defence against infective agents, which are themselves continually changing and adapting. HLA genes are reshuffled in each generation and the constantly changing resistance against infection in the reshuffling process has been proposed as the major evolutionary benefit of sex. Because MHC proteins bind epitopes in the molecular groove (Bjorksten groove), created by the β-pleated sheet of the heterodimer, polymorphisms in the genome determine the capacity to bind specific epitopes and present them to T cells. Epitopes that are not presented will not activate (and therefore effectively bypass) the immune response.

Allergens and low-molecular weight chemical haptens, which bind to host proteins, are taken up by dendritic cells, degraded into oligopeptides which are bound in the groove of MHC-2 proteins, expressed on the cell surface, and recognized by CD4+ T lymphocytes possessing the relevant TCR. Variation in the immunological response to inhaled allergens and haptens may therefore in part be determined by differences in HLA type. For this reason, studies of the molecular genetics in OA have to date focused on searching for associations between MHC Class 2 (HLA-DR, -DP, and -DQ) genes and the development of specific IgE antibody and asthma in those who are exposed to allergens and haptens in the workplace.

Before the advent of molecular techniques, HLA typing was undertaken serologically. The ability to distinguish HLA types by molecular methods—probing with sequence-specific oligonucleotides (SSOs) after amplification by polymerase chain reaction (PCR) or, more specifically, using sequence-specific primers (SSPs)—has increased considerably the number of different HLA types recognized and the accuracy of their identification. In addition, knowledge of the amino acid sequence of different HLA molecules has allowed the identification of specific amino acid substitutions in HLA molecules, which may be associated with susceptibility or resistance to a particular disease [see isocyanate-induced asthma and chronic beryllium disease (CBD) below].

Studies relating to the associations of disease with a particular HLA haplotype have usually been made by comparing the frequency of the HLA haplotype in patients with the disease, with the frequency in an appropriately matched referent group. The relative risk between the two groups can be expressed as an odds ratio and appropriate statistical tests can be applied. A significant association between the disease and HLA type may imply:

A Cause and Effect Relationship

The particular HLA type is a genetic determinant of the disease whose importance is reflected in the size of the odds ratio. An odds ratio in excess of 100 (e.g., ankylosing spondylitis and HLA-B27) implies the particular HLA type as a major genetic determinant of the disease. Odds ratios of this size are rare and weaker associations more usual. In these circumstances, the contribution of the particular HLA to the disease, although real, may be of less importance than other genes or environmental factors. The effect of multiple gene polymorphisms, however, can be cumulative.

Linkage Disequilibrium

Linkage disequilibrium takes place when two genes occur together more frequently than would be expected by chance. This is more likely to occur with HLA polymorphisms which can confer a selective advantage against infectious disease. For example, HLA-A1 and -B8 occur more frequently than would be expected by chance in North Europeans, possibly because this combination conferred protection against plague. An HLA type which is associated with a disease may, therefore, only be a marker for a polymorphism of another HLA gene with which it is in linkage disequilibrium.

Confounding

The association of the disease with HLA type reflects the association of HLA type with a particular ethnic or geographical group, which differs between the disease group and the referent group. As an illuminating example of such confounding, Lander and Schork (21) highlighted the association of HLA-A1 with the ability to use chop sticks in the population of San Francisco, a relationship more likely to reflect the higher prevalence of this polymorphism in Chinese than in Caucasians, than immunological determinism of agility in handling chopsticks. Referent groups need to be matched with the disease group or be capable of adjustment for factors which may confound HLA relationships that include social, geographical, and ethnic background.

Overestimating the High Probability of a Chance Association in Multiple Comparisons

The majority of studies which have explored associations between the HLA types and the disease have been "fishing expeditions" undertaken without a specific prior hypothesis. The probability of an association occurring by chance among the multiple comparisons made with different HLA types is predictably high. This problem can be overcome in at least two ways.

a. Applying Bonferroni's correction the P value of each test is multiplied by the number (λ) of comparisons made ($P' = \lambda P$). For example, where $P = 0.02$ and five comparisons have been made, Bonferroni's correction: $P = 0.02 \times 5 = 0.1$.

b. The results of the fishing expedition are regarded as hypothesis generating, from which a specific hypothesis informed by the results of the initial study may be tested in a hypothesis testing study in a second independent population.

ASSOCIATION STUDIES IN COMPLEX DISEASES

Linkage analyses and association studies are the most widely used methods to identify genetic determinants of complex diseases. Linkage analyses identify genes responsible for diseases with simple Mendelian inheritance, such as cystic fibrosis. However, the application of linkage analysis to complex disorders is very difficult because of genetic heterogeneity, incomplete penetrance, and gene-environment interactions. Association studies are usually performed to study the genetics of multifactorial diseases. The case–control study is the most widely used design for detecting common disease alleles with modest risk, in which the differences in allele or genotype frequencies between cases and controls are evaluated. However, the characteristics of complex diseases also limit the power of association studies. The general limitations for such studies are population stratification, small sample sizes, modest genetic effects, gene—environment interactions, the assessment of statistical significance, and multilocus effects. In addition, the difficulties in quantifying and characterizing exposure characteristics (length of exposure, onset of symptoms, etc.), intermediate phenotypes (such as IgE levels or airway responsiveness in the case of asthma), and multiple outcomes make association studies of complex traits a challenge (22–25).

In multifactorial diseases, the risk is often confounded by interactive and additive effects of genes and by interactions between genes and environmental or occupational factors as has been shown in the case of silicosis (26). Silicosis, an interstitial lung disease resulting from inhalation of crystalline silica, is characterized by chronic inflammation leading to severe pulmonary fibrotic changes. Proinflammatory cytokines, such as tumor necrosis factor (TNF) α and IL-1, have been implicated in the formation of these lesions and a strong association was found between the disease severity and TNFα-238 variant. Gene–gene interactions, including IL-1α +4845 plus TNFα-238 and IL-1RA +2018 plus TNFα-308, were associated with

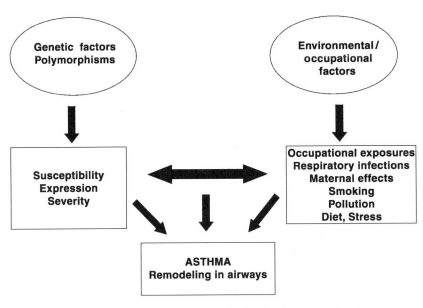

Figure 1   Gene–environment interactions in the development of asthma.

altered risk for silicosis ($P=0.04$ for both). Three-way interaction analysis between each gene–gene interaction and exposure showed that the prevalence of silicosis increases with increasing exposure, except in the case where both IL-1α +4845 and TNFα–308 minor variants are present (26,27). Figure 1 illustrates a similar inter- action model for asthma. Susceptibility genes are assumed not to confer a major risk for the disease; rather they act either alone or in combination with other genes to modify disease progression, severity, or resolution after exposure to triggering factors. The interaction between genes and exposure usually determine the onset or expression of disease. Gene–environment interactions may be measured by the different effects of an exposure on disease risk among individuals with different gen- otypes, or by the different effects of a genotype on disease risk among individuals with different exposures (28,29). In OA, the main factors that affect the onset of the symptoms are the types and intensity of allergen exposure. The higher the level of exposure, the more likely sensitization will develop and the less the genetic influ- ence. The genetic variations do not cause qualitative differences in the response, but rather induce a shift in the dose–response relationship (30). OA may be a good model for studying gene–environment interactions because the exposure, the time that individual became sensitized, and the interval between exposure and onset of clinical symptoms can be observed (31).

Occupational Asthma

Investigation of the genetic influences and of genetic–environmental interactions in the development of asthma and atopy in the general community is beset by consider- able difficulties. The problems of phenotype definition have already been described. In addition, there have to date been few identified polymorphisms associated with atopy or asthma. There is also a lack of accurate measures of exposure to relevant allergens in defined populations, necessary to assess exposure–response relationships and from these, genetic–environmental interactions.

OA overcomes many of these hurdles. Unambiguous case definition (phenotype) can be made on the basis of inhalation tests (for asthma) or serological tests for specific IgE or skin-prick test responses (for immunological sensitization). The disease occurs in identifiable and circumscribed populations, in well-defined and measurable circumstances of exposure.

The majority of reported cases of OA fulfill the criteria for a specific hypersensitivity response, implying the development of an immunological reaction to the responsible initiating agent. For most of the causes of hypersensitivity-induced OA, there is accompanying evidence of specific IgE antibody. This implies specific activation of TH2 lymphocytes with IL-4 and -5 generation. Specific IgE antibody has been identified for all high-molecular-weight proteins and for some low-molecular-weight chemicals (e.g., acid anhydrides, complex platinum salts, and reactive dyes). However, asthma caused by low-molecular-weight chemicals, such as isocyanates and plicatic acid, has been accompanied by specific IgE antibody, inconsistently, in a minority of cases. Examination of the airway mucosa in bronchial biopsies from patients with asthma induced by isocyanates and plicatic acid, however, has shown the presence of activated lymphocytes and eosinophils—a pattern of cellular infiltration characteristic of allergic asthma. Asthma in these cases may be the outcome of activated IL-5 but not IL-4 secreting TH2 lymphocytes.

HLA and High-Molecular-Weight Allergens

HLA association studies are likely to be most fruitful when studying immunological responses or diseases initiated by proteins with a limited number of epitopes. HLA molecules bind to and present single epitopes to T lymphocytes. Multiple epitopes are likely to be expressed by different HLA molecules diluting the strength of any individual HLA–epitope associations that may be important in disease etiology.

In their studies of the relationship of HLA types with specific IgE to purified short ragweed pollen allergens, Marsh et al. (32) found the strongest associations of the low-molecular-weight allergens—HLA-DR2.2 with specific IgE to Amb a V and HLA-DR5 and Amb a VI (33). The associations with high-molecular-weight allergens were weaker, probably reflecting the greater epitope density on high-molecular-weight proteins.

Possibly for this reason the majority of published studies of HLA associations in OA have been investigations of low-molecular-weight chemical sensitizers, which act as haptens and are probably a constituent of the epitope, potentially minimizing the number of epitopes, and therefore different HLA molecules, engaged in the immune response.

The majority of studies of OA caused by high-molecular-weight allergens have not found strong relationships. Three association studies have been reported of laboratory animal allergy and HLA. One study found the prevalence of HLA-DR4 and -B15 in 27 cases of laboratory animal allergy, which was about double that of normal controls, and of those drawn from the same workforce (34). In another study, Kerwin et al. (35) reported HLA restriction of human T lymphocyte responses, from nine mouse allergic patients, to mouse allergens (Mus m 1). There was an excess of HLA-DR4, -DR11, and -DRW17 in the nine cases as compared to 100 controls tested in the same laboratory. Both of these studies included only a small number of cases (27 and 9), and the first investigated the association of HLA with specific IgE to a complex mixture of high-molecular-weight protein allergens present in rat urine.

Table 1 Laboratory Animal Allergy. HLA: Sensitization and Symptoms (OR 95% CI[a])

	Sensitization	Work-related chest symptoms	Sensitization + work-related chest symptoms
HLA-DR7	1.82 (1.12–2.97)	2.96 (1.64–5.37)	3.81 (1.90–7.65)
HLA-DR3	0.55 (0.31–0.97)	0.71 (0.35–1.45)	0.57 (0.24–1.32)

[a]Adjusted for atopy, exposure, and site.
Abbreviations: CI, confidence interval; HLA, human leukocyte antigen; OR, odds ratio.
Source: From Ref. 36.

The third and considerably the largest reported study of HLA associations in laboratory animal allergy was of 109 cases with specific IgE to rat urine proteins and of 397 referents from six pharmaceutical companies in the United Kingdom. The cases and referents had worked with rats for a similar period, an average of eight years. Jeal et al. (36) found an increasingly strong association between HLA-DR7 and specific IgE to rat urine protein, work-related respiratory symptoms and work-related respiratory symptoms with specific IgE to rat urine protein. Individuals with specific IgE to rat urine protein were more likely than referents to be HLA-DR3 negative (Table 1).

Although the authors recognize that the findings should be considered as hypothesis generating, needing testing in a separate population, they do have biological plausibility. The lipocalin rat allergen (Rat n 1) binds with high affinity to hydrophobic ligands. Of seven amino acid residues in which HLA-DR3 and -DR7 differ in their hydrophobicity, six are hydrophobic in HLA-DR7 and hydrophilic in HLA-DR3. Pocket nine of the peptide-binding groove of the HLA molecule has three polymorphic residues (positions 9, 37, and 57), all of which are hydrophobic in HLA-DR7 and hydrophilic in HLA-DR3. Binding affinity for Rat n 1 could be increased by hydrophobic residues in pocket nine of HLA-DR7 and reduced by hydrophilic residues of HLA-DR3, plausibly, at least in part, explaining these differential HLA associations with allergy to rat urine proteins.

HLA and Low-Molecular-Weight Chemical Sensitizers

Low molecular chemical haptens have, at least in theory, the advantage for HLA association studies that if they are a constituent part of the "foreign" epitope, the potential for dilution of association by multiple epitopes is diminished. Certainly, the majority of association studies of HLA with the development of specific IgE or asthma have been reported for cases caused by low-molecular-weight chemicals.

Acid Anhydrides. Young et al. (37) reported an association between HLA-DR3 and the presence of specific IgE antibody to albumin conjugates of trimellitic anhydride (TMA) but not the closely related phthalic anhydride (PA). The 30 cases were chosen from acid anhydride workers identified from factory surveys or from clinical referrals as having specific IgE antibody to TMA, PA, or tetrachlorophthalic anhydride (TCPA). Twenty-eight (93%) cases had rhinitis, asthma, or both. The 30 referents were matched on type and duration of acid anhydride exposure such that they had an equal opportunity for developing specific IgE to anhydrides. Referents did not have specific IgE (identified by skin-prick test or RAST) to acid anhydrides or symptoms of rhinitis or asthma. Referents were also matched for atopy and smoking habit.

Table 2 HLA-DR3 Frequency in Cases and Referents Exposed to the Acid Anhydrides TMA, PA, and TCPA

Acid anhydride exposure	Cases DR3+	Referents DR3+	Odds ratio	p
TMA	8/11	2/14	16	<0.05
PA	2/12	2/14		
TCPA	5/7	0/0		
Total	15/30 (50%)	4/28 (14%)		

Abbreviations: HLA, human leukocyte antigen; PA, phthalic anhydride; TMA, trimellitic anhydride; TCPA, tetrachlorophthalic anhydride.
Source: From Ref. 37.

The frequency of HLA-DR3 in cases and referents exposed to the three anhydrides is shown in Table 2. After correction for multiple comparisons, HLA-DR3 was found significantly more frequently in the cases of TMA sensitization with an odds ratio of 16. Cases of PA sensitization, however, were no more likely to be HLA-DR3 positive than their referents. The proportion of TCPA cases that were HLA-DR3 positive (5/7) was similar to that of TMA (8/11), but unfortunately no referents were obtained for comparison.

The results of the study suggested HLA type to be important in determining the development of specific IgE to TMA, possibly TCPA, but not PA. The study, however, had no specific prior hypothesis and the association of specific IgE to TMA with HLA-DR3 requires testing in another population.

Isocyanates (and Beryllium). Isocyanate-induced asthma differs from the majority of cases of acid anhydride-induced asthma in the lack of a consistent accompaniment of specific IgE antibody. Although the explanation for the lack of specific IgE antibody to isocyanates may be technical, it suggests a possible differ-ence in the nature of the immunological response underlying the development of iso-cyanate-induced asthma. Nonetheless, the finding of activated lymphocytes and eosinophils in bronchial biopsies from cases suggests an immunological basis for the disease.

Bignon et al. (38) investigated HLA specificity in isocyanate-induced asthma and found an association of disease with HLA-DQB*0503 and an inverse relation-ship with HLA-DQB*0501 (Table 3). In a subsequent study, Balboni et al. confirmed these results in another population of isocyanate workers and observed that in the 57 position of HLA-DQB1, aspartic acid was present in HLA-DQB1*0503 and valine in HLA-DQB1*0501 (Table 4) (39). The observations suggested that the amino acid

Table 3 Isocyanate-Induced Asthma and HLA DQB1*0501 and *0503

	Isocyanate asthma	Referents	RR	p
HLA-DQB1	56	32		
*0501	1 (2%)	5 (16%)	0.14	<0.03
*0503	7 (13%)	0 (0)	9.8	<0.04

Abbreviations: HLA, human leukocyte antigen; RR, relative risk.
Source: From Ref. 38.

Table 4 Isocyanate-Induced Asthma and HLA-DQB Asp 57

HLA-B Asp 57 haplotypes	Isocyanate asthma	Referents
Asp 57+ homozygotes	17 (57%)	44 (32%)
Asp 57 heterozygotes	12 (40%)	73 (53%)
Asp 57− homozygotes	1 (3%)	21 (15%)
Total	30	138

Abbreviation: HLA, human leukocyte antigen.
Source: From Ref. 39.

present in residue 57 of HLA-DQB1 could be an important determinant of susceptibility to isocyanates in exposed workforces.

The importance of a specific amino acid substitution in an HLA molecule in determining the ability of an individual to present a hapten has also been suggested by Richeldi et al. (40) in relation to CBD. CBD, a disease very similar in its clinical manifestations to sarcoidosis, is characterized by the presence of hypersensitivity granuloma and proliferation of T lymphocytes from blood and bronchoalveolar lavage when incubated with beryllium salts. Richeldi et al. (40) demonstrated a strong association between the presence of glutamic acid in position 69 of the β1 chain of the HLA-DPB1 molecule and development of CBD in exposed workers. Of the 32 cases of CBD, 31 (97%) were HLA-DPB1* Glu 69 positive as compared to 27% of the 44 referents without CBD.

Complex Platinum Salts (and Beryllium Again). Complex platinum salts, of which ammonium hexachloroplatinate (ACP) is the most important, are essential intermediates in platinum refining. ACP is a potent cause of asthma, which is associated with an immediate skin-prick test response in the majority of cases.

In a case-referent study of the male workforce of a platinum refinery in South Africa, Newman Taylor et al. (41) found an excess of HLA-DR3 and a deficit of HLA-DR6 in skin-test positive cases as compared to referents, matched for intensity and duration of exposure and ethnic background. Stratifying those employed into "high" and "low" exposure jobs, the relative risk of a case being HLA-DR3 positive or HLA-DR6 negative was greater in the low than in the high exposure groups (Table 5).

These results suggest that in those occupationally exposed to ACP, genetic susceptibility is an important determinant of the development of sensitization

Table 5 HLA and Exposure Intensity vs. Sensitization to Complex Platinum Salts

	Cases, *n* (%)	Referents, *n* (%)	OR (95% CI)
HLA-DR3			
All	18 (41)	15 (26)	2.3 (1.0–5.6)
Low exposure	6 (55)	4 (22)	Infinite
High exposure	12 (36)	11 (28)	1.6 (0.6–4.1)
HLA-DR6			
All	16 (36)	34 (60)	0.4 (0.2–0.8)
Low exposure	2 (18)	12 (67)	0.1 (0.02–1.1)
High exposure	14 (42)	22 (56)	0.5 (0.2–1.3)

Abbreviations: HLA, human leukocyte antigens; OR, odds ratio; CI, confidence index.
Source: From Ref. 41.

and although the absolute risk of becoming a case is greater in the more heavily exposed, among those who were HLA-DR3 positive or -DR6 negative, the relative risk of becoming sensitized to ACP was markedly greater in those with lower exposure to ACP.

The other study that has investigated genetic environmental interactions is that reported by Richeldi et al. (42) of the risks of developing CBD in a factory workforce exposed to beryllium, in relation to intensity of exposure (using job title as a surrogate measure) and HLA-DPB1 Glu 69 (Table 6). On exposure to beryllium, 6 out of 127 cases (4.7%) developed CBD, the majority of cases (5/6) occurring among the machinists in the high-exposure group (ca. 0.9 μg/m³). Five cases occurred among the 41 HLA-DPB1 Glu 69 positive individuals (12.2%) and one case among 86 HLA-DPB1 Glu 69 negative individuals (1.2%), a 10-fold increased risk for HLA-DPB1 Glu 69 positive individuals. Because the number in the study population was small, it is difficult to interpret genetic environmental interactions with confidence, only one case of CBD occurring in a nonmachinist who was HLA-DPB1 Glu 69 positive. The results, however, indicate an exposure–response relationship overall and in the Glu 69 positive group. In contrast to the findings in the ACP population, the relative risk of developing CBD in Glu 69 positive individuals was greater at higher levels of exposure to beryllium.

Implications of HLA Associations

These HLA associations have clear biological implications. They provide substantial evidence for specific immunological response in the development of OA initiated by low-molecular-weight chemical sensitizers. This is of particular importance for iso-cyanate-induced asthma, where the absence of demonstrable specific IgE antibody has led to suggestions that the disease is not immunologically mediated. The clear evidence for HLA association, taken with the finding of infiltration by activated lym-phocytes and eosinophils in bronchial biopsies, provides coherent evidence for an immunological mechanism. In the case of acid anhydrides and complex platinum salts, where there is evidence for an exposure–response relationship, modified parti-cularly by smoking but also by atopy, the association of sensitization with HLA type identifies a further and important risk factor, whose magnitude may vary with the level of exposure.

Genetic markers, such as HLA polymorphisms, hold out the hope that they will allow identification of susceptible individuals. However, to date, as with asthma caused by agents such as laboratory animals and platinum salts, and atopy, the asso-ciation is not strong enough to be used as a discriminatory preemployment tool.

Table 6   Beryllium Exposure

	Machinist (0.9 μg/m³)	Non-machinist (0.3 μg/m³)	Total
HLA-DPB1 Glu 69 +ve	4/16 (25%)	1/25 (4%)	5/41 (12.2%)
HLA-DPB1 Glu 69 −ve	1/31 (3.2%)	0/55 (0%)	1/86 (1.2%)
Total	5/47 (10.6%)	1/80 (1.3%)	6/127 (4.7%)

Abbreviation: HLA, human leukocyte antigen.

Source: From Ref. 42.

In the best studied, and only replicated, example of HLA-DPB1 Glu 69 and CBD, although 25% to 30% of the beryllium-exposed population were Glu 69 positive and the disease virtually limited to Glu 69 positive individuals, only 12% of Glu 69 positive individuals developed disease. More than 85% (36/41) of the exposed individuals who were Glu 69 positive did not develop CBD, suggesting that while HLA type has an influence on the development of the disease, other genetic and environmental factors are at least as important. One of the factors described above was intensity of exposure to beryllium, but even among machinists (the high exposure group) only 10% overall and 25% who were Glu 69 positive developed CBD. Accurate prediction of individuals at risk of developing allergic lung disease, including OA, will have to await the identification of other relevant genetic polymorphisms, knowledge of which will need to be integrated into an understanding of exposure–response relationships, their modification by environmental (e.g., tobacco smoking) factors, and by the possibly varying influence of genetic susceptibility at different levels of exposure.

Association Studies in Asthma

Although MHC variants are strongly associated with asthma, genes which regulate inflammatory and allergic components are also involved. Many of these genes are found on chromosomes 5q31-q33, 6p21, 11q13, and 12q (22,43) including cytokines IL-4, -5, -9, -13, and TNFα, which are either determining or modifying factors in immunologic responses to asthma. Tumor growth factor (TGF)β1, IFNγ, IL-1β, IL-4 receptor α (IL-4Rα), IL-10, -12B, TNFα, and IL-13 are some of the candidate cytokine genes with known polymorphic variants involved in asthma and related phenotypes (44–50). Of these, TGFβ1, IL-4, -4Rα, -10, and -13 are more likely involved in the development of immune-mediated asthma while IFNγ, TNFα, IL-1β, and -12β are involved in inflammation. Recently, variations in other chromosomal regions have been associated with asthma phenotypes including toll-like receptor (TLR)–10, ADAM 33, CD14, monocyte chemoattractant protein–1 (MCP-1), and angiotensin-converting enzyme genes (51–54). Examples of single nucleotide polymorphisms (SNPs) associated with asthma or its partial phenotypes are given in Table 7.

The potential for gene–gene interactions in disease initiation and severity also exists for polygenic diseases such as asthma. For example, a significant gene–gene interaction exists between IL-4Rα (+478) and IL-13 (–1111), such that individuals homozygous for both the IL-4Rα variant and heterozygous or homozygous for the IL-13 variant are almost five times more likely to develop asthma than those without the genotype (55). In addition, individuals with the IL-4 590C and the IL-4Rα Arg551 genotype have been reported to have a higher risk of developing asthma (56). However, the role of these SNPs, and others with similar activities, has not been comprehensively examined in OA. As in other forms of asthma, inflammatory changes and allergen-specific T lymphocytes are found in the airways of many patients with OA, along with eosinophils, cytokines, and serum IgE antibodies (57–59). Thus, similar genetic associations as in immune-mediated asthma might be expected to occur in OA.

A role for low-penetrance genes in disease modification has been identified for OA. Oxidative stress is a major component of inflammation, and impaired ability to detoxify reactive oxygen species (ROS) may perpetuate the inflammatory processes and precipitate asthma symptoms (60). In this respect, genes coding for antioxidant enzymes such as glutathione S-transferases (GSTs) and N-acetyl transferase (NAT)

Table 7 Examples of Associations Between Polymorphisms and Asthma or Related Phenotypes in Different Populations

Gene	SNP position	Summary	References
IL-10	−627	−627A allele reported to be a risk factor of developing atopic asthma	(47)
IL-12B	−4237, −6402	−4237 and −6402 polymorphisms were associated with asthma severity-phenotype	(48)
IL-13	−1055	−1055TT genotype was found to be associated with the development	(50)
TLR-10	+1031, +2322	+1031 and +2322 SNPs were associated with physician-diagnosed asthma	(51)
ADAM 33	ST+7	ST+7 SNP was associated with asthma	(53)
IL-4Rα	S478P	Significant association was found between S478P and high IgE levels	(55)
TNFα	−308	Homozygosity for −308 allele was associated with increased risk of physician-diagnosed asthma	(79)
TGFβ	−509	−509 T variant was associated with asthma severity	(80)
IL-4	−589	−589T variant was associated with the development of asthma and the regulation of total serum IgE	(81)
IL-3	Ser27Pro	27 Pro allele showed protective effect on development of asthma in nonatopic subjects	(82)
GSTP1	Ile-105	Gene-environment interaction was reported between Ile-105 homozygotes and outdoor air pollution for childhood asthma	(83)
CD14	−159	−159T variant was associated with expression of a more severe asthma	(84)

Abbreviations: IL, interleukin; TLR, toll-like receptor; TNF, tumor necrosis factor; GST, glutathione S-transferases; TGF, tumor growth factor; CD, cytotoxic drug.

are strong candidates for OA association studies. GSTs play an important role in the protection of cells from ROS damage because they detoxify a wide variety of electrophiles such as lipid and DNA peroxides. GSTP, located on chromosome 11q13, provides more than 90% of the GST activity in the lung and contains two genetic polymorphisms: an A→G transition at nucleotide +313 that leads to the 105 Ile/ Val substitution, and a C→T transition at nucleotide +314. It has been demonstrated that the *val* variant alters specific activity and affinity for electrophilic substrates. For example, sevenfold greater catalytic activity for polycyclic aromatic hydrocarbon diol epoxides and a threefold lower activity for 1-chloro-2,4-dinitrobenzene were reported in individuals with the rare allele (61,62). An association was also found between the 105 *val* variant and lung cancer and COPD (63–65). Earlier, the

GSTP1 *val/val* genotype was reported to confer a sixfold lower risk of asthma (OR = 0.16; 95% CI: 0.05–0.55) and 10-fold lower risk (OR = 0.11, 95% CI: 0.02–0.50) for high IgE levels (60). Although it did not achieve statistical significance, a protective effect of *val/val* genotype was observed in TDI-induced asthma in subjects exposed to TDI for 10 or more years (OR = 0.23, 95% CI: 0.05–1.13) (66). In these studies the homozygosity for the *val* variant was lower in subjects with asthma (5.1%) after 10 years of TDI exposure than in those without asthma (18.8%). Although the sample size was low and statistical significance was not attained, this finding points to the importance of exposure intensity and other genetic factors in the development of asthma after short-term exposure (67). In another study, 182 diisocyanate-exposed workers were examined for GST polymorphisms (68). GSTM1 null and GSTM3 AA genotypes were related to late reactions in the specific bronchial provocation test, individually (OR = 2.82, 95% CI: 1.15–6.88 and OR = 3.75, 95% CI: 1.26–11.2, respectively) or in combination (OR = 11.0, 95% CI: 2.19–55.3). GSTM1 catalyzes the reaction of glutathione for a wide variety of organic compounds to form thioethers. The homozygosity for the GSTM1 null allele results in loss of gene function. Although relatively little is known about the role of the GSTM3 in enzyme metabolism, it is known to have overlapping substrate specificities with GSTM1 (69). GSTM1 null and the combination of GSTM1 null and GTM3AA genotypes were also reported to be related with lack of diisocyanate-specific IgE antibodies. Although the GSTP1 *val/val* genotype was associated with higher total serum IgE levels (OR = 5.46, 95% CI: 1.15–26.0), no statistically significant association was observed between GSTP1 genotypes and risk of diisocyanate-induced asthma. The difference in total serum IgE levels with respect to GSTP1 *val/val* genotype, compared to the data of Fryer et al. (60), may be explained by the small sample size, differences in the study populations, and the level and nature of exposure.

Like GSTs, there are large inter-individual variations in enzyme responses of NATs. NATs are involved in the deactivation of aromatic amines that can be formed from aromatic diisocyanates (70) and also play a role in the inactivation of proinflammatory cysteinyl leukotrienes which are potent mediators of airway narrowing (71). Polymorphisms in the NAT genes have been associated with lung cancer (72,73). The NAT1 variant, responsible for slow acetylation, was found to be associated with a 2.5-fold higher risk for developing diisocyanate-induced asthma (95% CI: 1.32–4.91) and 7.7-fold risk for developing TDI-induced asthma (95% CI: 1.18–51.6) (74). The presence of GSTM1 null and either NAT1 or NAT2 genotypes also conferred an increased risk (OR = 4.53; 95% CI: 1.76–11.6 and OR = 3.12; 95% CI: 1.11–8.78, respectively). Similar associations were also reported for the NAT1 and NAT2 slow acetylator genotypes (OR = 4.20; 95% CI: 1.51–11.6).

FUTURE DIRECTIONS

Meta-analyses of genetic association studies are currently underway to help identify susceptibility loci in candidate genes. Reports from multiple studies may help to establish genes with modest effects for multifactorial diseases such as asthma (75,76). Advance high-throughput technologies available for data generation and the amount and complexity of the data that can be obtained require the creation of new algorithms and methodologies for use in the computational interpretation and analysis of biological data. These advances could lead to better predictive models to incorporate genetic variability for human risk assessment (77).

The conduct of genetic studies raises the ethical, legal, and social implications of such research. The scientific profit from genetic research requires full integration of ethics components into the structure and functioning of genetic studies (78). The formulation and adoption of societal issues and widespread education are required to protect individuals against genetic-based discrimination or inappropriate use of the results (80). Despite the increasing availability of such data, there has been little effort to incorporate genetic information into the risk assessment process. Molecular epidemiology studies in workplace would provide more accurate information on the inter-individual variability that could be used in risk assessment and for improving the regulation and redefinition of acceptable exposure levels in the workplace. This information would also be useful in the development of more appropriate disease models that help to investigate disease risk, gene–environment interactions, and new therapeutic or treatment regimens.

REFERENCES

1. Cookson WO, Hopkin JM. Dominant inheritance of atopic immunoglobulin responsiveness. Lancet 1988; 1:86–88.
2. Sibbald B. Genetic basis of asthma. Semin Resp Med 1986; 7:307–315.
3. Jenkins MA, Hopper JL, Flander LB, Carlin JB, Giles GG. The associations between childhood asthma and atopy and parental asthma, hay fever and smoking. Paediatr Perinat Epidemiol 1993; 7:67–76.
4. Edfors-Lub ML. Allergy in 7000 twin pairs. Acta Allergol 1971; 26:249–285.
5. Hopper JL, Hannah MC, Macaskill GT, Matthews JD. Twin concordance for a binary trait: III A bivariate analysis of hay fever and asthma. Genet Epidemiol 1990; 7:277–299.
6. Harris JR, Magnus P, Samuelsen SO, Tambs K. No evidence for effects of family environment on asthma. A retrospective study of Norwegian twins. Am J Respir Crit Care Med 1997; 156:43–49.
7. Hanson B, McGue M, Roitman-Johnson B, Segal NL, Bouchard TJ, Blumenthal MN. Atopic and immunoglobulin E in twins reared apart and together. Am J Hum Genet 1991; 48:873–879.
8. Cooke RA, Vander Veer A. Human sensitization. J Immunol 1996; 1:201–305.
9. Schwarz M. Heredity in Bronchial Asthma. Copenhagen: Munksgaard Press, 1952.
10. Sibbald B, Horn MC, Brain EA, Gregg I. Genetic factors in childhood asthma. Thorax 1980; 35:671–674.
11. Cookson WOCM, Sharp PA, Faux JA, Hopkin JM. Linkage between immunoglobulin E responses underlying asthma and rhinitis and chromosome 11q. Lancet 1989; 1:1292–1295.
12. Young RP, Sharp PA, Lynch JR, et al. Confirmation of genetic linkage between atopic IgE responses and chromosome 11q. J Med Genet 1992; 29:236–238.
13. Cookson WOCM, Young RP, Sandford AJ. Maternal inheritance of atopic IgE responsiveness on chromosome 11. Lancet 1992; 340:381–384.
14. Sandford AJ, Shirakawa T, Moffatt MF, et al. Localization of atopy and β subunit of high affinity IgE receptor (FCERI) on chromosome 11q. Lancet 1993; 341:332–334.
15. Shirakawa T, Airong L, Dubowitz M, et al. Associations between atopy and variants of the β subunit of the high affinity immunoglobulin E receptor. Nat Genet 1994; 7:125–130.
16. Hall I, Faux J, Ryan G, et al. FCERI-β polymorphisms and risk of atopy in a general population sample. Brit Med J 1995; 311:776–779.
17. Lympany P, Welsh KI, Cochrane GM, Kemeny DM, Lee TH. Genetic analysis of the linkage between chromosome 11q and atopy. Clin Exp Allergy 1992; 22:1085–1092.

18. Rich SS, Roitman Johnson B, Greenberg M, Roberts S, Blumenthal MN. Genetic analysis of atopy in three large kindreds: no evidence of linkage to D11S 97. Clin Exp Allergy 1992; 22:1070–1076.

19. Marsh DG, Neely JD, Breazeale DR, et al. Linkage analysis of IL4 and other chromosome 5q 31.1 markers and total serum IgE concentrations. Science 1994; 264:1152–1156.

20. Postma DS, Bleeker ER, Alemung PJ, et al. Genetic susceptibility to asthma–bronchial hyperresponsivenes coinhertied with a major gene for atopy. N Engl J Med 1995; 333:894–900.

21. Lander ES, Schork NJ. Genetic dissection of complex traits. Science 1994; 265:2037–2048.

22. Palmer LJ. Linkages and associations to intermediate phenotypes underlying asthma and allergic disease. Curr Opin Allergy Clin Immunol 2001; 1:393–398.

23. Palmer LJ, Cookson WO. Using single nucleotide polymorphisms as a means to understanding the pathophysiology of asthma. Respir Res 2001; 2:102–112.

24. Mapp CE. The role of genetic factors in occupational asthma. Eur Respir J 2003; 22: 173–178.

25. Silverman EK, Palmer LJ. Case-control association studies for the genetics of complex respiratory diseases. Am J Respir Cell Mol Biol 2000; 22:645–648.

26. Yucesoy B, Vallyathan V, Landsittel DP, et al. Association of tumor necrosis factor-alpha and interleukin-1 gene polymorphisms with silicosis. Toxicol Appl Pharmacol 2001; 172:75–82.

27. Yucesoy B, Vallyathan V, Landsittel DP, et al. Polymorphisms of the IL-1 gene complex in coal miners with silicosis. Am J Ind Med 2001; 39:286–291.

28. Khoury MJ, James LM. Population and familial relative risks of disease associated with environmental factors in the presence of gene-environment interaction. Am J Epidemiol 1993; 137:1241–1250.

29. Ottman R. An epidemiologic approach to gene-environment interaction. Genet Epidemiol 1990; 7:177–185.

30. Kelada SN, Eaton DL, Wang SS, Rothman NR, Khoury MJ. The role of genetic polymorphisms in environmental health. Environ Health Perspect 2003; 111:1055–1064.

31. Frew AJ. What can we learn about asthma from studying occupational asthma? Ann Allergy Asthma Immunol 2003; 90:7–10.

32. Marsh DG, Friedhoff LR, Ehrhick-Kautzky E, Bias WB, Roebber M. Immune responsiveness to Ambrosia artemisi-ifolia (short ragweed) pollen allergen Amba V1(Rae 6) is associated with HLA DR5 in allergic humans. Immuno Genet 1987; 26:230–236.

33. Marsh DG, Hsu SH, Roebber M, et al. HLA-DW2: a genetic marker for human immune response to short ragweed pollen allergen Ra5.1. Response resulting primarily from natural antigenic exposure. J Exp Med 1982; 155:1439–1451.

34. Low B, Sjostedt L, Willirs S. Laboratory animal allergy-possible association with HLA B15 and DR4. Tissue Antigens 1988; 32:224–226.

35. Kerwin EM, Freed JH, Dresback JK, Rosenwagger LJ. HLA DR4 DRW 11 (15) and DR 17 (3) function as restriction elements for Mus m 1 allergic human T cells. J Allergy Clin Immunol 1993; 91:235.

36. Jeal H, Draper A, Jones M, et al. HLA associations with occupational sensitisation to rat lipocalin allergens : a model for other animal allergies? J Allergy Clin Immunol 2003; 111:795–799.

37. Young RP, Barker RD, Pile KD, Cookson WOCM, Newman Taylor AJ. The association of HLA DR3 with specific IgE to inhaled acid anhydrides. Am J Respir Crit Care Med 1995; 151:219–221.

38. Bignon JS, Aron Y, Ju LY, et al. HLA Class II alleles in isocyanates induced asthma. Am J Respir Crit Care Med 1994; 149:71–75.

39. Balboni A, Baricoidi OR, Fabbri LM, Gandini E, Ciaecia A, Mapp CE. Association between toluene diisocyanate induced asthma and DQB1 markers: a possible role for aspartic acid at position 57. Eur Respir J 1996; 9:207–210.

40. Richeldi L, Sorrentino R, Saltini C. HLA-DPB1 glutamate 69: a genetic marker of beryllium disease. Science 1993; 262:242.

41. Newman-Taylor AJ, Cullinan P, Lympany PA, Harris JM, Dowdeswell RJ, du Bois RM. Interaction of HLA phenotype and exposure intensity in sensitisation to complex platinum salts. Am J Respir Crit Care Med 1999; 160:435–438.

42. Richeldi L, Kreiss K, Mroz MM, Zhen B, Tartoni P, Saltini C. Interaction of genetic and exposure factors in the prevalence of berylliosis. Am J Ind Med 1997; 32:337–340.

43. Cookson WO. Asthma genetics. Chest 2002; 121:7S–13S.

44. Nakao F, Ihara K, Kusuhara K, et al. Association of IFN-gamma and IFN regulatory factor 1 polymorphisms with childhood atopic asthma. J Allergy Clin Immunol 2001; 107:499–504.

45. Karjalainen J, Nieminen MM, Aromaa A, Klaukka T, Hurme M. The IL-1beta genotype carries asthma susceptibility only in men. J Allergy Clin Immunol 2002; 109:514–516.

46. Cui T, Wu J, Pan S, Xie J. Polymorphisms in the IL-4 and IL-4R [alpha] genes and allergic asthma. Clin Chem Lab Med 2003; 41:888–892.

47. Hang LW, Hsia TC, Chen WC, Chen HY, Tsai JJ, Tsai FJ. Interleukin-10 gene-627 allele variants, not interleukin-1 beta gene and receptor antagonist gene polymorphisms, are associated with atopic bronchial asthma. J Clin Lab Anal 2003; 17:168–173.

48. Randolph AG, Lange C, Silverman EK, et al. The IL12B gene is associated with asthma. Am J Hum Genet 2004; 75:709–715.

49. Noguchi E, Yokouchi Y, Shibasaki M, et al. Association between TNFα polymorphism and the development of asthma in the Japanese population. Am J Respir Crit Care Med 2002; 166:43–46.

50. van der Pouw Kraan TC, van Veen A, Boeije LC, et al. An IL-13 promoter polymorphism associated with increased risk of allergic asthma. Genes Immun 1999; 1:61–65.

51. Lazarus R, Raby BA, Lange C, et al. TOLL-like receptor 10 genetic variation is associated with asthma in two independent samples. Am J Respir Crit Care Med 2004; 170:594–600.

52. Szalai C, Kozma GT, Nagy A, et al. Polymorphism in the gene regulatory region of MCP-1 is associated with asthma susceptibility and severity. J Allergy Clin Immunol 2001; 108:375–381.

53. Van Eerdewegh P, Little RD, Dupuis J, et al. Association of the ADAM33 gene with asthma and bronchial hyperresponsiveness. Nature 2002; 418:426–430.

54. Urhan M, Degirmenci I, Harmanci E, Gunes HV, Metintas M, Basaran A. High frequency of DD polymorphism of the angiotensin-converting enzyme gene in Turkish asthmatic patients. Allergy Asthma Proc 2004; 25:243–247.

55. Howard TD, Koppelman GH, Xu J, et al. Gene-gene interaction in asthma: IL4RA and IL13 in a Dutch population with asthma. Am J Hum Genet 2002; 70:230–236.

56. Lee SG, Kim BS, Kim JH, et al. Gene-gene interaction between interleukin-4 and interleukin-4 receptor alpha in Korean children with asthma. Clin Exp Allergy 2004; 34:1202–1208.

57. Bentley AM, Maestrelli P, Saetta M, et al. Activated T-lymphocytes and eosinophils in the bronchial mucosa in isocyanate-induced asthma. J Allergy Clin Immunol 1992; 89:821–829.

58. Park H, Jung K, Kim H, Nahm D, Kang K. Neutrophil activation following TDI bronchial challenges to the airway secretion from subjects with TDI-induced asthma. Clin Exp Allergy 1999; 29:1395–1401.

59. Malo JL, Chan-Yeung M. Occupational asthma. J Allergy Clin Immunol 2001; 108:317–328.

60. Fryer AA, Bianco A, Hepple M, Jones PW, Strange RC, Spiteri MA. Polymorphism at the glutathione S-transferase GSTP1 locus. A new marker for bronchial hyperresponsiveness and asthma. Am J Respir Crit Care Med 2000; 161:1437–1442.

61. Watson MA, Stewart RK, Smith GB, Massey TE, Bell DA. Human glutathione S-transferase P1 polymorphisms: relationship to lung tissue enzyme activity and population frequency distribution. Carcinogenesis 1998; 19:275–280.

62. Hu X, Xia H, Srivastava SK, et al. Activity of four allelic forms of glutathione S-transferase hGSTP1-1 for diol epoxides of polycyclic aromatic hydrocarbons. Biochem Biophys Res Commun 1997; 238:397–402.

63. Ishii T, Matsuse T, Teramoto S, et al. Glutathione S-transferase P1 (GSTP1) polymorphism in patients with chronic obstructive pulmonary disease. Thorax 1999; 54:693–696.

64. He JQ, Ruan J, Connett JE, Anthonisen NR, Pare PD, Sandford AJ. Antioxidant gene polymorphisms and susceptibility to a rapid decline in lung function in smokers. Am J Respir Crit Care Med 2002; 166:323–328.

65. Miller DP, Neuberg D, de Vivo I, et al. Smoking and the risk of lung cancer: susceptibility with GSTP1 polymorphisms. Epidemiology 2003; 14:545–551.

66. Mapp CE, Fryer AA, De Marzo N, et al. Glutathione S-transferase GSTP1 is a susceptibility gene for occupational asthma induced by isocyanates. J Allergy Clin Immunol 2002; 109:867–872.

67. Park HS, Frew AJ. Genetic markers for occupational asthma. J Allergy Clin Immunol 2002; 109:774–776.

68. Piirila P, Wikman H, Luukkonen R, et al. Glutathione S-transferase genotypes and allergic responses to diisocyanate exposure. Pharmacogenetics 2001; 11:437–445.

69. Hayes JD, Strange RC. Potential contribution of the glutathione S-transferase supergene family to resistance to oxidative stress. Free Radic Res 1995; 22:193–207.

70. Bolognesi C, Baur X, Marczynski B, Norppa H, Sepai O, Sabbioni G. Carcinogenic risk of toluene diisocyanate and 4,4′-methylenediphenyl diisocyanate: epidemiological and experimental evidence. Crit Rev Toxicol 2001; 31:737–772.

71. Devillier P, Baccard N, Advenier C. Leukotrienes, leukotriene receptor antagonists and leukotriene synthesis inhibitors in asthma: an update. Part I: synthesis, receptors and role of leukotrienes in asthma. Pharmacol Res 1999; 40:3–13.

72. Bouchardy C, Mitrunen K, Wikman H, et al. N-acetyltransferase NAT1 and NAT2 genotypes and lung cancer risk. Pharmacogenetics 1998; 8:291–298.

73. Hengstler JG, Arand M, Herrero ME, Oesch F. Polymorphisms of N-acetyltransferases, glutathione S-transferases, microsomal epoxide hydrolase and sulfotransferases: influence on cancer susceptibility. Recent Results Cancer Res 1998; 154:47–85.

74. Wikman H, Piirila P, Rosenberg C, et al. N-Acetyltransferase genotypes as modifiers of diisocyanate exposure-associated asthma risk. Pharmacogenetics 2002; 12:227–233.

75. Jacobs KB, Burton PR, Iyengar SK, Elston RC, Palmer LJ. Pooling data and linkage analysis in the chromosome 5q candidate region for asthma. Genet Epidemiol 2001; 21(suppl 1):S103–S108.

76. Wise LH. Inclusion of candidate region studies in meta-analysis using the genome screen meta-analysis method: application to asthma data. Genet Epidemiol 2001; 21(suppl 1): S160–S165.

77. Collins FS, Green ED, Guttmacher AE, Guyer MS. A vision for the future of genomics research. Nature 2003; 422:835–847.

78. Harris JR, Willemsen G, Aitlahti T, et al. Ethical issues and GenomEUtwin. Twin Res 2003; 6:455–463.

79. Albuquerque RV, Hayden CM, Palmer LJ, et al. Association of polymorphisms within the tumour necrosis factor (TNF) genes and childhood asthma. Clin Exp Allergy 1998; 28:578–584.

80. Pulleyn LJ, Newton R, Adcock IM, Barnes PJ. TGFbeta1 allele association with asthma severity. Hum Genet 2001; 109:623–627.

81. Kabesch M, Tzotcheva I, Carr D, et al. A complete screening of the IL4 gene: novel polymorphisms and their association with asthma and IgE in childhood. J Allergy Clin Immunol 2003; 112:893–898.

82. Park BL, Kim LH, Choi YH, et al. Interleukin 3 (IL3) polymorphisms associated with decreased risk of asthma and atopy. J Hum Genet 2004; 49:517–527.

83. Lee YL, Lin YC, Lee YC, Wang JY, Hsiue TR, Guo YL. Glutathione S-transferase P1 gene polymorphism and air pollution as interactive risk factors for childhood asthma. Clin Exp Allergy 2004; 34:1707–1713.

84. Sharma M, Batra J, Mabalirajan U, et al. Suggestive evidence of association of C-159T functional polymorphism of the CD14 gene with atopic asthma in northern and north-western Indian populations. Immunogenetics 2004; 56:544–547.

5
Pathophysiology

Piero Maestrelli
Department of Environmental Medicine and Public Health, University of Padova, Padova, Italy

Leonardo M. Fabbri
Section of Respiratory Diseases, Department of Oncology and Hematology, University of Modena, Modena, Italy

Cristina E. Mapp
Section of Hygiene and Occupational Medicine, Department of Clinical and Experimental Medicine, University of Ferrara, Ferrara, Italy

INTRODUCTION

Much of the significant progress in elaborating the complex pathophysiological pathways of asthma in the past 30 years can be attributed to collaborative interdisciplinary contributions of physiologists, pathologists, and immunologists/allergists. These investigators of the disease now agree that inflammation is the common denominator among the other pathologic hallmarks of asthma. The complex cascade of events associated with asthmatic inflammation has, largely, been demonstrated by the study of immunological or allergic asthma, utilizing either bronchoalveolar lavage (BAL), bronchial biopsies, induced sputum, or animal models. None of these advances would have been possible without access to sophisticated immuno-histological and molecular biology techniques.

Clinical, functional, and pathological alterations in occupational asthma (OA) are similar to those found in non-OA. Airway smooth muscle contraction and mucosal edema are probably the main causes of acute airflow obstruction. Chronic airflow obstruction may be due to increase of airway wall thickness caused by accumulation of inflammatory cells, edema, hypertrophy of airway smooth muscles, obstruction of airway lumen by exudate and/or mucus, and changes in the mechanical properties of the airway wall. Airway hyperresponsiveness (AHR), i.e., an excessive reaction to bronchoconstrictor stimuli, is the hallmark of both OA and non-OA. The pathogenesis of this AHR, which is generally long lasting and poorly reversible, remains unknown. By contrast, the transient increase of airway responsiveness observed during exacerbations of OA most often seems to be associated with an acute inflammatory reaction in the airways. The pathologic alterations of the airways in OA are characterized by infiltration of the airway mucosa by inflammatory cells, including eosinophils, mast cells, and activated lymphocytes. Subepithelial fibrosis is an end result of the inflammatory cascade that is rather specific for asthma. The relationship between these pathologic alterations and the clinical and functional features of asthma is only partially understood. In particular, the mechanisms of "induction" or sensitization by which many allergenic high-molecular-weight (HMW) occupational agents cause asthma parallel the events of nonoccupational allergen-induced immunoglobulin E (IgE)-mediated asthma. Induction mechanisms have not been well defined for many low-molecular-weight (LMW) agents, which cause OA, but do not consistently induce specific IgE, and for the agents causing irritant-induced asthma.

Although the pathogenetic basis of OA is closely interwoven with previous and current research of natural-occurring asthma, several cogent features of OA provide an optimal milieu for enhancing the global understanding of asthma in general. First, both immunologic (i.e., extrinsic) and nonimmunologic (i.e., intrinsic) asthma occur in occupational settings, and occasionally both forms of asthma may be concurrent. Thus, similarities and/or differences of pathogenetic mechanisms between these major categories of asthma may be directly observed. Second, in the case of immunologically induced asthma, immunopathogenesis can be investigated through various phases of the immune response: onset of sensitization, the latent period, the elicitation episode(s), and the effect of repetitive episodes. Similarly, the roles of epithelial cell injury, microvascular leakage, reflex, and pharmacologically mediated mechanisms can be explored in a systematic way. Finally, etiologic and/or inciting agents can be more easily identified than in non-OA. Taken together, these special attributes confer unique advantages on OA as an immunopathogenetic model for nonwork-related asthma. Most of what we know of the mechanisms of asthma has been obtained from studies of non-OA, as unfortunately not many mechanistic studies have been performed in OA. In this chapter, we therefore describe pathophysiologic mechanisms involved in both non-OA and OA. We also analyze these mechanisms with special emphasis on what can be learned from the similarities and the dissimilarities between these two types of asthma.

PATHOPHYSIOLOGICAL MECHANISMS COMMON TO NON-OA AND OA

Acute and Chronic Airway Narrowing

Airway narrowing may be due to airway smooth muscle contraction, airway wall inflammation, accumulation of fluid in the airway lumen, or loss of elastic support from lung parenchyma (1). Airway smooth muscle contraction and mucosal edema are probably the main causes of acute airflow obstruction during immediate asthmatic reactions, whereas late asthmatic reactions are also associated with accumulation of inflammatory cells and exudate in the airway walls and lumen (2). The relative proportion of airflow obstruction caused by each mechanism remains to be established.

Specific inhalation challenge testing is considered the "gold standard" for the confirmation of OA (Chapter 10) (3). After exposure, various temporal patterns of reactions can occur, including those of typical (immediate, late, and dual) and atypical (progressive, square waved, and prolonged immediate) reactions. Late asthmatic responses occur more commonly on inhalation challenge testing with LMW agents, but this may be a consequence of the single-dose challenge protocol that is commonly used, rather than being mediated by a different pathogenetic mechanism compared with the asthmatic reaction induced by HMW agents (4).

If exposure continues after diagnosis, OA persists or may even deteriorate as measured by tests of AHR and/or chronic airflow limitation (5–9). Interestingly, only about 10% of nonoccupational adult asthmatics fully recover from asthma in 25 years (10). It remains undetermined whether the low rate of recovery is a result of the persistence of exposure that induces symptoms or due to other reasons.

Chronic airflow obstruction may be due to increase of airway wall thickness from accumulation of inflammatory cells, edema, and increased mass of smooth muscle, airway-wall remodeling, obstruction of the airway lumen by exudate and/or mucus, and changes of elastic properties of the airway walls and/or loss of the interdependence between the airways and the surrounding parenchyma (1,2,11–13). In most asthmatic patients, the hypertrophy of airway smooth muscle is more pronounced in the central airways, but in a subgroup of patients, it is extended to peripheral bronchioles (14). Some studies showed that persistence of OA is associated with long-term airway inflammation, suggesting that once triggered, the inflammatory process in the airways may continue even without further exposure (15–18).

Airway Hyperresponsiveness

The principal feature that distinguishes asthmatic airways from normal ones is the excessive response to bronchoconstrictor stimuli, resulting in airway narrowing that far exceeds that which can be induced by the same stimuli in normal airways. AHR to either methacholine or histamine is the hallmark of both OA and non-OA (19–21). In subjects with OA, the degree of airway responsiveness to methacholine or histamine is usually, but not invariably, increased (22,23). Figure 1 illustrates the variability of peak expiratory flow (PEF) and the provocative dose of methacholine inducing a 20% fall in forced expiratory volume in one second ($PD_{20}FEV_1$) in a representative subject sensitized to toluene diisocyante (TDI). It is noteworthy that both parameters decrease after occupational exposure. Similarly, although AHR to methacholine or histamine may be normal prior to the diagnosis of OA in the laboratory, it usually increases (i.e., $PD_{20}FEV_1$ decreases) after a positive inhalation challenge with a sensitizing agent, particularly in subjects who develop a late asthmatic reaction (24,25). Clinical investigations indicate that the increase in AHR may begin as early as two hours after challenge test with either high- or low-molecular-weight sensitizing agents (26–28). The increase in airway responsiveness induced by sensitizing agents may last for days or even longer (25). Moreover, a decrease in $PD_{20}FEV_1$ may be the only residual effect of exposure to a sensitizing agent in a worker previously known to be sensitive to that agent (25). To summarize, these data suggest that AHR is one of the most important sequelae of OA (29) even if its significance in non-OA remains questionable (30). Indeed, Josephs et al. (29) showed that variation in AHR does not parallel changes in asthma severity, and that it might not be a valuable marker for monitoring the severity of asthma.

Workers with OA often demonstrate AHR even when they are asymptomatic. The AHR present during the asymptomatic stage of the disease seems to be long lasting and only partly reversible or irreversible even after treatment (6,8,9,18,31–34). The pathogenesis of such long lasting, poorly reversible AHR in OA remains unknown. By contrast, the transient increase in AHR occurring during or after an asthmatic reaction induced by specific inhalation challenge testing seems to be associated with an acute inflammatory reaction in the airways (35,36). However, Durham et al. (28) observed increases in histamine-induced airway responsiveness two to three hours after challenges with various occupational agents prior to the

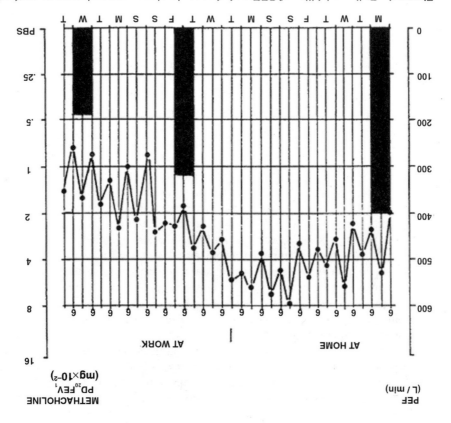

Figure 1 Daily variability of PEF and changes in airway responsiveness to methacholine expressed as provocative dose of 20% fall in the FEV_1 ($PD_{20}FEV_1$) in one subject with OA induced by isocyanates. Measurements were obtained during a week while the subjects were at work and, before, during a week while the subject was not working. *Abbreviations:* FEV_1, forced expiratory volume in one second; OA, occupational asthma; PEF, peak expiratory flow; M, T, W, T, F, S, S, days of the week.

influx of inflammatory cells in the airways, and suggested that the time course of the various components of the inflammatory response may be different (28).

Studies in patients with asthma suggest that AHR to an indirect stimulus of bronchoconstriction as adenosine 5'-monophosphate (AMP) is a better marker of bronchial inflammation than AHR to methacholine. In a follow-up study on occupational allergy in young adults, AMP hyperresponsiveness showed a stronger association with allergic rhinitis and asthma, and with blood eosinophilia than methacholine hyperresponsiveness, whereas the latter was more strongly related to a lower prechallenge level of FEV_1 (37). However, hyperresponsiveness to methacholine and to AMP were both predictors for development of nasal symptoms to occupational allergens in a follow-up study among laboratory animal workers and bakery apprentices (38).

MECHANISMS OF OA

Similar to non-work-related asthma, the signals that initiate and perpetuate OA are highly variable depending on the agent and the extent of exposure. High- and some low-molecular-weight substances typically induce Th2 cytokine/IgE-dependent

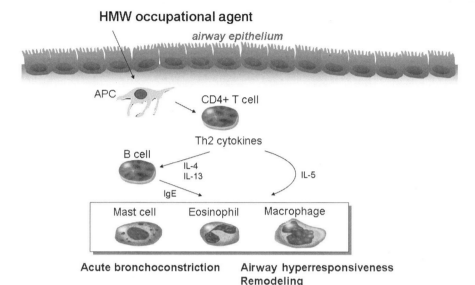

Figure 2 Schematic summary of possible mechanisms in OA induced by HMW agents. HMW agents are recognized by APC and mount a CD4-Type 2 response with production of specific IgE antibodies by IL-4/IL-13–stimulated B cells. Binding of IgE to their receptors and Th2 (IL-5) cytokines induce recruitment and activation of inflammatory cells. These cells (eosinophils, mast cells, macrophages, and activated lymphocytes) characterize airway inflammation, which contributes to the functional alterations of OA, i.e., acute and chronic airway narrowing and airway hyperresponsiveness. Subepithelial fibrosis due to thickening of the reticular basement membrane is considered a histopathological feature of OA. However, the role of this remodeling of the airways on lung function is obscure. *Abbreviations*: APC, antigen presenting cells; HMW, high molecular weight; IL, interleukin; OA, occupational asthma.

allergic (atopic) asthma (Fig. 2), while some chemicals (e.g., isocyanates and plicatic acid) may induce asthma in nonatopic individuals, through immunological mechanisms that may be independent of the classical IgE-mediated pathways (Fig. 3).

The mechanism of asthma induced by irritants is not known (39). Many reports indicate that unintentional high-level respiratory irritant exposures can induce new-onset asthma (40). As this type of OA occurs after inhalation of high levels of irritants, the main target for the initial injury could be the bronchial epithelium that becomes denudated and loses its protective properties. Consequences of the damage in the bronchial epithelium are the loss of relaxing factors derived from epithelium, the exposure of nerve endings leading to neurogenic inflammation, and the release of inflammatory mediators and cytokines following the nonspecific activation of mast cells (41). A further consequence of the disruption of the epithelium with the secretion of growth factors for epithelial cells, smooth muscle, and fibroblasts, together with matrix degradation, is a tissue regenerative and remodeling response (41,42). Although the onset of irritant-induced asthma is immediate and specific sensitization is not involved, an immunologic mechanism for the persistence of pathologic and functional changes cannot be excluded. The "Danger model" of immune response assumes that resting antigen-presenting cells can be activated by signals originating from injured cells in the immediate environment. These alarm signals may be recognized by receptors of innate immunity as CD14, toll-like

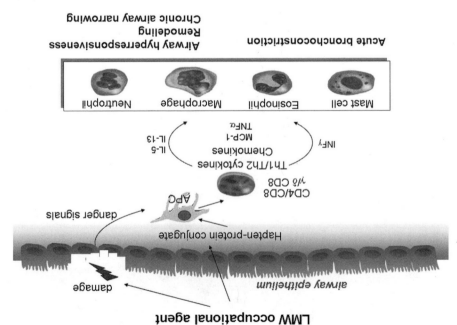

LMW occupational agent

damage

airway epithelium

danger signals

Hapten-protein conjugate

APC

CD4/CD8
γ/δ CD8

Th1/Th2 cytokines

IL-5
IL-13

Chemokines
MCP-1
TNFα

INFγ

Mast cell   Eosinophil   Macrophage   Neutrophil

Acute bronchoconstriction   Airway hyperresponsiveness
Remodeling
Chronic airway narrowing

Figure 3 Schematic summary of possible mechanisms in OA induced by LMW agents. Most LMW agents do not consistently induce specific IgE antibodies. The immune response may be initiated by recognition of LMW agent bound to protein by antigen presenting cells. In addition, danger signals originated by injury of bronchial epithelial cells may contribute to the activation of immunocompetent cells. In this case of OA, a mixed CD4-CD8 Type 2/Type 1 response or induction of γ/δ specific CD8 may play a role. Th2 (IL-5) and Th1 (IFN-γ) cytokines, and other proinflammatory chemokines MCP-1, TNF-α induce recruitment and activation of inflammatory cells. *Abbreviations:* IFN-γ, interferon-γ; LMW, low molecular weight; MCP-1, monocyte chemoattractant protein-1; TNF-α, tumor necrosis factor alpha.

receptors, and nucleotide-binding oligomerization domain (NOD) receptors (43). In subjects who develop irritant-induced asthma, alarm signals from damaged cells might in turn activate immuno-competent cells that drive the remodeling/hyperreactivity phenotype (Fig. 4).

In non-work-related asthma, it has been postulated that expression of Th2 cytokines, C–C chemokines, and IgE are similar in atopic and nonatopic forms of asthma (44–48). However, nonatopic asthma appears to have increased numbers of monocytes/macrophages, increased submucosal infiltration by CD68+ cells, and upregulation of the granulocyte macrophage-colony stimulating factor (GM-CSF) receptors on CD68+ cells (49–51). Although these sophisticated similarities and dissimilarities have not yet been fully explored in OA, new data concerning the roles of genetic predisposition and immunologic mechanisms in OA have been reported.

Genetic Aspects

Little is known about individual susceptibility to OA. A previous history of asthma is not significantly associated with OA. An underlying susceptibility to OA is likely to exist because only a proportion of workers exposed to similar exposures develop OA. Susceptibility has also been suggested by the observation that the time course

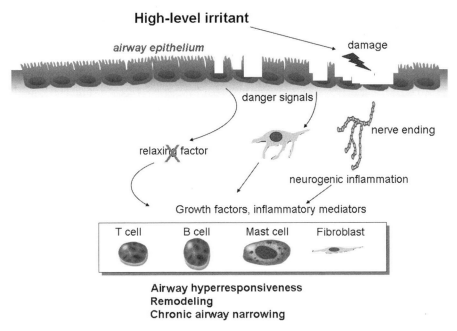

High-level irritant

Figure 4 Schematic summary of possible mechanisms in OA induced by exposure to high levels of respiratory irritants. Inhalation of irritants may damage airway epithelium. In subjects who develop irritant-induced asthma, alarm signals from damaged cells might in turn activate immunocomponent cells. Other consequences of the damage in the bronchial epithelium are the loss of relaxing factors derived from epithelium, the exposure of nerve endings leading to neurogenic inflammation, and the release of inflammatory mediators and cytokines following the nonspecific activation of mast cells. Secretion of growth factors for epithelial cells, smooth muscle, and fibroblasts, together with matrix degradation, may induce tissue regenerative and remodeling response. *Abbreviation*: OA, occupational asthma.

for the development of OA has the pattern of an epidemic curve, with a median period of about one year, consistent with the development of sensitization and asthma in a susceptible population.

Most reported genetic studies of OA have been performed on small sample sizes and, sometimes, the findings are unreplicated and fragmentary. Asthma is a complex disease in which combinations of multiple genetic and environmental factors are necessary for the expression of the phenotype. In detecting a gene–environment interaction, it is important to measure both the genotype and the environmental risk factor. Moreover, large sample sizes need to be used to detect interactions. Unfortunately, these steps, important for the study of complex diseases, i.e., asthma, are difficult to pursue in performing genetic studies on both OA and non-OA. However, the field of asthma genetics has advanced considerably in recent years with the cloning of two asthma genes, ADAM 33 and PHF11. This has generated new information and interest in the study of gene–gene interaction and in how linkage disequilibrium blocks and haplotypes can be used as functional units to pinpoint mutations and capture the relative risk of mutated genes in complex diseases such as asthma (52). Moreover, asthma is a phenotypically heterogeneous disorder, and the phenotypes of adult-onset asthma are still poorly understood (53). In this respect, OA offers the advantage of defining an accurate phenotype of the disease.

A number of studies have examined the role of gene coding for Class II human leukocyte antigen (HLA) and the development of OA. HLA Class II molecules are highly polymorphic, and are encoded by the major histocompatibility complex genes on chromosome 6p. They are plausible candidate genes that influence the development of a specific immunological response. Associations of OA with Class II molecules have been demonstrated for isocyanates, complex platinum salts, western red cedar, acid anhydrides, laboratory animal proteins, and natural rubber latex (54–56). Apparent discrepancies between HLA studies on isocyanate-induced asthma may be due to differences in study design and in selection of subjects. In a recent study, it has been shown that DQB1*501 is particularly frequent in subjects sensitized to organic acid anhydrides, indicating that the DQB1*501 gene confers susceptibility to develop specific IgE antibodies against organic acid anhydrides. It is of interest that the DQB1*501 is protective for other LMW agents such as isocyanates and plicatic acid, suggesting that different affinities for the corresponding specific Class II molecules may exist (55). A recent study of the association of HLA Class II genes with sensitization and development of symptoms to rat lipocalin allergens showed that approximately 40% of the subjects examined could be attributed to an HLA-DRB1*07 phenotype, whereas the attributable proportions for atopic status and daily exposure in an animal housing facility were 58% and 74%, respectively (56). Indeed, the conclusions are that genetic polymorphisms that code for HLA Class II genes may predispose to the development of OA to a number of agents. Moreover, HLA associations indicate a specific immunologic response in asthma induced by LMW agents. In isocyanate-induced asthma, the role of gene coding for Class I HLA has also been examined, and no significant associations have been found (57).

OA has been reported among aluminum-smelter potroom workers, although the mechanisms have not been clarified. A case–control study has examined whether polymorphisms were associated with the development of potroom asthma. Genotyping was performed for the beta2-adrenoreceptor, high affinity IgE receptor, and tumor necrosis factor (TNF), but no associations were found between potroom asthma case status and genotype (58).

Occupational sensitizers may cause oxidative stress, and defects in antioxidant defenses could contribute to the susceptibility to OA. In isocyanate-induced asthma, a role is played by the μ-class of the polymorphic glutathione-S transferase (GST) (59). More recently, it has been shown that homozygosity for the GSTP1*Val allele confers protection against asthma induced by exposure to TDI and AHR (60). This view is supported by the finding that the protective effect is more apparent with increasing duration of exposure. Our data also suggest that the GSTP1 Ile^{105}–Val^{105}, rather than the Ala^{114}–Val^{114}, substitution mediates the protective effect. Moreover, the association between the GSTP1 genotype and TDI-induced asthma was independent of atopy, sex, age, and smoking history. The ability to handle reactive oxygen species (ROS) and their products may be an important independent risk factor in determining development of airway inflammation leading to asthma. This study confirms previous data showing a strong association of GSTP1 genotypes with asthma and AHR in a cohort of English patients with atopic asthma, in whom the association of the GSTP1 genotype with asthma and AHR appeared independent of atopic status (61). Recently, a significant association between GSTP1 Ile^{105}Val polymorphism and susceptibility to asthma and a protective role for GSTP1 Val^{105} genotype have been reported in a study in Turkey, indicating similarities between OA induced by TDI and non-OA (62). The idea that GST genes are critical in the protection of cells from ROS, key components of inflammation, is supported by two studies published in 2004. The first, performed in Mexico City in an area with high ozone exposure, demonstrated that asthmatic children with a genetic deficiency of GSTM1 may be more susceptible to the deleterious effect of ozone on the small airways (63). The second, a randomized, placebo-controlled cross-over study, tested the hypothesis that GSTM1 and GSTT1 are key regulators of the adjuvant effects of diesel exhaust particles on allergic responses based on the hypothesis that particulate pollution may be associated with the occurrence of asthma and allergy (64). Patients sensitive to ragweed allergen were challenged intranasally with the allergen alone or with allergen plus diesel exhaust particles; polymorphisms of GSTM1 and GSTP1 modified the adjuvant effect of particles on allergic inflammation, with greater effects observed for both the GSTM1 null and GSTP1 I/I genotypes.

In addition to GST, N-acetyltransferase genotypes play a role in OA, where the N-acetyltranseferase slow acetylator genotypes posed a 7.77-fold risk of TDI asthma (65). On the other hand, TNFα A-308G is not associated with susceptibility or resistance to the development of TDI asthma (58). These results of genetic studies in isocyanate-induced asthma are consistent with the hypothesis that an immunologic mechanism may be involved in TDI-induced asthma. Indeed, several studies have demonstrated an association between certain haplotypes and individual responses to purified allergens and to other chemical sensitizers (e.g., acid anhydrides and platinum salts) believed to act by inducing specific IgE antibodies (66–68). However, OA induced by isocyanates and atopic asthma differs not only from some epidemiological points of view (e.g., isocyanate-induced asthma develops more often in nonatopic adult individuals and specific IgE antibodies are often absent, whereas atopic asthma develops in young atopic subjects and is invariably associated with specific IgE antibodies) but also in terms of its association with particular HLA class II alleles or haplotypes. While atopic asthma is associated with haplotype DR4, isocyanate-induced asthma is not. An immunologic mechanism in TDI-induced asthma is likely to occur because the clinical manifestations are similar to atopic asthma and, as in atopic asthma, the inflammatory response of the airways in TDI-induced asthma is characterized not only by increased numbers of mucosal eosinophils and mast cells, but also by persistent activation of lymphocytes and chronic expression of proinflammatory cytokines (69). The exact nature of the antigen that causes to sensitization to isocyanates is unknown. Isocyanates themselves may be involved in antibody binding or in the induction of structural changes or in an unidentified protein.

IgE-Mediated Allergy

Many occupational sensitizers, particularly HMW proteins and vegetable gums, are believed to act through an IgE-mediated reaction (Chapter 8). According to this mechanism, inhaled allergens gain access to the viable airway epithelium and engage and activate local dendritic cells so that allergen is transported to regional nodes and presented effectively to T lymphocytes. The cytokine milieu may determine whether T cell differentiation is biased toward a Th1 or Th2 response with IL-12 production leading to Th1 and IL-4/IL-13 to Th2 phenotype, respectively. Occupational allergens provoke the development of polarized immune responses that result in the development of Th2-type T lymphocytes, and the cytokine products of these cells facilitate the production of allergen-specific IgE antibody. Cross-link of allergens with specific IgE on the surface of mast cells, basophils, and possibly macrophages, dendritic cells, eosinophils, and platelets supports immediate-type allergic hypersensitivity responses (Fig. 2). HMW agents act as complete antigens and are therefore capable of cross-linking surface-bound IgE. However, LMW chemicals must first react with autologous or heterologous proteins to produce a complete allergen. The specific reaction between allergen and IgE gives rise to the cascade of events that is responsible for inflammatory cell activation with subsequent synthesis and/or release of a wide variety of preformed and newly formed inflammatory mediators, which then orchestrate the inflammatory reaction. Although other classes of antibodies have been hypothesized to have a role in asthma, substantive evidence for their participation is not available (70,71).

Antibody Studies in OA

Most OA studies have concentrated on antibody-mediated immunity. These consist of surveys using skin and/or in vitro antibody tests. Positive skin and specific immunoglobulin (IgE and IgG) tests have been shown to be present mainly in atopic subjects sensitized to HMW proteins, vegetable gums, and polysaccharides (72), but also in some subjects sensitized to LMW chemical agents (e.g., acid anhydride compounds, platinum salts, nickel, diisocyanates, and plicatic acid) (73–76). Positive skin tests against animal allergens, enzymes, egg white antigens, cereal flours, and plants, coffee, castor beans, and other HMW agents may be found from both in symptomatic and in some asymptomatic exposed workers (77–80). However, positive skin or IgE-specific in vitro tests (RAST) may precede respiratory sensitization, and skin test–positive asymptomatic patients should be monitored carefully by routine tests of pulmonary function or AHR.

Skin-prick tests against some HMW proteins (e.g., detergent enzymes and egg white antigens) are specific and/or sufficiently sensitive for the identification of occupational allergy in enzyme workers and egg processors (81,82). No special diagnostic or pathogenetic information is gained by the presence of specific IgG subclass antibodies (particularly the IgG4 reagin), which are equally distributed between exposed symptomatic and asymptomatic subjects (83,84).

Specific IgG antibodies are present in some subjects sensitized to diisocyanates with a positive inhalation challenge (75). However, specific IgG antibodies are also present in exposed workers with no history of asthma and negative inhalation challenges. The number of workers with specific IgG antibodies was no different in the groups with different types of asthmatic reactions (75). Additionally, the prevalence of specific antibody was different between subjects sensitized to different diisocyanate compounds. In contrast to TDI, MDI and HDI elicit specific antibody responses to both IgE and IgG isotypes in 36% and 80% of OA patients, respectively. Thus, the presence of elevated specific antibodies to HDI– and/or MDI–human serum albumin (HSA) conjugates in sera of diisocyanate workers has been found to be a specific but not a sensitive diagnostic marker of OA induced by either of these polyisocyanates (75,85).

In contrast to the variability of immune responsiveness in diisocyanate-exposed workers, investigations of acid anhydride–induced asthma have revealed that IgE-mediated immune responses may play a major role in the development of asthma. This may be due to the fact that various compounds in this class of chemicals [phthalic anhydride (PA), trimellitic anhydride (TMA), himic anhydride (HA), hexahydrophthalic anhydride (HHPA), tetrachlorophthalic anhydride (TCPA), and methyl tetrahydrophthalic anhydride (MTHPA)] readily form highly allergenic epitopes after conjugation of TMA, HA, HHPA, TCPA, and MTHPA with autologous human proteins. Cutaneous puncture tests with these reagents also have exhibited good diagnostic sensitivity (86). RAST cross-inhibition studies using sera of PA-, HHPA-, and HA-sensitized workers have demonstrated that antibody responses are heterogeneous. In some workers, specific IgE responses are directed primarily against the haptenic ligand (i.e., PA and HA) while in others IgE antibodies are directed against new antigenic determinants with no evidence of hapten specificity (87). Some TMA-exposed workers develop late respiratory and systemic symptoms that are associated with elevated serum-specific IgG antibodies to TMA–HSA (88). A few workers exposed to high concentrations of TMA fumes develop pulmonary hemorrhage and hemolytic anemia in association with high levels of IgG antibody (presumably Type 2-cytotoxicity–mediating antibody) to TMA–HSA (89–91). Specific IgE levels to TCPA–HSA antigens decline at a rate of half-life per year after cessation of exposure to this chemical, but cutaneous sensitivity persists for years (92). A systematic immunological investigation of acid anhydride chemicals demonstrated that ring structure, position of double bonds, and methyl group substitution may be critical determinants of IgE-mediated sensitization (93,94).

A special role for IgE-mediated immunopathogenesis has been demonstrated in workers exposed to chlorinated platinum salts. These workers exhibit positive prick tests to very dilute concentrations of these salts (95–98). Specific IgE tests also correlate with clinical respiratory symptoms (74). It has been shown that skin test–positive platinum workers have higher serum total IgE levels than skin test–negative platinum workers. Moreover, it was also observed that both high levels of IgE and cutaneous reactivity to platinum salt persisted four years after cessation of exposure (98).

Certain industrial agents may evoke antibody production, which may not correlate with clinical symptoms. Specific IgE antibodies against plicatic acid have been detected in both asthmatic and nonasthmatic workers exposed to red cedar. As the prevalence did not differ between the two groups, it was concluded that the presence of IgE may be a manifestation of work exposure, but its presence did not necessarily prove a cause–effect relationship with the subsequent development of OA (76). Similar results were observed in morphine production workers, many of who developed morphine-specific IgG antibodies, which did not correlate with symptomatic status (99). Thus, the latter reports, combined with the previous ones of the nonspecific nature of IgG antibodies in MDI workers, suggest that the presence of humoral antibodies, either IgE or IgG, may simply represent biologic markers of exposure.

From the previous discussion, it is apparent that the precise role of humoral antibodies in the pathogenesis of OA depends upon the intrinsic nature of the sensitizing agent or immunogen, the conditions of exposure, and the susceptibility of exposed workforce population. The presence of specific IgE antibodies may be highly diagnostic and prognostic in the case of HMW allergens and some LMW chemicals such as acid anhydrides and platinum salts. Under other circumstances, either specific IgE or IgG antibodies may be useful adjuncts in association with pulmonary function tests in following the evolutionary course of immunologically mediated asthma. Finally, when either specific IgE or IgG antibodies are present in both symptomatic and asymptomatic workers (i.e., MDI, plicatic acid, and morphine), their sole value may be as biologic markers of exposure.

IgE-Independent Cellular Immune Responses in OA

Evidence for the elicitation by respiratory chemical allergens of Th2-type selective response is derived from extensive studies in rodents (100–103), although there is reason to suppose that the same or similar responses may occur in humans also (104–106). The difficulty in translating these observations directly to humans is that there remains some uncertainty about a universal mandatory role for IgE antibody in the pathogenesis of occupational respiratory allergy to chemicals. Although confirmed chemical respiratory allergens can induce IgE antibody responses in exposed subjects, a number of investigations have found that a substantial proportion of symptomatic individuals lack demonstrable IgE antibody (85,107–109). IgE-dependent mechanisms may not explain all the manifestations of nonatopic (intrinsic) asthma or some forms of chemical-induced OA (e.g., toluene diisocyanate and western red cedar). Thus, Walker et al. (110) reported more pronounced activation of peripheral blood CD4+, CD8+, and memory T cells as well as high concentrations of IL-5, but not IL-4, in BAL fluid of intrinsic asthmatic patients. Concordant with these results were the findings of Del Prete et al. (111) and Maestrelli et al. (112) who observed that the majority of T cell clones derived from patients with TDI-induced asthma were CD8+ and capable of producing IL-5. These T lymphocytes may represent a CD3+/CD4-/CD8+ population expressing the γ/δ T-cell receptor (113,114). Interestingly, a small but significant proportion of T lymphocytes from peripheral blood of subjects with OA induced by red cedar produce IL-5 and IFNγ after stimulation with HSA–plicatic acid conjugate. This pattern of mixed Th1/Th2 cytokine productions is compatible with the nonatopic status and with the airway mucosa eosinophilia present in these subjects (115). In a recently developed model, female BALB/c mice were sensitized epicutaneously with HDI followed by intranasal challenge with HDI–mouse serum albumin (MSA) conjugate (116). Mice developed HDI-specific IgG antibodies as well as lymphocyte and eosinophil lung infiltrates. Inflammatory cells from the lung digest produced elevated levels of IL-5, IL-13, and IFNγ upon restimulation with HDI–MSA, indicating a mixed Th1/Th2 immune response as seen in humans (Fig. 3). Interestingly, the optimal sensitizing dose for antibody production was higher than that for airway inflammation and cytokine production. This finding is in concordance with that of Matheson et al. (117) suggesting that a different mechanism may dominate these outcomes. The role of CD4+ and CD8+ T lymphocytes was also investigated by Herrick et al. (118) showing that infiltration of eosinophils into the BAL fluid was markedly reduced in mice deficient in CD4+ T lymphocytes. This finding is consistent with the attenuated inflammatory response observed in IL-4 and -13 knockout mice (116). In contrast, mice deficient in CD8+ T lymphocytes showed a partial reduction in contact hypersensitivity, but no change in the presence of lung inflammatory cells. Together, these findings suggest a dominant role for CD4+ T lymphocytes and T_H2 immunity in HDI-induced lung inflammation. The strong influence of strain differences on the development of diisocyanate asthma in mice also shown by Herrick et al. (118) support the hypothesis of a genetic influence on the immune response to diisocyanate exposure and may help in explaining the discrepancies between animal and human studies. On repetitive antigenic stimulation in tissue culture of peripheral blood mononuclear cells from diisocyanate asthmatics, it was revealed that these cells synthesized TNFα, a non-IgE dependent proinflammatory cytokine, and the C-C chemokine, mononuclear chemoattractant protein-1 (MCP-1), but not IL-4 or -5 (119). Other examples of chemical-induced asthma associated with IgE-independent cellular immune responses have been observed (119–121). None of the above studies had addressed the possibility that local bronchial mucosal IgE-mediated processes could be involved in the absence of systemic IgE, as has been postulated to occur in nonoccupational intrinsic asthma (50). It is possible that the correlation between IgE antibody and occupational respiratory allergy is considerably closer than is sometimes assumed. This conclusion is based upon the fact that the circulating IgE antibodies may be missed for the following possible reasons: inappropriate analytical methods may have been used, analyses may have been conducted too long a period following last exposure, or levels of IgE antibody in target tissues may not be reflected by those in plasma. However, it must be acknowledged that, even if the association in humans between respiratory allergy to chemicals and IgE is somewhat stronger than has sometimes been reported, there may exist mechanisms of allergic sensitization that are independent of IgE antibody; this may be true especially of diisocyanates.

PATHOLOGIC FEATURES OF OA

There is overwhelming evidence, as demonstrated by sputum cytology, BAL, bronchial biopsies, surgical specimens, and postmortem lung tissue, that chronic inflammation is the hallmark of asthma and that variations of clinical activity of asthma are associated with the degree and type of airway inflammation (122–126). Similar findings occur in OA. Airway inflammation in all variants of asthma is thought to account for AHR and other sequelae, which result in airway limitation.

The pathology of one patient who died as a direct consequence of OA was remarkably similar to postmortem changes of non-OA. Thus, in one of these fatal cases associated with diisocyanate exposure, there was marked epithelial desquamation, an extensive layer of collagen beneath the true basement membrane, and massive infiltration of inflammatory cells, particularly eosinophils (127,128). In addition, the lungs showed edematous airways plugged by mucus, inflammatory cells, and exudate. However, this case presented during an extremely severe stage of the disease, and it is unclear to what extent these postmortem findings reflect the pathology of OA in living patients, especially those evaluated during periods of remission between asthma attacks.

Quantitative structural analysis of bronchial biopsies obtained from patients with OA induced by TDI showed an increased number of inflammatory cells as compared to biopsies of normal control subjects (Fig. 5) (129). It was also noted that eosinophils were increased in mucosal and submucosal layers while mast cells were increased only in the epithelium. Both cell types showed evidence of degranulation. In the immunochemistry survey of these specimens, both eosinophils and lymphocytes showed evidence of activation (105). Interestingly, the intercellular spaces between basal epithelial cells were increased. This morphologic finding is consistent with an abnormality of intercellular adhesion, which keeps basilar cells attached to each other and to columnar cells, thereby preventing epithelial desquamation, a characteristic feature of asthma (105,129,130). Glycoprotein adhesion molecules are also known to modulate the migration of inflammatory cells through endothelial intercellular spaces. Biopsy specimens also revealed that the thickness of the basement membrane was increased in the reticular layer (Fig. 5). This phenomenon has been demonstrated to be due to the deposition of interstitial cross-linked collagens (types I, III, and IV) produced by myofibroblasts and not deposition of collagen IV, which is one of the specific components of the "true" basement membrane (131–133). This observation has been made both in non-OA and OA (11,131–133).

Similar results have been obtained in bronchial biopsies from subjects sensitized to western red cedar (134). Somewhat different results have been obtained in biopsies from subjects who developed the reactive airways dysfunction syndrome after acute exposure to irritants: the airway epithelium is extensively damaged, the

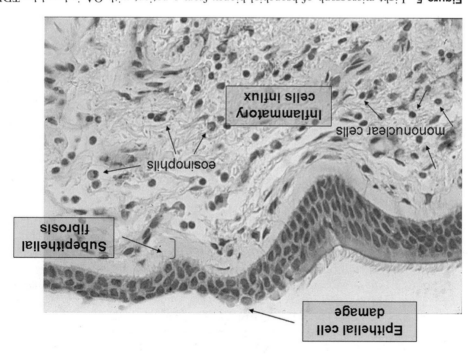

Figure 5 Light micrograph of bronchial biopsy from a patient with OA induced by TDI showing characteristic pathologic features. *Abbreviations:* OA, occupational asthma; TDI, toluene diisocyanate.

submucosa is infiltrated predominantly by mononuclear cells, and more importantly, the subepithelial fibrosis is more evident with a thickness of the reticular layer of the basement membrane that can reach 30 to 40 μm compared to 6 to 15 μm reported in isocyanate asthma and 3 to 8 μm in normal subjects (17,128,133,135).

Although cessation of exposure is not always associated with clinical improvement of OA, there may be improvement at the histopathologic level, as suggested by a decrease in the number of inflammatory cells in the airway mucosa, and by the reversal of the subepithelial fibrosis present at the time of diagnosis (16,17,133). Deposition of collagen beneath the bronchial epithelium has been described in young children with asthma, and even shortly after an allergen inhalation challenge, indicating that it may be an early change and not necessarily dependent on severe irreversible chronic asthma (136,137). This hypothesis is supported by the observation that subepithelial collagen thickening is reversible after cessation of exposure to occupational insults, and after treatment with inhaled steroids (16,17,138,139).

A correlation between indices of airway inflammation as assessed by inflammatory cell counts and/or activation status and severity of asthma has been reported (21). This concept has been recently challenged, taking into account the several studies showing either a weak or no correlation between airway inflammation and AHR (140). A weak but significant correlation between the thickness of the reticular layer of the basement membrane and the severity of asthma has been recently reported, suggesting a cardinal role of subepithelial fibrosis, one of the features of airway remodeling, as a contributor to progressive disease (141). These findings were similar to previous reports of cessation of workplace exposure in which reduction of subepithelial fibrosis and airway inflammation were associated with reduction of disease severity

(16,17). Interestingly, the decrease in thickness of the basement membrane reticular layer was also associated with a decrease in the number of fibroblasts in the submucosa. The relevance of airway inflammation in subjects with OA after cessation of exposure has been confirmed in a recent large follow-up study of 133 subjects with a prolonged mean period of follow-up of 8.7 years (18). The persistence of NSBH, found in 73% of subjects, was associated with more eosinophils and neutrophils in sputum.

The Phases of Airway Inflammation in Asthmatic Reactions

Early asthmatic reactions induced by allergens or occupational sensitizing agents are probably associated with smooth muscle contraction and/or edema induced by inflammatory mediators, but they are often not associated with an abundant inflammatory response; on the other hand, late asthmatic reactions induced by the same stimuli are associated with a prolific influx of inflammatory cells, which may release the inflammatory mediators responsible for the characteristic features of asthma (142,143). BAL samples obtained during various time intervals of late asthmatic reactions demonstrated a significant increase of neutrophils and/or eosinophils after exposure to TDI and plicatic acid, respectively (144,145). Histamine prostanoids, leukotrienes, and other inflammatory mediators have also been measured in BAL fluid during early asthmatic reactions induced by occupational and nonoccupational agents (141,142,146).

The source and nature of the chemotactic factors responsible for leukocyte infiltration in the airways are not known. However, metabolites of the lipoxygenase pathway of arachidonic acid have been identified in lavage supernatants obtained during asthma attacks induced by occupational agents (e.g., LTB4 after TDI challenge), which may be responsible for at least part of this chemotactic activity. BAL fluid obtained during asthmatic reactions induced by plicatic acid was found to contain clumps of ciliated epithelial cells, which were probably the result of epithelial desquamation (145). Because columnar epithelial cells adhere both to themselves and basal cells and/or basement membrane, epithelial cell desquamation and inflammatory cell infiltration imply changes in the adherence properties of the cells (147).

Histamine and leukotriene E4 (LTE4) are increased in bronchial lavage fluids sampled during early asthmatic reactions by plicatic acid (148). Urinary LTE4 is increased during early but not late asthmatic reactions induced by various occupational agents including diisocyanates in workers with OA (149). Taken together, these results suggest the importance of sulfidopeptide leukotrienes in asthmatic reactions (146,147) and the potential diagnostic utility of measuring urinary metabolites as an index of airway inflammation of asthma in general and OA in particular.

Cellular Components of Airway Inflammation

The chronic airway inflammation that characterizes asthma and its functional and clinical manifestations are most likely caused by complex interactions among inflammatory cells, structural cells, and nerves. The paracrine interaction between the various cells and nerves takes place through the synthesis and release of proinflammatory mediators and cytokines having different chemical structures. Among these cells T lymphocytes appear to orchestrate the inflammatory process (150). Eosinophils, mast cells, epithelial cells, and neutrophils appear to be the main effector cells that cause the characteristic manifestations of asthma through the release of their respective inflammatory mediators (i.e., smooth muscle contraction, mucus hypersecretion, plasma exudation with bronchial wall edema, and epithelial damage).

Noninvasive Assessment of Airway Inflammation

Analysis of induced sputum is a valid, reproducible method for studying airway inflammation instead of invasive diagnostic procedures, such as BAL and bronchial biopsies (151). In fact, in asthmatics, there is fairly good agreement between the eosinophil count in induced sputum and BAL and bronchial biopsy specimens (152). The test is relatively easy to perform. The patient inhales a hypertonic saline solution, which induces sputum production. Several studies have shown that sputum inflammatory indices such as eosinophils and eosinophil cationic protein are increased following exposure to common allergens and reduced on using corticosteroids (153–155). At 8 and 24 hours after inhalation challenge with diisocyanates, Maestrelli et al. (156) reported sputum eosinophilia in patients with early and late reactions (Fig. 6). Several subsequent studies confirmed the role of eosinophils in asthma induced by both HMW and LMW occupational agents (157–160). Interestingly, circadian variability in pulmonary function in asthma could be related to changes in airway eosinophil recruitment, as recently shown by sputum analysis (161). However, Obata et al. (159) and Lemiere et al. (160) confirmed the specificity of the changes in sputum eosinophils in OA by showing that exposure to occupational agents in asthmatics who were not sensitized to the agents, did not induce airway inflammation and did not change the sputum cell counts. Eosinophils are central inflammatory effector cells in OA. However, divergent results have also emerged. One study reports that the increase in sputum eosinophils was less in subjects with OA caused by LMW agents (162). The difference was not related to asthma severity. The authors speculated on the potential role of the degree of exposure (continuous exposure is prevalent in HMW OA, while intermittent exposure is more frequent in LMW OA). A different pathogenetic mechanism cannot, however, be ruled out. In another study, Lemiere et al. (163) found that the increase in the sputum eosinophil count was higher in subjects who had been exposed to LMW compounds than in subjects exposed to HMW compounds, at the same time after exposure.

In addition to methacholine responsiveness, changes in sputum eosinophil counts are satisfactory predictors of significant airway responsiveness to occupational agents

Sputum eosinophils

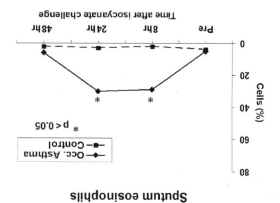

Figure 6 Time course of eosinophilic inflammation of the airways induced by exposure to isocyanates. Eosinophils were quantified in induced sputum before and 8, 24, and 48 hours after specific inhalation challenge in the laboratory in subjects with OA and in control subjects not exposed previously to isocyanates. *Abbreviation:* OA, occupational asthma. *Source:* Data from Ref. 156.

(164). Lemière et al. observed that eosinophils, eotaxin, and IL-5 were present in sputum on the day before an asthmatic reaction even though functional parameters (FEV_1 and PC_{20}) were unchanged (163). These findings were more pronounced after exposure to LMW agents than to HMW agents. The presence of sputum eosinophilia is useful not only in the clinical diagnosis of OA but also in disease monitoring. Chan-Yeung and coworkers showed that sputum eosinophils did not correlate with airway responsiveness but correlated inversely with FEV_1 (164). Analysis of induced sputum is helpful in the detection of occupational eosinophilic bronchitis which is characterized by cough on exposure to occupational agents, without any functional changes (165,166).

Exhaled nitric oxide (NO) levels are another tool in the investigation of OA and in the assessment of airway inflammation (167). Produced by various activated inflammatory cells, NO concentrations are elevated in the exhaled air from patients with asthma, and these high exhaled NO levels fall with corticosteroid therapy (168,169). A few occupational studies have investigated the role of exhaled NO in OA, but with inconsistent results (159,170,171). It has been suggested that measurement of exhaled NO can be used to indicate the development of airway inflammation accompanying late asthmatic reactions after specific inhalation challenges in patients with normal or slightly increased basal NO levels (172). The usefulness of exhaled NO in the investigation of OA is limited by factors affecting its determination, such as therapy with inhaled steroids and smoking. Thus, whereas the sensitivity of this measurement is high, its specificity is low.

Eosinophilic Bronchitis

Eosinophilic bronchitis has been described as a syndrome characterized by chronic cough and sputum eosinophilia, in the absence of demonstrable variable airflow limitation or nonspecific AHR (173). It has been suggested that eosinophilic bronchitis can be regarded as a variant syndrome of OA, when it develops as a consequence of work exposures (174,175). Eosinophilic bronchitis does not meet the current definition of OA, but it should be considered as an occupational respiratory disorder when work-related changes in sputum eosinophil counts are significant and reproducible (175). It is unknown whether eosinophilic bronchitis will progress to typical OA or if eosinophilic airway inflammation will persist when asthma symptoms and AHR have waned after cessation of exposure to the occupational allergen. Although it has been reported that patients with eosinophilic bronchitis may develop asthma or progressive chronic airflow limitation, the available data suggest that eosinophilic bronchitis is usually a benign and self-limiting disorder (176,177). Exposure to occupational agents such as natural rubber latex (NRL), mushroom spores, acrylates, and an epoxy resin has been reported to cause eosinophilic bronchitis (155,166,178,179). Drugs, e.g., bucillamine, may also induce eosinophilic bronchitis without concomitant alveolitis (180). Immunopathologic characterization was performed by studies in nonoccupational eosinophilic bronchitis. The immunohistochemical analysis of bronchial biopsy specimens from patients with asthma, patients with eosinophilic bronchitis, and normal control subjects revealed that both groups with disease had a similar degree of submucosal eosinophilia and thickening of the subepithelial collagen. However, the number of mast cells in the bundles of airway smooth muscle from subjects with asthma was significantly higher than that in subjects with eosinophilic bronchitis and in normal controls (181). In addition, the median concentration of exhaled nitric oxide was significantly higher in patients with eosinophilic bronchitis or asthma than in normal controls (182). Sputum eosinophil cationic protein and cysteinyl-leukotrienes concentrations were significantly higher in eosinophilic bronchitis and in asthma, compared with those in control subjects (183). However, in eosinophilic bronchitis, the mean concentrations of sputum histamine and sputum PGD_2 were significantly higher than in asthma. In addition, the concentration of tussive mediators were found to be elevated in induced sputum supernatants in patients with chronic cough caused by eosinophilic bronchitis (184). No substantial differences in the airway Th2 type cytokine expression was detected between patients with asthma and eosinophilic bronchitis (185,186).

Neutrophilic Inflammation in OA

Both human and animal studies suggest that long-term AHR which persists between asthmatic exacerbations is associated with mild airway inflammation, characterized by activation of T lymphocytes and increase in mast cells, eosinophils, and possibly macrophages, but not neutrophils. While several studies have shown a correlation between the number of eosinophils, mast cells, and/or epithelial cells in BAL and the severity of asthma (e.g., by symptom scores, airflow limitation, or AHR), only a few studies have reported a relationship between the severity of asthma and the number of neutrophils (187). Based on these observations, it would appear that neutrophils are not involved in the chronic airway inflammation associated with mild to moderate, stable asthma (188). By contrast, there is substantial evidence, particularly in humans, that neutrophils may be involved in exacerbations of asthma, particularly in the early stages of sudden and severe asthma exacerbations. The predominant involvement of neutrophils in some types of asthma exacerbations (i.e., induced by allergens, viral infections, or occupational sensitizers) suggests that different triggers of asthma may induce airway inflammation through different mechanisms (188).

OA exhibiting neutrophilic inflammation is less common, but has been described after exposure to LMW agents (189–192). Di Franco et al. (189) analyzed induced sputum cellularity in subjects with OA caused by either HMW or LMW compounds, who were still exposed to the offending agent. Compared with non-OA, the neutrophil percentage was significantly higher only in subjects with asthma due to LMW compound (189). In a study on subjects with OA for whom exposure had ceased, no differences in neutrophil counts were found in patients with OA that had been triggered by a range of agents (163). The discrepancies in the results of the different investigations were ascribed to the different techniques (BAL in this report versus induced sputum in others) or to exposure cessation. Anees et al. (190) identified an eosinophilic and a noneosinophilic variant of OA caused by LMW compounds. Eosinophilic inflammation was associated with more severe disease (lower $FEV_1\%$ predicted and greater methacholine reactivity) and greater bronchodilator reversibility, but did not correlate with the causative agent, duration of exposure, or magnitude of fall in PEF during work periods. Lack of bronchodilator reversibility in the latter suggests less bronchial smooth muscle involvement, which might occur if airway inflammation and remodeling are prevalent. This hypothesis is in line with the observation by Maghni et al. (18) in a long-term follow-up that a substantial proportion of inflammatory response in OA persistent after cessation of exposure appears to involve interleukin-8–mediated neutrophil influx or a mixed eosinophil–neutrophil response.

In the model of TDI-induced asthma, the role of neutrophils is unclear. Neutrophilia has been found in the BAL fluid of subjects with TDI-induced asthma, especially in those exhibiting a late asthmatic response after specific inhalation challenge. However, the concentrations of TDI used in the challenge were higher than those used in the studies that followed (144). In non-OA, the presence of neutrophils is considered a marker of the severity of the disease (193). What is unclear in OA is whether neutrophilia can also be considered a marker of severe disease due, perhaps, to higher levels of exposure, or whether, for unknown reasons, the same level of exposure may produce an inflammatory airway infiltrate in which eosinophils or neutrophils are the predominant cells (158,190). Lemière et al. (160) demonstrated that the increase in sputum neutrophil count after a positive specific inhalation challenge varied with the molecular weight of the compound. For example, sputum neutrophil counts were increased after exposure to isocyanates. Park et al. (191,194), by examining bronchial biopsies, serum, and induced sputum in TDI-induced asthma, found neutrophils to play a role. They proposed a role for IL-8 released after exposure to TDI, and they speculated that mast cells could be the origin of the neutrophil chemotactic activity found after TDI challenge (195). Similarly, in grain dust–induced asthma-like disorders, the number of neutrophils in the bronchial mucosa is higher than that in allergic asthma, and the levels of IL-8 in induced sputum increase significantly after inhalation challenge compared with baseline values (196). The actual cause for this entity is currently unknown. Endotoxin inhalation may reproduce some of the clinical, functional, and pathologic features of grain dust asthma-like disorder.

Reflex Mechanisms and Neurogenic Inflammation

The system of innervation of the airways is much more complex than was previously believed. In addition to the classic cholinergic and adrenergic mechanisms, nonadrenergic and noncholinergic (NANC) neural pathways have been described in human airways (197). The demonstration that an extensive network of nerve fibers contains potent peptides, in addition to classic neurotransmitters, has revived interest concerning the possible involvement of neurogenic inflammatory mechanisms in the pathogenesis of asthma (126).

Substance P (SP), neurokinin A (NKA), neurokinin B (NKB), calcitonin gene–related peptide (CGRP), and vasoactive intestinal peptide (VIP) are the chief neuropeptides that could be involved in the pathophysiology of asthma. Vasointestinal peptide has been localized in cholinergic nerves of the airways where it may act as a cotransmitter with acetycholine. It may therefore function as a counterbalancing bronchodilator to cholinergic bronchoconstriction. In addition to causing vagally mediated reflex bronchoconstriction, several irritants may stimulate sensory nerves (i.e., the nonmyelinated sensory C-fiber endings) to release SP and other related tachykinins, which have the remarkable ability to affect multiple cells in the airways, thereby provoking responses referred to as neurogenic inflammation (126,198).

Neurogenic inflammation and release of neuropeptides are well-established amplifying mechanisms in rodent models of airway inflammation and asthma. However, evidence that the same mechanisms are operative in human asthma, is much less convincing. Many neuropeptides, particularly NKA (199), SP, and CGRP, are localized in airway nerves and may participate in airway inflammation by causing or amplifying plasma exudation, mucus secretion, and recruitment and activation of inflammatory cells. Other neuropeptides (e.g., VIP) may exert the opposite effect and modulate asthmatic inflammation (126).

Neuropeptides elicit most of the characteristic features of asthma (i.e., cough, mucus secretion, smooth muscle contraction, plasma extravasation, and neutrophil adhesion). Neutral endopeptidase (NEP), an enzyme present on the surface of the cells containing receptors for neuropeptides, limits the concentration of neuropeptides that reach the receptors of the cell's surface by cleaving and inactivating them. This interaction modulates and inhibits neurogenic inflammation (126,198).

The neuropeptide found in highest concentration is VIP. It is found in efferent nerves of human lung and functions as a neurotransmitter of NANC inhibitory nerves. Although a primary defect of NANC innervation seems unlikely, airway inflammation may trigger a functional defect in this system. In asthmatic airways, inflammatory cells such as eosinophils, neutrophils, and mast cells may release a variety of peptidases (e.g., tryptase), which could inactivate VIP. The consequent, unchecked reflex cholinergic bronchoconstriction could contribute to the development of AHR associated with airway inflammation (110,199). However, local production of nitric oxide appears to be the main inhibitory mechanism of neurally mediated bronchoconstriction (200).

A striking increase of SP-like immunoreactive nerves and a decrease of VIP+ nerves has been reported in the airways of asthmatics in some studies, but not confirmed in others (201–204). The effects of tachykinins and tachykinin antagonists in man have not yet convincingly shown that neurogenic inflammation plays a significant role in airway inflammation in asthma (126).

Several nonspecific workplace stimuli (i.e., sulfur dioxide, dust, and cold air) may trigger reflex bronchoconstriction by stimulating the sensory receptors in the airways. This physiologic defense mechanism may trigger bronchoconstriction both in normal and asthmatic subjects. TDI has been shown to stimulate the release of both SP and CGRP; it also inhibits neutral endopeptidase in experimental animals and in vitro preparations (205,206). Thus, occupational stimuli that activate the "efferent" function of capsaicin-sensitive nerves and/or inhibit neutral endopeptidases could trigger neurogenic inflammation and precipitate asthma. Although this mechanism of action of isocyanates has been demonstrated in rats and guinea pigs, it has not been possible to prove its role in humans, and particularly in subjects with OA induced by isocyanates, in part due to the lack of specific antagonists (205).

Epithelial Disruption

Destruction or denudation of airway epithelium has important intermediate consequences in the pathophysiology of asthma. Damaged epithelium may generate arachidonic acid metabolic products such as 8,15-HETE neutrophil chemotactic factor (207). It has also been shown that epithelial-derived relaxant factors may modulate the bronchoconstricting effects of many exogenous and endogenous bronchoconstrictor substances (207). Widespread epithelial damage would result in deprivation of this regulating mechanism. Desquamation of the airway epithelium exposes afferent nerve endings, which are more readily stimulated to release SP and other neurotachykinins, the results of which have been discussed. If epithelial repair processes are delayed by excessive exposure to an environmental irritant or allergen, altered epithelial function could persist even after cessation of exposure.

Airway Microvascular Leakage

There is an increased concentration of albumin in the supernatant of BAL fluid obtained during late asthmatic reactions induced by occupational agents (e.g., isocyanates and plicatic acid) compared to the concentration of albumin present in atopic asthmatic patients after early asthmatic reactions or in normal subjects

(21,144). It has been suggested that the increased concentration of albumin in lavage supernatants reflects microvascular leakage and mucosal edema (2). Macromolecules of albumin leak through gaps between endothelial cells in postcapillary venules. They cross both endothelial and epithelial basement membranes and then accumulate in airway lumina. This process of plasma exudation is associated with significant movement of water, which causes mucosal edema and accumulation of exudate in the airway lumen (2). Airway edema and exudate in airway lumina have been observed in a subject with OA who died after exposure to the sensitizing agent at work (127). It is therefore apparent that the increased concentration of albumin and the cellular exudation occurring during asthmatic reactions induced by occupational agents, provide further compelling evidence that an acute inflammatory reaction of the airways is a sine qua non of active asthmatic reactions.

CONCLUSIONS

OA induced by HMW compounds and by some LMW occupational sensitizers (e.g., acid anhydrides and platinum halide salts) shares many characteristics with IgE-mediated asthma. In both, the responsible agent is known, and the predisposition of atopic subjects, the clinical presentation, the response to inhalation challenge in the laboratory and the response to antiasthma drugs, are remarkably similar. By contrast, many workers with OA induced by some LMW occupational agents, particularly TDI and plicatic acid, show no evidence of an IgE-mediated mechanism, and atopy is not a risk factor. The pathology of the airway mucosa in atopic, nonatopic, and other variants of OA is remarkably similar, suggesting similar terminal pathogenetic events for asthma independent of its causal agent. However, immunologic mechanisms of OA may have distinctive pathways, with IgE-mediated mechanisms more likely to be relevant for asthma induced by HMW and some LMW (e.g., acid anhydrides and platinum halide salts) agents, and cellular immune-mediated mechanisms for OA induced by other LMW occupational sensitizers (e.g., TDI and western red cedar).

Because most of the inducing occupational agents can be identified as immunogens, allergens, or irritants, OA is an ideal model for non-OA. The occupational venue enables long-term studies of the consequences of airway obstruction and bronchial hyperresponsiveness. Owing to the fact that diagnostic bronchial challenge is required more often in OA, there are increased opportunities for investigation of local, humoral, and cellular immune responses, airways microvascular leakage, irritant effects, and neurogenic inflammation.

DIRECTIONS FOR FUTURE RESEARCH

- Structure–function relationship to identify causal agents of OA
- Dose–response relationship between exposure to occupational agent and sensitization, and interaction with other factors such as smoking, viral infection, endotoxin, and other pollutants
- Role of airway inflammation and remodeling in the persistence of OA
- Mechanism of irritant-induced asthma using animal models or prospective studies of individuals at risk of exposure to irritants

ACKNOWLEDGMENTS

This work was supported by MIUR (PRIN 2003 and 2004), ARCA, Padova, Consorzio Ferrara Ricerche, Ferrara, and individual Grants MIUR ex-60% from Universities of Ferrara, Padova and Modena.

REFERENCES

1. Wiggs B, Moreno R, James A, Hogg J, Pare PD. A model of the mechanics of airway narrowing in asthma. In: Kaliner MA, Barnes PJ, Persson CGA, eds. Asthma: Its Pathology and Treatment. New York: Marcel Dekker, 1991:73–101.

2. Persson CGA. Microvascular–epithelial exudation of bulk plasma in airway defense, disease, and repair. In: Holgate ST, Busse WW, eds. Inflammatory Mechanisms in Asthma. New York, Basel, Hong Kong: Marcel Dekker, 1998 (Chapter 26).

3. Vandenplas O, Malo JL. Inhalation challenges with agents causing occupational asthma. Eur Respir J 1997; 10(11):2612–2629.

4. Stenton SC. Determinants of whether occupational agents cause early, late, or dual asthmatic responses. Occup Med 2000; 15:431–444.

5. Chan-Yeung M, Grzybowski S. Prognosis in occupational asthma (editorial). Thorax 1985; 40(4):241–243.

6. Allard C, Cartier A, Ghezzo H, Malo JL. Occupational asthma due to various agents. Absence of clinical and functional improvement at an interval of four or more years after cessation of exposure. Chest 1989; 96(5):1046–1049.

7. Cote J, Kennedy S, Chan-Yeung M. Outcome of patients with cedar asthma with continuous exposure. Am Rev Respir Dis 1990; 141(2):373–376.

8. Mapp CE, Corona PC, De Marzo N, Fabbri L. Persistent asthma due to isocyanates. A follow-up study of subjects with occupational asthma due to toluene diisocyanate (TDI). Am Rev Respir Dis 1988; 137(6):1326–1329.

9. Vedal S, Enarson DA, Chan H, Ochnio J, Tse KS, Chan-Yeung M. A longitudinal study of the occurrence of bronchial hyperresponsiveness in western red cedar workers. Am Rev Respir Dis 1988; 137(3):651–655.

10. Panhuysen CI, Vonk JM, Koeter GH, Schouten JP, van Altena R, Bleecker ER, Postma DS. Adult patients may outgrow their asthma: a 25-year follow-up study [published erratum appears in Am J Respir Crit Care Med 1997; 156(2 Pt 1):674]. Am J Respir Crit Care Med 1997; 155(4):1267–1272.

11. Redington AE, Howarth PH. Airway wall remodelling in asthma [editorial, see comments]. Thorax 1997; 52(4):310–312.

12. Redington AE, Sime PJ, Howarth PH, Holgate ST. Fibroblast and the extracellular matrix in asthma. In: Holgate ST, Busse WW, eds. Inflammatory Mechanisms in Asthma. New York, Basel, Hong Kong: Marcel Dekker, 1998:chapter 21.

13. Macklem PT. Mechanical factors determining maximum bronchoconstriction. Eur Respir J Suppl 1989; 6:516S–519S.

14. Ebina M, Yaegashi H, Chiba R, Takahashi T, Motomiya M, Tanemura M. Hyperreactive site in the airway tree of asthmatic patients revealed by thickening of bronchial muscles. A morphometric study. Am Rev Respir Dis 1990; 141(5 Pt 1):1327–1332.

15. Paggiaro PL, Paoletti P, Bacci E. Eosinophils in bronchoalveolar lavage (BAL) of patients with toluene diisocyanate (TDI) asthma after cessation of work. Chest 1990(98):536–542.

16. Saetta M, Maestrelli P, DiStefano A, et al. Effect of cessation of exposure to toluene diisocyanate (TDI) on bronchial mucosa of subjects with TDI-induced asthma. Am Rev Respir Dis 1992; 145(1):169–174.

17. Saetta M, Maestrelli P, Turato G, et al. Airway wall remodeling after cessation of exposure to isocyanates in sensitized asthmatic subjects. Am J Respir Crit Care Med 1995; 151(2 Pt 1):489–494.

18. Maghni K, Lemière C, Ghezzo H, Yuquan W, Malo J-L. Airway inflammation after cessation of exposure to agents causing occupational asthma. Am J Respir Crit Care Med 2003; 169:367–372.

19. Chan-Yeung M. Occupational asthma. Environ Health Perspect 1995; 6:249–252.

20. Venables KM, Chan-Yeung M. Occupational asthma. Lancet 1997; 349(9063):1465–1469.

21. O'Byrne PM. Mechanisms of airway hyperresponsiveness. In: Holgate ST, Busse WW, eds. Inflammatory Mechanisms in Asthma. New York, Basel, Hong Kong: Marcel Dekker, 1998 (chapter 34).

22. Hargreave FE, Ramsdale EH, Pugsley SO. Occupational asthma without bronchial hyperresponsiveness. Am Rev Respir Dis 1984; 130(3):513–515.

23. Mapp CE, Dal Vecchio L, Boschetto P, De Marzo N, Fabbri LM. Toluene diisocyanate-induced asthma without airway hyperresponsiveness. Eur J Respir Dis 1986; 68(2):89–95.

24. Mapp CE, Di Giacomo GR, Omini C, Broseghini C, Fabbri LM. Late, but not early, asthmatic reactions induced by toluene-diisocyanate are associated with increased airway responsiveness to methacholine. Eur J Respir Dis 1986; 69(4):276–284.

25. Cartier A, L'Archeveque J, Malo JL. Exposure to a sensitizing occupational agent can cause a long-lasting increase in bronchial responsiveness to histamine in the absence of significant changes in airway caliber. J Allergy Clin Immunol 1986; 78(6):1185–1189.

26. Thorpe JE, Steinberg D, Bernstein IL, Murlas CG. Bronchial reactivity increases soon after the immediate response in dual-responding asthmatic subjects. Chest 1987; 91(1):21–25.

27. Steinberg DR, Bernstein DI, Bernstein IL, Murlas CG. Prednisone pretreatment leads to histaminic airway hyporeactivity soon after resolution of the immediate allergic response. Chest 1989; 95(2):314–319.

28. Durham SR, Graneek BJ, Hawkins R, Newman-Taylor AJ. The temporal relationship between increases in airway responsiveness to histamine and late asthmatic responses induced by occupational agents. J Allergy Clin Immunol 1987; 79(2):398–406.

29. Josephs LK, Gregg I, Mullee MA, Holgate ST. Nonspecific bronchial reactivity and its relationship to the clinical expression of asthma. A longitudinal study. Am Rev Respir Dis 1989; 140(2):350–357.

30. Postma DS, Kerstjens HA. Characteristics of airway hyperresponsiveness in asthma and chronic obstructive pulmonary disease. Am J Respir Crit Care Med 1998; 158(5 Pt 3):S187–S192.

31. Banks DE, Rando RJ, Barkman HW Jr. Persistence of toluene diisocyanate-induced asthma despite negligible workplace exposures. Chest 1990; 97(1):121–125.

32. Padoan M, Pozzato V, Simoni M, et al. Long-term follow-up of toluene diisocyanate-induced asthma. Eur Respir J 2003; 21:637–640.

33. Maestrelli P, DeMarzo N, Saetta M, Boscaro M, Fabbri LM, Mapp CE. Effects of inhaled beclomethasone on airway responsiveness in occupational asthma. Am Rev Respir Dis 1993; 148:407–412.

34. Malo JL, Cartier A, Cote J, et al. Influence of inhaled steroids on recovery from occuptional asthma after cessation of exposure: an 18 month double-blind cross over study. Am Rev Respir Dis 1996; 153:953–960.

35. Lam S, LeRiche J, Phillips D, Chan-Yeung M. Cellular and protein changes in bronchial lavage fluid after late asthmatic reaction in patients with red cedar asthma. J Allergy Clin Immunol 1987; 80(1):44–50.

36. Chan-Yeung M, Leriche J, Maclean L, Lam S. Comparison of cellular and protein changes in bronchial lavage fluid of symptomatic and asymptomatic patients with red cedar asthma on follow-up examination. Clin Allergy 1988; 18(4):359–365.

37. De Meer G, Heederik D, Postma DS. Bronchial responsiveness to adenosine 5'-monophosphate and methacholine differ in their relationship with airway allergy and baseline FEV1. Am J Respir Crit Care Med 2002; 165:317–318.

38. De Meer G, Heederik D, Postma DS. Bronchial responsiveness to adenosine 5'-monophosphate and methacholine as predictors for nasal symptoms due to newly introduced allergens. A follow-up study among laboratory animal workers and bakery apprentices. Clin Exp Allergy 2003; 33:789–794.

39. Malo JL. Irritant-induced asthma and reactive airways dysfunction syndrome. Can Respir J 1998; 5:66–67.

40. Tarlo SM. Workplace irritant exposures: do they produce true occupational asthma? Ann Allergy Asthma Immunol 2003; 90(5 S2):19–23.

41. Gautrin D, Boulet LP, Boutet M, et al. Is reactive airways dysfunction syndrome a variant of occupational asthma? J Allergy Clin Immunol 1994; 93:12–22.

42. Lemiere C, Malo JL, Boutet M. Reactive airways dysfunction syndrome due to chlorine: sequential bronchial biopsies and functional assessment. Eur Respir J 1997; 10:241–244.

43. Matzinger P. The danger model: a renewed sense of self. Science 2002; 296:301–305.

44. Humbert M, Durham SR, Ying S, et al. IL-4 and IL-5 mRNA and protein in bronchial biopsies from patients with atopic and nonatopic asthma: evidence against "intrinsic" asthma being a distinct immunopathologic entity. Am J Respir Crit Care Med 1996; 154(5):1497–1504.

45. Humbert M, Ying S, Corrigan C, et al. Bronchial mucosal expression of the genes encoding chemokines RANTES and MCP-3 in symptomatic atopic and nonatopic asthmatics: relationship to the eosinophil-active cytokines interleukin (IL)-5, granulocyte macrophage-colony-stimulating factor, and IL-3. Am J Respir Cell Mol Biol 1997; 16(1):1–8.

46. Ying S, Humbert M, Barkans J, et al. Expression of IL-4 and IL-5 mRNA and protein product by CD4+ and CD8+ T cells, eosinophils, and mast cells in bronchial biopsies obtained from atopic and nonatopic (intrinsic) asthmatics. J Immunol 1997; 158(7):3539–3544.

47. Humbert M, Durham SR, Kimmitt P, et al. Elevated expression of messenger ribonucleic acid encoding IL-13 in the bronchial mucosa of atopic and nonatopic subjects with asthma. J Allergy Clin Immunol 1997; 99(5):657–665.

48. Humbert M, Corrigan CJ, Kimmitt P, Till SJ, Kay AB, Durham SR. Relationship between IL-4 and IL-5 mRNA expression and disease severity in atopic asthma. Am J Respir Crit Care Med 1997; 156(3 Pt 1):704–708.

49. Bentley AM, Menz G, Storz C, et al. Identification of T lymphocytes, macrophages, and activated eosinophils in the bronchial mucosa in intrinsic asthma. Relationship to symptoms and bronchial responsiveness. Am Rev Respir Dis 1992; 146(2):500–506.

50. Humbert M, Grant JA, Taborda-Barata L, et al. High-affinity IgE receptor (FcepsilonRI)-bearing cells in bronchial biopsies from atopic and nonatopic asthma. Am J Respir Crit Care Med 1996; 153(6 Pt 1):1931–1937.

51. Kotsimbos AT, Humbert M, Minshall E, et al. Upregulation of alpha GM-CSF-receptor in nonatopic asthma but not in atopic asthma. J Allergy Clin Immunol 1997; 99(5):666–672.

52. Halapi E, Hakonarson H. Recent development in genomic and proteomic research for asthma. Curr Opin Pulm Med 2004; 10:22–30.

53. Bel EH. Clinical phenotypes of asthma. Curr Opin Pulm Med 2004; 10:44–50.

54. Mapp CE, Beghe B, Balboni A, et al. Association between HLA genes and susceptibility to toluene diisocyanate induced asthma. Clin Exp Allergy 2000; 5:651–656.

55. Jones MG, Nielsen J, Welch J, et al. Association of HLA-DQ5 and HLA-DR1 with sensitisation to organic acid anhydrides. Clin Exp Allergy 2004; 34:812–816.

56. Jeal H, Draper A, Jones M, et al. HLA associations with occupational sensitisation to rat lipocalin allergens: a model for other animal allergies? J Allergy Clin Immunol 2003; 111:795–799.

57. Arnaiz NO, Kaufman JD, Daroowalla FM, Quigley S, Farin F, Checkoway H. Genetic factors in aluminium smelter workers. Arch Environ Health 2003; 58:197–200.

58. Beghe B, Padoan M, Moss CT, et al. Lack of association of HLA class I genes and TNF alpha-308 polymorphism in toluene diisocyanate-induced asthma. Allergy 2004; 59:61–64.

59. Piirila P, Wikman H, Luukkonen R, et al. Glutathione S-transferase genotypes in allergic responses to diisocyanate exposure. Pharmacogenetics 2001; 11:437–441.

60. Mapp CE, Fryer AA, De Marzo N, et al. Glutathione S-transferase GSTP1 is a susceptibility gene for occupational asthma induced by isocyanates. J Allergy Clin Immunol 2002; 109:867–872.

61. Fryer AA, Bianco A, Hepple M, Jones PW, Strange RC, Spiteri MA. Polymorphism at the glutathione S-transferase GSTP1 locus. A new marker for bronchial hyperresponsiveness and asthma. Am J Respir Crit Care Med 2000; 161:1437–1442.

62. Aynacioglu AS, Nacak M, Filiz A, Ekinci E. Roots Protective role of glutathione S-transferase P1 (GSTP1) Val105Val genotype in patients with bronchial asthma. Br J Clin Pharmacol 2004; 57:213–217.

63. Romieu I, Sienra-Monge JJ, Ramirez-Aguilar M, et al. Genetic polymorphism of GSTM1 and antioxidant supplementation influence lung function in relation to ozone exposure in asthmatic children in Mexico City. Thorax 2004; 59:8–10.

64. Gilliland FD, Li YF, Saxon A, Diaz-Sanchez D. Effect of glutathione-S-transferase M1 and P1 genotypes on xenobiotic enhancement of allergic responses: randomised, placebo-controlled crossover study. Lancet 2004; 363:119–125.

65. Wikman H, Piirila P, Rosenberg C, et al. N-acetyltransferase genotypes as modifiers of diisocyanate exposure-associated asthma risk. Pharmacogenetics 2002; 12:227–233.

66. Barnes KC, Marsh DG. The genetics and complexity of allergy and asthma. Immunol Today 1998; 19(7):325–332.

67. Young RP, Barker RD, Pile KD, Cookson OCM, Newman-Taylor AJ. The association of HLA-DR3 with specific IgE to inhaled acid anhydrides. Am J Respir Crit Care Med 1995; 151(1):219–221.

68. Newman Taylor AJ, Cullinan P, Lympany PA, Harris JM, Dowdeswell RJ, du Bois RM. Interaction of HLA phenotype and exposure intensity in sensitization to complex platinum salts. Am J Respir Crit Care Med 1999; 160(2):435–438.

69. Maestrelli P, Di Stefano A, Occari P, et al. Cytokines in the airway mucosa of subjects with asthma induced by toluene diisocyanate. Am J Respir Crit Care Med 1995; 151(3 Pt 1): 607–612.

70. Durham SR. Mechanisms of mucosal inflammation in the nose and lungs. Clin Exp Allergy 1998; 2:11–16.

71. Costa JJ, Galli SJ, Church MK. Mast cell cytokines in allergic inflammation. In: Holgate ST, Busse WW, eds. Inflammatory Mechanisms in Asthma. New York, Base, Hong Kong: Marcel Dekker, 1998:chapter 6.

72. Novey HS, Bernstein IL, Mihalas LS, Terr AI, Yunginger JW. Guidelines for the clinical evaluation of occupational asthma due to high molecular weight (HMW) allergens. Report of the Subcommittee on the Clinical Evaluation of Occupational Asthma due to HMW Allergens. J Allergy Clin Immunol 1989; 84(5 Pt 2):829–833.

73. Maccia CA, Bernstein IL, Emmett EA, Brooks SM. In vitro demonstration of specific IgE in phthalic anhydride hypersensitivity. Am Rev Respir Dis 1976; 113(5):701–704.

74. Biagini RE, Bernstein IL, Gallagher JS, Moorman WJ, Brooks S, Gann PH. The diversity of reaginic immune responses to platinum and palladium metallic salts. J Allergy Clin Immunol 1985; 76(6):794–802.

75. Cartier A, Grammer L, Malo JL, et al. Specific serum antibodies against isocyanates: association with occupational asthma. J Allergy Clin Immunol 1989; 84(4 Pt 1):507–514.

76. Tse KS, Chan H, Chan-Yeung M. Specific IgE antibodies in workers with occupational asthma due to western red cedar. Clin Allergy 1982; 12(3):249–258.

77. Cartier A, Malo JL, Forest F, et al. Occupational asthma in snow crab-processing workers. J Allergy Clin Immunol 1984; 74(3 Pt 1):261–269.

78. Mitchell CA, Gandevia B. Respiratory symptoms and skin reactivity in workers exposed to proteolytic enzymes in the detergent industry. Am Rev Respir Dis 1971; 104(1):1–12.

79. Karr RM. Bronchoprovocation studies in coffee worker's asthma. J Allergy Clin Immunol 1979; 64(6 pt 2):650–654.

80. Davison AG, Britton MG, Forrester JA, Davies RJ, Hughes DT. Asthma in merchant seamen and laboratory workers caused by allergy to castor beans: analysis of allergens. Clin Allergy 1983; 13(6):553–561.

81. Merget R, Stollfuss J, Wiewrodt R, et al. Diagnostic tests in enzyme allergy. J Allergy Clin Immunol 1993; 92(2):264–277.

82. Bernstein DI, Smith AB, Moller DR, et al. Clinical and immunologic studies among egg-processing workers with occupational asthma. J Allergy Clin Immunol 1987; 80(6): 791–797.

83. Tiikkainen U, Klockars M. Clinical significance of IgG subclass antibodies to wheat flour antigens in bakers. Allergy 1990; 45(7):497–504.

84. Popp W, Zwick H, Rauscher H. Short-term sensitizing antibodies in bakers' asthma. Int Arch Allergy Appl Immunol 1988; 86(2):215–219.

85. Tee RD, Cullinan P, Welch J, Burge PS, Newman-Taylor AJ. Specific IgE to isocyanates: a useful diagnostic role in occupational asthma. J Allergy Clin Immunol 1998; 101(5):709–715.

86. Nielsen J, Welinder H, Skerfving S. Allergic airway disease caused by methyl tetrahydrophthalic anhydride in epoxy resin. Scand J Work Environ Health 1989; 15(2): 154–155.

87. Bernstein DI, Gallagher JS, D'Souza L, Bernstein IL. Heterogeneity of specific-IgE responses in workers sensitized to acid anhydride compounds. J Allergy Clin Immunol 1984; 74(6):794–801.

88. Zeiss CR, Wolkonsky P, Pruzansky JJ, Patterson R. Clinical and immunologic evaluation of trimellitic anhydride workers in multiple industrial settings. J Allergy Clin Immunol 1982; 70(1):15–18.

89. Ahmad D, Morgan WK, Patterson R, Williams T, Zeiss CR. Pulmonary haemorrhage and haemolytic anaemia due to trimellitic anhydride. Lancet 1979; 2(8138):328–330.

90. Patterson R, Addington W, Banner AS, et al. Antihapten antibodies in workers exposed to trimellitic anhydride fumes: a potential immunopathogenetic mechanism for the trimellitic anhydride pulmonary disease—anemia syndrome. Am Rev Respir Dis 1979; 120(6):1259–1267.

91. Turner ES, Pruzansky JJ, Patterson R, Zeiss CR, Roberts M. Detection of antibodies in human serum using trimellityl-erythrocytes: direct and indirect haemagglutination and haemolysis. Clin Exp Immunol 1980; 39(2):470–476.

92. Venables KM, Topping MD, Nunn AJ, Howe W, Newman Taylor AJ. Immunologic and functional consequences of chemical (tetrachlorophthalic anhydride)-induced asthma after four years of avoidance of exposure. J Allergy Clin Immunol 1987; 80(2): 212–218.

93. Zhang XD, Lotvall J, Skerfving S, Welinder H. Antibody specificity to the chemical structures of organic acid anhydrides studied by in-vitro and in-vivo methods. Toxicology 1997; 118(2–3):223–232.

94. Zhang XD, Welinder H, Jonsson BA, Skerfving S. Antibody responses of rats after immunization with organic acid anhydrides as a model of predictive testing. Scand J Work Environ Health 1998; 24:220–227.

95. Cleare MJ, Hughes EG, Jacoby B, Pepys J. Immediate (type I) allergic responses to platinum compounds. Clin Allergy 1976; 6(2):183–195.

96. Venables KM, Dally MB, Nunn AJ, et al. Smoking and occupational allergy in workers in a platinum refinery. BMJ 1989; 299(6705):939–942.

97. Pepys J, Parish WE, Cromwell O, Hughes EG. Passive transfer in man and the monkey of Type I allergy due to heat labile and heat stable antibody to complex salts of platinum. Clin Allergy 1979; 9(2):99–108.

98. Baker DB, Gann PH, Brooks SM, Gallagher J, Bernstein IL. Cross-sectional study of platinum salts sensitization among precious metals refinery workers. Am J Ind Med 1990; 18(6):653–664.

99. Biagini RE, Klincewicz SL, Henningsen GM, et al. Antibodies to morphine in workers exposed to opiates at a narcotics manufacturing facility and evidence for similar antibodies in heroin abusers. Life Sci 1990; 47(10):897–908.

100. Ban M, Hettich D. Relationship between IgE positive cell numbers and serum total IgE levels in mice treated with trimellitic anhydride and dinitrochlorobenzene. Toxicol Lett 2001; 118:129–137.

101. Farraj AK, Harkema JR, Kaminski NE. Allergic rhinitis induced by intranasal sensitization and challenge with trimellitic anhydride but not with dinitrochlorobenzene or oxazolone in A/J mice. Toxicol Sci 2004; 79:315–325.

102. Dearman RJ, Warbrick EV, Skinner R, Kimber I. Cytokine fingerprinting of chemical allergens: species comparisons and statistical analyses. Food Chem Toxicol 2002; 40:1881–1892.

103. Hayashi M, Higashi K, Kato H, Kaneko H. Assessment of preferential Th1 or Th2 induction by low-molecular-weight compounds using a reverse transcription-polymerase chain reaction method: comparison of two mouse strains, C57BL/6 and BALB/c. Toxicol Appl Pharmacol 2001; 177:38–45.

104. Herrick CA, Das J, Xu L, Wisnewski AV, Redlich CA, Bottomly K. Differential roles for CD4 and CD8 T cells after diisocyanate sensitization: genetic control of TH2-induced lung inflammation. J Allergy Clin Immunol 2003; 111:1087–1094.

105. Bentley AM, Maestrelli P, Saetta M, et al. Activated T-lymphocytes and eosinophils in the bronchial mucosa in isocyanate-induced asthma. J Allergy Clin Immunol 1992; 89:821–829.

106. Maestrelli P, Occari P, Turato G, et al. Expression of interleukin (IL)-4 and IL-5 proteins in asthma induced by toluene diisocyanate (TDI). Clin Exp Allergy 1997; 27: 1292–1298.

107. Grammer L, Shaughnessy M, Kenamore B. Utility of antibody in identifying individuals who have or will develop anhydride-induced respiratory disease. Chest 1998; 114:1199–1202.

108. Vandenplas O, Malo JL, Saetta M, Mapp CE, Fabbri LM. Occupational asthma and extrinsic alveolitis due to isocyanates: current status and perspectives. Br J Ind Med 1993; 50:213–228.

109. Tarlo SM. Diisocyanate sensitization and antibody production. J Allergy Clin Immunol 1999; 103:739–741.

110. Walker C, Bode E, Boer L, Hansel TT, Blaser K, Virchow JC Jr. Allergic and nonallergic asthmatics have distinct patterns of T-cell activation and cytokine production in peripheral blood and bronchoalveolar lavage. Am Rev Respir Dis 1992; 146(1):109–115.

111. Del Prete GF, De Carli M, D'Elios MM, Maestrelli P, Ricci M, Fabbri L, Romagnani S. Allergen exposure induces the activation of allergen-specific Th2 cells in the airway mucosa of patients with allergic respiratory disorders. Eur J Immunol 1993; 23(7): 1445–1449.

112. Maestrelli P, Del Prete GF, De Carli M, et al. CD8 T-cell clones producing interleukin-5 and interferon-gamma in bronchial mucosa of patients with asthma induced by toluene diisocyanate. Scand J Work Environ Health 1994; 20(5):376–381.

113. Wisnewski AV, Cain H, Magoski N, Wang H, Holm CT, Redlich CA. Human gamma/delta T-cell lines derived from airway biopsies. Am J Respir Cell Mol Biol 2001; 24: 332–338.

114. Wisnewski AV, Herrick CA, Liu Q, Chen L, Bottomly K, Redlich CA. Human gamma/delta T-cell proliferation and IFN-gamma production induced by hexamethylene diisocyanate. J Allergy Clin Immunol 2003; 112:538-546.

115. Frew A, Chang JH, Chan H, et al. T-lymphocyte responses to plicatic acid-human serum albumin conjugate in occupational asthma caused by western red cedar. J Allergy Clin Immunol 1998; 101(6 Pt 1):841-847.

116. Herrick CA, Xu L, Wisnewski AV, Das J, Redlich CA, Bottomly K. A novel mouse model of diisocyanate-induced asthma showing allergic-type inflammation in the lung after inhaled antigen challenge. J Allergy Clin Immunol 2002; 109:873-878.

117. Matheson JM, Lemus R, Lange RW, Karol MH, Luster MI. Role of tumor necrosis factor in toluene diisocyanate asthma. Am J Respir Cell Mol Biol 2002; 27:396-405.

118. Herrick CA, Das J, Xu L, Wisnewski AV, Redlich CA, Bottomly K. Differential roles for CD4 and CD8 T cells after diisocyanate sensitization: Genetic control of TH2-induced lung inflammation. J Allergy Clin Immunol 2003; 111:1087-1094.

119. Lummus ZL, Alam R, Bernstein JA, Bernstein DI. Diisocyanate antigen-enhanced production of monocyte chemoattractant protein-1, IL-8, and tumor necrosis factor-alpha by peripheral mononuclear cells of workers with occupational asthma. J Allergy Clin Immunol 1998; 102(2):265-274.

120. Gallagher JS, Tse CS, Brooks SM, Bernstein IL. Diverse profiles of immunoreactivity in toluene diisocyanate (TDI) asthma. J Occup Med 1981; 23(9):610-616.

121. Shirakawa T, Morimoto K. Brief reversible bronchospasm resulting from bichromate exposure. Arch Environ Health 1996; 51(3):221-226.

122. Holgate ST. The cellular and mediator basis of asthma in relation to natural history. Lancet 1997; 350(2):SII5-119.

123. Boushey HA, Fahy JV. Basic mechanisms of asthma. Environ Health Perspect 1995; 6:229-233.

124. Holgate ST, Bradding P, Sampson AP. Leukotriene antagonists and synthesis inhibitors: new directions in asthma therapy. J Allergy Clin Immunol 1996; 98(1):1-13.

125. Li JT. Mechanisms of asthma. Curr Opin Pulm Med 1997; 3(1):10-16.

126. Barnes PJ. Airway neuropeptides and their role in asthma. In: Holgate ST, Busse WW, eds. Inflammatory Mechanisms in Asthma. New York, Basel, Hong Kong: Marcel Dekker, 1998:chapter 24.

127. Fabbri LM, Danieli D, Crescioli S, Bevilacqua P, Meli S, Saetta M, Mapp CE. Fatal asthma in a subject sensitized to toluene diisocyanate. Am Rev Respir Dis 1988; 137(6):1494-1498.

128. Saetta M, Di Stefano A, Rosina C, Thiene G, Fabbri LM. Quantitative structural analysis of peripheral airways and arteries in sudden fatal asthma. Am Rev Respir Dis 1991; 143(1):138-143.

129. Saetta M, Di Stefano A, Maestrelli P, et al. Airway mucosal inflammation in occupational asthma induced by toluene diisocyanate. Am Rev Respir Dis 1992; 145(1):160-168.

130. Montefort S, Roberts JA, Beasley R, Holgate ST, Roche WR. The site of disruption of the bronchial epithelium in asthmatic and non-asthmatic subjects. Thorax 1992; 47(7):499-503.

131. Montefort S, Djukanovic R, Roche WR, Holgate ST. Ciliated cell damage in the bronchial epithelium of asthmatics and non-asthmatics. Clin Exp Allergy 1993; 23(3):185-189.

132. Roche WR, Beasley R, Williams JH, Holgate ST. Subepithelial fibrosis in the bronchi of asthmatics. Lancet 1989; 1(8637):520-524.

133. Brewster CE, Howarth PH, Djukanovic R, Wilson J, Holgate ST, Roche WR. Myofibroblasts and subepithelial fibrosis in bronchial asthma. Am J Respir Cell Mol Biol 1990; 3(5):507-511.

134. Frew AJ, Chan H, Lam S, Chan-Yeung M. Bronchial inflammation in occupational asthma due to western red cedar. Am J Respir Crit Care Med 1995; 151(2 Pt 1):340-344.

135. Gautrin D, Boulet LP, Boutet M, et al. Is reactive airways dysfunction syndrome a variant of occupational asthma?. J Allergy Clin Immunol 1994; 93(1 Pt 1):12–22.

136. Barbato A, Turato G, Baraldo S, et al. Airway inflammation in childhood asthma. Am J Respir Crit Care Med 2003; 168:798–803.

137. Gizycki MJ, Adelroth E, Rogers AV, O'Byrne PM, Jeffery PK. Myofibroblast involvement in the allergen-induced late response in mild atopic asthma. Am J Respir Cell Mol Biol 1997; 16(6):664–673.

138. Trigg CJ, Manolitsas ND, Wang J, et al. Placebo-controlled immunopathologic study of four months of inhaled corticosteroids in asthma. Am J Respir Crit Care Med 1994; 150(1):17–22.

139. Olivieri D, Chetta A, Del Donno M, et al. Effect of short-term treatment with low-dose inhaled fluticasone propionate on airway inflammation and remodeling in mild asthma: a placebo-controlled study. Am J Respir Crit Care Med 1997; 155(6):1864–1871.

140. Crimi E, Spanevello A, Neri M, et al. Dissociation between airway inflammation and airway hyperresponsiveness in allergic asthma [see comments]. Am J Respir Crit Care Med 1998; 157(1):4–9.

141. Chetta A, Foresi A, Del Donno M, et al. Bronchial responsiveness to distilled water and methacholine and its relationship to inflammation and remodeling of the airways in asthma. Am J Respir Crit Care Med 1996; 153(3):910–917.

142. Peters SP, Shaver JR, Zangrilli JG, Fish JE. Airways responses to antigen in asthmatic and nonasthmatic subjects. In: Holgate ST, Busse WW, eds. Inflammatory Mechanisms in Asthma. New York, Basel, Hong Kong: Marcel Dekker, 1998 (chapter 7).

143. Sheth KK, Lemanske RF. The early and late asthmatic reaction to allergen. In: Holgate ST, Busse WW, eds. Inflammatory Mechanisms in Asthma. New York, Basel, Hong Kong: Marcel Dekker, 1998:chapter 34.

144. Fabbri LM, Boschetto P, Zocca E, et al. Bronchoalveolar neutrophilia during late asthmatic reactions induced by toluene diisocyanate. Am Rev Respir Dis 1987; 136(1): 36–42.

145. Chan-Yeung M, Lam S. Evidence for mucosal inflammation in occupational asthma. Clin Exp Allergy 1990; 20(1):1–5.

146. Zocca E, Fabbri LM, Boschetto P, et al. Leukotriene B4 and late asthmatic reactions induced by toluene diisocyanate. J Appl Physiol 1990; 68(4):1576–1580.

147. White SR, Leff AR. Epithelium as a target. In: Holgate ST, Busse WW, eds. Inflammatory Mechanism in Asthma. New York, Basel, Hong Kong: Marcel Dekker, 1998:chapter 23.

148. Chan-Yeung M, Chan H, Tse KS, Salari H, Lam S. Histamine and leukotrienes release in bronchoalveolar fluid during plicatic acid-induced bronchoconstriction. J Allergy Clin Immunol 1989; 84(5 Pt 1):762–768.

149. Manning PJ, Rokach J, Malo JL, et al. Urinary leukotriene E4 levels during early and late asthmatic responses. J Allergy Clin Immunol 1990; 86(2):211–220.

150. Larchè M, Robinson DS, Kay AB. The role of T lymphocytes in the pathogenesis of asthma. J Allergy Clin Immunol 2003; 111:450–463.

151. Djukanovic R, Sterk PJ, Fahy JV, Hargreave FE, eds. Standardized methodology of sputum induction and processing. Eur Respir J 2002; 20(suppl 37):1S–55S.

152. Maestrelli P, Saetta M, Di Stefano A, Calcagni PG, Turato G, Ruggieri MP, Roggeri A, Mapp CE, Fabbri LM. Comparison of leukocyte counts in sputum, bronchial biopsies and bronchoalveolar lavage. Am J Respir Crit Care Med 1995; 152:1926–1931.

153. Pizzichini E, Pizzichini MM, Efthimiadis A, Evans S, Morris MM, Squillace D, Gleich GJ, Dolovich J, Hargreave FE. Indices of airway inflammation in induced sputum: reproducibility and validity of cell and fluid-phase measurements. Am J Respir Crit Care Med 1996; 154:308–307.

154. Pavord ID, Pizzichini MM, Pizzichini E, Hargreave FE. The use of induced sputum to investigate airway inflammation. Thorax 1997; 52:498–501.

155. Kips JC, Kharitonov SA, Barnes PJ. Noninvasive assessment of airway inflammation in asthma. Eur Respir Mon 2003; 23:164–179.

156. Maestrelli P, Calcagni P, Saetta M, et al. Sputum eosinophilia after asthmatic responses induced by isocyanates in sensitized subjects. Clin Exp Allergy 1994; 24:29–34.

157. Lemière C, Pizzichini MM, Balkissoon R, et al. Diagnosing occupational asthma: use of induced sputum. Eur Respir J 1999; 13:482–488.

158. Lemière C, Romeo P, Chaboillez S, Tremblay C, Malo JL. Airway inflammation and functional changes after exposure to different concentrations of isocyanates. J Allergy Clin Immunol 2002; 110:641–646.

159. Obata H, Dittrick M, Chan H, Chan-Yeung M. Sputum eosinophils and exhaled nitric oxide during late asthmatic reaction in patients with western red cedar. Eur Respir J 1999; 13:489–495.

160. Lemière C, Chaboillez S, Malo JL, Cartier A. Changes in sputum cell counts after exposure to occupational agents: what do they mean? J Allergy Clin Immunol 2001; 107: 1063–1068.

161. Panzer SE, Dodge AM, Kelly EAB, Jarjour N. Circadian variation of sputum inflammatory cells in mild asthma. J Allergy Clin Immunol 2003; 111:308–312.

162. Sastre J, Vandenplas O, Park H-S. Pathogenesis of occupational asthma. Eur Respir J 2003; 22:364–373.

163. Lemière C, Chaboillez S, Trudeau C, Taha R, Maghni K, Martin JG, Hamid Q. Characterization of airway inflammation after repeated exposures to occupational agents. J Allergy Clin Immunol 2000; 106:1163–1170.

164. Chan-Yeung M, Obata H, Dittrick M, Chan H, Abboud R. Airway inflammation, exhaled nitric oxide, and severity of asthma in patients with western red cedar asthma. Am J Respir Crit Care Med 1999; 159:1434–1438.

165. Quirce S, Fernandez-Nieto M, de Miguel J, Sastre J. Chronic cough due to latex-induced eosinophilic bronchitis. J Allergy Clin Immunol 2001; 108:143.

166. Lemière C, Efthimiadis A, Hargreave FE. Occupational eosinophilic bronchitis without asthma: an unknown occupational airway disease. J Allergy Clin Immunol 1997; 100: 852–853.

167. Bates CA, Silkoff PE. Exhaled nitric oxide in asthma: from bench to bedside. J Allergy Clin Immunol 2003; 111:256–262.

168. Alving K, Weitzberg E, Lundberg J. Increased amount of nitric oxide in exhaled air of asthmatics. Eur Respir J 1993; 6:1368–1370.

169. Kharitonov S, O'Conor B, Evans D, Barnes P. Allergen-induced late asthmatic reactions are associated with elevation of exhaled nitric oxide. Am J Respir Crit Care Med 1995; 151:1894–1899.

170. Adisesh LA, Kharitonov SA, Yates DH, Snashell DC, Newman-Taylor AJ, Barnes PJ. Exhaled and nasal nitric oxide is increased in laboratory animal allergy. Clin Exp Allergy 1998; 28:876–880.

171. Olin AC, Ljungkvist G, Bake B, Hagberg S, Henriksson L, Toren K. Exhaled nitric oxide among pulpmill workers reporting gassing incidents involving ozone and chlorine dioxide. Eur Respir J 1999; 14:828–831.

172. Piipari R, Piirila P, Keskinen H, Tuppurainen M, Sovijarvi A, Nordman H. Exhaled nitric oxide in specific challenge tests to assess occupational asthma. Eur Respir J 2002; 20:1532–1537.

173. Gibson PG, Fujimura M, Niimi A. Eosinophilic bronchitis: clinical manifestations and implications for treatment. Thorax 2002; 57:178–182.

174. Quirce S. Eosinophilic bronchitis in the workplace. Curr Opin Allergy Clin Immunol 2004; 4:87–91.

175. Vandenplas O, Malo JL. Definitions and type of work-related asthma: a nosological approach. Eur Respir J 2003; 21:706–712.

176. Brightling CE, Woltmann G, Wardlaw AJ, Pavord ID. Development of irreversible airflow obstruction in a patient with eosinophilic bronchitis without asthma. Eur Respir J 1999; 14:1228–1230.

177. Hancox RJ, Leigh R, Kelly MM, Hargreave FE. Eosinophilic bronchitis. Lancet 2001; 358:1104.

178. Tanaka H, Saikai T, Sugawara H, Takeya I, Tsunematsu K, Matsuura A, Abe S. Work-place-related chronic cough on a mushroom farm. Chest 2002; 122:1080–1085.

179. Kobayashi O. A case of eosinophilic bronchitis due to epoxy resin system hardener, methl endo methylene tetrahydro phtalic anhydride. Arerugi 1994; 43:660–662.

180. Ogawa H, Fujimura M, Heki U, Kitagawa M, Matsuda T. Eosinophilic bronchitis presenting with only severe dry cough due to bucillamine. Respiratory Med 1995; 89: 219–221.

181. Brightling CE, Bradding P, Symon FA, Holgate ST, Wardlaw AJ, Pavord ID. Mast-cell infiltration of airway smooth muscle in asthma. N Eng J Med 2002; 346:1699–1705.

182. Brightling CE, Symon FA, Birring SS, Bradding P, Wardlaw AJ, Pavord ID. Comparison of airway immunopathology of eosinophilic bronchitis and asthma. Thorax 2003; 58:528–532.

183. Brightling CE, Ward R, Woltmann G, Bradding P, Sheller JR, Dworski R, Pavord ID. Induced sputum inflammatory mediator concentrations in eosinophilic bronchitis and asthma. Am J Respir Crit Care Med 2000; 162:878–882.

184. Birring SS, Parker D, Brightling CE, Bradding P, Wardlaw AJ, Pavord ID. Induced sputum inflammatory mediator concentrations in chronic cough. Am J Respir Crit Care Med. 2004; 169:15–19.

185. Gibson PG, Zlatic K, Scott J, Sewell W, Woolley K, Saltos N. Chronic cough resembles asthma with IL-5 and granulocyte-macrophage colony-stimulating factor gene expression in bronchoalveolar cells. J Allergy Clin Immunol 1998; 101:320–326.

186. Brightling CE, Symon FA, Birring SS, Bradding P, Wardlaw AJ, Pavord ID. T_H2 cytokine expression in bronchoalveolar lavage fluid T lymphocytes and bronchial submucosa is a feature of asthma and eosinophilic bronchitis. J Allergy Clin Immunol 2002; 110:899–905.

187. Tillie-Leblond I, Gosset P, Tonnel A-B. Inflammatory events in severe acute asthma. Allergy 2005; 60:23–29.

188. Fabbri LM, Boschetto P, Caramori G, Maestrelli P. Neutrophils and asthma. In: Holgate ST, Busse WW, eds. Inflammatory Mechanisms in Asthma. New York, Basel, Hong Kong: Marcel Dekker, 1998 (chapter 15).

189. Di Franco A, Vagaggini B, Bacci E, et al. Leukocyte counts in hypertonic saline-induced sputum in subjects with occupational asthma. Respir Med 1998; 92:550–557.

190. Anees W, Huggins V, Pavord ID, Robertson AS, Burge PS. Occupational asthma due to low molecular weight agents: eosinophilic and non-eosinophilic variants. Thorax 2002; 57:231–236.

191. Park H, Jung K, Kim H, Nahm D, Kang K. Neutrophil activation following TDI bronchial challenges to airway secretion from subjects with TDI-induced asthma. Clin Exp Allergy 1999; 29:1395–1401.

192. Jung KS, Park HS. Evidence for neutrophil activation in occupational asthma. Respirology 1999; 4:303–306.

193. Jatakanon A, Uasuf C, Maziak W, Lim S, Chung KF, Barnes PJ. Neutrophilic inflammation in severe persistent asthma. Am J Respir Crit Care Med 1999; 160:1532–1539.

194. Park HS, Hwang SC, Nahm DH, Yim HE. Immunohistochemical characterization of cellular infiltrate in airway mucosa of toluene diisocyanate-induced asthma. J Korean Med Sci 1998; 13:12–16.

195. Saite J, Banks DE, Lopez M, Barkman HW, Salvaggio JE. Neutrophil chemotactic activity in toluene diisocyanate (TDI)-induced asthma. J Allergy Clin Immunol 1990; 85: 567–572.

196. Park HS, Jung KS, Hwang SC, Nahm DH, Yim HE. Neutrophil infiltration and release of IL-8 in airway mucosa from subjects with grain dust-induced occupational asthma. Clin Exp Allergy 1998; 28:724-730.

197. Barnes PJ, Baraniuk JN, Belvisi MG. Neuropeptides in the respiratory tract. Part II. Am Rev Respir Dis 1991; 144(6):1391-1399.

198. Nadel JA. Neutral endopeptidase modulates neurogenic inflammation. Eur Respir J 1991; 4(6):745-754.

199. Heaney LG, Cross LJ, McGarvey LP, Buchanan KD, Ennis M, Shaw C. Neurokinin A is the predominant tachykinin in human bronchoalveolar lavage fluid in normal and asthmatic subjects. Thorax 1998; 53(5):357-362.

200. Barnes PJ. NO or no NO in asthma? Thorax 1996; 51(2):218-220.

201. Ollerenshaw SL, Jarvis D, Woolcock AJ, Sullivan CE, Scheibner T. Absence of immunoreactive vasoactive intestinal polypeptide in tissue from the lung of patients with asthma. N Engl J Med 1991(320):1244-1248.

202. Ollerenshaw SL, Jarvis D, Sullivan CE, Woolcock AJ. Substance P immunoreactive nerves in airways from asthmatics and nonasthmatics. Eur Respir J 1991; 4(6):673-682.

203. Lilly CM, Bai TR, Shore SA, Hall AE, Drazen JM. Neuropeptide content of lungs from asthmatic and nonasthmatic patients. Am J Respir Crit Care Med 1995; 151(2 Pt 1):548-553.

204. Howarth PH, Springall DR, Redington AE, Djukanovic R, Holgate ST, Polak JM. Neuropeptide-containing nerves in endobronchial biopsies from asthmatic and nonasthmatic subjects. Am J Respir Cell Mol Biol 1995; 13(3):288-696.

205. Mapp CE, Lucchini RE, Miotto D, et al. Immunization and challenge with toluene diisocyanate decrease tachykinin and calcitonin gene-related peptide immunoreactivity in guinea pig central airways. Am J Respir Crit Care Med 1998; 158(1):263-269.

206. Sheppard D, Thompson JE, Scypinski L, Dusser D, Nadel JA, Borson DB. Toluene diisocyanate increases airway responsiveness to substance P and decreases airway neutral endopeptidase. J Clin Invest 1988; 81(4):1111-1115.

207. O'Byrne PM. Leukotrienes in the pathogenesis of asthma. Chest 1997; 111(suppl 2):275-345.

6

Animal Models of Occupational Asthma: Tools for Understanding Disease Pathogenesis

Victor J. Johnson and Michael I. Luster
Toxicology and Molecular Biology Branch, Health Effects Laboratory Division, NIOSH/CDC, Morgantown, West Virginia, U.S.A.

INTRODUCTION

Occupational asthma is the most frequently reported occupational respiratory disease in industrialized nations, and numerous low-molecular-weight chemicals and high-molecular-weight proteins encountered in the workplace are known or suspected causative agents (1). Classical and novel animal models are being used to investigate exposure determinants, epitope identity, and the role played by the immune system in occupational asthma in order to recapitulate disease phenotype and further current understanding of its pathogenesis. Important aspects of exposure determinants that can be addressed and controlled using animal models include (*i*) relevant routes of exposure including respiratory and/or skin, (*ii*) exposure dose, (*iii*) exposure duration and frequency, and (*iv*) determination of relevant epitopes. In addition, well-defined genetics of animal models present unique opportunities for detailed investigations into pathogenic mechanisms through the use of transgenic models and antibody neutralization strategies. The data generated through the use of animal models is instrumental for risk assessment used to refine workplace exposure limits. Numerous guinea pig, rat, and mouse models of occupational asthma have been developed to address these issues. It is likely that key molecular and cellular events will be identified through the use of these models, potentially leading to new treatment modalities that may be specific for these classes of asthmogen and will aid in establishing more protective workplace exposure limits.

OCCUPATIONAL ASTHMA PRODUCED BY LOW-MOLECULAR-WEIGHT CHEMICAL HAPTENS

Among the major low-molecular-weight chemical classes known to induce occupational asthma, diisocyanates and organic acid anhydrides have been studied the most.

Diisocyanate Asthma

The Clinical Condition

Diisocyanates are highly reactive, low-molecular-weight chemicals that represent the leading cause of occupational asthma, a disease that accounts for nearly 10% of all adult-onset asthma (2). The three major diisocyanates encountered in the workplace include toluene diisocyanate (TDI), diphenyl-methane diisocyanate (MDI), and hexa-methylene diisocyanate (HDI), and all are used in a variety of industries including polyurethane foam manufacturing, auto body painting and repair, and plastics manu-facturing. It is estimated that as many as 5% of workers exposed to diisocyanates develop asthma and the disease may persist indefinitely, even in the absence of continued exposure.

Occupational asthma to diisocyanates is usually characterized by a variable lag period consisting of months to years of exposure prior to the development of symptoms (3). Once sensitized to diisocyanates, low-level exposures, even those below permissible workplace limits, can induce clinical onset of disease (4). Clinical expression of diisocya-nate asthma displays characteristics similar to those present in allergic asthma, suggest-ing common immunopathogenesis. These include development of immediate, late, or dual asthmatic responses following chemical exposure. In addition, patients often develop persistent airway hyperresponsiveness (AHR) to nonspecific stimuli that can last for years, even in the absence of continued exposure, and complete recovery of lung function may never be achieved (5–7). Recent evidence shows a correlation between recovery of AHR and persistence of eosinophilic inflammation in diisocya-nate asthma, persistent inflammation being associated with poor or no recovery (8). Pathological features of diisocyanate asthma also include goblet cell metaplasia, mucus hypersecretion, upper and lower respiratory tract inflammation consisting of leukocytic infiltration of the airway mucosa, and leukocyte extravasation leading to luminal eosinophilia and neutrophilia. There is also evidence that humans demon-strate airway remodeling in diisocyanate asthma, which is characterized by sub-epithelial thickening (collagen deposition) and fibrosis (9). Airway remodeling may be an important determinant for persistence of diisocyanate-induced asthma.

Despite the clinical similarities to allergic asthma, human data on the immune mechanisms of diisocyanate asthma highlight important differences between the two diseases. The immunopathogenesis of allergic asthma involves recruitment of CD4+ T lymphocytes to the lung and production of T-helper 2 (T_H2) type cytokines including interleukin (IL) -4, -5, and -13. CD4+ lymphocytes and T_H2 cytokines are integral to the development and severity of diisocyanate asthma, but recent evidence also points to an important role for CD8+ lymphocytes and T_H1 cytokines, including

Occupational asthma has also been reported in workers exposed to chemicals from wood products such as plicatic acid found in western red cedar resin. Low-molecular-weight chemicals are usually too small to be recognized by the immune system in their native form. As such, low-molecular-weight chemicals act as haptens that bind to host proteins, and result in new antigenic determinants capable of eliciting immune responses. Although some progress has been made, the nature of these conjugates in humans and the mechanisms underlying occupational asthma caused by low-molecular-weight chemicals, for the most part, remain to be elucidated. The following section will focus on the use of animal models of occupational asthma caused by low-molecular-weight chemicals, to further the understanding of disease pathogenesis.

IFNγ (10–12). Another difference between the etiopathogenesis of diisocyanate asthma and allergic asthma is the low prevalence of specific IgE antibodies in diisocyanate asthma. Specific IgE antibodies are only detectable in 5% to 30% of diisocyanate asthmatics, suggesting that other immune mechanisms may be responsible for disease progression (13,14).

Animal Models of Diisocyanate Asthma

Guinea Pig Models. The first animal studies of diisocyanate asthma were conducted in guinea pigs and identified this class of chemicals as respiratory toxins that are capable of producing acute airway irritation as well as sensitization. Guinea pig models display many of the clinical features of human diisocyanate asthma including AHR, epithelial injury, and neutrophilic inflammation (15–17). Guinea pig models also demonstrate airway eosinophilia and a late phase asthmatic reaction characteristic of human disease (18,19). The guinea pig has been used as a model to demonstrate that isolated airway exposure to TDI results in skin sensitization and that dermal exposure results in pulmonary hypersensitivity (20,21).

The classic guinea pig model developed by Karol involves inhalation exposure to vapor phase TDI (0–7.6 ppm) for three hours per day for five consecutive days followed by a three week–rest period prior to inhalation challenge with aerosolized TDI–guinea pig serum albumin (GPSA) conjugate (22,23). Additional animals were exposed to 20 ppb TDI for six hours per day for 70 days followed by TDI–GPSA challenge three weeks later. Subacute inhalation exposure (five days) at levels $\geq$120 ppb TDI were required for specific antibody production, the titer of which increased progressively with exposure concentrations above 120 ppb. Changes in pulmonary function were observed at $\geq$360 ppb TDI. Subchronic inhalation to low concentrations of TDI (20 ppb for 70 days) did not result in immune sensitization or altered lung function (22). Interestingly, higher TDI antibody titers in guinea pigs did not always correlate with changes in pulmonary function, suggesting that different mechanistic pathways are involved. Aoyama et al. (17) showed a similar relationship between immune sensitization and changes in pulmonary function following TDI vapor challenge. Their model also demonstrated that nonsensitizing concentrations of TDI were capable of eliciting pulmonary reactivity in previously sensitized guinea pigs. This is an important discovery and suggests that acceptable workplace atmospheres (<5 ppb for TDI) may result in potential life-threatening reactions in sensitized workers. In fact, workplace levels of TDI as low as 1 ppb have been shown to invoke respiratory distress in sensitized workers (24). Using a similar sensitization protocol, Raulf et al. (25) demonstrated elevated numbers of eosinophils and increased leukotrienes in the bronchoalveolar lavage fluid (BALF). Huang et al. (26) used the same model to demonstrate that exposure to TDI–GPSA conjugates stimulated histamine release from lung mast cells in guinea pigs when sensitized with TDI concentrations sufficient to elicit respiratory responses. The authors suggested that mast cell stimulation might underlie the different sensitivity of antibody and pulmonary responses.

Additional studies using guinea pigs investigated the effects of combined inhalation and intradermal exposure to diisocyanates. Pauluhn exposed guinea pigs to TDI by inhalation (0–7 ppm, three hours per day for five days), with or without intradermal injection of 0.3% TDI (27). Challenge consisted of TDI vapor or TDI–GPSA conjugates three weeks following initial exposure. Lower incidence and reduced intensity of respiratory responses were observed in guinea pigs challenged with TDI vapor compared to that observed after exposure to TDI-GPSA conjugate with an approximately equal TDI concentration. This suggests that only a portion of the reactions between TDI and biological molecules resulted in haptens capable of being recognized by the immune system. This notion is supported by the observation that TDI-GPSA was only one of several adducted proteins present in the BALF of guinea pigs following inhalation exposure (28). The TDI-albumin conjugates are known to cause sensitization, but the identity and immune reactivity of other conjugates formed in the lungs of guinea pigs are presently unknown (29). Exposure of guinea pigs to HDI following a similar sensitization/challenge paradigm demonstrated that both inhalation and intradermal exposure result in sensitization, although antibody and respiratory responses were greater following intradermal injection (30). Challenge with free HDI did not result in appreciable changes in respiratory parameters in contrast to the marked respiratory responses elicited by HDI-GPSA conjugates, similar to the observation made in experiments involving TDI and TDI–albumin conjugate. The authors suggested that the reaction of free HDI with the nasal mucosa may have effectively reduced the bronchial concentration below a threshold level required to provoke pulmonary responses in sensitized animals.

Guinea pigs have also been used to investigate the role of dermal and intradermal exposure in the development of diisocyanate asthma (18,21,27,30–32). In a model developed by Karol et al. (21) a single epicutaneous exposure to $50\,\mu L$ of TDI (1% to 100%; $25\,\mu L$ applied to two shaved dorsal sites) was followed two weeks later by a bronchial provocation challenge with TDI vapor and/or TDI–protein conjugates. Contact hypersensitivity and antibody production were consistently detected in animals sensitized with >10% TDI. Consistent with this finding, a single dermal exposure to MDI at concentrations as low as 10% resulted in a dose-dependent increase in specific antibody production (32). These models were able to demonstrate respiratory hypersensitivity following skin exposure in approximately 25% to 30% of the guinea pigs topically exposed to TDI or MDI, following inhalation challenge with the respective chemical.

The immunopathologic response in the lung to an inhalation challenge has been characterized in guinea pigs following intradermal injection of TDI (18). In this model, animals received intradermal injections of neat TDI ($50\,\mu L$ for every two dorsal sites) once a week for three weeks, followed seven days later by inhalation challenge with 5 to 20 ppb of TDI vapor. Challenged guinea pigs showed elevated TDI-specific antibodies and TDI challenge increased blood eosinophil numbers. Increased numbers of eosinophils and mast cells were observed in the submucosa and lamina propria of the airways as early as six hours postchallenge in sensitized animals. Pulmonary infiltration of $CD4^+$ lymphocytes was also evident and administration of anti–IL-5 antibody reduced eosinophil accumulation, supporting a role for T_H2 immunity in TDI asthma. Huang et al. (33) demonstrated that intradermal injection of neat TDI on days one and six resulted in TDI-GPSA specific and nonspecific AHR to methacholine in guinea pigs challenged with TDI-GPSA on day 21. In contrast to the intradermal model developed by Mapp et al. (18), increased eosinophils were not observed in this model. This may be related to slight variations in the frequency and timing of intradermal injection or the use of TDI vapor versus TDI-GPSA conjugates for challenge.

The guinea pig has also been used to study potential neurogenic mechanisms related to, or initiated by diisocyanate-induced inflammation in the lung. Intranasal application of 5% TDI for several weeks resulted in increased immunoreactivity of substance P (SP) and calcitonin gene–related peptide (CGRP) in the nasal mucosa concomitant with nasal allergy symptoms (34). Pretreatment of guinea pigs with capsaicin abrogated nasal allergy symptoms and pulmonary hyperreactivity to TDI (34,35). More recently, Mapp et al. (36) demonstrated decreased SP and CGRP immunoreactivity in the central airways of sensitized guinea pigs following TDI challenge. Together, these findings support a role for the interaction of neurogenic peptides and inflammatory mediators in TDI asthma.

Rat Models. Rat models have not received as much attention as guinea pig or murine models for studying the mechanisms of diisocyanate asthma, although rats have been used extensively to study the irritant effects of these chemicals. A model of phenyl isocyanate–induced asthma has been developed and displays airway inflammation characteristic of asthma (37). Wistar rats were exposed to nonirritating concentrations of phenyl isocyanate (0–10 mg/m^3) for six hours per day, five days a week, for two weeks. Although the rats did not receive a specific challenge, histopathological analysis revealed goblet cell metaplasia at concentrations >4 mg/m^3 in addition to smooth muscle hypertrophy, epithelial desquamation, mucus hypersecretion, and eosinophil infiltration at concentrations >7 mg/m^3. These characteristic features of asthmatic inflammation were accompanied by decreased forced expiratory flow and quasistatic lung compliance. The pathological changes in response to phenyl isocyanate were reversed within two months following the cessation of exposure. Because rats were not challenged in this study, phenyl isocyanate challenge following a rest period will be important to demonstrate the utility of this model for studying occupational asthma.

Wistar rats have also been used to study TDI asthma following intranasal exposure. Rats were exposed to 5 μL of 10% TDI applied to each nostril for seven consecutive days followed by nasal provocation challenge with 5 μL of 5% TDI one week later. Marked increases in eosinophils, lymphocytes, macrophages, and neutrophils were observed in the BALF of sensitized rats following challenge. TDI challenge also increased IL-4 and -6 levels in the BALF as well as eosinophil infiltration in the peripheral airways. This model lends support to the involvement of T_H2 immunity in the development of airway inflammation in TDI asthma. A similar nasal sensitization and challenge study design in Brown Norway rats showed increased histamine receptor and histamine decarboxylase expression in the nasal mucosa, suggesting that the histamine pathway may be important in the observed nasal allergy symptoms following TDI exposure (38,39).

Mouse Models. Mice offer the distinct advantage of a better-defined genome than guinea pigs or rats and the availability of antibody reagents and transgenic strains to investigate detailed mechanistic pathways. Early studies using murine models demonstrated the involvement of the immune system in immunological reactivity to diisocyanates, as topical exposure to TDI induced production of TDI-specific IgE antibodies and contact hypersensitivity (40–43). It was later shown that CD4$^+$ and CD8$^+$ T lymphocytes were important effector cells in these responses (44). However, these early models lacked evidence of respiratory inflammation. Recently, Scheerens et al. demonstrated that epicutaneous sensitization to TDI led to increased tracheal hyperreactivity to carbachol (45). Male BALB/c mice were exposed to 1% TDI epicutaneously on days 0 and 1, followed by intranasal challenge eight days later with 20 μL of 1% TDI. Importantly, lymphocyte involvement in the tracheal hyperreactivity was demonstrated by adoptive transfer experiments. Changing the sensitization schedule to six weeks, with skin exposure to TDI on days 0, 7, 14, 21, 28, and 35 followed by intranasal challenge, resulted in a more robust respiratory response (46). Necrosis was evident in nonsensitized mice, indicating that the airway pathology was likely owing to the irritancy of 1% TDI intranasal challenge. Lung inflammation, characteristic of diisocyanate occupational asthma in humans, was not evident. A significant contribution of this model was the demonstration that altering the length of sensitization and cumulative dose resulted in different immunological processes, which may help explain the diversity of symptoms exhibited in humans.

The role of inflammatory mediators in TDI-induced asthma was recently demonstrated using a murine model employing subcutaneous sensitization and inhalation challenge (47). Female C57BL/6 mice were sensitized by multiple subcutaneous injections of TDI (20 µL neat TDI, day 1; 20 µL of 20% TDI, days 4 and 11) and then challenged by inhalation with 100 ppb TDI vapor on days 20, 22, and 24. AHR to methacholine was accompanied by mucus metaplasia, inflammation, and cytokine expression in the airways. However, inflammation was evident only in the upper airways with lymphocyte and neutrophil infiltration and inflammatory cytokine expression in the nares and trachea, respectively. Matheson et al. (47) found that histopathological changes and inflammatory cell involvement were not evident in athymic mice, supporting the hypothesis that diisocyanate occupational asthma is dependent upon specific immunity. Using tumor necrosis factor α (TNFα)–deficient mice, Matheson et al. (48) identified TNFα as an integral proinflammatory cytokine in disease development. Interestingly, however, mice developed TDI-specific IgG antibodies regardless of their TNFα status, supporting the hypothesis that IgG antibodies are better markers of exposure than disease. Similarly, diisocyanate-specific IgG levels generally correlate better with exposure than disease in humans (49).

In recent studies, female BALB/c mice were sensitized epicutaneously with 0.1% or 1% HDI on days 0 and 7 followed by intranasal challenge with HDI–mouse serum albumin (MSA) (50 µL at 2 mg/mL) conjugate on days 14, 15, 18, and 19 (50). Mice developed HDI-specific IgG antibodies as well as lymphocyte and eosinophil lung infiltrates. Inflammatory cells from the lung digest produced elevated levels of IL-5, -13, and IFNγ upon restimulation with HDI-MSA, indicating a mixed T_H1/T_H2 immune response as seen in humans (10,51). The optimal sensitizing dose for antibody production was higher than that for airway inflammation and cytokine production. This finding is in concordance with that of Matheson et al. (48) suggesting that differing mechanism may be dominant in these outcomes. In addition to the dose, frequency of dermal exposure influences greatly respiratory responses to TDI in sensitized BALB/c mice (52). The role of CD4+ and CD8+ T lymphocytes was also investigated by Herrick et al. (53) who showed that the presence of eosinophils in the BALF was markedly reduced in mice deficient in CD4+ T lymphocytes, despite an intact contact hypersensitivity response. This finding is consistent with their previous work in which attenuated inflammatory responses were observed in IL-4 and -13 knockout mice (50). In contrast, mice deficient in CD8+ T lymphocytes showed a partial reduction in contact hypersensitivity, but no change in the presence of lung inflammatory cells. Together, these findings suggest a dominant role for CD4+ T lymphocytes and T_H2 immunity in HDI-induced lung inflammation. Herrick et al. (53) also showed an influence of mouse strain on the development of diisocyanate asthma in mice.

Lee et al. (54–56) developed a murine (BALB/c) model of TDI asthma using intranasal sensitization with 3% TDI given for two cycles of five daily instillations with a three week–rest period between each cycle, and inhalation challenge with

1% TDI a week later. This was the first model to demonstrate AHR following sensitization via the respiratory tract in mice. In addition, significant pathology in the lower airways was evident and was accompanied by a variety of inflammatory mediators. Administration of specific inhibitors of two of these mediators, vascular endothelial growth factor, or matrix metalloproteinase (MMP), markedly reduced the disease (55,56). Doxycycline, a tetracycline antibiotic capable of inhibiting MMPs, also reduced MMP-9 expression and disease pathogenesis following TDI challenge (57). More recently, this model was employed to demonstrate that TDI challenge decreased the lung ratio of MMP-9/tissue inhibitor of metallopro-teinase (TIMP)-1, starting at seven hours postchallenge and persisting for at least 72 hours (58). A balance between MMPs and their TIMP inhibitors is essential for maintenance of homeostasis of the lung's extracellular matrix, and these studies support the notion that there may be a disruption of this balance in the pathogenesis of occupational asthma.

To examine the pathophysiological responses in occupational asthma following inhalation exposure, the predominant route of exposure in the workplace, our labora-tory exposed C57BL/6J mice to 20 ppb TDI vapor via inhalation for four hours per day, five days a week for six weeks, followed 14 days later by a one-hour inhalation challenge with 20 ppb TDI. Challenge with TDI resulted in a marked increase in AHR to methacholine (59). Histopathological changes in the lung included goblet cell hyperplasia, epithelial damage, mucus hypersecretion, and eosinophilia. Serum levels of total IgE and TDI-specific IgG antibodies were elevated in sensitized mice, and serum transfer resulted in sensitivity to TDI challenge in naive animals. A role for IgE and possibly other reagenic antibodies was supported by the inability of TDI to sensitize FcErIg transgenic mice, which lack the γ-chain subunit of the FcγRI, FcγRIII and FcϵRI receptors and the inability of heat-treated serum to trans-fer disease to naive mice (59). Elevated expression of IL-4, -5, and IFNγ was observed in the lung, consistent with a mixed T_H1/T_H2 cytokine profile as suggested by findings in other animal models and humans (10,50,51,53). Interestingly, a single inhalation exposure to 500 ppb TDI, which represents an irritating concentration, for two hours followed two weeks later by 20 ppb TDI challenge resulted in an elevated nonspecific AHR and epithelial changes in the lung consistent with asthma, although there was a lack of eosinophils (59). This exposure paradigm was examined to deter-mine whether accidental spills in the workplace that cause respiratory irritation can lead to sensitization and the development of occupational asthma.

Adoptive transfer experiments were conducted using lymphocytes from TDI-sensitized mice to determine the role of specific immunity in the response to TDI (59). Airway reactivity was increased in naive mice that received unfractionated lymphocytes, purified B cells or purified T cells, from sensitized mice (59). That the isocyanate-induced occupational asthma involves a mixed T_H1/T_H2 phenotype was supported in studies using various transgenic mouse models sensitized to TDI sub-chronically, as described above. For example, IFNγ-deficient mice demonstrated a reduction in airway inflammation, serum antibody levels, and histopathological changes, but to a lesser degree than that observed in IL-4-deficient mice (60). In humans with occupational asthma, T_H2 cells comprise only a small portion of the sensitized T cells in the airways, with most cells representing a T_H1 phenotype. In fact, the majority of T cell clones derived from bronchial mucosa of patients with isocyanate-induced asthma present a CD8[+] phenotype, and produce IFNγ and IL-5 (12,61). In this respect, we observed that either CD8[+] or CD4[+] deficiency pre-vented TDI asthma following subchronic treatment (60).

Acid Anhydride Asthma

The Clinical Condition

Acid anhydrides are low-molecular-weight organic chemicals used in the production of alkyd, epoxy, and polyester resins for plastic and paint manufacturing. Acid anhydrides commonly encountered in the workplace include trimellitic anhydride (TMA), phthalic anhydride (PA), and maleic anhydride, as well as many derivatives of these compounds. Exposure to these agents can result in direct irritation, immunological respiratory hypersensitivity, or a combination of both (62). Direct irritant effects are usually associated with high exposure concentrations (62). Although workplace concentrations have been reduced in recent years, intermittent spikes in ambient levels in air can result in irritation despite the time-weighted average being within an acceptable range (62).

Respiratory hypersensitivity reactions to acid anhydrides include three clinically distinct syndromes: allergic asthma/rhinitis, late respiratory systemic syndrome, and pulmonary disease anemia (63). Sensitized workers present asthmatic symptoms including a T_H2 phenotype with early- and late-phase AHR and eosinophilic inflammation, with or without pulmonary hemorrhage. The particular syndrome presented in exposed workers is related to the nature of the immune response as well as the exposure route and concentration, with asthma resulting at lower concentrations. The immune response to acid anhydrides in humans includes the production of IgE and IgG antibodies specific for chemical–protein conjugates including haptenized serum albumin (64,65). Cell-mediated immune responses have also been reported in humans. It is thought that specific IgE antibody production and T_H2 cytokines are related to the asthma/rhinitis syndrome, whereas specific IgG antibody production and cell-mediated responses are related to the late respiratory systemic syndrome/hypersensitivity pneumonitis (63). As with other allergens, atopy and HLA genotype have been identified as important risk factors for the development of acid anhydride–induced asthma (66–68).

Animal Models of Acid Anhydride Asthma

Guinea Pig Models. Inhalation exposure to vapor and aerosol forms of acid anhydrides is a primary concern in the workplace. Guinea pigs have been shown to develop immunological sensitization following inhalation exposure. Homocytotropic antibodies were detected in the serum of guinea pigs exposed to atmospheres containing TMA dust (1–100 mg/m³) for three hours per day, for five consecutive days (69). Despite evidence of sensitization, inhalation challenge with TMA–GPSA failed to elicit changes in the respiratory rate in this model. In contrast, Pauluhn and Eben showed that challenge with TMA dust or TMA–GPSA induced an immediate change in the breathing pattern indicative of an early asthmatic response in guinea pigs sensitized to TMA via inhalation (70). The differences between the two studies may be related to the sensitization exposure paradigms employed. Exposure of guinea pigs to PA dust (0.5–5.0 mg/m³) through inhalation resulted in dose-dependent production of allergic IgG_{1a} antibodies with detectable antibodies present even at the lowest concentration tested (71). Challenge of sensitized animals with TMA–GPSA, but not TMA dust, resulted in changes in respiratory rate indicating a pulmonary hypersensitivity response. Pathological changes included hemorrhagic foci and alveolar hemorrhage, which were similar to changes observed in workers exposed to acid anhydrides.

The intradermal sensitization route was used in a number of guinea pig studies of acid anhydride respiratory effects. Hayes et al. (72) sensitized guinea pigs using intradermal injection of 0.1, 0.3, or 30% TMA in corn oil as an acute exposure or with four injections over two weeks. TMA-specific IgG_1 antibodies were detected in the serum of all animals receiving TMA, while no specific antibodies were detected in the control animals. Anaphylactic IgE antibodies, specific for TMA, were also present in the sera from low-dose sensitized guinea pigs (73). Challenge consisted of intravenous injection of TMA–GPSA, which resulted in elevated pulmonary inflation pressure in half of the sensitized guinea pigs. This study showed that guinea pigs exposed to either single or repeated low doses of TMA during sensitization had greater pulmonary responses to challenge than those sensitized with a high dose despite high antibody titers in the later group. Challenge with TMA–GPSA directly into the trachea resulted in immediate increases in lung resistance and significant microvascular leakage in low-dose sensitized animals (73). Inhalation challenge with TMA dust induced AHR to acetylcholine in high-dose sensitized animals, which was accompanied by eosinophil infiltration into the lung tissue and increased mucus secretion (74,75). A strong correlation between eosinophilia and AHR was shown after inhalation of TMA dust in guinea pigs that were sensitized via intramuscular injection of TMA–BSA (bovine serum albumin) in complete Freund adjuvant (76). Decreased respiratory rates were also evident following challenge with TMA or PA dust in animals sensitized to the respective chemical (31). Challenge with TMA dust, but not TMA–GPSA, induced mild changes in airway resistance and eosinophilia in lungs of nonsensitized guinea pigs, suggesting that challenge with protein-conjugated TMA may not accurately reflect occupational exposures (77).

Using a similar intradermal sensitization protocol including two doses of 0.3% TMA administered 24 hours apart, Arakawa et al. (78) showed that TMA-specific IgG_1 antibodies were elevated within two weeks following sensitization and remained elevated for more than eight weeks. Intratracheal challenge with TMA–GPSA induced plasma extravasation, evidenced by Evans blue dye leakage into the lung, which occurred as early as one week after sensitization and increased until eight weeks. In contrast, the challenge increased lung resistance as early as one week after sensitization, although this response declined with time following sensitization. Systemic antibody production correlated with changes in microvascular permeability, but not with airway resistance. These findings do not preclude the involvement of TMA-specific IgG in AHR because the administration of a combination of TMA-specific IgG_1 and IgG_2 antibodies to naive guinea pigs resulted in significant elevation of AHR following the TMA–GPSA challenge (79).

The role of inflammatory mediators and the complement system in acid anhydride–induced respiratory disease was studied using similar guinea pig models. Intravenous administration of antagonists of histamine, cyclooxygenase, platelet activating factor, lipoxygenase, or thromboxane synthase significantly attenuated changes in lung resistance following TMA–GPSA, whereas only inhibitors of histamine, cyclooxygenase, and lipoxygenase attenuated plasma extravasation. These results suggest that arachidonic acid metabolism may play different roles in the observed changes in lung resistance versus changes in microvascular permeability following acid anhydride exposure (80–82). Treatment with cyclosporine A during sensitization also attenuated changes in lung resistance and microvascular leakage (83). A similar model was employed to demonstrate a critical role for complement activation in disease pathogenesis. Elevated levels of the C3a complement activation product were evident in the lungs of sensitized guinea pigs following challenge with

TMA (84). Administration of cobra venom factor, a potent inhibitor of complement activation, markedly attenuated bronchoconstriction and microvascular leakage (85). Together, these observations suggest that complement activation is an important pathway involved in acid anhydride–induced respiratory disease.

Rat Models of Acid Anhydride Asthma. The pathogeneses of TMA-induced pulmonary hemorrhage and hypersensitivity pneumonitis have been investigated in Sprague-Dawley rats (86). Rats were exposed to dry TMA powder (0–300 mg/m^3) by inhalation, six hours per day, five days a week for two weeks. This exposure regimen resulted in elevated lung weights, grossly observable external hemorrhagic foci, alveolar hemorrhage, and pulmonary macrophage and leukocyte accumulation, all of which were dose-dependent and undetectable 12 days after exposure (86–88). Challenge on day 26 with TMA dust at the same concentration as the original exposure induced significant lung pathology although the severity was less than that observed after 10 days of exposure (86). IgG, IgA, and IgM antibodies specific for TMA–rat serum albumin (RSA) could be detected in the serum and BALF (88,89). Subsequent studies showed that specific antibody production was dependent on exposure dose and correlated with increases in lung weight and the number of hemorrhagic foci in the lung (90). Passive transfer of serum from sensitized rats into naive recipients resulted in lung injury following a single challenge with TMA (91). These studies suggest that lung pathology observed in this model is likely immunological in origin. It is important to note that chronic, low-dose inhalation exposure to naive rats can also lead to changes in respiratory physiology accompanied by eosinophilia and other asthma-associated pathology (92).

The Brown Norway rat, which is genetically predisposed to favor T$_H$2 responses, has also been used to study acid anhydride–related respiratory effects. A single intradermal injection of 0.3% TMA in corn oil resulted in immunological sensitization, as evidenced by elevated levels of TMA-specific IgG and IgE antibodies (93). Challenge of sensitized rats with aerosolized TMA–RSA resulted in eosinophil infiltration into the bronchial wall. Lungs from TMA sensitized rats also show epithelial lesions and a trend toward increased nonspecific AHR following a single challenge. Multiple challenges over a period of seven days resulted in increased levels of TMA-specific IgG antibodies in serum and a significant increase in nonspecific AHR. In fact, multiple challenges with 0.003% TMA–RSA produced a much greater pulmonary response than a single 0.03% challenge dose (94). Extending the challenge exposure to five days a week for nine weeks resulted in considerable airway remodeling characterized by airway wall thickening and luminal narrowing, goblet cell metaplasia, and smooth muscle thickening (95). This model reproduces many of the pathological features of human asthmatic response to TMA, making it suitable for the investigation of underlying mechanisms.

Direct contact with skin represents a substantial concern for workers exposed to acid anhydrides. As such, dermal application of dry TMA powder has been used to sensitize Brown Norway rats. Zhang et al. (96) applied dry TMA powder (0–20 mg) to the shaved back of rats followed by occlusion overnight on days 0, 7, 14, and 21. TMA–RSA specific IgG and IgE were detected in the serum of half of the rats exposed to 0.3 mg of TMA. All rats developed antibodies in a dose-dependent manner at exposures above this dose. The production of TMA-specific antibodies was also time dependent, appearing by day 14 and peaking by day 28. This model successfully demonstrated immunologic sensitization following dermal exposure to TMA, suggesting that this may be a potential route for human sensitization. More importantly, rats sensitized by the dermal route developed significant

TMA-specific early- and late-phase obstruction following a challenge with dry TMA powder via inhalation (97). A similar biphasic airway response can be observed in sensitized workers upon reexposure. Dermal sensitization and inhalation challenge has also been shown to induce eosinophil infiltration and goblet metaplasia in sensitized rats (92,98).

    Mouse Models. Numerous studies in mice show that dermal exposure results in immunologic sensitization characterized by IgG and IgE antibody production and predominantly T_H2 cytokine production in the draining lymph node, following dermal challenge (99–101). Nevertheless, little effort has been applied to developing murine models for acid anhydride–induced asthma. Inhalation exposure to 5 mg/m^3 of TMA for one hour per day for three days resulted in the production of specific IgE and IgG antibodies in BALB/c mice, although no measures of asthma were examined (102). Subsequently, Regal et al. (103) developed a model in which BALB/c mice were sensitized by intradermal injection of 3% TMA in corn oil on days 1 and 3, followed by an intratracheal boost with TMA–MSA (30 or 400 µg) on day 12 and subsequently challenged on days 19, 22, and 23 via the intratracheal route. This exposure paradigm resulted in lung inflammation dominated by eosinophils. With further characterization, this model may prove useful for determining mechanisms and mediators responsible for causing eosinophilia, characteristic of human occupational asthma induced by acid anhydride exposure.

Animal Models of Occupational Asthma to Other Low-Molecular-Weight Chemicals

Low-Molecular-Weight Chemicals Encountered in Lumber and Woodworking Industries

Occupational asthma from western red cedar is caused by plicatic acid present in the wood. Disease in workers is characterized by early, late, or biphasic asthmatic reactions that are associated with infiltration of eosinophils into the lung, although the mechanisms responsible remain to be elucidated (104). Chan et al. (105) immunized neonatal rabbits with plicatic acid–ovalbumin conjugates mixed with Al(OH)$_3$ using a vigorous regimen to produce specific IgE antibodies. In addition, immunized rabbits reacted to intravenous challenge with plicatic acid–protein conjugates with increases in respiratory frequency and pulmonary resistance, although these rabbits failed to respond to plicatic acid challenge by inhalation. In follow-up studies, guinea pigs were immunized to the plicatic acid–ovalbumin conjugate by intraperitoneal injection of 10 µg adsorbed to Al(OH)$_3$ once a month for six months (106). Sensitization allowed for the development of specific IgG$_1$ antibodies to plicatic acid in the serum and plicatic acid–mediated release of histamine and eicosanoids from mast cells obtained from the lungs. In addition, trachea isolated from sensitized guinea pigs demonstrated an IgG-dependent increase in contraction following treatment with plicatic acid.

OCCUPATIONAL ASTHMA TO HIGH-MOLECULAR-WEIGHT PROTEIN ALLERGENS

Unlike low-molecular-weight asthmogens, less effort has been devoted to establish and characterize animal models for high-molecular-weight occupational asthmogens, these usually being proteins. This is despite the fact that there is a considerable inci-dence of asthma in certain occupations involving materials such as latex and subtili-sin (proteolytic enzymes of bacterial origin found in detergents). This problem is probably as much because of the difficulties in establishing realistic exposure para-digms as to the fact that ovalbumin animal models have served well, from the point of view of mechanistic studies. In this respect, ovalbumin animal models have also been used to assess the "adjuvant" activity of many occupational and environmental pollutants such as ozone and diesel exhausts (107–112). Historically, guinea pig has been the animal of choice to identify respiratory protein allergens, although not necessarily related to asthma (113). This is because of the ease with which they become sensitized and respond to allergen challenge following inhalation or intratra-cheal instillation. Responses have been measured by relatively simple, nonspecific events such as monitoring labored breathing, to more complicated methods such as whole body plethysmography as well as assessment for changes in histology and biochemical mediators (21,70). Guinea pigs were used to identify the occupational allergen, subtilisin (114). In these studies, animals sensitized to 150 μg/m^3 subtilisin 15 minutes per day for five consecutive days demonstrated both immediate- and delayed-onset respiratory responses. Ritz et al. (115) and later Sarlo et al. (116) deve-loped an intratracheal model in guinea pigs using exposure levels of subtilisin similar to the then threshold limit value. The relative ability of proteins to give rise to the formation of anaphylactic antibody in the guinea pig has been used as an indicator of its ability to produce asthma, although its positive predictive value is inconclusive (113,116,117). Recently, an alternative model has been proposed, which assesses the formation of specific IgG$_1$ antibody in a mouse intranasal test, the assumption being that specific IgG$_1$ antibody is a surrogate for anaphylactic antibody in the mouse (117).

Although latex products have been used for over a century, latex allergies have received worldwide attention only during the last decade. Latex allergies include both allergic contact dermatitis and IgE-mediated pulmonary responses, although the latter is less common (118). Aamir et al. (119) first demonstrated that the cuta-neous response to latex proteins in guinea pigs is mediated by IgE and induced systemic anaphylaxis to latex proteins using a passive systemic anaphylaxis assay. Guinea pigs were also used initially to identify the most active (immunogenic) frac-tions from latex, which contains over 250 peptides (120). In mice, exposure to latex proteins through the respiratory tract results in elevated nonspecific AHR following nonspecific or latex-specific challenge and pulmonary histopathology consistent with the presence of eosinophils and dose-dependent increases in total IgE. The latter occurs independent of the exposure route (121–123). In a detailed study, Hardy et al. (124) observed that sensitization of mice with either Hev b 5, a major latex allergen, or latex glove protein extract by intraperitoneal injection resulted in a pat-tern of response similar to that which occurs following ovalbumin sensitization. This included antigen-specific IgE, eosinophilic pulmonary infiltration, elevated levels of IL-5 protein in lung lavage fluid, and epithelial cell mucus hypersecretion in the lung airways. Studies by Xia et al. (125) noted latex-specific IgE and IgG$_1$ antibodies, increased antigen-specific airway resistance, and histological evidence for eosinophi-lia, goblet cell metaplasia, and inflammatory cell infiltration, following intranasal challenge of BALB/c mice with latex proteins. Sensitization was induced by intrana-sal administration of 30 μg of latex proteins twice per week for four weeks. IgE-specific antibodies and eosinophils were absent in mice deficient in IL-4 following this exposure regimen (125).

SUMMARY AND FUTURE DIRECTIONS

Controversy surrounds the nature of the antigen, role of specific antibodies, and the role of T lymphocyte–subsets in orchestrating the pathophysiological response leading to occupational asthma. Animal models of occupational asthma share common features with human disease, although no single model recapitulates the disease in its entirety. Newer murine models of occupational asthma have made progress toward a more accurate representation of human exposure and disease. For example, mouse models of diisocyanate asthma have identified a role for both T_H1 and T_H2 cells as well as $CD4^+$ and $CD8^+$ T lymphocytes, and evidence now strongly suggests that reagenic antibodies provide a major contribution to disease outcome, indicating the need for better antibody detection systems in humans. Species differences in susceptibility to sensitization and clinical disease outcome strongly support the hypothesis of genetic predisposition to occupational asthma and support recent findings in human studies. Demonstration of sensitization in animal models at exposure concentrations below current exposure limits should be used to prompt reexamination of such limits. Continued use of animal models will enable the pursuit of novel findings from patient-oriented studies and will facilitate improvement of preventive, therapeutic, and diagnostic interventions aimed at improving worker safety and health.

REFERENCES

1. Lombardo LJ, Balmes JR. Occupational asthma: a review. Environ Health Perspect 2000; 108(suppl 4):697–704.
2. Gautrin D, Newman-Taylor AJ, Nordman H, Malo JL. Controversies in epidemiology of occupational asthma. Eur Respir J 2003; 22:551–559.
3. Liu Q, Wisnewski AV. Recent developments in diisocyanate asthma. Ann Allergy Asthma Immunol 2003; 90:35–41.
4. Lemiere C, Romeo P, Chaboillez S, Tremblay C, Malo JL. Airway inflammation and functional changes after exposure to different concentrations of isocyanates. J Allergy Clin Immunol 2002; 110:641–646.
5. Saetta M, Maestrelli P, Turato G, et al. Airway wall remodeling after cessation of exposure to isocyanates in sensitized asthmatic subjects. Am J Respir Crit Care Med 1995; 151:489–494.
6. Piirila PL, Nordman H, Keskinen HM, et al. Long-term follow-up of hexamethylene diisocyanate-, diphenylmethane diisocyanate-, and toluene diisocyanate-induced asthma. Am J Respir Crit Care Med 2000; 162:516–522.
7. Padoan M, Pozzato V, Simoni M, et al. Long-term follow-up of toluene diisocyanate-induced asthma. Eur Respir J 2003; 21:637–640.
8. Maghni K, Lemiere C, Ghezzo H, Yuquan W, Malo JL. Airway inflammation after cessation of exposure to agents causing occupational asthma. Am J Respir Crit Care Med 2004; 169:367–372.
9. Saetta M, Di Stefano A, Maestrelli P, et al. Airway mucosal inflammation in occupational asthma induced by toluene diisocyanate. Am Rev Respir Dis 1992; 145:160–168.
10. Lee M, Park S, Park HS, Youn JK. Cytokine secretion patterns of T cells responding to haptenized-human serum albumin in toluene diisocyanate (TDI)-induced asthma patients. J Korean Med Sci 1998; 13:459–465.
11. Lummus ZL, Alam R, Bernstein JA, Bernstein DI. Diisocyanate antigen-enhanced production of monocyte chemoattractant protein-1, IL-8, and tumor necrosis factor-alpha by peripheral mononuclear cells of workers with occupational asthma. J Allergy Clin Immunol 1998; 102:265–274.

12. Wisnewski AV, Herrick CA, Liu Q, Chen L, Bottomly K, Redlich CA. Human gamma/delta T-cell proliferation and IFN-gamma production induced by hexamethylene diisocyanate. J Allergy Clin Immunol 2003; 112:538–546.

13. Cartier A, Grammer L, Malo JL, et al. Specific serum antibodies against isocyanates: association with occupational asthma. J Allergy Clin Immunol 1989; 84:507–514.

14. Bernstein DI, Jolly A. Current diagnostic methods for diisocyanate induced occupational asthma. Am J Ind Med 1999; 36:459–468.

15. Karol MH, Stadler J, Magreni C. Immunotoxicologic evaluation of the respiratory system: animal models for immediate- and delayed-onset pulmonary hypersensitivity. Fundam Appl Toxicol 1985; 5:459–472.

16. Gordon T, Sheppard D, McDonald DM, Distefano S, Scypinski L. Airway hyper-responsiveness and inflammation induced by toluene diisocyanate in guinea pigs. Am Rev Respir Dis 1985; 132:1106–1112.

17. Aoyama K, Huang J, Ueda A, Matsushita T. Provocation of respiratory allergy in guinea pigs following inhalation of free toluene diisocyanate. Arch Environ Contam Toxicol 1994; 26:403–407.

18. Mapp CE, Lapa e Silva JR, Lucchini RE, et al. Inflammatory events in the blood and airways of guinea pigs immunized to toluene diisocyanate. Am J Respir Crit Care Med 1996; 154:201–208.

19. Niimi A, Amitani R, Yamada K, Tanaka K, Kuze F. Late respiratory response and associated eosinophilic inflammation induced by repeated exposure to toluene diisocyanate in guinea pigs. J Allergy Clin Immunol 1996; 97:1308–1319.

20. Ebino K, Ueda H, Kawakatsu H, et al. Isolated airway exposure to toluene diisocyanate results in skin sensitization. Toxicol Lett 2001; 121:79–85.

21. Karol MH, Hauth BA, Riley EJ, Magreni CM. Dermal contact with toluene diisocyanate (TDI) produces respiratory tract hypersensitivity in guinea pigs. Toxicol Appl Pharmacol 1981; 58:221–230.

22. Karol MH. Concentration-dependent immunologic response to toluene diisocyanate (TDI) following inhalation exposure. Toxicol Appl Pharmacol 1983; 68:229–241.

23. Karol MH. The development of an animal model for TDI asthma. Bull Eur Physio-pathol Respir 1987; 23:571–576.

24. Lemiere C, Romeo P, Chaboillez S, Tremblay C, Malo JL. Airway inflammation and functional changes after exposure to different concentrations of isocyanates. J Allergy Clin Immunol 2002; 110:641–646.

25. Raulf M, Tennie L, Potthast J, Marek J, Baur X. Cellular and mediator profile in bronchoalveolar lavage of guinea pigs after toluene diisocyanate (TDI) expo-sure. Lung 1995; 173:57–68.

26. Huang J, Aoyama K, Ueda A. Experimental study on respiratory sensitivity to inhaled toluene diisocyanate. Arch Toxicol 1993; 67:373–378.

27. Pauluhn J. Assessment of respiratory hypersensitivity in guinea pigs sensitized to toluene diisocyanate: improvements on analysis of respiratory response. Fundam Appl Toxicol 1997; 40:211–219.

28. Jin R, Day BW, Karol M. Toluene diisocyanate protein adducts in the bronchoalveo-lar lavage of guinea pigs exposed to vapors of the chemical. Chem Res Toxicol 1993; 6:906–912.

29. Chen SE, Bernstein IL. The guinea pig model of diisocyanate sensitization. I. Immuno-logic studies. J Allergy Clin Immunol 1982; 70:383–392.

30. Pauluhn J, Eidmann P, Mohr U. Respiratory hypersensitivity in guinea pigs sensitized to 1,6-hexamethylene diisocyanate (HDI): comparison of results obtained with the monomer and homopolymers of HDI. Toxicology 2002; 171:147–160.

31. Blaikie L, Morrow T, Wilson AP, et al. A two-centre study for the evaluation and validation of an animal model for the assessment of the potential of small molecular weight chemicals to cause respiratory allergy. Toxicology 1995; 96:37–50.

32. Rattray NJ, Botham PA, Hext PM, et al. Induction of respiratory hypersensitivity to diphenylmethane-4,4'-diisocyanate (MDI) in guinea pigs. Influence of route of exposure. Toxicology 1994; 88:15–30.

33. Huang J, Millecchia LL, Frazer DG, Fedan JS. Airway hyperreactivity elicited by toluene diisocyanate (TDI)-albumin conjugate is not accompanied by airway eosinophilic infiltration in guinea pigs. Arch Toxicol 1998; 72:141–146.

34. Kalubi B, Takeda N, Irifune M, et al. Nasal mucosa sensitization with toluene diisocyanate (TDI) increases preprotachykinin A (PPTA) and preproCGRP mRNAs in guinea pig trigeminal ganglion neurons. Brain Res 1992; 576:287–296.

35. Baur X, Marek W, Ammon J, et al. Respiratory and other hazards of isocyanates. Int Arch Occup Environ Health 1994; 66:141–152.

36. Mapp CE, Lucchini RE, Miotto D, et al. Immunization and challenge with toluene diisocyanate decrease tachykinin and calcitonin gene-related peptide immunoreactivity in guinea pig central airways. Am J Respir Crit Care Med 1998; 158:263–269.

37. Pauluhn J, Rungeler W, Mohr U. Phenyl isocyanate-induced asthma in rats following a 2-week exposure period. Fundam Appl Toxicol 1995; 24:217–228.

38. Kitamura Y, Miyoshi A, Murata Y, Kalubi B, Fukui H, Takeda N. Effect of glucocorticoid on upregulation of histamine H1 receptor mRNA in nasal mucosa of rats sensitized by exposure to toluene diisocyanate. Acta Otolaryngol 2004; 124:1053–1058.

39. Kitamura Y, Miyoshi A, Murata Y, Maeyama K, Takeda N, Fukui H. Increase in the level of histidine decarboxylase mRNA expression in nasal mucosa of rats sensitized by toluene diisocyanate. Inflamm Res 2004; 53(suppl 1):S13–S14.

40. Satoh T, Kramarik JA, Tollerud DJ, Karol MH. A murine model for assessing the respiratory hypersensitivity potential of chemical allergens. Toxicol Lett 1995; 78:57–66.

41. Tse CS, Chen SE, Bernstein IL. Induction of murine reaginic antibodies by toluene diisocyanate. An animal model of immediate hypersensitivity reactions to isocyanates. Am Rev Respir Dis 1979; 120:829–835.

42. Dearman RJ, Basketter DA, Kimber I. Variable effects of chemical allergens on serum IgE concentration in mice. Preliminary evaluation of a novel approach to the identification of respiratory sensitizers. J Appl Toxicol 1992; 12:317–323.

43. Dearman RJ, Spence LM, Kimber I. Characterization of murine immune responses to allergenic diisocyanates. Toxicol Appl Pharmacol 1992; 112:190–197.

44. Dearman R, Moussavi A, Kemeny D, Kimber I. Contribution of CD4+ and CD8+ T lymphocyte subsets to the cytokine secretion patterns induced in mice during sensitization to contact and respiratory chemical allergens. Immunology 1996; 89:502–510.

45. Scheerens H, Buckley TL, Davidse EM, Garssen J, Nijkamp FP, Van Loveren H. Toluene diisocyanate-induced in vitro tracheal hyperreactivity in the mouse. Am J Respir Crit Care Med 1996; 154:858–865.

46. Scheerens H, Buckley TL, Muis TL, et al. Long-term topical exposure to toluene diisocyanate in mice leads to antibody production and in vivo airway hyperresponsiveness three hours after intranasal challenge. Am J Respir Crit Care Med 1999; 159:1074–1080.

47. Matheson JM, Lange RW, Lemus R, Karol MH, Luster MI. Importance of inflammatory and immune components in a mouse model of airway reactivity to toluene diisocyanate (TDI). Clin Exp Allergy 2001; 31:1067–1076.

48. Matheson JM, Lemus R, Lange RW, Karol MH, Luster MI. Role of tumor necrosis factor in toluene diisocyanate asthma. Am J Respir Cell Mol Biol 2002; 27:396–405.

49. Redlich CA, Karol MH. Diisocyanate asthma: clinical aspects and immunopathogenesis. Int Immunopharmacol 2002; 2:213–224.

50. Herrick CA, Xu L, Wisnewski AV, Das J, Redlich CA, Bottomly K. A novel mouse model of diisocyanate-induced asthma showing allergic-type inflammation in the lung after inhaled antigen challenge. J Allergy Clin Immunol 2002; 109:873–878.

51. Lummus ZL, Alam R, Bernstein JA, Bernstein DI. Diisocyanate antigen-enhanced production of monocyte chemoattractant protein-1, IL-8, and tumor necrosis factor-[alpha]

by peripheral mononuclear cells of workers with occupational asthma. J Allergy Clin Immunol 1998; 102:265-274.

52. Vanoirbeek JA, Tarkowski M, Ceuppens JL, Verbeken EK, Nemery B, Hoet PH. Respiratory response to toluene diisocyanate depends on prior frequency and concentration of dermal sensitization in mice. Toxicol Sci 2004; 80:310-321.

53. Herrick CA, Das J, Xu L, Wisnewski AV, Redlich CA, Bottomly K. Differential roles for CD4 and CD8 T cells after diisocyanate sensitization: genetic control of TH2-induced lung inflammation. J Allergy Clin Immunol 2003; 111:1087-1094.

54. Lee KS, Jin SM, Kim HJ, Lee YC. Matrix metalloproteinase inhibitor regulates inflammatory cell migration by reducing ICAM-1 and VCAM-1 expression in a murine model of toluene diisocyanate-induced asthma. J Allergy Clin Immunol 2003; 111:1278-1284.

55. Lee Y, Song C, Lee H, et al. A murine model of toluene diisocyanate-induced asthma can be treated with matrix metalloproteinase inhibitor. J Allergy Clin Immunol 2001; 108:1021-1026.

56. Lee YC, Kwak Y-G, Song CH. Contribution of vascular endothelial growth factor to airway hyperresponsiveness and inflammation in a murine model of toluene diisocyanate-induced asthma. J Immunol 2002; 168:3595-3600.

57. Lee KS, Jin SM, Kim SS, Lee YC. Doxycycline reduces airway inflammation and hyper-responsiveness in a murine model of toluene diisocyanate-induced asthma. J Allergy Clin Immunol 2004; 113:902-909.

58. Lee KS, Jin SM, Lee H, Lee YC. Imbalance between matrix metalloproteinase-9 and tissue inhibitor of metalloproteinase-1 in toluene diisocyanate-induced asthma. Clin Exp Allergy 2004; 34:276-284.

59. Matheson JM, Johnson VJ, Vallyathan V, Luster MI. Exposure and immunological determinants in a murine model for toluene diisocyanate (TDI) asthma. Toxicol Sci 2004; 84:88-98.

60. Matheson JM, Johnson VJ, Luster MI. Immune mediators in a murine model for occupational asthma: studies with toluene diisocyanate. Toxicol Sci 2004; 84:99-109.

61. Maestrelli P, Del Prete GF, De Carli M, et al. CD8 T-cell clones producing interleukin-5 and interferon-gamma in bronchial mucosa of patients with asthma induced by toluene diisocyanate. Scand J Work Environ Health 1994; 20:376-381.

62. Venables KM. Low molecular weight chemicals, hypersensitivity, and direct toxicity: the acid anhydrides. Br J Ind Med 1989; 46:222-232.

63. Zhang XD, Siegel PD, Lewis DM. Immunotoxicology of organic acid anhydrides (OAAs). Int Immunopharmacol 2002; 2:239-248.

64. Griffin P, Allan L, Beckett P, Elms J, Curran AD. The development of an antibody to trimellitic anhydride. Clin Exp Allergy 2001; 31:453-457.

65. Zeiss CR. Advances in acid anhydride induced occupational asthma. Curr Opin Allergy Clin Immunol 2002; 2:89-92.

66. Gautrin D, Ghezzo H, Infante-Rivard C, Malo JL. Incidence and determinants of IgE-mediated sensitization in apprentices. A prospective study. Am J Respir Crit Care Med 2000; 162:1222-1228.

67. Barker RD, van Tongeren MJ, Harris JM, Gardiner K, Venables KM, Newman Taylor AJ. Risk factors for sensitisation and respiratory symptoms among workers exposed to acid anhydrides: a cohort study. Occup Environ Med 1998; 55:684-691.

68. Taylor AJ. HLA phenotype and exposure in development of occupational asthma. Ann Allergy Asthma Immunol 2003; 90:24-27.

69. Botham PA, Hext PM, Rattray NJ, Walsh ST, Woodcock DR. Sensitisation of guinea pigs by inhalation exposure to low molecular weight chemicals. Toxicol Lett 1988; 41:159-173.

70. Pauluhn J, Eben A. Validation of a non-invasive technique to assess immediate or delayed onset of airway hypersensitivity in guinea-pigs. J Appl Toxicol 1991; 11:423-431.

71. Sarlo K, Clark ED, Ferguson J, Zeiss CR, Hatoum N. Induction of type I hypersensitivity in guinea pigs after inhalation of phthalic anhydride. J Allergy Clin Immunol 1994; 94:747–756.

72. Hayes JP, Daniel R, Tee RD, Barnes PJ, Chung KF, Newman Taylor AJ. Specific immunological and bronchopulmonary responses following intradermal sensitization to free trimellitic anhydride in guinea pigs. Clin Exp Allergy 1992; 22:694–700.

73. Hayes JP, Lotvall JO, Baraniuk J, et al. Bronchoconstriction and airway microvascular leakage in guinea pigs sensitized with trimellitic anhydride. Am Rev Respir Dis 1992; 146:1306–1310.

74. Hayes JP, Daniel R, Tee RD, Barnes PJ, Taylor AJ, Chung KF. Bronchial hyperreactivity after inhalation of trimellitic anhydride dust in guinea pigs after intradermal sensitization to the free hapten. Am Rev Respir Dis 1992; 146:1311–1314.

75. Hayes JP, Kuo HP, Rohde JA, et al. Neurogenic goblet cell secretion and bronchoconstriction in guinea pigs sensitised to trimellitic anhydride. Eur J Pharmacol 1995; 292:127–134.

76. Obata H, Tao Y, Kido M, Nagata N, Tanaka I, Kuroiwa A. Guinea pig model of immunologic asthma induced by inhalation of trimellitic anhydride. Am Rev Respir Dis 1992; 146:1553–1558.

77. Larsen CP, Regal JF. Trimellitic anhydride (TMA) dust induces airway obstruction and eosinophilia in non-sensitized guinea pigs. Toxicology 2002; 178:89–99.

78. Arakawa H, Lotvall J, Kawikova I, et al. Airway allergy to trimellitic anhydride in guinea pigs: different time courses of IgG1 titer and airway responses to allergen challenge. J Allergy Clin Immunol 1993; 92:425–434.

79. Fraser DG, Graziano FM, Larsen CP, Regal JF. The role of IgG1 and IgG2 in trimellitic anhydride-induced allergic response in the guinea pig lung. Toxicol Appl Pharmacol 1998; 150:218–227.

80. Hayes JP, Lotvall JO, Barnes PJ, Newman Taylor AJ, Chung KF. Involvement of inflammatory mediators in the airway responses to trimellitic anhydride in sensitized guinea-pigs. Br J Pharmacol 1992; 106:828–832.

81. Arakawa H, Kawikova I, Skoogh BE, et al. Role of arachidonic acid metabolites in airway responses induced by trimellitic anhydride in actively sensitized guinea pigs. Am Rev Respir Dis 1993; 147:1116–1121.

82. Arakawa H, Lotvall J, Linden A, Kawikova I, Lofdahl CG, Skoogh BE. Role of eicosanoids in airflow obstruction and airway plasma exudation induced by trimellitic anhydride-conjugate in guinea-pigs 3 and 8 weeks after sensitization. Clin Exp Allergy 1994; 24:582–589.

83. Arakawa H, Andius P, Kawikova I, Skoogh BE, Lofdahl CG, Lotvall J. Treatment with cyclosporin A during sensitization with trimellitic anhydride attenuates the airway responses to allergen challenge three weeks later. Eur J Pharmacol 1994; 252: 313–319.

84. Larsen CP, Regal RR, Regal JF. Trimellitic anhydride-induced allergic response in the guinea pig lung involves antibody-dependent and -independent complement system activation. J Pharmacol Exp Ther 2001; 296:284–292.

85. Fraser DG, Regal JF, Arndt ML. Trimellitic anhydride-induced allergic response in the lung: role of the complement system in cellular changes. J Pharmacol Exp Ther 1995; 273:793–801.

86. Leach CL, Hatoum NS, Ratajczak HV, Zeiss CR, Roger JC, Garvin PJ. The pathologic and immunologic response to inhaled trimellitic anhydride in rats. Toxicol Appl Pharmacol 1987; 87:67–80.

87. Zeiss CR, Levitz D, Leach CL, et al. A model of immunologic lung injury induced by trimellitic anhydride inhalation: antibody response. J Allergy Clin Immunol 1987; 79:59–63.

88. Leach CL, Hatoum NS, Sherwood RL, Zeiss CR, Garvin PJ. Pulmonary cellular and antibody response to trimellitic anhydride inhalation. Inhal Toxicol 1989; 1:37–47.

89. Chandler MJ, Zeiss CR, Leach CL, et al. Levels and specificity of antibody in bronchoalveolar lavage (BAL) and serum in an animal model of trimellitic anhydride-induced lung injury. J Allergy Clin Immunol 1987; 80:223-229.

90. Zeiss CR, Leach CL, Levitz D, Hatoum NS, Garvin PJ, Patterson R. Lung injury induced by short-term intermittent trimellitic anhydride (TMA) inhalation. J Allergy Clin Immunol 1989; 84:219-223.

91. Leach CL, Hatoum NS, Ratajczak HV, Zeiss CR, Garvin PJ. Evidence of immunologic control of lung injury induced by trimellitic anhydride. Am Rev Respir Dis 1988; 137:186-190.

92. Pauluhn J. Respiratory hypersensitivity to trimellitic anhydride in Brown Norway rats: analysis of dose-response following topical induction and time course following repeated inhalation challenge. Toxicology 2003; 194:1-17.

93. Andius P, Arakawa H, Molne J, Pullerits T, Skoogh BE, Lotvall J. Inflammatory responses in skin and airways after allergen challenge in brown Norway rats sensitized to trimellitic anhydride. Allergy 1996; 51:556-562.

94. Cui ZH, Sjostrand M, Pullerits T, Andius P, Skoogh BE, Lotvall J. Bronchial hyperresponsiveness, epithelial damage, and airway eosinophilia after single and repeated allergen exposure in a rat model of anhydride-induced asthma. Allergy 1997; 52:739-746.

95. Cui ZH, Skoogh BE, Pullerits T, Lotvall J. Bronchial hyperresponsiveness and airway wall remodelling induced by exposure to allergen for 9 weeks. Allergy 1999; 54: 1074-1082.

96. Zhang XD, Murray DK, Lewis DM, Siegel PD. Dose-response and time course of specific IgE and IgG after single and repeated topical skin exposure to dry trimellitic anhydride powder in a Brown Norway rat model. Allergy 2002; 57:620-626.

97. Zhang XD, Fedan JS, Lewis DM, Siegel PD. Asthma like biphasic airway responses in Brown Norway rats sensitized by dermal exposure to dry trimellitic anhydride powder. J Allergy Clin Immunol 2004; 113:320-326.

98. Arts JH, Bloksma N, Leusink-Muis T, Kuper CF. Respiratory allergy and pulmonary irritation to trimellitic anhydride in Brown Norway rats. Toxicol Appl Pharmacol 2003; 187:38-49.

99. Dearman RJ, Warbrick EV, Humphreys IR, Kimber I. Characterization in mice of the immunological properties of five allergenic acid anhydrides. J Appl Toxicol 2000; 20:221-230.

100. Dearman RJ, Filby A, Humphreys IR, Kimber I. Interleukins 5 and 13 characterize immune responses to respiratory sensitizing acid anhydrides. J Appl Toxicol 2002; 22:317-325.

101. Plitnick LM, Loveless SE, Ladics GS, et al. Cytokine profiling for chemical sensitizers: application of the ribonuclease protection assay and effect of dose. Toxicol Appl Pharmacol 2002; 179:145-154.

102. Dearman RJ, Hegarty JM, Kimber I. Inhalation exposure of mice to trimellitic anhydride induces both IgG and IgE anti-hapten antibody. Int Arch Allergy Appl Immunol 1991; 95:70-76.

103. Regal JF, Mohrman ME, Sailstad DM. Trimellitic anhydride-induced eosinophilia in a mouse model of occupational asthma. Toxicol Appl Pharmacol 2001; 175:234-242.

104. Obata H, Dittrick M, Chan H, Chan-Yeung M. Sputum eosinophils and exhaled nitric oxide during late asthmatic reaction in patients with western red cedar asthma. Eur Respir J 1999; 13:489-495.

105. Chan H, Tse KS, Van Oostdam J, Moreno R, Pare PD, Chan-Yeung M. A rabbit model of hypersensitivity to plicatic acid, the agent responsible for red cedar asthma. J Allergy Clin Immunol 1987; 79:762-767.

106. Salari H, Howard S, Chan H, Dryden P, Chan-Yeung M. Involvement of immunologic mechanisms in a guinea pig model of western red cedar asthma. J Allergy Clin Immunol 1994; 93:877-884.

107. Depuydt PO, Lambrecht BN, Joos GF, Pauwels RA. Effect of ozone exposure on allergic sensitization and airway inflammation induced by dendritic cells. Clin Exp Allergy 2002; 32:391–396.

108. Neuhaus-Steinmetz U, Uffhausen F, Herz U, Renz H. Priming of allergic immune responses by repeated ozone exposure in mice. Am J Respir Cell Mol Biol 2000; 23:228–233.

109. Tsai JJ, Lin YC, Kwan ZH, Kao HL. Effects of ozone on ovalbumin sensitization in guinea pigs. J Microbiol Immunol Infect 1998; 31:225–232.

110. Fujimaki H, Ui N, Ushio H, Nohara K, Endo T. Roles of CD4+ and CD8+ T cells in adjuvant activity of diesel exhaust particles in mice. Int Arch Allergy Immunol 2001; 124:485–496.

111. Ichinose T, Takano H, Miyabara Y, Sadakaneo K, Sagai M, Shibamoto T. Enhancement of antigen-induced eosinophilic inflammation in the airways of mast-cell deficient mice by diesel exhaust particles. Toxicology 2002; 180:293–301.

112. Takano H, Ichinose T, Miyabara Y, Yoshikawa T, Sagai M. Diesel exhaust particles enhance airway responsiveness following allergen exposure in mice. Immunopharmacol Immunotoxicol 1998; 20:329–336.

113. Sarlo K, Karol M. Guinea pig predictive tests for respiratory hypersensitivity. In: Dean JH, Luster MI, Munson AE, Kimber I, eds. Immunotoxicology and Immunopharmacology. New York: Raven, 1994:703–720.

114. Thorne PS, Hillebrand J, Magreni C, Riley EJ, Karol MH. Experimental sensitization to subtilisin. I. Production of immediate- and late-onset pulmonary reactions. Toxicol Appl Pharmacol 1986; 86:112–123.

115. Ritz HL, Evans BL, Bruce RD, Fletcher ER, Fisher GL, Sarlo K. Respiratory and immunological responses of guinea pigs to enzyme-containing detergents: a comparison of intratracheal and inhalation modes of exposure. Fundam Appl Toxicol 1993; 21: 31–37.

116. Sarlo K, Fletcher ER, Gaines WG, Ritz HL. Respiratory allergenicity of detergent enzymes in the guinea pig intratracheal test: association with sensitization of occupationally exposed individuals. Fundam Appl Toxicol 1997; 39:44–52.

117. Blaikie L, Basketter DA. Experience with a mouse intranasal test for the predictive identification of respiratory sensitization potential of proteins. Food Chem Toxicol 1999; 37:889–896.

118. Meade BJ, Weissman DN, Beezhold DH. Latex allergy: past and present. Int Immunopharmacol 2002; 2:225–238.

119. Aamir R, Safadi GS, Mandelik J, et al. A guinea pig model of hypersensitivity to allergenic fractions of natural rubber latex. Int Arch Allergy Immunol 1996; 110:187–194.

120. Hunt LW, Boone-Orke JL, Fransway AF, et al. A medical-center-wide, multidisciplinary approach to the problem of natural rubber latex allergy. J Occup Environ Med 1996; 38:765–770.

121. Kurup VP, Kumar A, Choi H, et al. Latex antigens induce IgE and eosinophils in mice. Int Arch Allergy Immunol 1994; 103:370–377.

122. Thakker JC, Xia JQ, Rickaby DA, et al. A murine model of latex allergy-induced airway hyperreactivity. Lung 1999; 177:89–100.

123. Woolhiser MR, Munson AE, Meade BJ. Immunological responses of mice following administration of natural rubber latex proteins by different routes of exposure. Toxicol Sci 2000; 55:343–351.

124. Hardy CL, Kenins L, Drew AC, Rolland JM, O'Hehir RE. Characterization of a mouse model of allergy to a major occupational latex glove allergen Hev b 5. Am J Respir Crit Care Med 2003; 167:1393–1399.

125. Xia JQ, Rickaby DA, Kelly KJ, Choi H, Dawson CA, Kurup VP. Immune response and airway reactivity in wild and IL-4 knockout mice exposed to latex allergens. Int Arch Allergy Immunol 1999; 118:23–29.

7

Clinical Assessment and Management of Occupational Asthma

David I. Bernstein and Paloma Campo
Division of Allergy–Immunology, Department of Internal Medicine, College of Medicine, University of Cincinnati, Cincinnati, Ohio, U.S.A.

Xaver Baur
Department of Occupational Medicine, Ordinariat und Zentral Institut für Arbeitsmedizin Hamburg, Institute of Occupational Medicine, University of Hamburg, Hamburg, Germany

Illustrative Case History: A 31-year-old carpenter worked for seven years in a piano factory where he came in regular contact with wood dust of various tree species. He also regularly used glue that contained methylene diphenyl-diisocyanate (MDI). Wood planks were painted with the glue and then heated in an oven at 100°C. After two years at work, the carpenter developed cough, dyspnea, and urticaria during work, which improved when at home or on vacation. He also noticed conjunctival inflammation and rhinorrhea when planing mahogany and obeche wood. The worker was referred to an occupational health clinic for evaluation of suspected allergy to wood.

What studies and tests are needed to confirm the diagnosis and identify a causative agent?

INTRODUCTION

The initial assessment of an individual worker suspected of having occupational asthma (OA) should include a comprehensive occupational history, spirometry, and a search for potential causative agents in the workplace. Exposure assessment is an essential component of the overall evaluation of a patient suspected of OA. In this chapter, evaluation of OA due to suspected sensitizing agents is addressed. Since the last edition of this text, new biomarkers of inflammation [e.g., exhaled nitric oxide (eNO) and induced sputum] have been investigated as diagnostic aids for evaluation of OA, and some of these may prove to be useful. However, performing lung function studies at the work site and/or during specific inhalation challenge (SIC) testing remain(s) the essential tools for confirming the diagnosis of OA (1). Both traditional and novel diagnostic approaches are reviewed in this chapter. Finally, an evidence-based algorithm for clinical diagnosis of OA is presented.

Table 1   Key Elements of the Occupational History in the Evaluation of OA

Demographic information

Employment history
  Current department and jobs including dates begun, interrupted, and ended
  List all processes and substances used in the employee's work environment. A schematic
    diagram of the workplace is useful to track exposures emanating from immediate and
    adjacent work areas
  List prior jobs at current workplace with description of job, duration and materials used

Prior employment and job descriptions

Symptoms
  Categories
  Chest tightness, wheezing, cough, shortness of breath
  Nasal rhinorrhea, sneezing, lacrimation, and ocular itching
  Systemic symptoms: fever, arthralgias, myalgias
  Duration of symptoms
  Duration of employment at the current job prior to onset of symptoms
  Identify temporal pattern of symptoms in relationship to work
  Immediate onset beginning at work with resolution soon after coming home
  Delayed onset beginning 4–12 hrs after starting work or after coming home
  Immediate onset followed by recovery with symptoms recurring 4–12 hrs after initial
    work exposure
  Improvement away from work

Identify potential risk factors
  Current smoking status and candidate number of pack years
  Asthmatic symptoms preceding current work exposure
  Atopic status
  History of seasonal nasal or ocular symptoms
  Familial history of atopic disease
  Confirmation by percutaneous testing to a panel of common aeroallergens
  History of accidental exposures to substances (e.g., heated gas fumes or chemical spills)

Abbreviation: OA, occupational asthma.

THE OCCUPATIONAL HISTORY

It is essential to obtain a comprehensive and detailed occupational history of all patients presenting with work-related asthmatic symptoms. Failure of clinicians to recognize early manifestations can delay the diagnosis of OA for months or years. A physician, experienced in the evaluation of occupational diseases, is more likely to inquire about current and previous employment, workplace exposure to sensitizing agents, and work-related respiratory symptoms. A cursory interview is less informative than a structured occupational history that is designed to maximize the capture of essential data and minimize important omissions. Structured questionnaires supplement the physician's nondirected interview. An outline of essential data is shown in Table 1. An itemized questionnaire has been published that was developed conjointly by the University of Cincinnati Occupational Allergy Laboratory and the National Institute of Occupational Safety and Health (NIOSH) (2,3).

Employment and Exposure History

The employment history must be detailed and comprehensive (Table 1). All details of the worker's job must be documented, as should substances to which there is either direct or indirect exposure. The duration and nature of exposure to all agents currently or previously encountered at work should be recorded. Material safety data sheets, which must be supplied by employers in the United States, and any environmental monitoring reports if present, should be requested and studied in detail (4). Industrial hygiene sampling may provide information about the nature and magnitude of potential sources of exposure to suspect causative agents. The list of substances present in the workplace should be checked against a comprehensive list of agents known to cause OA (see Appendix). Such lists are posted on various web sites, which are cited in the Appendix. Failure to find citations for a suspected substance found in the workplace should not be a reason for its exclusion as a cause because new etiologic agents are continuously being recognized. It is important to document the efficiency of control and the secondary prevention measures such as general hygiene practice, ventilation systems, enclosure of hazardous processes, and the use of respiratory protective devices. All aspects of work processes must be thoroughly reviewed to identify jobs or tasks that could be associated with ambient exposure to aerosols, dusts, or fumes. Processes in adjacent work areas must also be reviewed, as indirect exposure to substances could be significant. All preceding jobs of the worker should be listed to determine if there was any prior exposure (and possibly sensitization) to agents similar or identical to those to which the worker is currently exposed. Workers should be queried about any encounter with accidental spills or exposure(s) to toxic chemicals, fumes, or smoke, which preceded the onset of asthma symptoms and which are known to initiate development of OA or reactive airways dysfunction syndrome (RADS) (5).

Medical History

A worker should be queried about rhinitis and conjunctival symptoms as well as lower respiratory symptoms experienced while at work. Work-related ocular (lacrimation, itching, or burning) and nasal symptoms (sneezing, rhinorrhea, and nasal congestion) that precede or coexist with asthma, are characteristic of immunoglobulin (Ig)E–mediated OA (6) and this is usually present in cases with OA induced by high-molecular-weight (HMW) allergens. In a survey of occupational rhinitis, conducted among workers with confirmed OA, Malo et al. (6) found that rhinitis symptoms were reported in more than 90% and conjunctivitis symptoms in 72% of workers. There was no difference between HMW and low-molecular-weight (LMW) agents in overall prevalence of symptoms, but rhinitis symptoms caused by HMW agents were more intense than those triggered by LMW agents. Prodromal rhinitis symptoms that preceded OA were seen less in cases caused by LMW agents (6).

Contact urticaria is quite frequently associated with sensitization to HMW allergen. Hives may precede or be manifested concomitantly in nearly all workers who develop rhinoconjuctival and asthma symptoms elicited by aerosolized natural rubber latex (NRL) allergens (70). Contact urticaria is common among sensitized laboratory animal workers, and in crab processing workers exposed to snow crab–allergens (11). Coughing while at work often precedes the onset of wheezing or dyspnea. For each symptom, the examining physician must inquire about the duration, time of onset after beginning the workshift, and if symptoms persist or resolve on weekends and vacations. It should also be determined whether each reported symptom or group of symptoms is temporally related to exposure to a substance(s) at work. The duration of the "latency period," or exposure to a substance in the workplace prior to the onset of asthmatic symptoms, should be quantified. A latency period from months to years is characteristic of IgE-mediated OA caused by HMW allergens as well as by certain reactive chemicals (e.g., acid anhydrides). Although rare, respiratory sensitization and OA may follow a chemical (e.g., diisocyanates) spill, a rare scenario in which there is no identifiable latency period (7).

Ocular burning, nasal stuffiness, rhinorrhea, and cough (and sometimes epistaxis) occurring after acute high-level exposure to inhaled chemical fumes or smoke, and in the absence of a latency period, are consistent with irritant-induced responses. Mild irritant symptoms quickly resolve after leaving the workplace. Less than 10% of incidental exposures to high-levels of irritants are followed by development of asthma (5). Diagnostic criteria for RADS are discussed and reviewed in Chapter 25. Cough or asthma that persists long after an acute exposure to an irritant at work should prompt consideration of RADS.

Resolution of respiratory symptoms on weekends or vacations is characteristic of OA as well as work-aggravated asthma provoked by a nonspecific irritant trigger, exercise, or physical stimuli (e.g., cold air) encountered at work. Moderate and severe OA in its advanced stages is characterized by continuous daytime and nocturnal asthmatic symptoms, which often persist on weekends, on vacation, or even months or years after leaving work, reflecting the persistence of nonspecific bronchial hyperresponsiveness. Chronic asthma may persist for months or years after cessation of workplace exposure to a sensitizer (8,9). Thus, the absence of symptomatic improvement following complete cessation of workplace exposure does not exclude a diagnosis of OA. Finally, the physician should inquire about factors that may identify risk factors for OA in individual workers. Smoking has been identified as a risk factor for OA in laboratory animal workers and snow crab–workers (10,11). Surprisingly, nonsmoking workers exposed to red cedar wood dust or diisocyanates are more likely to develop OA than their colleagues who smoke (12). In general, atopic workers are at greater risk than nonatopic workers for OA caused by sensitization to HMW protein allergens (e.g., laboratory animals, NRL, or microbial enzymes) (13,14). Atopic status is not generally considered a risk factor for OA due to reactive chemicals (3). However, Venables and coworkers reported that atopic smokers exposed to tetrachlorophthalic anhydride (TCPA) are more likely to exhibit elevated serum-specific IgE antibodies reactive with TCPA-human serum albumin (HSA) (15). Preexisting airway hyperresponsiveness has not been considered a risk factor for development of OA (12). However, in a prospective study of laboratory animal workers who underwent preemployment evaluations, Gautrin et al. (16) found that baseline methacholine responsiveness ($PC_{20} < 32$ mg/mL) was associated with subsequent development of OA among apprentices exposed to laboratory animals.

Physical examination is rarely helpful in evaluating OA unless wheezing is auscultated during or after the workshift. Because the chest examination is often normal, the absence of wheezing should not deter the clinician from insistently evaluating workers reporting asthmatic symptoms. Auscultation of inspiratory crackles should prompt evaluation for occupational pneumoconiosis, hypersensitivity pneumonitis, or congestive heart failure. In such cases, a chest X ray is required to exclude nonasthmatic cardiopulmonary disorders.

IMMUNOLOGIC ASSESSMENT

Although demonstration of allergic sensitization to a suspected causative agent is quite informative, such findings alone do not confirm OA. For HMW sensitizers, the skin-prick test is preferred because it is sensitive, rapid, and inexpensive. However, the capacity to conduct a skin test or measure specific IgE depends entirely upon availability of well-characterized test antigens. Unfortunately, standardized antigens are not commercially available in many countries. Because of the high sensitivity and negative predictive value (NPV), the skin-prick test can be used to exclude OA caused by HMW sensitizers. One example is nonammoniated latex (NAL), which was tested in the United States. NAL was shown in a multicenter study to posses both high sensitivity (99%) and specificity (100% μg/mL), at a test concentration of 100 μg/mL, in identifying health care workers with latex allergy (17). Using specific challenge testing as the diagnostic gold standard, Koskela et al. (18) reported that skin-prick testing with a 1:100 commercial bovine dander extract provided 100% NPV and 100% sensitivity and was therefore useful in evaluating OA.

Skin testing is rarely used for evaluating workers suspected of OA because of sensitization to reactive chemicals. Because of limited experience, the predictive values of such test antigens have not been well-defined (19). Positive skin-prick tests have been elicited with diisocyanate–HSA antigens in anecdotal case reports of OA, but skin testing has very low sensitivity for identifying workers with diisocyanate asthma (DA) (20). Skin-prick testing directly with chloramine T (sulfonechloramide) has been used to confirm sensitization to this bacteriocidal, disinfectant agent, in individual workers with confirmed OA (21,22). In platinum-refining workers, skin-prick testing with hexachloroplatinate salt solutions failed to exhibit adequate diagnostic sensitivity and specificity in identifying workers with OA confirmed by SIC testing (23).

In vitro radioallergosorbent test (RAST) or enzyme-linked immunosorbent assay (ELISA) methods are generally considered less sensitive but more specific than skin testing. However, due to improvements in assay technology, specific IgE assays have been improved during the past 10 years. Koskela et al. (18) studied the utility of bovine serum–specific IgE antibodies measured by quantitative fluoroenzymatic immunoassay (UniCAP[TM], Pharmacia Diagnostics, Kalamazoo, Michigan, U.S.A.). In studies of dairy farmers with positive SIC tests with bovine epidermal extract, a specific IgE level of greater than 5 IU/L possessed 82% sensitivity and 100% specificity for diagnosis of OA.

Cartier et al. (24) reported elevated serum-specific IgE and/or specific IgG binding (performed by ELISA) with diisocyanate–HSA antigens in 72% of workers in whom the diagnosis of OA was confirmed by SIC. The sensitivity of elevated serum-specific IgE was 31% and specificity was 97% for identifying workers with OA, whereas sensitivity and specificity for IgG was 72% and 76%, respectively. Measurements of serum-specific IgG_4 antibodies to chemical antigens have not been shown to be diagnostically useful. It has been suggested that serum-specific IgG responses to diisocyanate antigens primarily reflect exposure rather than disease (25). However, Park et al. (26) reported that elevations in specific IgG for toluene diisocyanate (TDI)-HSA exhibited 46% sensitivity and 92.3% specificity in identifying OA (confirmed with SIC testing) in exposed workers undergoing evaluation for DA. In this study, the authors found a higher prevalence of serum-specific IgG antibodies to TDI–HSA conjugates than that found for specific IgE in patients with TDI-induced asthma. Recently, it is recognized that the mode of antigen preparation can affect assay test characteristics. Wisnewski et al. (27) found that immunoassays performed with antigens prepared by exposing HSA to hexamethylene diisocyanate (HDI) chemical vapors were more highly associated with OA than those assays performed with chemicals–protein antigens prepared in liquid phase.

Some investigators have evaluated the diagnostic utility of specific cellular immune assays. Wisnewski et al. (28) evaluated in vitro lymphocyte proliferation to HDI antigens and discovered significant responses in HDI-exposed workers with OA as well as in asymptomatic exposed workers. Recently, other in vitro techniques measuring antigen-specific cellular responses have been investigated. An assay for measuring in vitro production of monocyte chemoattractant protein-1 (MCP-1) by mononuclear cells cocultured with diisocyanate-HSA antigens (29) was performed in 54 diisocyanate-exposed workers evaluated by SIC for DA. Production of MCP-1 was detected in 79% of the exposed workers with SIC confirmed DA; test specificity was 91%. Further studies of this assay in larger worker populations are required before this test can be adapted for clinical use.

EVALUATION OF OA WITH LUNG FUNCTION STUDIES

The role of lung function testing in the assessment of OA is discussed in Chapter 9. Baseline and postbronchodilator spirometry may reveal reversible airway obstruction and confirm asthma, but is not adequate for confirming OA. Spirometric measurements can also be recorded before and after the workshift to evaluate for work-related obstruction. Ideally, these measurements should be recorded over an entire workweek and during known exposure to the suspect causative substance(s). Unfortunately, there is no guarantee that substantial exposure to a suspect agent will occur on a particular workday. Cross-shift spirometry is considered an insensitive method for documentation of work-related asthma (30). An intrashift change in forced expiratory volume in one second (FEV_1) of 10% or greater is considered significant. It is more desirable to have a technician collect multiple measurements of FEV_1 before, during, and after the workshift and the results compared with control days, or on days at work when the agent is not used. If the latter approach is not feasible, workers can be instructed on self-collection of serial peak expiratory flow rates (PEFR) (12).

Serial Testing of PEFR and Methacholine PC_{20}

For unsupervised monitoring of lung function, Leroyer et al. (31) reported that the sensitivity and specificity of serial self-monitoring of PEFR is superior to self-collection of serial FEV_1 in correctly identifying OA confirmed by specific challenge testing. This finding was attributed to the supposition that lack of direct supervision had an adverse effect on the reliability of self-collected FEV_1 results. It is recommended that PEFR be collected daily every two to three hours if possible (although every four hours is adequate) for two weeks while at work, and for an additional two to three week period when away from work (32). Because the PEFR measurement is an effort-dependent maneuver, careful supervision and monitoring are required. Malo et al. (33) performed a study comparing self-reported peak flow rates with those recorded with an electronic device and found that reported values corresponded precisely to stored values only 52% of the time. Falsification of data, which commonly occurs, can to some extent be reduced by concurrent use of compact computerized devices, which store values and recording times on a memory chip (33–36).

Perrin et al. (37) evaluated the sensitivity and specificity of PEFR monitoring combined with bronchial responsiveness to histamine or methacholine PC_{20}, in comparison to the diagnostic standard SIC testing, in 61 workers undergoing evaluation for OA. PEFR data and PC_{20} values were interpreted by three blinded investigators and there was complete agreement in 78% of cases. Visual analysis of PEFR yielded sensitivity and specificity of 81% and 74%, respectively, and visual interpretation was superior to other analytic methods. Thus, global evaluation of the PEFR records by an experienced clinician is the best method for interpreting peak flow records (37,38). Methods of analysis and interpretation of PEFR data are reviewed extensively in Chapter 9. The presence of significant diurnal variability in PEFR ($\geq 20\%$) detected on days at work, but not on days off work, is consistent with OA. Differences in diurnal variability between workplace and home may not always be apparent in those workers who develop severe persistent OA in which symptoms may continue for months or years after the termination of workplace exposure. Because PEFR variability correlates with airway responsiveness, methacholine inhalation tests are often used to validate abnormal serial PEFR studies by obtaining methacholine PC_{20} on the last day of a PEFR recording at work and two to three weeks after the worker has been away from the work environment (39). A methacholine PC_{20} that increases at least threefold after a period of a few weeks away from work is considered significant (40).

SIC Testing

SIC testing is regarded as the gold standard for establishing OA. The SIC methods and indications are addressed in Chapter 10. Contraindications include other pulmonary diseases, cardiac disease, hypoxemia, and pregnancy. The tests should not be performed if asthma is unstable, or during or immediately after an acute respiratory infection. The SIC test should not be conducted if the baseline FEV_1 is less than 2 L. There are three types of SIC tests: (*i*) the workplace challenge, as already mentioned, which involves closely supervised and frequent monitoring of lung function (e.g., FEV_1) during and away from work exposure to the suspect substance(s); (*ii*) a laboratory challenge involving serial measurements of FEV_1 during simulation of a job or work task; and (*iii*) specific bronchial provocation testing in the laboratory where a challenge substance is generated in a controlled fashion and lung function closely monitored (1,41). Each of these approaches has advantages and disadvantages. During a workplace challenge where there are multiple substances in a given work environment, it may be impossible to identify the exact causative agent. Simulation of the work activity in a closed, well-ventilated chamber does not allow precise control of exposure to the test substance. A controlled specific bronchial provocation test offers relative safety in that aerosols, fumes, or powdered agents can be generated in a closed chamber and the amount of exposure can be regulated and closely monitored. Ideally, exposure to the test substance can be achieved safely at subirritant levels equivalent or below permissible exposure limits in the workplace. Whichever method is selected, lung function must also be monitored on a nonexposure control day. Trained and experienced personnel should perform specific challenge tests in a specialized center where there is adequate resuscitative equipment. It should be mentioned that a false negative SIC test could occur following prolonged absence from the workplace. In these cases, a twofold decrease in methacholine PC_{20}, despite a negative SIC test, could indicate that subsequent repeat SIC testing may become positive following reexposure to the challenge agent at work (42–44).

Based on controlled laboratory inhalation challenge studies, there are three common patterns of work-related asthmatic responses that include early asthmatic responses (EAR), isolated late asthmatic responses (LAR), and dual-phase asthmatic responses, i.e., both EAR and LAR (41). Dual and isolated EAR are quite character-istic of IgE-mediated OA due to HMW and some LMW sensitizers, but these can also occur in the absence of a demonstrable immunologic mechanism (45). An isolated LAR that begins 4 to 12 hours after starting the workshift is detected in about 40% of OA cases because of LMW compounds (e.g., red cedar, diisocyanates) (37).

NONINVASIVE MARKERS OF AIRWAYS INFLAMMATION

Measurement of Exhaled Nitric Oxide (eNO)

Exhaled NO is a noninvasive marker of airway inflammation which is easy to mea-sure and shows a positive correlation with induced sputum eosinophils (46–50). As shown in Figure 1, challenge testing with powdered allergenic latex gloves resulted in significant increases in eNO among NRL sensitized workers with specific nasal or bronchial responses to latex compared with nonsensitized workers, although these differences were noted at 22 hours after NRL glove challenge. Measurements of eNO levels are limited because of the inability to discriminate between those subjects with OA and occupational rhinitis, and because the eNO levels are decreased in smokers; increases in eNO are inhibited by corticosteroid treatment (51). Thus, this tool can only be used in corticosteroid naive workers.

Induced Sputum

Measurement of eosinophils in induced sputum samples has recently been applied to the evaluation of OA. Increases in sputum eosinophil counts have been observed

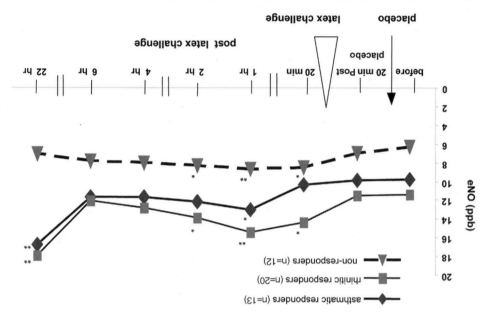

Figure 1 Courses of eNO postlatex allergen challenge of asthmatic responders, rhinitic responders, and nonresponders (mean values). $*p < 0.05$, $**p < 0.01$; eNO 22 hours post chal-lenge vs. respective baseline eNO. *Abbreviation:* eNO, exhaled nitric oxide.

after SIC with different occupational agents (52,53). Recently, Girard et al. (54) evaluated a group of 45 workers and demonstrated a significant change in sputum eosinophil counts in subjects with positive SIC, whereas such changes were not found in SIC negative workers (these workers developed mainly a neutrophilic inflammation). When combined with serial PEF monitoring, and with a cutoff of at least 1% increase in sputum eosinophils considered positive, the sensitivity and specificity of the combined methods for recognizing OA was 50% and 78%, respectively.

DIFFERENTIAL DIAGNOSIS

Many conditions that can be confused with OA must be considered in the differential diagnosis (3). A worker with preexisting asthma can experience bronchoconstriction triggered by nonspecific stimuli including chemical irritants, smoke, or physical factors (e.g., cold air) at work, and this condition would be aptly described as "work-aggravated asthma." Chronic obstructive pulmonary disease or COPD must be considered in workers with dyspnea at work, a condition that is recognized as an occupational disease in some countries. As with non-OA, vocal cord dysfunction, chronic bronchitis, bronchiolitis, pneumonia, pulmonary embolism, congestive heart failure, and other conditions should be considered. Bronchiolitis obliterans, a fibrotic obliterative disease of the terminal bronchioles and small airways, may follow exposure to toxic irritants, gases, or fumes (55). Affected individuals exhibit pulmonary infiltrates, evidence of airway obstruction as well as diffusion abnormalities. Occasionally, nonasthmatic pulmonary diseases such as pneumoconiosis or hypersensitivity pneumonitis can be mistaken for OA. Therefore, a chest roentgenogram and complete pulmonary function testing that includes the testing of lung volumes and diffusion capacity should be performed in all workers suspected of other occupational pulmonary disorders. Metal fume fever presents in welders of galvanized steel. In this disorder, flu-like symptoms, fever, and myalgias, accompanied by dyspnea and cough, continue for 24 to 48 hours after inhalation of fumes containing zinc oxide that is thought to induce lung macrophages to release lung cytokines including tumor necrosis factor-α (21,56,57). The organic dust toxic syndrome presumably is caused by release of endotoxins from microorganisms in grain or humidifiers.

GENERAL APPROACH TO THE CLINICAL ASSESSMENT OF OA

In the earlier editions of this text, a diagnostic algorithm for OA was introduced. Subsequently, the Canadian Thoracic Society published diagnostic guidelines for OA (58). This evidenced-based guideline closely corresponds with the algorithm previously published in *Asthma in the Workplace.*

A more recent guideline has been published by the American Thoracic Society (59). These documents emphasize the importance of evaluating workers for OA while they are still exposed in the work environment, so that essential measurements of lung function can be collected. In fact, these tests should be completed before advising an employee to leave work. Such studies may include methacholine inhalation testing, serial recording of PEFR, and a workplace challenge study. Therefore, it is essential that a worker remains at work until the OA evaluation is completed. This recommendation does not apply to high-risk workers with severe asthmatic symptoms that are consistently triggered at work, and they should be restricted from further exposure.

The clinical assessment of workers suspected of OA should be a stepwise approach. A comprehensive evaluation begins with a detailed medical and occupational history. Elicitation of detailed information pertaining to substances and processes in the workplace is crucial. If single or multiple causative agents are suspected, the clinician should pursue a thorough review of the medical literature and other data sources. As a resource, the editors of this book have provided a compendium of recognized causes of OA, and websites where exhaustive lists of etiologic agents can be found (see Appendix). It may be necessary to visit the plant or worksite and confer with industrial hygienists and safety personnel about the worker's exposure.

RATIONAL APPROACH FOR DIAGNOSING OA

Due to the complexity of modern work environments and the multitude of agents that are encountered by a worker, it can be very difficult to confirm OA and, at the same time, demonstrate causation by a specific agent. It is incumbent upon a consultant to objectively confirm OA because a diagnosis based on history alone is highly nonspecific (60). Although many clinics have intrinsic limitations that preclude immunologic testing to confirm sensitization to a occupational allergen or lack facilities required for specific inhalation testing, OA can be confirmed or excluded in most cases provided that the symptomatic worker is referred early, is still actively exposed, and consequently can be assessed while at work.

A logical diagnostic algorithm that is to be followed to assess OA at work is described in Figure 2. A very similar approach is recommended in the Canadian Guidelines (58). The diagnostic algorithm can be applied only in those workers who remain at work during the entire course of the evaluation. Two decision pathways are presented in the algorithm. The first describes evaluation in the workplace, whereas the second employs controlled specific inhalation testing in the laboratory. If causation by a HMW or LMW allergen is suspected (and if reliable test reagents are available), skin testing or in vitro serologic specific IgE assays are performed to confirm allergic sensitization. Demonstration of sensitization is useful to establish causation to an occupational allergen, when combined with work-related decrements in lung function that improve when away from exposure. A negative skin test, which has high NPV, may be used for excluding sensitization (and OA) due to a suspect HMW protein allergen (17,18).

As shown in Figure 2, the next essential step after obtaining a history and after immunologic testing is to objectively confirm or exclude asthma. This is achieved either by demonstrating reversibility in FEV_1 after bronchodilator treatment or by performing a methacholine test. Unfortunately, reversibility in lung function is often not demonstrable while away from work. In that case, methacholine testing should be performed either while at work or immediately after coming off the workshift at the end of the workweek, and after the worker has been exposed for at least two consecutive weeks. As shown in Figure 2, because of its high NPV, a normal methacholine test ($PC_{20} > 10$ mg/mL) in a symptomatic patient still exposed at work would exclude current asthma (and OA) (58). A positive methacholine test ($PC_{20} \leq 10$ mg/mL) does not establish a specific diagnosis of OA, and therefore must be followed by the monitoring of lung function while at work. To

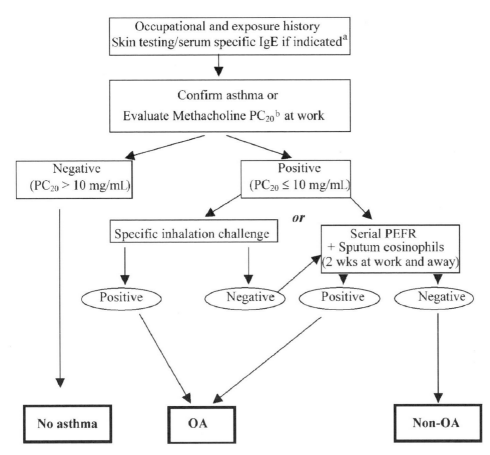

Figure 2 Algorithm for evaluation of OA. *Notes*: [a]A negative skin-prick test with a well-characterized allergen has high NPV and, in the evaluation of HMW allergens, excludes OA to that suspected allergen. [b]A negative methacholine text excludes current asthma and OA with a high degree of medical probability in a worker with current asthma symptoms who is actively exposed to causative agents. *Abbreviations*: HMW, high molecular weight; NPV, negative predictive value; OA, occupational asthma.

accomplish this, serial self-monitoring of PEFR for one to two weeks while at work and two to four weeks while away from work is recommended. OA can be diagnosed with a reasonable degree of medical certainty in workers with a positive methacholine test ($PC_{20} \leq 10$ mg/mL) and serial PEFR data plots compatible with OA, as determined by visual interpretation (i.e., reduced at work and improved at home or on weekends). As mentioned above, the validity of these tests can be confirmed by concurrently demonstrating a threefold fall in methacholine PC_{20} after two weeks of work exposure from preexposure baseline. If workers are not receiving treatment with inhaled corticosteroids, serial induced sputum eosinophils should be obtained in conjunction with PEFR studies and assessed after two weeks at work and two weeks after avoidance of exposure. As previously mentioned, this test can enhance sensitivity and specificity of serial PEFR studies (54).

Alternatively, a workplace challenge is preferable to self-monitoring of PEFR and this can be performed under the supervision of a nurse or a technician. A positive workplace challenge test confirms OA, whereas a test that fails to show a clear relationship between work exposure and reduced lung function is indicative of non-OA. If there is no consistent improvement in the PEFR while away from work, the worker most likely has non-OA. Prevarication of PEFR data, suboptimal technique, and poor adherence are the causes of concern, and there is good evidence showing that workers do not accurately record or report their PEFR readings obtained with portable devices (33). Therefore, whenever possible, an electronic device that records and stores PEFR values on a memory chip should be used.

As shown in Figure 2, an alternate approach for the evaluation of a worker with a positive methacholine test at work is to refer for SIC testing in a suitable laboratory. A SIC test performed in a controlled manner in the laboratory and resulted positive is diagnostic of OA, obviating the need for serial PEFR monitoring or a workplace challenge test. However, a negative laboratory SIC test does not always exclude OA. A false negative result could be attributable to the underestimation of the level or duration of exposure normally encountered and needed to elicit an asthmatic reaction. A negative result could also be due to incorrect identification of the causative agent. For these reasons, all such workers should continue to be monitored closely for PEFR for several weeks after returning to work. Serial PEFR studies that are not consistent with OA would confirm a negative specific inhalation test and definitively exclude OA. If PEFR study results are suggestive of OA even after a negative specific laboratory challenge, a closely supervised workplace challenge test should be performed to confirm OA. The methods for lung physiologic tests as well as their indications, advantages, and limitations are reviewed in other chapters.

OA due to a specific HMW allergen encountered in the work environment is established when there is: (i) history of work-related asthmatic symptoms associated with exposure to a substance which is known to cause OA, (ii) demonstration of significant decrements in lung function at work and improvement while away from work, (iii) positive methacholine test at work, and (iv) evidence of specific IgE-mediated sensitization to the suspect causative agent. The existence of a latency period ranging from months to years prior to the onset of symptoms is also supportive of the diagnosis. Thus, the presence of supportive historical and physiologic findings together with a positive skin-prick test is adequate for making a specific diagnosis of OA due to a HMW allergen (61). Specific bronchoprovocation testing may be considered in cases where there is uncertainty and where objective demonstration of bronchial sensitivity may be necessary to determine whether a worker must be restricted from exposure to the causative substance (1).

CLINICAL MANAGEMENT

In addition to modification of exposure to causative substances, OA is treated in an identical fashion to non-OA. This includes assessment for nonoccupational sensitizers (common aeroallergens) by skin testing and institution of appropriate environmental and pharmacotherapeutic interventions. Such treatment should follow the published asthma guidelines for addressing patients classified as episodic, mild persistent, moderate persistent, and severe asthma (62). Maestrelli et al. (63) demonstrated in a placebo-controlled study that inhaled beclomethasone diproprionate improved methacholine PC_{20} in subjects with TDI-induced asthma, but had no effect in reducing bronchial sensitivity to TDI. Thus, pharmacotherapy for OA should never be considered as a suitable substitute for effective exposure avoidance.

Complete restriction from further exposure to causative agents is usually necessary. Longitudinal studies of worker groups with confirmed OA, induced by diisocyanates and red cedar wood dust, indicate that an early diagnosis relative to the time of onset of asthma symptoms followed by prompt interventions (i.e., exposure cessation), results in favorable outcomes manifested by clinical improvement in asthma (3,8). In red cedar workers with OA, early recognition of symptoms and a preserved FEV_1 were favorable prognostic variables. Thus, an early diagnosis of OA followed by termination of further exposure is likely to prevent persistent morbidity and disability due to chronic asthma, and even asthma mortality. Anecdotal reports of work-related asthma deaths have been reported among symptomatic diisocyanate and bakery workers who remained in the workplace, emphasizing the folly of allowing sensitized workers with OA to remain in a hazardous work environment (64–66).

On the other hand, workers with RADS (irritant-induced asthma) or even work-aggravated asthma can usually continue to work provided adequate measures are implemented to prevent high-level exposure to irritants or triggers (e.g., cold air, tobacco smoke) encountered at work.

After the diagnosis of OA has been confirmed, the employer is required by the American Disabilities Act to institute a needed accommodation for the worker. This may involve interventions, which prevent exposure to levels that are less than the threshold limit value (TLV) recommended by NIOSH in the American Conference of Governmental Industrial Hygienists (ACGIH). Accommodating an employee with work-related asthma may involve use of protective equipment (e.g., respirators) during short-term unavoidable exposures. However, the long-term use of respirators to prevent exposure to sensitizers is generally not effective (58). Once an exposure restriction has been implemented, all workers with OA who continue to work in the same workplace should undergo periodic medical evaluations. Subsequent evidence of deterioration in asthma symptoms or lung function should prompt complete removal of the worker from the workplace followed by medical surveillance. It is likely that strict environmental controls in terms of ideal ventilation systems and respiratory equipment can reduce the incidence of OA but seldom can these completely prevent development of OA.

Identification of a sentinel case of OA in a specific work environment obligates the consultant to consider other employees at risk. Interactions with physicians at the plant or industrial hygiene personnel may lead to specific changes in the work process (e.g., improved ventilation) aimed at reducing exposure to a causative agent. Worker screening and surveillance programs can be implemented if necessary.

Immunomodulation has been investigated as a treatment modality for some causes of OA. Wahn and Siraganian reported improvement in allergic respiratory symptoms among laboratory animal workers receiving immunotherapy with purified rodent proteins (67). Sastre et al. (68) conducted a double-blind, placebo-controlled study of health care workers with NRL allergy, using standardized latex extract. Specific immunotherapy led to a significant reduction in bronchial and nasal symptoms in the treated group documented during the SIC, compared with the placebo, although there were no significant differences in the magnitude of decrease in FEV_1. Significant reductions in percutaneous reactivity to the NRL extract, and decreased responses to the NRL glove use tests were observed in the NRL-treated group compared to placebo. Another placebo-controlled study of NRL immunotherapy in 17 health care workers failed to show significant reduction in asthma symptoms,

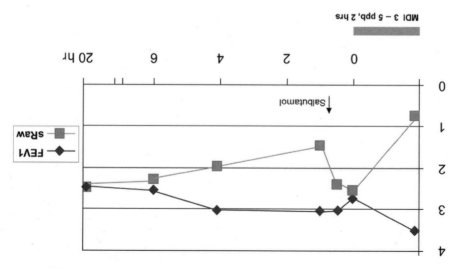

MDI 3 – 5 ppb, 2 hrs

Figure 3 SIC test to MDI in a piano factory worker. *Abbreviations:* MDI, methylene diphenyl-diisocyanate; SIC, specific inhalation challenge.

although rhinitis and cutaneous symptoms related to NRL exposure improved in the treated subjects (69).

Evaluation and Discussion of Illustrative Case History (page 161): Lung function testing of a worker measured after three days at work revealed an FEV_1/FVC ratio of 66% and the airway resistance was 0.54 kPa × s/L (normal less than 0.30). Lung function improved after two days away from work, to FEV_1/FVC ratio of 77%, as did the airway resistance (0.34 kPa × s/L). Skin-prick testing to common aeroaller-gens was positive to grass pollen and house-dust mite *Dermatophagoides pteronyssinus* with no reactivity to wood dust extracts. Serum-specific IgE reactive with MDI-HSA antigens was elevated. The worker returned for SIC testing with MDI (3–5 ppb) that led to a dual-asthmatic response (Fig. 3). Specific challenge tests were negative to mahogany and obeche wood dust samples collected from the workplace. Because a diagnosis of OA due to diisocyanates was established, the worker was advised to leave his job at the piano factory; he requested for and received workers compensation, and subsequently was retrained as a computer specialist. One year later, the patient was asymptomatic with normal lung function parameters.

The history in this worker was suggestive of occupational rhinitis and conjunctivitis and work-related asthma. As shown in the diagnostic algorithm (Fig. 2), the presence of asthma was initially confirmed by demonstrating reversible airway obstruction. Immunologic tests were useful in confirming atopy, in excluding percutaneous sensitization to wood dusts, and in demonstrating specific IgE reactive with MDI-HSA. Despite the fact that lung function was decreased at work, there was uncertainty about which agent was causative. Therefore, in this case, specific challenge testing was indicated which clearly established that MDI, a component of the glue, caused OA and excluded the wood dusts as etiologic agents. This diagnostic assessment was later validated by an excellent outcome documented one year later when the worker returned with no symptoms and with normal lung function. The latter experience underlines the need to establish a timely diagnosis while the worker is still at work and of prompt termination of exposure to the causative substance.

This is a rare presentation of DA, which appears to be IgE-mediated and associated with occupational urticaria.

DIRECTIONS OF FUTURE RESEARCH

- Immunologic diagnosis is hindered by lack of standardized occupational allergens and test protocols. Multicenter, interlaboratory studies will be required to standardize and validate in vitro assays, skin test protocols, and test antigens.
- SIC, the diagnostic gold standard for OA, is not widely available. Future investigations of studies performed in the workplace could identify alternative tests that are predictive of OA.

REFERENCES

1. Cartier A, Bernstein IL, Burge PS, et al. Guidelines for bronchoprovocation on the investigation of occupational asthma. Report of the Subcommittee on Bronchoprovocation for Occupational Asthma. J Allergy Clin Immunol 1989; 84(5 Pt 2):823–829.
2. Smith AB, Castellan RM, Lewis D, Matte T. Guidelines for the epidemiologic assessment of occupational asthma. Report of the Subcommittee on the Epidemiologic Assessment of Occupational Asthma, Occupational Lung Disease Committee. J Allergy Clin Immunol 1989; 84(5 Pt 2):794–805.
3. Bernstein DI, Korbee L, Stauder T, et al. The low prevalence of occupational asthma and antibody-dependent sensitization to diphenylmethane diisocyanate in a plant engineered for minimal exposure to diisocyanates. J Allergy Clin Immunol 1993; 92(3): 387–396.
4. Bernstein JA. Material safety data sheets: are they reliable in identifying human hazards? J Allergy Clin Immunol 2002; 110(1):35–38.
5. Sallie B, McDonald C. Inhalation accidents reported to the SWORD surveillance project 1990–1993. Ann Occup Hyg 1996; 40(2):211–221.
6. Malo JL, Lemiere C, Desjardins A, Cartier A. Prevalence and intensity of rhinoconjunctivitis in subjects with occupational asthma. Eur Respir J 1997; 10(7):1513–1515.
7. Perfetti L, Brame B, Ferrari M, Moscato G. Occupational asthma (OA) with sensitization to diphenylmethane diisocyanate (MDI) presenting at the onset like a reactive airways dysfunction syndrome (RADS). Am J Ind Med 2003; 44(3):325–328.
8. Chan-Yeung M, MacLean L, Paggiaro PL. Follow-up study of 232 patients with occupational asthma caused by western red cedar (*Thuja plicata*). J Allergy Clin Immunol 1987; 79(5):792–796.
9. Moller DR, Brooks SM, McKay RT, Cassedy K, Kopp S, Bernstein IL. Chronic asthma due to toluene diisocyanate. Chest 1986; 90(4):494–499.
10. Venables KM, Upton JL, Hawkins ER, Tee RD, Longbottom JL, Newman Taylor AJ. Smoking, atopy, and laboratory animal allergy. Br J Ind Med 1988; 45(10):667–671.
11. Cartier A, Malo JL, Forest F, et al. Occupational asthma in snow crab-processing workers. J Allergy Clin Immunol 1984; 74(3 Pt 1):261–269.
12. Chan-Yeung M. Occupational asthma. Chest 1990; 98(suppl 5):148S–161S.
13. Sjostedt L, Willers S. Predisposing factors in laboratory animal allergy: a study of atopy and environmental factors. Am J Ind Med 1989; 16(2):199–208.
14. Liss, GM, Sussman GL, Deal K, et al. Latex allergy: epidemiological study of 1351 hospital workers. Occup Environ Med 1997; 54(5):335–342.

15. Taylor AJ, Venables KM, Durham SR, Graneek BJ, Topping MD. Acid anhydrides and asthma. Int Arch Allergy Appl Immunol 1987; 82(3-4):435-439.

16. Gautrin D, Infante-Rivard C, Ghezzo H, Malo JL. Incidence and host determinants of probable occupational asthma in apprentices exposed to laboratory animals. Am J Respir Crit Care Med 2001; 163(4):899-904.

17. Hamilton RG, Adkinson NF Jr. Diagnosis of natural rubber latex allergy: multicenter latex skin testing efficacy study. Multicenter Latex Skin Testing Study Task Force. J Allergy Clin Immunol 1998; 102(3):482-490.

18. Koskela H, Taivainen A, Tukiainen H, Chan HK. Inhalation challenge with bovine dander allergens: who needs it? Chest 2003; 124(1):383-391.

19. Bernstein DI, Zeiss CR. Guidelines for preparation and characterization of chemical-protein conjugate antigens. Report of the Subcommittee on Preparation and Characterization of Low Molecular Weight Antigens. J Allergy Clin Immunol 1989; 84(5 Pt 2): 820-822.

20. Liss GM, Bernstein DI, Moller DR, Gallagher JS, Stephenson RL, Bernstein IL. Pulmonary and immunologic evaluation of foundry workers exposed to methylene diphenyldiisocyanate (MDI). J Allergy Clin Immunol 1988; 82(1):55-61.

21. Dijkman JH, Vooren PH, Kramps JA. Occupational asthma due to inhalation of chloramine-T. I. Clinical observations and inhalation-provocation studies. Int Arch Allergy Appl Immunol 1981; 64(4):422-427.

22. Bourne MS, Flindt ML, Walker JM. Asthma due to industrial use of chloramine. Br Med J 1979; 2(6181):10-12.

23. Merget R, Schultze-Werninghaus G, Bode F, Bergmann EM, Zachgo W, Meier-Sydow J. Quantitative skin prick and bronchial provocation tests with platinum salt. Br J Ind Med 1991; 48(12):830-837.

24. Cartier A, Grammer L, Malo JL, et al. Specific serum antibodies against isocyanates: association with occupational asthma. J Allergy Clin Immunol 1989; 84(4 Pt 1): 507-514.

25. Lushniak BD, Reh CM, Bernstein DI, Gallagher JS. Indirect assessment of 4,4'-diphenylmethane diisocyanate (MDI) exposure by evaluation of specific humoral immune responses to MDI conjugated to human serum albumin. Am J Ind Med 1998; 33(5):471-477.

26. Park HS, Kim HY, Nahm DH, Son JW, Kim YY. Specific IgG, but not specific IgE, antibodies to toluene diisocyanate-human serum albumin conjugate are associated with toluene diisocyanate bronchoprovocation test results. J Allergy Clin Immunol 1999; 104(4 Pt 1):847-851.

27. Wisnewski AV, Stowe MH, Cartier A, et al. Isocyanate vapor-induced antigenicity of human albumin. J Allergy Clin Immunol 2004; 113(6):1178-1184.

28. Wisnewski AV, Herrick CA, Liu Q, Chen L, Bottomly K, Redlich CA. Human gamma/delta T-cell proliferation and IFN-gamma production induced by hexamethylene diisocyanate. J Allergy Clin Immunol 2003; 112(3):538-546.

29. Bernstein DI, Cartier A, Cote J, et al. Diisocyanate antigen-stimulated monocyte chemoattractant protein-1 synthesis has greater test efficiency than specific antibodies for identification of diisocyanate asthma. Am J Respir Crit Care Med 2002; 166(4): 445-450.

30. Burge PS. Single and serial measurements of lung function in the diagnosis of occupational asthma. Eur J Respir Dis Suppl 1982; 123:47-59.

31. Leroyer C, Perfetti L, Trudeau C, L'Archeveque J, Chan-Yeung M, Malo JL. Comparison of serial monitoring of peak expiratory flow and FEV1 in the diagnosis of occupational asthma. Am J Respir Crit Care Med 1998; 158(3):827-832.

32. Malo JL, Cote J, Cartier A, Boulet LP, L'Archeveque J, Chan-Yeung M. How many times per day should peak expiratory flow rates be assessed when investigating occupational asthma? Thorax 1993; 48(12):1211-1217.

33. Malo JL, Trudeau C, Ghezzo H, L'Archeveque J, Cartier A. Do subjects investigated for occupational asthma through serial peak expiratory flow measurements falsify their results? J Allergy Clin Immunol 1995; 96(5 Pt 1):601–607.
34. Quirce S, Contreras G, Dybuncio A, Chan-Yeung M. Peak expiratory flow monitoring is not a reliable method for establishing the diagnosis of occupational asthma. Am J Respir Crit Care Med 1995; 152(3):1100–1102.
35. Henneberger PK, Stanbury MJ, Trimbath LS, Kipen HM. The use of portable peak flowmeters in the surveillance of occupational asthma. Chest 1991; 100(6):1515–1521.
36. Tarlo SM, Broder I. Outcome of assessments for occupational asthma. Chest 1991; 100(2):329–335.
37. Perrin B, Lagier F, L'Archeveque J, et al. Occupational asthma: validity of monitoring of peak expiratory flow rates and non-allergic bronchial responsiveness as compared to specific inhalation challenge. Eur Respir J 1992; 5(1):40–48.
38. Moscato G, Godnic-Cvar J, Maestrelli P. Statement on self-monitoring of peak expiratory flows in the investigation of occupational asthma. Subcommittee on Occupational Allergy of European Academy of Allergy and Clinical Immunology. J Allergy Clin Immunol 1995; 96(3):295–301.
39. Cartier A, Pineau L, Malo JL. Monitoring of maximum expiratory peak flow rates and histamine inhalation tests in the investigation of occupational asthma. Clin Allergy 1984; 14(2):193–196.
40. Crapo RO, Casaburi R, Coates AL, et al. Guidelines for methacholine and exercise challenge testing-1999; This official statement of the American Thoracic Society was adopted by the ATS Board of Directors, Jul 1999. Am J Respir Crit Care Med 2000; 161(1):309–329.
41. Pepys J, Hutchcroft BJ. Bronchial provocation tests in etiologic diagnosis and analysis of asthma. Am Rev Respir Dis 1975; 112(6):829–859.
42. Vandenplas O, Delwiche JP, Jamart J, Van de Weyer R. Increase in non-specific bronchial hyperresponsiveness as an early marker of bronchial response to occupational agents during specific inhalation challenges. Thorax 1996; 51(5):472–478.
43. Lemiere C, Cartier A, Dolovich J, et al. Outcome of specific bronchial responsiveness to occupational agents after removal from exposure. Am J Respir Crit Care Med 1996; 154(2 Pt 1):329–333.
44. Sastre J, Fernandez-Nieto M, Novalbos A, De Las Heras M, Cuesta J, Quirce S. Need for monitoring nonspecific bronchial hyperresponsiveness before and after isocyanate inhalation challenge. Chest 2003; 123(4):1276–1279.
45. Burge PS. Occupational asthma in electronics workers caused by colophony fumes: follow-up of affected workers. Thorax 1982; 37(5):348–353.
46. Payne DN, Adcock IM, Wilson NM, Oates T, Scallan M, Bush A. Relationship between exhaled nitric oxide and mucosal eosinophilic inflammation in children with difficult asthma, after treatment with oral prednisolone. Am J Respir Crit Care Med 2001; 164(8 Pt 1):1376–1381.
47. Kharitonov SA, O'Connor BJ, Evans DJ, Barnes PJ. Allergen-induced late asthmatic reactions are associated with elevation of exhaled nitric oxide. Am J Respir Crit Care Med 1995; 151(6):1894–1899.
48. Gratziou C, Lignos M, Dassiou M, Roussos C. Influence of atopy on exhaled nitric oxide in patients with stable asthma and rhinitis. Eur Respir J 1999; 14(4):897–901.
49. Thomassen MJ, Raychaudhuri B, Dweik RA, et al. Nitric oxide regulation of asthmatic airway inflammation with segmental allergen challenge. J Allergy Clin Immunol 1999; 104(6):1174–1182.
50. Lim S, Jatakanon A, Meah S, Oates T, Chung KF, Barnes PJ. Relationship between exhaled nitric oxide and mucosal eosinophilic inflammation in mild to moderately severe asthma. Thorax 2000; 55(3):184–188.
51. Baur X, B.L. Latex allergen exposure increases exhaled nitric oxide in patients with stable asthma and rhinitis. Eur Resp J. In press.

52. Obata H, Dittrick M, Chan H, Chan-Yeung M. Sputum eosinophils and exhaled nitric oxide during late asthmatic reaction in patients with western red cedar asthma. Eur Respir J 1999; 13(3):489–495.

53. Youakim S. Work-related asthma. Am Fam Physician 2001; 64(11):1839–1848.

54. Girard F, Chaboillez S, Cartier A, et al. An Effective Strategy for Diagnosing Occupational Asthma: Use of Induced Sputum. Am J Respir Crit Care Med 2004; 170(8):845–850.

55. Epler GR, Colby TV. The spectrum of bronchiolitis obliterans. Chest 1983; 83(2):161–162.

56. Blanc PD, Boushey HA, Wong H, Wintermeyer SF, Bernstein MS. Cytokines in metal fume fever. Am Rev Respir Dis 1993; 147(1):134–138.

57. Malo JL, Cartier A. Occupational asthma due to fumes of galvanized metal. Chest 1987; 92(2):375–377.

58. Tarlo SM, Boulet LP, Cartier A, et al. Canadian Thoracic Society guidelines for occupational asthma. Can Respir J 1998; 5(4):289–300.

59. Guidelines for assessing and managing asthma risk at work, school, and recreation. Am J Respir Crit Care Med 2004; 169(7):873–881.

60. Malo JL, Ghezzo H, L'Archeveque J, Lagier F, Perrin B, Cartier A. Is the clinical history a satisfactory means of diagnosing occupational asthma? Am Rev Respir Dis 1991; 143(3):528–532.

61. Bardy JD, Malo JL, Seguin P, et al. Occupational asthma and IgE sensitization in a pharmaceutical company processing psyllium. Am Rev Respir Dis 1987; 135(5):1033–1038.

62. National Asthma Education and Prevention Program. Expert Panel Report: Guidelines for the Diagnosis and Management of Asthma Update on Selected Topics-2002; J Allergy Clin Immunol 2002; 110(suppl 5):S141–S219.

63. Maestrelli P, De Marzo N, Saetta M, Boscaro M, Fabbri LM, Mapp CE. Effects of inhaled beclomethasone on airway responsiveness in occupational asthma. Placebo-controlled study of subjects sensitized to toluene diisocyanate. Am Rev Respir Dis 1993; 148(2):407–412.

64. Ehrlich RI. Fatal asthma in a baker: a case report. Am J Ind Med 1994; 26(6):799–802.

65. Fabbri LM, Danieli D, Crescioli S, et al. Fatal asthma in a subject sensitized to toluene diisocyanate. Am Rev Respir Dis 1988; 137(6):1494–1498.

66. Carino M, Aliani M, Licitra C, Sarno N, Ioli F. Death due to asthma at workplace in a diphenylmethane diisocyanate-sensitized subject. Respiration 1997; 64(1):111–113.

67. Wahn U, Siraganian RP. Efficacy and specificity of immunotherapy with laboratory animal allergen extracts. J Allergy Clin Immunol 1980; 65(6):413–421.

68. Sastre J, Fernandez-Nieto M, Rico P, et al. Specific immunotherapy with a standardized latex extract in allergic workers: a double-blind, placebo-controlled study. J Allergy Clin Immunol 2003; 111(5):985–994.

69. Leynadier F, Herman D, Vervloet D, Andre C. Specific immunotherapy with a standardized latex extract versus placebo in allergic healthcare workers. J Allergy Clin Immunol 2000; 106(3):585–590.

70. Bernstein DI, Karnani R, Biagini RE, et al. Clinical and occupational outcomes in health care workers with natural rubber latex allergy. Ann Allergy Asthma Immunol 2003; 90:209–213.

8

Immunological and Inflammatory Assessments

Catherine Lemiere
Department of Chest Medicine, Sacré-Cœur Hospital, Montreal, Quebec, Canada

Raymond E. Biagini
Biomonitoring and Health Assessment Branch, Robert A. Taft Laboratories, NIOSH/CDC, Cincinnati, Ohio, U.S.A.

C. Raymond Zeiss
Allergy/Immunology Division, Northwestern/Feinberg School of Medicine, Chicago, Illinois, U.S.A.

INTRODUCTION

A 30-year-old man was employed for five years in a platinum refinery. Two years after starting this work, he noticed shortness of breath, chest tightness, wheezing, and a persistent dry cough as well as nasal symptoms—such as runny, stuffy nose and sneezing—when at work. These symptoms improved substantially on weekends. His physical examination and chest radiograph were normal. Allergy skin-prick tests (SPTs) to 19 common extracts were negative. His treatment consisted of the use of an albuterol inhaler as needed, budesonide nasal spray $200\,\mu g/day$, and antihistamines. When at work, he had severe dyspnea; chest tightness; dry cough; wheezing; runny, stuffy nose; and sneezing, and normal spirometry and airway responsiveness. After three weeks off work, he did not complain of any remaining respiratory symptoms. SPTs with platinum salts could not be interpreted reliably, because the subject was taking antihistamines. Radioallergosorbent test (RAST) to platinum salts showed platinum salt–specific immunoglobulin E (IgE). After two weeks at work, induced sputum cell counts showed eosinophilic inflammation (sputum eosinophils: 10%) that decreased after two weeks away from work (sputum eosinophils: 1%). Serial peak expiratory flow (PEF) monitoring did not show any difference between the periods at work and away from work. Methacholine PC_{20} was greater than $16\,mg/mL$ after two weeks at work.

  The next sections discuss the different tests that can be performed to make a diagnosis in this patient. This chapter addresses the current methods for performing an immunological assessment by skin testing and by serological assays, and also describes the role of noninvasive assessment of airway inflammation by sputum cell counts.

IMMUNOLOGICAL ASSESSMENT BY SKIN TESTS

Immunologic assessment of individuals with suspected occupational asthma (OA) by skin testing has been an important tool in the diagnosis of OA, as exemplified by the classic work of Dr. J. Pepys on industrial enzymes in the detergent industry and platinum salts in the refining industry (1,2).

A number of recent excellent reviews on OA and on the epidemiology of asthma in the workplace describe the extensive number and diversity of important occupational allergens (3–9). The examples of occupational agents that have been assessed by skin testing and other diagnostic studies are listed in Table 1 (10–64).

Demonstration of skin test reactivity indicates that the worker has become sensitized to low- or high-molecular-weight allergen in the work environment and is not by itself diagnostic of OA as discussed elsewhere in this volume. The immediate wheal and flare reaction induced by prick or intradermal skin tests to occupational allergens is associated with an underlying IgE antibody–mediated response, which can also be confirmed by specific IgE in vitro assays as discussed below.

Two types of skin tests are employed, the SPT and the intradermal test, with the prick test having safety and specificity and the intradermal test having greater sensitivity, when done with appropriate positive (histamine) and negative (saline) controls. The SPT is usually performed with antigen concentrations between 1 and 10 mg/mL, approximating 10,000 allergy units/mL, while the intradermal tests are conducted at 100- to 1000-fold lower concentrations.

The low-molecular-weight chemical allergens need to be coupled to appropriate carrier molecules to become complete occupational allergens. Although the classic methods of conjugation, in which the reactive chemical is added to a purified protein carrier such as human serum albumin in solution, have served well, newer methods of conjugation, such as the use of isocyanate vapors to haptenize human albumin, may lead to improved diagnostic skin test reagents (65,66).

The acid anhydrides are prototypic, low-molecular-weight, reactive chemical reagents, which have been shown to form bonds in vivo with specific amino acids on the protein carrier molecules in nasal lavage fluid (67). In addition to anhydride hapten specificity, the coupling of anhydrides to human carrier proteins can induce new antigenic determinants (NAD) and elicit specific antibody responses. These new determinants are characterized for specificity with the chemical hapten, but may not be sufficient to completely define the determinant (68). These new determinants are most likely the result of a conformational change in the protein carrier molecule induced by the adducted hapten.

New biochemical techniques allow the detection of anhydride-adducted proteins in human biologic fluids that have added quantitative precision to the assessment of inhalation exposures encountered by workers in the industrial setting (69). These techniques should allow a better understanding of the exposure–response relationships that lead to immunologic sensitization as determined by in vitro and in vivo tests.

IMMUNOLOGICAL ASSESSMENT BY SEROLOGICAL ASSAYS

History

The first evidence that there was a key serum factor important in allergy (found during a blood transfusion) was obtained in 1919, when a case of asthma caused

Table 1 Examples of Etiologic Agents in Occupational Asthma

Agents	Skin test	Immunoassay	Broncho-provocation	References
Arthropods	+	+	+	11
Azodicarbonamide	+	+	+	12
B. subtilis enzymes	+	+	+	13,14
Buckwheat	+	+	+	15,16
Carmine dye	+	+	+	17
Castor bean	+	+	ND	18
Chloramine-T	+	+	+	19
Chromate	+	+	+	20,21
Clam	+	+	+	22
Coffee bean	+	+	+	23
Coriander (nutmeg shell and paprika)	+	+	+	24
DTFB	ND	+	ND	25
Dimethylethanolamine	ND	ND	+	26
Dyes, textile	+	+	+	27
Egg	+	+	+	28,63
Fennel seed	+	+	+	29
Garlic	+	+	+	30
Grasshoppers	+	+	+	31
Hog trypsin	+	+	+	35
HDI	ND	+	+	32
HHPA	+	+	ND	33,34
Laboratory animals	+	+	ND	36
Latex	+	+	+	37
Locusts	+	+	ND	38
Maple wood dust	+	+	+	39
Mealworm	+	+	+	40
MDI	+	+	+	32,41,64
Mite (red spider mite)	+	+	+	42
Mushroom	+	ND	+	43
Nickel	+	+	+	21,44,45
Papain	+	+	+	46
Pancreatic extract	+	ND	+	47
Penicillin	+	ND	+	48
Penicillamine	+	+	+	49
PA, TCPA	+	+	+	50,51
PA	+	+	+	52
Platinum	+	+	+	53,54
Protease bromelain	+	+	+	55
Senna	+	+	+	56
Shrimp	+	+	+	22
Spiramycin	+	+	+	57
TDI	ND	+	+	58,59
TMA	+	+	+	60
Wheat flour components	+	+	+	15,61,62

Abbreviations: DTFB, diazonium tetrafluoroborate; HDI, hexamethylene diisocyanate; HHPA, hexahydrophthalic anhydride; MDI, diphenylmethane diisocyanate; PA, phthalic anhydride; TCPA, tetrachlorophthalic anhydride; TDI, toluene diisocyanate; TMA, trimellitic anhydride; ND, not defined.

by allergy to horse dander was described (70). Praunsitz and Küstner (71) performed their famous passive transfer of a positive skin test, later called the PK test, in 1921. This serum factor was later called reagin. However, despite efforts during the next 40 years, little progress was achieved with regard to isolation and characterization of reagin. In the late 1960s, Ishizaka et al. (72) and Johansson (73) identified the serum factor capable of mediating allergic reactivity as IgE.

Immunoglobulin E

Human IgE is an immunoglobulin of approximately 190,000 Da that circulates in the blood as a monomer. Its concentration in serum is highly age dependent, and it constitutes approximately 0.0005% of the total serum immunoglobulins in adults. The level of total serum IgE is commonly reported in kilo international units per liter (kIU/L) based on the 75/502 IgE standard from the World Health Organization. Conversion of serum IgE levels to mass per volume (µg/L) units is accomplished by multiplying the kIU/L value by 2.4 (1 kIU/L = 2.4 µg/L) (74). The Fc portion of this reaginic antibody attaches to Fc receptors on the surface of target cells, tissue mast cells, and circulating basophils, leaving the F(ab)2 portion of the molecule available to bind with its homologous antigen. The variable region of IgE has an estimated 10^6 to 10^8 antigen-binding specificities (75). Subsequent allergen exposure causes mast cell surface–bound IgE antibody to be cross-linked, leading to an increase in intracellular calcium, and the release of preformed mediators (e.g., histamine and proteases) and newly synthesized lipid-derived mediators (e.g., leukotrienes and prostaglandins) (74). These mediators induce the physiological and anatomical changes ranging from allergic rhinitis, acute allergic urticaria (hives), and extrinsic bronchial asthma, to generalized anaphylactic shock (76).

Measurement of IgE

The discovery of the role of IgE in clinical allergy subsequently resulted in a new generation of in vitro diagnostic assays to measure serum levels of allergen-specific IgE. The first immunoassays (radioimmunosorbent test or paper radioimmunosorbent test, named as such because paper discs were used as the solid support) were developed to quantitate the serum concentration of total IgE and used radioactive iodine ^{125}I as labels. Total serum IgE is currently the only diagnostic allergy test that is regulated under the Federal Clinical Laboratory Improvement Act of 1988 (CLIA-88). Total IgE is almost exclusively measured by a 2-site (capture and detection antibody), noncompetitive immunometric (labeled antibody) assay in which a solid-phase antihuman IgE is used to bind IgE from human serum. Following removal of unbound serum proteins, a second antihuman IgE that is labeled with a radionuclide, enzyme, or fluorophor detects bound IgE. Removal of unbound detection antibody is followed by development and quantitation of the response signal. The quantity of the final assay response signal (counts per minute bound, optical density, fluorescence signal, etc.) measured is proportional to the amount of human IgE that is bound in the middle of the sandwich between the capture and detection antibodies (Fig. 1). The analytical sensitivity of most total serum IgE assays is 0.5 to 1 µg/L (74). In normal individuals, IgE is usually present at low levels where 130 ng/mL represents the upper limit of the normal range. However, a significant number of asymptomatic normal individuals, patients with parasitic diseases, and patients with depressed cell-mediated immunity exceed this level. Also, some

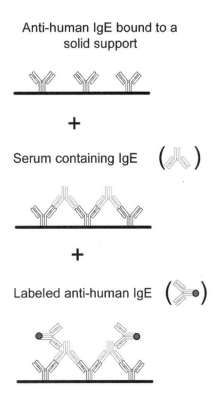

Anti-human IgE bound to a
solid support

+

Serum containing IgE

+

Labeled anti-human IgE

Resultant bound label read
in a fluorimeter,
spectrophotometer or
radioactivity counter

Figure 1 Radioimmunosorbent test (RIST). Antihuman IgE is bound to a solid support, serum is added, and unbound serum proteins are removed. Labeled antihuman IgE is added and the resultant labeled complex measured.

allergic (atopic) persons may exhibit normal total IgE test results in the presence of elevated levels of specific IgE. Although the total serum IgE level is considered useful in the evaluation of an allergic patient, it is more important to demonstrate the presence of allergen-specific IgE in a patient's serum (77).

Measurement of Specific IgE

Allergen-specific IgE was first measured using the RAST in 1967, so called because the secondary antibody was labeled with ^{125}I and an allergen or allergens were bound to an activated (cyanogen bromide) solid support (Sephadex) (77). In brief, a RAST test consists of specific allergen(s) which are bound to a solid-phase support (paper, microtiter well, glass, polystyrene, magnetized beads, or some other surface). Patient serum containing both allergen specific and nonspecific total IgE is incubated with the solid phase material, allowing reaction of the specific IgE in the patient's sample. Excess serum and nonallergen specific IgE is then washed away. Labeled polyclonal or monoclonal antihuman IgE antibody (^{125}I) is added. During this second incubation period, a sandwich complex of allergen-specific IgE and labeled anti-IgE is formed. A subsequent wash removes unbound labeled antibody. Measurement of the remaining labeled anti-IgE is directly proportional to the patient's allergen-specific IgE (Fig. 2).

The acronym RAST in reality refers only to a test where a radionuclide is used as the label for anti-IgE. Numerous other systems using differing solid supports and differing detection systems (various polyclonal and monoclonal anti-IgE detection antibodies) and labels have been described, such as enzyme allergosorbent test, basically an enzyme linked immunosorbent assay, fluorescence enzyme immunoassay, fluorescence allergosorbent test, etc. Examples of indicator systems (labels) used in RAST are I^{125} for radioimmunoassay systems and alkaline phosphatase, horse radish peroxidase, or urease for enzyme-based immunoassay systems. These assays have been automated to the extent that assay precision and reproducibility have been improved [second]-(Pharmacia CAP System) and third-generations (DPC Immulite)] to the level where some IgE antibody assays on autoanalyzers require only singlicate measurements for accurate results (74). In the present chapter, RAST is used to refer to all the specific anti-IgE assays. Systems for measuring specific IgE reactive with

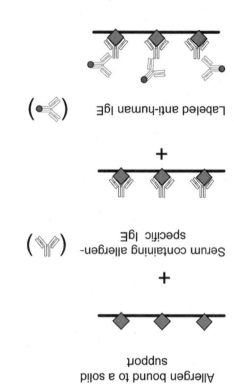

Allergen bound to a solid
support

+

Serum containing allergen-
specific IgE   ( )

+

Labeled anti-human IgE ( )

Resultant bound label read
in a fluorimeter,
spectrophotometer or
radioactivity counter

Figure 2 Radioallergosorbent test (RAST). Allergen is bound to a solid support, serum is added, and unbound serum proteins are removed. Labeled antihuman IgE is added and the resultant labeled complex measured.

multiple allergens simultaneously have also been described (78,79). There are also cell based and other technologies for the detection of allergen-specific IgE antibody. These include the measurement of allergen-induced mediator release [histamine and cysteinyl leukotriene C4 (LTC4)], flow cytometric basophil activation assays (CD63 and CD209), etc. These assays, although having great promise, are generally considered as research applications at the present time (80).

The Food and Drug Administration (FDA) defines a RAST test under 21CFR866.5750 as a immunological test system that consists of the reagents used to measure, by immunochemical techniques, the allergen antibodies (antibodies which cause an allergic reaction) specific for a given allergen. Measurement of specific allergen antibodies may aid in the diagnosis of asthma, allergies, and other pulmonary disorders. Some commercial RAST tests are FDA cleared or approved as in vitro diagnostic devices (IVD) through a process known as premarket notification [510(k) program] based on the Medical Device Amendments of 1976 (81). Many RAST tests are 510K cleared as being essentially equivalent to previously cleared assays. The FDA 510K online database (FDA product code "DHB") lists 214 510K cleared RAST tests and/or systems yielding FDA-cleared tests for literally hundreds of environmental, occupational, and food allergens. It should be pointed out that FDA clearance does not guarantee diagnostic performance. In 1996, the FDA introduced a new IVD classification category called analyte-specific reagents (ASR) (81). The FDA defines ASRs as "antibodies, both polyclonal and monoclonal, specific receptor proteins, ligands, nucleic acid sequences, and similar reagents which, through specific binding or chemical reaction with substances in a specimen, are intended for use in a diagnostic application for identification and quantification of an individual chemical substance or ligand in biological specimens." In essence, the FDA recognized ASRs as the active ingredients of in-house tests, which when used in combination with general purpose reagents (such as buffers or reactive materials without specific intended uses) and general purpose laboratory instruments, could be the basis for an assay developed and used by a single laboratory. In addition to those tests to which the regulatory oversight of the FDA applies, laboratories may develop and use in-house tests that are not regulated. Although tests may be useful as a tool in the diagnosis of disease, the responsibility for validation of the test falls to the laboratory developing the test. There are no "rules" for validation of these tests; however, at a minimum such validation should address evaluation of solid-phase binding of antigen or antibody, primary and secondary incubation antibody times, the effect of interfering substances, and nonspecific binding. When developing an assay to determine whether elevated concentrations of allergen-specific IgE are present in a cohort compared with a control population, great care must be exercised in selection of an appropriate control group.

Appropriate comparison groups would generally consist of persons without identifiable excessive exposure to the allergen that is of concern among the "exposed" group. By evaluating clinical samples among the test ("exposed") and comparison ("unexposed") groups, it may be possible to determine whether a statistically elevated concentration of allergen-specific IgE is diagnostically meaningful (82,83).

Many occupational allergens are low-molecular-weight compounds which are not complete antigens (e.g., isocyanates, anhydrides, etc.) (84,85). In vivo, their first interaction is with a native human macromolecule (such as albumin) leading to recognizable epitopes, either on the hapten–protein conjugate or through interaction of the hapten with the constituitive macromolecule leading to the formation of NAD (84). Care must be taken when synthesizing these hapten–protein conjugates for in vitro serologic testing, as the synthesized hapten–protein conjugates may not be equivalent to those formed in vivo. The National Committee for Clinical Laboratory Standards (NCCLS) is an international, interdisciplinary, nonprofit, standards-developing, educational organization that promotes the development and use of voluntary consensus standards and guidelines within the health care community. The NCCLS has published a guideline that addresses evaluation methods and analytical performance characteristics of immunological assays for human IgE measurements (86).

Interpretation of In Vitro IgE Tests

Determination of specific IgE antibodies to known allergens by SPT or in vitro tests is an important component of an appropriate systematic clinical evaluation for many common medical conditions, including, for example, rhinitis, sinusitis, and reactions related to food allergies (87,88). Contraindications to SPT include generalized skin disease or the inability to discontinue antihistamine use; in these cases, in vitro assays for specific IgE may be useful. In addition, up to 60% of positive SPT results to foods and up to 50% of positive SPT results to latex do not reflect symptomatic allergy (89,90). Clinical accuracy is the basic ability to discriminate between two subclasses of subjects where there is some clinically relevant reason to do so. This concept of clinical accuracy refers to the quality of the initial classification of the subjects based on a diagnostic discriminator. The accuracy of the probing provided by the discriminator is the basis of any comparisons of the usefulness of diagnostic testing. Receiver operating characteristics (ROC) curves is one method to analyze the efficiency of this probing (91,92). ROC plots graphically display the entire spectrum of a test's performance for a particular sample group by demonstrating the ability of a test to discriminate between alternative states of health. The points along the ROC curve represent the sensitivity–specificity pairs corresponding to all possible decision thresholds for defining a positive test result. ROC curves yield a simple graphical method to evaluate the trade-offs obtained between sensitivity and specificity across all test cut offs yielding the possibility to determine, with some confidence, the accuracy of the diagnostic tests used to dichotomize subjects. Choosing the optimal decision is a trade-off between optimizing sensitivity and specificity. For example, sera collected from 311 subjects (131 latex puncture skin test (PST) positive and 180 PST negative) were analyzed for latex-specific IgE antibodies using three FDA-cleared assays. Diagnostic accuracy was evaluated using ROC curves in relation to the subjects' PST status and the results of the immunoassays. ROC areas under the curve (AUCs) based on PST for the three diagnostic tests were 0.858 ± 0.024, 0.869 ± 0.024, and 0.924 ± 0.017. One system had a significantly greater AUC based on PST than those observed for the other two ($p < 0.05$). When the diagnostic tests were probed as to the cutoffs giving maximal diagnostic efficiency compared to PST, two tests yielded values of less than 0.35 kU/L of allergen IgE, while the other yielded 0.11 kU/L. The diagnostic efficiencies based on PST at these cutoffs were 87.1%, 88.1%, and 88.7%, respectively (92). Likelihood ratios of a positive test (LR+) and the likelihood ratio of a negative test (LR−) can also be calculated from diagnostic sensitivity and specificity where LR+ = sensitivity/(1−specificity) and LR− = (1 − sensitivity)/(specificity).

The optimal decision thresholds obtained in this type of analysis are selected assuming that the cost of a false-positive result and the cost of a false-negative result were equal, but this may not be the case in some clinical applications. The optimal decision threshold for a specific clinical application involves a number of factors that are not properties of the testing system; rather they are properties of the clinical application. These include prevalence, the outcomes and the relative values of those outcomes, the costs to the patient and others of incorrect classification (false positive and false negative classifications), and the costs and benefits of various interventions. These characteristics interact with the test results to affect usefulness. Methods for determining the optimal decision threshold based on the prevalence and the costs of incorrect classification have been developed (92). In general, a higher decision threshold is preferred if the prevalence is low or if the cost of a false positive result is greater than the cost of a false negative result. A lower decision threshold is preferred if the prevalence is high or if the cost of a false negative result is greater than the cost of a false positive result. These data assume that sensitivity and specificity are inherent properties of the test and thus, independent of prevalence. Although this is generally assumed to be the case, sensitivity and specificity may vary among different subpopulations and thus, are dependent on the composition of the population under study (93). Unlike sensitivity and specificity, diagnostic efficiency is dependent on disease prevalence and the prevalence in the study sample may not be representative of the prevalence in the target population in some clinical applications; thus, the diagnostic efficiencies reported for the assays cannot be generalized to other clinical applications. Another disadvantage of comparing diagnostic efficiencies of different tests is that two tests may have the same diagnostic efficiency, but perform quite differently. For example, one test may result in many false positives and few false negatives, whereas another test may result in many false negatives but few false positives. ROC analyses also provide support for the hypothesis that IgE antibody assays can detect different subsets of IgE antibody of a given specificity; possibly as a result, clinical tests intended for disease diagnosis may not perform optimally when used in low prevalence populations for a condition such as IgE sensitization (94). Clinical tests (such as RAST) are optimized for use in evaluating patient populations where there is usually a high pretest probability for the condition of interest. Assuming constant sensitivity and specificity, the higher the true prevalence of a condition, the more accurately a test will identify the prevalence of that condition in a population. If a condition is present at low prevalence, a larger proportion of test positives will be false positives, resulting in poor positive predictive value of the test and overestimation of prevalence (92,95,96).

NONINVASIVE ASSESSMENT OF AIRWAY INFLAMMATION

Use of Sputum Cell Counts as a Noninvasive Assessment of Airway Inflammation

Induced sputum analysis is a reproducible, valid, responsive, and noninvasive method for studying airway inflammation. It comprises two steps: sputum induction and processing. Sputum induction involves inducing sputum production by inhalation of a hypertonic saline solution. A task force composed of experts in the field of sputum analysis have tried to standardize the methods for inducing and processing sputum under the auspices of the European Respiratory Society (97,98). Their conclusions are summarized in a supplement of the European Respiratory Journal (97,98).

Several methods for inducing sputum have been proposed using different types of nebulizers with different outputs. The nebulizer output and inhalation time can influence the sputum cell count and fluid phase measurements (99). An ultrasonic nebulizer with an output of at least 1 mL/min achieves a high success rate (97).

Different methods have been proposed to process induced sputum. Some methods use the entire sample collected, whereas others select denser portions from the expectorated sample using an inverted microscope. Both methods have advantages and disadvantages. The whole selection method is quicker and does not necessitate an inverted microscope, but the reading of the slides may be more difficult especially when there is a high squamous cell contamination. Indeed, the reproducibility of cell counts seems to be lower when the squamous cell contamination exceeds 20% of all recovered cells (100). Although one study reported a higher percentage of eosinophil count on using the method of selecting denser portions of sputum compared with the method using the entire sample, the differential cell counts obtained after processing the entire sputum samples or selected samples have been reported to be similar in others (101–103). One method or the other can be used reliably, but it is important to remember that these two methods are not interchangeable. The same method should always be followed within the same study. The different steps of sputum processing according to the Sputum Task Force are described in Figure 3 (98). The reproducibility of sputum cell count has been clearly demonstrated for different-ial cell counts in healthy subjects, asthmatics, and smokers. Compared with healthy subjects, asthmatics had increased sputum cell counts for eosinophils, metachro-matic cells, and neutrophils as well as for markers of inflammatory cell activation (104). It has been demonstrated in several studies that sputum inflammatory indices such as eosinophils and eosinophil cationic protein are increased by exposure to common allergens or by reduction of steroid treatment whereas treatment with cor-icosteroids leads to a reduction in these indices (105–112). There is also evidence that the use of sputum eosinophils improves the management of asthma by decreasing the number of asthma exacerbations (113).

Changes in Sputum Cell Counts After Exposure to Occupational Agents in the Laboratory

The changes in airway inflammation have mainly been assessed after exposure to occupational agents in the laboratory. In the majority of cases, sputum eosinophilia has been observed after exposure to occupational agents. Indeed, sputum eosinophils have been shown to increase after exposure to both high- and low-molecular-weight agents such as isocyanates, red cedar, or cyanoacrylate (109,114–117). However, there are examples where exposure to occupational agents can predominantly induce a sputum neutrophilia. Increase in sputum neutrophils has been observed mainly after exposure to isocyanates, but also after exposure to other agents, for example, metalworking fluid or grain dust (118–121). The type of asthmatic reaction and the intensity of airway inflammation induced by exposure to isocyanates can be influenced by the concentration and the length of exposure to these agents (122). Indeed, isocyanate-induced asthma seems to be enhanced when isocyanates are generated at low concentrations for a long period of time, compared to when they are generated at a higher concentration for a shorter duration of exposure.

Changes in Sputum Cell Counts After Exposure to Occupational Agents at the Workplace

Only a few studies have investigated the changes in induced sputum at the workplace. Subjects with OA and asthmatics without OA working in the same environment were investigated during periods at work and away from work (123). Sputum induction

(A)   **(B)**

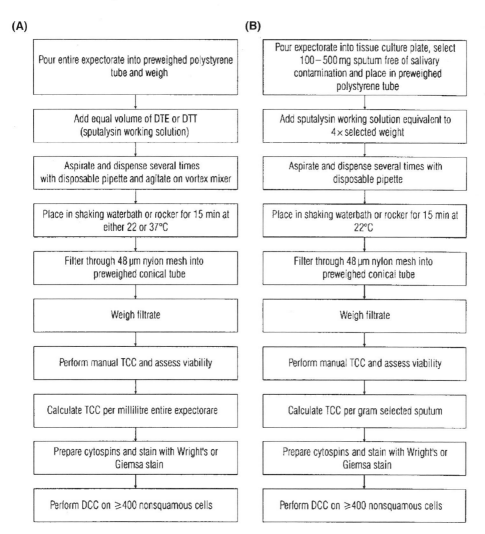

Figure 3 Sputum processing method for: (**A**) entire sputum and (**B**) selected sputum. *Abbreviations*: DCC, differential cell count; DTE, dithioerythritol; DTT, dithiothreitol; TCC, total cell count. *Source*: From Ref. 98.

was performed at the end of these periods. The subjects with OA had an increase in sputum eosinophils when at work, which resolved when they were removed from their workplace, whereas asthmatics, without OA working in the same environment, did not show any change in airway inflammation. Another study investigated the changes in induced sputum in 38 subjects with OA caused by exposure to low-molecular-weight agents while working (124). The diagnosis of OA was confirmed by PEF monitoring in 36 subjects. Twelve of them also underwent specific inhalation challenge (SIC), which were positive. Only 14 had sputum eosinophils greater than 2.2%, when at work. The authors reported that subjects had sputum neutrophilia (59% of neutrophils), but there was no comparison with periods away from work. A subject exposed to metalworking fluid was reported to have marked increase in neutrophils when at work, which resolved after periods away from work (120). The sputum findings were mirrored by corresponding changes in spirometry and PC_{20} methacholine.

Recently, the addition of sputum cell counts to the monitoring of PEF was shown to increase the specificity of this test compared with SIC by 18% [range (r): 13.7–25.5] or 26.8% (r: 24.8–30.4) depending on whether an increase of sputum eosinophils greater than 1% or 2% when at work was considered significant (125). When at work, subjects with positive SIC had a significant increase in sputum eosinophils, whereas the group with a negative SIC had higher neutrophils compared with the periods away from work. The mechanisms explaining the neutrophilic inflammation are unclear, but may be due to an irritant effect of agents at the workplace, in asthmatic subjects. Further research is needed to assess to which extent neutrophilic inflammation can be influenced by smoking, inhaled corticosteroid treatment, or exposure to irritant agents in subjects with work-aggravated asthma.

Occupational Eosinophilic Bronchitis

The analysis of induced sputum has led to the identification of a condition causing chronic cough without airflow limitation or airway hyperresponsiveness. This condition, called "eosinophilic bronchitis," was originally described in 1989 (126). The exposure to occupational agents can also cause eosinophilic bronchitis. This condition was initially reported in a subject who developed respiratory symptoms upon exposure to cyanoacrylates and was labeled "occupational eosinophilic bronchitis" (127). Exposure to cyanoacrylate during periods of occupational exposure was shown to induce eosinophilic bronchitis without any change in forced expiratory volume in one second (FEV_1) or PC_{20}; this condition resolved when the patient was away from work and recurred when she returned to the workplace. Sputum eosinophilia was also induced by the exposure to cyanoacrylate in the laboratory. Since this first report was published, eosinophilic bronchitis has been reported after exposure to a number of occupational agents such as latex, mushroom spores, and lysozyme (128–131). This condition is likely to be underestimated, because analysis of induced sputum is not routinely performed in many centers. However, this test should be done when respiratory symptoms, mainly cough, are exacerbated in the workplace in spite of normal airway responsiveness and normal FEV_1. Although it is unknown whether subjects with occupational eosinophilic bronchitis will go on to develop OA if they stay exposed to the offending agent, it would seem medically prudent to remove them from the workplace.

DISCUSSION OF ILLUSTRATIVE CASE HISTORY

The clinical case presented at the beginning of this chapter illustrates the importance of a thorough immunological assessment to confirm the sensitization to an occupational agent. It also emphasizes the importance of suspecting an occupational eosinophilic bronchitis, when there is no evidence of asthma when the subject is working.

The sensitization can be detected by SPTs, which are the most sensitive tests to detect the sensitization to an allergen. However, there are situations where SPT cannot be performed. Indeed, there are no allergenic extracts available for testing the majority of low-molecular-weight agents. In the present case, OA due to platinum salts is clearly IgE dependent and allergenic extracts for platinum salts are available. However, SPT cannot be interpreted reliably when subjects are taking antihistamines or are experiencing dermographism. In these situations, RAST can demonstrate the presence of specific IgE directed against the suspected occupational agent.

This clinical case also highlights the need for investigating airway inflammation at work and away from work to explore the possibility of an occupational eosinophilic bronchitis when there is no objective evidence of asthma. Indeed, the subject discussed here was sensitized to platinum salts, complained of respiratory symptoms, but did not show any objective feature of asthma—no airflow limitation, no PEF variability, normal PC_{20}—when at work. In these conditions, eosinophilic bronchitis is suspected. Performing sputum induction after periods at work and away from work is the easiest way to confirm this diagnosis.

DIRECTIONS OF FUTURE RESEARCH

- Immunologic testing that assesses IgE-mediated sensitization to occupational allergens depends on availability of well-characterized test allergens. There is a critical need to produce standardized occupational allergens that can be immunologically characterized and then shared between those groups employing in vivo or in vitro tests in assessing OA.
- Laboratories utilize a variety of specific IgE and IgG immunoassay protocols. Multicenter validation studies are needed to determine which assays and antigens exhibit optimal performance in identifying those workers with OA. Adaption of common antigens and protocols by different laboratories would allow for meaningful interpretation of results obtained in individual workers and in large cohorts.

REFERENCES

1. Murdoch RD, Pepys J, Hughes EG. IgE antibody responses to platinum group metals: a large scale refinery survey. Br J Ind Med 1986; 43(1):37–43.
2. Pepys J. Allergic asthma to *Bacillus subtilis* enzyme: a model for the effects of inhalable proteins. Am J Ind Med 1992; 21:587–593.
3. Malo JL, Lemiere C, Gautrin D, Labrecque M. Occupational asthma. Curr Opin Pulm Med 2004; 10(1):57–61.
4. Meredith S. Reported incidence of occupational asthma in the United Kingdom, 1989–1990. J Epidemiol Commun Health 1993; 47(6):459–563.
5. Wild LG, Lopez M. Occupational asthma caused by high-molecular-weight substances. Immunol Allergy Clin North Am 2003; 23(2):235–250, vii.
6. Bernstein DI. Occupational asthma caused by exposure to low-molecular-weight chemicals. Immunol Allergy Clin North Am 2003; 23(2):221–234, vi.
7. Tilles SA, Jerath-Tatum A. Differential diagnosis of occupational asthma. Immunol Allergy Clin North Am 2003; 23(2):167–176, v.
8. Copilevitz C, Dykewicz M. Epidemiology of occupational asthma. Immunol Allergy Clin North Am 2003; 23(2):155–166.
9. Sastre J, Vandenplas O, Park HS. Pathogenesis of occupational asthma. Eur Respir J 2003; 22(2):364–373.
10. Grammer LC, Patterson R. Immunologic evaluation of occupational asthma. In: Bernstein IL, Chan-Yeung M, Malo JL, Bernstein DI, eds. Asthma in the Workplace. 2nd ed. New York: Marcel Dekker Inc., 1999:159–171.

11. Cipolla C, Lugo G, Sassi C, et al. A new risk of occupational disease: allergic asthma and rhinoconjunctivitis in persons working with beneficial arthropods. Int Arch Occup Environ Health 1996; 68(2):133–135.

12. Kobayashi S. Occupational asthma due to inhalation of pharmacological dusts and other chemical agents with some reference to other occupational asthmas in Japan. Allergology Proceedings of the VIII International Congress of Allergology, Tokyo, October, 1973–1974; Excerpta Medica, Ams:124–132.

13. Slavin RG, Lewis CR. Sensitivity to enzyme additives in laundry detergent workers. J Allergy Clin Immunol 1971; 48(5):262–266.

14. Pepys J, Wells ID, D'Souza MF, Greenberg M. Clinical and immunological responses to enzymes of *Bacillus subtilis* in factory workers and consumers. Clin Allergy 1973; 3(2):143–160.

15. Sutton R, Skerritt J, Baldo B, Wrigley C. The diversity of allergens involved in bakers' asthma. Clin Allergy 1984; 14:93–107.

16. Park H, Nahm D. Buckwheat flour hypersensitivity: an occupational asthma in a noodle maker. Clin Exp Allergy 1996; 26:423–427.

17. Quirce S, Cuevas M, Olaguibel J, Tabar A. Occupational asthma and immunologic responses induced by inhaled carmine among employees at a factory making natural dyes. J Allergy Clin Immunol 1994; 93:44–52.

18. Thorpe SC, Kemeny DM, Panzani RC, McGurl B, Lord M. I. Allergy to castor bean. II. Identification of the major allergens in castor bean seeds. J Allergy Clin Immunol 1988; 82(1):67–72.

19. Blasco A, Joral A, Fuente R, Rodriguez M, Garcia A, Dominguez A. Bronchial asthma due to sensitization to chloramine T. J Investig Allergol Clin Immunol 1992; 2(3): 167–170.

20. Card WI. A case of asthma sensitivity to chromates. Lancet 1935; 2:167–170.

21. Novey H, Habib M, Wells I. Asthma and IgE antibodies induced by chromium and nickel salts. J Allergy Clin Immunol 1983; 72:407–412.

22. Desjardins A, Malo J, L'Archevêque J, Cartier A, McCants M, Lehrer S. Occupational IgE-mediated sensitization and asthma due to clam and shrimp. J Allergy Clin Immunol 1995; 96:608–617.

23. Karr R. Bronchoprovocation studies in coffee worker's asthma. J Allergy Clin Immunol 1979; 64:650–654.

24. Sastre J, Olmo M, Novalvos A, Ibanez D, Lahoz C. Occupational asthma due to different spices. Allergy 1996; 51:117–120.

25. Luczynska C, Hutchcroft B, Harrison M, Dorman J, Topping M. Occupational asthma and specific IgE to diazonium salt intermediate used in the polymer industry. J Allergy Clin Immunol 1990; 85:1076–1082.

26. Vallieres M, Cockcroft D, Taylor D, Dolovich J, Hargreave F. Dimethyl ethanolamine-induced asthma. Am Rev Respir Dis 1977; 115:867–871.

27. Nilsson R, Nordlinder R, Wass U, Meding B, Belin L. Asthma, rhinitis, and dermatitis in workers exposed to reactive dyes. Br J Ind Med 1993; 50:65–70.

28. Bernstein J, Kraut A, Bernstein D, et al. Occupational asthma induced by inhaled egg lysozyme. Chest 1993; 103:532–535.

29. Schwartz H, Jones R, Rojas A, Squillace D, Yunginger J. Occupational allergic rhinoconjunctivitis and asthma due to fennel seed. Ann Allergy Asthma Immunol 1997; 78:37–40.

30. Lemiere C, Cartier A, Lehrer SB, Malo JL. Occupational asthma caused by aromatic herbs. Allergy 1996; 51(9):647–649.

31. Soparkar G, Patel P, Cockcroft D. Inhalant atopic sensitivity to grasshoppers in research laboratories. J Allergy Clin Immunol 1993; 92:61–65.

32. Grammer L, Harris K, Malo J-L, Cartier A, Patterson R. The use of an immunoassay index for antibodies against isocyanate human protein conjugates and application to human isocyanate disease. J Allergy Clin Immunol 1990; 86:94–98.

33. Moller D, Gallagher J, Bernstein D, Wilcox T, Burroughs H, Bernstein I. Detection of IgE-mediated respiratory sensitization in workers exposed to hexahydrophthalic anhydride. J Allergy Clin Immunol 1985; 75:663–672.

34. Grammer L, Shaughnessy M, Lowenthal M, Yarnold P. Risk factors for immunologically mediated respiratory disease from hexahydrophthalic anhydride. JOM 1994; 36:642–646.

35. Colten H, Polakoff P, Weinstein S, Strieder D. Immediate hypersensitivity to hog trypsin resulting from industrial exposure. N Engl J Med 1975; 292:1050–1053.

36. Newill CA, Eggleston PA, Prenger VL, et al. Prospective study of occupational asthma to laboratory animal allergens: stability of airway responsiveness to methacholine challenge for one year. J Allergy Clin Immunol 1995; 95:707–715.

37. Brugnami G, Marabini A, Siracusa A, Abbritti G. Work-related late asthmatic response induced by latex allergy. J Allergy Clin Immunol 1995; 96:457–464.

38. Burge P, Edge G, O'Brien I, Harries M, Hawkins R, Pepys J. Occupational asthma in a research centre breeding locusts. Clin Allergy 1980; 10:355–363.

39. Reijula K, Kujala V, Latvala J. Sauna builder's asthma caused by obeche (*Triplochiton scleroxylon*) dust. Thorax 1994; 49:622–623.

40. Bernstein D, Gallagher J, Bernstein I. Mealworm asthma: clinical and immunologic studies. J Allergy Clin Immunol 1983; 72:475–480.

41. Littorin M, Truedsson L, Welinder H, Skarping G, Martensson U, Sjoholm AG. Acute respiratory disorder, rhinoconjunctivitis and fever associated with the pyrolysis of polyurethane derived from diphenylmethane diisocyanate. Scand J Work Environ Health 1994; 20(3):216–222.

42. Delgado J, Gomez E, Palma JL, et al. Occupational rhinoconjunctivitis and asthma caused by *Tetranychus urticae* (red spider mite). A case report. Clin Exp Allergy 1994; 24:477–480.

43. Symington I, Kerr J, McLean D. Type I allergy in mushroom soup processors. Clin Allergy 1981; 11:43–47.

44. McConnell L, Fink J, Schlueter D, Schmidt M. Asthma caused by nickel sensitivity. Ann Int Med 1973; 78:888–890.

45. Malo J, Cartier A, Doepner M, Nieboer E, Evans S, Dolovich J. Occupational asthma caused by nickel sulfate. J Allergy Clin Immunol 1982; 69:55–59.

46. Novey H, Keenan W, Fairshter R, Wells I, Wilson A, Culver B. Pulmonary disease in workers exposed to papain: clinico-physiological and immunological studies. Clin Allergy 1980; 10:721–731.

47. Hill D. Pancreatic extract lung sensitivity. Med J Aust 1975; 2(14):553–555.

48. Davies R, Hendrick D, Pepys J. Asthma due to inhaled chemical agents: ampicillin, bensyl penicillin, 6 amino penicillanic acid and related substances. Clin Allergy 1974; 4:227–247.

49. Lagier F, Cartier A, Dolovich J, Malo J-L. Occupational asthma in a pharmaceutical worker exposed to penicillamine. Thorax 1989; 44:157–158.

50. Grammer LC, Harris KE, Chandler MJ, Flaherty D, Patterson R. Establishing clinical and immunologic criteria for diagnosis of occupational immunologic lung disease with phthalic anhydride and tetrachlorophthalic anhydride exposures as a model. J Occup Med 1987; 29(10):806–811.

51. Venables K, Topping M, Nunn A, Howe W, Newman-Taylor A. Immunologic and functional consequences of chemical (tetrachlorophthalic anhydride)-induced asthma after four years of avoidance of exposure. J Allergy Clin Immunol 1987; 80:212–218.

52. Maccia C, Bernstein I, Emmett E, Brooks S. In vitro demonstration of specific IgE in phthalic anhydride hypersensitiviy. Am Rev Resp Dis 1976; 113:701–704.

53. Cromwell O, Pepys J, Parish W, Hughes E. Specific IgE antibodies to platinum salts in sensitized workers. Clin Allergy 1979; 9:109–117.

54. Biagini R, Bernstein I, Gallagher J, Moorman W, Brooks S, Gann P. The diversity of reaginic immune responses to platinum and palladium metallic salts. J Allergy Clin Immunol 1985; 76:794–802.

55. Gailhofer G, Wilders-Truschnig M, Smolle J, Ludvan M. Asthma caused by bromelain: an occupational allergy. Clin Allergy 1988; 18:445–450.

56. Helin T, Makinen-Kiljunen S. Occupational asthma and rhinoconjunctivitis caused by senna. Allergy 1996; 51:181–184.

57. Davies R, Pepys J. Asthma due to inhaled chemical agents—the macrolide antibiotic Spiramycin. Clin Allergy 1975; 1:99–107.

58. Butcher B, O'Neil C, Reed M, Salvaggio J. Radioallergosorbent testing of toluene diisocyanate-reactive individuals using p-tolyl isocyanate antigen. J Allergy Clin Immunol 1980; 66:213–216.

59. Butcher BT, Karr RM, O'Neil CE, et al. Inhalation challenge and pharmacologic studies of toluene diisocyanate (TDI)—sensitive workers. J Allergy Clin Immunol 1979; 64:146–152.

60. Zeiss CR, Levitz D, Chacon R, Wolkonsky P, Patterson R, Pruzansky JJ. Quantitation and new antigenic determinant specificity of antibodies induced by inhalation of trimellitic anhydride in man. Int Arch Allergy Appl Immunol 1980; 61(4):380–388.

61. Block G, Tse K, Kijek K, Chan H, Chan-Yeung M. Baker's asthma. Clin Allergy 1983; 13:359–370.

62. Houba R, Heederik D, Doekes G, vanRun P. Exposure-sensitization relationship for alpha-amylase allergens in the baking industry. Am J Resp Critic Care Med 1996; 154:130–136.

63. Bernstein DI, Smith AB, Moller DR, et al. Clinical and immunologic studies among egg-processing workers with occupational asthma. J Allergy Clin Immunol 1987; 80:791–797.

64. Liss GM, Bernstein DI, Moller DR, Gallagher JS, Stephenson RL, Bernstein IL. Pulmonary and immunologic evaluation of foundry workers exposed to methylene diphenyldiisocyanate (MDI). J Allergy Clin Immunol 1988; 82(1):55–61.

65. Zeiss C, Patterson R, Pruzansky J, Miller M, Rosenberg M, Levitz D. Trimellitic anhydride-induced airway syndromes: clinical and immunologic studies. J Allergy Clin Immunol 1977; 60:96–103.

66. Wisnewski AV, Stowe MH, Cartier A, et al. Isocyanate vapor-induced antigenicity of human albumin. J Allergy Clin Immunol 2004; 113(6):1178–1184.

67. Kristiansson MH, Lindh CH, Jonsson BA. Correlations between air levels of hexahydrophthalic anhydride (HHPA) and HHPA-adducted albumin tryptic peptides in nasal lavage fluid from experimentally exposed volunteers. Rapid Commun Mass Spectrom 2004; 18(14):1592–1598.

68. Liss G, Bernstein D, Moller D, Gallagher J, Stephenson R, Bernstein I. Pulmonary and immunologic evaluation of foundry workers exposed to methylene diphenyldiisocyanate (MDI). J Allergy Clin Immunol 1988; 82:55–61.

69. Kristiansson MH, Lindh CH, Jonsson BA. Determination of hexahydrophthalic anhydride adducts to human serum albumin. Biomarkers 2003; 8(5):343–359.

70. Ramirez MA. Horse asthma following blood transfusion: a case report. JAMA 1919; 73:984–985.

71. Prausnitz O, Küstner H. Studien über die Überempfindlichkeit. Zentralb Bacteriol 1921; 1:160.

72. Ishizaka K, Ishizaka T, Terry WD. Antigenic structure of gamma-E-globulin and reaginic antibody. J Immunol 1967; 99(5):849–858.

73. Johansson S. Raised levels of a new immunoglobulin class (IgND) in asthma. Lancet 1967; 2:951–953.

74. Hamilton RG, Adkison NF Jr. Clinical laboratory assessment of IgE-dependent hypersensitivity. J Allergy Clin Immunol 2003; 111(suppl 2):S687–S701.

75. Kohler G. Frequency of precursor cells against the enzyme beta-galactosidase: an estimate of the BALB/c strain antibody repertoire. Eur J Immunol 1976; 6(5):340–347.

76. Trout DB, Page EH. Fungal exposure and lower respiratory illness in children. Am J Respir Crit Care Med 2004; 169(8):969–970.

77. Wide L, Bennich H, Johansson S. Diagnosis of allergy by an in-vitro test for allergen antibodies. Lancet 1967; 2:1105–1107.
78. Brown CR, Higgins KW, Frazer K, et al. Simultaneous determination of total IgE and allergen-specific IgE in serum by the MAST chemiluminescent assay system. Clin Chem 1985; 31(9):1500–1505.
79. Fulton RJ, McDade RL, Smith PL, Kienker LJ, Kettman JR. Advanced multiplexed analysis with the FlowMetrix system. Clin Chem 1997; 43(9):1749–1756.
80. Hamilton RG, Franklin AN Jr. In vitro assays for the diagnosis of IgE-mediated disorders. J Allergy Clin Immunol 2004; 114(2):213–225.
81. Gutman S. The role of Food and Drug Administration regulation of in vitro diagnostic devices—applications to genetics testing. Clin Chem 1999; 45(5):746–749.
82. Trout DB, Seltzer JM, Page EH, et al. Clinical use of immunoassays in assessing exposure to fungi and potential health effects related to fungal exposure. Ann Allergy Asthma Immunol 2004; 92(5):483–491.
83. Biagini RE, Driscoll RJ, Bernstein DI, et al. Hypersensitivity reactions and specific antibodies in workers exposed to industrial enzymes at a biotechnology plant. J Appl Toxicol 1996; 16(2):139–145.
84. Biagini RE, Bernstein DI, Gallagher JS, et al. Immune responses of cynomolgus monkeys to phthalic anhydride. J Allergy Clin Immunol 1988; 82:23–29.
85. Bernstein DI, Jolly A. Current diagnostic methods for diisocyanate induced occupational asthma. Am J Ind Med 1999; 36(4):459–468.
86. NCCLS. Evaluation methods and analytical perfomance characteristics of immunological assays for human immunoglobulin E (IgE) antibodies of defined allergen specificities approved guideline. NCCLS, 1997.
87. Sampson HA. Food allergy. J Allergy Clin Immunol 2003; 111(suppl 2):S540–S547.
88. Dykewicz MS. Rhinitis and sinusitis. J Allergy Clin Immunol 2003; 111(suppl 2): S520–S529.
89. Sampson HA. Food allergy. JAMA 1997; 278(22):1888–1894.
90. Arellano R, Bradley J, Sussman G. Prevalence of latex sensitization among hospital physicians occupationally exposed to latex gloves. Anesthesiology 1992; 77(5):905–908.
91. NCCLS. Assessment of clinical accuracy of laboratory tests using receiver operating characteristic (ROC) plots. Approved guideline. NCCLS document GP10-A, 1998.
92. Biagini RE, Krieg EF, Pinkerton LE, Hamilton RG. Receiver operating characteristics analyses of Food and Drug Administration-cleared serological assays for natural rubber latex-specific immunoglobulin E antibody. Clin Diagn Lab Immunol 2001; 8(6):1145–1149.
93. Begg CB. Biases in the assessment of diagnostic tests. Stat Med 1987; 6(4):411–423.
94. Metz CE. Basic principles of ROC analysis. Semin Nucl Med 1978; 8(4):283–298.
95. Yeang HY. Prevalence of latex allergy may be vastly overestimated when determined by in vitro assays. Ann Allergy Asthma Immunol 2000; 84(6):628–632.
96. Meade BJ, Weissman DN, Beezhold DH. Latex allergy: past and present. Int Immunopharmacol 2002; 2(2–3):225–238.
97. Paggiaro PL, Chanez P, Holz O, et al. Sputum induction. Eur Respir J Suppl 2002; 37:3S–8S.
98. Efthimiadis A, Spanevello A, Hamid Q, et al. Methods of sputum processing for cell counts, immunocytochemistry and in situ hybridisation. Eur Respir J Suppl 2002; 37:19S–23S.
99. Belda J, Hussack P, Dolovich M, Efthimiadis A, Hargreave FE. Sputum induction: effect of nebulizer output and inhalation time on cell counts and fluid-phase measures. Clin Exp Allergy 2001; 31(11):1740–1744.
100. Louis R, Shute J, Goldring K, et al. The effect of processing on inflammatory markers in induced sputum. Eur Respir J 1999; 13(3):660–667.
101. Spanevello A, Beghe B, Bianchi A, et al. Comparison of two methods of processing induced sputum: selected versus entire sputum. Am J Respir Crit Care Med 1998; 157(2):665–668.

102. Pizzichini E, Pizzichini MM, Efthimiadis A, Hargreave FE, Dolovich J. Measurement of inflammatory indices in induced sputum: effects of selection of sputum to minimize salivary contamination. Eur Respir J 1996; 9(6):1174–1180.

103. Gershman N, Wong H, Liu J, Mahlmeister M, Fahy J. Comparison of two methods of collecting induced sputum in asthmatic subjects. Eur Respir J 1996; 9:2448–2453.

104. Pizzichini E, Pizzichini MM, Efthimiadis A, et al. Indices of airway inflammation in induced sputum: reproducibility and validity of cell and fluid-phase measurements. Am J Respir Crit Care Med 1996; 154:308–317.

105. Pizzichini E, Pizzichini MM, Efthimiadis A, et al. Changes in the cellular profile of induced sputum after allergen-induced asthmatic responses. Am Rev Respir Dis 1992; 145:1265–1269.

106. Fahy J, Liu J, Wong H, Boushey H. Analysis of cellular and biochemical constituents of induced sputum after allergen challenge: a method for studying allergic airway inflammation. J Allergy Clin Immunol 1994; 93:1031–1039.

107. Wong BJ, Dolovich J, Ramsdale EH, et al. Formoterol compared with beclomethasone and placebo on allergen-induced asthmatic responses. Am Rev Respir Dis 1992; 146:1156–1160.

108. Pizzichini MM, Kidney JC, Wong BJ, et al. Effect of salmeterol compared with beclomethasone on allergen-induced asthmatic and inflammatory responses. Eur Respir J 1996; 9:449–455.

109. Maestrelli P, Calcagni PG, Saetta M, et al. Sputum eosinophilia after asthmatic responses induced by isocyanates in sensitized subjects. Clin Exp Allergy 1994; 24:29–34.

110. Gibson P, Wong B, Hepperle M, et al. A research method to induce and examine a mild exacerbation of asthma by withdrawal of inhaled corticosteroid. Clin Exp Allergy 1992; 22:525–532.

111. Gibson P, Hargreave F, Girgis-Gabardo A, Morris M, Denburg J, Dolovich J. Chronic cough with eosinophilic bronchitis: examination for variable airflow obstruction and response to corticosteroid. Clin Exp Allergy 1995; 25:127–132.

112. Pizzichini MM, Pizzichini E, Clelland L, et al. Sputum in severe exacerbations of asthma: kinetics of inflammatory indices after prednisone treatment. Am J Respir Crit Care Med 1997; 155(5):1501–1508.

113. Green RH, Brightling CE, McKenna S, et al. Asthma exacerbations and sputum eosinophil counts: a randomised controlled trial. Lancet 2002; 360(9347):1715–1721.

114. Lemiere C, Chaboillez S, Malo JL, Cartier A. Changes in sputum cell counts after exposure to occupational agents: What do they mean? J Allergy Clin Immunol 2001; 107(6):1063–1068.

115. Alvarez MJ, Estrada JL, Gozalo F, Fernandez-Rojo F, Barber D. Oilseed rape flour: another allergen causing occupational asthma among farmers. Allergy 2001; 56(2):185–188.

116. Obata H, Dittrick M, Chan H, Chan-Yeung M. Sputum eosinophils and exhaled nitric oxide during late asthmatic reaction in patients with western red cedar asthma. Eur Respir J 1999; 13:489–495.

117. Quirce S, Baeza ML, Tornero P, Blasco A, Barranco R, Sastre J. Occupational asthma caused by exposure to cyanoacrylate. Allergy 2001; 56(5):446–449.

118. Park H, Jung K, Kim H, Nahm D, Kang K. Neutrophil activation following TDI bronchial challenges to the airway secretion from subjects with TDI-induced asthma. Clin Exp Allergy 1999; 29(10):1395–1401.

119. Lemiere C, Romeo P, Chaboillez S, Tremblay C, Malo JL. Airway inflammation and functional changes after exposure to different concentrations of isocyanates. J Allergy Clin Immunol 2002; 110(4):641–646.

120. Leigh R, Hargreave FE. Occupational neutrophilic asthma. Can Respir J 1999; 6(2):194–196.

121. Park HS, Jung KS, Hwang SC, Nahm DH, Yim HE. Neutrophil infiltration and release of IL-8 in airway mucosa from subjects with grain dust-induced occupational asthma. Clin Exp Allergy 1998; 28(6):724–730.

122. Lemiere C, Romeo P, Chaboillez S, Tremblay C, Malo JL. Airway inflammation and functional changes after exposure to different concentrations of isocyanates. J Allergy Clin Immunol 2002; 110(4):641–646.
123. Lemiere C, Pizzichini MM, Balkissoon R, et al. Diagnosing occupational asthma: use of induced sputum [see comments]. Eur Respir J 1999; 13(3):482–488.
124. Anees W, Huggins V, Pavord ID, Robertson AS, Burge PS. Occupational asthma due to low molecular weight agents: eosinophilic and non-eosinophilic variants. Thorax 2002; 57(3):231–236.
125. Girard F, Chaboillez S, Cartier A, et al. An effective strategy for diagnosing occupational asthma: use of induced sputum. Am J Respir Crit Care Med 2004; 170(8): 845–850.
126. Gibson P, Dolovich J, Denburg J, Ramsdale E. Chronic cough: eosinophilic bronchitis without asthma. Lancet 1989; 334:1346–1348.
127. Lemiere C, Efthimiadis A, Hargreave FE. Occupational eosinophilic bronchitis without asthma: an unknown occupational airway disease. J Allergy Clin Immunol 1997; 100 (6 Pt 1):852–853.
128. Quirce S, Swanson MC, Fernandez-Nieto M, De las HM, Cuesta J, Sastre J. Quantified environmental challenge with absorbable dusting powder aerosol from natural rubber latex gloves. J Allergy Clin Immunol 2003; 111(4):788–794.
129. Tanaka H, Saikai T, Sugawara H, et al. Workplace-related chronic cough on a mushroom farm. Chest 2002; 122(3):1080–1085.
130. Escudero C, Quirce S, Fernandez-Nieto M, Miguel J, Cuesta J, Sastre J. Egg white proteins as inhalant allergens associated with baker's asthma. Allergy 2003; 58(7):616–620.
131. Quirce S. Eosinophilic bronchitis in the workplace. Curr Opin Allergy Clin Immunol 2004; 4(2):87–91.

9

Physiological Assessment: Serial Measurements of Lung Function and Bronchial Responsiveness

P. Sherwood Burge
Occupational Lung Disease Unit, Birmingham Heartlands Hospital, Birmingham, U.K.

Gianna Moscato
Allergy and Immunology Unit, Fondazione Salvatore Maugeri, IRCCS, Scientific Institute of Pavia, Pavia, Italy

Anthony Johnson
Research and Education Unit, Workers' Compensation (Dust Diseases) Board, Sydney, New South Wales, Australia

Moira Chan-Yeung
Occupational and Environmental Lung Disease Unit, Respiratory Division, Department of Medicine, University of British Columbia and Vancouver General Hospital, Vancouver, British Columbia, Canada

INTRODUCTION

Occupational asthma (OA) is suspected in a person when respiratory symptoms improve on days away from work or during holidays. The diagnosis needs objective confirmation as the history lacks sufficient specificity; objective tests confirm OA in a little over 50% of those with suggestive symptoms. Tests available include bronchial responsiveness either as single measurement while being exposed or changes that occur after the exposure is stopped, measurement of lung function before and after exposure or over time, or serial frequent measurements several times daily over a few weeks, and specific bronchial provocation tests. There has been a recent systematic review of the literature (1).

DIURNAL VARIATION IN AIRWAYS CALIBER

The spontaneous diurnal variation in airways caliber is fundamental for understanding the physiological measurements of lung function in relationship to work. There is a spontaneous diurnal rhythm (for instance, in peak flow) that can be demonstrated in the majority of normal population, but is exaggerated in people with asthma (2). The lowest readings are usually around the time of waking; there is then an improvement for six to eight hours followed by a subsequent decline until sleeping, with a further decline overnight. The trigger for the diurnal variation appears to be sleep stage, airway caliber being reduced during periods of REM sleep, particularly during narrative dreams. Any reaction at work will be superimposed on this diurnal variation. The relationship between work and sleep can be altered substantially by shift work. Most day-workers and workers on early shifts (for instance 6 A.M. to 2 P.M.) wake shortly before going to work. The first few hours at work will therefore coincide with the period of improving lung function. The effects of an immediate reaction is then to blunt the rise in peak flow rather than to cause any fall, as shown in Figure 1 (3). Workers on afternoon shifts (for instance, 2.00 P.M. to 10.00 P.M.) usually wake substantially before going to work and go to sleep shortly after returning from work. This results in the occupational exposure coinciding with the declining phase of lung function. Immediate reactions are usually more obvious on such shifts. The patterns of sleep in night workers is highly variable and usually changes between the days at work and days away from work. Some have long periods without sleep and some sleep more than once per 24 hours. As each period of sleep is usually associated with a morning (or more properly, waking) dip, the patterns of reaction can then be complex. The diurnal variation usually resets itself within 24 hours of a change in sleep pattern (for instance, working nights), unlike the diurnal variations of cortisol and adrenaline, which take a longer time to reset.

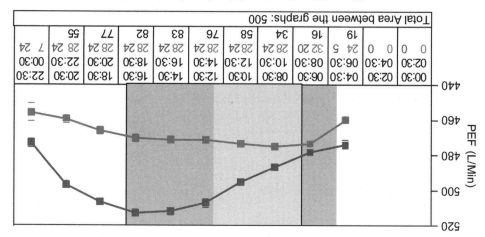

Average Hour for Rest and Day Shift days

	00:30	02:30	04:30	06:30	08:30	10:30	12:30	14:30	16:30	18:30	20:30	22:30
	02:30	04:30	06:30	08:30	10:30	12:30	14:30	16:30	18:30	20:30	22:30	00:30
	0	0	0	0	19	16	34	58	76	83	82	77	55
	0	0	5	24	32 20	28 24	28 24	28 24	28 24	28 24	28 24	28 24	7 24

Total Area between the graphs: 500

Time of Day, Number of Readings And Areas (Day Shift) (Rest)

Figure 1 Two hourly plot of peak expiratory flow in a foundry core shop worker with incidental exposure to diphenylmethane diisocyanate in the cold box process, also exposed to phenol formaldehyde and furanes. He has occupational asthma. The shaded area is at work on the lower trace. The record shows a diurnal variation of 8% on the day at home, with the best reading at 4 P.M. On the workday, the diurnal variation is 3% and the best values are between 9 A.M. and 11 A.M. (with earlier waking). The work exposure has blunted the rise in peak flow.

BEFORE AND AFTER SHIFT MEASUREMENTS

There have been many attempts to document OA from before- and after-shift measurements. They are surprisingly difficult to carry out, i.e., to make the first reading before any work exposure and the last reading at the end of work exposure. Great care is needed to prevent indirect work exposure, for instance, during clocking on, changing, etc., which often involves walking through an area of exposure. Most studies have looked at the whole workforce and tried to document the changes between different exposure groups. The changes seen are usually exceedingly small (in the order of 100 to 200 mL over an eight-hour shift) and are rarely standardized for the time of waking (4–10). It has often been impossible to differentiate those with and without OA from these measurements. In a study of electronics workers exposed to colophony, FEV_1 fell by more than 10% in 16 out of 48 workers having symptoms of OA and two out of 43 asymptomatic workers (11). In a similar study of pharmaceutical manufacturers exposed to psyllium, three out of five workers with OA and 7 out of 13 without OA had similar changes (12), and none of the three workers having OA caused by spiramycin had a 10% postshift fall in FEV_1 (13). The systematic reviews were unable to find sufficient data to calculate sensitivity and specificity of any given cross-shift change in lung function (1). This method cannot be recommended for the validation of OA.

LONGITUDINAL MEASUREMENTS OF LUNG FUNCTION

Many surveillance schedules require serial measurements of lung function in workers who are exposed to occupational allergens such as isocyanates; these records are rarely standardized for time of day or recent exposure. An assumption is made that workers whose lung function falls between measurements are those developing OA. In practice, the intrasubject variability over periods of months is large, such that changes in FEV_1 of at least 400 mL between measurements are seen in workers without sensitization. Figure 2 shows supervised measurement of FEV_1 taken six to nine months apart in workers exposed to isocyanates. There are workers who show a fall of at least 20% (some also show a rise up to 20%) between the two measurements. The distribution of the results is normal, the outliers represent the tails of the normal distribution. This type of surveillance provides a good measure of the mean change in FEV_1. It is good for looking at the longitudinal decline in a group, but is a poor method for picking out individuals developing symptoms, for which a surveillance questionnaire is much better. There is some evidence that those without OA having jobs that involve exposure to occupational allergens show an accelerated loss of FEV_1. Serial measurements form the best means of detecting such an accelerated loss. It is difficult to calculate longitudinal changes in FEV_1 with less than five year's data (or three years' if decline exceeds 150 mL/yr). There are also problems when measurements are made in young workers, as the FEV_1 increases up to the age of about 25, and in the absence of smoking or other damage, has a plateau before declining at around 30 mL/yr from the age of about 35. An example of OA detected (somewhat belatedly) from accelerated declines in FEV_1 is shown in Figure 3.

SERIAL MEASUREMENTS OF PEAK EXPIRATORY FLOW

Patterns of Asthma in the Workplace

The response to occupational allergens was first documented with bronchial provocation testing following single exposures of short duration. Immediate, late, dual, or

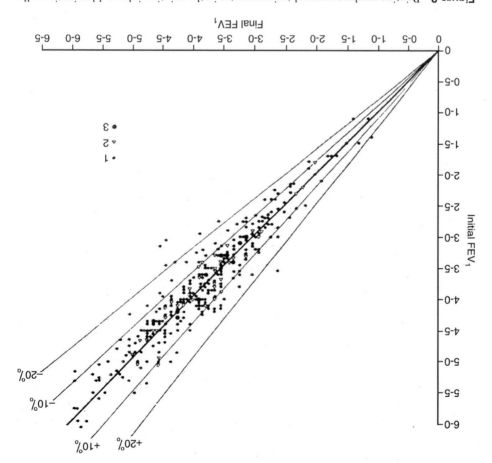

Figure 2 Printing workers exposed to isocyanates in the printing inks and laminating adhesives had measurements of FEV$_1$ twice at six to nine months apart as part of a surveillance scheme. The initial and final reading for each worker is compared. There are five workers whose FEV$_1$ has declined more than 20% between the two measurements (and two who have improved by more than 20%). The plot shows a normal distribution of results, and not a bimodal distribution, which would be needed to identify workers with occupational asthma from such records (there were 13 workers challenge positive for isocyanates in the factory, the two with the largest falls on this plot had negative isocyanate challenges as expected). (The symbols 1–3 show data points with 1, 2, and 3 identical results.)

recurrent reactions may follow a single exposure. In the work situation, exposure usually continues for eight hours or more, each day of the week. The descriptions of the patterns of response to these types of exposure awaited the development of portable peak flow meters, because lung function measurements are needed throughout the working day and in the evening at home, as well as on the days away from work for their elucidation (14–16). With regular daily exposure, the pattern of response depends principally on the rate of recovery. The following patterns can be recognized.

Hourly Pattern

The pattern of response using hour-by-hour records depends on the relationship between the time of exposure to the occupational allergen and the individual worker's underlying diurnal variation.

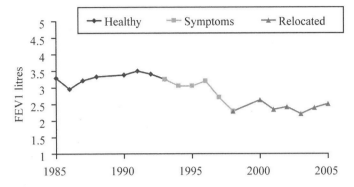

Figure 3 Annual measurements of FEV_1 in a breakfast cereal manufacturer sensitised to thiamine sprayed onto the cereals. The plot starts with eight years when he was exposed to thiamine and was asymptomatic with little change in FEV_1. This is followed by five years after developing work-related asthmatic symptoms when his FEV_1 fell by 200 mLs per year. During the final six years, he was relocated away from thiamine when his FEV_1 decline returned to normal albeit at a lower level than before.

Immediate Reactions. Immediate reactions start within an hour of coming to work. They usually progress hour by hour at work. They may show an improvement during a period away from work, for example, the mid-day break, and usually improve shortly after leaving work. Lung function often returns to normal by the following morning.

Late Reactions. On a morning shift, late reactions do not start until leaving work. The reactions progress in the evening after work and often wake the workers from sleep. Lung function measurements taken at the time of leaving work are often better than that on arriving at work, and many workers say they are not worse at work (but are much better on days away from work). Recovery is rarely complete by the following morning, and reactions usually progress from day to day.

The Flat Reaction. After repeated exposures, deterioration usually ceases and the stage of a relatively fixed airway obstruction is reached with little diurnal variation and little obvious reaction to work exposure. It may take many days away from work for such reactions to resolve. Workers are often identified as having fixed airway obstruction at this stage, which develops commonly with regular exposure to agents such as isocyanates and wood dusts. Similar changes are seen in workers on early shifts with immediate reactions, where the decline caused by work is equivalent to the increase that would have occurred if there had been no work exposure.

The occupational exposure is rarely the only provoker of asthma in a sensitized worker. Once OA develops, reactions usually occur to other nonspecific stimuli, particularly to exercise and infection. If travel to and from work requires exercise (for instance, riding on a bicycle), the reactions to exercise may be superimposed on those caused by work exposures.

Diurnal Variation in Peak Flow

Asthma is traditionally associated with increased diurnal variation. There is, however, no standard method for calculating the diurnal variation, and no clear distinction between asthma and normality. Asthma, by definition, is a variable condition, so a normal diurnal variation measured over a few weeks does not exclude the diagnosis. Population studies have generally shown that the diurnal variation is best expressed as the daily maximum minus the daily minimum divided by the daily mean. This calculation has problems when subjects with reduced peak flow are studied, as the random and systematic variations in the measurements account for increasing percentages as the mean peak flow decreases. When the mean peak flow is below the predicted level, the diurnal variation is best expressed as a percentage of the predicted value. In patients with chronic obstructive airway disease, this method is least correlated with absolute peak flow (17).

An increased diurnal variation is usually seen in those with immediate and late reactions, but is usually lost in those with flat reactions. Increased diurnal variation (for instance, a diurnal variation in peak flow of >20%) is not always seen in workers with OA, but can often be demonstrated by taking the worker away from exposure for a number of days. In other situations, very small deteriorations at work occur with low diurnal variation. This may be because of a number of situations, which include an irritant effect superimposed on a predominantly nonasthmatic airflow obstruction, very low levels of exposure in a sensitized asthmatic wearing good respiratory protection, or a flat reaction in a sensitized worker with severe occupational exposure. They can only be differentiated by removing the worker from exposure.

The diurnal variation in lung function can be studied by trying to fit a cosine wave to the observed data, and performing tests to see if the data conforms to this pattern (2). A 24-hour cosinor analysis can be done on the majority of peak flow records from normal subjects and asthmatics. From the analysis, the amplitude and time of the peak (acrophase) and mesor (a measure of the mean) can be calculated. A study in electronic workers with colophony OA showed that the amplitude decreased from 29% to 19%, when comparing the five-day workweek with five-day periods off work; the acrophase was at 1524 hours away from work and 1144 hours at work, and treatment with cromoglycate or corticosteroids postponed the acrophase by about 90 minutes. It should be possible to fit cosinor rhythms to whole workweeks; this has, however, proved less successful (3). The ability to fit symmetrical cosine waves depends on the number of readings available per 24 hours; the fewer the readings, the better the statistical fit. The discrepancy is because of the actual asymmetry of the rise and fall, which is lost with fewer readings.

Day by Day Reactions

The patterns of reaction which can be readily identified are as follows:

Equivalent Daily Deterioration. In this situation the deterioration each day is similar on each day of exposure (Fig. 4). Recovery is usually rapid on days away from work and is usually complete before the next day's exposure. Such reactions are common with laboratory animal workers and with colophony. Variations of this are associated with the flat hourly pattern.

Progressive Daily Deterioration. This is the commonest reaction to most occupational agents, following repeated exposure, and may take several days of exposure before becoming readily identifiable. This condition is usually associated with incomplete recovery the following morning and frequently with nocturnal wakening (Fig. 5). They are common following exposure to wood dust and isocyanates amongst others. The pattern from week to week depends on whether recovery is complete during rest days or not. If a two-day rest period occurs, recovery taking up to three days is compatible with repeated patterns on a week by week basis.

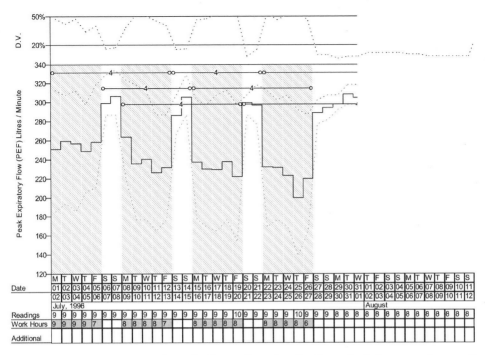

Figure 4 Daily PEF pattern from the Oasys plotter in a hard metal grinder exposed to metal working fluids. The upper panel shows the daily diurnal variation in PEF, the central panel shows the daily maximum (*top line*), mean (*middle line*) and minimum (*bottom line*) PEF. The days at work have a shaded background and the days off work have a clear background. There is equivalent deterioration on each work day with recovery on days away from work, which is usually greater on the second day away from work. The bottom panel shows the number of days making up each day's mean (9–10 in this case showing two-hourly readings). The record shows clear occupational asthma. Cobalt was shown to be the cause by finding a positive skin prick test to cobalt chloride, a positive immediate reaction on specific challenge testing and finding high levels of urinary cobalt following a day at work (23.5 μg/L).

If recovery takes three days, the first day at work is usually better than the days away from work, with deterioration occurring subsequently. If recovery takes more than three days with a two day break, then the next work period starts from a lower baseline, so that deterioration may occur week by week.

   First Day Worst and Midweek Deterioration.   There are a few situations where deterioration is maximal on the first day with subsequent recovery despite continuing exposure. This situation is classically seen in byssinosis (Fig. 6) and is also seen in other situations where microbial aerosols are found, such as aerosols from used coolant oils and from humidifiers in ventilation systems (18,19). However, in all these situations, some workers have progressive daily deterioration, the usual pattern when hypersensitivity is the cause, probably implying that different individuals can react to the same agent in different ways. In a small study of workers with OA, working in a building that had a contaminated humidifier in the air conditioning system, positive skin-prick tests to an extract from the humidifier were only seen in workers with progressive daily deterioration (19). A variant of first day deterioration is that which progresses for the first two to three days after work, and then improves despite continuing exposure. It probably has the same underlying mechanism

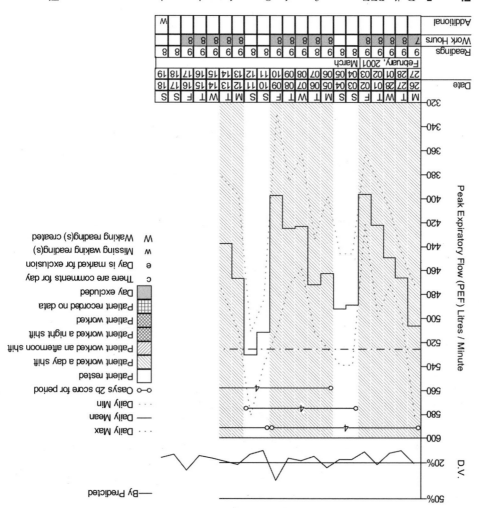

Figure 5 Daily PEF pattern from the Oasys plotter in a maintenance carpenter. The upper panel shows the daily diurnal variation in PEF, the central panel shows the daily maximum (*top line*), mean (*middle line*) and minimum (*bottom line*) PEF. The days at work have a shaded background and the days off work have a clear background. There is progressive daily deterioration on each work period with recovery on days away from work, which is usually greater on the second day away from work. The bottom panel shows the number of days making up each day's mean (8–9 in this case showing two-hourly readings). The record shows clear occupational asthma. MDF was shown to be the cause by finding a positive late asthmatic reaction on specific challenge testing.

and implies the development of tolerance to repeated exposures, such as that occurring with endotoxins.

Portable Measuring Devices in OA

The ideal device should be robust, small, and light, should be easy to calibrate, be stable over a period of weeks, have a linear response, and include a logging device to record at least the time, date, and measurement of lung function. It should also

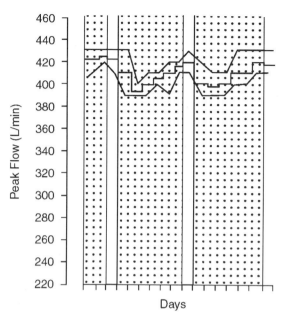

Figure 6 Plot of daily maximum (*top line*), mean (*middle line*), and minimum (*bottom line*) peak flow in a 64-year-old stripper and grinder with 46 years exposure to cotton dust. Days at work have a shaded background, days away from work a clear background. Symptoms of byssinosis developed after 42 years of exposure. The record shows a low diurnal variation throughout, never exceeding 6%. There is a deterioration on the second day in the first work-week and a deterioration on the first day in the second workweek, with recovery during each workweek despite continuing exposure. There is a clear work effect with improvement or deterioration on all of the four possible occasions; the changes are however very small. Such records are often seen in byssinotics, but also occur in workers exposed to "standard" occupational sensitizers, the significance of this type of record is unclear.

be able to make an assessment of the adequacy of the quality of the expiratory maneuver. Several meters measure FEV_1 more reliably than peak flow meters; meters with pneumotachographs often lose calibration if not used for more than four weeks, and do not perform well when cold (for instance, when kept in a car in a cold winter). In practice, it is very difficult to obtain reliable, repeated measurements of vital capacity, as this causes substantial discomfort at the end of even one day's recording. There is some evidence that peak flow readings are about 30 L/min lower when unsupervised (20), and that some workers improve in the first few days of a record because of a learning effect. Workers should be trained in peak flow measurement, should make at least three readings on each occasion, and record the maximum. If the best two peak flow readings are not within 20 L/min of each other, further readings should be made.

Peak flow measurement was chosen for serial patient measurement because of the availability of portable meters, rather than on any physiological advantage of PEF over FEV_1. Portable logging FEV_1 meters are now available, giving a choice in the parameter for measurement. Studies comparing PEF with FEV_1 are compounded by the different methods of measuring used in each. The original Wright peak flow meter, and those modelled on it (the Mini-Wright, Vitalograph, and Ferraris meters) have all been found to be nonlinear when calibrated with a computer-controlled syringe, which delivers air in the form of a forced expiration (21). The meters over-read by about 70 L/min at about 300 L/min, and under-read at flows greater than 600 L/min. The consequence depends on the range of PEF recorded by the individual; the greatest increases in diurnal variation seen in patients whose readings are around 300 L/min. This nonlinearity has been corrected in the meters now used in most countries. Some peak flow meters are unable to record high flows (e.g., the Assess), and the analysis is flawed if the worker can exceed the maximum value of the meter (22).

There is no reason why the percentage change in PEF should be the same as the percentage change in FEV_1. The PEF is mainly a measure of the large airways, but the FEV_1 has a greater component derived from the small airways. There is some evidence that the measurements FEV_1 shows more sensitivity in detecting late rather than early asthmatic reactions following bronchial provocation testing (23). A comparison of FEV_1 and PEF measured with a Mini–Wright or Assess meter showed a poor correlation. The easy-one also under-reads peak flow in those with a short rise time. In one study, the median fall in FEV_1 (27%) was greater than the median fall in PEF (17%), following challenges selected to have a >15% fall in FEV_1 (24). Another study found that the differences were similar in challenges affecting predominately large airways, and those induced by allergen affecting all airways (25). Two studies have compared FEV_1 and PEF, using the same instrument away from the hospital. On using the Micromedical diarycard (with a turbine), the mean diurnal variation was found to be the same for PEF (12.9%) and FEV_1 (12.1%). The turbine does not have the same error profile as the original Wright meter (26). Serial measurements of PEF and FEV_1 were obtained from the VMX (using a pressure transducer) and analyzed for occupational effect by experts. The sensitivity was 60% when the PEF plots were used and 50% when the FEV_1 plots were used. The specificity was 91 % for both sets when compared with specific provocation tests (27). On current evidence, both PEF and FEV_1 are suitable for unsupervised monitoring; PEF should be linearized before analysis if a nonlinear meter is being used. It should be easier to retrospectively check the quality of the blow from meters that store flow/volume data.

Frequency of Measurement

Serial PEF measurements were originally described following hourly readings that were made from the time of waking to that of sleeping in workers who kept records over many weeks (14,15). In most situations, they can conveniently be done every two hours rather than on an hourly basis. However, if the records are carried out less frequently than this, there may be one or no readings during the work period, and immediate reactions at work may be missed; they are also more likely to give isolated low readings (e.g., following exercise) and readings that are more variable (28). Expert interpretation of occupational effect using the readings that were taken every four hours rather than those taken every two hours decreased the sensitivity from 73% to 61%, when compared with that observed on using specific challenges (29). Measurements made every four hours are optimal for the calculation of diurnal variation; fewer readings tend to underestimate the changes, and more frequent readings do not increase precision (30). It is important to make the first reading on waking, including on rest days, and to strive for reproducibility. The complete method for performing these tests has been described (31).

Assessment of Serial Peak Flow Records

Initial attempts were made to analyse these records statistically. An analysis of variance using the model Glim 3 was performed on each record separately. Estimates with their standard errors were derived from the effects of (*i*) work exposure or rest day, (*ii*) treatment, and (*iii*) number of hour of the day (from waking). *F* tests were performed separately on the work type in effect. As this was a nonorthogonal analysis, the factor being assessed was run after the other factors. For work type the effects of treatment and time of day preceded the assessment of work effect. Table 1 shows the number of records showing a significantly positive *F* test in the groups of workers exposed to either colophony in the electronics industry or isocyanates in the printing of flexible packaging, who also underwent occupational type challenges (32). The statistical analysis was clear when the visual inspection of the record was clear. It had a number of substantial limitations. The treatment taken was often increased on days at work. Running the effect of treatment before the effect of work reduced the significance of the work effect. This particularly applied to the colophony-exposed workers, who mostly recovered quickly after leaving work. Those who were exposed to isocyanate during their work frequently took a long time to recover when away from work. The statistical analysis depended substantially on the number of days that recording were made when from work, as the first few days away from work were frequently worse than the first days at work. The statistical results were often positive in those with negative challenges, mostly in workers where the differences between work days and rest days were extremely small in absolute terms, but were consistent in statistical terms. This sometimes resulted because of a lower reading that was recorded at the time of waking in workers who were getting up earlier on work days than on rest days. It is clear from these results that any statistical analysis will have to be more sophisticated.

Rule-based systems establish criteria for a work effect, for example, the number of times a given decrease in PEF occurs on work and rest days. Although some success has been reported, there are two problems with this approach (33–35). Basing diagnosis on a specific percentage of fall in PEF will produce bias in those with a low peak flow for other reasons, such as smoking, but also in those who need an extended time away from work for recovery (18). Criteria based on percentage falls in PEF are again very dependent on the accuracy and linearity of the peak flow meters used. Some studies have used more sophisticated statistical methods. Henneberger et al. (36) used *t*-tests to compare the mean peak flow and mean diurnal

Table 1   Results of Analysis of Variance

Significant *F* tests for work effect	Bronchial provocation test result	
	Positive	Negative
Colophony exposure—no treatment	15/15	2/6
Colophony exposure with steroid or DSCG treatment	6/15	–
Isocyanate exposure	5/6	5/8

Note: The significance of the work effect is tested after adjusting for treatment and time-of-day effects. The number of records showing a significantly positive *F* test in groups of workers exposed to either colophony in the electronics industry or isocyanates in the printing of flexible packaging, who also had occupational type challenges.

Abbreviation: DSCG, disodium cromoglycate.

variation of work days versus rest days. Compared with the visual interpretation of the record by three experts, mean peak flow had a sensitivity of 86% and specificity of 71%; for the diurnal variation, sensitivity was 43% and specificity 86%. Although the number of subjects was small, the method of plotting the peak flow was not stated and two types of peak flow meters were used. Perrin et al. (37) used a number of statistical indices, but found none as satisfactory as visual interpretation of the record. The Italian working group on peak flow measurement also used several indices of daily and day-to-day variability (25). They found that the mean peak flow, the coefficient of variation, and the maximum amplitude were all statistically different on days at work when compared with the readings obtained on days away from work for those with OA but not for those with nonoccupational asthma. The same group later commented that using the same indices as that for peak flow monitoring allowed the detection only of typical cases of OA (38).

Plotting of Serial Records

Peak flow records are usually plotted serially, predominantly to document the response to treatment, i.e., to look for progressive change over time. Occupational records plotted in this way are difficult to interpret, unless the changes are obvious. The differences related to work exposure can be seen more easily by plotting the daily maximum, mean, and minimum peak flow, as illustrated in Figures 4 through 7. Days at work are differentiated from days away from work by background shading. To maximize the difference between the days at and the days away from work, the workday starts with the first reading at work and finishes with the last reading before work the following day. In this way, the morning dip is included with the previous day. It is very important to include a waking value in each day's plot, and to make sure that records are made on waking, on days away from work, because a delay after waking can increase the peak flow and occasionally produce artificial improvement on restdays (39). Taking readings in workers changing shifts is more complicated. Those starting work, say at 2.00 P.M, would have the 2.00 P.M. reading as the first reading of that workday, and the readings will be taken continuously in regular intervals until 1 P.M. of the following day, even if it was a rest day (when the 2:00 P.M. to bedtime readings on the first rest day would not be included in the plot).

The original analyses of these records were designed to be specific, rather than sensitive. The criteria for a positive record were identified as the deterioration in at least three-fourths of the workweeks and improvement in at least three-fourths of the periods off work. For those with long time periods (taking more than three days to improve when away from work), two periods of deterioration and one period of improvement (or vice versa) were required (Fig. 7). The sensitivity and specificity of peak flow records assessed in this way are shown in Table 2. The records had acceptable sensitivity when no prophylactic treatment was taken, but had a serious lack of sensitivity when corticosteroids of cromoglycate were used regularly. In these circumstances, the changes in peak flow are much smaller, and it sometimes also requires a larger than usual exposure to result in a breakthrough of the asthma. The records that were difficult to assess were those showing small absolute changes, or changes that are irregular. It is likely that the above criteria for a positive record can be relaxed without lack of specificity.

Using the Oasys-2 expert system, adequate sensitivity (78.1%) and specificity (91.8%) was achieved when the record had at least four readings per day,

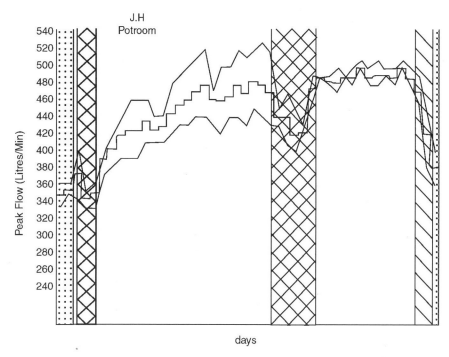

Figure 7 Plot of daily maximum (*top line*), mean (*middle line*), and minimum (*bottom line*) peak flow in a prebake pot operator from an aluminium foundry. Days at work have a shaded background, days away from work a clear background (dots: morning shift; cross hatch: night shift; diagonal lines: afternoon shift). The diurnal variation in peak flow during the first work periods does not exceed 10%; however, it increases during the three weeks away from work to reach 17%, and decreases again on return to work. There is deterioration in all of the four work-periods and improvement in all of the three periods away from work. Before the holiday the absolute changes are very small (about 20 L/min). The substantial improvement on holiday favors asthma with sensitization rather than the result of the known irritants at work superimposed on unrelated chronic airflow obstruction. The methacholine PC_{20} was 11.4 µmol before the holiday and 77.5 µmol before return to work. Although both are within the normal range, the significant improvement again favors occupational asthma.

Table 2 Sensitivity and Specificity of Visual Assessments of Plotted PEF Records and Specific Provocation Testing, Compared with a Diagnosis Based on the Subsequent Course of the Disease with Prolonged Follow-Up

	Isocyanate exposure		Colophony exposure	
	Sensitivity	Specificity	Sensitivity	Specificity
Specific challenge	82	100	100	67
Serial PEF; no prophylaxis	100	80	77	100
Serial PEF; on steroids or cromoglycate			44	—

Note: Subjective assessments required changes related to work/rest on >75% of periods.
Abbreviation: PEF, peak expiratory flow.

periods at work lasting at least three days, and at least five changes between consecutive days at work and away from work (about three weeks). Records that failed at least one of these quality standards had reduced sensitivity (63.6%) and specificity (83.3%) (40).

Other works have shown that visual inspection of the records is more helpful than statistical testing (41). Perrin et al. (37) prospectively studied 61 subjects with suspected OA using serial peak flow readings, methacholine responsiveness before and after a period off work, and specific bronchial provocation testing. They took the specific provocation test as the gold standard and compared the peak flow record assessed by three people, to that analyzed statistically. They excluded seven peak flow records, which were regarded as inadequate for making firm conclusions. The sensitivity and specificity of their analyses are shown in Table 3. Subjective assessment of the records achieved 87% sensitivity (by undefined criteria) and 84% specificity. A 3.2-fold change in methacholine responsiveness while off work was 48% sensitive and 64% specific, while the best statistical analysis achieved 76% sensitivity and 58% specificity. Agreement between readers is important, but not always appreciated. In studies to date looking at relatively clear-cut cases, Liss and Tarlo, for example, quoted agreement as measured by a kappa score of 0.62 to 0.83 for inter-reader agreement, while Malo et al. (29) quoted intrareader agreement as 83% to 100% (35). Using a wide range of equivocal and clear-cut records, seven experts had a median kappa value of 0.84 when deciding whether a peak flow record was more or less likely to show an occupational effect (42). The same experts had less agreement on the presence or absence of asthma from the same plots (kappa 0.58). As expected there was less agreement for the records showing less clear-cut changes. Experts were less certain than they were on using Oasys-2 (underscoring compared to Oasys-2), a system with > 90% specificity.

Oasys-2 is a computer-based pattern recognition system developed for the identification of work effects in serial peak flow records and has the advantage of complete repeatability. It is designed to detect an occupational effect rather than OA (43). The analysis splits the record up into a series of overlapping elements containing either a period at work, a period away from work, and a period at work (a work-rest-work complex), or its counterpart, a rest-work-rest complex. Discriminant analyses have been developed to mimic the effects of an expert, and tested against a

Table 3 Sensitivity and Specificity of Measures Taken from Serial Plots of Peak Flow and Measurements of Methacholine Reactivity Before and After a Period of at Least Two Weeks Off Work, Compared with Specific Bronchial Provocation Tests, Used as the Gold Standard

	Sensitivity (%)	Specificity (%)
Visual inspection of peak flow plot	87	84
Methacholine PC_{20} >3.2-fold change	43	65
Mean peak flow lower at work	76	58
Maximum peak flow lower at work	44	81
Minimum peak flow lower at work	57	81
Three workdays with mean peak flow >2 SD of values away from work	52	22

Note: The work period was two weeks unless obvious deterioration occurred earlier. Results from the Montreal group.
Source: From Ref. 37.

wide range of workers records. The sensitivity and specificity improve with more frequent readings, the absence of isolated workdays, and records of at least three weeks duration, as noted above.

The interpretation of equivocal records can be enhanced by including measurements of nonspecific bronchial responsiveness, before and after a two-week period away from exposure (44,45), or after removal from exposure (46). A fourfold increase in the dose of histamine or methacholine required to drop the FEV_1 by 20% after a period without exposure increases the probability of occupational asthma. Failure to show an improvement in nonspecific reactivity, or measurements within the normal range at work are, however, relatively frequent in workers with genuine OA (47).

It is unclear as yet whether these records can differentiate between irritant and allergic asthmatic reactions, largely owing to the problems of differentiating between these types of mechanisms using other criteria. There are some workers who have quite large day to day changes at work, with very low diurnal variations throughout. It seems unlikely that smooth muscle constriction in the bronchi is a prominent feature in this type of reaction. Large diurnal variations can certainly be caused by nonallergic mechanisms, for instance, the classical asthmatic reaction to exercise. Identifications of patterns of reactions from serial peak flow records does allow the separation of reactions into different groups suitable for mechanistic evaluation. A study of workers with asthma caused by low-molecular-weight agents showed no relationship between the magnitude of diurnal variation or mean PEF falls on workdays and the presence or absence of sputum eosinophilia, increased nonspecific reactivity, atopy, smoking, or treatment (48).

Confounding Factors

The control for confounding factors is fundamental before any meaningful analysis of work effect can be done. Varying treatment is the most difficult to control for, and is best eliminated by making the PEF record while on the same treatment throughout. The effect of bronchodilator use can be minimized by making readings before inhalation. Without control, some individuals will increase treatment in anticipation of, or following, deterioration at work, thereby minimizing any change in PEF. If less treatment is taken on days away from work, the maximum PEF may be lower; this combined with an increase in the minimum daily PEF on the same days should alert the reporter to the problem (16). Periods on and off corticosteroids need analyzing separately. Respiratory infections are the most serious, as they can cause large changes in PEF. If the worker takes time off with the infection, it appears that the period away from work is worse than the period at work. A worker may be more susceptible (because of the effects of the infection) or less susceptible (because of the effects of treatment) to the effects of the working environment for some time after the acute infection. Upper respiratory tract infections can produce effects as large as those caused by work, with a maximum mean fall in PEF of around 20%, lasting for an average of seven days (49). The most appropriate solution is to remove the part of the record affected by respiratory infection. There can be problems with differentiating between respiratory infection and occupational rhinitis when symptoms alone are used. Previously normal workers who develop OA also develop wheeze with nonspecific triggers such as exercise, perfumes, cold air, etc., causing the PEF to drop. Provided that the recording is long enough it is unlikely that confounding will occur. The possible exception is exercise, which may be a fundamental part of some jobs; in such cases it may be impossible to separate the effects of sensitization and exercise from PEF records alone.

Exposure to the offending agent is usually not measured and is likely to vary from day to day. Days when exposure is known not to occur should be analyzed as days away from exposure. Varying daily exposure is likely to be a major determinant of the inconsistent work effects seen in some records.

Practical Aspects

Obtaining records that are suitable for analysis involves repeated and usually unsupervised exposures to a work environment which may be causing OA. It is clearly not suitable for workers with anaphylactic type reactions, for whom carefully controlled bronchial provocation testing with suitable minute levels of exposure are more appropriate, if a specific diagnosis is required. Serial peak flow measurement requires commitment from workers, and is difficult to achieve in some workplaces where full respiratory protection is required. It is usually possible to make recordings on waking, on arrival at work, during each formal rest period at work, on leaving work, at home after work, and on retiring to bed. Such records are unlikely to be evenly spaced in time; this probably does not matter when there are at least four readings per day (although it provides a problem for spectral analysis) (50). It is best to aim for readings that are recorded every two hours, particularly in those with mild reactions or those whose peak flow pattern is chaotic. After sending instruction through by post, 56% of patients referred to a specialist clinic returned records, increasing to 85% after personal instruction (51). The requirement of three consecutive workdays is the most frequent reason for failing quality standards, and the requirement for readings that are recorded every two hours are the most easily obtained. Most workers who fail to keep an adequate record transcribed manually also fail to produce adequate records with a logging meter. Some workers keep much better records on workdays than rest days. Rest day records are often the most important, as there are usually fewer of them. Some workers seem to take amazingly few days off work and for them records over annual holidays are often required.

Records may be compounded when workers make up the readings, or record them inaccurately. Twenty one subjects, eight of whom had OA, were asked to keep two-hour measurements of PEF using a VMX meter (fairly bulky), for a mean of 36 days. There was some entry for 80% of the possible two-hour measurements; of these 69% were recorded by hand and logged by the meter, 3% logged but not hand recorded, and 28% recorded by hand and not logged (and probably invented) (52). The hand record differed from the logged record by more than 20 L/min for 11% of readings, and the timing differed by more than one hour for 29% of the readings. Those seeking compensation kept records less satisfactorily. Similar results were obtained in a study of 13 workers investigated for OA; 11% of recordings had different values between the manual and logged readings, 13% had differences in timing, and 20% had manual readings which were not logged. When the subjects were asked to keep six readings a day for an average of 23 days, there was a logged entry for 97% of the required times (53). The records from these two studies were pooled for an assessment of expert interpretation. Experts found it easier to agree about the interpretation of the hand records rather than the logged records, but also diagnosed OA more often from the hand records. Records from the less compliant were more difficult to interpret (52). Some have interpreted the inaccuracy of the hand records over the logged record as invalidating the diagnosis of occupational asthma using this method (53). The sensitivities of the assessments ranging from 69% to 100% and the specificity ranging from 84% to 100% described above include the presumably prefabricated and mistimed readings, suggesting that the method is robust enough to cope with these inaccuracies.

SERIAL MEASUREMENTS OF NONALLERGIC BRONCHIAL RESPONSIVENESS

Asthma is characterized by nonallergic bronchial hyperresponsiveness (NBHR). It is not surprising that most patients with symptomatic OA demonstrate evidence of NBHR irrespective of the causative agent (54–57). It is not clear whether NBHR is a predisposing risk factor for developing OA or occurs as a consequence of OA. In a study of four western red cedar workers, NBHR developed along with the development of asthma and was not present in any of the workers beforehand (58). In another study of laboratory animal workers (59), the development of chest symptoms was associated with an increase in NBHR after 18 months of exposure and correlated with the intensity of exposure. The level of preemployment NBHR did not predict sensitization. The results of these two studies suggest that development of NBHR is the result of sensitization and not a predisposing factor. However, in a more recent prospective study of apprentices exposed to laboratory animals, preexisting NBHR ($PC_{20} < 32$ mg/mL methacholine) carried a relative risk of 2.5 (95% CI: 1.0–5.8) for developing probable OA (60).

Rationale for Measurement of NBR in the Diagnosis of OA

There are several important observations of NBR in patients with OA that render its measurement potentially useful in the assessment and diagnosis of OA. First, while symptomatic patients with OA have NBHR, their NBHR improves and may even return to normal after the cessation of exposure to the offending agent (56,61–66). The speed with which NBHR returns to normal is highly variable. In a study of snowcrab workers with OA, NBHR was found to be significantly improved by the first follow-up assessment at a mean of 12.8 months after leaving work (56). The plateau for improvement occurred at about two years. In a recent report of 48 subjects with OA examined 8.9 years on average after the exposure had ceased, there was significant improvement in NBHR when compared with another group of subjects for whom exposure had ceased less than five years before, suggesting that improvement in NBHR may occur beyond two years (67). However, NBHR may not improve after the cessation of exposure in some types of OA (62,68). For example, in a group of platinum workers with OA, no improvement in BHR occurred after an average of 19 months (range 1–77 months) away from exposure even though 29% of them ceased to have asthmatic symptoms (62). In another group of patients with diisocyanate-induced asthma, NBHR did not change during follow up in most subjects even when specific challenges became negative (63). The likelihood of NBHR returning to normal after the exposure has ceased appears to depend on the degree of airflow obstruction, the degree of BHR, and the duration of exposure to the offending agent at the time of diagnosis (64,65,69). Early diagnosis and early removal from exposure is associated with NBHR returning to normal. Treatment with inhaled beclomethasone for five months after removal from exposure has been shown to significantly reduce the degree of NBHR in toluene diisocyanate–induced asthma in a placebo-controlled trial (70).

Second, after returning to normal, NBHR may recur in conjunction with symptoms of asthma on re-exposure to the offending agent (71). Thus serial measurements of NBHR at work and away from work may be another objective test to demonstrate work-relatedness of asthma in addition to serial measurement of PEF, which is largely dependent on the compliance of the patients.

Third, the induction of a late or dual asthmatic reaction after specific challenge testing is often associated with an increase in NBHR (72,73). In some subjects, NBHR may increase after specific inhalation challenge testing, in the absence of a significant change in the FEV_1. This observation can be an early and sensitive marker of a specific bronchial response to occupational agents, especially in subjects removed from workplace exposure for a long time. It is an indicator that subjects will likely react to the specific agent at the next or subsequent dose of challenge testing (74).

Fourth, the degree of specific responsiveness to an occupational agent on challenge testing is directly correlated with the degree of NBHR (75). This observation is particularly useful in the assessment of patients with OA caused by low-molecular-weight compounds when skin testing with the relevant agent is not possible to determine the initial concentration that can be safely used in specific inhalation challenge tests. When a patient has a high degree of NBHR, it is important to start inhalation testing using a very low dose of the specific agent.

Methods of Measurement of NBR

Nonallergic bronchial responsiveness can be evaluated using a number of stimuli, including methacholine, histamine, adenosine, cold air, hyperventilation, or hypoosmolar or hyperosmolar stimuli. Histamine and methacholine are the most common agents employed because the method of challenge testing has been standardized and guidelines for performing such testing have been published by the American Thoracic Society (76). Methacholine or histamine may be administered in two ways, either by a timed period of tidal breathing of aerosols of known concentration (77) or controlled inhalation of discrete doses, for example, the rapid method of Yan et al. (78). The time between dosages is one minute for the Yan method (78) and about five minutes for most others (77–79). The response is usually measured as the percentage change in the FEV_1 from baseline. This is then plotted against the log of concentration or dose. The dose plotted may be either cumulative or noncumulative. Doubling doses of histamine at one-minute intervals produces a cumulative effect, whereas when histamine or methacholine is being given in doubling doses at five-minute intervals, there is no significant cumulative effect. The position of the resulting curve indicates the sensitivity of the airways to the provoking agent. The result is usually reported as the dose or concentration that causes a 20% fall in FEV_1, $PD_{20}FEV_1$, or $PC_{20}FEV_1$. Values for $PD_{20}FEV_1$ or $PC_{20}FEV_1$ are reproducible to within 1.5 to 2 doubling doses (80,81). Results from the tidal breathing method are usually reported as $PC_{20}FEV_1$. In adults, histamine and methacholine appear to be equipotent in asthmatics (82). The dose-response curve in asthmatics is characterized by a shift to the left and an increased maximal response when compared those with normal subjects (83).

The degree of NBHR in the population is log-normally distributed (84). An arbitrary cutoff must therefore be selected in defining an abnormal test, for example, a PD_{20} FEV_1 of 3.9 to 7.8 μmol or a $PC_{20}FEV_1$ of 8 to 16 mg/mL. Cutoff points have been selected so as to be highly sensitive, including all asthmatics, but have moderate specificity. In population samples, the prevalence of asthma is usually <10%. When BHR is measured in such samples, because of its high sensitivity but moderate specificity, it has a high negative predictive value for symptoms (99–100%), but a low positive predictive value (25–35%) (85). Cockcroft et al. (86) performed histamine challenge tests on 500 randomly selected university students. They concluded that a PC_{20} greater than 8 mg/mL virtually rules out current symptomatic asthma, and a PC_{20} below 1 mg/mL is diagnostic of current symptomatic asthma, whereas values between 1 and 8 mg/mL are borderline.

NBHR is present in almost all subjects with current symptomatic asthma. Mild degree of NBHR is found in some subjects with rhinitis but without chest symptoms and in some asymptomatic individuals (87). The measurement of HBHR is helpful when correlated with symptoms. Thus, in subjects with atypical chest symptoms and normal spirometry, the presence of NBHR increases the likelihood of asthma. In subjects with current chest symptoms, the absence of NBHR excludes the diagnosis of asthma in most cases (provided there is no other reason for the lack of NBHR, such as high dose of steroids). However, some symptomatic subjects may not have NBHR within the usual asthmatic range, but on exposure to the offending agent, develop reduction in lung function and increase in symptoms.

Technical factors may influence measurement of NBHR; the most important is nebulizer output. The nebulizer's output should be calibrated regularly at two- to three-month intervals (76). Several subject factors also influence measurement of NBHR, and the most important one is the prechallenge FEV_1 (88). Other factors include recent exposure to allergens (69,92) or occupational sensitizers (89–91), time of the day, recent respiratory infections, and acute exacerbations of asthma. H_1 inhibitors block the effect of histamine, and anticholinergic drugs block the effect of methacholine. All bronchodilators inhibit the effects of histamine and methacholine (93). These drugs should be withheld for an appropriate length of time before the challenge tests (76). Methacholine or histamine challenge test should not be done when the baseline FEV_1 is below 70% of predicted, as the results are difficult to interpret (94,95).

The Role of Measurement of NBHR in the Management of OA

Diagnosis of Asthma

The first step in the diagnosis of OA is to determine whether the patient has asthma. A normal NSBH does not exclude the diagnosis of OA, particularly when the subjects are being tested after they have been away from work (54). In some patients with early OA, NBHR may return to normal within a short period of time without exposure, which can be as short as one to two days (73). There are a large number of studies using different methods of measurement of NBHR from many centers, showing that NBHR may be normal in 5% to 40% of patients with positive specific challenge tests (96–105). Nevertheless, measurement of NBHR should be done as part of the investigation of a patient with OA for its various other roles as discussed below.

Assessment of Work Relatedness

Serial measurements of NBHR have been recommended to supplement serial measurements of PEF in assessment of work-relatedness of asthma, as the latter test is entirely dependent on the patient's effort and has been shown to be unreliable at

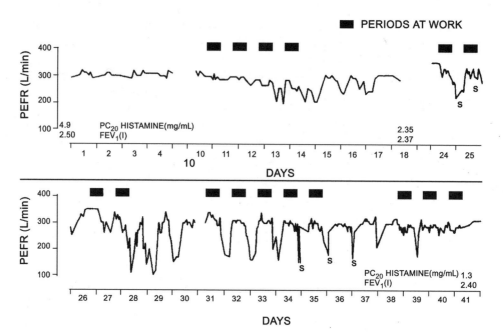

Figure 8 Serial daily change in PEFRs demonstrating significant fluctuations on return to work without recovery on weekends. PC_{20} results and baseline FEV_1 are presented. S is the inhaled salbutamol (200 μg) used. *Abbreviation*: PEFR, peak expiratory flow rate. *Source*: From Ref. 105.

times (53). In a study of western red cedar workers, the sensitivity and specificity of changes in PC_{20} alone for the diagnosis of OA were 62% and 78%, respectively, using the results of the specific challenge test as the gold standard (41). Perrin et al. (37) studied a group of patients with OA caused by other agents and reported a sensitivity of 48% and a specificity of 64% using a 3.2-fold change in NBHR as the criteria; using a twofold change in NBHR, the sensitivity increased to 67% but the specificity reduced to 64%. The addition of measurement of BHR did not improve the diagnostic accuracy of serial measurements of PEF. While it is easier to demonstrate an increase in NBHR when the patient is exposed to the allergen or chemical sensitizer in the work place, it is less easy to demonstrate a decrease in BHR when the patient is away from work as it may take a long time before NSBH improves (54,92). The demonstration of appropriate changes in BHR, together with appropriate changes in serial monitoring of PEF, confirms the work relationship (Fig. 8).

NBHR in the Diagnosis of Reactive Airways Dysfunction Syndrome

One of the main characteristics of the syndrome is the development of NBHR which persists after one single exposure to a high level of toxic gases and fumes. The presence of NBHR is crucial to the diagnosis of this condition as specific challenge test and re-exposure to reproduce the symptoms are not feasible. In one report, persistence of BHR was found up to 13 years after the initial episode (106). A longitudinal study of firefighters who experienced massive exposure to airborne particulates at the World Trade Centre sites found that the development and persistence of BHR and reactive airway dysfunctional syndrome were strongly and independently associated with exposure intensity (107).

Determination of Initial and Subsequent Doses of Occupational Agents for Specific Challenge Tests

Specific challenge tests, while very useful in establishing work-relatedness of asthma, have to be performed with care to avoid the induction of anaphylaxis or a severe attack of asthma. When the occupational agent is a high-molecular-weight allergen and an extract is available for skin tests, the initial concentration to use for specific challenge test can be determined by skin testing. Cockcroft et al. (108) recommended that the initial concentration of the high-molecular-weight allergen to be used for inhalation challenge test should be three to four doubling dilutions below the predicted allergen PC_{20} (the dose of allergen that induces a 20% fall in FEV_1). The allergen PC_{20} is predicted from the formula $\log_{10}$ allergen $PC_{20} = 0.68 \log_{10} (PC_{20} \times SS)$, where SS is the skin sensitivity, which is defined as the lowest allergen dilution that gives a wheal 2-mm in diameter (the mean of two perpendicular measurements on each of the two duplicate prick tests). However, when the occupational agent is a low-molecular-weight compound such as diisocyanate and plicatic acid, skin testing is usually negative. Measurement of BHR is essential before specific challenge testing. Patients with a high degree of BHR should be challenged very cautiously by starting at a very low concentration of the specific agent to avoid severe reactions.

Inhalation challenge tests with low-molecular-weight agents induce isolated late asthmatic reactions frequently. Specific challenge tests with diisocyanates are time consuming. To avoid serious reactions, the duration of exposure or the nonirritative concentrations (5–20 ppb) is usually increased stepwise over several days. When no airflow obstruction is detected at eight hours after the specific challenge testing, it is useful to determine the level of BHR. If the PC_{20} decreases in the absence of airflow obstruction, it is likely that the patient may react to the next dose (either increased concentration or increased duration of exposure) of the specific agent the following day. False negative results can be avoided in the absence of significant changes in FEV_1 after specific challenge testing with diisocyanates, by monitoring of BHR before and after specific challenge testing (109).

Assessment of Respiratory Impairment/Disability in OA

Measurement of NBHR has been found to correlate with various parameters for assessment of asthma severity such as diurnal variation of peak flow rates (110), asthma symptom scores (111), and the minimum medication requirement necessary to achieve control of symptoms (112). Thus measurement of the degree of BHR adds another dimension in the objective assessment of respiratory impairment in OA as discussed in the chapter on impairment assessment (113,114). As improvement in BHR may occur after two years of being away from exposure, it may be necessary to have periodic reassessment of impairment after the initial evaluation for permanent respiratory impairment carried out at two years.

SUMMARY

Self-recorded lung function always lacks credibility to the sceptic. Logging meters overcome some of the problems. Such meters should record all blows and provide quality control in real time so that the worker knows whether further blows are required. The meters should obviously be technically satisfactory and linear. In our experience, compliance with logging meters is often less than that with conventional peak flow meters. Many logging meters are heavier, and some are quite complicated.

Many require a FEV_1 maneuver, which can be more difficult. However, even in the case of a positive pattern, PEF cannot relate symptoms to a specific agent. Thus it is not useful in etiological diagnosis, except when there is a clear demonstration of specific sensitization to agents present at work (115).

Serial measurement of NBHR is helpful when there are appropriate changes in NBHR together with appropriate changes in serial monitoring of PEF.

Measurement of NBHR is also mandatory for the diagnosis of reactive airway dysfunction syndrome or irritant-induced asthma and is very helpful in assessing the dose of occupational agent for specific inhalation testing especially for low-molecular-weight agents.

DIRECTIONS FOR FUTURE RESEARCH

- Further work is needed on the analysis of long periods off work in serial PEF monitoring. If significant improvement occurs during a two- to four-week period off work, with deterioration on return to work, OA is likely whatever the rest of the record shows.
- Further analysis of the diurnal variation changes and average hourly plots of serial PEF measurement may produce better diagnostic accuracy.
- Study of the serial PEF changes from irritant reactions and to distinguish them from those caused by hypersensitivity.
- Recommendations for analysis and interpretation of PEF records during treatment should be developed.
- Prospective studies to determine whether NBHR predisposes to the development of OA and/or is a consequence of the disease.
- Study the mechanisms for persistence of NBHR in patients with OA after removal from exposure to the offending agent.

REFERENCES

1. Nicholson PJ, Cullinan P, Newman Taylor AJ, Burge PS, Boyle C. Evidence based guidelines for the prevention, identification and management of occupational asthma: Evidence review and recommendations. Occup Environ Med 2005; 62:290–299.
2. Hetzel MR, Clark TJH. Comparison of normal and asthmatic circadian rhythms in peak expiratory flow rate. Thorax 1980; 35:732–738.
3. Randem B, Smolensky MH, Hsi B, Albright D, Burge PS. Field survey of circadian rhythm in PEF of electronics workers suffering from colophony-induced asthma. Chronobiol Int 1987; 4:263–271.
4. do Pico GA, Reddan W, Anderson S, Flaherty D, Smally E. Acute effects of grain dust exposure during a work shift. Am Rev Respir Dis 1983; 128:399–404.
5. Enarson DA, Vedal S, Chan-Yeung M. Fate of grainhandlers with bronchial hyperreactivity. Clin Invest Med 1988; 11:193–197.
6. Gee JB, Morgan WKC. A 10 year follow-up study of a group of workers exposed to isocyanates. J Occup Med 1985; 27:15–18.
7. Krumpe PE, Finley TN, Martinez N. The search for expiratory obstruction in meat wrappers studied on the job. Am Rev Respir Dis 1979; 119:611–618.
8. Liss GM, Bernstein DI, Moller DR, Gallagher JS, Stephenson RL, Bernstein IL. Pulmonary immunologic evaluation of foundry workers exposed to methylene diphenyldiisocyanate (MDI). J Allergy Clin Immunol 1988; 82:55–61.

9. Moller DR, Gallagher JS, Bernstein DI, Wilcox TG, Burroughs HE, Bernstein IL. Detection of IgE mediated respiratory sensitisation in workers exposed to hexahydrophthalic anhydride. J Allergy Clin Immunol 1985; 75:663–672.

10. Orford RR, Wilson JT. Epidemiologic and immunologic studies in processors of the king crab. Am J Industr Med 1985; 7:155–169.

11. Burge PS, Perks WH, O'Brien IM, et al. Occupational asthma in an electronics factory; a case control study to evaluate aetiological factors. Thorax 1979; 34:300–307.

12. Bardy J-D, Malo J-L, Seguin P, et al. Occupational asthma and IgE sensitisation in a pharmaceutical company processing psyllium. Am Rev Respir Dis 1987; 135:1033–1038.

13. Malo J-L, Cartier A. Occupational asthma in workers of a pharmaceutical company processing spiramycin. Thorax 1988; 43:371–377.

14. Burge PS, O'Brien IM, Harries MG. Peak flow rate records in the diagnosis of occupational asthma due to colophony. Thorax 1979; 34:308–316.

15. Burge PS, O'Brien IM, Harries MG. Peak flow rate records in the diagnosis of occupational asthma due to isocyanates. Thorax 1979; 34:317–323.

16. Burge PS. Single and serial measurements of lung function in the diagnosis of occupational asthma. Eur J Respir Dis Suppl 1982; 123:47–59.

17. Weir DC, Burge PS. Measures of reversibility in response to bronchodilators in chronic airflow obstruction: relation to airway calibre. Thorax 1991; 46:43–45.

18. Robertson AS, Weir DC, Burge PS. Occupational asthma due to oil mists. Thorax 1988; 43:200–205.

19. Burge PS, Finnegan M, Horsfield N, et al. Occupational asthma in a factory with a contaminated humidifier. Thorax 1985; 40:248–254.

20. Gannon PFG, Dickinson S, Hitchings D, Burge PS. Quality of self recorded peak expiratory flow. Thorax 1993; 48:1062.

21. Miller MR, Dickinson SA, Hitchings DJ. The accuracy of portable peak flow meters. Thorax 1992; 47:904–909.

22. Shapiro SM, Hendler JM, Ogirala RG, Aldrich TK, Shapiro MB. An evaluation of the accuracy of Assess and MiniWright peak flowmeters. Chest 1991; 99:358–362.

23. Berube D, Cartier A, L'Archeveque J, Ghezzo H, Malo J-L. Comparison of peak expiratory flow rate and FEVl in assessing bronchomotor tone after challenges with occupational sensitizers. Chest 1991; 99:831–836.

24. Giannini D, Paggiaro PL, Moscato G, et al. Comparison between peak expiratory flow and forced expiratory volume in one second (FEVl) during bronchoconstriction induced by different stimuli. J Asthma 1997; 34:105–111.

25. Paggiaro PL, Moscato G, Giannini D, et al. The Italian working group on the use of peak expiratory flow rate (PEFR) in asthma. Eur Respir Rev 1993; 3:438–443.

26. Bright P, Burge PS. Comparison of mean daily diurnal variation in PEF and FEVl. Am J Respir Crit Care Med 1997; 155:A137.

27. Leroyer C, Perfetti L, Trudeau C, Ghezzo H, Chan-Yeung M, Malo J. Comparison of PEF and FEV1 monitoring with specific inhalation challenge in the diagnosis of occupational asthma. Am J Respir Crit Care Med 1997; 155:A137.

28. Blainey AD, Ollier S, Cundell D, Smith RE, Davies RJ. Occupational asthma in a hairdressing salon. Thorax 1986; 41:42–50.

29. Malo JL, Cote J, Cartier A, Boulet LP, L'Archeveque J, Chan-Yeung M. How many times per day should peak expiratory flow rates be assessed when investigating occupational asthma? Thorax 1993; 48:1211–1217.

30. Gannon PF, Newton DT, Pantin CF, Burge PS. Effect of the number of peak expiratory flow readings per day on the estimation of diurnal variation. Thorax 1998; 53:790–792.

31. Bright P, Burge PS. The diagnosis of occupational asthma from serial measurements of lung function at and away from work. Thorax 1996; 51:857–863.

32. Burge PS. Prolonged and frequent recording of peak expiratory flow rate in workers with suspected occupational asthma due to colophony or isocyanate fumes. MSc thesis, London School of Hygiene, 1978.

33. Smith AB, Bernstein DI Aw T-C, et al. Occupational asthma from inhaled egg protein. Am J Industr Med 1987; 12:205–218.

34. Cartier A, Bernstein IL, Burge PS, et al. Guidelines for bronchoprovocation on the investigation of occupational asthma. J Allergy Clin Immunol 1989; 84:823–829.

35. Liss GM, Tarlo SM. Peak expiratory flow rates in possible occupational asthma. Chest 1991; 100:63–69.

36. Heinneberger PK, Stanbury MJ, Trimbath LS, Kipen HM. The use of portable peak flow meters in the surveillance of occupational asthma. Chest 1991; 100:1515–1521.

37. Perrin B, Lagier F, L'Archeveque J, et al. Occupational asthma: validity of monitoring of peak expiratory flow rates and nonallergic bronchial responsiveness as compared to specific inhalation challenge. Eur Respir J 1992; 5:40–48.

38. Giannini D, di Pede F, Moscato G, et al. Sensitivity of peak flow monitoring to detect occupational asthma in relationship with specific bronchial challenge. Eur Respir J 1994; 7:312s.

39. Venables KM, Davison AG, Browne K, Newman Taylor AJ. Pseudo-occupational asthma. Thorax 1989; 44:760–761.

40. Gannon PFG, Newton DT, Belcher J, Pantin CF, Burge PS. Development of OASYS-2: a system for the analysis of serial measurement of peak expiratory flow in workers with suspected occupational asthma. Thorax 1996; 51:484–489.

41. Cote J, Kennedy S, Chan-Yeung M. Sensitivity and specificity of PC20 and peak expiratory flow rate in cedar asthma. J Allergy Clin Immunol 1990; 85:592–598.

42. Baldwin DR, Gannon PFG, Bright P, et al. Interpretation of occupational peak flow records: level of agreement between expert clinicians and Oasys-2. Thorax 2002; 57:860–864.

43. Gannon PFG, Newton DT, Belcher J, Pantin CF, Burge PS. Development of OASYS-2: a system for the analysis of serial measurement of peak expiratory flow in workers with suspected occupational asthma. Thorax 1996; 51:484–489.

44. Cartier A, Pineau L, Malo J-L. Monitoring of maximum expiratory peak flow rates and histamine inhalation tests in the investigation of occupational asthma. Clin Allergy 1984; 14:193–196.

45. Kongerud J, Soyseth V, Burge PS. Serial measurements of peak expiratory flow and responsiveness to methacholine in the diagnosis of aluminium potroom asthma. Thorax 1992; 47:292–297.

46. Malo J-L, Cartier A, Ghezzo H, Lafrance M, McCants M, Lehrer SB. Patterns of improvement in spirometry, bronchial hyperresponsiveness, and specific IgE antibody levels after cessation of exposure in occupational asthma caused by snow-crab processing. Am Rev Respir Dis 1988; 138:807–812.

47. Burge PS. Non-specific hyperreactivity in workers exposed to toluene diisocyanate, diphenyl methane diisocyanate and colophony. Eur J Respir Dis 1982; 123(63 suppl):91–96.

48. Anees W, Huggins V, Pavord I, Robertson AS, Burge PS. Occupational asthma due to low molecular weight agents: eosinoiphilic and non-eosinophilic variants. Thorax 2002; 57:231–236.

49. O'Brien C, Bright P, Nicholson C, Burge PS. Pattern of peak expiratory low response to upper respiratory tract infections in asthmatics. Eur Respir J 1995; 19(suppl 8):272.

50. Belcher J, Hampton JS, Tunicliffe Wilson G. Parameterisation of continuous time autoregressive models for irregularly sampled time series data. Appl Stat 1993.

51. Huggins V, Anees W, Pantin CFA, Burge PS. Improving the quality of peak flow measurements for the diagnosis of occuapational asthma. Occup Med 2005; 55: 385–388.

52. Malo JL, Carrier A, Ghezzo H, Chan-Yeung M. Compliance with peak expiratory flow readings affects the within-and between-reader reproducibility of interpretation of graphs in subjects investigated for occupational asthma. J Allergy Clin Immunol 1996; 98:1132–1134.

53. Quirce S, Contreras G, Dybuncio A, Chan-Yeung M. Peak expiratory flow monitoring is not a reliable method for establishing the diagnosis of occupational asthma. Am J Respir Crit Care Med 1995; 152:1100–1102.
54. Lam S, Wong R, Chan-Yeung M. Nonspecific bronchial reactivity in occupational asthma. J Allergy Clin Immunol 1979; 63:28–34.
55. Burge PS. Occupational asthma in electronics workers caused by colophony fumes: follow-up of affected workers. Thorax 1982; 37:348–353.
56. Malo JL, Cartier A, Ghezzo H, Lafrance M, McCants M, Lehrer SB. Patterns of improvement in spirometry, bronchial hyperresponsiveness, and specific IgE antibody levels after cessation of exposure in occupational asthma caused by snow-crab processing. Am R Respir Dis 1988; 138:807–812.
57. Graneek BJ, Durham SR, Newman Taylor AJ. Late asthmatic reactions and changes in histamine responsiveness provoked by occupational agents. Bull Eur Physiopathol Respir 1987; 23:577–581.
58. Chan-Yeung M, Desjardins A. Bronchial hyperresponsiveness and level of exposure in occupational asthma due to western red cedar (*Thuja plicata*). Serial observations before and after development of symptoms. Am R Respir Dis 1992; 146:1606–1609.
59. Renstrom A, Malmberg P, Larsson K, Larsson PH, Sundblad BM. Allergic sensitization is associated with increased bronchial responsiveness: a prospective study of allergy to laboratory animals. Eur Respir J 1995; 8:1514–1519.
60. Gautrin G, Infante-Rivard C, Ghezzo H, Malo JL. Incidence and host determinants of probable occupational asthma in apprentices exposed to laboratory animals. Am J Respir Crit Care Med 2001; 163:899–904.
61. Saric M, Marelja J. Bronchial hyperreactivity in potroom workers and prognosis after stopping exposure. Brit J Ind Med 1991; 48:653–655.
62. Merget R, Reineke M, Rueckmann A, Bergmann EM, Schultze-Weminghaus G. Nonspecific and specific bronchial responsiveness in occupational asthma caused by platinum salts after allergen avoidance. Am J Respir Crit Care Med 1994; 150:1146–1149.
63. Paggiaro PL, Vagaggini B, Dente FL, et al. Bronchial hyperresponsiveness and toluene diisocyanate. Long-term change in sensitized asthmatic subjects. Chest 1993; 103:1123–1128.
64. Chan-Yeung M, Lam S, Koerner S. Clinical features and natural history of occupational asthma due to western red cedar (*Thuja plicata*). Am J Med 1982; 72:411–415.
65. Chan-Yeung M, MacLean L, Paggiaro PL. Follow-up study of 232 patients with occupational asthma caused by western red cedar (*Thuja plicata*). J Allergy Clin Immunol 1987; 79:792–796.
66. Lemiere C, Cartier A, Dolovich J, et al. Outcome of specific bronchial responsiveness to occupational agents after removal from exposure. Am J Respir Crit Care Med 1996; 154:329–333.
67. Perfetti L, Cartier A, Ghezzo H, Gautrin D, Malo J-L. Follow-up of occupational asthma after removal from or diminution of exposure to the responsible agent: relevance of the length of the interval from cessation of exposure. Chest 1998; 114:398–403.
68. Pisati G, Zedda S. Outcome of occupational asthma due to cobalt hypersensitivity. Sci Environ 1994; 150:167–171.
69. Mapp CE, Corona PC, De MN, Fabbri L. Persistent asthma due to isocyanates. A follow-up study of subjects with occupational asthma due to toluene diisocyanate (TDI). Am R Respir Dis 1988; 137:1326–1329.
70. Maestrelli P, De MN, Saetta M, Boscaro M, Fabbri LM, Mapp CE. Effects of inhaled beclomethasone on airway responsiveness in occupational asthma. Placebo-controlled study of subjects sensitized to toluene diisocyanate. Am Rev Respir Dis 1993; 148:407–412.
71. Banks DE, Rando RJ. Recurrent asthma induced by toluene diisocyanate. Thorax 1988; 43:660–662.
72. Fabbri LM, Picotti G, Mapp CE. Late asthmatic reactions, airway inflammation and chronic asthma in TDI sensitized subjects. Eur Respir J 1991(suppl 13):2.

73. Malo JL, Ghezzo H, L'Archeveque J, Cartier A. Late asthmatic reactions to occupational sensitizing agents: frequency of changes in nonspecific bronchial responsiveness and of response to inhaled beta 2-adrenergic agent. J Allergy Clin Immunol 1990; 85:834–842.

74. Vandenplas O, Delwiche JP, Jamart J, Van de Weyer R. Increase in non-specific bronchial hyperresponsiveness as an early marker of bronchial response to occupational agents during specific inhalation challenges. Thorax 1996; 51:472–478.

75. Lam S, Tan F, Chan H, Chan-Yeung M. Relationship between types of asthmatic reaction, nonspecific bronchial reactivity, and specific IgE antibodies in patients with red cedar asthma. J Allergy Clin Immunol 1983; 72:134–139.

76. American Thoracic Society. Guidelines for methacholine and exercise challenge testing-1999. Am J Respir Crit Care Med 2000; 161:309–329.

77. Cockcroft DW, Killian DN, Mellon JJA, Hargreave FE. Bronchial reactivity to inhaled histamine: a method and clinical survey. Clin Allergy 1977; 7:235–243.

78. Yan K, Salome C, Woolcock AJ. Rapid method for measurement of bronchial responsiveness. Thorax 1983; 38:760–765.

79. Chai H, Fair R, Froehlich LA, et al. Standardization of bronchial inhalation challenge procedures. J Allergy Clin Immunol 1975; 56:323–327.

80. Chinn S, Britton JR, Burney PG, Tattersfield AE, Papacosta AO. Estimation and repeatability of the response to inhaled histamine in a community survey. Thorax 1987; 42:45–52.

81. Peat JK, Salome CM, Bauman A, Toelle BG, Wachinger SL, Woolcock AJ. Repeatability of histamine bronchial challenge and comparability with methacholine bronchial challenge in a population of Australian school children. Am R Respir Dis 1991; 144:338–343.

82. Salome CM, Schoeffel RE, Woolcock AJ. Comparison of bronchial reactivity to histamine and methacholine in asthmatics. Clin Allergy 1980; 10:541–546.

83. Woolcock AJ, Salome C, Yan K. The shape of the dose-response curve to histamine in asthmatics and normal subjects. Am R Respir Dis 1984; 130:71–75.

84. Peat JK, Unger WR, Combe D. Measuring changes in logarithmic data, with special reference to bronchial responsiveness. J Clin Epidemiol 1994; 47:1099–1108.

85. Backer V. Bronchial hyperresponsiveness in children and adolescents. Dan Med Bull 1995; 42:397–409.

86. Cockcroft DW, Murdock KY, Berscheid BA, Gore BP. Sensitivity and specificity of histamine PC20 determination in a random selection of young college students. J Allergy Clin Immunol 1992; 89:23–30.

87. Varpela E, Laitinen LA, Keskinen H, Korhola O. Asthma, allergy and bronchial hyperreactivity to histamine in patients with bronchiectasis. Clin Allergy 1978; 8:273–280.

88. Ulrik CS. Bronchial responsiveness to inhaled histamine in both adults with intrinsic and extrinsic asthma: the importance of prechallenge forced expiratory volume in 1 second. J Allergy Clin Immunol 1993; 91:120–126.

89. van der Heide S, de Monchy JG, de Vries K, Bruggink TM, Kauffman HF. Seasonal variation in airway hyperresponsiveness and natural exposure to house dust mite allergens in patients with asthma. J Allergy Clin Immunol 1994; 93:470–475.

90. Cartier A, Thomson NC, Frith PA, Roberts R, Hargreave FE. Allergen-induced increase in bronchial responsiveness to histamine: relationship to the late asthmatic response and change in airway caliber. J Allergy Clin Immunol 1982; 70:170–177.

91. Cockcroft DW, Ruffin RE, Dolovich J, Hargreave FE. Allergen-induced increase in non-allergic bronchial reactivity. Clin Allergy 1977; 7:503–513.

92. Cartier A, L'Archeveque J, Malo JL. Exposure to a sensitizing occupational agent can cause a long-lasting increase in bronchial responsiveness to histamine in the absence of significant changes in airway caliber. J Allergy Clin Immunol 1986; 78:1185–1189.

93. Hargreave FE, Dolovich J, Boulet LP. Inhalation provocation tests. Sem Respir Med 1983; 4:224–236.

94. American Academy of Asthma, Allergy and Immunology. Diagnosis and evaluation in Practice parameters for the diagnosis and treatment of asthma. J Allergy Clin Immunol 1995; 96:737–738.

95. Martin RJ, Wanger JS, Irvin CG, Bucher Bartelson B, Cherniack RM. Methacholine challenge testing: safety of low starting FEV1. Chest 1997; 112:53–56.

96. Vandenplas O, Binard-Van Cangh F, Brumagne A, et al. Occupational asthma in symptomatic workers exposed to natural rubber latex: evaluation of diagnostic procedures. J Allergy Clin Immunol 2001; 107(3):542–547.

97. Vandenplas O, Delwiche IP, Evrard G, et al. Prevalence of occupational asthma due to latex among hospital personnel. Am J Respir Crit Care Med 1995; 151(l):54–60.

98. Merget R, Dierkes A, Rueckmann A, Bergmann EM, Schultze-Weminghaus G. Absence of relationship between degree of nonspecific and specific bronchial responsiveness in occupational asthma due to platinum salts. Eur Respir J 1996; 9(2): 211–216.

99. Merget R, Schultze-Weminghaus G, Bode F, Bergmann EM, Zachgo W, Meier-Sydow J. Quantitative skin prick and bronchial provocation tests with platinum salt. Br J Ind Med 1991; 48(12):830–837.

100. Tarlo SM, Broder I. Outcome of assessments for occupational asthma. Chest 1991; 100(2):329–335.

101. Anees W, Huggins V, Pavord ID, Robertson AS, Burge PS. Occupational asthma due to low molecular weight agents: eosinophilic and non-eosinophilic variants. Thorax 2002; 57(3):231–236.

102. Lemiere C, Weytjens K, Cartier A, Malo JL. Late asthmatic reaction with airway inflammation but without airway hyperresponsiveness. Clin Exp Allergy 2000; 30(3):415–417.

103. Baur X, Huber H, Degens PO, Allmers H, Ammon J. Relation between occupational asthma case history, bronchial methacholine challenge, and specific challenge test in patients with suspected occupational asthma. Am J Ind Med 1998; 33(2):ll4–122.

104. Moscato G, Dellabianca A, Vinci G, Candura SM, Bossi MC. Toluene diisocyanate-induced asthma: clinical findings and bronchial responsiveness studies in 113 exposed subjects with work-related respiratory symptoms. J Occup Med 1991; 33(6):720–725.

105. Malo JL, Ghezzo H, L'Archeveque J, Lagier F, Perrin B, Cartier A. Is the clinical history a satisfactory means of diagnosing occupational asthma? Am Rev Respir Dis 1991; 143(3):528–532.

106. Piirila PL, Nordman H, Korhonen OS, Winblad I. A thirteen-year follow-up of respiratory effects of acute exposure to sulfur dioxide. Scand J Work Environ Health 1996; 22:191–196.

107. Banauch GI, Alleyne D, Sanchez R, et al. Persistent hyperreactivity and reactive airway dysfunction in firefighters at the World Trade Centre. Am J Respir Crit Care Med 2003; l68:54–62.

108. Cockcroft DW, Murdock KY, Kirby J, Hargreave F. Prediction of airway responsiveness to allergen from skin sensitivity to allergen and airway responsiveness to histamine. Am R Respir Dis 1987; 135:264–267.

109. Sastre J, Fernandez-Nieto M, Novalbos A, De Las Heras M, Cuesta J, Quirce S. Need for monitoring nonspecific bronchial hyperresponsiveness before and after isocyanate inhalation challenge. Chest 2003; 123:987–989.

110. Ryan G, Latimer KM, Dolovich J, Hargreave FE. Bronchial responsiveness to histamine: relationship to diurnal variation of peak flow rate, improvement after bronchodilator, and airway calibre. Thorax 1982; 37:423–429.

111. Makino S. Clinical significance of bronchial sensitivity to acetylcholine and histamine in bronchial asthma. J Allergy 1966; 38:127–142.

112. Juniper EF, Frith PA, Hargreave FE. Airway responsiveness to histamine and methacholine: relationship to minimum treatment to control symptoms of asthma. Thorax 1981; 36:575–579.

113. Chan-Yeung M, Becklake M, Bleecker ER, et al. Impairment of men and women for work: Some scientific issues and evaluation. Am R Respir Dis 1987; 136:1052–1054.
114. American Thoracic Society. Guidelines for the evaluation of impairment/disability in patients with asthma. Am J Respir Crit Care Med 1993; 147:1056–1061.
115. Moscato G, Godnic-Cvar J, Maestrelli P, Malo J-L, Burge PS, Coifman R. Statement on self monitoring of peak expiratory flow in the investigation of occupational asthma. Official Statement. Eur Respir J 1995; 8:1605–1610.

10
Occupational Challenge Tests

Olivier Vandenplas
Department of Chest Medicine, Mont-Godinne Hospital, Catholic University of Louvain, Yvoir, Belgium

André Cartier and Jean-Luc Malo
Department of Chest Medicine, Université de Montréal and Sacré-Cœur Hospital, Montreal, Quebec, Canada

INTRODUCTION—HISTORICAL BACKGROUND

Charles Blackley was the first researcher reported to have performed inhalation challenges using common allergens (1). In 1952, Herxheimer documented the occurrence of late reactions, which have been the subject of numerous studies in the last few years because they are related to the development of bronchial inflammation and "eosinophilic bronchitis," a characteristic of asthma (2). The occurrence of these late reactions after exposure to common allergens was later confirmed by other investigators (3). Based on the work of Helge Colldahl in Stockholm (4), Citron and Pepys described dual reactions in the case of other immunologically mediated bronchoalveolar reactions such as allergic bronchopulmonary aspergillosis (5), farmers' lung (6), and bird fancier's lung (7). In 1970, Professor Pepys suggested the use of specific inhalation tests in the investigation of occupational asthma (OA). As Professor Pepys wrote in a letter:

> The next development was in occupational asthma. We did not know how to test by aerosol inhalation with agents such as TDI etc. or with potentially irritant or extremely potent allergens such as the platinum salts.
>
> The answer to this was the patient with severe asthma clearly related to his work. He made the boats for the Oxford and Cambridge boat race and used a two part polyurethane/TDI marine varnish. As soon as I heard this, he was asked to provide these two separate materials which are mixed together prior to use. The first day, he painted on a slab of wood with the polyurethane with no effect, whereas the mixture tested in the same way the next day elicited asthmatic reactions. This was the answer to the problem and the origin of simulated "occupational type" provocation tests, in other words a piece, and usually a very, very small piece of real life as a highly analytical, precise, and reproducible form of testing. There can be no objections to this if carried out properly since it is no different from the work exposure.

Originally, these tests were carried out in the corridors of the Brompton hospital with people walking about. A well-ventilated cubicle in a room was later made available. A series of reports were published beginning in 1972, dealing with dusts, powders, fumes, gaseous emanations, and aerosols (8–11). For these tests, subjects were asked to reproduce their usual work in a small cubicle under close supervision and with functional assessment. A summary of the proposals for the tests was later published (12). At that time, occupational inhalation challenges (OIC) in the laboratory were the only objective way to confirm that asthma was caused by an agent present in the workplace. Since then, other means such as the monitoring of peak expiratory flows (PEF) at work and away from work (13) have been proposed. There are several summary publications and statements that give general guidelines for the investigation of OA (14–21). For most investigators, OIC, either in the laboratory or at the workplace, is still the gold standard against which other means should be compared. There are reviews on the use of these tests in the investigation of OA (22–24), and guidelines have been issued by the American Academy of Allergy and Clinical Immunology (25) and the European Respiratory Society (26). A recent report focuses on the low occurrence of exaggerated bronchoconstriction and of associated factors (27).

PURPOSE AND JUSTIFICATION FOR THE TESTS

The purpose of occupational challenge tests (OCT) is to explore, through a direct observational approach, the causal relationship between exposure to occupational agents and asthma. This aim is in keeping with the definition of immunological (or allergic) OA (see Chapter 1), which implies that agents causing immunological OA should be able to induce the development of the characteristic features of asthma, including variable airflow limitation, nonspecific bronchial hyperresponsiveness (NSBH), and airway inflammation. Advances in understanding the pathophysiological mechanisms of asthma in recent years have clearly outlined the importance of distinguishing between agents that cause airway inflammation and NSBH, described as "inducers," and those that trigger airway narrowing in subjects with NSBH without inducing airway inflammation, referred to as "inciters" (28). Conceptually, only inducers can be considered as causing asthma, because they induce not only airflow obstruction but also cause airway inflammation and NSBH, whereas inciters increase the frequency of asthma symptoms in those with preexisting or coincidental asthma.

Differentiating immunological OA from work-aggravated asthma is relevant not only for scientific reasons, but also for medical, preventive, and medicolegal purposes. Immunological OA may require complete removal from workplace exposure, because persistence of exposure to sensitizing agents can result in the progressive worsening of the characteristic features of asthma and long-term functional impairment (29). Such therapeutic and preventive options are associated with tremendous professional, financial, and social consequences (29). In contrast, asthma symptoms triggered by physical stimuli or irritant substances at work could be managed at a lower societal cost by reducing the levels of irritants to within acceptable limits at work and/or by optimizing antiasthma treatment. Accepting exacerbation of asthma symptoms at work as an occupationally induced disease would have a considerable financial and psychosocial impact. Nevertheless, there is substantial evidence that the relationship between asthma and workplace exposure is currently assessed using objective tests in only a minority of subjects experiencing work-related asthma symptoms. This relationship is ascertained in less than one-third of reports to surveillance programs and claims notified to compensation agencies (30–32). Epidemiological data indicate that approximately 10% of adult asthma is attributable to the work environment (33). However, only a low proportion (generally less than 50%) of subjects who experience exacerbation of asthma symptoms at work demonstrate objective evidence of asthma worsening when they are exposed to the suspected agent at their workplace or in the laboratory (34–36).

Diagnosing OA cannot be based solely on documenting the presence of asthma and workplace exposure to agents known to cause asthma, because both are common occurrences in the general population. The level of evidence required for establishing a diagnosis OA may, however, vary according to the purposes and circumstances. Diagnosing OA for clinical or medicolegal purposes requires the highest level of reliability, as it is associated with considerable medical and socioeconomic consequences. The requirements for workplace surveillance programs and epidemiological investigation may be less demanding than for medical evaluation, although the validity of the inferences that can be drawn from the findings depends largely on the accuracy of the criteria used for case identification (37). A number of procedures can be used for investigating OA, including the clinical history, assessment of NSBH, and immunological tests (20). None of these tests taken alone allows for diagnosing OA with a sufficient level of confidence, although a combination of these tests in a stepwise approach can make the diagnosis of OA likely or very likely. The major rationale for performing OCT is that this experimental approach remains the most reliable procedure to document organ-specific responsiveness to an occupational agent in a given individual. OCT allows for the precise identification of the agent causing OA, which is important to give proper advice to affected workers and employers. OCT could also be included as the final confirmatory step in surveillance programs and epidemiological surveys of OA in high-risk workplaces. In addition, OCT can be used to assess the efficacy of preventive measures and protective devices. For instance, bronchial response to latex gloves with low protein content has been assessed using OCT in allergic health-care workers (38). Combining OCT with quantitative assessment of airborne agents could help to determine the level that elicits reactions in already sensitized subjects and could be used as a guide to establish permissible exposure levels at work (39).

In conclusion, OCT represent an important tool to confirm the diagnosis of OA, to identify new agents responsible for asthma, to identify the agent responsible for asthma when there are multiple possible agents in the workplace, and for exploring the mechanisms leading to asthmatic reactions (see below). In the case they are available in a specialized center, they should be preferred to other means to confirm work-related asthma.

PERFORMING THE TEST

OCTs have to be carried out with great precautions. However, in a large series of subjects who underwent OCT recently at Sacré-Coeur Hospital, the occurrence of exaggerated bronchoconstriction defined by changes in forced expiratory volume in one second (FEV_1) equal to or greater than 30% was low (immediate reactions in 18 out of 95 or 19% of subjects who underwent challenges with the closed-circuit equipment and 16 out of 43 or 37% of subjects who had tests with the realistic approach) (27). Specific challenge tests should consequently be carried out in specialized centers by trained personnel under the close supervision of physicians who have expertise in this field. The centers performing such tests should do a sufficient number of tests each year so as to offer efficient service and maintain their expertise in the field. The tests can be performed on an outpatient basis. Subjects come to the hospital laboratory in the morning and leave in the late afternoon. If the induced airway obstruction is still present at the end of the day, the physician should ensure that the subject responds to an inhaled beta-2 adrenergic agent before he or she is discharged. The subject should know how to use an inhaled beta-2 adrenergic agent at home when needed and should have rapid access to medical treatment if required. If the response to bronchodilators at the end of the day is insufficient, the subject should be kept in hospital for further observation and the asthmatic reaction must be treated accordingly, with bronchodilators and steroids.

Stability of Asthma and Need for Medication

As shown in Table 1, it is important to first ensure that the asthmatic is in a reasonably steady state. This is done by monitoring airway caliber on a control day with no exposure. FEV_1 fluctuations should be less than 10% throughout an observation period of eight hours. Ideally, all bronchodilator and anti-inflammatory medications should be withheld before the challenge. However, this is often not possible in moderate to severe asthmatic subjects where large fluctuations in FEV_1 can occur spontaneously. Short-acting inhaled beta-2 adrenergic agents should be stopped at least eight hours before the challenge, whereas long-acting beta-2 adrenergic agents and sustained-release theophylline preparations should be withheld at least 48 hours

Table 1 Scheme for Performing Specific Inhalation Challenges on the Control Days

Day 1: Control day	Day 2: Control day of exposure
Aim	Aim
Make sure asthma is stable	Make sure subjects do not react to a control agent
Prerequisite	Prerequisite
Stop inhaled beta-2 adrenergic agent 8 hrs, oral sustained-release theophylline 48 hrs before, inhaled or oral antiinflammatory preparation in the morning of the test	Same as for day 1 + baseline FEV_1 is $\pm$ 10% of baseline FEV_1 on day 1
Procedure	Procedure
Baseline spirometry, oral temperature, WBC, and FEV_1 every 10 mins in the first hr, every 30 mins for the second hour and hourly for 7–8 hrs; oral temperature hourly	Exposure for 30–120 mins to a control agent (examples: lactose if the causal agent if flour, other wooddust if it is a wooddust, diluent of isocyanates, etc.); same monitoring as for day 1; no PC_{20} at the end of the day.
PC_{20} at the end of the day	
PEFR monitoring in the evening at home	
If: baseline FEV_1 <2 L and/or FEV_1 fluctuations >10%, improve asthma treatment and postpone tests	If: changes in FEV_1 >10%, same management as for day 1

before the challenge. However, some subjects may require continuous use of theophylline and beta-2 adrenergic preparations if their asthma proves too unstable. The same applies to anti-inflammatory medications. If a subject takes these drugs to control asthma, the total dose should be administered at the end of each challenge day, but at least eight hours before the next challenge. Although it cannot be excluded that the use of antiasthma medication can reduce the magnitude of bronchoconstriction, challenges in subjects on such preparations performed in this way have elicited positive reactions.

Functional Tests

Forced Expiratory Volume in One Second

The FEV_1 is still regarded as the gold standard for assessing airway caliber for nonspecific and specific inhalation challenges. It has the advantage of being easy to perform, both for the technician and the subject. It also requires only portable and relatively inexpensive instruments. From a physiological point of view, it reflects the presence of large and small airway obstruction. However, it is effort-dependent and requires a satisfactory collaboration from the subject. It is also influenced by volume history (i.e., the inspiratory maneuver from tidal volume breathing to total lung capacity), which can provoke bronchodilatation. This has been described both for nonspecific challenges using pharmacological agents (40–42) and hyperventilation of unconditioned air (43,44). This effect also occurs with allergen challenges (45). Forced expiratory maneuvers can cause bronchoconstriction in subjects with enhanced bronchial responsiveness (46).

Baseline FEV_1 should be equal to or greater than two liters for reasons of safety and proper interpretation of the test. Fluctuations in FEV_1 on the control day should not exceed 10% (Table 1). To be considered positive, investigators generally require a fall of 20% or more in FEV_1 at the time of an immediate reaction with progressive recovery in the first hour, or a sustained fall in FEV_1 of at least 20% in the case of nonimmediate reactions, provided that such changes are absent on the day of exposure to the control product.

Other Functional Tests

Other tests have been proposed. PEF can be obtained with cheaper apparatus and has a reproducibility that is little less than FEV_1. However, this test is even more effort-dependent than the FEV_1 and we have shown that it is less sensitive to detect a late asthmatic reaction (47), although it is equally sensitive and specific in the case of immediate reactions (48). Forced expiratory flow (FEF) rates in the middle-half of the forced vital capacity (FEF 25% to 75%) and flow rates derived from the lower-half of the expiratory flow–volume curve, which are not effort-dependent, have also been proposed; however, these tests have poor reproducibility and the interpretation of what constitutes significant changes is questionable. Tests that do not require maximum inspiratory breathing maneuvers for assessing airway resistance/conductance in a body plethysmograph or using the oscillometry methodology have been proposed as well and are particularly useful in the case of intermediate changes (15% to 20%) in FEV_1 (49). However, the relative advantage of these tests because they are not affected by breathing maneuver is greatly counterbalanced by the fact that they have a less satisfactory reproducibility in a challenge situation (50). They also require more expensive and cumbersome equipment and cannot be proposed if the monitoring of spirometry is carried out at the workplace.

Assessment of Nonspecific Bronchial Responsiveness

Assessment of nonspecific bronchial responsiveness using pharmacological agents such as histamine or methacholine should be carried out at the end of the control day (Table 1). It is useful to assess the level of bronchial responsiveness of the airways before the test, as this is one of the predictors of a response to a specific agent (51–53). A negative pharmacological test does not exclude the possibility of OA; indeed, some workers may have ended exposure a long time before the assessment and show brisk changes in airway responsiveness after exposure to a specific agent (54–56). It is also an indication of whether a longer exposure should be considered. It has been demonstrated that changes in nonspecific bronchial responsiveness can occur when no significant changes in spirometry occurred; a longer exposure to the suspected agent can later reveal the bronchospastic reaction (57). Vandenplas et al. identified five subjects who failed to react to an occupational agent in terms of changes in FEV_1, but had changes in responsiveness to histamine at the end of the day. They reacted to the agent when exposure was prolonged on subsequent days (58). Similar conclusions were also reached by Sastre et al. in the case of challenges with isocyanates (59).

An increase in nonallergic bronchial responsiveness classically occurs after late reactions but not after immediate asthmatic reactions (52). However, this is not constant (60). Indeed, we showed that 41 out of 101 (41%) subjects with late reactions and 11 out of 63 (17%) subjects with isolated immediate reactions demonstrated a 3.2-fold or greater change in the provocative concentration of histamine or methacholine, causing a 20% fall in FEV_1 (PC_{20}) from baseline (61). The usefulness of monitoring PC_{20} before and after specific challenges has been confirmed in two studies. Changes in PC_{20} may precede changes in airway caliber and can be considered as an early marker of subsequent changes in airway caliber (58,59).

Other Assessments

Although the subject is discharged at the end of the day, he or she can continue measuring PEF during the evening of the test or during the night, whenever required. This will enable the investigator to know on the following day whether airway obstruction occurred after the subject left the hospital. However, when changes in FEV_1 are less than 10% at eight hours after the end of exposure test, in our experience, significant changes in PEF do not occur later in the evening or at night.

Oral temperature is recorded hourly, to document any possible hypersensitivity pneumonitis, which can accompany asthmatic reactions in some instances (62). In an analysis of 317 subjects who had positive reactions to occupational agents, we showed that 5% of reactions were accompanied by fever; these occurred with late reactions and they were accompanied by blood neutrophilia (61). Blood is drawn at the beginning and the end of the first day and then after a same time interval or the following morning (which is even more sensitive) (63) when challenges are positive. The occurrence of eosinophilia or leukocytosis can then be demonstrated. The serum can also be stored for immunological tests (specific IgE and/or IgG) when applicable.

In recent years, the investigation of inflammation using noninterventional tools has progressed considerably with the addition of examination of exhaled NO and induced sputum to the diagnostic means in OA (35,64). Changes in sputum eosinophils and/or neutrophils at the end of a day of exposure to a sensitizing agent can significantly add to the diagnostic validity of specific inhalation challenges (65).

DURATION AND SCHEDULE OF EXPOSURE AND MONITORING SPIROMETRY

Spirometry should be assessed for at least eight hours, i.e., every 10 minutes for the first hour, every 30 minutes for the second hour and then on an hourly basis. After a control day to ensure functional stability, subjects should be exposed to a control substance (lactose in the case of an agent in powder form such as flours, pharmaceutical products, etc.) or a control vapor, aerosol, or fume. In the specific case of polyisocyanates, this can be the chemical normally mixed with isocyanate in the two- or three-system component (Table 1).

The duration and intensity of the initial exposure to the suspected offending agent should be dictated by clinical history; if there is any indication of a severe immediate reaction, a short exposure under controlled conditions should be considered. The level of bronchial obstruction and responsiveness should also help in determining the duration and level of the initial exposure. We would normally start exposure to isocyanates for five minutes (total duration) on the first day if the PC_{20} is ≥ 0.25 mg/mL but for only one minute if it is lower. The principle is to draw a dose–response curve by increasing the duration and/or concentration of exposure. In our experience, it is always preferable to start with the following durations: 1 breath, 10 seconds, 30 seconds, 1 minute, 5 minutes, etc. (Table 2). For agents likely to cause immediate reactions such as high-molecular-weight agents (flour, psyllium, animal dander, etc.), the increase in duration of exposure can be progressive until an immediate reaction occurs. For agents likely to cause isolated late reactions, such as western red cedar and polyisocyanates, a total initial exposure of one to five minutes (depending on the history and level of nonspecific responsiveness) done progressively as for high-molecular-weight agents should be considered for the first day of exposure, increasing it from 15 from 30 minutes and then up to two hours the following two days. This gradual increase in exposure intervals can be modified, especially if there is evidence that the onset of an asthmatic reaction has been induced by monitoring PC_{20} at the end of the day.

It has been shown that it is neither the concentration nor the duration of exposure per se but the dose (i.e., concentration × duration of exposure) (66) that determines the magnitude of the asthmatic reaction.

METHODOLOGY

Nature of the Agent

Water-Soluble High-Molecular-Weight Allergens

Some antigens like flour (67) or snow-crab extracts (68) can be diluted in water and the concentration assessed. These testing solutions should be compared and assayed under the conditions recommended for commercial allergenic extracts. Materials are prepared by extraction into phenolated saline solution. The preferred technique of assuring stabilization is to use lyophilized extracts, which are reconstituted with

Table 2 Scheme for Performing Specific Inhalation Challenge Tests to the Possible Causal Agent

Active day(s): Day 3 and subsequent days

Aim
  Verify if subjects show a significant reaction (changes in $FEV_1 \geq 20\%$) after exposure to the suspected agent
Prerequisite
  Same as for day 2
Procedure
  Progressive exposure with in-between functional assessments *high molecular weight agent*, IgE mediated mechanism, expect immediate reaction: progressive exposure: one breath, 10 sec, 20 sec, 30 sec, 2 min, 5 min, 30 min, etc. for a total of 2 hrs; *low-molecular-weight agent*: exposure for one breath, 10 sec, 20 sec, 30 sec (total one min) on the first day, 1, 2, and 2 min (total = 5 min) on the second day, 5, 10, and 15 min (total = 30 min) on the third day and 15, 15, 30, 30, and 30 min (total = 2 hrs) on the last day; assess FEV_1 immediately and 10 min after each exposure period; if changes <10%, continue with the proposed protocol; if changes >10%, repeat a similar period of exposure as the previous one; if changes $\geq 20\%$, stop exposure
If positive reaction
  Repeat PC_{20} at the end of the day or in the following morning provided FEV_1 is back to baseline; if significantly lower than on day 1, treat with anti-inflammatory preparation; repeat PC_{20} until it is back to baseline
If late reaction
  Administer inhaled beta-2 adrenergic agent; if FEV_1 back to ±10% baseline 15–20 mins later, discharge with advice to subject that inhaled beta-2 adrenergic agent may be required in the evening or night; if FEV_1 not back to baseline, administer oral steroids and discharge; see the subject on the following day to make sure FEV_1 is back to baseline; follow-up required if not;
If negative test
  Repeat PC_{20} at the end of the day; if no significant change, no further exposure; if significantly lower PC_{20}, increase duration of exposure to a maximum of 4 hrs on the following day.

phenolated saline diluent prior to use. All reconstituted extracts should be stored at 4°C, and allergy extracts diluted to 1:1000 or higher should be discarded after one month. The concentration of allergy extracts to be used for aerosolized bronchial challenges is expressed as either weight per volume (w/v) or protein nitrogen units/mL (PNU/mL). In some cases it may be desirable to determine biologic allergen activity (allergy units).

Before attempting OCT with these solutions, a skin prick test should be done to assess the threshold concentration, which is expressed as that dilution of test allergen that gives a 3-mm wheal. The first inhalational test dose should be threefold dilutions below the calculated skin dose. As for common allergens, the idea is to assess the concentration of the occupational sensitizer required to give a 20% fall in FEV_1 for suspected immediate reactions by determining the PC_{20} and the wheal diameter of the allergen with skin prick testing (69,70).

Test aerosols may be administered by continuous aerosol generation and tidal breathing or individual breaths drawn from a hand-operated nebulizer. The output of the nebulizer, which is the principal technical determinant of the response, should be assessed as for nonspecific inhalation challenges (see Chapter 9). When either the intermittent (71) or continuous (72) aerosol generation methods are used, doses of allergens can be expressed in inhalation units. One inhalation unit equals one breath of 1/5000 (w/v) dilution of one breath of 100 PNU/mL (a protein solution with 1 µg protein nitrogen/mL). In the intermittent method, the subject inhales five breaths of allergen solution, beginning with the most dilute and proceeding to the most concentrated (1:100 or 5000 PNU/mL) (71). FEV_1 is measured immediately and 10 minutes after each dose challenge. The test proceeds in this manner until there has been at least a 20% fall in FEV_1 from baseline or when the most concentrated dose has been nebulized.

The results of aerosolized provocation tests are expressed on a log-linear paper, the dose of allergen being plotted on the logarithmic abscissa and the FEV_1 response in linear units on the ordinate. As for pharmacological agents, sensitivity to the allergen is determined by the provocation dose causing a 20% fall in FEV_1 (PC_{20}).

Agents in Powder or Dust Form

It was originally suggested by Pepys and Hutchcroft (12) that these agents be tipped from one tray to another in a challenge room that is well ventilated, thereby preventing against contamination of the laboratory and sensitization of the personnel. Models of well-ventilated rooms have been proposed by others (73). However, this method does not allow for monitoring of the concentration of particles in the air. There should be provision to keep the levels of dust below the threshold limit value, short-term exposure limit (TLV-STEL) set by the American Conference for Governmental Industrial Hygienists (ACGIH). An apparatus has been developed that makes exposure to steady and low concentrations of particles possible and permits monitoring of the diameter of the particles (Fig. 1) (74–76). It is important that a significant percentage of particles be <10 µm (respirable dusts). Dose–response curves can be obtained by increasing the duration or concentration of exposure (Fig. 2). This apparatus has the advantage of making the procedure safe, as subjects are exposed to low levels of dusts in a progressive way. Furthermore, it can distinguish satisfactorily between irritant and sensitizing reactions; irritant reactions are unlikely to occur if TLV-STEL concentrations are used. This apparatus can be used for different types of dust: flour, sawdust (including western red cedar), pharmaceutical powders, guar gum, etc. There is no contamination of the air in the room where the apparatus is located. If the test is negative after two hours of exposure using this apparatus, we would perform the test in the realistic way as proposed by Pepys and Hutchcroft (12) for two hours so as to ensure that the test is negative. We have shown that intermediate changes in FEV_1 (15% to 20%) using the apparatus were followed by changes equal or greater than 20%; when the realistic approach was used on the next day, this occurred in only 2% of subjects.

Polyisocyanates

On the control day (second day of the challenge tests), the isocyanate subjects are exposed to the control chemical (the chemical that is usually mixed with polyisocyanates) for a total of 15 minutes in a challenge room. For hexamethylene diisocyanate (HDI), the most frequently used isocyanate incorporated into paints for cars, airplanes, etc., the control chemical is an enamel containing aromatic hydrocarbons, ketones, aliphatic ester, and ether ester; for diphenylmethane diisocyanate (MDI) that is used in making molds and in the plastics industry, various aromatic

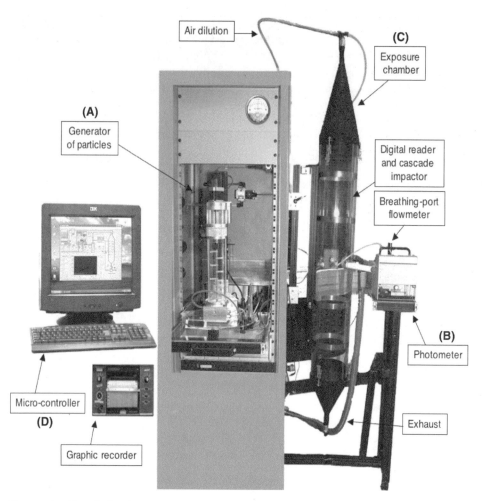

Figure 1 Closed-circuit apparatus for inhalation challenges in the specific case of dry particles. The following components are shown: (**A**) generation device for dry aerosol; (**B**) photometer from which concentration is derived; (**C**) exposure chamber; (**D**) self-control computerized feedback (left end side).

hydrocarbons and fluorocarbons are used. For toluene diisocyanate (TDI), used mainly in the preparation of foam, we use a commercial preparation made of polyol (99%) and aliphatic amine (1%) as the diluent. On the third and subsequent days if required, subjects are exposed to polyisocyanates in one of the following ways: (*i*) for TDI, approximately 100 mL of pure commercial TDI (80% 2,4-TDI and 20% 2,6-TDI) is deposited in a small cup, (*ii*) for HDI, the commercial preparation the subject is exposed to at work (from 20% to 75% of HDI/HDI biuret, depending on the product), is nebulized with the diluent (1:3 concentration) using a nebulizer, (*iii*) for MDI, the commercial preparation containing 40% to 50% MDI and 50% to 60% polymethylene polyphenyl isocyanate is heated in a metal cup to approximately 80°C. On the isocyanate challenge day(s), subjects are asked to remain in the challenge room for progressively longer periods of time: one breath, 15 and 45 seconds for a total of one minute on the first day (if the PC_{20} is ≤ 0.25mg/mL and/or there is a history of an important reaction), one minute, two minutes, and

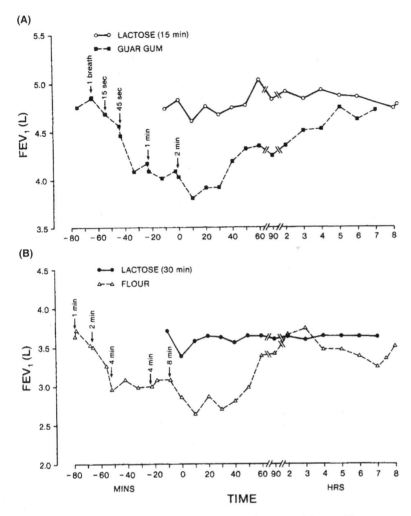

Figure 2 Examples of dose–response curves for two subjects with guar gum (*top panel*) and flour (*lower panel*) for consecutive exposures (*shown*) on the same day. The falls in FEV_1 are progressive. "0" time corresponds to the end of last exposure. *Abbreviation*: FEV_1, forced expiratory volume in one second. *Source*: From Ref. 75.

another two minutes for a total of five minutes on the second day (this can be done on the first day if the PC_{20} is >0.25mg/mL and there is no clinical history pointing to a severe reaction on exposure), and total periods varying from 15 to 120 minutes on subsequent days.

Challenges with isocyanates and other agents in vapor, powder, or gas form have so far been performed in relatively large challenge rooms (77). These rooms are well ventilated with a circuit near the ceiling. By controlling the ventilation in the room, the technician can stabilize the concentration of isocyanates in the challenge room (that is monitored continuously with a MDA-7100 or a GMD monitor) and keep it below 20 ppb (TLV-STEL). The technician has a direct view of the monitor's digital reading. Humidity is kept at 50% in the challenge room (the reading of isocyanates by the MDA-7100 monitor is affected by humidity) and there is a

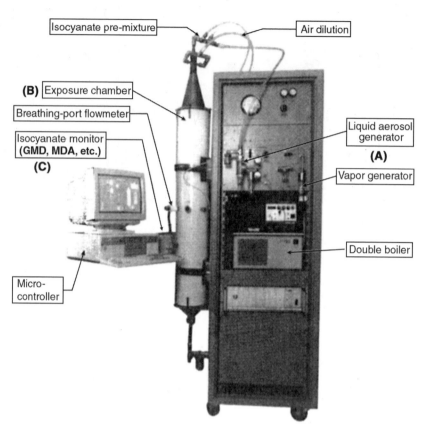

Figure 3 Closed-circuit apparatus for inhalation challenges with isocyanates in liquid and vapor forms in three parts: (**A**) the liquid or vapor generator on the right; (**B**) the exposure chamber in the centre; (**C**) the recording instruments (i.e. the isocyanate monitor) on the left.

ventilator in the challenge room to homogenize the isocyanate in the air. An improved closed-circuit mixing chamber was designed in conjunction with engineer Yves Cloutier of the Institut de Recherche en Santé et Sécurité du travail du Québec (IRSST) for polyisocyanates and other agents (Fig. 3) (78). This circuit is similar to what is described above for agents in powder or dust form. Isocyanate can be generated in vapor and aerosol. Continuous recording of the isocyanates is possible and concentrations can be kept stable at ±2 ppb. Preset levels of isocyanates are generated by adjusting the airflow to a small receptacle containing the isocyanate, which can be heated if needed (in the case of HDI or MDI). The isocyanate is inhaled through an orofacial mask in the middle of an exposure tube. The expelled air is filtered through charcoal. A similar procedure can be used for other agents existing in the vapor form, such as formaldehyde (79) and glutaraldehyde.

In summary, challenge rooms have evolved from the one originally proposed by Pepys and Hutchcroft (12) to more sophisticated versions still based on relatively large chambers, and more recently, to small closed-circuit chambers, which present the advantage of a more precise and stable generation of the agent with a significantly lower frequency of exaggerated bronchoconstriction than that seen on using the realistic methodology (27).

Duration of Exposure

It remains unknown how long a subject should be exposed to a product before the test is considered negative. It is our experience that subjects have to be exposed for periods up to two hours before the test can be considered negative. We have even documented cases where subjects had to be exposed for four hours (80). However, in general, an asthmatic reaction can be documented after exposure for a maximum period of two hours; this was the case in 14 of 15 subjects in whom specific inhalation challenges were repeated two years or more after cessation of exposure (81). When there is a negative test, subjects have to return to the work place where PEF are serially monitored. This may happen when subjects have been away from work for too long (82,83). OCTs are then repeated in the laboratory if returning to work provokes an exacerbation of asthma accompanied by changes in PEF. As mentioned above, exposure needs to be prolonged in subjects who only show changes in bronchial responsiveness to document changes in airway caliber.

PATTERNS OF REACTION

In clinical practice, specific inhalation challenges are generally considered positive when there is a sustained fall in FEV_1 of 20% or more from the prechallenge value in the

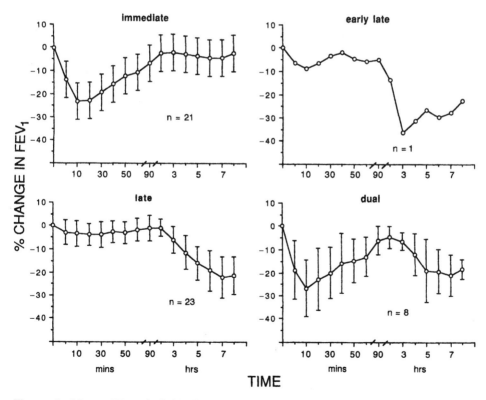

Figure 4   Mean $\pm$ SD or individual values of the % change in FEV_1 (*on the ordinate*) as a function of time since exposure (*on the abscissa*) for the four typical patterns of reactions (see text for definition). The number of subjects for each pattern is shown. *Abbreviation:* FEV_1, forced expiratory volume in one second. *Source:* From Ref. 85.

absence of significant ($\geq 10\%$) changes after exposure to a control product. Changes of 15% to 19% remain open to interpretation. Typical patterns of reaction have been summarized by Pepys and Hutchcroft (12). Figure 4 illustrates these reactions.

The immediate reaction is characterized by a brisk onset at a maximum of 10 to 20 minutes after exposure ends and lasting for one to two hours. These reactions respond well to bronchodilator therapy and are assumed to be harmless as they cause no inflammation, but they can actually be the most dangerous because they can be unpredictable, particularly in subjects for whom skin testing with the suspected agent is not possible. By contrast, late reactions are the cause of airway inflammation, but are easy to manage because there is plenty of time to intervene (see below). When the history is highly suggestive of severe acute reactions with greatly enhanced bronchial responsiveness ($PC_{20} \leq 0.25$ mg/mL), it is important to start inhalation challenge test with a very low concentration and for only one breath. In this instance, an indwelling intravenous catheter should be placed for immediate administration of bronchodilators and a beta-2 adrenergic solution should be ready for inhalation along with oxygen.

Late reactions develop slowly and progressively either one to two hours ("early late") or four to eight hours (late) after exposure. They may be accompanied by fever [this being documented in approximately 5% of cases (61)] and general malaise. Unlike immediate reactions, they cause eosinophilia (63). If they have fever, this may be accompanied by leukocytosis (61). Contrary to popular belief, they generally respond well to inhaled beta-2 adrenergic agents (61). In the event of a late reaction, an inhaled beta-2 adrenergic agent should be administered and confirmation that the FEV_1 is $\geq 90\%$ baseline should be shown before the subject is discharged. The patient should receive precise instructions on how relapsing bronchoconstriction, monitored at home with portable instruments assessing PEF and/or FEV_1, should be managed after leaving the laboratory. Anti-inflammatory preparations (inhaled or oral, depending on the severity of the reaction) can be given for two weeks. Bronchial responsiveness to methacholine or histamine and induced sputum can then be reassessed, making sure it is back to baseline.

Dual reactions are a combination of immediate and late reactions. Atypical reactions principally after exposure to polyisocyanates have been reported (84–86). In a group of 23 subjects who had positive reactions to isocyanates, it was found that 30% had atypical reactions (Fig. 5) (87). They were mainly of the progressive type (starting within minutes after exposure ended, progressing to a maximum seven to eight hours later). A previously unrecognized square-waved reaction (no recovery between the immediate and late components of the reaction) was also described. "Progressive recovery" patterns were also seen where subjects had maximum bronchoconstriction immediately after exposure, but functional recovery took seven to eight hours. We have described in the recent past patterns of reactions to increasing day-to-day doses of isocyanates. Although the most common pattern is linear (i.e., progressively day-to-day increasing reactions), we also found other patterns, i.e., minimal effect followed by a brisk change, significant changes followed by a plateau effect, and biphasic, i.e., significant change followed by a reduction in the effect and significant change on the last day of exposure (86).

Available information regarding the validity of procedures that can be used for diagnosing OA is summarized in Table 3. Studies have consistently found that the clinical history is a sensitive but not a specific tool for identifying OA. Interestingly, the presence or absence of typical symptoms such as improvement away from work is not a satisfactory index for the presence of OA, probably because workplace exposure to irritants is likely to trigger nonspecific symptoms in subjects with asthma, simulating

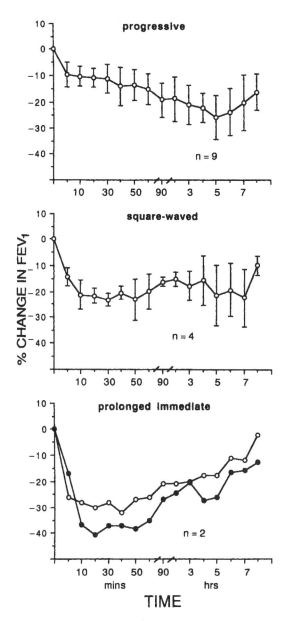

Figure 5 Mean ± SD or individual values of the % change in FEV₁ (*on the ordinate*) as a function of time since exposure (*on the abscissa*) for the three atypical patterns of reactions (see text for definition). The number of subjects for each pattern is shown. *Abbreviation*: FEV₁, forced expiratory volume in one second. *Source*: From Ref. 87.

true OA. Assessment of NSBH can be used to confirm the presence of asthma, although NSBH may be absent in subjects with OA, particularly when they are evaluated after removal from exposure. This measurement is more useful for excluding OA, because the absence of NSBH within 24 hours from a work exposure makes the diagnosis of OA exceedingly unlikely. Documentation of immunological sensitization to occupational agents does not necessarily imply that the target organ (i.e., the airways) is involved, because specific IgE antibodies can be present

Table 3 Validity of Diagnostic Procedures as Compared with Occupational Challenge Tests

Diagnostic procedures/ occupational agents	Positive OCT/ performed OCT[a]	Sensitivity (%)	Specificity (%)	References
Clinical history				
Various agents	75/162	87	27	(34)
Isocyanates, latex, flour	40/204	80	55	(88)
Latex	12/62	92	32	(88)
Latex	31/45	87	14	(89)
Latex	19/30	89	50	(39)
Baseline NSBH				
Isocyanates	34/63	68	69	(90)
Isocyanates, latex, flour	40/204	72	51	(88)
Latex	31/45	90	7	(89)
Latex	19/30	90	10	(39)
Bovine dander	11/27	82	65	(91)
Immunological tests				
Enzymes[b]	13/42	100	93	(92)
Enzymes[c]	13/42	62	96	(92)
Latex[b]	31/45	100	21	(89)
Latex[b]	19/30	100	20	(39)
Latex[c]	19/30	95	40	(39)
Flour (wheat and rye)[b]	62/98	56	94	(93)
Flour (wheat and rye)[c]	62/98	71	70	(93)
Bovine dander[b]	11/27	100	50	(91)
Bovine dander[c]	11/27	82	100	(91)
Isocyanates[c]	29/62	31	97	(94)
Isocyanates[c]	58/101	28	91	(95)
Clinical history and NSBH				
Isocyanates, latex, flour	40/204	65	75	(88)
Clinical history and immunological tests				
Latex[b]	31/45	94	36	(89)
Baseline NSBH and immunological tests				
Latex[b]	19/30	84	70	(39)
PEF monitoring				
Red cedar	14/23	86	89	(96)
Various agents	25/61	81	74	(102)
Monitoring of PEF and NSBH				
Red cedar (23)	14/23	92	67	(96)
Various agents	25/61	84	61	(102)

[a]Number of positive OCTs out of the total number of OCTs performed.
[b]Skin-prick tests.
[c]Measurement of specific IgE antibodies.
Abbreviations: OCT, occupational challenge test; PEF, peak expiratory flow; NSBH, nonspecific bronchial hyperresponsiveness.

in asymptomatic exposed workers (97). Immunological testing is often limited by the lack of commercially available standardized reagents (93). For most low-molecular-weight agents, the presence of specific IgE has been documented in only a small subset of affected workers (97). Available diagnostic procedures should be combined in a stepwise approach (98), although the predictive value of combined tests has been hardly evaluated. In the investigation of OA exposed to latex, it has been shown that combining skin-prick tests to latex with the clinical history does not improve substantially the positive predictive value of the history alone (from 75% to 76%), while the negative predictive value increases from 50% to 71% (89). Quirce et al. (39) found that the combination of the clinical history with assessment of NSBH provides a positive predictive value of 84% and a negative predictive value of 70% for identifying latex-induced OA.

The causal relationship between the exposure to occupational agents and the development of asthma can be assessed directly either through serial measurements of PEF at work and away from work (99,100) or through OCT in the laboratory or at the workplace. PEF monitoring has a sensitivity of 81% to 86% and a specificity of 74% to 86% as compared to OCT (96,101). Combining PEF monitoring with assessment of work-related changes in NSBH increases sensitivity only slightly (84–92%), but decreases specificity (61–67%), as compared with PEF alone (96,101). When the advantages and practical limitations of PEF monitoring are carefully weighted (99), it becomes apparent that OCT should be preferred to PEF in the following settings: (*i*) the worker has been removed from his or her work and cannot be returned to work on a trial basis; (*ii*) the worker is exposed to a known agent at work and facility is available for performing the tests safely and reliably; (*iii*) the clinical history suggests that exposure to the workplace is associated with severe asthmatic reactions; (*iv*) the causal agent has to be precisely identified to implement appropriate preventive strategies; and (*v*) the suspected agent has never been reported as causing OA. In the remaining circumstances, PEF recording could be used as a first line procedure.

PITFALLS

False-Positive Results

Bronchoconstriction owing to a nonspecific irritant effect (which does not fit the definition of OA) can occur in subjects with marked NSBH or unstable asthma. Most controlled experiments in asthmatic volunteers have failed to demonstrate a physiologically relevant effect of exposure to irritant substances at permissible levels (28,101–107), although some individuals may develop minimal changes in airway caliber (103,104,108). Nevertheless, available data suggest that some irritant substances, such as sulfur dioxide (109) and chlorine (110), could induce transient decrements in lung function in asthmatic subjects at lower levels than in those without NSBH. Immediate bronchial responses to irritant stimuli cannot be easily distinguished from those caused by sensitizing agents, because their temporal patterns are very similar. Nevertheless, the occurrence of such "irritant" reactions can be prevented, or at least identified, during OCT. The subjects should be monitored during a control day to ensure that they are in a stable functional state. Exposure to a control "irritant" substance (lactose for powders, diluents for paints and resins, etc.) is important to identify nonspecific bronchial responses. Monitoring of changes in NSBH and sputum cell counts may provide further evidence that bronchial responses result from "sensitizing" mechanisms (60,107). Using devices that allow for measuring and regulating the concentrations of the products generated during OCT in the laboratory could further prevent the occurrence of irritant reactions.

False-Negative Results

There are several reasons for a false-negative OCT. First, the subject has not been tested with the agent that actually caused their asthma. Carroll et al. (111) reported an interesting case of a subject who became sensitized to a product used in a nearby plant rather than to the agent worked with. The subject may have been challenged with the wrong physical or chemical form of the product (e.g., isocyanate monomers instead of polymers) (112). Also, specific bronchial reactivity to the causal agent may decrease after removal from exposure for a long time (82,83), although recent studies have shown that complete loss of specific bronchial reactivity is a rare occurrence (82,113). These potential causes of false-negative OCT can be substantially minimized by taking a careful occupational history and by challenging the subjects for prolonged periods. Post-challenge changes in the level of NSBH (58) or in the number of sputum eosinophils are more sensitive than changes in airway caliber in detecting bronchial responses to occupational agents (114). Changes in these indices should lead to repeat challenge exposure before excluding the diagnosis of OA. In addition, when an OCT is negative in the laboratory, provisions should be made to return the subject to his normal workplace while serial monitoring of PEF is done. As soon as changes in PEF or bronchial responsiveness are demonstrated, OCT should be repeated in the laboratory or at the workplace.

Adverse Effects

OCTs carry only minimal risk of inducing severe asthmatic reactions as long as safety requirements are stringently respected (see safety measures above), exposure to occupational agents is progressively increased, and bronchial response is carefully monitored. More than 1500 subjects have been challenged with various agents at the Hôpital du Sacré-Coeur of Montreal; only one subject developed a severe immediate reaction that required temporary intubation and recovered completely over a three-hour period (115). It has been recently demonstrated that closed-circuit equipments substantially reduce the risk of eliciting exaggerated immediate bronchoconstriction (i.e., a fall in FEV_1 of more than 30%) (38% of subjects exposed with "realistic" methods in comparison to 19% of subjects exposed with the closed-circuit methodology) (27). As regards non-immediate reactions, the proportion of subjects developing exaggerated bronchoconstriction was also lower with the closed-circuit devices (37%) than with the realistic procedures (48%), although the difference did not reach statistical significance. That the protective effect of the closed-circuit methodology was significantly more pronounced in subjects with higher levels of NSBH is noteworthy. OCTs have also been documented as inducing transient exacerbation of asthma with recurrent nocturnal symptoms (116). It is our experience that only a low proportion (less than 5%) of subjects with positive OCT experience mild worsening of their asthma symptoms for a few days after challenge exposure. For those subjects who demonstrate late asthmatic reactions, initiating or increasing inhaled steroids for a short period could be indicated to prevent the associated increase in inflammatory processes and bronchial hyperresponsiveness. Cutaneous and anaphylactic reactions have occasionally been reported during OCTs (117). Accordingly, skin contact with occupational agents should be reduced as much as possible during inhalation challenges, by using protective clothes or closed-circuit delivery systems.

OCTs are often discussed on ethical grounds. However, Pepys gave the following outline: "One of the primary obligations of the clinician in asthma, as in any other disease, is to make a precise etiologic diagnosis. This is particularly relevant to allergic disorders, in which avoidance of the causative agent may terminate or reduce the disorder... Failure to do the tests (OCT) could be regarded as an act of omission" (12). The possibility of inducing or increasing sensitization to occupational agents in workers by OCT has been raised as an ethical issue. However, it can be argued that the usual workplace exposure is much more prolonged than that produced in the context of OCT. In addition, Kurtz et al. (118) have recently shown that repeated challenge exposures to latex do not cause an increase in immunological reactivity to this agent. On the other hand, inadvertent exposure to occupational agents can induce sensitization of the personnel in charge of OCTs. These tests should, therefore, be performed in enclosed cubicles equipped with effective exhaust ventilation systems or by using closed-circuit equipments to avoid exposure to technicians.

Practical Limitations

Many physicians are reluctant to carry out OCT because the procedure is time-consuming and expensive. The cost of OCT is, however, largely overweighed by the financial consequences of falsely negative and falsely positive diagnoses of OA for the workers, employers, and health care–insurance organizations, and society. The major practical issue is that the facility and expertise for performing OCT are currently not widely available. A recent survey of pulmonary, allergy, and occupational medicine residency programs in the United States and Canada showed that OCT was available in only 16% of training programs and the procedure was used in 11% of the patients investigated for OA (119).

OCT in the laboratory should not be considered a pragmatic approach when: (*i*) no agent known as causing OA has been identified in the subject's workplace, (*ii*) the subject is exposed to multiple agents that are known as potential cause of OA, and (*iii*) the mode of exposure at work cannot be reliably reproduced in the laboratory when complex industrial processes are involved. In these settings, OCT can be done at the workplace. This procedure should include supervised measurements of spirometry during both a control day in the laboratory and exposure at the usual work. OCT at the workplace may not be ideal because there is no control over exposure (at times, the exposure is intermittent and the worker may not be well exposed to the sensitizing agent if it is unknown; at other times, he or she may be exposed to very high levels) and it may be difficult to exclude an irritant reaction. Workplace OCTs have practical limitations, because it may be difficult to obtain the employer's authorization and to perform the tests under the conditions of exposure that prevailed when the subject developed work-related asthma. In addition, these tests are more expensive than OCT in the laboratory, as a technician is required for a single test outside of the hospital setting.

OCT IN THE CASE OF ALVEOLITIS

Occasionally, exposure to an occupational agent can cause alveolitis or hypersensitivity pneumonitis. Cases of alveolitis after exposure to polyisocyanates have been described by several authors (62,120–122). Criteria for defining a positive "alveolar" reaction have been described by Hendrick et al. (123). This includes a body temperature $>37.2°C$, an increase in circulating neutrophils of $2500/mm^3$ or more, and a fall in forced vital capacity of 15% or more. Diffusing capacity and changes in lung subdivisions proved to be too insensitive to be useful. These tests can be per-formed in the laboratory or at the workplace, and the value of other tools (chest examination and radiograph, in vitro tests for cell-mediated immunity, bronchoal-veolar lavage, lung biopsy, and therapeutic trial) has been reviewed elsewhere (124).

OCT WITH OCCUPATIONAL AGENTS AS A RESEARCH TOOL

OA is a satisfactory model of asthma. Therefore, OCT may lead to interesting obser-vations on the pathophysiology of asthma. Fabbri et al. (125) have shown that both neutrophils and eosinophils were involved in late asthmatic reactions caused by poly-isocyanates, as demonstrated by bronchoalveolar lavage at different time intervals after exposure. The same group of investigators later showed that only beclometha-sone was effective in preventing changes in bronchial responsiveness following exposure to isocyanates (126). Lam et al. (127) have demonstrated an increase in eosinophils in the bronchoalveolar lavage after late reactions caused by plicatic acid. Urinary leukotrienes were shown in the case of immediate reactions to common and occupational agents (128). Multiple studies summarized elsewhere have evaluated the efficacy of antiasthma drugs in suppressing asthmatic reactions following exposure to occupational agents (12). OCT can therefore be useful in improving our understanding of the pathophysiology of asthma.

CONCLUSION AND RESEARCH NEEDS

It is our opinion that OCT in investigating OA should still be regarded as the gold stan-dard for confirming the diagnosis. Since the proposal of these tests by Professor Pepys in the 1970s, attempts have been made to improve the methodology of the test from a functional and exposure point of view. These efforts that should be intensified are aimed at offering a more precise diagnosis of OA and a more appropriate advice to the employee and employer. Recent studies have also shown that they should not be considered as dangerous provided that rigorous procedure and methodology are followed. Information on the cost-effectiveness of these tests should be obtained. These tests can also be helpful as a research tool because human asthma is a better model than various types of bronchial hyperresponsiveness that have been induced in animals.

ACKNOWLEDGMENTS

The authors would like to thank Lori Schubert and Katherine Tallman for reviewing the manuscript.

REFERENCES

1. Aas K. The Bronchial Provocation Test. Springfield, IL: Charles C Thomas Publisher, 1975.
2. Herxheimer H. The late bronchial reaction in induced asthma. Int Arch Allergy Appl Immunol 1952; 3:323–328.

3. Dominjon-Monnier F, Carton J, Guibert L, Burtin P, Brille D, Kourilsky R. Épreuves ventilatoires aux extraits de moisissures atmosphériques. Rev Franç Mal Resp 1962; 2:191–202.

4. Colldahl H. A study of provocation test on patients with bronchial asthma. Acta Allergol 1952; 5:133–142.

5. Pepys J, Riddell RW, Citron KM, Clayton YM, Short EI. Clinical and immunologic significance of *Aspergillus fumigatus* in the sputum. Am Rev Respir Dis 1959; 80:167–180.

6. Pepys J, Jenkins PA. Precipitin (F.L.H.) test in farmer's lung. Thorax 1965; 20:21–35.

7. Hargreave FE, Pepys J, Longbottom JL, Wraith DG. Bird breeder's (fancier's) lung. Lancet 1966; 1:445–449.

8. Pickering CAC, Batten JC, Pepys J. Asthma due to inhaled wood dusts—western red cedar and iroko. Clin Allergy 1972; 2:213–218.

9. Pepys J, Pickering CAC, Terry DJ. Asthma due to inhaled chemical agents—tolylene di-isocyanate. Clin Allergy 1972; 2:225–236.

10. Pickering CAC. Inhalation tests with chemical allergens: complex salts of platinum. Proc Roy Soc Med 1972; 65:272–274.

11. Davies RJ, Hendrick DJ, Pepys J. Asthma due to inhaled chemical agents: ampicillin, bensyl penicillin, 6 amino penicillanic acid and related substances. Clin Allergy 1974; 4:227–247.

12. Pepys J, Hutchcroft BJ. Bronchial provocation tests in etiologic diagnosis and analysis of asthma. Am Rev Respir Dis 1975; 112:829–859.

13. Burge PS, O'Brien IM, Harries MG. Peak flow rate records in the diagnosis of occupational asthma due to colophony. Thorax 1979; 34:308–316.

14. Chan-Yeung M, Lam S. Occupational asthma. Am Rev Respir Dis 1986; 133:686–703.

15. Pauli G, Bessot JC, Dietemann-Molard A. L'asthme professionnel: investigations et principales étiologies. Occupational asthma: investigations and aetiological factors. Bull Eur Physiopathol Respir 1986; 22:399–425.

16. Chan-Yeung M, Malo JL. Occupational asthma. Chest 1987; 91:130S–136S.

17. Chan-Yeung M. Occupational asthma update. Chest 1988; 93:407–411.

18. Bernstein DI, Cohn JR. Guidelines for the diagnosis and evaluation of occupational immunologic lung disease: preface. J Allergy Clin Immunol 1989; 84:791–793.

19. Ad hoc Committee on Occupational Asthma of the Standards Committee Canadian Thoracic Society. Occupational asthma: recommendations for diagnosis, management and assessment of impairment. CMAJ 1989; 140:1029–1032.

20. Chan-Yeung M, Malo JL. Occupational asthma. N Engl J Med 1995; 333:107–112.

21. Malo JL, Yeung M Chan. Occupational asthma. J Allergy Clin Immunol 2001; 108: 317–328.

22. Spector SL. Provocative Challenge Procedures: Bronchial, Oral, Nasal and Exercise. Boca Raton, FL: CRC Press, 1983.

23. Malo JL, Cartier A. Bronchoprovocation testing. In: Harber P, Schenker MB, Balmes JR, eds. Occupational and Environmental Respiratory Disease. St. Louis: Mosby, 1996:55–66.

24. Vandenplas O, Malo JL. Inhalation challenges with agents causing occupational asthma. Eur Respir J 1997; 10:2612–2629.

25. Cartier A, Bernstein IL, Burge PS, et al. Guidelines for bronchoprovocation on the investigation of occupational asthma. Report of the subcommittee on bronchoprovocation for occupational asthma. J Allergy Clin Immunol 1989; 84:823–829.

26. Sterk PJ, Fabbri LM, Quanjer PH, et al. Airway responsiveness. Standardized challenge testing with pharmacological, physical and sensitizing stimuli in adults. Report working party standardization of lung function tests European community for steel and coal. Official statement of the European Respiratory Society. Eur Respir J suppl 1993; 16:53–83.

27. Malo JL, Cartier A, Lemière C, et al. Exaggerated bronchoconstriction due to inhalation challenges with occupational agents. Eur Respir J 2004; 23:300–303.

28. Vandenplas O, Malo JL. Definitions and types of work-related asthma: a nosological approach. Eur Respir J 2003; 21:706–712.

29. Vandenplas O, Toren K, Blanc P. Health and socioeconomic impact of work-related asthma. Eur Respir J 2003; 22:689–697.

30. Henneberger PK, Stanbury MJ, Trimbath LS, Kipen HM. The use of portable peak flowmeters in the surveillance of occupational asthma. Chest 1991; 100:1515–1521.

31. Ameille J, Pauli G, Calastreng-Crinquand A, et al. ONAP and the corresponding members of the reported incidence of occupational asthma in France, 1996–99. Occup Environ Med 2003; 60:136–142.

32. Gannon PFG, Burge PS. A preliminary report of a surveillance scheme of occupational asthma in the West Midlands. Br J Ind Med 1991; 48:579–582.

33. Blanc PD, Toren K. How much asthma can be attributed to occupational factors? Am J Med 1999; 107:580–587.

34. Malo JL, Ghezzo H, L'Archevêque J, Lagier F, Perrin B, Cartier A. Is the clinical history a satisfactory means of diagnosing occupational asthma?. Am Rev Respir Dis 1991; 143:528–532.

35. Lemière C, Pizzichini MMM, Balkissoon R, et al. Diagnosing occupational asthma: use of induced sputum. Eur Respir J 1999; 13:482–488.

36. Tarlo SM, Leung K, Broder I, Silverman F, Holness DL. Asthmatic subjects symptomatically worse at work: prevalence and characterization among a general asthma clinic population. Chest 2000; 118:1309–1314.

37. Banks DE. Use of the specific challenge in the diagnosis of occupational asthma: a 'gold standard' test or a test not used in current practice of occupational asthma? Curr Opin Allergy Clin Immunol 2003; 3:101–107.

38. Vandenplas O, Delwiche JP, Depelchin S, Sibille Y, Weyer Vande R, Delaunois L. Latex gloves with a lower protein content reduce bronchial reactions in subjects with occupational asthma caused by latex. Am J Respir Crit Care Med 1995; 151:887–891.

39. Quirce S, Swanson MC, Fernández-Nieto M, Heras de las M, Cuesta J, Sastre J. Quantified environmental challenge with absorbable dusting powder aerosol from natural rubber latex gloves. J Allergy Clin Immunol 2003; 111:788–794.

40. Nadel JA, Tierney DF. Effect of a previous deep inspiration on airway resistance in man. J Appl Physiol 1961; 16:717–719.

41. Fish JE, Kelly JF. Measurements of responsiveness in bronchoprovocation testing. J Allergy Clin Immunol 1979; 64:592–596.

42. Sestier M, Pineau L, Cartier A, Martin RR, Malo JL. Bronchial responsiveness to methacholine and effects of respiratory manoeuvres. J Appl Physiol 1984; 56:122–128.

43. Lim TK, Pride NB, Ingram RH Jr. Effects of volume history during spontaneous and acutely induced air-flow obstruction in asthma. Am Rev Respir Dis 1987; 135:591–596.

44. Malo JL, L'Archevêque J, Cartier A. Comparative effects of volume history on bronchoconstriction induced by hyperventilation and methacholine in asthmatic subjects. Eur Respir J 1990; 3:639–643.

45. Fish JE, Ankin MG, Kelly JF, Peterman VI. Comparison of responses to pollen extract in subjects with allergic asthma and nonasthmatic subjects with allergic rhinitis. J Allergy Clin Immunol 1980; 65:154–161.

46. Gayrard P, Orehek J, Grimaud CH, Charpin J. Mechanisms of the bronchoconstrictor effects of deep inspiration in asthmatic patients. Thorax 1979; 34:234–240.

47. Bérubé D, Cartier A, L'Archevêque J, Ghezzo H, Malo JL. Comparison of peak expiratory flow rate and FEV1 in assessing bronchomotor tone after challenges with occupational sensitizers. Chest 1991; 99:831–836.

48. Weytjens K, Malo JL, Cartier A, Ghezzo H, Delwiche JP, Vandenplas O. Comparison of peak expiratory flows and FEV_1 in assessing immediate asthmatic reactions due to occupational agents. Allergy 1999; 54:621–625.

49. Larbanois A, Delwiche JP, Jamart J, Vandenplas O. Comparison of FEV_1 and specific airway conductance in assessing airway response to occupational agents. Allergy 2003; 58:1256–1260.

50. Dehaut P, Rachiele A, Martin RR, Malo JL. Histamine dose–response curves in asthma: reproducibility and sensitivity of different indices to assess response. Thorax 1983; 38:516–522.

51. Killian D, Cockcroft DW, Hargreave FE, Dolovich J. Factors in allergen-induced asthma: relevance of the intensity of the airways allergic reaction and non-specific bronchial reactivity. Clin Allergy 1976; 6:219–225.

52. Cartier A, Thomson NC, Frith PA, Roberts R, Hargreave FE. Allergen-induced increase in bronchial responsiveness to histamine: relationship to the late asthmatic response and change in airway caliber. J Allergy Clin Immunol 1982; 70:170–177.

53. Lam S, Tan F, Chan G, Chan-Yeung M. Relationship between types of asthmatic reaction, nonspecific bronchial reactivity, and specific IgE antibodies in patients with red cedar asthma. J Allergy Clin Immunol 1983; 72:134–139.

54. Banks DE, Barkman HW Jr, Butcher BT, et al. Absence of hyperresponsiveness to methacholine in a worker with methylene diphenyl diisocyanate (MDI)-induced asthma. Chest 1986; 89:389–393.

55. Mapp CE, Vecchio L Dal, Boschetto P, Marzo N De, Fabbri LM. Toluene diisocyanate-induced asthma without airway hyperresponsiveness. Eur J Respir Dis 1986; 68:89–95.

56. Hargreave FE, Ramsdale EH, Pugsley SO. Occupational asthma without bronchial hyperresponsiveness. Am Rev Respir Dis 1984; 130:513–515.

57. Cartier A, L'rchevêque J, Malo JL. Exposure to a sensitizing occupational agent can cause a long-lasting increase in bronchial responsiveness to histamine in the absence of significant changes in airway caliber. J Allergy Clin Immunol 1986; 78:1185–1189.

58. Vandenplas O, Delwiche JP, Jamart J, Weyer Van de R. Increase in non-specific bronchial hyperresponsiveness as an early marker of bronchial response to occupational agents during specific inhalation challenges. Thorax 1996; 51:472–478.

59. Sastre J, Fernandez-Nieto M, Novalbos A, Heras De Las M, Cuesta J, Quirce S. Need for monitoring nonspecific bronchial hyperresponsiveness before and after isocyanate inhalation challenge. Chest 2003; 123:1276–1279.

60. Malo JL, Ghezzo H, L'Archevêque J, Cartier A. Late asthmatic reactions to occupational sensitizing agents: frequency of changes in nonspecific bronchial responsiveness and of response to inhaled beta-2 adrenergic agent. J Allergy Clin Immunol 1990; 85:834–842.

61. Lemière C, Gautrin D, Trudeau C, et al. Fever and leucocytosis accompanying asthmatic reactions due to occupational agents: frequency and associated factors. Eur Respir J 1996; 9:517–523.

62. Malo J-L, Ouimet G, Cartier A, Levitz D, Zeiss R. Combined alveolitis and asthma due to hexamethylene diisocyanate (HDI), with demonstration of crossed respiratory and immunologic reactivities to diphenylmethane diisocyanate (MDI). J Allergy Clin Immunol 1983; 72:413–419.

63. Durham SR, Kay AB. Eosinophils, bronchial hyperreactivity and late-phase asthmatic reactions. Clin Allergy 1985; 15:411–418.

64. Obata H, Cittrick M, Chan H, Chan-Yeung M. Sputum eosinophils and exhaled nitric oxide during late asthmatic reaction in patients with western red cedar asthma. Eur Respir J 1999; 13:489–495.

65. Girard F, Chaboillez S, Cartier A, et al. An effective strategy for diagnosing occupational asthma: use of induced sputum. Am J Respir Crit Care Med. 2004; 170:845–850.

66. Vandenplas O, Cartier A, Ghezzo H, Cloutier Y, Malo JL. Response to isocyanates: effect of concentration, duration of exposure, and dose. Am Rev Respir Dis 1993; 147:1287–1290.

67. Block G, Tse KS, Kijek K, Chan H, Chan-Yeung M. Baker's asthma. Clin Allergy 1983; 13:359–370.

68. Cartier A, Malo JL, Ghezzo H, McCants M, Lehrer SB. IgE sensitization in snow crab-processing workers. J Allergy Clin Immunol 1986; 78:344–348.

69. Cockcroft DW, Ruffin RE, Frith PA, et al. Determinants of allergen-induced asthma: dose of allergen, circulating IgE antibody concentration, and bronchial responsiveness to inhaled histamine. Am Rev Respir Dis 1979; 120:1053–1058.

70. Cockcroft DW, Murdock KY, Kirby J, Hargreave F. Prediction of airway responsiveness to allergen from skin sensitivity to allergen and airway responsiveness to histamine. Am Rev Respir Dis 1987; 135:264–267.

71. Chai H, Farr RS, Froehlich LA, et al. Standardization of bronchial inhalation challenge procedures. J Allergy Clin Immunol 1975; 56:323–327.

72. Cockcroft DW, Killian DN, Mellon JJA, Hargreave FE. Bronchial reactivity to inhaled histamine: a method and clinical survey. Clinical Allergy 1977; 7:235–243.

73. Salvaggio JE, Butcher BT, O'Neil CE. Occupational asthma due to chemical agents. J Allergy Clin Immunol 1986; 78:1053–1058.

74. Cloutier Y, Lagier F, Lemieux R, et al. New methodology for specific inhalation challenges with occupational agents in powder form. Eur Respir J 1989; 2:769–777.

75. Cloutier Y, Malo JL. Update on an exposure system for particles in the diagnosis of occupational asthma. Eur Respir J 1992; 5:887–890.

76. Cloutier Y, Lagier F, Cartier A, Malo JL. Validation of an exposure system to particles for the diagnosis of occupational asthma. Chest 1992; 102:402–407.

77. Butcher BT. Inhalation challenge testing with toluene diisocyanate. J Allergy Clin Immunol 1979; 64:655–657.

78. Vandenplas O, Malo JL, Cartier A, Perreault G, Cloutier Y. Closed-circuit methodology for inhalation challenge tests with isocyanates. Am Rev Respir Dis 1991; 145:582–587.

79. Lemière C, Cloutier Y, Perrault G, Drolet D, Cartier A, Malo JL. Closed-circuit apparatus for specific inhalation challenges with an occupational agent, formaldehyde, in vapor form. Chest 1996; 109:1631–1635.

80. Cartier A, Chan H, Malo JL, Pineau L, Tse KS, Chan-Yeung M. Occupational asthma caused by Eastern white cedar (*Thuja occidentalis*) with demonstration that plicatic acid is present in this wood dust and is the causal agent. J Allergy Clin Immunol 1986; 77:639–645.

81. Lemière C, Cartier A, Dolovich J, et al. Outcome of specific bronchial responsiveness to occupational agents after removal from exposure. Am J Respir Crit Care Med 1996; 154:329–333.

82. Cartier A, Malo JL, Forest F, et al. Occupational asthma in snow crab-processing workers. J Allergy Clin Immunol 1984; 74:261–269.

83. Butcher BT, O'Neil CE, Reed MA, Salvaggio JE, Weill H. Development and loss of toluene diisocyanate reactivity: immunologic, pharmacologic, and provocative challenge studies. J Allergy Clin Immunol 1982; 70:231–235.

84. Séguin P, Allard A, Cartier A, Malo JL. Prevalence of occupational asthma in spray painters exposed to several types of isocyanates, including polymethylene polyphenylisocyanates. JOM 1987; 29:340–344.

85. Zammit-Tabona M, Sherkin M, Kijek K, Chan H, Chan-Yeung M. Asthma caused by diphenylmethane diisocyanate in foundry workers. Clinical, bronchial provocation, and immunologic studies. Am Rev Respir Dis 1983; 128:226–230.

86. Malo JL, Ghezzo H, Elie R. Occupational asthma caused by isocyanates: Patterns of asthmatic reactions to increasing day-to-day doses. Am J Respir Crit Care Med 1999; 159:1879–1883.

87. Perrin B, Cartier A, Ghezzo H, et al. Reassessment of the temporal patterns of bronchial obstruction after exposure to occupational sensitizing agents. J Allergy Clin Immunol 1991; 87:630–639.

88. Baur X, Huber H, Degens PO, Allmers H, Ammon J. Relation between occupational asthma case history, bronchial methacholine challenge, and specific challenge test in patients with suspected occupational asthma. Am J Ind Med 1998; 33:114–122.

89. Vandenplas O, Cangh F Binard-Van, Brumagne A, et al. Occupational asthma in symptomatic workers exposed to natural rubber latex: Evaluation of diagnostic procedures. J Allergy Clin Immunol 2001; 107:542–547.

90. Karol MH, Tollerud DJ, Campbell TP, et al. Predictive value of airways hyperresponsiveness and circulating IgE for identifying types of responses to toluene diisocyanate inhalation challenge. Am J Respir Crit Care Med 1994; 149:611–615.

91. Koskela H, Taivainen A, Tukiainen H, Chan HK. Inhalation challenge with bovine dander allergens: who needs it? Chest 2003; 124:383–391.

92. Merget R, Stollfuss J, Wiewrodt R, et al. Diagnostic tests in enzyme allergy. J Allergy Clin Immunol 1993; 92:264–277.

93. Sander I, Merget R, Degens PO, Goldscheid N, Bruning T, Raulf-Heimsoth M. Comparison of wheat and rye flour skin prick test solutions for diagnosis of baker's asthma. Allergy 2004; 59:95–98.

94. Cartier A, Grammer L, Malo JL, et al. Specific serum antibodies against isocyanates: association with occupational asthma. J Allergy Clin Immunol 1989; 84:507–514.

95. Tee RD, Cullinan P, Welch J, Burge PS, Newman-Taylor AJ. Specific IgE to isocyanates: a useful diagnostic role in occupational asthma. J Allergy Clin Immunol 1998; 101:709–715.

96. Côté J, Kennedy S, Chan-Yeung M. Sensitivity and specificity of PC 20 and peak expiratory flow rate in cedar asthma. J Allergy Clin Immunol 1990; 85:592–598.

97. Sastre J, Vandenplas O, Park HS. Pathogenesis of occupational asthma. Eur Respir J 2003; 22:364–373.

98. Moscato G, Malo JL, Bernstein D. Diagnosing occupational asthma: how, how much, how far? Eur Respir J 2003; 21:879–885.

99. Moscato G, Godnic-Cvar J, Maestrelli P, Malo JL, Burge PS, Coifman R. Statement on self-monitoring of peak expiratory flows in the investigation of occupational asthma. J Allergy Clin Immunol 1995; 96:295–301.

100. Hankinson JL. Beyond the peak flow meter: Newer technologies for determining and documenting changes in lung function in the workplace. Occup Med State of the Art Rev 2000; 15:411–420.

101. Perrin B, Lagier F, L'Archevêque J, et al. Occupational asthma: validity of monitoring of peak expiratory flow rates and non-allergic bronchial responsiveness as compared to specific inhalation challenge. Eur Respir J 1992; 5:40–48.

102. Harving H, Korsgaard J, Dahl R. Low concentrations of formaldehyde in bronchial asthma: a study of exposure under controlled conditions. Br Med J 1986; 293:310.

103. Green DJ, Sauder LR, Kulle TJ, Bascom R. Acute response to 3.0 ppm formaldehyde in exercising healthy nonsmokers and asthmatics. Am Rev Respir Dis 1987; 135: 1261–1266.

104. Luca S De, Caire N, Cloutier Y, Cartier A, Ghezzo H, Malo J-L. Acute exposure to sawdust does not alter airway calibre and responsiveness to histamine in asthmatic subjects. Eur Respir J 1988; 1:540–546.

105. Harving H, Dahl R, Mølhave L. Lung function and bronchial reactivity in asthmatics during exposure to volatile organic compounds. Am Rev Respir Dis 1991; 143:751–754.

106. Beach JR, Raven J, Ingram C, et al. The effects on asthmatics of exposure to a conventional water-based and a volatile organic compound-free paint. Eur Respir J 1997; 10:563–566.

107. Lemière C, Chaboillez S, Malo JL, Cartier A. Changes in sputum cell counts after exposure to occupational agents: what do they mean? J Allergy Clin Immunol 2001; 107:1063–1068.

108. Vandenplas O, Delwiche JP, Staquet P, et al. Pulmonary effects of short-term exposure to low levels of toluene diisocyanate in asymptomatic subjects. Eur Respir J 1999; 13:1144–1150.

109. Committee of the Environmental and Occupational Health Assembly of the American Thoracic Society. Health effects of outdoor air pollution. Am J Respir Crit Care Med 1996; 153:3–50.

110. D'Alessandro A, Kuschner W, Wong H, Boushey HA, Blanc PD. Exaggerated responses to chlorine inhalation among persons with nonspecific airway hyperreactivity. Chest 1996; 109:331–337.

111. Carroll KB, Secombe CJP, Pepys J. Asthma due to non-occupational exposure to toluene (tolylene) di-isocyanate. Clin Allergy 1976; 6:99–104.

112. Vandenplas O, Cartier A, Lesage J, et al. Prepolymers of hexamethylene diisocyanate (HDI) as a cause of occupational asthma. J Allergy Clin Immunol 1993; 91:850–861.

113. Lemière C. Persistence of bronchial reactivity to occupational agents after removal from exposure and identification of associated factors. Ann Allergy Asthma Immunol 2003; 90(suppl):52–55.

114. Lemière C, Chaboilliez S, Trudeau C, et al. Characterization of airway inflammation after repeated exposures to occupational agents. J Allergy Clin Immunol 2000; 106: 1163–1170.

115. Cartier A, Malo JL, Dolovich J. Occupational asthma in nurses handling psyllium. Clin Allergy 1987; 17:1–6.

116. Cockcroft DW, Hoeppner VH, Werner GD. Recurrent nocturnal asthma after bronchoprovocation with western red cedar sawdust: association with acute increase in non-allergic bronchial responsiveness. Clin Allergy 1984; 14:61–68.

117. Romano C, Sulotto F, Pavan I, Chiesa A, Scansetti G. A new case of occupational asthma from reactive dyes with severe anaphylactic response to the specific challenge. Am J Ind Med 1992; 21:209–216.

118. Kurtz KM, Hamilton RG, Schaefer JA, Primeau MN, Adkinson NF Jr. Repeated latex aeroallergen challenges employing a hooded exposure chamber: safety and reproducibility. Allergy 2001; 56:857–861.

119. Ortega HG, Weissman DN, Carter DL, Banks D. Use of specific inhalation challenge in the evaluation of workers at risk for occupational asthma. Chest 2002; 121:1323–1328.

120. Charles J, Bernstein A, Jones B. Hypersensitivity pneumonitis after exposure to isocyanates. Thorax 1976; 31:127–136.

121. Fink JN, Schlueter DP. Bathtub refinisher's lung: an unusual response to toluene diisocyanate. Am Rev Respir Dis 1978; 118:955–959.

122. Baur X, Dewair M, Rommelt H. Acute airway obstruction followed by hypersensitivity pneumonitis in an isocyanate (MDI) worker. J Occup Med 1984; 26(4):285–287.

123. Hendrick DJ, Marshall R, Faux JA, Krall JM. Positive "alveolar" responses to antigen inhalation provocation tests: their validity and recognition. Thorax 1980; 35:415–427.

124. Richerson HB, Bernstein IL, Fink JN, et al. Guidelines for the clinical evaluation of hypersensitivity pneumonitis. J Allergy Clin Immunol 1989; 84:839–844.

125. Fabbri LM, Boschetto P, Zocca E, et al. Bronchoalveolar neutrophilia during late asthmatic reactions induced by toluene diisocyanate. Am Rev Respir Dis 1987; 136:36–42.

126. Mapp C, Boschetto P, Vecchio L Dal, et al. Protective effect of antiasthma drugs on late asthmatic reactions and increased airway responsiveness induced by toluene diisocyanate in sensitized subjects. Am Rev Respir Dis 1987; 136:1403–1407.

127. Lam S, LeRiche J, Phillips D, Chan-Yeung M. Cellular and protein changes in bronchial lavage fluid after late asthmatic reaction in patients with red cedar asthma. J Allergy Clin Immunol 1987; 80:44–50.

128. Manning PJ, Rokach J, Malo J-L, et al. Urinary leukotriene E_4 levels during early and late asthmatic responses. J Allergy Clin Immunol 1990; 86:211–220.

11

Environmental Monitoring: General Considerations, Exposure–Response Relationships, and Risk Assessment

Mark Nieuwenhuijsen
Division of Primary Care and Population Health Sciences, Department of Epidemiology and Public Health, Imperial College London, London, U.K.

Xaver Baur
Department of Occupational Medicine, Ordinariat und Zentral Institut für Arbeitsmedizin Hamburg, Institute of Occupational Medicine, University of Hamburg, Hamburg, Germany

Dick Heederik
Division of Environmental and Occupational Health, Institute for Risk Assessment Sciences, University of Utrecht, Utrecht, The Netherlands

INTRODUCTION—MONITORING GENERAL CONSIDERATIONS

Personal exposure monitoring involves the monitoring of people's personal exposure rather than environmental media around them, that is, environmental monitoring, for example, in the case of occupational airborne allergen measurements, attaching an exposure monitor to the person rather than placing a sampler in the area where they work. Personal exposure monitoring is widely accepted as the most appropriate way of environmental sampling in occupational epidemiology (1,2).

Exposure to any substances is characterized by its nature (e.g., its chemical form or particle size), the concentration, duration, and frequency of contact. Estimates of these characteristics can generally be obtained instrumentally (i.e., using a monitoring device), via questionnaires, through direct observation, or through the use of biomarkers. The emphasis in the first section of this chapter is on the measurement of personal exposure with instruments; these provide information mainly on the level of exposure.

Personal monitoring is generally labor intensive, costly, and may be difficult to carry out. These factors restrict its use, even though the information obtained is generally more informative and relevant than other approaches, depending on the circumstances, and increase the scientific value of epidemiological studies. It is generally not possible to carry out personal monitoring on a very large number of people. A more efficient use may be to develop and/or validate (statistical) exposure models in a representative sample and/or time period of the population under study (3–5).

Once the decision has been made to use personal monitoring for an epidemiological study, a comprehensive sampling strategy needs to be designed and carried out, and the results needs to be interpreted. In the process, a number of choices need to be made which will fundamentally affect the way in which the study is carried out, and the reliability and interpretation of the results. These include whether to adopt a group or individual sampling approach, the number of measurements needed, the duration of monitoring and appropriate averaging time, the type of monitor or method to be used, and how the data will be analyzed, interpreted, and used for the epidemiological study. Crucial to these choices is the fact that, in most circumstances, marked variation occurs in exposure levels, both over time for any individual and between individuals for any given time. Thus, a single "best estimate" of the average exposure level may not be sufficient; instead, data are needed on levels of variations in exposure. The challenge is to design a strategy that incorporates the variability to the advantage of the epidemiological study and in the most efficient way while attempting to avoid potential bias.

Group vs. Individual Approach

Two main approaches are available, (*i*) the individual approach and (*ii*) the group approach, but task-based approaches have also been suggested. In the individual approach, every member of the population is monitored either once or repeatedly, and data are obtained at the individual level. In the group approach, the group is first split into smaller subpopulations based on specific determinants of exposure. In occupational epidemiological studies, exposure groups may be defined a priori on the basis of (*i*) work similarly, i.e., having the same job title and/or carrying out similar work, (*ii*) similarity with respect to particular substances, and (*iii*) similarity of environmental conditions, e.g., process equipment and ventilation. The underlying assumption is that subjects within each exposure group experience similar exposure characteristics, including exposure levels and variation. Subsequently, a representative sample of members from each exposure group is monitored, either once or repeatedly. If the aim is to estimate mean exposure, the average of the exposure measurements is then assigned to all the members in that particular exposure group. (Where a sufficient number of samples have been taken in a population, the exposure group could be divided afterwards into subpopulations based on statistical analysis on those samples.)

Where possible, repeated measurements on individuals should be taken. This enables the estimation of the within and between subject variance in the individual approach and within and between subject variance and between group variance in the group approach, which can be used to optimize exposure–response relationships (2,6).

Number of Subjects and Measurements

The number of subjects to be measured and the number of measurements to be taken on each subject depend on the chosen strategy and the distribution of the variability in exposure across the population. In the case of the individual approach, every subject will be monitored. Repeated measurements are highly recommended so that the within and between subject variance can be estimated, and reduce attenuation in health risk estimates. The number of repeated measurements required can be estimated, and is dependent on the ratio of within and between subject variance and the level of attenuation (7). In the group approach, the number of measurements depends on ratio of the between group variance (or between subpopulation variance) and between and within group variance, and the required precision of the estimated mean for each group (8,9). The number of measurements required for a certain precision can be calculated in various ways, for example:

$$n = \left(\frac{t * \text{CV}}{E}\right)^2$$

where n is the number of samples, t, the t-distribution value for the chosen confidence level and n_0-1 degrees of freedom (e.g., 1.96 for 95% confidence, infinite degrees of freedom), CV, the coefficient of variation (e.g., in geometric standard deviation/in geometric mean), and E is the chosen level of error (0.1 for 10% variation around the mean).

It is important to note that repeated measurements on individuals contribute less to the overall precision of the exposure group mean.

Loomis et al. (10) reported a more practical approach. They designed a study with a fixed target measurement size, based on considerations of precision and feasibility. They aggregated jobs into three levels of presumed exposure. The number of measurements for each job was weighted such that the presumed medium and high exposure groups were respectively sampled with three times and five times the frequency of the low exposure group. Because the variance increases with an increase in exposure level, a greater number of measurements were needed in the more highly exposed groups to meet the desired precision criterion. The measurements were distributed within these levels in proportion to the relative size of the various companies involved. Workers were selected randomly, and those in the medium and high exposure groups were monitored twice on randomly selected days. To be able to take so many measurements they send out the sampler through the mail.

The number of measurements can be increased by sending out (passive) samplers rather than handing them out or by self-monitoring (10,11). In this way the number of measurements can be increased even though the method(s) may not be reliable. The benefits of a larger number of samples however may outweigh the loss in reliability. However, this approach has technical limitation, because passive samples are only available for a limited number of chemical agents and have not been developed for the analysis of high-molecular-weight sensitizers.

Whatever the approach, to avoid bias and to fulfill the assumptions of statistical programs, subjects and measurements should be selected randomly.

Duration of Sampling

The duration of the sampling period (or averaging period) depends, among others, on the health outcome of interest in the epidemiological study, the detection limits of the measurement technique, and the level of the pollutant in the environment. Relatively long sampling times may also be necessary for less sensitive measurement and analysis techniques to make sure that enough material is collected. In the latter case the duration can be shortened if the flow rate of the sampler is increased, but this may also introduce other problems such as the increase in weight of the sampler. In general, the variance of the exposure measurements decreases with increasing monitoring time (12,13).

Chronic disease outcomes (e.g., the effects of potential carcinogens on cancer prevalence) generally require long sampling durations (many hours to days). Studies of acute disease outcomes (e.g., relationships between ammonia and irritant effects) require shorter sampling durations (minutes to less than an hour).

At times it may not be known what the sampling duration should be, and short- and long-term sampling may need to be carried out. Flour and its additives such as fungal α-amylase are well known causes of bakers' asthma. Little is known about the duration, frequency, and levels of exposure required for the development of bakers' asthma (or other causes), i.e., it is unknown whether short-term peak exposure levels or long-term exposure levels (work shift) may be responsible for it, although more recent studies have shown exposure–response relationships with work shift levels (see later). In a recent epidemiological study in bakeries and flour mills (14,15), a group-based and a task-based approach were used to characterize exposure. Personal exposure measurements of total dust were taken on a representative sample within each group for a whole work shift and during tasks that were expected to have high dust exposure and analyzed gravimetrically and for flour aeroallergen levels in the laboratory with an immunoassay (16–18).

They presented full shift and highest exposed task levels of dust and flour aeroallergen in the main exposure groups in bakeries and flour mills. Short-term exposure levels during certain tasks were considerably higher than average full shift levels. For example, flour millers experienced a 15-fold greater dust exposure level during spillage clean up compared to their full shift average exposure. Frequency and duration of peak levels differed, for example, some peaks occurred a few times during a day and others a few times a month.

In the bakeries and flour mills no correlation existed between duration of exposure and intensity indices of exposure (peak and average) for both dust and flour aeroallergen, suggesting that these can be used as independent exposure indices in the epidemiological analysis (18). Moderate to good correlation existed between the various intensity measures of exposures for both dust and flour aeroallergen. Good correlations existed between measures of exposure to dust and measures of exposure to flour aeroallergen. Because the exposure variables were fairly well correlated, only full shift dust measurements were used in the epidemiological analysis, and exposure–response relationships were demonstrated (14,15).

Active or Passive Sampling

To take personal airborne samples, equipment is needed which is light enough to be carried around without undue inconvenience to the subject and which will not significantly alter their usual behavior patterns. The sampler should be placed such that it takes a sample of the inhaled air of the subject, often referred to as the breathing zone (within around 30 cm of the nose and the mouth). Both active and passive samplers are available for this purpose.

For active sampling, air is drawn by a sampling pump through a collection unit, e.g., a sampling head with a filter inside for particulate matter, or a Tenax tube for VOCs. The sampling flow rate is dependent on the requirements of the collection unit and may vary from less than 100 mL/min for gas sampling to over 4 L/min or more for particulate matter sampling. The exposure concentration in air is determined by dividing the difference in the measured amount of the substance before and after the sampling period (e.g., for particulate matter, the weight on the filter before and after sampling, adjusted for blanks), by the volume of air (in m^3) drawn through the collection unit. The volume of air is the duration of air multiplied by the flow rate. Active sampling is generally used in workplace sampling, partly because of the relatively short sampling duration (up to eight hours per day).

Passive sampling is based on the principle of diffusion and does not require a sampling pump. It is widely used for gaseous substances, such as NO_2. Passive samplers for particulates are in the design stage (19). A problem in sampling environmental pollutants using passive samplers is that the concentrations of pollutants present are often low, relative to the detection limits of the samplers. This implies the need for relatively long sampling durations and means that the samplers typically provide measures of long-term average concentrations only (e.g., over a week or longer period). There are also problems of accuracy and precision. On the other hand, passive sampling is generally less labor intensive and costly than active sampling. This provides the possibility of taking more measurements for the same cost and of carrying out relatively intense spatial and temporal sampling (e.g., for use of estimating variance components). Recent advances in the design of passive samplers, the application of strict sampling protocols (including repeat measurements at each site), and the use of validation studies comparing passive samplers with more conventional methods offer scope to improve the performance of passive sampling.

Continuous or Average Sampling

Depending on the collection unit used, exposure measurements can take the form of either continuous readings or an average over the sampling period. Continuous measurements are provided by direct reading instruments, such as the MINIRAM, TSI DustTrak ($PM_{2.5}$), TSI P-Trak (ultrafine), and GRIMM monitor for particulate sampling and the Langan CO Enhanced Measurer T15 monitor for CO. They can be useful for the study of acute health effects. Wegman et al. (20) used the MINIRAM to successfully examine the acute effects of dust in an occupational epidemiological study.

Information from direct reading instruments can be stored in data loggers and downloaded to a computer, where they can be graphed and analyzed. Although direct reading instruments can provide a very informative picture of the variation in exposure over the sampling period (Fig. 1), they are relatively rarely used for epidemiological studies. The instruments are often expensive; they are sometimes not very specific, and accurate calibration is of considerable importance. Also, in case of chronic disease, short-term variations in exposure may not be considered important. More commonly monitoring is aimed at providing estimates of average concentrations over a measurement period, e.g., a work shift (approximately eight hours), a day, or a few days. Only one concentration value is obtained per measurement period. As noted above, time-averaged data of this type are provided by both passive and active monitors.

Health-Based Size Selective Sampling

Over the years epidemiological studies have examined the health effects of airborne particulates. The health hazard from airborne particulates varies with its nature, i.e., physical, chemical, toxicological, and/or biological properties. An important property is the aerodynamic diameter, which determines how deeply the particle is likely to penetrate into the respiratory system. Particles have thus been categorized according to which region they are likely to reach in the respiratory system; to measure different size fractions, a personal sampler with different sampling

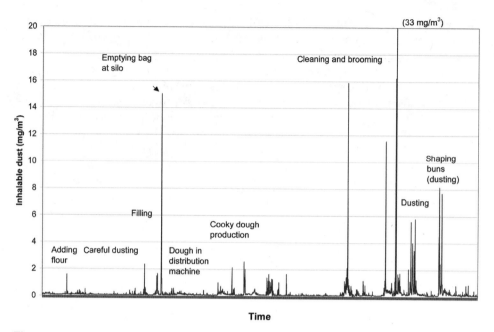

Figure 1 Measurement of the dust exposure pattern over a working day in workers of a bakery. The peak exposures are clearly visible. Some peaks involve pure enzyme dust that reaches levels of several tens of milligrams during a few minutes. *Source*: Courtesy of N. de Pater, TNO, Zeist, The Netherlands.

heads is needed (2). The inhalable particle fraction is the fraction that enters the nose and the mouth, and has a 50% cut point diameter of 100 µm. For example, an IOM sampler can be used to measure this at a flow rate of 2 L/min (21). Other samplers widely used like the German GSP and the Dutch PAS6 sampling head have been compared in validation studies, and some results are discussed in Kenny et al. (22). The inhalable dust fraction is often measured in the workplace, but rarely in the general environment. The thoracic fraction is the fraction that enters the thorax, and has a 50% cut point diameter of 10 µm; it is therefore often referred to as PM_{10}. The PM_{10} is often measured in the general environment, but rarely in the workplace. The respirable fraction is the fraction that enters the lungs (the alveolar region). This has a 50% cut point diameter of 4 µm, and can be measured with special cyclones. $PM_{2.5}$, particles with a 50% cut off diameter of 2.5 µm, is the fraction that penetrates deep into the alveolar region. A personal cascade impactor such as the eight-stage Sierra Marple 298 separates particulate matter by aerodynamic diameter and can be used to estimate the particle size distribution during the entire monitoring period, but tends to require higher particulate matter concentrations to collect enough matter on the different stages (23,24). This impactor was used in the study of occupational asthma mentioned above and most of the particles belonged to the extra thoracic fraction (Table 1).

Identifying Determinants of Exposure and Building Exposure Models

As mentioned before, taking personal measurements may not be the most cost effective approach to obtain exposure estimates. An alternative approach could be

Table 1 Particle Size Distribution by Mass (%) in Bakeries and Flour Mills Taken with an Eight-Stage Personal Cascade Impactor

50% cut of diameter (μm)	Packing areas		Dough brake	
	Dust	FA	Dust	FA
21.3	56.2	41.9	55.9	34.0
14.8	23.8	26.9	30.7	41.1
9.8	10.4	11.5	5.6	16.0
6.0	4.7	10.5	2.4	5.5
3.5	1.8	3.0	1.0	0.5
1.55	0.6	1.5	1.0	0.7
0.93	0.6	1.3	1.0	0.7
0.52	0.6	1.2	1.4	0.7
0.05	1.3	2.2	1.0	0.7

Abbreviation: FA, flour aeroallergen.
Source: From Ref. 24.

to administer questionnaires containing questions on potential or known major determinants of exposure to all the subjects in an epidemiological study, and conduct personal monitoring and apply regression techniques in a proportion of the study subjects to build a stochastic model that can be applied to all the subjects, by combining the regression coefficients from the model and the information from the questionnaire data (3–5,25).

The regression model can be described as follows:

$$\ln(C_{ij}) = \beta_0 + \beta_i \text{var}_i + \cdots + \beta_j \text{var}_j + E$$

whereby $\ln(C_{ij})$ denotes the natural logarithm of the concentration, β_0, the intercept which can be interpreted as the background level, β_x, the regression coefficient of potential determinants var_x from the questionnaire, which estimates the magnitude of the exposure effect, and E denotes a random variable with mean 0, often called the error term.

The application of linear regression models will be illustrated by an example of the effect of farm characteristics on endotoxin concentrations among pig farmers, where personal exposure measurements were taken on two days, and diaries were filled out on 14 days (4). In the study among 198 Dutch pig farmers the effect of endotoxins exposure on lung function was evaluated. Exposure to inhalable dust containing endotoxins was determined by means of personal sampling. Measurements for eight hours were conducted for each participant during one shift in summer and one shift in winter. The farmers were requested to complete a diary on time spent in different activities during the day of the measurements and the following six days. In addition, farm characteristics of all breeding compartments were registered during a walk-through survey. Information was recorded on number of animals, feeding methods, heating and ventilation, type of floor, bedding material, and degree of contamination. A linear regression model was fitted, based upon all factors that showed a significant effect. In the model outdoor temperature, 12 farm characteristics, and eight activities in pig farming explained about 37% of the variation in log-transformed time-weighted average exposure to endotoxins. The intercept in the statistical model corresponded roughly to $80\,\text{ng/m}^3$, indicating that the background endotoxin concentration in these pig farms was relatively high compared with the overall average concentration of $129\,\text{ng/m}^3$. The activities with the largest contribution to the predicted endotoxin exposure were teeth cutting ($\beta = 0.51$) and ear tagging ($\beta = 0.43$), and the most important farm characteristic was the presence of a convex floor ($\beta = -0.22$).

The regression coefficients from the two measurement days were applied to the diary data from the days that no measurements were taken to obtain improved estimates of personal exposure due to the larger number of observations available (14 vs. 2). The authors showed an improved exposure–response relationship using this approach.

This approach is now used in a health surveillance system covering more than 16,000 allergen exposed flour millers and bakers in the Netherlands. The participants receive a short questionnaire with three questions on the sector of industry they work in, their job title, and the tasks they perform on a regular basis. Information from an earlier exposure survey was used in which more than 600 wheat flour allergen and fungal α-amylase measurements were taken. These measurements were used to evaluate the relationship between allergen exposure and sector of industry, job title, and tasks. The regression model obtained was used to estimate the exposure for each of the 16,000 workers included in the health surveillance system. Details about the models used are described in the literature (26).

Further Laboratory Analysis

Not only the particulate mass and size may be important in the development of adverse health effects but also the composition of the particulates. It is therefore often useful to analyze particulate samples for their biological and elemental composition. A range of techniques are available for further analysis, including X-ray fluorescence, inductively coupled plasma-mass spectrometry, gas chromatography–mass spectrometry, GC-FID, GFAAS, immunoassays, electron scanning microscopy, or reflectance methods. Further information on these techniques can be found in analytical chemistry books. Results of immunoassays measuring flour aeroallergen are given in Tables 1 through 3 and will also be discussed in chapter 17.

EXPOSURE–RESPONSE RELATIONSHIPS

Theoretical Considerations

Exposure to environmental aeroallergens causes Th2-dependent sensitization which follows exposure–response relationships (2,42,43). The same is true for endpoint responses (symptoms and diseases) if sensitized subjects are re-exposed to the sensitizing allergen. In addition to the dose, the concentration (e.g., in ng/m^3) or the product of intensity and duration of exposure should also be considered. Different multiple regression models from the generalized linear model family are being used in different epidemiological designs to calculate measures of association such as the Cox proportional hazard model in cross-sectional or longitudinal studies (44), to calculate, respectively, Prevalence Ratio's and Relative Risks. Logistic regression models are usually applied in case control studies and cross-sectional studies to calculate Odds Ratios. For risk assessment purposes, Relative Risks or its closest estimate is to be preferred.

Table 2 Studies of Exposure–Response Relationships of Occupational and Environmental Inhalant Allergens

Allergen	Source	Exposure evaluation	No. of subjects	Lowest observed effective allergen level	Exposure–response relation
Flour dust	Houba et al. (27)	Air concentration	230	1–2.4 mg/m³	Sensitization
	Musk et al. (28)	Air concentration	279	1.7 mg/m³	Sensitization, symptoms, PD_{20}
α-Amylase	Houba et al. (29)	Air concentration	178	0.25 ng/m³	Sensitization
Alkalase	Cullinan et al. (30)	Air concentration	350	<5 ng/m³	Sensitization, asthma
Red cedar	Noertjojo et al. (31)	Air concentration	243	0.2–0.4 mg/m³	Lung function decline
Natural rubber latex	Baur (32)	Air concentration	145	0.6 ng/m³	Sensitization, symptoms
Cow, Bos d 2	Hinze et al. (33)	Room dust	40	1–29 µg/dust	Sensitization
Rat urinary prot	Cullinan et al. (14)	Questionnaire, air conc.	323	0.1–68 µg/m³	Symptoms
Midge, Chi t 1–9	Liebers et al. (34)	Questionnaire	184	>5 mg/month	Sensitization
Acid anhydrides	Venables (35)	Air concentration	Review	0.3–1.7 mg/m³	Symptoms
TCPA	Liss et al. (36)	Air concentration	52	0.1–0.39 mg/m³	Symptoms
TMA	Boxer et al. (37)	Air concentration	17	0.82 mg/m³	Symptoms, sensitization
TMA	Barker et al. (38)	Air concentration	49	<0.04 mg/m³	Symptoms, sensitization
Isocyanates	Baur et al. (39)	Air concentration	84	5–10 ppb	Symptoms, lung function decline
Colophony	Burge et al. (40)	Air concentration	88	<0.01 mg/m³	Asthma, lung function decline
Platinum salts	Calverley et al. (41)	Air concentration	78	≤2 µg/m³	Sensitization, asthma

Abbreviations: PD_{20}, provocative dose of methacholine producing a 20% decrease in forced expiratory volume in one second; TCPA, tetrachlorophthalic anhydride; TMA, trimelletic anhydride.

Table 3 Mandatory Medical Surveillance Programs for Occupational Airways Sensitizers and Dust as an Instrument of Health-Based Institutional Policies in Germany

Airways sensitizer	NOAEL	OEL	Criterion of mandatory medical surveillance	
			Concentration	Listed exposures
Flour	0.5–1 mg/m³	4 mg/m³	>4 mg/m³(i.d.)	
Cereals/feed		4 mg/m³	>4 mg/m³(i.d.)	
Hardwood dust	<0.2 mg/m³	2 mg/m³	>2 mg/m³(i.d.)	
Latex	0.5 ng/m³			>30 µg/g (protein/rubber)
Laboratory animals	<0.1 ng EQ/m³			Lab animal confinement and/or skin contact skin or airway exposure
Isocyanates	<0.05 mg/m³	0.02–0.07 mg/m³	>0.05 mg/m³	
Epoxy resins	<0.01 mg/m³	0.04–1 mg/m³		
Welding fumes			>3 mg/m³(i.d.)	
Platinum salts	<0.002 mg/m³	0.002 mg/m³	>0.002 mg/m³(i.d.)	
Beryllium	<0.002 mg/m³		>0.005 mg/m³(i.d.)	
Inhalable dust	4 mg/m³	10 mg/m³	>10 mg/m³(i.d.)	
Respirable dust	1.5 mg/m³	3 mg/m³	>3 mg/m³	

Abbreviations: NOAEL, no observed adverse effect levels; OEL, occupational exposure limit; i.d., inhalable dust.

A major issue is the exposure assessment in epidemiological studies. The first epidemiological studies that described exposure–response relationships for allergens have not always presented the available information in an optimal way. Usually exposure categories were distinguished, but average exposure levels were not always given for each exposure category. Moreover, there is a general problem with harmonization of assays used to measure allergens exposure, and this complicates comparison of study results and pooling or summarizing of findings from different studies.

For a few years, we see application of smoothing approaches, for instance by using semi-parametric GAM models to explore the shape of the exposure–response relationship in greater detail. Discussion of the details of this approach is beyond the scope of this chapter, but use of these models in analyzing exposure sensitization relationships for wheat flour and house dust mite allergen suggest that no exposure threshold exists below which no excess risk can be observed. These models have also shown that in some studies flattening of exposure–response relationships may occur, or even a bell shape. Figure 2 shows exposure–response relationships for wheat flour and sensitization based on two different studies in four different industrial sectors (26). It is unlikely that the heterogeneity in response is the result of biological phenomena, but it is more likely explained by differences in health worker effect between the studies.

Epidemiological studies including quantitative measurement of molecularly characterized allergens in the range of ng/m^3 on the one hand and antibody responses and symptoms (diseases) on the other hand allow one to estimate exposure–response relationships. The shape of such exposure–response relationships may differ from substance to substance and may be steeper for atopic subjects and smokers compared to nonatopics and nonsmokers (Fig. 3). At present, reliable data

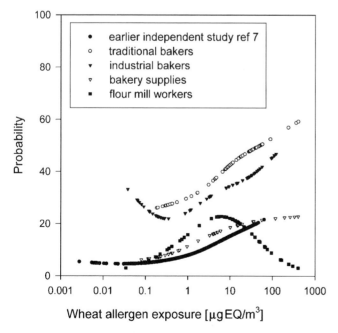

Figure 2 Wheat sensitization (probability) as a function of exposure to inhalable dust by sector of industry, based on actual measured wheat allergens ($\mu gEQ/m^3$) on a log scale, together with the relationship as published in an independent study. *Source*: From Refs. 26, 27.

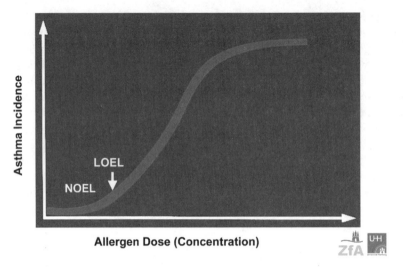

Figure 3   Theoretical exposure–response curve for asthma-inducing occupational sensitizers.

are mainly from bakeries, laboratory animal facilities, the health care sector, and enzyme-detergent manufactory plants.

Flour

Measurements of inhalable dust concentrations in bakeries were calculated by several groups using personal or area dust samplers (14,16,27,28,45). Concentrations varied considerably and were partly above $30 \, \text{mg/m}^3$. As published by Houba et al. (27), Heederik and Houba (43), Musk et al. (29), and Cullinan et al. (14), flour dust concentrations as low as 1 to $2.5 \, \text{mg/m}^3$ are associated with a significantly elevated risk of sensitization to wheat allergens. Using logistic or linear regression, Musk et al. (28) studying 279 workers of a modern bakery found immediate-type skin-prick test responses to wheat as well as symptoms, lung function decrease, and bronchial reactivity related to current or past exposure. Similarly, Heederik and Houba (43) clearly demonstrated dose–response relationships between cumulative wheat allergen load on the one hand and sensitization and asthma on the other. More important than total dust is the concentration of flour antigens which only shows an approximate relationship to total dust (1 mg of bakery dust referred to 2.4–6 µg wheat allergens) (16).

The TLV-TWA currently proposed by ACGIH (46) for inhalable flour dust is $0.5 \, \text{mg/m}^3$. The Dutch Expert Committee on Occupational Standards (DECOS) suggested a cumulative inhalable flour dust exposure of $11.97 \, \text{mg/year/m}^3$ (43).

Enzymes

Another important bakery allergen is fungal α-amylase, derived from *Aspergillus oryzae.* It is widely used as a baking additive. Air concentrations in bakeries are in the ng/m^3 range. Approximately 20% of symptomatic bakers are sensitized to this enzyme (47).

A study of 178 Dutch bakers performed by Houba et al. (29) reveals dose–response relations with an increased frequency of sensitization at $\geq 0.25 \, \text{ng/m}^3$ already. This effect is much more pronounced in atopics than in nonatopics.

In the late 1960s, the introduction of alkaline heat-stable enzymes (proteases, amylase, and cellulase) in the detergent industry was associated with estimated enzyme air concentrations in the workplace of approximately $300 \, \text{ng/m}^3$ and higher. Forty percent to 50% of the workers were sensitized and developed asthma and/or rhinitis. A follow-up of 1642 workers from 1968 until 1975 showed increased exposure (based on dustiness of job) and atopy to be related with increased incidences of sensitization with the highest proportion of sensitization within the first two years of observation (48). In the meantime, mainly due to enzyme encapsulation, exposures have been reduced to less than $15 \, \text{ng/m}^3$. This drop is reported to be associated with less than a 20% sensitization of the plant population over a period of 10 years and an annual incidence of less than 3% (49,50).

Cullinan et al. (30), however, found 19% of detergent workers exposed to enzymes (geometric mean: $4.25 \, \text{ng/m}^3$) to be sensitized; 16% had work-related respiratory symptoms. In this study seven out of a subgroup of 74 subjects who started working three years ago were sensitized (five to protease and/or amylase; four to cellulase), and seven of them noticed work-related symptoms of the upper-respiratory tract or chest. Due to these rather high prevalences, the authors concluded that enzyme encapsulation alone is not sufficient to prevent enzyme-induced allergy and asthma. In 2005 ACGIH (46) published a TLV-STEL-C (ceiling) of $0.06 \, \mu\text{g/m}^3$ for the bacterial protease subtilisin.

Wood Dust

Vedal et al. (51) and Noertjojo et al. (31) investigated sawmill workers exposed to western red cedar dust. In the longitudinal study of Noertjojo et al. (31), three exposure groups were differentiated: low ($0.2 \, \text{mg/m}^3$), medium (0.2–$0.4 \, \text{mg/m}^3$), and high ($>0.4 \, \text{mg/m}^3$). An exposure-related significant annual decline in forced vital capacity (FVC) was found. Similarly, Vedal et al. (51) observed that forced expiratory volume in one second (FEV_1) and FVC deteriorations were inversely related to the wood dust load.

Natural Rubber Latex

Gloves made by natural rubber latex, the milky fluid from the rubber tree *Hevea brasiliensis*, have become a major cause of immediate-type allergic skin diseases, asthma, and rhinitis among health care workers since the 1990s. These latex protein allergens also adhere to the cornstarch powder and cotton fluffs (32) of gloves which function as airborne allergen carriers. High concentrations of this allergenic powder may occur in surgery rooms and intensive care units. Approximately 60 allergens were found in two-dimensional immunoelectrophoresis of latex (52), and so far, 13 allergens (Hev b 1–13) have been described on the molecular level. Hev b 1, 3, and 5 are found in glove powder.

Health care workers, who require latex gloves and working around them, have on an average risk of 3% to 20% to become sensitized to latex.

As a surrogate for latex exposure, Tarlo et al. (53), Heese et al. (54), and Levy et al. (55) used the duration of training of dental students. All three studies showed an increase in latex sensitization parallel with exposure.

In spina bifida children, who need multiple surgeries and have frequent direct internal or mucosal contact with latex medical devices, such as bladder catheters, the number of operations indicating a cumulative latex allergen dose correlates with the frequency of latex sensitization which may exceed 60% (56–58).

Our own study of 145 health care workers showed that sensitization to latex (observed in 22 cases) occurred only in hospital rooms with a latex allergen concentration of more than $0.5\,ng/m^3$ (59,60). Furthermore, several intervention studies with hospital conversion from powdered to nonpowdered low-protein gloves or to synthetic gloves were associated with a decrease of new cases (61,62).

Cow Allergen

Cow allergens are a major cause of respiratory allergies of farmers (63–65). Hinze et al. (33) investigated 40 dairy farmers and analyzed dust samples from their living rooms. Thresholds of 1 to $20\,\mu g$ (atopics) and 25 to $50\,\mu g$ (nonatopics) of the major cow allergen Bos d 2 per gram dust were found to be significantly associated with IgE levels of greater than $0.7\,kU/L$ in atopics and nonatopics. Rautiainen et al. (66) reported that the level of antibodies to bovine epithelial allergens among exposed subjects reflects the level of clinical allergies.

Rat Urinary Aeroallergen

Prevalence of rat allergy among laboratory animal workers range from 12% to 31% (67). Already in 1981, Schumacher et al. (68) comparing areas with low rat allergen levels (mean: $9.6\,ng/m^3$) with those of high levels described clear dose–response relationships for rhinitis and bronchial asthma. Cullinan et al. (14), Nieuwenhuijsen et al. (69,70), and Hollander et al. (71) used highly specific immunoassays for the quantification of rodents' urinary allergens in workplace atmospheres. Cross-sectional studies revealed that the exposure levels to rat urinary aeroallergens (range 0 to $>1.25\,ng\ EQ/m^3$) correlated with the frequency of positive skin test results as well as with upper- and lower-respiratory responses. Atopic workers had a more than threefold increased sensitization risk at low allergen levels than nonatopics. Data were consistent in all three aforementioned studies (72).

Similar results have been reported for mouse allergens/urinary proteins (67,73). The recent publication of Nieuwenhuijsen et al. (70) describes the clearest exposure–response relationship for the intensity of exposure ($\mu g/m^3$) among sensitized subjects, whereas weekly duration or the product of intensity and weekly duration of exposure produced less clear results (Fig. 4).

Soybean

Outbreaks of epidemic asthma were reported in several harbor cities during unloading of ships which are associated with liberation of soybean hull allergens. Sensitization as well as symptoms (in sensitized subjects) were dose and atopy dependent (74).

Chironomid Hemoglobins

Dried red mosquito larvae of nonbiting midges (Chironomidae) frequently used by fish hobbyists contain hemoglobins (Chi t 1–9) which are highly allergenic. They were identified as the first structurally defined allergens (75). We could demonstrate an association between the degree of exposure as calculated by frequency and

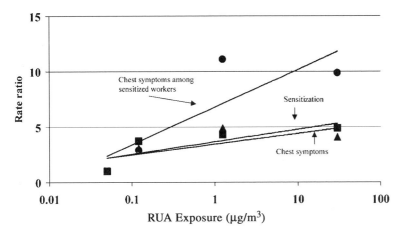

Figure 4 Exposure–response relations for chest symptoms (*triangles*), skin-prick test (*squares*), and sensitized chest symptoms (*circles*), including a best fit line. *Source*: From Ref. 70.

amount of material handled and symptoms as well as IgE-mediated sensitization. Asthma was significantly more often observed in heavily exposed workers of fishfood factories (16/85) than in moderately exposed fish hobbyists (25/205) (76). Furthermore, asthmatic symptoms were associated with high levels of specific IgE antibodies to Chi t 1–9 (34).

Acid Anhydrides

Acid anhydrides, a class of chemical agents frequently used in the production of resins and plastics, were found to cause respiratory symptoms in the mg/m^3 range (35,37,38). Barker et al. (38) who investigated 506 acid anhydride workers described work-related respiratory symptoms and elevated prevalence of sensitization related to increasing full shift exposures; exposure–response relations were consistent with trimellitic anhydride (TMA) at concentrations from less than 0.01 to greater than $0.04\,mg/m^3$ and were not modified by smoking and atopy.

Liss et al. (36) also found a high prevalence of work-related airway complaints (27–39%) in workers with contact to tetrachlorophthalic anhydrides (TCPA); the prevalence decreased significantly when TCPA was reduced from 0.21 until 0.30 to $0.1\,mg/m^3$. A corresponding effect was observed by Bernstein et al. (77) for TMA which was reduced from 0.82 until $2.1\,mg/m^3$ to 0.01 until $0.03\,mg/m^3$. The latter study also showed a decrease in the number of workers with specific IgE antibodies.

Present OELs range from 0.04 [TMA, TLV-STEL-C (ceiling) by ACGIH $0.04\,mg/m^3$] to 1.2 (maleic anhydride, TLV-TWA by ACGIH $0.41\,mg/m^3$) to $2\,mg/m^3$ (phthalic anhydride, TLV-TWA by ACGIH 1 ppm) (46).

Isocyanates

Isocyanates have been increasingly used for production of polyurethane foam, elastomers, adhesives, varnishes, coatings, insecticides, and many other products. These highly reactive chemicals have become number one of occupational airway sensitizers in several western countries.

As an example of a recent study the work of Petsonk et al. (78) should be mentioned which evaluated respiratory health in a new wood products manufacturing plant using MDI and its prepolymer. In the follow-up survey including 178 employees, 15 out of 56 workers (27%) in areas with the highest potential exposures to liquid isocyanates (vs. 0 out of 43 workers in the lowest potential exposures) had an onset of asthma-like symptoms. Forty-seven percent of workers with MDI skin staining versus 19% without skin staining developed such symptoms which were associated with variable airflow limitation and specific IgE to MDI-HSA. Our cross-sectional studies performed in two factories showed significantly fewer symptomatic subjects in comparison to the group exposed to 5 to 10 ppb MDI, lung function impairments and specific IgE antibodies in the group exposed to less than 5 ppb TDI (79).

As already shown by several other authors, it should be mentioned, however, that only a minority of symptomatic isocyanate workers showed IgE antibodies to diisocyanate–HSA conjugates (39,80–84).

Several authors observed isocyanate exposure–dependent declines in lung function in the OEL range (85–88).

It is worth mentioning that in most western countries OELs for diisocyanates have been stipulated at 10 ppb. This value seems to be too high. According to literature, 5 or 2.5 ppb would be a health-based level (89,90). OELs for isocyanates should consider gaseous as well as aerosol forms and also the increasingly used polyisocyanates which cause the same disorders as diisocyanates. Moreover, the prevention of isocyanate skin contact is obviously also an effective measure to reduce the risk of respiratory disorders.

TLV-TWA currently proposed by ACGIH (46) are as follows: TDI 0.005 ppm (TLV-STEL 0.02 ppm), MDI 0.005 ppm, HDI 0.005 ppm.

Colophony

Burge et al. (40) studied 88 factory employees manufacturing flux-cored solder and being exposed to colophony fumes generated at 140°C. Airborne colophony levels in the workplace were measured spectrophotometrically at 455 nm, and three grades of exposure could be defined with medium levels of $1.92 \, mg/m^3$ (six workers), $0.02 \, mg/m^3$ (14 workers) and $<0.01 \, mg/m^3$ (68 workers). Occupational asthma was present in 21% of the two groups with higher exposure and in 4% of the lowest exposure group. Moreover, mean values of FEV_1 and FVC dropped with increasing exposure. The authors conclude that sensitization to colophony will not be prevented unless exposure is kept well below the present threshold limit value and that the whole resin acid rather than decomposition products (aldehydes) causes asthma. The authors therefore suggest that the threshold limit value at 140°C should be based on the resin acid content of colophony fume and not on the aldehyde content.

Platinum Salts

Calverley et al. (41) performed a prospective cohort study comprising 78 new recruits to a platinum refinery. Thirty-four of them worked in high exposure production areas (27% of samples $>2 \, \mu g/m^3$; TLV) and 44 in low exposure nonproduction services (all samples $<2 \, \mu g/m^3$). After two years, 32% of the subjects were found to be platinum salt–sensitive; 28% had positive skin-prick tests to platinum salt as well as work-related symptoms and 13% had work-related symptoms only. Multivariate analyses showed that the risk of sensitization was six times greater at high exposures than at low intensity exposures (after adjustment for smoking). Furthermore, the risk of sensitization was about eight times higher for smokers than for nonsmokers. Bolm-Audorff et al. (91) identified sensitization and respiratory symptoms even at concentrations lower than $0.1\,\mu g/m^3$, whereas Merget and Schulze-Werninghaus (92) observed no symptoms at $0.01\,\mu g/m^3$.

Table 3 provides an overview of the mandatory surveillance programs in Germany.

RISK ASSESSMENT

Exposure standards for the air in the work environment have been proposed that have been derived by applying classical risk assessment approaches, based on obtaining lowest observed adverse effect levels or no observed adverse effect levels

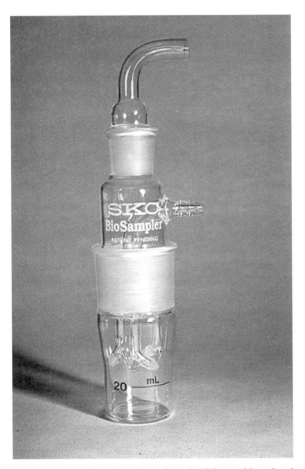

Figure 5 An isocyanate-exposed worker is equipped with a midget impinger such as these are shown for sampling isocyanate vapor and particulates filled during the performance of a specific task (sampling time 30 minutes maximally). The impinger is filled with di-*n*-butylamine in toluene to dissolve and stabilize the isocyanates. Samples can be analyzed by LC–MS. *Abbreviation*: LC–MS, liquid chromatography in combination with mass spectrometry. *Source*: Photo courtesy of Pronk, TNO and IRAS, Zeist and Utrecht, The Netherlands.

(NOAELs). Several examples of this approach exist: In the United States the ACGIH, for instance, has adopted a threshold limit value for inhalable flour dust of $0.5\,mg/m^3$ averaged over an eight hour work shift (46). In Sweden a standard has been adopted of $3\,mg/m^3$ over eight hours. All these values are either based on no adverse effect levels that have been obtained from the literature or are values that took these NOAELs as starting point, with changes made on the basis of technical feasibility. However, these approaches have limitations because some more recent studies suggest that an exposure threshold for the exposure, below which symptoms or sensitization does not occur, cannot be established (43). An entirely different approach has been followed by the DECOS. This concluded that on the basis of a reanalysis of a Dutch epidemiological study, no NOAEL can be defined, because the risk increases with increasing exposure, and no exposure threshold is observable (43). They therefore calculated the excess risk at a range of exposure levels, using the exposure–response relationship observed, assuming a baseline sensitization rate of 4% to wheat allergens in the general population. An uncertainty factor of two was applied for variation of the allergen content of wheat flour. Excess sensitization risks of 1% and 10% occur at exposure levels of 0.12 and $1.2\,mg/m^3$. Detailed knowledge of exposure–response relationships and application in risk assessment approaches will allow strategic planning of preventive measures taking into account cost-effect relations as well as ethical aspects.

REFERENCES

1. Nieuwenhuijsen MJ. Exposure assessment in occupational epidemiology: measuring present exposures with an example of occupational asthma. Int Arch Occup Environ Health 1997; 70:295–308.
2. Nieuwenhuijsen MJ, ed. Exposure Assessment in Occupational and Environmental Epidemiology. Oxford University Press, 2003 (ISBN 0-19-852861-2).
3. Hornung RW, Greife AL, Stayner LT, et al. Statistical model for prediction to ethylene oxide in an occupational mortality study. Am J Ind Med 1994; 125:825–836.
4. Preller L, Kromhout H, Heederik D, Tielen MJ. Modeling long-term average exposure in occupational exposure–response analysis. Scand J Work Environ Health 1995; 21:504–512.
5. Burstyn I, Kromhout H, Kauppinen T, Heikkilä, P, Boffetta P. Statistical modeling of the determinants of historical exposure to bitumen and polycyclic aromatic hydrocarbons among paving workers. Ann Occup Hyg 2000; 44:43–56.
6. Loomis D, Kromhout H. Exposure variability: concepts and applications in occupational epidemiology. Am J Ind Med 2004; 45:113–122.
7. Liu K, Stamler JA, Dyer A, McKeever P, McKeever P. Statistical methods to assess and minimize the role of intra individual variability in obscuring the relationship between dietary lipids and serum cholesterol. J Chronic Dis 1978; 31:399–418.
8. Kromhout H, Heederik D. Occupational epidemiology in the rubber industry; implications of exposure variability. Am J Ind Med 1995; 27:171–185.
9. Kromhout H, Tielemans E, Preller L, Heedrik D. Estimates of individual dose from current measurements of exposure. Occup Hyg 1996; 3:23–29.
10. Loomis DP, Kromhout H, Peipins LA, Kleckner RC, Iriye R, Savitz DA. Sampling design and field methods of a large randomized, multisite survey of occupational magnetic field study. Appl Occup Environ Hyg 1994; 9:49–56.
11. Liljelind IE, Rappaport SM, Levin JO, Stromback AE, Sunesson AL, Jarvholm BG. Comparison of self-assessment and expert assessment of occupational exposure to chemicals. Scand J Work Environ Health 2001; 27:311–317.

12. Coenen W. Beschreibung des zeitlichen verhaltens von schadtstoffkonzentrationen durch einen stetigen Markow-process. Staub-Reinhalt Luft 1976; 31:16–23.
13. LeClare PC, Breslin AJ, Ong LDY. Factors affecting the accuracy of average dust concentration measurements. Am Ind Hyg Assoc J 1969; 30:386–393.
14. Cullinan P, Lowson D, Nieuwenhuijsen MJ, et al. Work related symptoms, sensitisation and estimated exposure in workers not previously exposed to flour. Occup Environ Med 1994; 51:579–583.
15. Cullinan P, Cook A, Nieuwenhuijsen MJ, et al. Allergen and dust exposure as determinants of work-related symptoms in a cohort of flour-exposed workers; a case-control analysis. Ann Occup Hyg 2001; 45:97–103.
16. Nieuwenhuijsen MJ, Sandiford C, Lowson D, et al. Dust and flour aeroallergen in flour mills and bakeries. Occup Environ Med 1994; 51:584–588.
17. Nieuwenhuijsen MJ, Sandiford CP, Lowson D, et al. Peak exposure levels for dust and flour aeroallergen in flour mills and bakeries. Ann Occup Hyg 1995; 39:193–201.
18. Nieuwenhuijsen MJ, Lowson D, Venables KM, Newman Taylor AJ. Correlation between different measures of exposure in a cohort of bakery workers and flour millers. Ann Occup Hyg 1995; 39:291–298.
19. Brown RC, Wake D, Thorpe A, Hemingway MA, Roff MW. Preliminary assessment of a device for passive sampling of airborne particulate. Ann Occup Hyg 1994; 38:303–318.
20. Wegman DH, Eisen EA, Woskie SR, Hu X. Measuring exposure for the epidemiologic study of acute effects. Am J Ind Med 1992; 21.
21. Mark D, Vincent JH. A new personal sampler for airborne total dust in workplaces. Ann Occup Hyg 1986; 30:89–102.
22. Kenny LC, Aitken R, Chalmers C, et al. A collaborative European study of personal inhalable aerosol sampler performance. Ann Occup Hyg 1997; 41:135–153.
23. Marple VA, Rubow KL, Turner W, Sprengler JD. Low flow rate sharp cut impactors for indoor air sampling design and calibration. JAPCA 1987; 37:1303–1307.
24. Sandiford CP, Nieuwenhuijsen MJ, Tee RD, Newman Taylor AJ. Determination of the size of airborne flour particles. Allergy 1994; 12:891–893.
25. Nieuwenhuijsen MJ, Gordon S, Harris J, et al. Determinants of airborne allergen exposure in an animal house. Occup Hyg 1995; 1:317–324.
26. Peretz C, Pater N, de Monchy J, Oostenbrink J, Heederik D. Assessment of exposure to wheat flour and the shape of the relationship with specific sensitisation. Scand J Work Environ Health 2005; 31:65–74.
27. Houba R, Heederik D, Doekes G. Occupational exposure limit for wheat flour dust in the Netherlands. Zbl Arbeitsmed 1998; 48:485–487.
28. Musk AW, Venables KM, Crook B, et al. Respiratory symptoms, lung function and sensitivity to flour in a British bakery. Br J Ind Med 1989; 46:636–642.
29. Houba R, Heederik DJJ, Doekes G, van Run PEM. Exposure–sensitisation relationship for α-amylase allergens in the baking industry. Am Respir Crit Care Med 1996; 154:130–136.
30. Cullinan P, Harris JM, Newman Taylor AJ, et al. An outbreak of asthma in a modern detergent factory. Lancet 2000; 356(9245):1899–1900.
31. Noertjojo HK, Dimich-Ward H, Peelen S, Dittrick M, Kennedy SM, Chan-Yeung M. Western red cedar dust exposure and lung function: a dose–response relationship. Am J Respir Crit Care Med 1996; 154:968–973.
32. Baur X. Cotton fluffs as latex allergen carriers in a glove factory. J Allergy Clin Immunol 2003; 111(1):177–179.
33. Hinze S, Bergmann KC, Løwenstein H, Nordskov Hansen G. Differente Schwellenwertkonzentrationen für Sensibilisierungen durch das Rinderhaarallergen Bos d 2 bei atopischen und nicht-atopischen Landwirten. Pneumologie 1996; 50:177–181.
34. Liebers V, Hoernstein M, Baur X. Humoral immune response to the insect allergen Chi t I in aquarists and fish-food factory workers. Allergy 1993; 48:236–239.
35. Venables KM. Low molecular weight chemical hypersensitivity and direct toxicity: the acid anhydrides. Br J Ind Med 1989; 46:222–232.

36. Liss GM, Bernstein D, Genesove L, Roos JO, Lim J. Assessment of risk factors for IgE-mediated sensitisation to tetrachlorophthalic anhydride. J Allergy Clin Immunol 1993; 92:237–247.

37. Boxer MB, Grammer LC, Harris KE, Roach DE, Patterson R. Six-year clinical and immunologic follow-up of workers exposed to trimellitic anhydride. J Allergy Clin Immunol 1987; 80:147–152.

38. Barker RD, van Tongeren MJA, Harris JM, Gardiner K, Venables KM, Newman Taylor AJ. Risk factors for sensitisation and respiratory symptoms among workers exposed to acid anhydrides: a cohort study. Occup Environ Med 1998; 55:684–691.

39. Baur X, Marek W, Ammon J, Czuppon AB. Respiratory and other hazards of isocyanates. Int Arch Occup Environ Health 1994; 66:141–152.

40. Burge PS, Edge G, Hawkins R, White V, Taylor AJ. Occupational asthma in a factory making flux-cored solder containing colophony. Thorax 1981; 36:828–834.

41. Calverley AE, Rees D, Dowdeswell RJ, Linnett PJ, Kielkowski D. Platinum salt sensitivity in refinery workers: incidence and effects of smoking and exposure. Occup Environ Med 1995; 52:661–666.

42. Baur X, Chen Z, Liebers V. Exposure–response relationships of occupational inhalative allergens. Clin Exp Allergy 1998; 28:537–544.

43. Heederik D, Houba R. An exploratory quantitative risk assessment for high molecular weight sensitizers: wheat flour. Ann Occup Hyg 2001; 435(3):175–185.

44. Cox DR. Regression models and life-tables (with Discussion). J R Stat Soc B 1972; 34:187–220.

45. De Zotti R, Bovenzi M. Prospective study of work-related respiratory disease in trainee bakers. Occup Environ Med 2000; 57:58–61.

46. American Conference of Governmental Industrial Hygienists, ed. TLVs® and BEIs®. Cincinnati: ACGIH®, 2005.

47. Baur X, Degens P, Sander I. Baker's asthma: still among the most frequent occupational respiratory disorders. J Allergy Clin Immunol 1998; 102:984–997.

48. Juniper CP, How MJ, Goodwin BFJ, Kinshott AK. Bacillus subtilis enzymes: a 7-year clinical epidemiological immunological study of an industrial allergen. J Soc Occup Med 1977; 27:3–12.

49. Schweigert MK, MacKenzie DP, Sarlo K. Occupational asthma and allergy associated with the use of enzymes in the detergent industry: a review of the epidemiology, toxicology and methods of prevention. Clin Exp Allergy 2000; 30:1511–1518.

50. Sarlo K, Kirchner DB. Occupational asthma and allergy in the detergent industry: new developments. Curr Opin Allergy Clin Immunol 2002; 2(2):97–101.

51. Vedal S, Chan-Yeung M, Enarson D, et al. Symptoms and pulmonary function in western red cedar workers related to duration of employment and dust exposure. Arch Environ Health 1986; 41:179–183.

52. Posch A, Chen Z, Wheeler, Dunn MJ, Raulf-Heimsoth M, Baur X. Characterization and identification of latex allergens by two-dimensional electrophoresis and protein microsequencing. J Allergy Clin Immunol 1997; 99:385–395.

53. Tarlo S, Sussman GL, Holness DL. Latex sensitivity in dental students and staff: a cross-sectional study. J Allergy Clin Immunol 1997; 99:396–401.

54. Heese A, Peters KP, Koch HU, Hornstein OP. Allergien gegen Latexhandschuhe. Allergologie 1995; 18(9):358–365.

55. Levy DA, Charpin D, Pecquet C, Leynadier F, Vervloet D. Allergy to latex. Allergy 1992; 47:579–587.

56. Chen Z, Cremer R, Baur X. Latex allergy correlates with operation. Allergy 1997; 52:873.

57. Niggemann B, Buck D, Michael T, Wahn U. Latex provocation tests in patients with spina bifida: Who is at risk of becoming symptomatic? J Allergy Clin Immunol 1998; 102:662–670.

58. Yassin MS, Sanyurah S, Lierl MB, et al. Evaluation of latex allergy in patients with meningomyelocele. Ann Allergy 1992; 69:207–211.

59. Baur X. Measurement of airborne latex allergens. Methods 2002; 27:59–62.
60. Baur X, Chen Z, Allmers H. Can a threshold limit value for natural rubber latex airborne allergens be defined? J Allergy Clin Immunol 1988; 101:24–27.
61. Allmers H, Brehler R, Chen Z, Raulf-Heimsoth M, Fels H, Baur X. Reduction of latex aeroallergens and latex-specific IgE antibodies in sensitised workers after removal of powdered natural rubber latex gloves in a hospital. J Allergy Clin Immunol 1998; 102:841–846.
62. Tarlo SM, Easty A, Eubanks K, et al. Outcomes of a natural rubber latex control program in an Ontario teaching hospital. J Allergy Clin Immunol 2001; 108:628–633.
63. Terho EO, Husman K, Vohlonen I, Rautalahti M, Tukiainen H. Allergy to storage mites or cow dander as a cause of rhinitis among Finnish dairy farmers. Allergy 1985; 40(1):23–26.
64. Terho EO, Vohlonen I, Husman K, Rautalahti M, Tukiainen H, Viander M. Sensitization to storage mites and other work-related and common allergens among Finnish dairy farmers. Eur J Respir Dis Suppl 1987; 152:165–174.
65. Virtanen T, Vilhunen P, Husman K, Mantyjarvi R. Sensitization of dairy farmers to bovine antigens and effects of exposure on specific IgG and IgE titers. Int Arch Allergy Appl Immunol 1988; 87(2):171–177.
66. Rautiainen M, Virtanen T, Ruoppi P, Nuutinen J, Mantyjarvi R. Humoral responses to bovine dust in dairy farmers with allergic rhinitis. Acta Otolaryngol Suppl 1997; 529:169–172.
67. Bush RK, Wood RA, Peyton AE. Laboratory animal allergy. J Allergy Clin Immunol 1998; 102:99–112.
68. Schumacher MJ, Tait BD, Holmes MC. Allergy to murine antigens in a biological research institute. J Allergy Clin Immunol 1981; 68:310–318.
69. Nieuwenhuijsen MJ, Putcha V, Gordon S. Exposure response relationships in laboratory animal workers. GSF—National Research Center for Environment and Health, ISEE 2001. Thirteenth Conference of the International Society for Environmental Epidemiology. Garmisch-Partenkirchen: Neuherberg, 2001:A18.
70. Nieuwenhuijsen MJ, Putcha V, Gordon S, et al. Exposure–response relations among laboratory animal workers exposed to rats. Occup Environ Med 2003; 60:104–108.
71. Hollander A, Heederik D, Doekes G. Respiratory allergy to rats: exposure–response relationships in laboratory animal workers. Am J Respir Crit Care Med 1997; 155: 562–567.
72. Heederik D, Venables KM, Malmberg P, et al. Exposure–response relationships for work-related sensitization in workers exposed to rat urinary allergens: results from a pooled study. J Allergy Clin Immunol 1999; 103:678–684.
73. Thulin H, Björkdahl M, Karlsson AS, Renström A. Reduction of exposure to laboratory animal allergens in a research laboratory. Ann Occup Hyg 2002; 46(1):66–68.
74. Codina R, Ardusso L, Lockey F, Crisci C, Bertoya N. Sensitization to soybean hull allergens in subjects exposed to different levels of soybean dust inhalation in Argentina. J Allergy Clin Immunol 2000; 105:570–576.
75. Baur X, Aschauer H, Mazur G, Dewair M, Prelicz H, Steigemann W. Structure, antigenic determinants of some clinically important insect allergens: chironomid hemoglobins. Science 1986; 233:351–353.
76. Baur X, Liebers V. Insect hemoglobins (*Chi t* I) of the Diptera family Chironomidae are relevant environmental, occupational, and hobby-related allergens. Int Arch Occup Environ Health 1992; 64:185–188.
77. Bernstein DI, Roach DE, McGrath KG, Larsen RS, Zeiss CR, Patterson R. The relationship of airborne trimellitic anhydride concentrations to trimellitic anhydride-induced symptoms and immune responses. J Allergy Clin Immunol 1983; 72:709–713.
78. Petsonk EL, Wang ML, Lewis DM, Siegel PD, Husberg BJ. Asthma-like symptoms in wood product plant workers exposed to methylene diphenyl diisocyanate. Chest 2000; 118:1183–1193.

79. Latza, U, Baur X, Malo J-L. Isocyanate-induced health effects. In: Bakke JV, Norén JO, Thorud S, Aasen TB, eds. International Consensus Report on Isocyanates—Risk Assessment and Management, Appendices 10.2.1. Gjovik: Norwegian Labour Inspection Authority, 2002:37–51 (http://www.arbeidstilsynet.no/publikasjoner/rapporter/rapportleng.html).

80. Cartier A, Grammer L, Malo LJ, et al. Specific serum antibodies against isocyanates: association with occupational asthma. J Allergy Clin Immunol 1989; 84:507–514.

81. Grammer LC, Eggum P, Silverstein M, Shaughnessy MA, Liotta JL, Patterson R. Prospective immunologic and clinical study of a population exposed to hexamethylene diisocyanate. J Allergy Clin Immunol 1988; 82:627–633.

82. Karol MH. Concentration-dependent immunologic response to toluene diisocyanate (TDI) following inhalation exposure. Toxicol Appl Pharmacol 1983; 68:229–241.

83. Keskinen H, Tupasela O, Tikkainen U, Nordman H. Experiences of specific IgE in asthma due to diisocyanates. Clin Allergy 1988; 18:597–604.

84. Zammit-Tabona M, Sherkin M, Kijek K, Chan H, Chan-Yeung M. Asthma caused by diphenylmethane diisocyanate in foundry workers. Clinical, bronchial provocation and immunologic studies. Am Rev Respir Dis 1983; 128:226–230.

85. Peters JM. Cumulative pulmonary effects in workers exposed to tolyene (sic) diisocyanate. Proc R Soc Med 1970; 63:372–375.

86. Wegman DH, Peters JM, Pagnotto L, Fine LJ. Chronic pulmonary function loss from exposure to toluene diisocyanate. Br J Ind Med 1977; 34(3):196–200.

87. Diem JE, Jones RN, Hendrick DJ, et al. Five-year longitudinal study of workers employed in a new toluene diisocyanate manufacturing plant. Am Rev Respir Dis 1982; 126:420–428.

88. Omae K, Higashi T, Nakadate T, Tsugane S, Nakaza M, Sakurai H. Four-year follow-up of effects of toluene diisocyanate exposure on the respiratory system in polyurethane foam manufacturing workers. II: Four-year changes in the effects on the respiratory system. Int Arch Occup Environ Health 1992; 63:565–569.

89. Baur X. Occupational asthma due to isocyanates. Lung 1996; 174:23–30.

90. Bernstein DI, Korbee L, Stauder T, et al. The low prevalence of occupational asthma and antibody-dependent sensitisation to diphenylmethane diisocyanate in a plant engineered for minimal exposure to diisocyanates. J Allergy Clin Immunol 1993; 92:387–396.

91. Bolm-Audorff U, Bienfait HG, Burkhard J, et al. Prevalence of respiratory allergy in a platinum refinery. Int Arch Occup Environ Health 1992; 64:257–260.

92. Merget R, Schulze-Werninghaus G. Untersuchungen über allergische Reaktionen bei Exposition gegen Platinverbindungen. In: GSF: Forschungsverbund Edelmetallemissionen, Abschlussbericht, München, 1997.

12

Quantification of Bio-Active Protein Aerosols

Mark C. Swanson
Mayo Foundation, Rochester, Minnesota, U.S.A.

Dick Heederik
Division of Environmental and Occupational Health, Institute for Risk Assessment Sciences, University of Utrecht, Utrecht, The Netherlands

INTRODUCTION

Within the last 10 years a comprehensive understanding evolved regarding the nature and importance of bio-aerosol exposures and their relationship to allergic lung disease. A major factor contributing to the dearth of this knowledge prior to this time was the inability to characterize the toxic and immunologic potency of these aerosols. Progress and advancement in particle collection methods and immunochemistry have allowed characterization of complex mixtures of pathogenic and proteinaceous material. Although light microscopy facilitated morphologic identification of particulates (molds, pollen, fungi) and yielded some semi-quantitative data, there was a void in our understanding of aerosol potency and intensity until immunochemical methods were developed and applied in aero-biological studies. These studies included particle sizing, and distribution and quantification of the concentration of asthmagenic bio-aerosols. It became evident that even bio-aerosols comprising relatively large identifiable particulates (greater than 10 μm; pollens, mold, and fungi) contained smaller particle fractions which also conferred even more antigenic activity to the respiratory mucosa. These early studies elucidated the importance of immunochemical measurement of natural and man-made bio-aerosols. The general principles of industrial and environmental hygiene also apply in all respects to allergens, just as they do to any airborne toxic agents. Differences in application of these general principles to occupational asthma (OA) arise from the requirement for specialized sampling and assay techniques and from the fact that often not all workers are affected by the illness. Workers who develop lung hypersensitivity to airborne antigens develop symptoms and other signs often after exposure to very low concentrations of the agent that have no or little effect on other workers. Identification of offending agents and clinical evaluation of patients are considered in Chapters 7 and 16–24. This chapter summarizes the methods of air sampling and quantitative immunoassay, the principles for devising means of reducing the concentration of allergens in the air, and the procedures for follow-up monitoring to assure that measures undertaken to control exposure continue to be effective.

EXPOSURE ASSESSMENT IN THE EVALUATION OF OA

Identification of an occupation as being the source of OA has historically started with workers' or physicians' suspicions that asthma symptoms are temporally related to an occupational exposure of an aerosolized material that is a known or possible allergen. This suspicion is usually followed up by a survey of the workers. Instruments used typically include symptom diaries, spirometry, serial peak flow measurements, and skin or serological tests for IgE antibodies to the allergen. For investigation of individual cases, inhalation challenge tests are often applied to confirm that the suspected allergenic material which evoked IgE antibody actually can cause an asthmatic response (1,2). A necessary additional link in the chain of evidence that a suspected allergen is the cause of occupational asthma is measurement of the allergen in the air at the worksite. This is useful when the allergen is not known, the environment of interest has not been evaluated earlier, and control measures have to be considered. Knowledge of the concentration encountered at work also allows correlation of the exposure at work with an inhalation challenge test in the laboratory.

PURPOSE OF AIR SAMPLING

Source and Dispersion of Allergen in the Worksite

Planning a specific sampling protocol depends on the objectives of the investigation and management of the problem. In the initial phase of investigation of a plant or process suspected of being the source of occupational asthma, it is useful to confirm that the putative allergen does actually become airborne and to determine its approximate concentration at various locations within the work environment. Often the manufacturing equipment, operation, or activity responsible for aerosolizauon of the allergen is self-evident. There are other circumstances in which a closer evaluation of the situation through personal work-shift or task sampling will localize the time and place of the exposure and permit design of more precise and cost-effective control measures.

Dispersion of Allergen to Surrounding Areas in the Community

Cases of asthma from castor bean allergy have occurred in residents living downwind from castor bean processing plants in Ohio, South Africa, France, and Brazil (3–5). These observations suggest that allergen can escape the confines of the plant and affect nearby residents. More serious epidemics of asthma occurred during the 1980s in Barcelona, Spain (6,7). On epidemic days, as many as 100 patients sought treatment for acute, severe asthma at hospitals in Barcelona. Several patients died. Epidemiological investigation identified a point source of the epidemic in the harbor on days when soybeans were being unloaded at a soybean processing plant and weather conditions favored a slow drift of dust from the harbor over the populous part of the city. The affected patients had IgE antibody to soybean dust. On the epidemic days, high concentrations of soybean sterols and low molecular mass glycopeptide allergens from soybean hulls were found in the air over the city (8,9). After equipment was installed to control dust emission, the epidemics ceased and allergen was present in the air in only low concentrations. This aeroallergen was also found in significant concentrations around the port of New Orleans (10). Outdoor industrial dispersion of yeast (11) and snow crab (12) aerosols have also been documented. Individuals who live near grain elevators or cotton mills have developed asthma suspected of being due to allergy to these dusts, but this situation has not yet been fully investigated.

Risk Assessment

The primary purpose of measurement of occupational allergens is to evaluate the presence of specific hazards and estimate risk in the working environment. A distinction is made between the concentration that sensitizes initially and the concentration that provokes symptoms in workers already sensitized. The issues associated with risk assessment are discussed elsewhere.

Evaluation of Exposure Control

After changes to reduce the exposure have been made, a schedule of periodic air sampling is desirable to assure that the changes have been successful in achieving the goals. When the control strategy depends upon scheduled housekeeping, cleaning, or equipment maintenance, periodic monitoring is necessary to assure that the program is functioning. This has proven very useful in Barcelona where soybean handling and dust containment is critical (13).

PROTOCOLS FOR MONITORING OCCUPATIONAL EXPOSURE

Measurement Scheme

A schedule of air sampling at the place of maximum concentration should be established to assure that the control measures are effective when they are installed and continue to be effective during production or regular operation. This is particularly important when control depends upon proper housekeeping and equipment maintenance. The optimum sampling procedure will vary with the particular circumstances. It may include area or personal sampling and may be periodic or continuous. The concentration of any biological agent can be measured in the air, provided a reliable reference standard of the agent and specific antisera are available.

Methods

The principles for measuring bioaerosols are the same as those for measuring any chemical substance. Only the method of the assay differs. If it is desired to quantify the amount of viable microorganisms in the air, either culture techniques or counting particles deposited on a microscope slide using morphological criteria for identification are preferred. These techniques not only are very sensitive because a few colony forming units per cubic meter can easily be detected, but also allow taxonomic classification (14). Limitations are that the measured concentration depends heavily on aspects of the measurement process such as sampling time, sampling medium, incubation time, temperature, etc. Results therefore always require detailed documentation of the methods applied and circumstances during sampling. Airborne or settled dust components of microbial agents (i.e., gram-negative bacteria, gram-positive bacteria, and fungi) can be assayed for endotoxin using a Limulus amebolysates technique (15), $\beta(1\rightarrow3)$ glucans, peptidoglycans, muramic acid either by using immunoassays or sensitive chemical methods such as liquid and/or gas chromatography mass spectrometry. The following section will describe methods for quantifying non-viable proteins derived from microorganisms, plant material, or animals (16–19).

Air Sampling Volume and Sampling Time

Depending on the concentration of an airborne allergen, the volume of air that will allow sufficient allergen to be collected for accurate analysis may vary from 0.5 to 1000 m^3. If flow rates are fixed, the run times are varied to accommodate the required collection volume. Sampling time depends on the purpose of the exposure assessment strategy. Longer sampling periods have the disadvantage of lessened ability to correlate temporal changes in concentration with specific activities that generate exposure but the precision of the assessment is higher. On the other hand, personal samplers are often used in epidemiological studies and are usually applied for a period that is considered representative for an eight-hour workshift. The exposure data obtained allow estimation of long term average exposures that can be correlated to health endpoints.

Area Sampling

Properly located area samplers operated at flow rates of 1 to 3 L/sec provide samples large enough to quantify low concentrations of allergens believed to be clinically significant in relatively short collection periods (1–2 hours). Area sampling is a suitable way to provide information about the general presence or absence of exposure and to confirm the identity of the agent. In addition, area sampling allows comparison of different parts of the plant and changes in concentration over time in the same location. Being relatively simple and unobtrusive, it is suitable for long-term monitoring of the success of control measures. Area sampling can also yield relatively high amounts of well-defined dust samples, which are often necessary in the early stages of assay development. Automated samplers have been designed with programmable filter-changing devices to simplify collection of sequential samples and minimize human error.

Particle Sizing

The behavior of aerosols inhaled into the lung depends upon their aerodynamic properties, which in turn depend upon their size, density, and shape (20). Deposition of particles along the airways is not only determined by these aerodynamic properties, but is also influenced by the rate of airflow and patterns of respiration. For example, during nasal breathing, particles of 20 μm aerodynamic diameter and larger (such as pollen grains) are virtually all removed on the turbinates. About half the particles of size 5 μm and smaller pass through the nose into the thoracic airways. Particles with aerodynamic diameter less than 10 μm are considered "respirable." Aerodynamic diameter, or "mean mass aerodynamic diameter," is calculated from the particles' terminal settling velocity by comparison with spheres of unit density and is a function of the shape, size, and density of the aerosol particles. Aerosols generated by nebulizers for therapy and aerosols used experimentally to study deposition and clearance are more or less unit density spheres, but occupational dusts often have complex fibrous shapes and may form irregular, noncompact aggregates. Thus, their behavior is not determined solely by their size or density. Particles can deposit in the airways in four ways: sedimentation, inertial impaction, interception, and diffusion. Sedimentation by gravity depends upon the density and diameter of the particles, and for particles that are more or less spherical, sedimentation is the chief means of deposition in large airways. Inertial impaction occurs when the direction of the airstream is changed by curving or branching. The particles tend to follow the original path of the airstream and deposit on the epithelium through inertia. In the airways, inertial impaction is the chief means of deposition in the nose and is important in the central airways where flow rates are high. Interception is an important mechanism of deposition of fibrous particles and other particles of irregular shape. Long fibers less than 3 µm in diameter and as long as 200 µm tend to stay oriented longitudinally in the air-stream and can penetrate deeply into the lung. Alveolar deposition of asbestos fibers is an example. Diffusion, the chief way gases react with the airways, is responsible for deposition of submicrometer-sized particles. Most particles of this size are expelled in the expired air, however. Thus, it is often of interest to determine the particle size and aerodynamic behavior of allergenic aerosols. Anderson cascade impaction heads for high-volume samplers are available for this purpose (Fig. 1). Figure 2 illustrates the morphology of particles separated by this device after several hours of operation in a rat animal care room. Note especially the filaments, presumably rat hairs that have penetrated to the final stage with spherical particles smaller than the diameter of the fiber. The amount of allergen or medication carried in a droplet of 5 µm is 1000-fold more than that in a droplet 10 times smaller, 0.5 µm so it is more valuable to know the total amount of allergen in various aerodynamic sizes than the number of particles.

An important property of particulate matter is the aerodynamic diameter. The aerodynamic diameter determines how far a particle penetrates into the respiratory

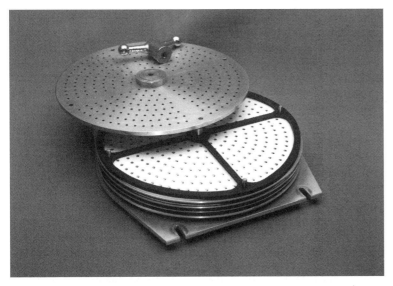

Figure 1 Model GMW 65000 Andersen cascade impaction particle sizing head for collection of particles in defined size ranges (Andersen Samplers, Atlanta, Georgia, U.S.A.).

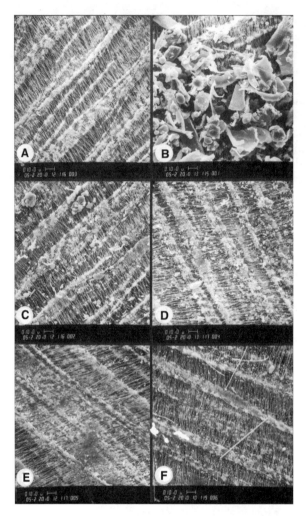

Figure 2 Scanning electron photomicrographs ($\times 500$) of PTFE media supporting sized particles from different mean mass aerodynamic diameter size ranges. (**A**) not exposed; (**B**) $> 9.4\,\mu m$; (**C**) $9.4\text{--}4.5\,\mu m$; (**D**) $4.5\text{--}2.7\,\mu m$; (**E**) $2.7\text{--}1.6\,\mu m$; (**F**) $< 1.6\,\mu m$. Note the fibers (probably hair) collected along with particles $< 1.6\,\mu m$. These fibers have oriented themselves in such a way as to attain a mean mass aerodynamic diameter similar to small particles. *Abbreviation*: PTFE, polytetrafluoroethylene.

system and where it will get deposited. Particles can be distinguished by the region which they are likely to reach in the respiratory system. These regions are defined as respirable dust, thoracic dust, and inhalable dust. The inhalable particle fraction is the fraction that enters the nose and the mouth, and has a 50% outpoint diameter of 100 μm. Different samplers have been developed that measure this fraction, in Europe the IOM-(U.K.), the PAS6-(The Netherlands), and GSP-(Germany) sampler are widely used and have been validated in wind tunnel experiments (21). Inhalable dust sampling is less common in the United States, but samplers such as the button sample are available. These samplers can be used to measure inhalable dust at flow rates between 2 and 3.5 L/min. This fraction is often measured in the workplace, but rarely in the general environment (22). The thoracic fraction is the fraction that enters the thorax, and has a 50% cut point diameter of 10 μm; it is therefore often referred to as PM10 and is often measured in the general environment, but rarely in the workplace. The respirable fraction is the fraction that enters the lungs (the alveolar region). This fraction has a 50% cut point diameter of 4 μm, and can be measured with special cyclones. Traditionally this fraction has been measured in mines where a risk of developing pneumoconiosis existed. PM2.5, particles with a 50% cut off diameter of 2.5 μm, is the fraction that penetrates deep into the alveolar region. Other, more expensive sampler configurations exist, such as the eight stage Andersen cascade impactor that separates particulate matter by mean mass aerodynamic diameter. These samplers can be used to estimate the particle size distribution. Their detection limit is higher because the dust is distributed over different stages. For studies on rhinitis and asthma, measurement of the personal inhalable dust fraction is most appropriate.

Personal Sampling

Equipment that samples the air in the personal breathing zone (1–5 Lpm) is useful for defining the particular tasks in the job that are associated with heavy, and therefore hazardous, exposure. Particle sizing may be accomplished with Sierra Marple® 298 personal cascade impactors. Recently, a nasal sampler has been developed and used for measurement of allergens in the respired air-stream (23). This miniature slit sampler captures particulates by impaction on a tape inside the sampler and is promoted as an alternative to conventional active air sampling that makes use of sampling heads and filtering techniques. New, more convenient silicon nasal filters have been developed and have been utilized for measurement of several domestic allergens and rat and latex allergen particulates in the work environment (23–26). After collection, allergen-containing particles were identified and counted with immuno-staining techniques, in addition to conventional extraction and immuno-chemical analysis of the allergen content. Sampling times are usually short, ranging between 10 and 60 minutes, and the collection is driven by the subject's inhalation pattern. Although collection of particles below 5 μm seems not very efficient (24), the correlation between results obtained by the nasal sampler and conventional samplers is relatively high ($r^2 = 0.8$, Pearson) (25,26). Accurate comparisons cannot always be made because the sampled volume is not known for the nasal sampler and thus units in which the exposure is expressed differ (allergen/nostril for the nasal sampler versus allergen concentration/m^3 for a conventional dust sampler). Comparisons have focused on correlations between measurement techniques while systematic differences that are present seem to be ignored (25,26). Issues that require further evaluation are the effect of mouth breathing on the sampling efficiency, and sampling efficiency in relation to particle size. The detection limit for allergen assessment in combination with nasal sampling is lower when immunostaining techniques are being used (27,28). It may be as low as a few particulates or in the low picogram range. A major application of the nasal sampler is in places where conventional sampling equipment cannot be used, is inconvenient to use, or where measurement of tasks and activities of short duration is required. Renström et al. (25) used the nasal sampler very elegantly to evaluate the protective effect of face masks in laboratory animal facilities. Such sampling also allows evaluation of the success of changes in manufacturing equipment, ventilation, air filtration, and job performance at particular sites or tasks. Either area sampling or personal sampling allows estimation of time-weighted average of exposure. It is not yet established, however, whether brief, heavy exposures are more likely to cause disease than prolonged, light exposures, so it is not clear whether time-weighted averages carry the same biological significance for allergen exposures as they do for toxin exposure.

Filter Medium and Sample Preparation

Proper filter medium is essential for success. The filter should offer low resistance to the air being sampled, yet have efficient capture and retention of respirable particles. It should not denature the protein, it should not adsorb the allergen, but permit high yields of recovery, and it should allow extraction of the allergen in small volumes (1 mL or less) so that concentration of the extract is not needed. Concentration adds to the cost of the assay and may cause loss of allergen through denaturation or adsorption. Polytetrafluoroethylene (PTFE, or Teflon^{TM}) has proven to be a very satisfactory filter medium. However, as with all collection media, validation studies are needed for their use in different environments. During the process of development and validation of an assay for a new allergen, it is desirable to determine the stability of the allergen on the filter and the efficiency of the extraction procedure. Although rigorous determinations have been done for only a few allergens, it appears that exposed dry filters can be stored for several months at $-20°C$ without significant loss of allergen. Exceptions seem to be some enzymes, for which the reactivity rapidly decreases over a period of weeks after sampling and dry storage at $-20°C$. After extraction, many allergens are unstable in aqueous solutions, partly because of inherent instability, and partly because of enzymatic activity of proteases in the solution. Lyophilization is an appropriate means of stabilizing some extracts, but some allergens are denatured by freeze drying. It is most practical to preserve the reference standard and filter extracts in a 50% glycerinated buffer at $-20°C$.

IMMUNOASSAYS

Two-Site Assays

For most applications, two-site assays or sandwich assays are the simplest to perform and the most sensitive (Fig. 3). They have the additional advantage over inhibition assays of being accurate over a broad range of protein concentrations. Thus, it is usually not necessary to perform a preliminary assay to determine the appropriate sample dilution. The assay is performed in microtiter wells that have been designed to adsorb proteins efficiently, and are supplied by a range of commercial firms (i.e., Immulon II or IV$^®$ microtiters, DYNEX Technologies Inc., Chantilly, Virginia, U.S.A.). The serum or ascites fluid containing the polyclonal or monoclonal capture antibody is diluted in 20 to 200 mM carbonate buffer at pH 9.2, and 100 µL added to wells of the microtiter plate, which is then incubated at room temperature in a humid chamber and the wells washed. The appropriate antibody dilution must be determined for each new assay system to provide conditions of antibody excess. The albumin and other nonspecific proteins in the serum or ascites fluid usually suffice to block all remaining protein-binding sites on the plate. This needs to be confirmed experimentally for each system. The next step adds an aliquot of the air sample extract, an internal standard, and dilutions of the reference standard antigen preparation to respective wells. After a second incubation and washing, the detection antibody is added. This antibody can be tagged with radiolabel, fluorophore, or chromophore for detection. After the third incubation, the wells are washed and

2-Site Radioimmunoassay

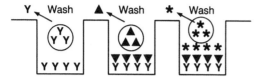

Y Antibodies (antigen specific)

▲ Antigens (allergens)

✱ Radioisotopic tracers
      (labeled purified antibodies)

Figure 3 Two-site RIA for airborne allergens. (*Left*) A capture antibody (monoclonal if available, or polyclonal animal or human IgG antibody) to the allergen is absorbed nonspecifically to plastic micro-liter plates. (*Center*) Either known amounts of the allergen standard or the unknown sample is added. Allergen binds to the antibody. (*Right*) A radio-iodinated antibody (either a monoclonal antibody to a second epitope on the allergen molecule or affinity-purified polyclonal IgG) is added and binds to a second site on the allergen. *Abbreviations*: IgG, immunoglobulin; RIA, radio-immunoassay.

counted. In addition to two-site monoclonal assays and polyclonal assays using affinity-purified antibody, it is possible to use an animal polyclonal antiserum for capture and a human IgE antibody–containing serum for detection. The amount of IgE antibody bound to the plate in this sandwich assay is measured with labeled anti-IgE. The results are calculated using a log-logit–transformed least-squares regression equation. In graphic terms, the x-axis is designated $\log_{10}$ of the antigen concentration. The y-axis is designated $\log_{10}$ of the percent of the maximum of the total counts bound, where

$$y = \mathrm{Ln}\left(\frac{\text{binding}/\text{binding}_{\text{max}}}{1 - \text{binding}/\text{binding}_{\text{max}}}\right)$$

Concentrations of the unknown are then interpolated from the standard regression curve (29). Although the example cited involves radio-tagged reagents, the assays may be designed as fluorescent, chemoluminescent, or colorometric.

Inhibition Assays

Inhibition assays are used when only a single antibody is available. The first step is to prepare a solid-phase allergen. Although cyanogen-activated paper discs, microcrystalline cellulose, or Sepharose® can be used to prepare the solid phase, the Immulon® wells described above are more convenient, reproducible, and sensitive. The optimum adsorption conditions of protein concentration and buffer strength and pH must be determined for each new allergen system. After the allergen has been adsorbed, the remaining protein-binding sites on the well surface are blocked with an inert protein such as human albumin. Then the concentration of antiserum needed for maximum antibody-binding should be determined for each serum pool. It is important that the amount of allergen adsorbed on the plate is adequate and oriented properly so that sufficient antibody is bound to give a strong signal. A reference curve of inhibition by serial dilutions of the reference allergen standard is constructed, and the results of individual samples are calculated along with an internal standard. After the details of the assay conditions have been established, fresh antigen-coated plates should be prepared for each batch of assays. Fifty microliters of the air sample extract (an internal standard or dilutions of the reference allergen extract are used to construct the standard curve) and 50 μL of antiserum are added to duplicate wells. After overnight incubation in a humid chamber at room temperature, the wells are washed and the detection reagent is added. For IgG antibody, this reagent can be a monoclonal antibody to the gamma chain or staphylococcus protein A; for IgE it is an affinity-purified rabbit antibody to the Fc$_\epsilon$ chain. After the final incubation and washing, the wells are counted. If the allergen concentration falls outside the range of the inhibition assay, it should be repeated with appropriate dilutions of the sample. The results are calculated using a log-linear transformation where the x-axis is designated log of the antigen concentration and the y-axis percent inhibition. Percent inhibition is defined as counts bound when the antigen standard or unknown is mixed with the antibody pool subtracted from counts bound by the antibody pool alone, divided by the counts bound by the antibody pool, all multiplied by 100.

Amplification Procedures

The sensitivity of an immunoassay can be increased several fold by amplifying the detection step with a biotin–avidin reaction. The detection antibody is biotinylated instead of being iodinated, and the final detection reagent is radio-iodinated or enzyme-conjugated streptavidin. This amplification of sensitivity may be useful for personal sampling studies in which only small air volumes can be collected.

Allergen Reference Standards

A desirable goal for expressing allergen concentrations would be a purified protein standard for each allergen in question and monoclonal antibodies to the allergen. Unfortunately, this goal is at present unrealistic, so it is necessary to settle for less rigorous reference preparations. Choice of a working standard depends upon the circumstances. If the allergen is a single protein such as papain, the standard may be a purified protein and the results can be expressed in mass units. More often the exposure involves complex dusts such as humidifier sludge, grain dust, or rat urine, which are mixtures of many allergenic molecules from several different microbial, plant, or animal sources. In such cases it is necessary to prepare a reference extract of the crude material that is used or generated as a result of the occupation and is likely to be the source of the allergen exposure (30–33). It is also useful to confirm that this material is a good source of the relevant allergens by immunoblotting because many sources contain a complex mixture of proteins. Results of the assay can be expressed in terms of the protein content of this extract or in terms of some arbitrary unit assigned to the reference preparation.

Antibody Source

Several kinds of antibodies are suitable for immunoassays. When they are available, two monoclonal antibodies directed to different epitopes on an allergenic molecule are useful. One antibody serves as a capture antibody; the other, after signal tagging (radio-, fluoro- or chromo-labeling), serves as detecting antibody. A high-titer polyclonal animal or human antiseram can also be adapted to a two-site assay, or can be used for inhibition assays. For the two-site assay, the whole serum can serve as the capture antibody, and the affinity-purified antibody from it serves as the detection antibody. In monoclonal systems, unfractionated mouse ascites fluid serves well for capture antibody, but the detection antibody should be purified by a protein A column. One advantage of the monoclonal system is that the antibody is available in unlimited amounts as long as the clone is maintained. An advantage of the animal or human IgG system over the human IgE system is that the serum can be diluted 100- or 1000-fold, so a reasonable-sized serum collection will suffice for many assays. The antibody, stored at −70°C, remains stable for many years. For some applications it is best to employ human IgE antibody. It may be the only antiserum available and provides assurance that the substance causing the disease is being measured when the identity of the allergenic molecules is uncertain or the dust contains a complex mixture of allergens. If a human IgE system is adopted for the study, it is desirable to obtain a large pool, at least 500 mL from each of 5 to 10 donors, to assure sufficient antibody to complete the entire project. A conceptual issue that has not been resolved is that monoclonal antibodies are directed to a single allergen or epitope determinant. Complex mixtures, i.e., extracts from plant material such as wheat and latex, contain a range of different allergens. When the ratio of the different allergen concentrations is not constant for different wheat species or latex samples, polyclonal antibodies may be preferable because they capture a whole range of different allergens to which workers are exposed. Validation studies must be performed that give insight into the variability of allergen content for one allergen relative to the others present in the extract (immunoblotting).

Quality Control

Although all the usual laboratory quality control procedures apply, some are particularly worth mentioning. The air samplers must be calibrated and the flow rate determined under the actual conditions of operation. Because calculation of the results is based on the volume of air drawn through the filter, it is also critical that the duration of the sampling period be accurately recorded. Precise records of extraction volumes as well as test volumes for air samples are required for proper dilution and aliquot factors to be used for final calculations of allergen units per cubic meter of air. Because degradation of the reagents can lead to serious error in results, appropriate controls must be used in every assay. For samples batched together in a single assay, an internal standard is included to demonstrate consistent assay performance with respect to previous assays. For samples taken over extended periods and groups of them assayed in several assays, control standards are needed for the assay performance and accuracy of the assay from time to time with respect to sample quantification.

Few studies are available that evaluate the comparability of immunoassays that have been used to measure aeroallergen concentrations (34–39). The most detailed comparison has been made as part of a collaborative European project (35,37). Methods to measure rat and mouse urinary aeroallergens of three institutes were compared by comparing parallel ambient air inhalable dust samples from animal facilities. Median rat allergen concentrations obtained with a competitive inhibition radio-immunoassay (RIA) method were a higher magnitude compared to the concentrations measured by enzyme immunoassay (EIA) methods. The difference between the two EIA methods was considerably smaller. Differences were even smaller for measured mouse allergen concentrations. Type of elution buffer and antibodies used were identified as the two major factors that caused the observed differences between sandwich assays. Variation in antibody specificity or in allergenic epitopes in the air samples, as well as standards used (purified allergens, crude extract) contribute to this quantitative divergence. Despite the systematic differences, correlation between allergen concentrations measured with different assays was high. So, these systematic differences are not necessarily problematic, as long as one knows which laboratory has done analyses, with which assay, and with which reference exposure data, comparisons have to be made. The comparisons become problematic when exposure standards are proposed without mentioning a measurement system with which to make valid comparisons. The optimal circumstances under which quantitative immunoassay of allergens is performed occur when the allergen has been identified, and when purified, allergen and monoclonal or polyclonal antibodies against the allergen are available. However, in the case of a simple sort of "hands on" hygiene survey, this is not necessary to reduce exposure and evaluate the effectiveness of the exposure reductions. Under conditions where larger populations are at risk, and exposure reduction will take more time, standardization of the allergen assay method could be considered.

New Measurement Technologies

Recently, assays have been developed for use in the field because all reagents are combined on carrier materials. An example is the one-step lateral flow immunoassays for the detection of house dust mite or other allergens such as mouse urinary allergens (Fig. 4). Allergenic material was sampled on filters by air flow or was wiped from surfaces, extracted in an appropriate buffer, and directly applied to the sample window

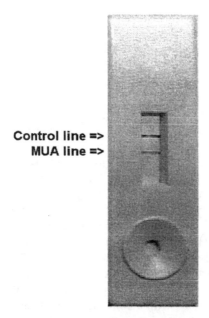

Control line =>
MUA line =>

Figure 4 One-step lateral flow immunoassay for the detection of MUA. Allergenic material was sampled on filters by air flow or wiped from surfaces, extracted in an appropriate buffer, and directly applied to the sample window of the device. Dependent on the allergen concentration results were visible in 10 to 30 minutes. *Abbreviation*: MUA, mouse urinary allergen.

of the device. Depending on the allergen concentration, results were visible in 10 to 30 minutes because gold or carbon particulates are being released. These approaches are useful for simple evaluation of the presence of allergen in product samples such as the presence of fungal α-amylase in bakery products. Although these assays might be used semi-quantitatively, they are best used for demonstration, teaching, and dissemination purposes. They should not be used for quantitative exposure assessment in combination with self-assessment of exposure by lay exposure assessors.

MEASUREMENTS TO CONTROL EXPOSURE TO OCCUPATIONAL ALLERGENS

The aim of controlling exposure is, of course, to reduce the concentration of the allergen in the air below the level that causes disease. In principle, two levels of allergen need to be considered: the level that initiates the sensitization in the first place and the level that elicits reactions in already sensitized subjects. Unfortunately, reliable information about either of these levels is still unavailable for most allergens, but it appears that in general, sensitizing levels are considerably higher and that occasional very high levels (for example, spills of toluene diisocyanate) are particularly likely to sensitize. After sensitization has occurred, much lower allergen levels can elicit reactions. For diisocyanates and similar chemicals, the eliciting level is of the order of 1 to 30 ng/m^3. From what we know about protein allergens, they appear to fall in this order of magnitude. Therefore, the goal of allergen abatement is to control both the occasional peak concentrations and the usual steady-state concentration. Preventing spills or other accidental reasons for occasional high concentrations is usually a matter of following proper operating procedures and proper maintenance of the manufacturing, cleaning, and air-handling equipment. The steady-state concentration of any indoor air pollutant is determined by ratio between the rate of production of the pollutant and the rate of its removal (40). The general mass balance equation describing the ratio is:

$$C_{ss}=PQ_vC_o+S(E_vQ_v+K+NE_dQ_d)^{-1}$$

Where C_{ss} represents steady-state concentration, the numerator represents the rate of generation of allergen, the denominator the rate of removal. PQ_vC_o is the outdoor source term; P is an empirically derived penetration factor which, for respirable-sized particles, can be assumed to be 1. Q_v equals ventilation rate; C_o is outdoor concentration. For most occupational allergens the outdoor source term is zero. S is indoor source substance generation rate. It has two components—de novo generation into the air and resuspension of settled allergen from dust. E_vQ_v is removal by ventilation. E_v is ventilation efficiency, calculated from the ratio of the concentration in the exhaust air to concentration in the occupied space divided by a mixing factor. In spaces where air is recirculated and mixing is good, E_v can reasonably be assumed to be one. Q_v is ventilation rate. K is natural decay rate (settling for particulates). NE_dQ_d is removal rate by air cleaning; N is cleaner removal efficiency. E_d is device ventilation efficiency analogous to E_v; Q_d is device flow rate. Reduction in steady-state concentrations can be achieved by three different strategies: prevent or reduce aerosolization at the source, increase ventilation and air filtration, and use personal respiratory protective equipment. Choice of one of these strategies or of a combination of them depends on the particular situation.

Prevent Aerosolization of the Allergen as the Source

From the above considerations, it is apparent that the most desirable means of controlling exposure is to eliminate the antigen at the source. Sometimes, it is possible to substitute a non-allergenic material, or it may be possible to substitute a less volatile chemical, for example, MDI for TDI in polyurethane processes. Sometimes the source of the allergen is some contaminating agent that can be removed. For example, an outbreak of hypersensitivity pneumonitis occurred among employees of nylon-manufacturing plants who worked in areas supplied by air from a chilled water cooling and humidification system. They and most of their fellow workers developed antibody to antigens extracted from the slime growing in the water reservoirs of this system. Inhalation challenge with these antigen preparations reproduced an acute episode of the disease (18,41). A number of engineering changes were made, including carefully controlled chlorination of the water. The slime was eradicated. Airborne concentrations of the slime antigens declined rather slowly because of considerable residual material in inaccessible ducts, but eventually the concentration inside the plant was reduced and the goal of keeping indoor concentrations lower than those outdoors was achieved. Parenthetically, these antigens that arise from a variety of organisms are ubiquitous, being detectable in low concentrations in outdoor air, stagnant water, and soil. After these changes were effected, no new cases of hypersensitivity pneumonitis developed, and newly hired workers did not develop antibody, although the original workers' antibody levels declined very slowly. From these observations, it is possible to estimate roughly the minimum allergen concentrations required to sensitize [100–1000 ng/m^3] and to elicit symptoms [1–10 ng/m^3]. Eradication of the source was possible in this and in similar cases because the antigen was not necessary to the purpose of the plant (42).

When the allergen is an integral part of the product, such as *Bacillus subtilis* enzyme in the detergent industry (43), eradication is not an option, and other means of reducing the amount of airborne allergen must be sought. In one instance, to reduce the concentration of the enzyme, the process used the enzyme encapsulated in granular form to reduce dust generation, and although it was not possible to eliminate the allergen from the air entirely, concentrations were reduced (44). However, measurable amounts remained in submicrometer-sized particles, and a few cases of occupational asthma occurred in employees who continued to work in a well-controlled environment. Newly hired workers may develop positive skin tests to the enzyme. This instance of occupational asthma illustrates the difficulty of recommending permissible exposure limits for allergens because of the wide variation, among individuals, of the concentration that elicits sensitization and provokes symptoms.

Sometimes the allergen is a component of the product. This is the case with natural rubber proteins associated with powdered latex examination gloves. Health care environments using powdered latex gloves will likely have measurable concentrations of natural rubber allergens in the air. The measured concentrations vary up to 1000-fold. This is a situation where the source can be eliminated, modified, or selected. The allergens are carried on cornstarch particles and become airborne during donning and removal of the gloves. Allergic sensitization to these rubber proteins has been recognized in significant numbers of health care workers who developed sinusitis and asthma. Concentrations in 10 medical center worksites where rubber gloves were frequently used ranged from 13 to 121 ng/m^3 and in areas where rubber gloves were seldom or never used ranged from 0.3 to 1.8 ng/m^3. Concentrations in operating suites ranged from 53 to 2080 ng/m^3. Personal breathing zone concentrations for health care workers in high rubber glove use areas ranged from 8 to 974 ng/m^3. Aeroallergen concentrations in nine dental offices, all using powdered gloves, ranged from 2 to 52 ng/m^3 (45). Particle sizing for natural rubber allergens demonstrated allergen distribution throughout all particle sizes, but predominantly in particles greater than 7 µm, mass median aerodynamic diameter. Although most of the allergen is carried on large particles, the amount of allergen that is carried on smaller particles is sufficient to provoke asthma and lower respiratory symptoms in sensitized individuals. The use of powder-free gloves is an obvious solution to eliminate airborne exposure. Measurement of allergen content in latex gloves and selecting low-allergen gloves for use is another option (46).

Improve Ventilation and Air Filtration

In some occupations, the source of allergen generation cannot be controlled. One example is laboratory animal handling, where the source is the animal itself—chiefly its urine (47,48). In this occupation, ventilation and filtration techniques are controls that are feasible. Measurements indicate that male mice, rats, and guinea pigs shed very large amounts of urinary allergens into the air, about 2, 20, and 200 ng/min/ animal, respectively. In a typical rat care room housing 250 to 300 rats with ventilation above the recommended ventilation rate of 15 changes of air per hour, the concentration of rat urinary protein allergen ranged around 200 ng/m^3. In a room with only 30 animals and relatively low concentrations of allergen, doubling the air-exchange ratio by recirculating air through a high-efficiency particulate arrestance or arrestor (HEPA) filter reduced the concentration in half. But in a similar room with 300 animals, the HEPA filter had a negligible effect because the total allergen production rate was very high, about 6 mg/min. To effectively reduce the steady-state allergen concentration in such a room required increasing the filtration with laminar flow, HEPA-filtered isolation cages (Fig. 5) to 172 changes of air per hour. This is about 100 times the air-exchange rate in most homes and offices. Particle sizing using the Andersen impaction head allowed assessment of the distribution

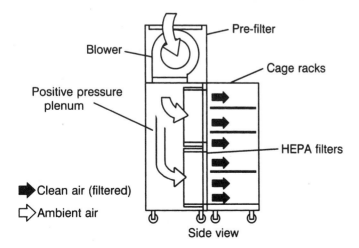

Figure 5 Schematic design of a laminar flow, HEPA-filtered small animal isolation racking system (Forma Scientific, Mallinckrodt, Marietta, Ohio, U.S.A.).

of allergens in particles of defined size ranges. Allergen was found in all particle size ranges (Fig. 2) (48). Sampling with a different device and assay yielded similar results (49).

Area air sampling is useful for confirmation and identification of possible air quality problems, but sometimes the data may mislead the investigator as to actual individual exposure during particular tasks. Even when an indoor environment can be defined and steady-state air concentrations measured, an individual's exposure within that work environment may vary considerably. Studies involving animal handlers, both laboratory technicians and animal care workers, have illustrated this point very well. Area samples were taken in animal housing rooms and personal samples were taken during full work shifts and during discrete tasks that were 15 minutes to $1\frac{1}{2}$ hours in duration. The personal samples included times in the animal rooms exclusively as well as times outside these confines. In general, time-weighted average exposures calculated from the area and full shift samples indicate similar values. However, discrete task samples frequently indicate much heavier exposures, up to an order of magnitude or more. When monitoring a worker performing a specific duty, important information is obtained regarding procedures, task related equipment, and actual task performance simply by the personal exposure an individual receives. From this information, recommendations about procedural changes and equipment modifications can be made objectively and with confidence. For example, this was the case when some workers emptied the bedding into open, unvented garbage cans and received substantial exposure, while others used HEPA-filtered waste disposal stations and their exposures were below limits of detection (Fig. 6).

When it appears that it will not be feasible to reduce airborne allergen by increasing ventilation or air filtration rates, workers can use individual protective equipment (50). Masks or laminar flow helmets have been reported to reduce allergic symptoms and anecdotally are useful in many situations (Fig. 7). Also, it is possible to provide work stations with airflow characteristics that minimize exposure during

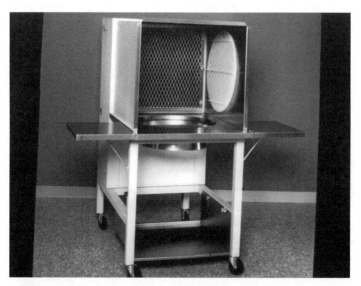

Figure 6 HEPA-filtered waste disposal station found effective at reducing animal allergen exposure of animal caretakers (Forma Scientific, Mallinckrodt, Marietta, Ohio, U.S.A.).

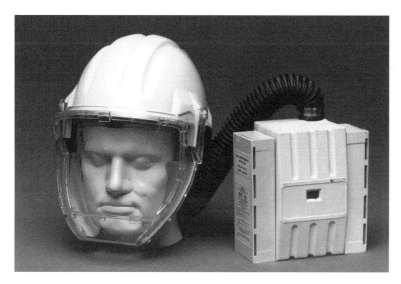

Figure 7 HEPA-filtered laminar flow helmet for protection against airborne particulates which include allergens (Racal Airstream, Frederick, Maryland, U.S.A.).

specific tasks. In theory, at least, full protective equipment with an outside air supply could be useful but does not seem a practical solution.

In summary, the principles of dealing with working environments where occupational respiratory disease occurs are no different when the disease is asthma than when the disease is pneumoconiosis or any other respiratory illness. Choice of abatement strategies depends upon the particular process, the physical structure of the equipment, and the rate of aerosolization of the allergen. When feasible, primary effort should be placed on preventing aerosolization. Increased ventilation and air filtration are feasible only when allergen production rate is low or localized to areas where exhaust fans can remove or capture the allergen before it reaches the workers' breathing zone. Masks or other personal respiratory protective equipment may be useful in circumstances of unavoidable exposure.

Illustrations of Application

We have mentioned several applications above, but two additional examples illustrate other points. Employee exposure to the enzyme papain in a meat-portioning facility caused allergic symptoms and asthma in some workers. In this case, a single, relatively pure and defined protein was the aeroallergen of interest. For this purpose, a commercially available rabbit antibody specific for papain proved useful. This polyclonal antibody was adsorbed to the surface of plastic microtiter wells and was used as a capture antibody. The specific antibodies were isolated by affinity column chromatography and radio-labeled for papain detection in a two-site sandwich assay. The approach yielded a specific, highly sensitive assay for papain capable of measuring picogram quantities of the enzyme. This allowed collection of personal air samples and effective measurement of papain exposure during discrete tasks. Although most personal exposures were in hundreds of nanograms per cubic meter, some ranged upward well into micrograms per cubic meter of air. Area air samples demonstrated low nanogram to microgram quantities of papain and on the whole indicated widespread distribution of the enzyme throughout the plant. Task sampling effectively identified personnel and certain tasks as the main sources of allergen dispersion. Interestingly, one of the most effective exposure control measures was frequent changing of work clothing (51).

Another example illustrates the problem more than the solution. Workers in plants where raw eggs are processed into liquid or powdered egg products may develop asthma from allergy to inhaled egg white protein (52,53). These plants process 1.5 million eggs a day. In a continuous operation the eggs are cracked, the shells blown away, and the whites separated from the yolk. Liquid whole egg or the separated egg white and yolk are pumped to refrigerated storage. Subsequently, the liquid is pumped through high-pressure spray nozzles into a drying oven. The dried product is picked up by a vacuum and transported to a cyclone separator, sifted, and packaged. Workers are exposed to aerosolized liquid egg products in the transfer and breaker rooms and to powdered egg yellow or white dust in the packaging room. Immunoassay of air samples in such a plant showed extraordinarily high levels of egg protein, hundreds of micrograms per cubic meter of air for ovalbumin, ovomucoid, and lysozyme (54). In this application, quantification of separate and specific egg white components is possible from a simple air sample. Worker's sera containing specific IgE are used in inhibition assays allowing quantification of many individual egg protein components making up a total airborne allergen load rarely ever seen. The concentrations of these egg proteins are so high that an air sample taken in a worker's bedroom demonstrated a level of 50 ng/m^3 of ovalbumin. This allergen was carried home on the worker's clothing. Concentrations of various allergens in other work environments are listed in Table 1. In egg-processing plants, appropriate means of reducing exposure have not yet been devised. The plants

Table 1 Maximum Concentrations of Aeroallergens in Various Locations[a]

Agent	Concentration (μg/m^3)	Location
Micropolyspora faeni	2700.000	Dairy bam during bedding chopping
Thermoactinomyces vulgaris	187.000	Dairy bam during bedding chopping
Aspergillus fumigatus	1.200	Quiet dairy bam in winter
Lolium perennae	0.085	Quiet dairy bam in winter
Lepidoglyphus destructor (storage mite)	12.000	Quiet dairy bam in winter
MUP	0.060	Animal quarters
Rattus norvegicus urinary protein	1.200	Animal quarters
Guinea pig urinary protein	17.000	Animal quarters
Bos domesticus epithelium	16.000	Quiet dairy bam in winter
Egg albumin	360.000	Egg-processing plant
Papain	5.000	Meat-processing plant
Esperase	0.180	Detergent-packing plant
Humidifier slime protein	15.000	Nylon-production plant
Natural rubber protein (latex)	1.000	Surgical suite
	10.000	Rubber glove manufacturing
Chionoecetes opilis (snow crab)	25.000	Processing vessel

[a]All data are from the same laboratory using standardized assays.
Abbreviation: MUP, mouse urinary protein.

supply filtered air in the breaking and packaging rooms to maintain positive pressure in accordance with U.S. Department of Agriculture guidelines. Total dust levels are often in accord with accepted values for nontoxic nuisance dusts, but are clearly much too high for a potent allergen. Even increasing ventilation 10-fold is not likely to be able to keep up with this extraordinary source. Major changes in the design of the egg cracking and transferring equipment will be required to prevent aerosolization of the egg proteins into the working environment.

CONCLUSIONS

Immunochemical methods have been developed for measuring exposure to allergenic protein aerosols. When applied to the workplace setting, such methods have been utilized to monitor exposure to occupational allergens in a variety of industries and have been successful in providing insight into the relevant determinants of exposure. Data generated from future studies which should include detailed exposure assessment may help establish permissible exposure limits that prevent respiratory sensitization in workers and allow evaluation of the efficacy of industrial hygiene or process modification measures aimed at reducing airborne exposure to a sensitizing substance. Given the proper tools and their correct implementation, useful methods of ensuring safe and healthy environments will continue to be possible with the immuno-aerobiological tools we have learned to use.

DIRECTIONS OF FUTURE RESEARCH

It is anticipated that future research will include:

- Refinement(s) of protein allergen detection by nasal sampling
- Personal exposure by measuring allergen in nasal lavage or breath condensate samples
- Determination of cumulative dose requirements for induction and elicitation of allergic sensitivity by properly designed epidemiologic surveillance studies, utilizing personal and area sampling among apprentices and newly hired workers in industries where exposure to highly allergenic substances is likely
- Qualitative and semiquantitative sampling (via ambient air and settled dust) for unsuspected allergen contaminants (e.g., cat dander brought into an office environment by workers having pets) and surrounding community (e.g., aerobiologic dissemination from industrial sources)
- Validated methods to sample allergen(s) on workers' personal clothing and to determine how much is transported from work to other sites

REFERENCES

1. Novey H, Bernstein I, Mihalas L, Terr A, Yunginger JW. Guidelines for the clinical evaluation of occupational asthma due to high molecular weight (HMW) allergens. Report of the Subcommittee on the Clinical Evaluation of Occupational Asthma due to HMW allergens. J Allergy Clin Immunol 1989; 85(5):829–833.

2. Bush R, Kagen S. Guidelines for the preparation and characterization of high molecular weight allergens used for the diagnosis of occupational lung disease. Report of the Subcommittee on Preparation and Characterization of High Molecular Weight Allergens. J Allergy Clin Immunol 1989; 85(52):814–819.

3. Figley K, Elrod R. Endemic asthma due to castor bean dust. J Am Med Assoc 1928; 90:79–82.

4. Ordman D. An outbreak of bronchial asthma in South Africa affecting more than 200 persons, caused by castor bean dust from an oil-processing factory. Int Arch Allergy Appl Immunol 1955; 7:10–24.

5. Mendes E, Ulhoa Cintra A. Collective asthma, simulating an epidemic, provoked by castor bean dust. J Allergy 1954; 25:253–259.

6. Anto J, JS. Asthma Collaborative Group of Barcelona Apoint-source asthma outbreak. Lancet 1986; (1):900–903.

7. Anto J, Sunyer J, Rodriguez-Rosin R, Search-Cervera M, Vasquez L. Community outbreaks of asthma and the toxic epidemiological committee associated with the inhalation of soybean dust. N Engl J Med 1989; 320:1097–1102.

8. Anto J, Grimalt J, Aceves M, Reed C. Outbreak of asthma associated with soybean dust. N Engl J Med 1990; 321:1128 (letter).

9. Rodrigo MJ, Morell F, Helm R, et al. Identification and partial characterization of the soybean-dust allergens involved in the Barcelona asthma epidemic. J Allergy Clin Immunol 1990; 85:778–774.

10. Li J, Swanson M, Rando R, et al. Soybean aeroallergen around the Port of New Orleans: a potential cause of asthma. Aerobiologica 1996; 12:173–176.

11. Preller L, Hollander A, Heederik D, BB. Potentially allergenic airborne particles in the vicinity of a yeast and penicillin production plant. JAPCA 1989; 39:1094–1097.

12. Swanson M, Pelley B, Helleur R, et al. Airborne concentrations of asthmagenic snow crab proteins immunochemically quantified for Canadian shore stationed processing facilities. In: Safety Net Conference: A Community Research Alliance on Health & Safety in Marine and Coastal Work. Memorial University of Newfoundland, St. John's, 2003.

13. Villalbi J, Plasencia A, Manzanera R, Armengol R, Anto J. The collaborative and technical support groups for the study of soybean asthma in Barcelona. Epidemic soybean asthma and public health: new control systems and initial evaluation in Barcelona. J Epidemiol Commun Health 2004; 58:461–465.

14. Solomon W. Airborne microbial allergens: Impact and risk assessment. Toxicol and Health 1990; 6:309–324.

15. Milton D, Gere R, Feldman H, Greaves I. Endotoxin measurement: aerosol sampling and application of a new limulus method. Am Ind 1990; 51:331–337.

16. Swanson M, Agarwal M, Reed C. An immunochemical approach to indoor aeroallergen quantitation with a new volumetric air sampler. Studies with mite, roach, cat, mouse and guinea pig antigens. J Allergy Clin Immunol 1985; 76:724–729.

17. Reed C, Swanson M, Agarwal M, Yunginger J. Allergens that cause asthma. Identification and quantification. Chest 1985; 87:40S–44S.

18. Reed CE, Swanson MC, Lopez M, et al. Measurement of IgG antibody and airborne antigen to control an industrial outbreak of hypersensitivity pneumonias. J Occup Med 1983; 25:207–210.

19. Campbell A, Swanson M, Reed C, May J, Pratt D. Aeroallergens in dairy barns near Cooperstown, NY and Rochester, MN. Am Rev 1989; 140:317–320.

20. Parkes W. Occupational Lung Disorders. London: Butterworths, 1982.

21. Kenny LC, Aitken R, Chalmers C, et al. A collaborative European study of personal inhalable aerosol sampler performance. Ann Occup Hyg 1997; 41:135–153.

22. Air sampling instruments. ACGIH, Cincinnati, Ohio, 2001.

23. O'Meara T, De Lucca S, Sporik R, Graham A, Tovey E. Detection of inhaled cat allergen. Lancet 1998; 351:1488–1489.

24. Graham A, Pavlicek P, Sercoambe J, Savier M, Tovey E. The nasal air sampler: a device for sampling inhaled aeroallergens. Ann Allergy Asthma Immunol 2000; 84:599–604.

25. Renström A, Karlsson A-S, Tovey E. Nasal sampling used for the assessment of occupational allergen exposure and the efficacy of respiratory protection. Clin Exp Allergy 2002; 32:1769–1775.

26. Poulos L, O'Meara T, Hamilton R, Tovey E. Inhaled latex allergen. J Allergy Clin Immunol 2002; 109:701–706.

27. Holmquist L, Vesterberg O. Luminiscence immunoassay of pollen allergens on air sampling polytetrafluoroethylene filters. J Biochem Biophys Meth 1999; 41:49–60.

28. Holmquist L, Vesterberg O. Miniaturized direct on air sampling filter quantification of pollen allergens. J Biochem Biophys Meth 2000; 42:111–114.

29. Rodbard D, Hutt D. Statistical analysis of radioimmunoassay and immunoradiometric (labeled antibody) assays: A generalized weighted, iterative, least squares method for logistic curve filling. In: Symposium on Radioimmunoassays and Related Procedures in Medicine. Vienna: International Atomic Energy Agency; 1984:165–192.

30. Schroeckenstern D, Meier-Davis S, Yunginger J, Bush R. Allergens involved in occupational asthma caused by baby's breath (Gypsophilia paniculata). J Allergy Clin Immunol 1990; 86:189–191.

31. Sutton R, Skerritt J, Baido B, Wrigley C. The diversity of allergens involved in bakers' asthma. Clin Allergy 1984; 14:93–107.

32. Davison A, Britton M, Foffester J, Davies R, Hughes D. Asthma in merchant seamen and laboratory workers caused by allergy to castor beans: Analysis of allergens. Clin Allergy 1983; 13:553–561.

33. Baur X, Weiss W, Sauer W, et al. Backmiittel als Miturasche des Backerasthmas. Deutsch Med Wochenschr 1988; 113:1275–1278.

34. Gordon S, Tee R, Lowson D, Newman Taylor A. Comparison and optimization of filter elution methods for the measurement of airborne allergens. Ann Occup Hyg 1992; 36:575–587.

35. Hollander A, Gordon S, Renstrom A, et al. Comparison of methods to assess airborne rat and mouse allergen levels. I. Analysis of air samples. Allergy 1999; 54:142–149.

36. Renstrom A, Larsson P, Malmberg P, Bayard C. A new amplified monoclonal rat allergen assay used for evaluation of ventilation improvements in animal rooms. J Allergy Clin Immunol 1997; 100:649–655.

37. Renstrom A, Gordon S, Hollander A, et al. Comparison of methods to assess airborne rat or mouse allergen levels: II Factors influencing antigen detection. Allergy 1999; 54:150–157.

38. Zock J-P, Hollander A, Doekes G, Heederik D. The influence of different filter elution methods on the measurement of airborne potato antigens. Am Ind Hyg Assoc J 1996; 57:567–570.

39. Lillienberg L, Baur X, Doekes G, et al. Comparison of four methods to assess fungal alpha-amylase in flour dust. Ann Occup Hyg 2000; 44:427–433.

40. Offerman F, Girman J, RG S. Recent advances in health sciences and technology. In: Indoor Air: Proceedings of the 3rd International Conference on Indoor Air Quality and Climate; 1984:257–261.

41. Stricker WE, Layton J, Homburger HA, et al. Immunologic response to aerosols of affinity-purifiedantigen in hypersensitivity pneumonitis. J Allergy Clin Immunol 1986; 78:411–416.

42. Woodward E, Friedlander B, Lesher R, Font W, Kinsey R, Heame F. Outbreak of hypersensitivity pneumonitis in an industrial setting. JAMA 1988; 259:1965–1969.

43. Ingram J, Dunnette S, Gleich G. Immunochemical quantitation of an airborne proteolytic enzyme, esperase TM, in a consumer products factory. Am Ind Hyg Assoc J 1986; 47:136–143.

44. Liss G, Kontinsky, Gallagher J, Melius J, Brooks S, Bernstein I. Failure of enzyme encapsulation to prevent sensitization of workers in the dry bleach industry. J Allergy Clin Immunol 1984; 73:348–355.
45. Swanson M, Yunginger J, Reed C. Immunochemical quantification of airborne natural rubber allergen in medical and dental office buildings. In: Maroni M. ed. Ventilation and Indoor Air Quality in Hospitals: Kleuver Academic Publishers, 1996:251–262.
46. Yunginger J, Jones R, Fransway A, Kelso J, Wamer M, Hunt L. Extractable latex allergens and proteins in disposable medical gloves and other rubber products. J Allergy Clin Immunol 1994; 93:836–840.
47. Newman Taylor A, Longbottom J, Pepys J. Respiratory allergy to urine proteins of rats and mice. Lancet 1977; 2:847–849.
48. Swanson M, Campbell A, O'Hollaren M, Reed C. Role of ventilation, air filtration and allergen production rate in determining concentrations of rat allergens in the air of animal quarters. Am Rev Respir Dis 1991; 141:1578–1581.
49. Platts-Mills T, Heyman P, Longbottom J, Wilkins S. Airborne allergens associated with asthma: Particle size canying dust mite and rat allergens measured with a cascade impactor. J Allergy Clin Immunol 1986; 77:850–857.
50. Muller-Wening D, Repp H. Investigation on the protective value of breathing masks in farmer's lung using an inhalation provocation test. Chest 1989; 95:100–105.
51. Swanson M, Boiano J, Galson S, Grauvogel L, Reed C. Immunochemical quantification and particle size distribution of airborne papain in a meat portioning facility. J Am Ind Hyg Assoc 1992; 53:1–5.
52. Smith AB, Bernstein DI, Aw TC, et al. Occupational asthma from inhaled egg protein. Am J Ind Med 1987; 12:205–218.
53. Bernstein DI, Smith AB, Moller DR, et al. Clinical and immunological studies among egg-producing workers with occupational asthma. J Allergy Clin Immunol 1987; 80:791–797.
54. Halverson P, Swanson M, Reed C. Occupational asthma in egg crackers is associated with extraordinarily high airborne egg allergen concentrations. J Allergy Clin Immunol 1988; 81:321.

13
Environmental Monitoring of Chemical Agents

Jacques Lesage
Laboratory Services and Expertise, Institut de Recherche Robert-Sauvé en Santé et en Sécurité du Travail, Montreal, Quebec, Canada

Guy Perrault
Consultation en R and D et Expertise en SST, Laval, Quebec, Canada

INTRODUCTION

The fact that asthmatic reactions may be induced and elicited by low and, on occasion, extremely low concentrations of a given substance has given occupational asthma (OA) its own place in industrial hygiene, where the classical notions of time-weighted average (TWA) exposure, short-term exposure limits (STEL), and ceiling limits have been treated as more or less irrelevant. In the case of OA, emphasis has been laid on the identification of the causative agents and subsequent hygiene control so that subjects with OA are no longer exposed to the causal agent (1–3).

The rapid increase in new cases of OA, the number of agents causing asthma (4,5) over the past few decades, and the distinction, in recent years, between work-related asthma in two categories of workers, namely those with preexisting asthma that was aggravated by work [i.e., work-aggravated asthma (WAA)] and those with work-related new onset asthma (NOA) (6) have emphasized the need for establishing methods to quantify worker exposure to both environmental and occupational agents. First, there is justification for verifying whether workers are exposed to a specific agent in the workplace. Second, surveillance and prevention of exposure are required to ensure that workers do not develop OA and that workers with OA are no longer exposed to the causal agent or are only exposed to the agent in a much lower concentration (7,8). Third, laboratory or workplace confirmation of OA is relevant for medical or medicolegal reasons. In all these instances, it is important to obtain information on the nature and concentrations of the agent(s) (9,10).

OA agents are generally classified as low- and high-molecular-weight agents. The latter generally cause sensitization through immunologic means. The mechanism of OA caused by low-molecular-weight agents, which are a growing cause of work-related asthma, is usually unknown. Two main approaches have been adopted for exposure assessment—immunoassays (11–14) and chemical assays. This chapter is devoted to the assessment of exposure to low-molecular-weight asthma agents both in the air and in biological matrices, by chemical assays.

MONITORING METHODS

This section will briefly review the main analytical methods used in the maintenance of industrial hygiene to identify and evaluate the presence of chemicals in workplaces. The main route of absorption of chemicals is inhalation; this emphasizes the role of methods of determination of the concentration of chemicals in the air or a few possibilities of biological exposure monitoring in asthma prevention. Each method includes a sampling and an analytical protocol. Most methods can be used for personal monitoring or area sampling. The main sampling and instrumental techniques will be described briefly and separately. However, all these techniques have to be used in accordance with an environmental sampling strategy that takes into account factors related to the nature and toxicology of the suspected contaminants and the characteristics of the worksite. Because asthma induction by skin absorption has been mentioned in a few scientific articles (15,16), the sampling and characterization of chemicals on surfaces will also be mentioned.

Sampling Techniques

The first point to consider before choosing a sampling technique is the route of absorption of the chemicals into the human body, namely inhalation, absorption through the skin, or ingestion. In the case of asthma, the main and well-documented route of absorption is inhalation. Consequently, sampling and analysis of air samples will constitute a large part of this section. Surface sampling will be briefly mentioned in the prevention of absorption through the skin. Finally, biological exposure monitoring will be mentioned as a means of obtaining an overall evaluation of the dose absorbed by the worker through different possible routes, for special cases.

Air

The first steps in analyzing an air sample are to collect the pollutant in such a way as to be able to carry it to the laboratory for further characterization, and to determine the volume of air from which this pollutant was obtained. In industrial hygiene and environmental analysis, several sampling techniques are used in most cases where a direct- or continuous-reading instrument is not available or is not adaptable to the sampling strategy.

In ambient air, a chemical pollutant can be present as a gas, vapor, or aerosol (mist or dust). Sampling of gases is routinely done in plastic, teflon, or aluminum bags filled by a pump. The flow and time of operation of the pump provide the volume of air necessary to calculate the concentration in parts per million (ppm) or milligram per cubic meter (mg/m^3) of air. These bags are then sent to the laboratory for qualitative or quantitative analysis. A variety of solid containers made of glass, plastic, or metals are also available. These containers can be filled by flushing them with the air to be collected if they have an inlet and an outlet valve, or by placing the container under vacuum and filling it by opening only one valve equipped with a flow controller (Simon, Farant, private communication). Sampling in bags or containers is limited to the sampling of stable gaseous products that do not chemically react with, physically diffuse through, or adsorb on the bag or the container material.

Sampling of volatile organic compounds as vapors or gases is usually performed by adsorption of the compounds on a solid sorbent such as activated charcoal, tenax, silica gel, XAD-2, etc. These adsorbents are chosen on the basis of their adsorption efficiency for a given compound or mixture of compounds and their ease of desorption by a suitable solvent before analysis. Solid sorbents can be used with an active or a passive sampling train.

In active sampling, the solid adsorbent is generally placed in a glass tube, and held at the inlet and the outlet of the tube by a fiberglass wool or polyurethane plug. This tube is then connected to a pump to draw a known quantity of air through the tube. The sample adsorbed on the sorbent is then sent to a laboratory to be desorbed and analyzed.

In passive sampling, the solid sorbent is placed in a cup and held in place by a layer of material permeable to organic vapors. Sampling is then the result of the diffusion of the sample from the air, where it is at a certain concentration, to the inside of the passive sampler, where it is at a much lower concentration. It is then captured on the solid sorbent, and the entire sampling train (badge) is sent to the laboratory for analysis (Fig. 1). The sampling rate constant of a passive sampler has to be predetermined in a generation chamber with the expected air concentration of the given organic compounds. This predetermined value is then combined with the sampling duration to obtain the air volume.

The use of bubblers (or impingers) containing liquid, for sampling vapors and aerosols, is on the decline. Bubblers are made of glass, plastic, or teflon, and are filled with an absorbing liquid to collect the sample. Spillproof versions are available for personal sampling and are well accepted by workers. The bubbler is connected to a pump to draw a measured volume of air through the solvent. The pollutant is dissolved in the solvent, and the entire impinger or bubbler is sent to the laboratory for analysis (Fig. 2).

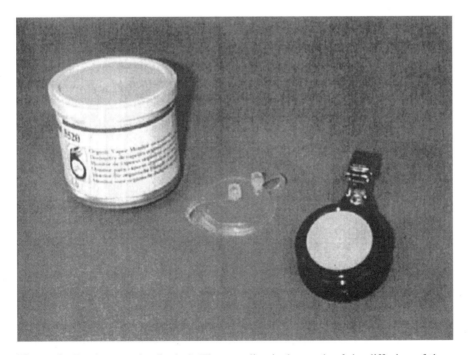

Figure 1 Passive sampler (badge). The sampling is the result of the diffusion of the sample from the air to the inside of the badge.

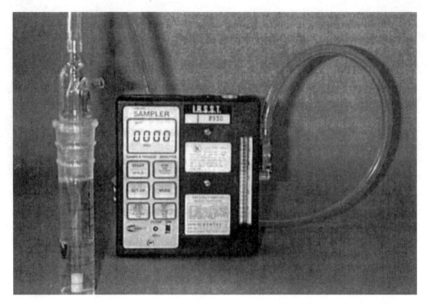

Figure 2 Sampling train with an impinger to collect vapors and aerosols in an absorbing liquid.

Aerosols, mists, or dusts are often sampled on filters (or membranes) composed of teflon, mixed cellulose esters, polyvinyl chloride, fiberglass, silver, and other materials. Filters are available in various pore sizes and are selected on the basis of the application. The choice of filter is dictated by the requirements of the analytical methods. For sampling, the filter is placed in a plastic cassette of 37, 25, or 13 mm diameter. The cassette containing the filter is then connected to a pump to aspirate the air through the filter on which the dust or mist will be collected. The cassette is then sent to the laboratory for analysis. For most cases of asthma prevention, sampling for inhalable dust (17) (Fig. 3) (also referred to incorrectly as total dust) is recommended for collecting the portion of the aerosol that can be inhaled by the worker and can be deposited anywhere in the respiratory tract (18). In the absence of wind, inhalable dust can be collected at a flow rate of 2 L/min in a filter cassette having an opening of at least 15 mm. Respirable dust, the portion of the aerosol that can be deposited in the gas-exchange region of the lung, including the respiratory alveoles, bronchioles, and associated ducts, can be sampled through a cyclone (median cut-size aerodynamic diameter: 4 μm) with a filter cassette (Fig. 4).

Surface

To prevent skin absorption, two surface sampling techniques can be used to detect possible contamination of work surfaces by chemical agents. The first technique consists of placing the substance to be identified in contact with a selectively reactive compound. The product resulting from the reaction between both chemical substances should develop coloration visible to the human eye. This technique has been used mainly for the detection of heavy metals, amines, and isocyanates. This technique has limitations in terms of specificity and quantitative evaluation but offers the advantage of an immediate on-site response to allow screening or immediate

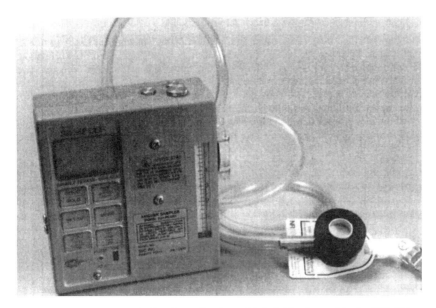

Figure 3 Sampling train for the collection of inhalable dust with the NR-701 personal dust sampler designed by the Institute of Occupational Medicine in Edinburgh, Scotland.

correction to avoid skin contamination with active agents. The second technique is a wipe test with an adsorbent material to collect the chemicals present on the work surface. The adsorbent material is then sent to the laboratory for identification and quantitative analysis.

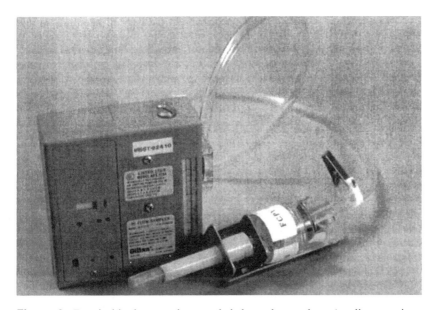

Figure 4 Respirable dust can be sampled through a cyclone (median cut-size aerodynamic diameter 4 μm) with a filter cassette.

Biological Exposure Monitoring

The biological exposure monitoring is a measure of the contaminant itself, or one of its metabolites, or any other biological parameter in a biological matrix (mainly blood, urine, and exhaled air). It gives an evaluation of the internal dose that has been absorbed by an individual worker, taking into account the characteristics of the worker's job, the process, the worker's individual parameters (age, sex, body mass, etc.), as well as the various routes of absorption, mainly by inhalation and through the skin.

All urine or blood samples for biological exposure monitoring must be collected by qualified medical personnel using state-of-the-art precautions to protect the worker and ensure the quality of the sample. For each contaminant, the sampling protocol has to take into account the objective of the monitoring, the requirements of the analytical technique, the integrity of the sample, and the sampling time. Results can be interpreted when the relationship between the internal dose and the biological effects has been established; this relationship has not been established for many contaminants. In asthma, metabolites of isocyanates and anhydrides are being studied for biological exposure monitoring.

Analytical Techniques

Gas Chromatography

Gas chromatography (GC) is essentially an analytical technique to achieve the chromatographic separation of mixtures of organic compounds in the gas phase and the quantitative assessment of each constituent. The instrumental protocol starts with the injection of a small sample of a gas or a vapor into an inert gas flow. This injected gas or vapor is carried by the flow of inert gas to a chromatographic column on which it will be separated into its different constituents. In brief, chromatographic separation depends on the boiling point or vapor pressure of each organic compound and the type of adsorbents in the chromatographic column. At the end of the column, the sample is carried by the gas flow to a detector that should have a response proportional to the concentration of the sample. Many different types of detectors can be chosen based on their sensitivity, specificity, or generality of application. Each constituent of the sample is identified by comparing its retention time (time from the injection of the sample until the response of the detector) to the retention time of a pure standard. Rather complex mixtures can be efficiently and rapidly analyzed using this instrumental technique.

Samples for GC analysis are generally collected in aluminum bags or on solid sorbents. GC can be used as a direct-reading instrument to monitor the concentration of a pure organic compound or well-identified mixtures of two or three organic compounds in a generation chamber. Portable instruments are available for use in the field by qualified technicians.

High-Performance Liquid Chromatography

Approximately 85% of all organic compounds cannot be analyzed by GC either because of their extremely low volatility or their high thermolability. In these cases, high-performance liquid chromatography (HPLC) is often used.

In HPLC, a liquid sample (a pure compound or a solution) is injected into the flow of a carrier liquid to be transported through a chromatographic column. Mixtures of organic compounds are separated by the diffusion of the analyte from the eluting solvent to the columns with a solid adsorbent. Each separated component is then detected by an appropriate detector giving a response that is proportional to the concentration of each compound. As in GC, each constituent of a mixture can be identified by comparing its retention time to the retention time of a reference compound. A choice of eluting solvents, chromatographic columns, and more or less specific detectors can be adapted to various analytical protocols.

For HPLC analysis, air samples are usually collected on solid sorbents, impingers, or filters. The requirement of injecting the sample as a liquid limits the practical use of HPLC to laboratory analysis of samples collected in workplaces or in generation chambers.

Atomic Spectrometric Methods

Atomic absorption spectrophotometry (AAS) is essentially a quantitative analytical technique for metallic atoms. In treatment of OA, it can be particularly useful in the analysis of metallic atoms such as Pb, Cu, Zn, Cd, Ni, Cr, Co, etc. The principle of the analytical technique is the absorption of light with wavelengths specific to the emission spectra of the vaporized atom. The intensity of this absorption can be measured by a photometric detector or a spectrophotometer.

Air samples for AAS are usually collected as fumes, dusts, or mists on a filter or a membrane. The filter is then digested by appropriate acids to destroy the filter material and dissolve the collected fumes or dusts. The resulting solution is vaporized using a flame or another heating device (graphite furnace) and irradiated by light of appropriate wavelength from a hollow cathode lamp.

AAS has good sensitivity and specificity, but it only analyzes one element at a time or a given number of elements (six to eight) in sequence. The results are given as the total metallic atoms contained in the sample without specification of derivatives or oxidation states. Atomic emission is used for applications where a multi-element technique is required; inductively coupled plasma (ICP) atomic emission or ICP with mass spectrometry (MS) (i.e., ICP–MS) is then recommended.

Spectrometry

Spectrometry covers a wide range of analytical techniques based on the principle of the interaction of electromagnetic radiation with matter. In the electromagnetic radiation spectrum, the ranges of ultraviolet (UV), visible, and infrared (IR) radiation are of special interest in the analysis of low-molecular-weight compounds in air. Techniques operating in the visible range of electromagnetic radiation are routinely used in clinical as well as environmental laboratories mainly because of their wide applicability resulting from the transformation of the sample into colored derivatives and the simplicity of the instrumentation, resulting in low cost and ease of operation. The formation of colored derivatives is often used for identification of surface contamination.

A spectrometer's operating principle is based on the absorption, by the sample, of electromagnetic radiation of specific wavelengths from a light source, which is usually a tungsten lamp in the visible range. The absorption of light, which is measured and quantified by an appropriate detector such as a phototube, is proportional to the concentration of the analyte (Beer's Law).

Generally, air samples, for analysis by visible spectrometry, are collected in impingers containing a solution of the derivative necessary for direct preparation of the colored compound that will be quantified. Direct-reading instruments using this technique have been developed for the analysis of a given analyte in a small volume of a derivatizing solution or on treated paper tapes.

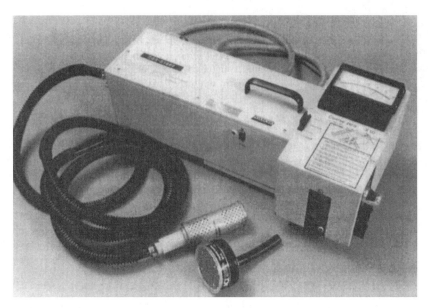

Figure 5 Example of an IR direct-reading instrument (Miran 103) that can be used in the field or in a chamber. *Abbreviation*: IR, infrared.

IR Spectrophotometry

The basic principle of IR spectrophotometry is identical to the absorption of electromagnetic radiation in visible spectrometry, except that the range of sources of electromagnetic radiation is in the IR region between 400 and 4000 cm^{-1}. IR spectrophotometry is mainly used to characterize pollutants but can also be effective in quantifying concentrations. The IR absorption of light at certain wave numbers is specific to the presence of functional groups in the molecules, such as ketones, esters, alcohols, isocyanates, organic acids, anhydrides, amines, alkanes, alkenes, alkynes, etc. This provides useful information in the characterization of families of contaminants, and in identifying pure compounds especially for a region of the absorption spectrum containing many discrete absorption lines, which are said to be the fingerprint of each organic compound. The intensity of absorption at a given wave number can be used to quantify specifically a pure pollutant or a pollutant in a mixture of other organic compounds that do not contain the functional group absorbing the IR radiation.

Analysis by IR can be performed on solids, liquids, or gases as long as they are transparent to IR radiation or suited for reflectance (solid sample), giving the technique a wide range of applicability. Gaseous samples can be monitored continuously in the atmosphere or in a generation chamber. Field instruments are available and routinely used in the field by industrial hygienists (Fig. 5).

Ion Chromatography

Ion chromatography (IC) is similar to HPLC, and separates by chromatography, mixtures carried by a liquid flow. IC, however, is particularly useful for analyzing inorganic ions, cations, or anions in solution (usually in water).

In this case, the analyte solution is injected into the liquid flow and is transported through an ion-exchange column where the various ions are separated. The separated constituents in solution are then treated in a suppressor and converted into strong acids or bases, which are detected and quantified by a conductivity or electrochemical cell.

In preparing for the IC technique, air samples are collected in impingers, on filters or on solid sorbents. As with HPLC, this technique is limited from a practical standpoint to the laboratory analysis of samples collected in the field or in generation chambers.

Mass Spectrometry

Mass spectrometry (MS) is used to identify and quantify components of complex mixtures. Its principle consists of ionizing the analyte in a source, of fragmenting molecular ions, and of analyzing specific molecular or fragmented ions according to their mass to charge ratio (m/z). This technique is often used as a specific detector with a gas chromatograph (GC–MS), HPLC (HPLC–MS), or ICP (ICP–MS) to identify the components of a complex mixture that are separated by GC or HPLC before being introduced into the ionization source of the mass spectrometer. The information generated by MS is equivalent to a fingerprint of an unknown sample, allowing the sample to be identified without using a reference compound. The technique has been developed for gaseous, liquid, or solid samples.

More sophisticated techniques consist of selecting a parent ion followed by a subsequent fragmentation to generate specific daughter ions. These techniques, referred to as MS–MS or as a double MS, improve the specificity and sensitivity of MS applied to the measurement of a component in a complex matrix. Some sophisticated installations can perform continuous monitoring in the field or in a generation chamber.

Other Methods

X-ray diffractometry has applications in the identification and quantification of dust constituents. It is limited, however, to crystalline compounds such as some metallic oxides. Polarized light microscopy can be used to identify solid compounds (guar gum).

EXPOSURE EVALUATION STRATEGY AS RELATED TO OA

A variety of exposure limit values have been developed by different organizations or national regulatory agencies to protect workers from the toxicological effects of uncontrolled exposure to chemical contaminants. The threshold limit values (TLV^{R}) proposed by the American Conference of Governmental Industrial Hygienists (ACGIH) have gained worldwide recognition for their quality and their acquisition by consensus. In the ACGIH list of TLVs, long-term exposure to low concentrations of contaminants resulting in chronic toxicological consequences has led to the notion of TWA values, below which there will be no deleterious effects on the health of a normal worker exposed for eight working hours, five days a week, over his lifetime. Acute exposure to relatively high concentrations of a contaminant for a short period of time, causing immediate toxicological reactions such as irritation, chronic or irreversible tissue damage, or necrosis, is prevented by the observance of STEL or ceiling limits.

Most of these thresholds can be scientifically supported by or extrapolated from animal or in vitro toxicological tests. A few have been proven by epidemiological studies. However, these exposure limits are often suspected of being inadequate in the prevention of OA where individual susceptibility could play an important role in the sensitizing process. It could then be assumed that the protection of a sensitized worker suffering from WAA or NOA for a given agent would require compliance with a much lower exposure limit than for unaffected workers to prevent the evolution to chronicity. These considerations placed the emphasis on the identification and quantification of sensitizing and irritating agents in the workplace at very low concentrations close to the background values of the general environment. Conversely, it could be argued that there is a certain exposure limit that prevents most unaffected workers from becoming sensitized and developing NOA. This existence of a sensitizing threshold has not yet been scientifically proven, but the risk of developing OA has been shown to be related to the degree of exposure (19–21), even though studies continue to clarify the contributions of the duration of exposure (3), individual susceptibility, and routes of absorption.

EXAMPLES OF EVALUATION OF EXPOSURE TO SPECIFIC SENSITIZING AGENTS

Isocyanates

Analytical methods to determine air concentrations of diisocyanates have been extensively reviewed by Dharmarajan et al. (22), Brown et al. (23), and Lesage and Perrault (24). Most methods have been developed for impinger sampling and subsequently modified for sampling on adsorbent tubes or filters impregnated with a derivative reagent (Table 1). Analytical methods are, in general, spectrometry for determining all isocyanate groups, and HPLC with a UV detector for specific analysis of a given diisocyanate molecule such as 2,4-toluene diisocyanate (2,4-TDI). Recently, a new analytical method using HPLC–MS gives a better sensitivity and specificity in diisocyanate and polyisocyanate determination (25). It should be noted that aliphatic compounds and cycloalkanes, for example, hexamethylene diisocyanate (HDI) and methylene bis(4-cyclohexylisocyanate), can be detected by the UV spectroscopy detector only after derivatization with a UV absorbing compound such as 9-(N-methyl aminomethyl) anthracene (MAMA) (Table 1).

A few recent publications have presented efforts to achieve lower limits of detection by optimizing the derivatization reaction to make the resulting compound sensitive to a specific detector such as the electron capture detector of a gas chromatograph, or the fluorescence or the MS detector of an HPLC. Karlsson et al. (32) have reported a limit of detection (LOD) of 0.5 to $0.8\,\mu g/m^3$ for TDI and HDI using HPLC-UV, and a lower limit of $0.1\,\mu g/m^3$ by HPLC–MS for 1,6-HDI. The same group of researchers (33) has published an LOD of $0.1\,\mu g/m^3$ for 2,4- and 2,6-TDI with the electrochemical detector of an HPLC (33). Simon and Moulut (34), and Schmidtke and Seifert (35) have adapted the 1-(2-methoxyphenyl) piperazine method to tube sampling. The quantification of isocyanate prepolymers to the methods, and an LOD of $1\,ng/m^3$ with the electrochemical detector has been achieved by the same group of researchers. Other groups are working on the development of new derivative agents such as 1-(9-anthracenylmethyl) piperazine (MAP) (36,37).

Lesage et al. have reported an LOD of $1\,\mu g/m^3$ with a double-filter cassette for separating and trapping isocyanate monomers and oligomers before their analysis by HPLC (38,39). This group has also developed, using the same sampler, an analytical

Table 1 Sampling and Analysis of Diisocyanates in the Air

Reagent	Sampling technique	Analytical technique	LOD[a] ($\mu g/m^3$)
MOPIP[c] (26)	Impinger (toluene) solid sorbent impinger/ solid sorbent	HPLC/UV/ electrochemical	0.1
MOPIP/MAMA[b] (27–30)	Double-filter cassette	HPLC/UV/ fluorescence	0.6
MAP[d] (31)	Impinger (butylbenzoate) solid sorbent impinger/solid sorbent	HPLC/UV/ fluorescence	1.7
DBA[e] (32)	Impinger (toluene)	HPLC–MS	0.2

[a]$0.015\,m^3$ air sample.
[b]9-(*N*-methylaminomethyl)anthracene.
[c]1-(2-methoxyphenyl)piperazine.
[d]1-(9-anthracenylmethyl)piperazine.
[e]Dibutylamine.
Abbreviations: HPLC, high-performance liquid chromatography; LOD, limit of detection; MS, mass spectrometry; UV, ultraviolet.

method with an HPLC coupled to a double mass spectrometer. The LOD observed is $0.04\,ng/m^3$ for TDI. The double-filter cassette also has the possibility of separating the aerosol into its liquid (mist) and vapor phases. Other techniques have been suggested for achieving this separation (40,41).

During thermal degradation, polyurethanes can regenerate isocyanates. Particular attention must be paid to the sampling of these isocyanates because they can differ from the isocyanates contained in the polyurethane formulations. For example, Boutin et al. observed the emission of aliphatic and alkenyl monoisocyanates during the pyrolysis (42) and combustion (43) of an HDI-based car paint.

Biological exposure monitoring has been tested using albumin adducts in plasma (44) and their corresponding diamine in plasma and urine (45). These studies have not yet reached the stage of being applicable to the monitoring of worker exposure to isocyanates.

Three types of direct-reading instruments based on colorimetry, ion mobility, and gravimetry are commercially available. These instruments are used for active-air sampling and passive dosimetry. Their main characteristics are summarized in Table 2. These instruments are suitable for monitoring diisocyanate concentrations in a generation chamber or at a worksite where the diisocyanates have been identified

Table 2 Diisocyanate Determination by Direct-Reading Instruments

Instrument	Analytical technique	LOD (ppm)	Response time
Impregnated paper tape active sampling	Visible spectrometry	0.002	2–5 min
Impregnated paper tape passive sampling	Colorimetry	0.01	60 min
Dräger	Ion mobility	0.001	40 sec

Abbreviation: LOD, limit of detection.

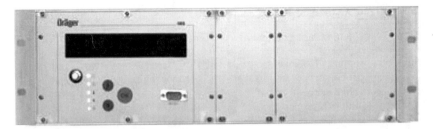

Figure 6 Example of an ion-mobility-spectrometer (Dräger IMS 5000) for the determination of TDI in air. *Abbreviation*: TDI, toluene diisocyanate.

by another technique. It is also recommended that the effect of humidity and of other air pollutants on instrument response be considered (Figs. 6 and 7). A coated piezoelectric detector (46) with a range of detection of 3 to 24 particles per billion (ppb) could be promising for application in a direct-reading instrument. The new instrument from Dräger, based on ion mobility, has been commercialized. It has an application range of 1 to 100 ppb. However this instrument is calibrated only for TDI.

For surfaces contaminated by isocyanate, a wipe test has been developed by Colorimetric Laboratories Inc. under the trade name of SWYPE. This product can be used for surface and skin contamination detection to identify exposures that contribute to dermal absorption. Research on this technique is continuing to increase its specificity and sensitivity.

In summary, many sampling and analytical methods are now available to determine the concentrations of diisocyanates in the air with the sensitivity required for detecting low-concentration or short-duration exposures. Research is continuing

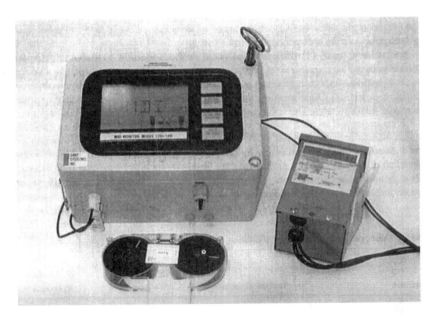

Figure 7 Example of a direct-reading instrument (GMD RIS) for continuous monitoring of isocyanates. *Abbreviation*: GMD RIS, Gesellschaft für Mathematik und Datenverarbeitung remote intelligence sensor.

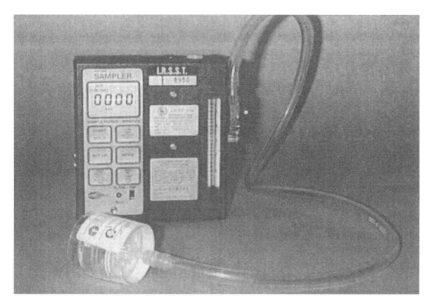

Figure 8 A sampling cassette (ISO-CHEK®) designed to collect diisocyanates as a vapor and aerosol fraction. A first Teflon filter collects the isocyanates that are present in the air as aerosols, while a second pretreated glass-fiber filter traps all vapor isocyanates.

to further improve the LOD to reach the no observed adverse effect level which is respectively 0.001 and 0.002 mg/m^3 for HDI and TDI. Direct-reading instruments are also available to monitor exposure to monomer diisocyanates. The applicability of these instruments to different diisocyanates can still be improved as well as their response to simple interferences such as humidity. Research efforts are now devoted to the representative sampling of mists containing isocyanate monomers and oligomers and to the analysis of polyisocyanate prepolymers (Fig. 8).

Acid Anhydrides

Methods for the sampling and analysis of hexahydrophthalic and methylhexahydrophthalic, acetic, phthalic, trimellitic, maleic, and methyltetrahydrophthalic anhydrides have been described (47–49). The air concentration of anhydrides is often determined by sampling a known volume of air through a collecting device to trap the organic aerosol. The anhydride is then hydrolyzed to the corresponding diacid or derivatized to a diester, extracted with an aqueous ammonia solution, and analyzed by HPLC with a UV detector. A method developed for hexahydrophthalic and methylhexahydrophthalic anhydride (48) and methyltetrahydrophthalic anhydride uses (49) a sorbent tube or a bubbler for collecting the sample, and GC with flame ionization detector or GC–MS for the analysis. The LOD is then 0.2 μg/m^3. For phthalic and trimellitic anhydrides, Occupational Safety and Health Administration (OSHA) has recommended sampling on two glass fiber filters coated with veratrylamine/di-*n*-octylphthalate and analysis by HPLC-UV (50). National Institute for Occupational Safety and Health (NIOSH) has recommended a GC method for trimellitic anhydride after sampling on a PVC filter and an HPLC-UV method for maleic anhydride after collection in a bubbler (47). The GC method should be adaptable to most organic anhydrides that can be volatilized without decomposition.

Biological exposure monitoring by analyzing hexahydrophthalic and methyl-hexahydrophthalic acids (51) and methyltetrahydrophthalic acid in urine has been described. Total plasma protein adducts of hexahydrophthalic and methylhexa-hydrophthalic anhydrides are reported to be excellent biomarkers of long-term exposure (52).

A direct-reading instrument for monitoring organic anhydride concentrations in a generation chamber could be based on IR spectrophotometry but has not been described in the scientific literature. Dedicated gas chromatographs could be set up for monitoring organic anhydrides with sufficiently high vapor pressure.

Formaldehyde and Other Aldehydes

Various methods have been used to determine the concentration of formaldehyde and other aldehydes in the air. The subject was reviewed in 1985 by Kennedy et al. (53) who listed the chromotropic acid, pararosaniline, 2,4-dinitrophenylhydra-zine (2,4-DNPH), 3-methyl-2-benzothiazolinone hydrazone (MBTH), Girard T reagent, hydrazine, and N-benzylethanolamine (BEA) methods. Most of these methods have been adapted to sampling with impingers (bubblers), adsorbent tubes, or passive samplers. Table 3 summarizes the reported performance of each method. The interferences given in this table refer to the application as a colorimetric technique. The pararosaniline, 2,4-DNPH, and BEA methods have been adapted to analytical techniques such as GC and HPLC to improve their specificity and sensitivity. OSHA (54) and NIOSH (55) recommend sampling on an XAD-2 sorbent tube coated with 2-(hydroxymethyl) piperidine (HMP) and analysis by GC or GC–MS, or 2,4-DNPH coated on a silica gel sorbent and analyzed by HPLC-UV. The 2-(hydroxymethyl) piperidine reacts with formaldehyde to form an oxazolidine derivative similar to that in the BEA method, and the 2,4-DNPH reacts to give a hydrazone derivative. Methods based on the same derivatives for the identification (screening) and quantification of many aldehydes simultaneously present in a work environment are described in NIOSH Method 2539 (Aldehydes, screening) published in 1994.

Formaldehyde can also be released from textiles or wood. A method has been developed for formaldehyde on dust, which requires the sampling of inhalable dust on a filter, extraction, derivatization with 2,4-DNPH, and analysis by HPLC (56).

Table 3 Analytical Methods for Formaldehyde in the Air

Methods	Sampling volume (L)	LOD (mg/m^3)	Interference
Chromotropic acid	60	0.025	Phenol and alcohols
Pararosaniline[a]	60	0.030	Aldehydes
2,4-DNPH[a]	30	0.002	Aldehydes and ketones
Girard T	18	0.300	Aldehydes
MBTH[a]	250	0.008	Aldehydes and ketones
Hydrazine	30	0.010	Specific by polarography
BEA	38	0.050	Specific by GC
HMP	10	0.300	Specific by GC

[a]Colorimetric method.
Abbreviations: BEA, N-benzylethanolamine; 2,4-DNPH, 2,4-dinitrophenylhydrazine; GC, gas chromatography; HMP, 2-(hydroxymethyl)piperidine; LOD, limit of detection; MBTH, 3-methyl-2-benzothiazolinone hydrazone.

Vairavamurthy et al. (57) have reviewed the determination of aldehydes in the atmospheric environment. They cite methods similar to the ones already mentioned for the work environment and some direct-reading instruments. However, these direct-reading spectroscopic instruments require long optical paths and are not easily applicable in a work environment. Another family of instruments uses colorimetric methods for quasicontinuous monitoring of formaldehyde (58). These instruments have the same problems with interference as other colorimetric techniques. A final family of instruments can be used in well-controlled atmospheres such as a generation chamber; these instruments are based on IR or UV spectroscopy (57). A direct-reading passive badge for glutaraldehyde and formaldehyde monitoring has been described with a LOD of 0.04 ppm for an eight-hour sampling (59).

In summary, the analytical techniques for formaldehyde and glutaraldehyde are well developed and are adaptable to a wide range of air concentrations. Many of these methods are adaptable to the analysis of other aldehydes, but methods for other aldehydes have not reached the same level of development as those for formaldehyde. Direct-reading instruments for the work environment are available and easy to use but are plagued with many types of interference. However, it should be remembered that formaldehyde and other aldehydes are often used as indicators (tracers) of worker exposure to complex mixtures of decomposed organic products of combustion or high temperature processes. These exposures are extremely complex, containing hundreds of products, many of which could be asthma-inducing agents. For this reason, Boutin et al. (60) developed a systematic approach for studying the thermal degradation of organic materials—whether natural or synthetic—in the laboratory. This approach can be used to identify the constituents of complex thermal degradation effluents. From this identification, tests can be done on sensitization by suspected sensitizing agents or mixtures of sensitizing agents.

Amines

The analytical techniques reported in the past 15 years use gas or liquid chromatography for the analysis of airborne volatile amines sometimes collected in impingers, but as often as possible in sorbent tubes or on treated filters. Table 4 summarizes the most recent publications on the analysis of aliphatic amines in the air, and Table 5, those for aromatic amines.

Many different analytical methods for analyzing amines in the air have been published. In general, the low limits of detection required by the application to OA are attainable only with methods in which the amine group is derivatized by attaching a moiety that is very sensitive to the detector of the analytical technique. The derivatization technique is not as easy, however, in the case of tertiary amines. These methods are limited to the straight application of GC or HPLC with a specific nitrogen-detector or a detector sensitive to quaternary amines for analysis by IC, but such methods have not yet been validated. Further studies are required before biological exposure monitoring by measurement of adduct formation can be considered as a tool in human studies (61).

Colophony and Fluxes

This natural complex pine resin is largely composed of acidic resins of which abietic acid is the main constituent. Colophony can be used in two different applications,

Table 4 Sampling and Analysis of Aliphatic Amines in the Air

Methods (Refs.)	Sampling	Analysis	Sampling volume (L)	LOD (mg/m^3)
Underivatized[a] (62–64)	Silica gel adsorbent	GC	20	0.1
Polymeric anhydride[b] (65–67)	Silica gel adsorbent	HPLC		1 μg
Naphthyl isothiocyanate[b] (68–70)	Adsorbent or filter	HPLC	15	0.01
m-Toluyl chloride[b]	Silica gel adsorbent	HPLC	60	0.1
	H$_3$PO$_3$ coated annular denuder	HPLC	30	0.001
Hexanesulfonic acid[c]	Impinger	IC	5–300	0.2–0.6[d]

[a]Primary, secondary, and tertiary amines.
[b]Primary and secondary amines.
[c]Methylethanolamine, diethanolamine, and triethanolamine.
[d]Lower limit of working range; better suited to area sampling than to personal sampling.
Abbreviations: GC, gas chromatography; HPLC, high-perfomance liquid chromatography; LOD, limit of detection; IC, ionic chromatography.

depending on whether it is heated below (as in paint and varnish application) or above its decomposition temperature of about 200°C (as in welding).

A method has been published for analyzing abietic acid and dehydroabietic acid in technical products (76). In this paper, reference is made to other methods such as GC and HPLC in effluents, shellac, and tall oil. However, measurements of abietic acid concentrations in the air when colophony is used do not seem to have been published.

In soldering or other similar uses, colophony is heated to high temperature and partly decomposed into fumes containing CO, CO$_2$, methane, ethylene, methanol, isopropyl alcohol, ketones, aldehydes, hydrocarbons, and terpenes. Historically,

Table 5 Sampling and Analysis of Aromatic Amines in the Air

Methods (Refs.)	Sampling	Analysis	Sampling volume (L)	LOD (mg/m^3)
Underivatized[a]	Silica gel adsorbent (71)	GC	3–150[c]	1.3–9[c,d]
	Filters and adsorbent tube (72)	GC	500	0.005–0.080[c]
Acetic anhydride[b] (73)	Acid-coated glass-fiber filter	HPLC	200	1.8–4.5[c,d]
Pentafluoropropionic anhydride[b] (74)	Acid-coated glass-fiber filter	GC–MS	500	0.001
Heptafluorobutyryl chloride[b] (75)	HCl bubbler	GC	1	0.0002

[a]Primary, secondary, and tertiary amines.
[b]Primary amines.
[c]Depending on the given amine.
[d]Low values in the working range.
Abbreviations: GC, gas chromatography; HPLC, high-performance liquid chromatography; LOD, limit of detection; MS, mass spectrometry.

because of the complexity of the mixture, formaldehyde has been used as a tracer to monitor exposure, even though it has been shown (77) to be a minor component of the soldering fumes. Obviously, such results should not be used to extrapolate on a dose–effect relationship with formaldehyde. Sampling of total fumes with determination of their concentration by gravimetry could be used for an overall evaluation of all fumes and dust produced during soldering. This method, while being relatively simple and economical, is uninformative due to its lack of specificity and its high LOD.

Metals

The concentration of airborne metals or inorganic metallic compounds is usually determined by sampling inhalable dust on a filter and analyzing its metallic content by AAS, ICP, or a variety of other techniques. For metals that have been reported as causing sensitization (Pt, Co, W, Ni, and Cr), industrial hygiene samples are collected on mixed cellulose ester filters and analyzed by atomic emission spectroscopy (AES) or ICP-AES. Using AAS, the LOD has been reported as being $0.011 \, mg/m^3$ for a 180-L sampling volume (78), and with ICP, $0.005 \, mg/m^3$ for a 500-L sampling volume (79). Because of the variation in carcinogenicity of some of their derivatives, Cr and Ni are often analyzed by analytical methods that can specify the oxidation state of the metallic elements, such as sampling on filter, and analysis by colorimetry or by IC. However, there is no published information on the variation in sensitization potency of different derivatives of Cr and Ni.

Other Substances

In the assessment of industrial hygiene, the sampling and analytical methods for other substances are well developed and could be used for OA studies. Methacrylates have been sampled on thermal desorption tubes with Tenax and analyzed by GC (80). Inorganic acids can be sampled on silica gel tubes and analyzed by IC. Fibers can be collected on filters, identified, and analyzed by transmission electron microscopy. Cutting oils such as mineral oils could be sampled on filters and analyzed by IR spectrometry for low-molecular-weight constituents. Soluble metal-working fluids could be subjected to sampling and analysis of the amines or nitroso derivatives that they may contain. However, the presence of microorganisms should also be considered. Compounds such as azobisformamide, chloramine T, ammonium persulfate, diazonium salts, and dyes would require extensive efforts in analytical method development.

CONCLUSION AND RESEARCH NEEDS

Although not exhaustive, this review of the chemical monitoring of agents that induce OA emphasizes the progress being made in developing highly sensitive detection methods for certain compounds such as diisocyanates, formaldehyde, and anhydrides. When a low-molecular-weight compound is identified or suspected as an asthma agent, it is possible to develop analytical methods that will meet the stringent requirements of low concentration detectability and short exposure duration applicable to the evaluation of OA. Analytical methods covering a wider range of applications than the routinely used methods validated for industrial hygiene, and sampling strategies adapted to establish dose–effect relationships both for the sensitization and the eventual evolution to chronicity of sensitized workers, should improve the prevention of OA. The monitoring of some families of compounds such as amines and aldehydes (other than formaldehyde) has not been significantly improved in the last five years.

The monitoring of chemical agents by direct-reading instruments is achievable in generation chambers used to perform the specific bronchoprovocation of individuals (Chapter 10). In this application, the atmosphere to be tested should have been chemically predefined; this allows the use of specialized instruments tailored to the specific requirements of the provocation test underway. Direct-reading instruments have to be used with caution on worksites because of the variability in the environments and the complexity of the matrices from other pollutants, which can cause interference.

Biological exposure monitoring and early indicators of lesion (not covered in this chapter) suggest future medical surveillance applications. However, these tests have still not been validated for use in managing asthma prevention.

REFERENCES

1. Bernstein L. Occupational asthma. Clin Chest Med 1981; 2(2):255–272.
2. Parkes WR. Occupational Lung Disorders. 3d ed. Oxford: Butterworth-Heinemann Ltd., 1994:717.
3. Malo JL, Chan-Yeung M. Occupational asthma. J Allergy Clin Immunol 2001; 108: 317–328.
4. Malo JL. Compensation for occupational asthma in Quebec. Chest 1990; 98:236S–239S.
5. Nordman H. Occupational asthma: time for prevention. Scand J Work Environ Health 1994; 20:108–115 (special issue).
6. Goe SK, Henneberger PK, Reilly MJ, et al. A descriptive study of work aggravated asthma. Occup Environ Med 2004; 61:512–517.
7. Wagner JR, Wegman DH. Occupational asthma: prevention by definition. Am J Ind Med 1998; 33:427–429.
8. National Institute for Occupational Safety and Health (NIOSH). National Occupational Research Agenda. Asthma and chronic obstructive pulmonary disease. 1996; 10–11.
9. Bush RK. Occupational asthma from vegetable gums (editorial). J Allergy Clin Immunol 1990; 86:443–444.
10. Cloutier Y, Lagier F, Lemieux R, Blais MC, Cartier A, Malo JL. Improved methodology for specific inhalation challenges with occupational agents in powder form. Eur Respir J 1989; 2:769–777.
11. Reed EC, Swanson MC, Yuginger JW. Measurements of allergen concentration in the air as an aid in controlling exposure to aeroallergens. J Allergy Clin Immunol 1986; 78: 1028–1030.
12. Newman-Taylor A, Tee RD. Environmental and occupational asthma: exposure assessment. Chest 1990; 98:209S–211S.
13. Grammer LC, Shaughnessy MA, Henderson J, et al. A clinical and immunologic study of workers with trimellitic-anhydride-induced immunologic lung disease after transfer to low exposure jobs. Am Rev Respir Dis 1993; 148:54–57.
14. Cullinan P, Lowson D, Nieuwenhuijsen MJ, et al. Work related symptoms, sensitisation, and estimated exposure in workers not previously exposed to flour. Occup Environ Med 1994; 51:579–583.
15. Rattray NJ, Botham BA, Hext PM, et al. Induction of respiratory hypersensitivity to diphenylmethane-4,4′diisocyanyate (MDI) in guinea pigs. Influence of route of exposure. Toxicology 1994; 88:15–30.

16. Piirila P, Estlander T, Keskinen H, et al. Occupational asthma caused by triglycidyl isocyanurate (TGIC). Clin Exp Allergy 1997; 25:510–514.

17. American Conference of Governmental Industrial Hygienists (ACGIH). Particle Size-Selective Sampling in the Workplace, Cincinnati, OH, 1985:4.

18. American Conference of Governmental Industrial Hygienists (ACGIH). 2004 TLVs and BEIs, Cincinnati, OH, 1996.

19. Bernstein JA. Overview of diisocyanate Occupational asthma. Toxicology 1996; 111: 181–189.

20. Baur X. Occupational asthma due to isocyanates. Lung 1996; 174:23–30.

21. Rosqvist S, Nielsen J, Welinder H, Rylander L, Lindh CH, Jönsson BA. Exposure-response relationships for hexahydrophthalic and methylhexahydrophthalic anhydrides with total plasma protein adducts as biomarkers. Scand J Work Environ Health 2003; 29(4):297–303.

22. Dharmarajan V, Lingg RD, Booth KS Hackathorn DR. Recent developments in the sampling and analysis of isocyanates in air. ASTM Special Technical Publication #957, Philadelphia, 1987; 190–202.

23. Brown RH, Ellwood PA, Groves JA, Robertson SM. New methods for the determination of airborne isocyanates. London: Occupational Hygiene Laboratory, 1987:1–8.

24. Lesage J, Perrault G. Caractérisation physique et chimique de l'exposition des travailleurs aux isocyanates. Annexe au rapport de recherche. Institut de recherche en santé et en sécurité du travail, Montréal, Canada, 1989.

25. Gagné S, Lesage J, Ostiguy C, Van Tra H. Determination of unreacted 2,4-toluene diisocyanate (2,4TDI) and 2,6-toluene diisocyanate (2,6TDI) in foams at ultratrace level by using HPLC-CIS-MS-MS. Analyst 2003; 128(12):1447–1451.

26. Health and Safety Executive (HSE). Methods for the determination of hazardous substances. 3d ed. Organic Isocyanates in Air Method 25/3, Sheffield, England, 1999.

27. Institut de recherche Robert-Sauvé en santé et en sécurité du travail (IRSST). Analyse du diisocyanate d'hexaméthylène-1,6 (HDI) dans l'air sous forme gazeuse, 3rd ed. Canada: Montréal, 1999; 224–233.

28. Institut de recherche Robert-Sauvé en santé et en sécurité du travail (IRSST). Analyse du diisocyanate d'hexaméthylène-1,6 (HDI) dans l'air sous forme aérosol, 2nd ed. Canada: Montréal, 1999; 234–242.

29. American Society for Testing and Materials (ASTM). Standard test method for determination of gaseous hexamethylene diisocyanate (HDI) in air with 9-(N-methylaminomethyl) anthracene method (MAMA) in the Workplace, Method D6562-00, West Conshohocken, PA, 2000.

30. American Society for Testing and Materials (ASTM). Standard test method for determination of 2,4-toluene diisocyanate (2,4-TDI) and 2,6-toluene diisocyanate (2,6-TDI) in Air (with 9-(N-methylaminomethyl)anthracene method) (MAMA) in the workplace, Method D5932-96, West Conshohocken, PA, 2000.

31. National Institute for Occupational Safety and Health (NIOSH). Manual of Analytical Methods, 4th ed., Isocyanates, Total (MAP), Method 5525, Cincinnati, OH, 2003.

32. Karlsson D, Spanne M, Dalene M, Skarping G. Determination of complex mixtures of airborne isocyanates and amines: Part 4. Determination of aliphatic isocyanates as dibutylamine derivatives using liquid chromatography and mass spectrometry. Analyst 1998; 123:117–123.

33. Dalene M, Mathiasson L, Skarping G, Sango C, Sandstrom JF. Trace analysis of airborne aromatic isocyanates and related aminoisocyanates and diamines using high-performance liquid chromatography with ultraviolet and electrochemical detection. Chromatography 1988; 20:469–481.

34. Simon P, Moulut O. Separation of the urea piperazine derivatives of polyisocyanate monomers and prepolymers by normal phase chromatography. J Liq Chromatogr 1988; 11:2071–2089.

35. Schmidtke F, Seifert B. A highly sensitive high-performance liquid chromatographic procedure for the determination of isocyanates in air. Fresenius J Anal Chem 1990; 336: 647–654.

36. Streicher RP, Arnold JE, Ernst MK, Cooper CV. Development of a novel derivatization reagent for the sampling and analysis of total isocyanate groups in air and comparison of its performance with that of several established reagents. Am Ind Hyg Assoc J 1996; 57:905–913.

37. Rudzinski WE, Norman S, Dahlquist B, et al. Evaluation of 1-(9-anthracenylmethyl) piperazine for the analysis of isocyanates in spray-painting operations. Am Ind Hyg Assoc J 1996; 57:914–917.

38. Lesage J, Goyer N, Desjardins F, Vincent JY, Perrault G. Workers' exposure to isocyanates. Am Ind Hyg Assoc J 1992; 53:146–153.

39. Lesage J, Perrault G. Sampling Device and Method for its Use. U.S. patent #4,961,916; October 9, 1990, Canadian patent #1299114, July 21, 1992.

40. Rando RJ, Poovey, HG. Dichotomous sampling of vapor and aerosol of methylene-bis-(phenylisocyanate) [MDI] with an annular diffusional denuder. Am Ind Hyg Assoc J 1994; 55:716–721.

41. Streicher RP, Kennedy ER, Lorberau CD. Strategies for the simultaneous collection of vapours and aerosols with emphasis on isocyanate sampling. Analyst 1994; 119:89–97.

42. Boutin M, Lesage J, Ostiguy C, Bertrand MJ. Comparison of EI and metastable atom bombardment ionization for the identification of polyurethane thermal degradation products. J Anal Appl Pyrolysis 2003; 70:505–517.

43. Boutin M, Lesage J, Ostiguy C, Pauluhn J, Bertrand MJ. Identification of the isocyanates generated during the thermal degradation of a polyurethane car paint. J Anal Appl Pyrolysis 2004; 71:791–802.

44. Lind P, Dalene M, Lindstrom V, Grubb A, Skarping G. Albumin adducts in plasma from workers exposed to toluene diisocyanate. Analyst 1997; 122:151–154.

45. Dalene M, Skarping G, Lind P. Workers exposed to thermal degradation products of TDI- and MDI-based polyurethane: biomonitoring of 2,4-TDA, 2,6-TDA, and 4,4'-MDA in hydrolyzed urine and plasma. Am Ind Hyg Assoc J 1997; 58:587–591.

46. de Andrade JF, Fatibello-Filho O, Suleiman AA, Guilbault GG. A coated piezoelectric crystal sensor for the determination of 2,4-toluene diisocyanate in air. Anal Lett 1989; 22:2601–2611.

47. National Institute for Occupational Safety and Health (NIOSH). Manual of Analytical Methods, Cincinnati, OH. Method 3512 (Maleic anhydride), 3506 (Acetic anhydride) and 5036 (Trimellitic anhydride). http://www.cdc.gov/niosh/nmam/method-4000.html.

48. Nielsen J, Welinder H, Jönsson B, Axmon A, Rylander L, Skerfving S. Exposure to hexahydrophthalic and methylhexahydrophthalic anhydrides—dose-response for sensitisation and airway effects. Scand J Work Environ Health 2001; 27(5):327–334.

49. Drexler H, Jönsson BAG, Göen T, Nielsen J, Lakemeyer M, Welinder H. Exposure assessment and sensitisation to organic anhydrides. Int Arch Occup Health 2000; 73: 228–234.

50. Occupational Safety and Health Administration. Chemical Data for Workplace Sampling & Analysis: OSHA's, Method 90, Phthalic anhydride (October 1991) and Method 98, Trimellitic anhydride (November 1992). http://www.osha.gov/dts/sltc/methods/organic/org090/org090.html.

51. Jönsson B, Lindh C. Determination of hexahydrophthalic and methylhexahydrophthalic acids in urine by gas chromatography-negative-ion chemical ionisation mass spectrometry. Chromatographia 1996; 42:647–652.

52. Rosqvist S, Johannesson G, Lindh C, Jönsson B. Total plasma protein adducts of allergenic hexahydrophthalic and methylhexahydrophthalic anhydrides as biomarkers of long-term exposure. Scand J Work Environ Health 2001; 27(2):133–139.

53. Kennedy ER, Teass AW, Gagnon YT. Industrial hygiene sampling and analytical methods for formaldehyde. In: Tureski V, ed. Formaldehyde: Analytical Chemistry and Technology. Washington, D.C.: American Chemical Society, 1985.

54. Occupational Safety and Health Administration. Chemical Data for Workplace Sampling & Analysis: OSHA's Chemical Information File, Method OSHA 52, 1996.

55. National Institute for Occupational Safety and Health (NIOSH). Manual of Analytical Methods, 3rd ed. Formaldehyde Method 2541, 2016, 2018, 2039 (2003) Cincinnati, OH, 1994.

56. National Institute for Occupational Safety and Health (NIOSH). Manual of Analytical Methods. 3rd ed. Method 5700, Cincinnati, OH, 1994.

57. Vairavamurthy A, Roberts JM, Newman L. Methods for determination of low molecular weight carbonyl compounds in the atmosphere: a review. Atmos Environ 1992; 26A: 1965–1993.

58. American Conference of Governmental Industrial Hygienists (ACGIH). Air Sampling Instruments for Evaluation of Atmospheric Contaminants. 7th ed. ACGIH, Cincinnati, OH, 1989:549–573.

59. Kirollos KS, Mihaylov GM, Chapman KB. Direct-read, Passive, Glutaraldehyde STEL Monitoring System. U.S. patent # 5364593.

60. Boutin M, Lesage J, Ostiguy C, Bertrand MJ. Investigating the thermal degradation of polymers: a systematic approach. Appl Occup Environ Hyg 2003; 18:724–728.

61. Wilson PM, La DK, Froines JR. Hemoglobin and DNA adduct formation in Fischer-344 rats exposed to 2,4- and 2,6-toluene diamine. Arch Toxicol 1996; 70:591–598.

62. Blome H, Hennig M. Dosage des amines aliphatiques et aromatiques dans l'air. Cahier de notes domcumentaires de l'Institut national de recherche en sécurité. N.D 1984; 1572:122–186.

63. Andersson B, Andersson K. Air sampling of N-methylmorpholine on solid sorbent and determination by capillary gas chromatography and a nitrogen-phosphorus detector. Anal Chem 1986; 58:1527–1529.

64. National Institute for Occupational Safety and Health (NIOSH). Manual of Analytical Methods. 4th ed. Amines, aliphatic Method 2010 Cincinnati, OH, 1994.

65. Chou TY, Colgan T, Kao DM, Krull IA. Pre-chromatographic derivatization of primary and secondary amines with a polymeric anhydride for improved high-performance liquid chromatographic detection. J Chromatogr 1986; 367:335–344.

66. Gao CX, Krull IS, Trainor UM. Determination of volatile amines in air by on-line solid-phase high-performance liquid chromatography with ultraviolet and fluorescence detection. J Chromtogr 1989; 463:192–200.

67. Jedrzejczak K, Gaind VS. Polymers with reactive functions as sampling and derivatizing agents. Part 1. Effective sampling and simultaneous derivatization of an airborne amine. Analyst 1990; 115:1359–1362.

68. Levin JO, Andersson K, Fängmark I, Hallgren C. Determination of gaseous and particulate polyamines in air using sorbent and filter coated with naphthylisothiocyanate. Appl Ind Hyg 1989; 4:98–100.

69. Levin JO, Lindhal R, Andersson K, Hallgren C. High-performance liquid chromatographic determination of diethylamine in air using diffusive sampling and thiourea formation. Chemosphere 1989; 18:2121–2129.

70. Levin JO, Andersson K, Hallgren, C. Determination of monoethanolamine and diethanolamine in air. Ann Occup Hyg 1989; 33:175–180.

71. National Institute for Occupational Safety and Health (NIOSH). Manual of Analytical Methods. 3d ed. Amines, Aromatic. Method 2002, Cincinnati, OH, 1994.

72. Otson R, Leach JM, Chung TK. Sampling of airborne aromatic amines. Anal Chem 1987; 50:58–62.

73. Gunderson EC, Anderson CC. A sampling and analytical method for airborne m-phenylenediamine (MPDA) and 4,4'-methylenedianiline (MDA). Am Ind Hyg Assoc J 1988; 49: 531–538.

74. Roussel R, Gaboury A, Larivière C. Aromatic amines in the workplace of an aluminum smelter. In: Rooy EL, ed. Light Metals. Warrendale, Pennsylvania: The Minerals, Metals & Materials Society, 1991:503–507.

75. Meddle DW, Smith AF. Field method for the determination of aromatic primary amines in air. Part I. Generation of standard atmospheres of amines. Analyst 1981; 106:1082–1087.

76. Ehrin E, Karlberg AT. Detection of rosin (colophony) components in technical products using an HPLC technique. Contact Dermatitis 1990; 23:359–366.

77. Cassebras M, Rolin A. Fils à souder à flux incorporé. Nuisances chimiques lors de la mise en oeuvre. Cahier des notes documentaires de l'Institut National de Recherche en Sécurité (France). ND 1984; 1492:116–184.

78. Institut de recherche en santé et en sécurité du travail (IRSST). Méthodes analytiques. Méthodes 2-2 (Co), Méthodes 3-1 (Cr), Méthodes 10-2 (Ni), Montréal, Canada, 1990.

79. National Institute for Occupational Safety and Health (NIOSH). Manual of Analytical Methods, 4th ed., Elements by ICP. Method 7300, Cincinnati, OH, 1994.

80. Henriks-Eckerman ML, Alanko K, Jolanki R, Kerosmo H, Kanerva L. Exposure to airborne methacrylates and natural rubber latex allergens in dental clinics. J Environ Monit 2001; 3:302–305.

14

Medicolegal Aspects, Compensation Aspects, and Evaluation of Impairment/Disability

I. Leonard Bernstein
Division of Allergy–Immunology, Department of Internal Medicine, College of Medicine, University of Cincinnati, Cincinnati, Ohio, U.S.A.

Helena Keskinen
Finnish Institute of Occupational Health, Helsinki, Finland

Paul D. Blanc
Division of Occupational and Environmental Medicine, Department of Medicine, University of California–San Francisco, San Francisco, California, U.S.A.

Moira Chan-Yeung
Occupational and Environmental Lung Disease Unit, Respiratory Division, Department of Medicine, University of British Columbia and Vancouver General Hospital, Vancouver, British Columbia, Canada

Jean-Luc Malo
Department of Chest Medicine, Université de Montréal and Sacré-Cœur Hospital, Montreal, Quebec, Canada

INTRODUCTION—BACKGROUND

As a prelude to a discussion of compensation issues specifically concerned with occupational asthma (OA), it is useful to review how occupational diseases per se evolved from the pre-eminence of injury as a raison d'être for workers' disability and compensation. The concept of protecting workers from the consequences of occupational disease—as contrasted to occupational injury—is a relatively recent development among industrial countries. In the late 19th century, middle European countries, starting with Switzerland, Germany, and Austria, began to compensate workers for work-related injuries (1). Similar legislation appeared in Britain in the first decade of the 20th century. This change is reflected in the transformation of the names given to agencies that are responsible for compensation. For example, in Quebec, the first name of the agency was Commission of Labor Injuries ("Commission des accidents de travail"), and it was only in 1980 that the name of the agency became Commission of Health and Security at Work ("Commission de la santé et sécurité du travail") (2). In the United States, workers' compensation legislation was under the purview of individual states, thereby resulting in a heterogeneity of disease definitions, covered diseases, exposure criteria, and other inconsistencies that still exist. Apart from three separate federal systems administered under the Federal Coal Mine Health and Safety Act of 1969, the Longshoreman's and Harbor Worker's Compensation Act, and the Federal Employees Compensation Act, there are no uniform governmental standards in the United States to guide individual state compensation disability programs. The first compensation laws adopted by individual states restricted compensation to those diseases caused by accidental injuries. These were modeled after the original British Workers' Compensation Statute of 1897. Massachusetts was the first state to extend legislation allowing for the compensation of "nontraumatic" occupational diseases. In 1920, New York State adopted the first schedule of compensable occupational diseases (3,4). California rapidly followed suit, and by the early 1930s, most states had passed workers' compensation laws concerning occupational diseases, although few of these provided broad coverage for many of the occupational diseases then being reported.

The impetus for compensation coverage of respiratory diseases was heightened in the early 1930s by the large number of claims for dust-induced diseases, particularly silicosis in coal mining and subsequently asbestosis in producing countries such as Canada (1). In that economically depressed era, many large suits were being awarded through the common law tort system. Coincidentally, the public was alerted to a major industrial disease calamity, which occurred when hundreds of workers succumbed to fatal doses of inhaled silica dust such as in a tunneling project at Gauley Bridge, West Virginia (5,6). Similar events were reported in other industrial countries. These disasters catalyzed lobbying by both employers and unions for legislative compensation relief in several states and countries, which subsequently culminated in special workers' compensation legislation dealing specifically with pneumoconiotic disease such as the "dust funds" in the United States (7). Although there subsequently was considerable variability in the recognition of other types of occupational legislation from country to country, from state to state, or from province to province, by 1978 every state in the United States had provided workers' compensation for disability resulting from this category of disease (5). Thus the thrust of workers' compensation disease legislation was focused primarily on dust-induced entities such as silicosis and asbestosis as well as respiratory conditions due to toxic agents. The possibility that OA might also require special legislative attention had not yet surfaced in most states and countries. Given that asthma had long been considered a benign "stressed-induced" condition by comparison with other chest diseases such as dust-induced pneumoconiosis that often led to respiratory failure and death, compensation for OA was neglected for many years. For years, it was common medical opinion that workers could not be affected with OA if they were not exposed to a dusty environment at work. In this context, bringing, for example, the rather new message that nurses working in "clean" hospitals could often be affected with OA seemed a rather challenging opinion.

As occupational diseases were gradually incorporated into the matrix of industrial compensation, it became apparent—in contrast to occupational injuries—that the legislative approach to such problems would be greatly influenced by special circumstances leading to the illness (1). For conditions such as asthma, specific etiological factors cannot always be demonstrated, and multiple-factor causality (e.g., interaction with atopy, cigarette smoking) frequently complicated the situation. To address these issues, special schedules or tables of specific diseases, occupations, and etiological agents were established by Euro-Canadian compensation agencies as well as several states in the United States. Because such lists were deemed to be overly restrictive and were generally not amended in a timely manner when new scientific evidence mandated a change, many agencies eventually abandoned the use of scheduling for occupational diseases. It seems reasonable to abandon referral to lists of at risk occupations and causal agents (it is indeed not because workers have asthma and they are exposed to an agent present on a list that this means they suffer from OA), provided that diagnostic tools allow for establishing the relationship of exposure to an agent or in a workplace and onset of asthma. Today, when expensive and sophisticated diagnostic methods are available for most health conditions, OA too often remains undiagnosed and incorrectly or insufficiently investigated by clinical and functional means (8). Medicolegal decisions are often made without objective medical evidence. Unfortunately, this is often the case in countries where the medicolegal system is more legal than medical.

When diagnostic approaches are inaccurate and not readily available outside large centers or recognition of the work relatedness of a presenting condition by the medical community is poor, occupational disease may not be identified and therefore not reported with all the health consequences of worsening of asthma (9). On the other hand, ignorance about appropriate diagnostic techniques necessary to confirm a disease may result in unwarranted claims and socioeconomic consequences of advising workers to leave their workplace. "Pragmatic" interactions of socioeconomic and political stresses may result in restriction of the scope of coverage or the clinical recognition of a particular occupational disease (10). The following definition of occupational disease used by the Nebraska compensation system contains many elements in common with other state definitions: "The term 'occupational disease' shall mean only a disease which is due to causes and conditions which are characteristic of and peculiar to a particular trade, occupation, process, or employment, and shall exclude all ordinary diseases of life to which the general public are exposed" (3).

Exacerbation or acceleration of preexisting conditions adds to the complexity of what constitutes an occupational disease. If a disease is rare and is due to a claimant's allergy in combination with workplace exposures, it will usually be held to be work related if the "increased exposure occasioned by employment in fact brought on the disease" (3). Placing time limitations on occupational diseases may overlook certain diseases (e.g., asbestos-induced mesothelioma), which develop only after a lengthy latency period, a situation which is frequent in the case of OA with a latency period. Many state laws also stipulate that the worker must have been on the job for a "somewhat extended period." Finally, the definition of an occupational disease often includes a minimum exposure rule in an attempt to exclude the frequently confounding variable of a concurrent "ordinary life disease." This situation is of concern in cases of irritant-induced asthma (IIA) which may occur at the time of a very first exposure in a workplace due to an inhalational accident. Many of the above issues impact on the diagnosis of OA and will be discussed in greater detail in the following section.

CURRENT STATE OF THE COMPENSATION SYSTEM FOR ASTHMA IN THE UNITED STATES

In the United States, the principle underlying workers' compensation is that of a "no-fault insurance system" in which employees waive their common law right to sue their employers for damages in exchange for income, medical benefits, and rehabilitation services paid for by private or state government insurers (5).

Regulations and policies governing compensation for OA vary from state to state. Reliable prevalence and incidence statistics are not available for most states. This is chiefly due to the varied manner in which workers' compensation programs define OA and the fact that most states do not keep accurate statistics of asthma as a distinct disease entity. The majority of states employ the American National Standards Institute (ANSI) nature of disease coding as specified by the supplementary data system of disease reporting instituted by the United States Department of Labor. Under this coding system, asthma is included with a number of other unrelated diseases such as influenza, bronchitis, emphysema, and pneumonia. Currently, ANSI specifies two codes for asthma embedded within broad classes of disease: (i) systemic poisoning (from inhalation, ingestion, etc.) (code 274), and (ii) conditions of the respiratory system (code 572). Thirty-one states maintain workers' compensation claims in machine-readable format that would permit retrieval of asthma data if there were a single code for that condition (7). With appropriate coding, compensation claims have proven to be a valuable tool for occupational disease surveillance (11,12). Secondary data sources such as death certificates and hospital discharge summaries have not served as reliable sources of disability induced by OA (7,13,14).

A retrospective analysis of the 1978 Social Security Disability Survey yielded interesting data about the contribution of workplace exposures to the prevalence of asthma in adults (15). In this study, an affirmative response to the question, "Was this condition caused by bad working conditions, such as noise, heat, or smoke?", met the case definition of work relatedness for any given disease. This question was asked for each identified condition in the survey so as not to create bias, and the questionnaire elicited information concerning the respondent's occupational history. The presence of asthma coupled with an affirmative answer to the question quoted above was accepted as occupationally related asthma for the epidemiological purpose of this study. Seventy-two (1.2%) of 6063 respondents, or 15.4% of all those with asthma attributed asthmatic symptoms to workplace exposures. These subjects were older and included more men, cigarette smokers, and former smokers. The relative risk for occupationally attributed asthma was elevated among industrial and agricultural workers as compared to white-collar and service occupations. Analysis of disability benefit status among various cohorts of this survey did not indicate that this method of analysis introduced major reporting bias. It was therefore concluded that the high prevalence of occupationally self-attributed asthma in this study was a valid observation.

Estimated prevalence and risk factors of OA were recently identified for both work-related wheezing and asthma as part of the third National Health and Nurition Examination Survey (NHANES), 1988–1994 (16). The questionnaire of this study included 28 major industries. These industry codes were specific for this study and cannot be extrapolated with the database of the National Occupational Exposure Survey (NOES) which utilized a Standard Industrial Classification index (17). In the NHANES study population the estimated prevalences of work-related asthma and work-related wheezing were 3.7% and 11.5%, respectively. Twofold or greater increases in odds ratios of work-related asthma were found for many industries but were significantly increased only for the entertainment industry (16). With respect to work-related wheezing, significant increases of odds ratios were shown for agriculture, forestry and fishing, construction, electrical machinery, repair services, and lodging places. Of particular interest in this study were exposures in entertainment (art media, stage settings, productions, makeup, and photographic chemicals) and educational (indoor allergens) industries.

Individual annual reporting systems from states that acquire such information have demonstrated different associations (18). For example, in California, among the estimated annual rate of 75 cases of OA/million workers, janitors/cleaners and firefighters had reporting ratios of 625/million and 300/million, respectively. In addition, half of all work-related asthma cases were associated with agents not known to be allergens.

Annual prevalence data of OA derived from workers' compensation claims are just beginning to appear from several states that are recollating OA cases from Doctors' First Report Forms or that are participating in the sentinel event notification system for occupational risks (SENSOR) instituted by the National Institute for Occupational Safety and Health (NIOSH) in 1987 (Table 1) (14,19). Wisconsin, New York, and Colorado participated in SENSOR from 1987 to 1992. Massachusetts, Michigan, and New Jersey have been in the program from 1987 to the present while California has been a participant since 1992. Although there is a considerable variation among states reporting these data, it is interesting that the number of reported cases of OA and reactive airways dysfunction syndrome (RADS) has exceeded the total number of dust diseases of the lungs in the United States, as self-reported by respondents in the 1988 National Health Interview Survey (NHIS) (20). The OA database contained in Table 1 illustrates how difficult it is to make interstate comparisons. For example, the marked trend of reduced OA reports from New Jersey has not occurred in the other states, although there may be a leveling-off trend. Asthma case data for California are based on Doctors' First Reports of Occupational Injury of Illness Forms. In Massachusetts and New Jersey, workers' compensation cases are based upon physician reports and hospital discharge data. The data shown for Michigan are based on physician reports, hospital discharge information, worker's compensation claims, regulatory agency information, and index case follow-up investigations. Table 2 is a compilation of the most frequently reported agents associated with new onset asthma as reported by the four current SENSOR programs (California, Massachusetts, Michigan, and New Jersey) from 1993 to 2003. Particularly noteworthy are the relatively high number of asthma cases associated with indoor pollutants and cleaning materials. Although the SENSOR system was not designed to be a comprehensive surveillance system, it has led to reports of previously unrecognized causes of OA (21). Moreover, the use of surveillance data may have been instrumental in detection of additional symptomatic coworkers and inadequate work practices. The goal of the current four state SENSOR program is to develop a prototypic surveillance system which could be used as a model for other states and territories (21).

MEDICOLEGAL DEFINITIONS OF OA

Many of the key problems associated with the definition of occupational disease also apply to OA (1). These include (*i*) multiple causality, (*ii*) availability of reliable objective tests, (*iii*) distinguishing between elicitation of OA (preexisting) and induction of OA (persistent), and (*iv*) variability of legal adjudication of OA claims.

Multiple Causality

Etiological factors are not always readily identifiable, especially by nonoccupationally trained, primary care practitioners. Under these circumstances, several U.S.

Table 1 Number of Cases of OA and RADS by State—California, Massachusetts, Michigan, and New Jersey SENSOR WRA Programs, 1988–2003

Year	California[a] OA	RADS	Massachusetts[b] OA	RADS	Michigan[c] OA	RADS	New Jersey[d] OA	RADS
1988	–	–	–	–	31	1	23	–
1989	–	–	–	–	63	5	26	3
1990	–	–	–	–	144	8	40	9
1991	–	–	–	–	115	16	44	3
1992	–	–	–	–	150	18	30	6
1993	139	11	45	–	176	19	65	26
1994	131	9	39	–	152	13	32	6
1995	143	5	37	24	127	17	31	7
1996	142	7	48	–	155	11	31	5
1997	136	10	54	5	162	16	35	9
1998	134	12	29	6	147	9	28	1
1999	138	10	31	1	141	12	3	0
2000	232	11	26	7	164	17	6	1
2001	256	9	34	4	139	18	5	0
2002	193	9	20	3	127	18	7	2
2003	(117)	(11)	(29)	(10)	(81)	(4)	6	1
Subtotals	1761	104	392	60	2,074	202	412	79
Totals	1865		452		2,276		491	

Note: This table includes provisional surveillance data as of December 2003. Data for 2003 are incomplete for several states. The OA cases included in this table represent OA and RADS cases that are identified by the state-based SENSOR asthma programs. Except for Michigan they do not include WEA (pre-existing asthma that has been exacerbated by exposures encountered in the workplace). –, Case counts not available for the specified year. Values inside parenthesis indicate data incomplete for the specified years.
[a]California data are based on DFR of occupational injury or illness.
[b]Massachusetts data are based on physician reports and cases identified through hospital discharge data. Potential cases from hospital discharge data have primary or secondary discharge diagnoses coded to ICD-9 493 (asthma) and report worker's compensation as the expected payer or ICD-9 506 (respiratory conditions due to chemical fumes and vapors) regardless of who the expected payer is.
[c]Michigan data are physician reports, hospital discharge information, worker's compensation claims, information obtained from regulatory agencies (Miner's Safety and Health Administration and the Occupational Safety and Health Administration), and index case follow-up investigations where coworkers of the index case are administered a symptom questionnaire that is reviewed by a physician. Coworkers with symptoms of work-related asthma are sent letters by the surveillance program informing of their questionnaire findings and encouraging them to seek medical evaluation of their symptoms. Hospital discharge data are searched for the same criteria used by New Jersey and Massachusetts.
[d]New Jersey data are based on physician reports and hospital discharge data. Hospital discharge data are searched for the same criteria as used by Michigan and Massachusetts.
Abbreviations: OA, occupational asthma; RADS, reactive airways dysfunction syndrome; WRA, work-related asthma; DFR, doctor's first reports; SENSOR, sentinel event notification system for occupational risks; WEA, work exacerbated asthma; ICD, international classification of disease.
Source: The information in this table was kindly supplied by the following agencies and professionals: California SENSOR WRA Program: Jennifer Flattery, MPH and Robert Harrison, M.D., MPH. Massachusetts SENSOR WRA Program: Elise Pechter, DPH and Letitia Davis, ScD. Michigan SENSOR WRA Program: Kenneth E. Rosenman, M.D. New Jersey SENSOR WRA Program: Katharine McGreevy, Ph.D. and David Valiante, MS.

Table 2   The 10 Most Frequent Reported Agents Associated with New Onset OA and RADS in Four SENSOR States, 1993–2003

Agents	Number of cases
Indoor pollutants	1047
Chemicals, NOS[a]	850
Polyisocyanates	350
Cleaning products	349
Metals and metal fluids	248
Smoke, NOS[a]	206
Exhaust fumes	133
Welding fumes	131
Dust, NOS[a]	124
Formaldehyde	84

[a]Not otherwise specified.
Abbreviations: OA, occupational asthma; RADS, reactive airways dysfunction syndrome; SENSOR, sentinel event notification system for occupational risks.
Source: The information in this table was kindly supplied by the following agencies and professionals: California SENSOR WRA Program: Jennifer Flattery, MPH and Robert Harrison, M.D., MPH. Massachusetts SENSOR WRA Program: Elise Pechter, DPH and Letitia Davis, ScD. Michigan SENSOR WRA Program: Kenneth E. Rosenman, M.D. New Jersey SENSOR WRA Program: Katharine McGreevy, Ph.D. and David Valiante, MS.

databases could provide essential information (NOES and NHANES). In addition, both workers and physicians need to be aware that they are entitled to have access to Material Safety Data Sheets on all substances to which they are exposed in the workplace.

Availability of Reliable Objective Tests

As discussed in more detail under *Impairment*, objective tests are essential for fair and objective evaluation of disability and adjudication of worker's compensation claims.

Preexistent and Persistent Asthma

Preexisting asthma may be exacerbated by conditions or substances at work. Exacerbation of asthma must clearly be distinguished from chronic, low-level exposure to specific sensitizers in the workplace or from IIA (or RADS) secondary to acute toxic exposures to nonsensitizing irritants such as gases and chemicals (21). Whether it is appropriate to include exacerbation of preexisting asthma in the disease category of OA is largely unsettled in the United States. Under the terms of the nosologic classification of OA described in Chapter 1, elicitation of symptoms by substances in the workplace in patients with preexisting asthma would be considered work-exacerbated asthma (WEA) (Chapter 26) and not in conformity with the definition of OA, which has to be induced de novo by work exposures to sensitizing or irritant substances. Many would argue that the designation of "preexisting" should require even further qualification (e.g., should this term include or exclude childhood asthma with complete remission since the childhood experience?). Some states (e.g., Pennsylvania, Michigan, and New York) clearly allow exacerbation of preexistent asthma as a compensable condition, but many states do not (5). However, under most circumstances, if aggravating stimuli are asthmogenic, it must be ascertained that they are peculiar to the workplace and not commonplace in the nonwork environment (1). In addition, a worker who is aware of preexisting asthma induced by known environmental insults (e.g., pollen) should not knowingly attempt to work under conditions that could predictably involve increased exposure to prior known allergens (22). Some states impose specified time limitations on occupational diseases (i.e., a worker would have to be exposed to a substance in a certain worksite for a given period of time, or at the other end of the spectrum, a claim would not be considered timely if there was a long latency period between initial exposure and first onset of symptoms) (5). Either situation could be unfair to a worker who develops occupationally induced airway obstruction and bronchial hyperresponsiveness. In the case of IIA, only a brief exposure is required and this could conceivably occur on the first or second day of work. On the other hand, it is not uncommon for workers in some industries (i.e., bakers) to work for many years before they actually develop symptoms due to one or more ingredients in flour. Another confounding variable is the increasing recognition that certain forms of OA, including IIA, may continue unabated for many years after cessation of exposure (23–28). Thus, the failure to improve or revert to normal status after the worker has been removed from the workplace is no longer a valid reason for a determination that the asthma was nonoccupational (29).

Despite the marked disparity in disposition of claims between OA and WEA among various Workers' Compensation Boards (WCBs), several groups of investigators have analyzed comparative data of these two specific entities. In Ontario, a Canadian province which approves awards for both OA and WEA, retrospective analysis of 469 occupationally related awards from 1984 to 1988 revealed an almost equal distribution between OA ($N = 235$) and WEA ($N = 234$) (30). The chief distinguishing feature between these groups was the clearing of symptoms in a shorter period of time in WEA, most probably a reflection of transient symptoms related to spills or temperature exposures to irritants. For workers with WEA, the most frequent triggers were paints, dust, and fumes (30). In the United States, SENSOR programs have provided a similar database but somewhat different results (31). Of 1101 cases of work-related asthma reported to SENSOR between 1993 and 1995, there were 891 (80.9%) and 210 (19.1%) cases of OA and WEA, respectively. Among the individuals whose WCB applications had been decided, there was a little difference between two groups in the percentage of claims awarded (77% for OA; 72% for WEA). This suggests a more lenient policy of WCBs in the four SENSOR states. It was also noted that the highest annual incidence rate for WEA was among workers within the public administration industry, which includes fire and police protection workers. Inasmuch as WEA is recognized under the mantra of OA in some states and countries, surveillance, prevention, and rehabilitation of WEA should be considered obligatory in the administrative mission of compensation.

Legal Adjudication of OA in the United States

While many states in the past have sought to limit the scope of compensation coverage for dust and respiratory diseases, restrictive regulations have not yet affected the diagnosis of OA. Some states still make it possible to include asthmatic disease under injury provisions (1). However, disputed questions of OA including formidable ones of diagnosis, causality, and disability are usually decided by litigation in an adversarial proceeding (5). Evidence from lay and expert witnesses is presented to adjudicators appointed by the compensation board. Because asthma may often be related to nonworkplace life exposures, tobacco smoking, and numerous irritants, it is estimated that 90% of these claims are litigated, often without success. Thus, of 242 workers' compensation claims filed for illnesses involving the respiratory system in the state of Washington for the period 1984 to 1988, 87 (36%) were rejected. This rate of rejection was higher than the average rate of rejection both for occupational diseases (18%) and for occupational injuries (4%). Those disease categories with the highest rates of rejection were those with the least well-developed diagnostic guidelines such as mental disorders (79%) and neoplasia (67%) (32). In some cases the success of this litigation often depends upon objective proof of causation, which in the case of OA may require controlled bronchial challenges. However, other factors such as the experience of the diagnosing physician with the rules of the compensation system may be a factor in the success of the claim (32).

Once a claim is allowed, complete medical care is provided and medical expenses are paid by either the self-insured employer or the state compensation fund for workers qualified under the respective programs (5). In most states, workers' compensation wage replacement equals two-thirds of workers' predisability wages but no more than a maximum determined from the statewide average weekly wage for the duration of disability. Compensation is provided for proven objective disability, not for impairment. Providing less than the complete compensation of wage loss is felt to serve as an incentive for healthy workers to avoid workplace injury and disease and for diseased workers to return to work, if at all possible. A particularly troubling feature of workers' compensation for occupational diseases in general is the small proportion (5%) of individuals who have a severe disability that resulted from a job-related exposure and rely on this system for benefits. According to a nationwide survey of disabled and nondisabled adults whose disability was the result of a job-related disease, the four primary sources of support were social security (53%), pensions (21%), veterans' benefits (17%), and public welfare (16%). It appears that the "safety net" in the United States may be social security, pension, and welfare systems (33). Rehabilitation and retraining programs are integral components of all state industrial programs. In the case of asthma, rehabilitation must be carried out with the goal of providing an environment free of future exposure to specific allergens and nonspecific aggravating agents.

Cost effective administration of any workers' compensation system requires adoption of a proactive rather than reactive attitude toward OA. Recognizing the potential hazards of specific agents [e.g., diisocyanates (DIISO)] and spills of many toxic agents, workers' compensation systems should expand efforts to emphasize the economic and worker health advantages of instituting appropriate exposure protection for OA and WEA (34). Educational programs should also be enhanced to encourage both worker and employer about the need for close medical surveillance and thorough diagnosis as soon as symptoms occur. Finally, once asthma occurs and compensation has been awarded, employees must receive adequate medical services and intensive counseling about not returning to work in their former employment. From the worker's point of view, well-structured and effective rehabilitation and educational (if necessary) programs are essential components of a disabled worker's health and economic readjustment.

OUTCOMES OF WORKERS COMPENSATED FOR WORK-RELATED ASTHMA

Approved worker's compensation claims are readily accessible as a reliable source of data relevant to outcome research of OA. These data have been utilized to determine risk of hospitalization, mortality, comparison of subgroups (i.e., OA vs. WEA), OA induced by specific agents, employability, and financial status of disabled workers.

Compared to a cohort of workers with musculoskeletal injuries, OA workers were more likely to be hospitalized for all causes [adjusted relative risk (RR 1.4), cardiovascular disease (RR 1.4), respiratory disease (RR 5.4), and asthma (RR 28)] (35). Those workers hospitalized for asthma were less likely to have had isocyanate-induced asthma compared to other asthma inducers. This was attributed to early diagnosis of the disease and removal from long-term exposure of workers to this chemical. Using the same worker's compensation OA database, there was a trend toward an excess risk of death from respiratory disease (RR 2.6) and, surprisingly, ischemic heart disease (RR 2.8) (36).

A retrospective analysis of worker's compensation claims of workers with sensitizer-induced OA and WEA revealed several interesting findings when accepted claims were reassessed two years after initial adjudication (37). Although complete clearing of asthma occurred in only 19%, 47% of workers had milder asthma. The prognosis was worse in workers exposed to spills without prior history of disease compared to OA and no prior history of asthma. Subsequently, a reanalysis of the same worker's compensation data set in another independent study revealed an important distinguishing feature between WEA (with previous asthma) and IIA (37,38). Workers identified as IIA had more prolonged symptoms after the exposure and were less likely to have returned to the same work environment as workers with WEA (30,37,38). A separate subanalysis of the same asthma workers' compensation cohort specifically with respect to DIISO claims was also reported (39). Compared to other causes of OA, these workers demonstrated shorter latent periods before onset, shorter duration of symptoms before diagnosis, and less atopic susceptibility. After a two-year reassessment, 73% of DIISO workers improved compared to 56% of OA induced by other agents. The better outcome of DIISO asthma was attributed to both early diagnosis and early removal from further exposure.

Compensation of OA claims has serious consequences for future income and financial status (40,41). For those workers filing a claim and receiving compensation, the risk of unemployment was as high as 54% (41). This was attributed to the relatively low level of education among workers who developed OA in this database. Not surprisingly, compensation was associated with loss of income because compensation rates are well below a worker's job income, and retraining possibilities for a new occupation are poor, especially in older workers (40,41).

THE INTERNATIONAL PERSPECTIVE

Reliance upon schedules or lists of covered diseases distinguishes workers' compensation systems in the United States from those in some industrialized countries in Europe (and some provinces in Canada) where compensation is allowed for all occupationally related diseases (1). In those countries relying upon schedules, if a claimant develops a disease within the scope of an approved schedule, there is a strong presumption that compensation will be allowed. On the other hand, if a worker claims for a disease not on the list, the presumption against compensation for that disease usually directs the worker to seek other sources of social assistance. In the United Kingdom and France, schedules are also used. Illustrations of representative lists of agents/exposures associated with OA in the United Kingdom and France are shown in Table 3 (42,43). Although the use of such restrictive lists of

Table 3 Agents Causing OA in the United Kingdom and France

United Kingdom
Platinum salts
Isocyanates
Epoxy resins
Colophony fumes
Proteolytic enzymes
Laboratory animals and insects
Grain (or flour dust)
Miscellaneous[a]
France
Aromatic amines (no. 13)
Phosphates, pyrophosphates, thiophophates (no. 34)
Tropical woods (no. 47)
Aromatic and alicyclic amines (no. 49)
Phenylhydrazine (no. 50)
Isocyanates (no. 62)
Enzymes (no. 63)

[a]Any occupational agent can be included if objective proof of causality is determined.
Abbreviation: OA, occupational asthma.
Source: Refs. 42, 43.

covered exposures may at first glance appear to be a harsh method of dealing with the socioeconomic hardships of an occupational disease, most of the countries in Western Europe and provinces in Canada have well-developed secondary sources of health and disability insurance that compensate at levels comparable to those if industrial compensation was allowed. To assure an even-handed approach when compensation is based upon restrictive lists of diseases, it is essential that these lists be upgraded at frequent intervals to accommodate the rapid pace of medical advancement in the field of OA. Inequalities in such systems could arise if, despite evolving medical evidence, legislative upgradings fail to materialize due to sociopolitical forces. However, as mentioned above, the great equalizer of these compensation systems outside the United States appears to be that sick and disabled workers have readily available alternative benefits (e.g., national health insurance, etc.) that may be equal to or only slightly less than workers' benefits (1). While these safety nets provide for greater opportunity for "full" compensation for the disabled worker, the true costs of occupational disease to industry are shifted to other insurance schemes. Questions of compensation faced by adjudication of industrial claims are less dramatic and compelling when an alternative compensation system is so readily available. In general, the experiences thus far in such countries suggest that when there are no disincentives to contesting a worker's claim, the incidence of occupational disease claims is not necessarily higher than in privately insured systems, particularly in regard to serious claims (1).

    Apart from the generally agreed upon use of specific lists for the presumptive diagnosis of OA, compensation systems outside the United States have considerable heterogeneity (1). Many of the international compensation systems have been discussed in a review and are summarized in Table 4 (34). In France, workers with occupational diseases have been compensated since 1919. Two official lists exist: one for farms and one for general employers. There is a table for each work-related disease, which includes a list of symptoms, an indication of workplaces where subjects may

Table 4 Review of Systems and Compensation for OA in Various Countries

	Who administers?	Who pays?	Is occupational asthma compensated?	Who examines cases?	How is the diagnosis made?	No. of cases per year	Permanent disability allocated?
Australia	Cases handled by court	Private insurers	Yes	Specialist	Multiple means	?	Yes
Belgium	National agency	Employers	Yes	Board of specialists	Multiple means	?	Yes
Brazil	National agency	Employers and government	Yes	Physician designated by the national agency	Multiple means	?	Yes
Bulgaria	National	Employers	Yes	Board of specialists	Multiple means	?	Yes
Canada							
Quebec	Agency	Employers	Yes	Specialists	Multiple means	50–70	Yes
Ontario	Agency	Employers	Yes	Specialists	Multiple means	60–80 (+60–80 cases of aggravation of asthma)	?
Finland	National agency	Employers/insurers	Yes	Specialists	Multiple means	304 (yr 2002)	Yes
France	Regional agencies	Employers	Yes	Social security practitioners	Multiple means	?	Yes
Italy	National	Employers	Yes	Board of specialists	Multiple means	167 (yr 2003)	Yes
New Zealand	National	Employers	Yes	Agency physician and claimant's M.D.	Variable	?	Yes

Norway	National agency and private insurance (compulsory)	Employers and private insurers	Yes	Specialist	Multiple means	174 (yr 2000)	Yes
Romania	National agency	Employers	Yes	Board of specialists	Multiple means	?	Yes
South Africa	National agency, mutual associations, major towns	Employers	Yes	Claimant's physician, medical advisory, panel	Multiple means	247 (yr 2002–2003)	Yes
South Korea	National agency	Employers and private insurers	Yes	Specialists	Multiple means	121/440,000 workers (yrs 1998–2002)	Yes
Spain	Governmental agency	Employer and governmental agency	Yes	Board of specialists	Multiple means	258–294 (yrs 2000–2003)	Yes
The Netherlands	No specific system	Employers and employees	No official acceptance	Board of chest physicians	Multiple means	?	No
United Kingdom	Governmental agency	General taxation	Yes	Career specialists for assessing occupational diseases	Variable	293 (yr 1991)	"prescribed disease provisions"
United States	No-fault insurance system	Employers	Yes	Variable (states)	Variable (states)	?	?

be exposed, and the minimum exposure (44). Compensation is awarded only if the symptoms and workplace are listed in the table. If a worker has a proven but unlisted occupational disease, for which compensation is not allowed, a claim must be made through a judiciary procedure. This is a rare occurrence, due to the complexity of the legal process. The listing system does not recognize all occupational diseases because they cannot be updated at regular intervals (43). In Belgium, compensation of occupational diseases is completely separated from that due to accidents in the workplace. The Belgian system removes the controversy between employers and workers over complex questions of etiology, diagnosis, and preexisting conditions by totally separating the financing of compensation and payment of benefits. Although asthma is not on the Belgian schedule of occupational illnesses, it is treated as an occupational disease when it occurs in workers exposed to certain hazards appearing in the schedule. However, some of these cases, such as exposure to flax, are conditioned by minimum exposure. Denmark now has a "mixed" private and state insurance system. Although compensation for asthma is usually linked to specified occupations or exposure, it is also recognized that disability may occur as a result of exposure to substances not on the current schedule. The Danish system is almost completely nonadversarial because there are ample social alternatives for workers with illnesses that are not compensable. The Workers' Compensation Program has been completely abolished in the Netherlands. If a worker is unable to return to work within one year, or his disability limits his ability to earn income, he is entitled to disablement insurance, which continues until he is fully cured, dies, or reaches the age of 65, at which time other pension arrangements supervene. How this broad and permissive program affects claims for OA is not yet clear.

In Finland all employees are insured in private insurance companies against occupational diseases. Of the self-employed workers, agricultural workers are entitled to compensation for an occupational disease. Voluntary insurance can be taken by other self-employed workers. An occupational disease is defined as "a disease caused mainly by a physical factor, a chemical substance, or a biological agent encountered in the work done under the contract of employment or as an 'agricultural entrepreneur.'" The diagnosis "requires such medical examination where there is sufficient knowledge on exposure in the work and where in the case of occupational diseases, a specialist in the field is in charge." A disease is to be deemed as occupational when the factor "is present in a person's work to such an extent that its exposure effect is sufficient to cause the disease in question, unless it is stated that the disease has been clearly caused by exposure outside the work." Table 5 gives figures for the number of new cases of OA with the type of agents. The diagnosis of OA in Finland is carried out by lung specialists in the central or university hospitals where the workers are usually sent by the plant physician. The Finnish Institute of

Table 5 Number of Cases of OA in Finland and Types of Agents

Year	1995	1996	1997	1998	1999	2000	2001	2002
New OA cases (total)	412	404	340	250	292	276	271	302
Cases caused by organic agents	334	343	289	212	234	213	206	222
Cases caused by chemicals	78	65	51	38	58	63	65	80

Abbreviation: OA, occupational asthma.

Occupational Health (FIOH) can also be consulted. The approximate annual number of new cases of OA reported to the Register of Occupational Diseases has been close to 400 but diminished lately (Table 5) (45). About 20% of these have been investigated at FIOH. A diagnosis of OA is made in about every third person investigated at FIOH for this suspected disease. When an occupational disease is suspected by a physician familiar with the exposure in the workplace, the insurance company is obligated to pay for the necessary diagnostic investigation. If the disease is accepted as occupational, the worker is entitled to several types of compensation, which are better than those obtained from national health insurance for a nonoccupational disease. This policy, combined with the fact that the investigations are free of charge, may create an increased incentive for the worker to claim occupational disease. Future costs of the disease, including medications, doctor's fees, travel expenses, rehabilitation programs as well as sick leave compensation, are totally paid. When the worker transfers to another, more suitable job without harmful exposure, but with a lower salary, the difference is largely compensated. If an occupational disease causes a permanent disability of more than 10%, a lump sum estimated to cover the harm caused by the disease is additionally paid according to the extent of the disability. When the occupational disease causes total disability, the pension granted will be higher (85% of the former salary) than that awarded for nonoccupational disability (60%). According to the statistics supplied to the Register of Occupational Diseases by insurance companies, about 80% of the claims for OA are accepted and compensated. A Finnish statistical review of occupational diseases is compiled every year. A synopsis in English is available from the Finnish Institute of Occupational Health (Helsinki, Finland) (46).

Several Canadian compensation programs have eliminated the adversarial approach in etiology and diagnosis. In all provinces, these issues are assigned to professionals representing neither the plaintiff nor the defendant (34). Thus, each case is decided solely on the merits of the exposure conditions and objective evidence of the disease. Prior experience with a similar administrative system had been gained in Quebec. Suspected cases of OA are referred for further investigation to specialists working in facilities devoted to such evaluations, one in Quebec City, the other in Montreal, the two centers accounting for a total of approximately four million workers. It is felt that two centers are sufficient to maintain the quality of the expertise without delays. Occupational claims comparing changes in number of claims in Quebec from 1988 to 2002 (Table 6) suggest that there has been a stability in asthma claims compared to claims for diseases related to asbestos exposure that have increased (due to mesotheliomas and bronchial cancers) and due to silica dust exposure that have decreased. Table 7 shows the distribution of agents that caused OA for the same years. There has been a reduction in the number of cases of OA due to isocyanates around 1995.

Determination of compensation costs in the Canadian provinces is based on a two-tier system (47). The first level provides for income replacement indemnity and complete costs for rehabilitation. Because many patients with OA are young, rehabilitation is mandatory. The process generally lasts one to two years. The second tier is based on permanent disability indemnity. The criteria used for determination of permanent disability are baseline bronchial obstruction, the degree of bronchial hyperresponsiveness, and the need for medication (47). These criteria are also the ones identified and proposed by organizations (48,49).

It is possible that removal of the adversarial status for compensation of occupational disease may be a disincentive for employers' responsibilities for assuring healthy and safe workplaces. This is particularly germane to workplaces representing a clearly excessive risk for OA, where the need for remedial industrial engineering

Table 6 New Cases of Compensated Occupational Lung Diseases in Quebec, 1988–2002

	1988	1989	1990	1991	1992	1993	1994	1995	1996	1997	1998	1999	2000	2001	2002
Asthma															
With LP	79	54	58	70	51	61	59	40	59	48	53	50	56	70	57
RADS	8	8	7	5	10	2	3	2	0	4	2	5	5	7	1
Total	87	62	65	75	61	63	62	42	59	52	55	55	61	77	58
Asbestos-related	77	57	53	76	66	61	71	70	113	84	84	99	116	108	132
Silicosis	40	31	42	45	25	38	27	18	26	24	38	21	29	19	28

Abbreviations: LP, latency period; RADS, reactive airways dysfunction syndrome.

Table 7 Principal Etiological Agents of OA[a]

	Year															
Agent	1988	1989	1990	1991	1992	1993	1994	1995	1996	1997	1998	1999	2000	2001	2002	Total
Isocyanates	17	17	18	23	16	25	8	7	11	7	8	9	12	11	10	199
Flour	10	9	9	16	5	9	11	8	13	9	6	12	11	5	8	141
Wood dusts	12	6	6	5	3	8	3	1	6	6	7	2	7	8	5	85
Seafood	7	2	2	7	0	2	9	2	2	5	4	6	3	8	6	65
Metals	4	3	3	6	6	4	4	1	6	2	3	5	3	5	2	57
Resins, glues	0	1	4	4	3	4	5	5	4	1	3	6	2	5	1	48
Cereals	9	3	3	2	2	1	4	1	3	3	4	1	2	7	3	48
Animals	3	2	3	3	4	2	5	1	3	0	6	3	0	3	1	39
Drugs	6	5	3	2	1	1	1	0	1	2	0	0	0	2	0	24

[a]Total for years 1988–2002 and grand total, Québec Workers' Compensation Board.
Abbreviation: OA, occupational asthma.

and more intensive medical surveillance is absolutely compelling. Unfortunately, a meta-analysis addressing this issue under adversarial and nonadversarial compensation systems has not yet been accomplished.

ASSESSMENT OF IMPAIRMENT/DISABILITY

Introduction

Asthma is a chronic condition that is relatively common among adults. Moreover, asthma prevalence and incidence span the years of working age, making it a disease particularly relevant to the question of work disability. In contrast, for example, chronic obstructive pulmonary disease (and especially emphysema) may be associated with greater physiologic compromise, but tends to be manifest only in later adulthood, nearer the age of declining labor force participation. Thus the interplay between impairment and disability in airway disease can be driven by a number of factors, including the demographic features of disease, temporal trends in incidence and prevalence over time, disease severity, and the spectrum of activities over which limitations or disability is being assessed.

Based on U.S. National Health Interview Survey (NHIS) data, 3.3% of U.S. adults aged 35 to 64 and 4.2% aged 15 to 34 report an episode of asthma or an asthma attack in the previous year, accounting for more the 6,650,000 persons with this condition (19). Based on NHIS data, the overall prevalence among adults appears to have stabilized since the mid-1990s, after a period of steep increases. Using a broader definition of disease, the Behavioral Risk Factor Surveillance System (BRFSS) has currently estimated that 7.2% of U.S. adults over age 18 have physician diagnosed asthma, with a stable estimate over two years (2000–2001). The proportion was 5.1% among males and 9.1% among females (50,51).

Of adults with asthma, the relative proportion reporting limitation and disability has remained stable over time, but is substantial. In 1994 to 1996, based on NHIS data, 14.6% of persons over age 18 with asthma reported activity limitations, compared to 14.4% in 1980 to 1982. The BRFSS estimates a higher proportion of those with asthma reporting activity limitation at 28%. The estimated number of asthma-related work absence days per year has been stable at 2.5 days per adult-asthma year; the total number of missed days, commensurate with temporal trends, has more than doubled over the same period, going from 6.2 to 14.5 million, based on the NHIS. Although all these data are specifically derived from the U.S. surveys, the overall pattern of asthma as a common adult disease with a heavy burden of limitations, at work and in general, appears to be relevant internationally as well.

Going from the population-based perceptive to the level of the individual person troubled by asthma, questions of impairment and disability are far more complex than may be suggested by standardized case definitions and structured surveys yielding prevalence rates and estimates of trends over time. Assessing impairment and disability can take the clinician into unfamiliar territory, dealing with an odd language filled with subjective qualifiers and driven by seemingly arcane definitions. In this domain, relying solely on "objective" physiologic signposts is unlikely to provide sufficient guidance; information frequently must be drawn from multiple disciplines including sociology, psychology, economics, and the law. This chapter is intended to systematically address the key issues in the evaluation of impairment and disability and in the medicolegal interface relevant to asthma in the workplace with the goal of orienting the clinician to this complex and challenging area of practice.

Definitions of Impairment and Disability

Clinicians frequently confuse the basic concepts of "impairment" and "disability," mistakenly using these two distinct terms loosely and interchangeably. They are interrelated, but are defined by fundamentally different criteria and serve very different purposes. This confusion is further magnified by "handicap," which refers to the degree to which the person with an impairment leading to disability adapts to this status. Although handicap is relevant to the impact of asthma at work and outside of work, it does not lie in the standard clinical evaluation of asthma and will not be addressed further here.

The concept of impairment is the more straightforward of the two. In general clinical terms, impairment refers to a decrement in function below an expected norm. In lung disease, especially in asthma, functional impairment is quantified as deficit determined through physiologic testing. Needless to say, there are multiple approaches to the physiological testing of lung function, both at rest and at exercise. Key modalities of testing relevant to impairment will be discussed in greater detail in the following pages. Although the correct performance of such testing demands rigorous quality control and the interpretation of results of testing requires nuanced expertise, its basic premise is familiar and intuitive. Physiological quantification of impairment simply presumes that an expectation of function can be set and that anything falling short of this constitutes a measured decrement.

Disability, as opposed to impairment, is another matter altogether. It is not that the former is "objective" and the latter "subjective," a commonly used dichotomization that provides little useful insight. Rather, the challenge is that disability, by definition, is relative rather than absolute. The relative nature of disability derives from the heterogeneous activities to which it applies. This subsumes a wide spectrum of human actions, including vocations (salaried or unsalaried), basic activities of daily living, and other pursuits, some of which have come to be characterized "valued life activities" because of their pivotal link to quality of life (QOL).

Work disability represents a specific subset of disability subsumed under a category of compromised capacity for employment. The relative nature of work disability in asthma is easy to highlight by example. A person who develops exercise-induced asthma may become disabled at a job that requires running up and down the stairs; an identical twin with the same physiological impairment would not be disabled in a sedentary job. A similar scenario can be drawn of a person with asthma exacerbated by temperature changes whose job as a butcher involves frequent cold air challenges in the meat locker. More saliently, a person specifically sensitized may be disabled in a job where the offending agent cannot be removed.

Work-related disability is further complicated because the nature of the employment itself may promote limitations. This can be derived not only from its physical attributes but also from the structure and organization of work. Jobs with little scheduling flexibility, for example, may lead to disability in asthma because frequently missed days are not tolerated. In contrast, a person with asthma of the very same degree of severity and "limitation" might be able to continue at the job under conditions that allowed self-scheduled telecommuting and more flexible work hours.

Just as limitation can be gauged by multiple parameters of physiological assessment, work disability can be quantified by a wide range of measures. This can include disease-related complete cessation of work, change in job or job duties, lost workdays (whole or in part), or decreased productivity on the job. It is clear from the nature of these outcomes that they typically derive from report by the person with disease, not the treating clinician, another sharp demarcation from the process of establishing limitation.

Maintaining clear and distinct definitions of "impairment" and "disability" is crucial to developing a consistent and stepwise approach to clinically assess the impact of disease on the day-to-day life, at work and at home, of the person with asthma. These definitions are also critical to the medical–legal interface of clinical care and workers' compensation and other social insurance support for the disabled patient.

General Principles in Assessment of Impairment and Existing Guidelines

Impairment assessment of respiratory disease requires the establishment of a medical diagnosis and the evaluation of the degree of impairment arising from the disorder. The following procedures are recommended.

History and Physical Examination

It is generally agreed that the assessment of respiratory impairment should be informed by physiologic testing rather than relying solely on symptoms or physical findings. Nonetheless, history and physical examination should be integral parts of the assessment. Dyspnea is a key symptom but reflects variable individual responses to a given degree of physiological abnormality. In addition dyspnea can be influenced by factors unrelated to the extent of lung disease, such as preoccupation with health, socioeconomic status, educational background, and physical fitness of the individual. Although there is some correlation between breathlessness and fall in expiratory flows in asthma, there is wide interindividual variation (52). Moreover, in asthma, dyspnea can be highly variable from time to time. Finally, although dyspnea is a symptom which is examined for all types of respiratory conditions, symptoms such as coughing, chest tightness, and, more specifically, wheezing are as relevant in asthma as they may more specifically reflect the degree of bronchial hyperresponsiveness than dyspnea, especially when these symptoms occur in certain circumstances such as after exercise, inhalation of cold air, laughing, and exposure to irritants.

Wheezing but also reduction in breath sounds should be sought on physical examination. Reduction in breath sounds reflects the degree of hyperinflation and air trapping, a common and sensitive physiological abnormality in asthma. In the case of subjects with more severe asthma, signs such as increased respiratory rate, use of accessory muscles, etc. can be present.

Chest Radiograph

Chest radiographs are irrelevant in stable asthma and are generally done only to exclude other chest conditions. Chest radiographic findings correlate poorly with physiological findings in diseases of airflow limitation such as chronic bronchitis and asthma. For some subjects, especially those with a history of chronic smoking, a high resolution CT scan might be indicated to exclude the possibility of concurrent emphysema. In asthma, CT scan may show increased thickness of the bronchial wall and, in severe airway disease, imbalance between ventilation and perfusion (mosaic perfusion) on expiratory views.

Physiological Measurements

Lung function tests are pivotal in determining the nature and the degree of the physiologic abnormality. They are essential in assessing the presence of impairment and in assessing its severity. Spirometry and the measurement of diffusing capacity are tests accepted by several professional societies for impairment evaluation (53,54). Measurement of nonallergic bronchial hyperresponsiveness has been accepted as an integral part of evaluation for subjects with asthma by the 1993 American Thoracic Society guidelines and, more recently, by the American Medical Association (AMA) (48,49). It is usually recommended that the patient should be evaluated after he or she has received "optimum therapy" or is in "optimal health," although no definition of optimal therapy or optimal health is given in these guidelines.

Spirometry

Spirometry is a well-standardized and simple test. Guidelines for spirometry include recommendations on equipment, methods of calibration, measurement of height, techniques of test performance, and strategies for interpretation of spirometric measurement have been published (55,56). Adequate consistency, i.e., the two best values must be within 5% of each other, is required. Paradoxically, the inability to achieve adequate consistency may be an indicator of the presence of disease, or it may represent poor technical or patient effort. Because poor reproducibility may represent disease, it may be necessary to present the data from several variable trials and comment on this factor rather than simply reject the results altogether (57). For impairment evaluation, only two parameters are specified in standard guidelines: forced expiratory volume in one second (FEV_1) and forced vital capacity (FVC) and their ratio (53,54,58,59).

When airflow obstruction is present (FEV_1/FVC is below 75%), the measurements should be repeated after the administration of an inhaled bronchodilator. A significant increase is defined as an increase in FEV_1 or FVC of greater than 12% (increase of 200 mL or greater) from the baseline as the presence of airway reversibility suggestive of asthma (56). In patients with asthma, the postbronchodilator response is used in the rating of respiratory impairment.

Measurement of NSBH

Nonspecific bronchial hyperresponsiveness (NSBH) is a hallmark of asthma and imparts a certain degree of functional impairment in these subjects. Measurement of NSBH has been included in impairment evaluation in subjects with asthma by the American Thoracic Society and the AMA (48,49). Methacholine and histamine challenge tests have been recommended for measurement of NSBH. Because the degree of NSBH is correlated with airway caliber, it is difficult to interpret the results of testing conducted on subjects with airflow obstruction (FEV_1 <70% predicted). The degree of bronchodilator response may be used as a surrogate measure of the degree of NSBH in these subjects (48). For subjects with FEV_1 between 70% and 80% of the predicted value, both bronchodilator response and methacholine or histamine challenge test could be used.

Exercise Tests

The majority of patients do not require exercise testing in impairment evaluation because there is a well-documented relationship between FEV_1, D_{LCO}, oxygen consumption, and work capacity (54). Exercise testing is indicated only when there is reason to believe that routine lung function tests may have underestimated impairment.

Exercise testing in such cases is used to determine whether a person is impaired and whether the impairment is due to a respiratory disorder. In subjects with asthma, exercise testing is sometimes indicated to assess bronchoconstriction in evaluation of impairment/disability which might occur in jobs requiring heavy exertion (54).

Measurement of the Diffusing Capacity

Measurement of the diffusing capacity of the lung for carbon monoxide (D_{LCO}) is a useful test in impairment evaluations in subjects with other types of lung diseases, but it is not useful in subjects with asthma. The test requires careful attention to detail standardization (60). The test result is dependent on hemoglobin concentration; results should be adjusted for hemoglobin concentration if the subject is anemic (61). It should also be adjusted for alveolar volume. Smokers should be told to refrain from smoking for 12 hours before the test; otherwise blood carboxyhemoglobin has to be measured for adjustment of back diffusion because of high levels of carbon monoxide in the blood.

Arterial Blood Gas Measurement

Because of its invasive nature, arterial blood gas analysis is not often used in impairment evaluation. For most individuals with obstructive lung disease, exercise capacity correlates better with FEV_1 than arterial partial pressure of oxygen (PO_2) (62).

Controversial Aspects of Impairment/Disability Evaluation

Normality of Lung Function Measurements

Although clear guidelines for maximal impairment (100%) are available, rating of partial impairment is difficult. This is partly due to difficulties of defining "normality" and of scaling between normality and total impairment.

The results of lung function tests are dependent on certain demographic characteristics, such as gender, age, height, and race. Prediction equations vary due to several reasons. These include differences in techniques, the population selected for the study, and mathematical models used to study the relationship between the predictors and lung function.

There are also several means of comparing individual results with those of the reference population. The decision of where and how to draw the line between "normal" and "abnormal" pulmonary functions is subject to disagreement. Lung function values may be expressed either as a percentage of the reference value or as deviations from the reference values in terms of standard deviation or standard error. The use of 80% of the reference value as the demarcation between normal and abnormal lung function has been widely accepted. However, this method tends to overestimate the prevalence of abnormalities in older individuals (63). The most recent recommendation is to define abnormality as values outside 95% confidence limits (56). Certain ethnic/racial groups such as Hispanics, Asians, and blacks may have smaller lung volumes than whites of the same age and height. Frequently a 10% to 15% correction factor is applied for race correction, but there is no standard formula in this regard (56). It is best for each laboratory to establish its own set of reference values, rather than using those generated by others not only because of equipment and technical differences but also racial differences.

Grading Impairment

As noted previously (see Definitions), impairment refers to a functional deficit. Such deficits can be based on well-delineated and expected normal physiologic values; it may be logical to attempt quantification of impairment in numeric terms. The AMA Guidelines for Evaluation of Permanent Impairment are often employed by practitioners as a primary source of guidance in matters related to impairment classification (49).

Table 8 shows the 1993 ATS guidelines. It incorporates into impairment classification three distinct components: FEV_1, degree of airflow reversibility or nonspecific bronchial responsiveness, and, most importantly, medication reliance, along with proposed criteria for estimating the severity of asthma (64). In this schema, a person with normal airflow and a mild degree of bronchial hyperresponsiveness (PC_{20} 2–8 mg/mL), but requiring daily inhaled and systemic corticosteroids to achieve that level of function, would still be placed in impairment class II (0 being no impairment and V being maximal impairment) (48). This approach acknowledges the need to rely on more than one factor to categorize impairment, but is still limited in scope.

Assessing Work Ability and Disability

Narrowly viewed, the medical evaluation process only grades impairment and does not directly quantify disability. The U.S. insurance system, both public (workers' compensation and Social Security) and private sectors, adjusters, or claim examiners "rate" disability through an independent process that heavily weights the medical component of impairment. Internationally, parallel processes are commonly used.

Table 8 American Thoracic Society Guidelines for Impairment/Disability in Patients with Asthma

Score	FEV_1	Post-bronchodilator reversibility of FEV_1 or degree of hyperresponsiveness		Minimum medication need
		% FEV_1 change	PC_{20} mg/mL	
0	>lower limit of N	<10	>8	No medication
1	70% to lower limit of N	10–19	$8 \rightarrow 0.5$	Occasional (not daily) BDT or cromolyn
2	60–69	20–29	$0.5 \rightarrow 0.125$	Daily BDT or cromolyn or low dose (<800 µg) beclomethasone or equivalent
3	50–59	≥30	≤0.125	Daily high dose (>800 mg) beclomethasone or equivalent or occasional course (1–3/yr) of oral steroids
4	<50	–	–	Daily high dose beclomethasone or equivalent and daily oral steroids

Impairment class 0: total score = 0; class I: total score = 1–3; class II: total score = 4–6; class III: total score = 7–9; class IV: total score = 10–11; class V: asthma not controlled despite maximal treatment.
Abbreviations: N, normal; BDT, bronchodilator treatment.
Source: From Ref. 64.

Thus the medical evaluation directly feeds into the determination of disability. Moreover, a variety of other data noted in the medical record beyond physiological impairment may be used to modify disability assessments. Actions taken by the health care provider may lead to modified duty or even complete work cessation regardless of how a disability is proportionally "rated." For these reasons the health care provider plays a key role in the disability process.

In theory, assessing work fitness is a cornerstone of occupational health practice. Classically, work demands have been quantified in terms of oxygen consumption on a job-specific basis and the individual screened by exercise testing to evaluate the ability to meet those demands. Leaving aside the fact that much of the established guidelines on job-specific demands are no longer applicable to current work life, there is little in this approach that is relevant to asthma in the workplace.

For asthma in the workplace, the critical factor is avoiding known triggers. As discussed elsewhere, the preferred prevention strategy is work process changes that remove or enclose the offending agent. This is usually beyond the control of the clinician forced to approach the problem from the starting point of the individual rather then the workplace as a whole. The usual action is a "work restriction" meant to eliminate or ameliorate exposure. In some cases this may be straightforward in a large workplace with many jobs physically separated from each other and involving distinct duties. For example, a university-employed laboratory animal handler who develops asthma from rat allergen may be reassigned to a position that no longer involves such contact. It should be remembered, however, that if a pay cut results or if job advancement is slowed this, is a manifestation of work disability.

In many cases work restrictions are not so clear cut, for example, if a specific trigger cannot be identified or in a case where exposure is ubiquitous, at least at levels sufficient to evoke an anamuestic response (e.g., a facility using isocyanates). IIA may be less problem ridden from the point of view of work restriction, because ongoing hyperresponsiveness should not be driven by low-level exposure, and work practices should be such as to prevent nonspecific irritation in all employees. Nonetheless, there is evidence that for some irritants, the airways of persons with asthma may respond at lower levels than do those of persons without hyperresponsiveness. An overly broad work restriction that cannot be feasibly implemented (e.g., "no exposure to any gas, dust, fumes, or vapors") is highly likely to result in work disability. In the United States, the Americans with Disabilities Act mandates that reasonable accommodations be made for employees with impairments, which presumably applies to asthma as well, although this is an area of evolving case law. There is little comparable legislation in EU or elsewhere.

Beyond work ability specific to asthma, other factors related to health and wellbeing should be addressed in an assessment of work ability and fitness because these factors will impact any disability assessment guided by the medical record. Obviously, other cardiopulmonary conditions are highly relevant, but so too are conditions of other systems, including psychiatric disorders (moreover, many somatoform disorders may include respiratory symptoms). In addition, psychosocial factors such as education and prior job training do fall under the purview of a complete assessment.

Assessing work ability and fitness should be a systematic and rigorous process that takes into account the multifactorial nature of disability. Consistent with this view, the ATS noted in its 1993 position paper on impairment and disability of asthma that "The rating of impairment is within the jurisdiction of the physician's expertise to quantitate. However, the determination of disability also requires consideration of many nonmedical variables. Physicians have considerable knowledge about how impairment impacts their patients' lives. Therefore it is important for physicians to identify all the individual factors modifying the impact of impairment on the patients' lives for administrators who determine compensation."

Asthma-Specific QOL

QOL, as a general construct, refers to the individual's perception of his/her position in life on a broad range of issues; health-related QOL (HRQOL) focuses on factors of QOL related to health (both physical and mental) and disease states. This includes aspects of physical status and symptoms, emotional wellbeing, and social functioning. Thus HRQOL is directly related to both impairment and disability, but it is not synonymous with either. Disease-specific HRQOL refers to symptoms and other ways that a discrete condition may affect QOL. For asthma, assessing disease-specific HRQOL can emphasize symptoms such as wheeze and shortness of breath, attitudes toward inhaler or other medication use, and avoidance of asthma triggers.

Correlations between the HRQOL and physiological measurements of impairment are often weak; this has been shown specifically to be the case with HRQOL and lung function measures (65,66). This can be a strength rather than a weakness in HRQOL, because it supports the view that this dimension of health is different than narrowly defined limitation.

A number of measures have been developed to assess HRQOL. Measures of "generic" HRQOL address a spectrum of health and disease and are not specific to any one condition. For this reason they can be used to compare across different diseases (OA vs. work-related musculoskeletal disease, for example) or can be used to assess deviation from the normal values of the population at large. The SF-36 [Medical Outcomes Study (MOS) Short-Form 36] is the most widely used generic HRQOL measure, including application to airway disease (both asthma and COPD) (67). The SF-36 is composed of 36 items in eight domains (physical functioning; role limitations due to physical health problems; role limitations due to emotional problems; body pain; social functioning; general mental health; vitality, energy, or fatigue; and general health perceptions). There is also a widely used shorter 12-item version (SF-12) (68). Other widely used generic HRQOL measures that have been applied to lung disease include the 38-item Nottingham Health Profile and the extensive 136-item Sickness Impact Profile (69,70).

There are two asthma-specific HRQOL instruments in wide usage. Juniper's Asthma QOL Questionnaire (AQLQ) is a 32-item measure covering symptoms, emotions, exposure to environmental stimuli, and activity limitations (71). This questionnaire asks respondents to identify specific activities that are affected by their asthma, which can include employment, but may not as the respondent chooses. There is also a shorter 15-item version of the AQLQ (MiniAQLQ) that includes only standardized questions (72). This includes work or, if the respondent is not employed, another major life activity. Although not applied specifically to OA, these characteristics of the AQLQ batteries would be likely to impact their applicability in this arena. The Marks AQLQ is a 20-item scale that includes items in four domains: breathlessness and physical restrictions, mood disturbance, social disruption, and concern for health (73,74). This measure does not include work impairment.

In addition to these asthma-specific measures, there are also lung-disease HRQOL measures that are meant to span a variety of respiratory conditions including but not limited to asthma. The most widely known of these is the 76-item

St. George's Respiratory Questionnaire which addresses symptoms, activities that cause or are limited by breathlessness, social functioning, and psychological impacts of disease (75). More recently the same group has developed a 20-item Airways Questionnaire (76). This battery does include an item specific for breathlessness during work activities.

Generic or disease-specific HRQOL measures are not routinely used in disability assessments in the one-on-one clinical context. They are gaining increasing importance, however, in the general epidemiological study of chronic diseases in relation to disability, including asthma. In occupational health research, HRQOL tools have been relatively underutilized (77). In the future, it is likely that measuring HRQOL will become more prominent in both clinical and research practices relating to occupational airway disease.

Impairment Assessment in Asthma and OA

General Principles

As discussed elsewhere, upon establishment of the diagnosis, the subject should be considered 100% impaired on a permanent basis for the job which caused the illness and for other jobs entailing exposure to the same causative agent. Impairment assessment of respiratory diseases requires the establishment of a medical diagnosis and the evaluation of the degree of impairment arising from the disorder. The following procedures are recommended.

Symptoms (frequency, degree of limitation of activities, and frequency of acute exacerbations) should be explored. Although the severity of symptoms should be considered in the assessment of disability, symptomatology is subjective and can be biased by the desire of getting rewarding financial compensation or by the fear of losing one's livelihood. The need of medication as set by the treating physician is a generally satisfactory means in reflecting the severity of asthma (78). Information on the nature of usual medication and of the compliance of subjects in taking this medication can also be checked. The degree of impairment should also be supported by objective means represented by physiologic parameters. The number of visits to the emergency room due to asthma does not satisfactorily reflect the severity of asthma. Such visits may reflect an asthmatic condition that is not being adequately treated on a chronic basis, reflecting poor access to routine care, or may indeed indicate severe disease. Exercise testing and assessment of lung volumes and diffusing capacity are not helpful in assessing impairment in OA although they may be helpful in excluding other reasons for dyspnea or chest symptoms, whether occupationally or non occupationally related.

Timing of Evaluation

Some "permanent stationary status" should be determined at the time of diagnosis to protect the employee and make him eligible to readaptation programs. A reassessment should be carried out afterwards. As discussed in Chapters 7 and 25, subjects with OA may be left with symptoms, bronchial obstruction, and NSBH after leaving exposure. Although it has been shown that a plateau of improvement is achieved approximately two years after leaving exposure in snow crab–induced asthma, the improvement continues after this landmark, though at a slower pace (79–81). Therefore, although it seems relevant to assess subjects two years after stopping exposure, there are instances in which the improvement will continue after this interval.

Re-evaluation may therefore be necessary after the initial two-year time interval, depending on the clinical course of each individual.

Possible deterioration of asthma after stopping exposure can exist but this phenomenon would be related to respiratory infections or other triggers. It is worth mentioning that subjects with OA do not appear to be at increased risk of becoming sensitized to common aeroallergens after stopping exposure (82). By contrast, at the time of exposure, 24% of subjects who were exposed to laboratory animals and who developed sensitization on skin testing also became sensitized to at least one ubiquitous allergen (83).

Stability of Asthma

Subjects should be assessed at a time the asthmatic condition is under reasonable control while on the lowest amount of medication. It may be necessary to assess the stability of asthma by monitoring peak expiratory flow (PEF) for a period of time. Increased fluctuations in PEF are usually associated with a heightened degree of NSBH (84). PEF monitoring for assessment of OA (Chapter 9) and non-OA has been plagued by the lack of patient compliance and possibly falsification of data (85,86). Fortunately, the use of computerized recorders obviates the latter issue. If the subject's asthma is not under good control, the assessment should be postponed. The criteria for good asthma control and the method of achieving good control should follow guidelines (87).

There may be a few patients with severe asthma in whom is difficult to achieve completely good control even over a period of months. In this situation, evaluation for permanent impairment should be done even though the disease is partly controlled.

Assessment of Spirometry and Bronchial Responsiveness

Spirometry and NSBH are the two parameters important in impairment evaluation in patients with asthma. Spirometry should be done before and after the inhalation of a beta-2 agonist. Anti-inflammatory drug should be taken as usual on the day of evaluation. The American Thoracic Society guidelines that have been recently endorsed by the AMA recommend the use of postbronchodilator FEV_1 and FVC for the grading of respiratory impairment (48,49). This intention is surely reasonable in subjects taking long acting beta-2 agonists that lessen the degree of diurnal variation in lung function considerably. However, it may not be in subjects not taking such medication. A marked degree of reversibility after the administration of an inhaled bronchodilator usually represents an inadequate control requiring adjustment of medication by the treating physician. Measurement of NSBH should be carried out after bronchodilator medications have been withheld for recommended periods (88).

Proposed Grading of Impairment

Scales assessing impairment use three parameters: need for medication, spirometry, and NSBH (48,49,89). In a similar way as scales have been proposed and used in respiratory impairment evaluation for standard pneumoconiosis, scales have been designed for asthma and OA using the above parameters. Table 9 is an example of such a scaling system which has been used in Quebec since 1984. The between-physician reproducibility in assessing the impairment (%) is satisfactory. Moreover, the scale has a satisfactory "content validity" as the degree of impairment reflects an

Table 9 Quebec Scaling System for Assessment of Disability for OA

Class	Level of bronchial obstruction	Level of bronchial responsiveness	Need for medication	% Disability
1	0	0	None	0
2A	0	1	None	5
2B	0	1	BDT prn	8
2C	0	1	BDT reg	10
2D	0	2	None	10
2E	0	2	BDT reg or prn	13
2F	0	3	BDT reg or prn	15
3A	1	1	BDT reg or prn	18
3B	1	2	BDT reg or prn	20
3C	1	3	BDT reg or prn	25
4A	2	1–2	BDT reg or prn	28
4B	2	3	BDT reg or prn	33
5A	3	1–2	BDT reg or prn	50
5B	3	3	BDT reg or prn	60
6	4	1–2–3	BDT reg or prn	100
			With oral steroids and with or without inhaled steroids to be added:	
			Inhaled steroid	3
			Oral steroid	10

Level of bronchial obstruction:
  0: FEV_1 (% pred) and/or FEV_1/FVC (% pred) >85% pred
  1: FEV_1 (% pred) and/or FEV_1/FVC (% pred) = 71–85% pred
  2: FEV_1 (% pred) and/or FEV_1/FVC (% pred) = 56–70% pred
  3: FEV_1 (% pred) and/or FEV_1/FVC (% pred) = 40–55% pred
  4: FEV_1 (% pred) and/or FEV_1/FVC (% pred) <40% pred.
Level of bronchial hyperresponsiveness:
  0: PC_{20} >16 mg/mL
  1: PC_{20} = 2–16 mg/mL
  2: PC_{20} = 0.25– mg/mL
  3: PC_{20} = 0.25 mg/mL.
Abbreviations: BDT, bronchodilator treatment; OA, occupational asthma; FEV_1, forced expiratory volume in one second; FVC, forced vital capacity.

impairment which might be judged to be equivalent in a subject with an interstitial lung disease. Another type of scale ("horizontal type") proposed by the American Thoracic Society and the AMA uses similar criteria (Table 8) (48,49).

Summary

In this section, we have brought arguments for justifying the need of assessing permanent impairment/disability in OA after removal from exposure to the causal agent on the grounds that subjects with OA are often left with permanent asthma. We have also made the point that criteria used for other pulmonary diseases do not apply to asthma, therefore justifying independent criteria and scales based on these criteria. The criteria should include need for medication, spirometry, and bronchial responsiveness. The assessment should be carried out at a time asthma is reasonably stable and when recovery of bronchial responsiveness is still at its fastest rate, i.e., approximately two years after removal from exposure (81).

RECOMMENDATIONS FOR THE FUTURE

Based on the increased volume of medical research and literature concerning OA, it has been predicted that asthma will surpass pneumoconiosis as the leading cause of respiratory disability in workers (22). In 1989 a program for the surveillance of work-related and occupational respiratory disease (SWORD) was established in the United Kingdom. With chest and occupational physicians as the reporting units, 554 cases of OA were identified in the first year of the SWORD project as compared to 322 cases of pneumoconiosis (90). These data have since been extended to include IIA occurring after inhalation accidents (91). These now comprise 10% of all reported occupational lung diseases. Data being assessed in the United States by the SENSOR project states suggest that a similar shift may have already occurred in some localities (Table 2). Confirmation of this trend will not be possible by analysis of current statistical data collected by compensation systems in individual states because asthma is classified with a miscellaneous group of unrelated pulmonary problems. However, workers' compensation claims could constitute a significant database for detection, surveillance, and prevention of workplace asthma provided individual states, provinces, and nations reach agreement about defining, classifying, and coding OA.

All would agree that OA is characterized by reversible narrowing of the lower airways with various degrees of airway hyperresponsiveness induced by exposure to work-related substances. However, there is still considerable controversy about whether such substances should be limited to sensitizing agents. Because many proven causes of asthma are due to nonsensitizing agents (e.g., polyvinyl chloride fumes, products of aluminum smelting) or accidental spills (RADS), it would seem unwise to restrict the definition to sensitizers. To resolve this issue there will have to be compromise on a subclassification of OA, which will encompass sensitizing, toxic irritating, and nontoxic irritating substances at work. In Germany, OA is distinguished as either allergic or irritative. If this system were universally adopted, it would then be possible to utilize Doctors' First Reports of OA, as is the case in California, where there appears to be an increasing trend of reported OA cases from 1983 to the present. Recognition of asthma as an occupational disease entity would also encourage standardized diagnostic coding and adoption of the International Classification of Disease nomenclature. If these changes were incorporated into the reporting systems of various workers' compensation agencies, it would then be possible to compare and analyze outcome experiences, monitor trends, and target workplace inspections to prevent work-related asthma.

Implementation of these goals in the United States requires a concerted effort and cooperation among individual state health departments and bureaus of workers' compensation. Appropriate federal agencies, such as NIOSH and the Bureau of Labor Statistics, have an important role in standardizing disease definitions, coding, and reporting. NIOSH has initiated the process by the SENSOR program (14,19). One of the by-products of this program has been the development of a universally applicable surveillance case definition of OA. With validation and modification of this case definition, state health departments will begin to access reliable data concerning OA from primary or selected groups of health providers. A partially successful attempt has already been made to validate a proposed surveillance case definition of OA, and case definition modifications have been suggested (92). A subsequently revised surveillance case definition was presented (14). The use of a consistent case definition by all state WCBs coupled with consistent coding of OA claims will allow for a more accurate determination of the incidence and prevalence of this condition.

An interesting set of tentative principles for reforming disability legislation in the United States was proposed in 1981 by the Ad Hoc Committee on Disability Legislation of the American Thoracic Society Scientific Assembly on Environmental and Occupational Health. This committee suggested that respiratory disability should be determined by qualified professionals from the fields of law, education, economics, and the health sciences. Further, it recommended that decisions regarding causation should encompass all available scientific data, including the results of appropriate epidemiological studies. These features have already been incorporated into several Euro-Canadian models of workers' compensation for OA, but it appears that reform of current workers' compensation disability plans in the United States will be a more arduous process (34).

SUMMARY

Workers' compensation is a "no-fault insurance system" in which employees waive their common law right to sue their employers for damages in exchange for income, medical benefits, and rehabilitation services paid for by private or state government insurers. Regulations and policies governing compensation for OA vary from state to state, province to province, and country to country. This variation is due to different ways of defining OA. Annual workers' compensation claims for OA are increasing. Many industrialized countries allow compensation for OA on the basis of schedules or lists of covered diseases. Further attempts to establish a uniform compensation system for OA will have to address multiple causality of asthma, difficulty of diagnosis, and methods to assess aggravating factors in the workplace. Finally, because OA may often cause the persistence of asthma even after removal from exposure, there should be provision to offer compensation for possible permanent impairment/disability using available scales.

REFERENCES

1. Barth PS, Hunt HA. Worker's Compensation and Work-Related Illnesses and Disease. Cambridge, MA: MIT Press, 1982.
2. Pontaut A. Santé et sécurité. Boréal Express, Montreal, 1985.
3. Larson A. Workers' Compensation Law: Cases, Materials and Text. New York: Matthew Bender & Company, 1990.
4. U.S. Chamber of Commerce. Analysis of Workers Compensation Laws. Washington, D.C., 1990.
5. Richman SI. Why change? A look at the current system of disability determination and workers' compensation for occupational lung disease. Ann Intern Med 1982; 95:774–776.
6. Cherniack M. The Hawks Nest Incident: America's Worst Industrial Disaster. New Haven, CT: Yale University Press, 1986.

7. Muldoon JT, Wintermeyer LA, Eure JA, et al. Occupational disease surveillance data sources. Am J Pub Health 1987; 77:1006–1008.
8. Ameille J, Pauli G, Calastreng-Crinquand A, et al. ONAP and the corresponding members of the reported incidence of occupational asthma in France, 1996–99. Occup Environ Med 2003; 60:136–142.
9. Rosenstock L, Hagopian A. Occupational medicine: too long neglected. Ann Intern Med 1987; 95:774–776.
10. Rosenstock L, Hagopian A. Ethical dilemmas in providing health care to workers. Ann Intern Med 1987; 107:575–580.
11. Kleinman GD, Cant SM. Occupational disease surveillance in Washington. JOM 1978; 20:750–754.
12. Melius JM, Sestito JP, Seligman PJ. Occupational disease surveillance with existing data sources. AJPH 1989; 79(S):46–52.
13. Freund E, Seligman PJ, Chorba TL, Safford SK, Drachman JG, Hull SF. Mandatory reporting of occupational diseases by clinicians. MMWR 1990; 39:19–28.
14. Matte TD, Hoffman RE, Rosenman KD, Stanbury M. Surveillance of occupational asthma under the SENSOR model. Chest 1990; 98:173S–178S.
15. Blanc P. Occupational asthma in a national disability survey. Chest 1987; 92:613–617.
16. Arif AA, Whitehead LW, Delclos GL, Tortolero SR, Lee ES. Prevalence and risk factors of work related asthma by industry among United States workers: data from the third national health and nutrition examination survey (1988–94). Occup Environ Med 2002; 59:505–511.
17. Seta JA, Young RO, Pedersen DH. Compendium III. The United States national exposure survey (NOES) data base. In: Bernstein IL, Chan-Yeung M, Malo JL, Bernstein DI, eds. Asthma in the Workplace. 2nd ed. New York: Marcel Dekker Inc., 1999:721–728.
18. Reinisch F, Harrison RJ, Cussler S, et al. Physician reports of work-related asthma in California, 1993–1996. Am J Ind Med 2001; 39:72–83.
19. Mannino DM, Homa DM, Akinbami L, Moorman JE, Gwynn C, Redd SC. Surveillance for asthma—United States, 1980–1999. MMWR 2002; 51:SS1–SS13.
20. U.S. Department of Health and Human Services Public Health Service, Centers for Disease Control and Prevention, National Institute for Occupational Safety and Health. Work-related lung disease surveillance report, Morgantown, WV, 1994, 128; Tables 9, 10, Other Lung Conditions, Morbidity.
21. Reilly MJ, Rosenman KD, Watt FC, et al. Surveillance for occupational asthma—Michigan and New Jersey, 1988–1992. MMWR 1994; SS-1:9–17.
22. Richman SI. Legal treatment of the asthmatic worker: a major problem for the nineties. J Occup Med 1990; 32:1027–1031.
23. Adams WGF. Long-term effects on the health of men engaged in the manufacture of toluene di-isocyanate. Br J Ind Med 1975; 32:72–78.
24. Moller DR, Brooks SM, McKay RT, Cassedy K, Kopp S, Bernstein IL. Chronic asthma due to toluene diisocyanate. Chest 1986; 90:494–499.
25. Paggiaro PL, Loi AM, Rossi O, et al. Follow-up study of patients with respiratory disease due to toluene diisocyanate (TDI). Clin Allergy 1984; 14:463–469.
26. Chan-Yeung M, Lam S, Koerner S. Clinical features and natural history of occupational asthma due to western red cedar (thuja plicata). Am J Med 1982; 72:411–415.
27. Burge PS. Occupational asthma in electronics workers caused by colophony fumes: follow-up of affected workers. Thorax 1982; 37:348–353.
28. Hudson P, Cartier A, Pineau L, Lafrance M, St-Aubin JJ, Dubois JY, Malo JL. Follow-up of occupational asthma caused by crab and various agents. J Allergy Clin Immunol 1985; 76:682–687.
29. Lass N, Arion H, Sahar J. Medico-legal aspects of occupational asthma. Ann Allergy 1971; 29:573–577.
30. Chatkin CJM, Tarlo SM, Liss G, Banks D, Broder I. The outcome of asthma related to workplace exposures. Chest 1999; 116:1780–1785.

31. Goe SK, Henneberger PK, Reilly MJ, et al. A descriptive study of work exacerbated asthma. Occup Environ Med 2004; 61:512–517.
32. Blessman JE. Differential treatment of occupational disease versus occupational injury by Workers' Compensation in Washington state. JOM 1991; 33:121–126.
33. United States Department of Labour. An interim report to congress on occupational diseases. Washington, D.C., 1980.
34. Dewitte JD, Chan-Yeung M, Malo JL. Medicolegal and compensation aspects of occupational asthma. Eur Respir J 1994; 7:969–980.
35. Liss GM, Tarlo SM, Macfarlane Y, Yeung KS. Hospitalization among workers compensated for occupational asthma. Am J Respir Crit Care Med 2000; 162:112–118.
36. Liss GM, Tarlo SM, Banks D, Yeung KS, Schweigert M. Preliminary report of mortality among workers compensated for work-related asthma. Am J Ind Med 1999; 35:465–471.
37. Tarlo SM, Liss G, Corey P, Broder I. A workers' compensation claim population for occupational asthma. Chest 1995; 107:634–641.
38. Henneberger PK, Derk SJ, Davis L, et al. Work-related reactive airways dysfunction syndrome cases from surveillance in selected US States. J Occup Environ Med 2003; 45:360–368.
39. Tarlo SM, Banks D, Liss G, Broder I. Outcome determinants for isocyanate induced occupational asthma among compensation claimants. Occup Environ Med 1997; 54:756–761.
40. Gannon PFG, Weir DC, Robertson AS, Burge PS. Health, employment, and financial outcomes in workers with occupational asthma. Br J Ind Med 1993; 50:491–496.
41. Ameille J, Parion JC, Bayeux MC, et al. Consequences of occupational asthma on employment and financial status: a follow-up study. Eur Respir J 1997; 10:55–58.
42. Hendrick DJ, Fabbri L. Compensating occupational asthma. Thorax 1981; 36:881–884.
43. Gervais P, Rosenberg N. Aspects médico-légaux internationaux de l'asthme professionnel. Rev Mal Respir 1988; 5:491–495.
44. www.asthmanet.com.
45. Karjalainen A, Kurppa K, Virtanen S, Keskinen H, Nordman H. Incidence of occupational asthma by occupation and industry in Finland. Am J Ind Med 2000; 37:451–458.
46. www.occuphealth.fi.
47. Malo JL. Compensation for occupational asthma in Quebec. Chest 1990; 98:236S–239S.
48. American Thoracic Society. Guidelines for the evaluation of impairment/disability in patients with asthma. Am Rev Respir Dis 1993; 147:1056–1061.
49. Cocchiarella L, Andersson GBJ, eds. Guides to the Evaluation of Permanent Impairment. 5th ed. Chicago, IL: American Medical Association, 2001.
50. Self-reported asthma prevalence among adults—United States, 2000. MMWR 2001; 50:682–686.
51. Self-reported asthma prevalence and control among adults—United States, 2002. MMWR 2003; 52:381–384.
52. Boulet LP, Cournoyer I, Deschesnes F, Leblanc P, Nouwen A. Perception of airflow obstruction and associated breathlessness in normal and asthmatic subjects: correlation with anxiety and bronchodilator needs. Thorax 1994; 49:965–970.
53. American Thoracic Society. Evaluation of impairment/disability secondary to respiratory disease. Am Rev Respir Dis 1982; 126:945–951.
54. American Thoracic Society. Evaluation of impairment/disability secondary to respiratory disorders. Am Rev Respir Dis 1986; 133:1205–1209.
55. American Thoracic Society. Standardization of spirometry. Am J Respir Crit Care Med 1995; 152:1107–1136.
56. American Thoracic Society. Lung function testing: selection of reference values and interpretation strategies. Am Rev Respir Dis 1991; 144:1202–1218.
57. Becklake MR. Epidemiology of spirometric test failure. Br J Ind Med 1990; 47:73–74.
58. Balmes JR, Barnhart S. Evaluation of respiratory impairment/disability. In: Murray JF, Nadel JA, ed. Textbook of respiratory medicine. 2nd ed. Philadelphia: WB Saunders Co., 1994:920–942.

59. Haber L. Disabling effects of chronic disease and impairments. J Chronic Dis 1971; 24:469–487.
60. Society American Thoracic. Single breath carbon monoxide diffusing capacity (transfer factor): recommendations for a standard technique. Am Rev Respir Dis 1987; 136:1299–1307.
61. Dinakara P, Blumental WS, Johnston RF, Kauffman LA, Solnick PB. The effects of anaemia on pulmonary diffusing capacity with derivation of a corrected equation. Am Rev Respir Dis 1970; 102:965–969.
62. Morgan WKC, Zaldivar GL. Blood gas analysis as determinant of occupationally related disability. J Occup Med 1990; 135:440–443.
63. Harber P, Schnur R, Emery J, Brooks S, Ploy-Song-Sang Y. Statistical "biases" in respiratory disability determination. Am Rev Respir Dis 1992; 128:413–418.
64. National Institutes of Health National Heart, Lung and Blood Institute. Global initiative for asthma (GINA). Global strategy for asthma management and prevention. NHLBI/SHO workshop report. National Institutes of Health publication, no. 95–3659, 1995.
65. Juniper EF, Guyatt GH, Ferrie PJ, Griffith LE. Measuring quality of life in asthma. Am Rev Respir Dis 1993; 147:832–838.
66. Juniper EF. Quality of life in adults and children with asthma and rhinitis. Allergy 1997; 52:971–977.
67. Ware JE, Snow KK, Kosinski M, Gandek B. SF-36 Health Survey. Manual and Interpretation Guide. Boston, MA: The Health Institute, New England Medical Center, 1993.
68. Ware JE, Kosinski M, Keller SD. SF-12: How to Score the SF-12 Physical and Mental Health Summary Scales. 2nd ed. Boston, MA: The Health Institute, New England Medical Center, 1995.
69. Hunt SM, McEwan J, McKenna SP. Measuring health status: a new tool for clinicians and epidemiologists. J R Coll Gen Practice 1985; 35:185–188.
70. Bergner M, Bobbitt RA, Carter WB, Gilson BS. The sickness impact profile: development and final revision of a health status measure. Med Care 1981; 19:787–805.
71. Juniper EF, Guyatt GH, Epstein RS, Ferrie PJ, Jaeschke R, Hiller TK. Evaluation of impairment of health-related quality of life in asthma: development of a questionnaire for use in clinical trials. Thorax 1992; 47:76–83.
72. Juniper EF, Guyatt GH, Cox MF, Ferrie PJ, King DR. Development and validation of the mini asthma quality of life questionnaire. Eur Respir J 1999; 14:32–38.
73. Marks GB, Dunn SM, Woolcock AJ. An evaluation of an asthma quality of life questionnaire as a measure of change in adults with asthma. J Clin Epidemiol 1993; 46(10):1103–1111.
74. Katz PP, Eisner MD, Henke J, Smith S, Shiboski S, Yelin EH, Blanc PD. The Marks Asthma Quality of Life Questionnaire: further validation and examination of responsiveness to change. J Clin Epidemiol 1999; 52:667–675.
75. Jones PW, Quirk FH, Baveystock CM. The St. George's Respiratory Questionnaire. Respir Med 1991; 85(suppl):25–31.
76. Barley EA, Wuirk FH, Jones PW. Asthma health status measurement in clinical practice: validity of a new short and simple instrument. Respir Med 1998; 92:1207–1214.
77. Blanc PD. Why quality of life should matter to occupational health researchers. Occup Environ Med 2004; 61:571.
78. Blanc PD, Cisternas M, Smith S, Yelin EH. Asthma, employment status, and disability among adults treated by pulmonary and allergy specialists. Chest 1996; 109:688–696.
79. Malo JL, Cartier A, Ghezzo H, Lafrance M, Mccants M, Lehrer SB. Patterns of improvement of spirometry, bronchial hyperresponsiveness, and specific IgE antibody levels after cessation of exposure in occupational asthma caused by snow-crab processing. Am Rev Respir Dis 1988; 138:807–812.
80. Perfetti L, Cartier A, Ghezzo H, Gautrin D, Malo JL. Follow-up of occupational asthma after removal from or diminution of exposure to the responsible agent. Chest 1998; 114:398–403.

81. Malo JL, Ghezzo H. Recovery of methacholine responsiveness after end of exposure in occupational asthma. Am J Respir Crit Care Med 2004; 169:1304–1307.
82. Perfetti L, Hébert J, Lapalme Y, Ghezzo H, Gautrin D, Malo JL. Changes in IgE-mediated allergy to ubiquitous inhalants after removal from or diminution of exposure to the agent causing occupational asthma. Clin Exp Allergy 1998; 28:66–73.
83. Nguyen B, Ghezzo H, Malo JL, Gautrin D. Time course of onset of sensitization to common and occupational inhalants in apprentices. J Allergy Clin Immunol 2003; 111: 807–812.
84. Ryan G, Latimer KM, Dolovich J, Hargreave FE. Bronchial responsiveness to histamine: relationship to diurnal variation of peak flow rate, improvement after bronchodilator, and airway calibre. Thorax 1982; 37:423–429.
85. Verschelden P, Cartier A, L'Archevêque J, Trudeau C, Malo JL. Compliance with and accuracy of daily self-assessment of peak expiratory flows (PEF) in asthmatic subjects over a three month period. Eur Respir J 1996; 9:880–885.
86. Moscato G, Godnic-Cvar J, Maestrelli P, Malo JL, Burge PS, Coifman R. Statement on self-monitoring of peak expiratory flows in the investigation of occupational asthma. J Allergy Clin Immunol 1995; 96:295–301.
87. International consensus report on the diagnosis and management of asthma. Clin Exp Allergy 1992; 22(suppl 1).
88. American Thoracic Society. Guidelines for methacholine and exercise challenge testing. Am J Respir Crit Care Med 1999; 161:309–329.
89. Occupational asthma: recommendations for diagnosis, management and assessment of impairment. Ad hoc committee on occupational asthma of the Standards Committee, Canadian Thoracic Society. Can Med Assoc J 1989; 140:1029–1032.
90. Meredith SK, Taylor VM, McDonald JC. Occupational respiratory disease in the United Kingdom 1989: a report to the British Thoracic Society and the Society of Occupational Medicine by the SWORD project group. Br J Ind Med 1991; 48:292–298.
91. McDonald JC, Keynes HL, Meredith SK. Reported incidence of occupational asthma in the United Kingdom, 1989–97. Occup Environ Med 2000; 57:823–829.
92. Klees JE, Alexander M, Rempel D, et al. Evaluation of a proposed NIOSH surveillance case definition for occupational asthma. Chest 1990; 98:212S–215S.

15
Prevention and Surveillance

Gary M. Liss
Gage Occupational and Environmental Health Unit, Department of Public Health Sciences, University of Toronto, and Occupational Health and Safety Branch, Ontario Ministry of Labour, Toronto, Ontario, Canada

Henrik Nordman
Department of Occupational Medicine, Finnish Institute of Occupational Health, Helsinki, Finland

Susan M. Tarlo
Gage Occupational and Environmental Health Unit, Departments of Medicine and Public Health Sciences, University of Toronto, and The Asthma Centre, Toronto Western Hospital, University Health Network, Toronto, Ontario, Canada

David I. Bernstein
Division of Allergy–Immunology, Department of Internal Medicine, College of Medicine, University of Cincinnati, Cincinnati, Ohio, U.S.A.

Case History: A 28-year-old hematology laboratory technician was seen in December 1990 with a two-year history of contact dermatitis while using the powdered latex gloves at work that were in general use at the time, followed by development of contact urticaria. She had previously had an anaphylactic episode while at work in 1988 and again during a cesarean section in 1989. She subsequently had less severe episodes of urticaria and angioedema at work with mild asthmatic and allergic rhinitis responses, which occurred even while she avoided personal contact with latex products at work (using nonlatex gloves) in 1992. Her symptomatic episodes were objectively documented, and she had a strongly positive skin test response to natural rubber latex (NRL) extract. Measurement of airborne NRL became nondetectable after the use of powder-free latex gloves in her laboratory. Her symptoms cleared, enabling her to continue work in the same environment with personal NRL avoidance.

INTRODUCTION—PREVENTION

Given that occupational asthma (OA) is one of the most common occupational lung diseases, with the burden of illness accounting for approximately 10% of all adult-onset asthma (1,2), and that it is largely preventable, it is clear that the role of prevention deserves emphasis.

Consideration will be given in turn to approaches for primary, secondary, and tertiary prevention. Where appropriate, these will be applied to the subgroups of OA: irritant OA [which accounts for approximately 10% of all OA and includes reactive airways dysfunction syndrome (RADS)] (3–5), and asthma caused by specific sensitization to a workplace agent (accounting for 80–90% of OA).

PRIMARY PREVENTION

Given that secondary and tertiary prevention of OA are not usually satisfactory, a stronger effort needs to be made on primary prevention. The most effective means of primary prevention of OA is by control of occupational exposure to respiratory sensitizers by reduction of exposure to the causative substance(s). Broad categories of measures include the following:

1. Reducing exposure (most important): This can be accomplished in a number of ways including (*i*) substitution of a recognized harmful agent with one that is less harmful; (*ii*) improved ventilation; (*iii*) automation of process (e.g., robotics); (*iv*) enclosure; (*v*) modification of the process or agent to reduce risk of sensitization; and (*vi*) dust reduction techniques, housekeeping, and work practices.
2. Identifying highly susceptible workers and locating them in areas without exposure to known sensitizers; limiting exposure to potential respiratory irritants for those with pre-existing asthma to reduce work-related aggravation of asthma.
3. Administrative controls to reduce the number of workers exposed or the duration of exposure, e.g., job rotation, rest periods, shift or location changes where fewer people are working with sensitizers or irritant exposures.
4. Personal protective equipment (for the worker) includes respirators, gloves, goggles, coveralls, etc.
5. Education of school children (and workers during the preplacement process) regarding risks, e.g., atopic children regarding risks of animal exposure, prior to entering the workforce.

Irritant-Induced OA

Irritant-induced asthma as currently understood results from acute exposure to an expected respiratory irritant (3,4). This is usually an accidental workplace occurrence, as in a spill or fire. Appropriate measures of occupational hygiene such as containment measures "at the source" (isolation/enclosure), ventilation measures "along the path to the worker," and appropriate respiratory protective devices "at the worker" may prevent some cases of irritant-induced asthma. As an example, the lack of usage of appropriate respiratory protection among firefighters working at the site of the World Trade Center collapse has been suggested to be a significant factor contributing to the relatively high prevalence of irritant-induced asthma and airway hyperresponsiveness in these workers following inhalation of high concentrations of alkaline respirable dust (6,7).

Lowering exposure to concentrations of respiratory irritant agents benefits workers with coincidental asthma by reducing the likelihood of work-related aggravation of asthma. The induction of asthma by chronic moderate or low exposures to respiratory irritants is suggested by epidemiologic studies but to date is unproven. If confirmed, there would be an additional potential primary preventive role for limiting such exposures.

Sensitizer-Induced OA

Host Factors

Because sensitization and OA from occupational agents occur in a minority of exposed workers (5% or less in many studies), host susceptibility factors are present. These include specific genotypes for which to date there is limited information (8), atopy, and smoking history, as previously reviewed (9). The importance of underlying atopy appears to be greatest in those who become sensitized by an IgE antibody–mediated response, particularly to high-molecular-weight (HMW) allergens such as animal proteins and plant products (9–11). However the high prevalence of atopy in the general population (around 20% or higher in some studies), compared with the relatively low risk of occupational sensitization, precludes this from being a useful determinant of employment, i.e., there is a low predictive value, and it would exclude many who would not develop OA. Similarly although smoking has been a significant risk factor for laboratory animal asthma, and the most significant associated host factor in sensitization to some occupational agents such as complex platinum salts and acid anhydrides (12,13), nevertheless the high proportion of the working age population who still smoke precludes this from usefulness in pre-employment screening to determine employment. Thus these factors cannot be justifiably used to prevent individuals from working in jobs that may lead to OA. Nevertheless, physicians caring for older children who are presensitized to workplace allergens or who have asthma and allergic diseases may offer useful advice to their patients regarding careers in which underlying allergy increases the risks for work-related sensitization, e.g., to NRL or to animal proteins (14).

Exposure Factors

For immunologic sensitization to occur to a specific workplace agent, there clearly has to be an exposure to that agent. In addition it has been shown for some agents and recently reviewed by Baur (15) and by Bush (16) that there is an exposure–response relationship between exposure and risk of OA; that is, the higher the exposure levels to a sensitizer, the greater the proportion of exposed workers who will become sensitized (16–18). As an example, we reported that among diisocyanate-using companies, those with workers who had claims accepted for OA due to diisocyanates were more likely to have measured concentrations of diisocyanates above 0.005 ppm than companies which did not have workers with claims over a four-year period (17).

An effective primary prevention measure would therefore be to avoid use of known sensitizers in a workplace (elimination), or to reduce the exposure levels to a minimum (isolation/control at source), aiming for levels which are not likely to induce sensitization except in those with the strongest genetic susceptibility. Unfortunately this may not be possible in many workplaces.

An example where this strategy has been very effective is the case of sensitization and occupational allergy including OA to NRL (19–24). This was recognized to be common in health care workers and other workers with exposure to powdered NRL gloves in the early 1990s (25–31). Factors thought to have increased the risk for sensitization at that time include increased glove usage with universal precautions to prevent infection with blood-borne pathogens in health care workers, resulting increased production of NRL gloves with increased tapping of rubber trees which may have altered proteins in the rubber latex, reduced leaching out of proteins from gloves during manufacture, and possibly earlier usage of gloves after manufacture. The NRL proteins became airborne in association with glove donning, generating powder in particles of a size which could be inhaled and lead to respiratory allergic manifestations (inhalation as well as cutaneous routes of exposure). These factors may have contributed to increased exposure to NRL proteins by those wearing NRL gloves, and recognition of NRL allergy and asthma increased markedly during this time.

Following understanding of the problem, recommendations were made to change to non-NRL gloves wherever possible, and to reduce the powder and the NRL protein content of NRL gloves if these needed to be used. Such changes have been associated with significant reductions in airborne dust and protein concentrations, declines in the incidence of NRL allergy and asthma as reflected in hospital series, and in compensation data and national figures, reported from Ontario (Canada) and Germany (21–24) (Fig. 1).

Removal of a sensitizer from the workplace and substitution with a nonsensitizing and nontoxic agent is an ideal approach that may not often be practical. The experience with NRL has shown however that where complete removal is not feasible, changes to minimize exposure, such as currently occurs in many areas with NRL glove use (by use of minimal powder and low-protein gloves), are likely to reduce, if not completely eliminate, sensitization (23,24).

A further example of primary prevention is the encapsulation of detergent enzymes (process modification; isolation) to reduce exposure (32,33). This was very successful when first introduced and as recently reviewed in a large company with associated medical surveillance measures (33). In contrast, introduction of new enzymes into a plant and failure of both primary and secondary prevention measures led to further "outbreaks" of sensitization and OA (34). The use of robots (automation), in addition to separated and ventilated areas as well as appropriate respiratory protective devices for workers with unavoidable intermittent potential exposures,

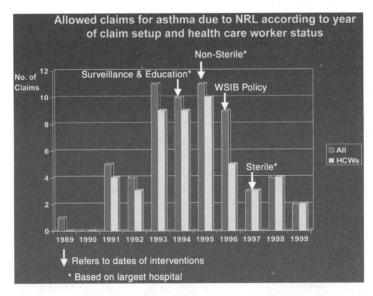

Figure 1 Allowed claims for asthma due to NRL in Ontario, Canada, according to year of claim setup and health care worker status. *Abbreviation*: NRL, natural rubber latex. *Source*: From Ref. 23.

in plants manufacturing polyurethane foam, has coincided with declining rates of sensitization to diisocyanates as suggested by compensation rates in Ontario (35). However there is no direct evidence to determine whether these changes or other temporally associated interventions have been responsible.

Substitution of occupational sensitizers with newer chemicals, which may not cause sensitization, might be effective, but there is currently no accurate method of determining the potential of new agents to cause human sensitization, despite the ability to obtain suggestive information from animal studies (36,37). The introduction of less volatile or more complex forms of some sensitizers such as prepolymeric diisocyanates requires further investigation to determine relative rates of human sensitization.

Although primary prevention by complete avoidance of respiratory sensitizers is an ideal intervention, it is clearly not feasible in many settings such as bakeries and animal care facilities. However, even in these settings, reduction of exposure sufficient to significantly reduce risks of sensitization can be feasible as described in laboratory care facilities and suggested for bakeries (16,38). The aim in these settings is to reduce the exposure to the lowest feasible level, but currently there is no known exposure concentration (other than zero) that will prevent sensitization in highly susceptible workers. The introduction of a surveillance program for diisocyanates in Ontario in 1983 (Ontario Ministry of Labour, 1983) included monitoring of diisocyanate concentrations in the workplace with a maximum allowable eight hour TWA of 5 ppb. The combination of this monitoring of workplace exposures and a medical surveillance program (see section "Secondary Prevention") was associated with a decline in new diisocyanate-related OA compensation claims (35). However, it could not be determined from the information available whether the decline was due to reduced exposure via primary prevention measures, i.e., increased use of robots and better worker education as to appropriate protective respirator use. The reduction may have also been attributable to secondary preventive measures such as institution of surveillance programs that detect early OA and result in prompt removal of affected workers from diisocyanate exposure.

SECONDARY PREVENTION

Definition: Medical surveillance (as distinguished from public health surveillance) has been defined as the serial performance of an observation or test used to detect evidence of a disease process that can be altered by appropriate intervention; it is a method of secondary prevention (39). The purpose of a medical surveillance program is to periodically evaluate the health status of the entire workforce in relation to the work environment, with the following objectives: (*i*) to recognize changes in health among groups of workers whenever possible before clinically important adverse health outcomes occur in individuals; (*ii*) to identify potentially hazardous working conditions using grouped health and environmental information; and (*iii*) to evaluate the effectiveness of exposure controls through the ongoing collection and analysis of the relevant data. To assure adequate monitoring of the health of the workforce, the overall surveillance program should periodically evaluate medical data in relation to industrial hygiene and other exposure information.

The major goal of medical surveillance programs in general is to detect workers with disease early in its course and thereby ultimately prevent its progression, to moderate or even to severe stage, with increasing morbidity and disability, and/or to be followed by appropriate intervention to prevent further cases in coworkers or future workers (secondary leading to primary prevention).

In the context of OA, the purpose of a medical surveillance (secondary prevention) program is to detect indicators of early sensitization or changes of sensitizer-induced OA workers with disease early in its course before there is progression or permanent asthma in addition to the potential to link with appropriate interventions to prevent further cases. This does not apply to irritant-induced asthma because the disease process starts with one or more high irritant exposures. It is also possible that medical surveillance may prevent rare fatal acute asthmatic episodes that have been associated with exposure to certain agents (e.g., diisocyanates) (40–42).

Rationale for Medical Surveillance

In the past, the inclusion of medical surveillance or monitoring programs has been recommended by various authors (43) and particularly in the context of exposure to isocyanates (44,45). In Ontario, Canada, and in the United Kingdom, inclusion of provision for surveillance in regulations has been instituted without reference to their rationale or effectiveness (46,47). A consensus statement in 1995 suggested that "routine surveillance be performed in all workers with exposure to agents known to cause asthma, and especially if cases of work-related asthma have occurred at a particular worksite" (48).

The main rationale for medical surveillance is the considerable *indirect* evidence that once OA has developed in a worker, the outcome is best with early diagnosis, early removal from exposure to the causative agent, and milder asthma at the time of removal from exposure (49–51). Despite this rationale underpinning recommendations in support of medical surveillance, the overall effectiveness of such programs has been assessed only rarely. That is, until recently, there was little or no direct evidence demonstrating that groups undergoing medical surveillance actually have better outcomes as compared with groups not subjected to this maneuver.

Some Examples

Medical surveillance programs for OA typically include a symptom questionnaire, skin-prick testing (if the sensitizer is a HMW allergen for which skin testing can detect specific IgE antibodies), and spirometry. Although there is some support for the effectiveness of such programs in some settings (32,33,35,52), it is often difficult to determine which component of the program is effective and what is the optimum frequency of delivering such programs.

An example of such a program for which skin testing has been feasible and which appears to have been very successful is in the detergent enzyme industry (32,33,53). The medical surveillance program for workers with enzymes that has been recommended includes periodic questionnaires, skin-prick tests (SPTs) with a dilute solution of the enzyme, and spirometry every six months for two years and then yearly (53). As with other HMW occupational allergens, upper respiratory allergic symptoms often precede the onset of or coincide with allergic asthma from the sensitizer. Workers who developed symptoms suggestive of an allergic upper or lower respiratory response at work and who had a positive skin test to the enzyme solution were moved away from further exposure in one company, and rates of OA in this setting significantly declined in temporal association with this program (33). Workers who developed upper respiratory symptoms only were removed temporarily until investigation was conducted.

Similarly a medical surveillance program for workers exposed to complex platinum salts has been reported to be very effective (54). A positive SPT to complex platinum salts has been found to be highly predictive of the development of later OA if exposure is continued (100% developed work-related symptoms in some studies). Therefore, those found to have a positive skin test on surveillance have been removed early from further exposure. Limitations of these programs are that the outcomes are usually compared to historical experience, rather to a concurrent setting not undergoing medical surveillance; so, one cannot separate the role of parallel hygiene and engineering control measures.

In the case of low-molecular-weight sensitizers such as diisocyanates, the immunologic mechanism is less clear. Only a minority of those with OA from sensitization to diisocyanates have been demonstrated to have serum IgE antibodies to diisocyanates with currently available methods of detection (55). In addition, the development of work-related nasal symptoms is not known to be a sensitive or specific marker of development of OA in this setting. Therefore medical surveillance programs for diisocyanates to date have relied on symptom questionnaires and spirometry, with referral for more specific testing based on these results. The program which was mandated by the Ontario Ministry of Labour (46) in the province of Ontario, Canada, required exposure monitoring, and also required a medical questionnaire administered every six months and performance of spirometry if indicated by questionnaire and at least every 24 months. Referral for further medical assessment was to be made if asthma-like symptoms were reported or if the spirometry showed that the forced expiratory volume in one second (FEV_1) or forced vital capacity (FVC) had declined at least 15% from previous results. No medical surveillance programs are mandated in Ontario for other asthmagens.

Unfortunately there was no prospective evaluation of this program when it was introduced. Retrospective evaluation has suggested benefit from some component of the program. Review of workers' compensation data has shown that in the period after introduction of the program, annual claims accepted for diisocyanate-induced asthma initially rose, consistent with increased case finding, then fell below baseline, suggesting a true reduced incidence (35), while claims due to other causes also rose and then remained stable. In addition, the compensation claimants with accepted diisocyanate-induced OA during the period before the program was likely to be fully in effect had a longer duration of work-related symptoms before diagnosis was made and had markers of more severe asthma (35), showing a temporal relationship between earlier diagnosis of asthma at a milder stage with introduction of the medical surveillance program. Also as compared with OA due to other causes, those with OA due to diisocyanates had a shorter duration with symptoms before diagnosis, milder asthma, and were less likely to be hospitalized (56).

However it remains possible that the earlier diagnosis may have resulted from other factors such as better knowledge of OA by family physicians and pulmonary physicians during the later time period or better education of workers with potential diisocyanate exposure so that they may have sought medical attention for work-related symptoms at an earlier stage. An analysis of companies known to be in compliance with the program showed an earlier diagnosis of OA (mean: 1.7 years) compared with those not known to be in compliance (mean: 2.7 years), and a trend to better outcome (49).

Education of Workers

Given that the prognosis in OA is related to early removal from exposure and shorter duration of time with symptoms, it is possible that education directed to workers may be an area for intervention to achieve prevention. This issue may fall under the rubric of primary (57) as well as secondary prevention. To explore barriers to (and delays in) diagnosis of OA from the worker perspective, Poonai et al. (58) undertook a pilot study in Ontario, Canada, involving structured telephone interviews with 42 patients referred to a tertiary level OA center for evaluation of OA from 1997 to 2002. The mean time to diagnosis was 4.9 years (3.4 years after excluding four outliers). On average, the patients waited 7.4 months before discussing the work relation of the symptoms with a physician, and the main self-reported reasons for this delay were lack of enquiry about work relatedness by the primary care physician (in 41%) and fear of losing work time (37%).

Socioeconomic factors that were significantly associated with *increased time to diagnosis* were *lower* level of education and *lower* household income before diagnosis. This investigation highlighted clues for possible intervention to remove barriers in diagnosis including physician education to increase awareness with regard to questions asked when taking a history with symptoms suggestive of asthma to initiate timely management, and education of workers by their employers regarding potential sensitizers in their work environment (which should be occurring by law already in many jurisdictions). In addition, it appears that those with lower education and income need special attention to navigate the social and health care systems. These factors were largely confined to the *time to diagnosis*. Further investigation is needed to explore factors associated with delay in the initial step of workers discussing (work-related) symptoms with their primary care provider.

Which Component of OA Surveillance Programs May Be Responsible?

Questionnaires: Although these studies have suggested a benefit from the program, it was difficult to determine which component was responsible. A small analysis of the relative role of spirometry as part of this surveillance program in one polyurethane foam–making company (59), showed a high proportion of false positive responses among those who had apparent spirometric changes in the absence of asthma symptoms on questionnaire (and spirometry did not add benefit to the questionnaire). Conversely, in a two-year longitudinal study (60), a study of 243 workers with low level MDI exposure followed with annual questionnaires, spirometry, and methacholine testing of workers reporting lower respiratory symptoms, three new cases of OA were identified. One of the three reported no respiratory symptoms and was initially identified by a decreased FEV_1 on screening spirometry. Once identified, asthma remitted in all cases one year after diagnosis and after removal from further MDI exposure. Similarly, in a medical surveillance program of a bakery (61), screening questionnaires were found to have a significant number of false negative reports, and the addition of an objective test has been advised wherever possible. The difference in these reports may in part reflect the lack of job security among those reporting symptoms in the bakery in contrast to the foam-making company (59) where transfer to areas away from diisocyanate exposure was feasible.

How Valid Are Questionnaires/Symptoms?: Malo et al. (62) reported that diagnoses derived from an occupational questionnaire failed to correctly identify workers with OA in whom the diagnosis was confirmed by specific bronchoprovocation testing. It tended to be relatively sensitive but not specific and performed better in excluding, rather than confirming the presence of OA, thus underscoring the need for objective confirmation.

More recently, Meijer et al. (63) attempted to develop a strategy for health surveillance based on answers to questionnaire items and exposure measurements to find predictors for the estimation of probability of sensitization to workplace allergens, using findings from a previous study of laboratory animal workers. In an initial diagnostic model, five questionnaire items (gender, wheeze, allergic symptoms during work, allergic symptoms during last year, and working for more than 20 hours per week with rats) were used to divide the population into high and low probability of being sensitized. Compared to those with a low score, workers with a high probability of sensitization at baseline showed high rates of work-related allergic symptoms (although this was included in the model as a predictor), doctor's visits, and lung function loss. They also developed a prognostic model to predict sensitization among those with an initial low probability of sensitization (80% of the original population). This model included four questionnaire items: less than four years of employment, symptoms suggesting atopy, work-related allergic symptoms, and working 12 or more hours per week, and predicted significantly higher rates of future allergic respiratory symptoms and asthmatic attacks.

Tests of Nonspecific Bronchial Hyperresponsiveness: Tests of nonspecific bronchial hyperresponsiveness (NSBH) (e.g., the methacholine inhalation test) are impractical for screening entire worker populations owing to the nonspecificity of these tests. There is no convincing evidence that pre-employment testing of NSBH can predict subsequent development of OA. However, in workers in whom the pre-test probability of OA is high (i.e., workers with positive SPTs and/or a history compatible with OA), methacholine testing is very useful. If a symptomatic worker is unresponsive to methacholine ($PC_{20} > 10 \, mg/mL$) while still actively exposed at work, asthma and OA can be excluded with a high degree of medical certainty (60,70). This is not actually part of the screening/medical surveillance process, but rather part of the confirmatory process.

Immunological Tests: When appropriate, detection of specific IgE by serological immunoassay or skin testing with occupational allergens may serve as useful screening tools. This may be particularly relevant for HMW proteinaceous allergens. Sensitivity of the SPT with protein allergens (e.g., natural enzymes, natural latex protein, and psyllium allergens) has been validated using specific inhalation testing as the gold standard for diagnosis of OA. These studies indicate that the prick test is an excellent tool for surveillance of IgE-mediated forms of OA (including platinum salts as a LMW exception) because its sensitivity equals or approaches 100%. In vitro measurements of serum specific IgE (e.g., RAST) to natural protein allergens are approximately 20% to 40% less sensitive than the SPT in detecting allergic sensitization and, therefore, should not be considered as a suitable alternative to skin testing for medical surveillance of worker populations (64,65). Within populations of detergent workers regularly exposed to microbial enzymes, serial skin testing can be used to screen for new cases of sensitization but also as a means to assess the effectiveness of industrial hygiene measures that are intended to reduce dermal and inhalational exposure to enzymes.

Recommendations

Should Medical Surveillance Be Conducted?: There is evidence from Ontario, Canada, based on nonrandomized studies, that OA has been diagnosed earlier and with better outcome in those exposed to an asthmagen for which medical surveillance was provided and among workers at companies with surveillance programs in place. Recent guidelines prepared by the British Occupational Health Research Foundation (66) concluded that "Health surveillance can detect OA at an earlier stage of disease and outcome is improved in workers who are included in a health surveillance program" referring to the Ontario experience (35). However, the quality of the available evidence was rated relatively low (one star out of a maximum of three) by the RCGP three star system (denoting "limited or contradictory evidence") and three (maximum 1) on the revised SIGN grading system denoting nonanalytic studies, e.g., case reports, case series.

Timing Considerations (*if one agrees that medical surveillance should be conducted*): In general, the majority of cases arise during the first two years of exposure. Malo et al. (67) and Chan-Yeung and Malo (68) pointed out that for LMW sensitizers, the symptoms often appear early in the course of exposure (perhaps in the first year), so surveillance should be instituted relatively quickly or more often. As for HMW agents, work-related asthma symptoms may, on average, take longer to appear, so that surveillance efforts should be spread out over longer intervals but also initiated immediately after the onset of exposure.

TERTIARY PREVENTION

Tertiary prevention is aimed at limiting medical impairment among those with established OA.

1. For those with *irritant-induced asthma*, it has been suggested that early treatment with oral corticosteroids may improve long term prognosis (69). However this is based only on a few case reports. For patients with persistent asthma induced by irritants, standard asthma management modalities such as patient education, limitation of nonoccupational irritant exposure, and relevant allergen exposure as well as pharmacologic management as for nonoccupational asthmatics should be utilized (70,71). Depending on the severity of asthma, subsequent job modification and/or occupational hygiene measures may be needed to reduce exposure to potential respiratory irritants to avoid resulting aggravation of asthma symptoms.

2. For workers with *sensitizer-induced OA*, the best prognosis generally requires complete avoidance of re-exposure to the sensitizing occupational agent and any immunologically cross-reacting agents, in addition to standard asthma management. Very low levels of NRL allergens may be tolerated by health care workers with NRL-induced OA (72), such as by avoidance of personal use of NRL products and use by coworkers when needed of only low-protein, powder-free NRL gloves. Residual powder should be removed from floors, furniture surfaces, and ceiling plenums. However the continuing presence of potential low exposures to airborne NRL allergen requires ongoing individual monitoring of the sensitized worker to ensure that there is no further work relationship of asthma. Reduction in occupational allergen concentrations to levels $<1\,\text{ng/m}^3$ has been shown to create an environment where NRL sensitized health care workers with OA can work safely (73,74).

In general the sensitized worker is advised to completely avoid further areas of exposure to the sensitizer. Nevertheless a few reports have indicated that use of an air-supply helmet respirator for occasionally needed work in areas of potential exposure can safely prevent asthma exacerbation (75,76).

At this time, specific allergen immunotherapy is not a standard treatment for OA. Early reports have suggested that it might be of some effect for allergy to NRL (77), but larger studies are needed.

Case Revised: The case at the beginning of the chapter illustrates principles of tertiary prevention, for a patient in whom the diagnosis of OA has been made, but in addition the interventions also illustrate primary preventive strategies by reduction of NRL exposure even for nonsensitized workers (78).

PUBLIC HEALTH SURVEILLANCE

Continuous surveillance of data relevant to morbidity for OA is essential for development of preventive public health strategies. This includes the systematic collection of data on incidence and causes of disease. Apart from public health strategies, the data also provide occupational health personnel, practitioners as well as clinicians, with valuable information. From a preventive point of view, incidence of OA is more important than prevalence. Prevalence is a function of frequency of occurrence of new cases and duration of disease. As symptoms often continue for several years, prevalence of OA is greater than incidence. Moreover, as duration of symptoms of OA varies, prevalence figures are difficult to interpret (79).

Surveillance data may be obtained using various sources: (*i*) reporting schemes collecting data on sentinel cases, (*ii*) occupational disease registers, (*iii*) statutory data on medical, medical–legal, and compensation, (*iv*) specific incidence studies in high-risk work environment, and (*v*) population studies on incidence of asthma in relation to occupation. All these sources are useful for the comprehensive understanding the overall picture of OA.

Sentinel Reporting Schemes

In the United States, NIOSH has instituted the Sentinel Event Notification System for Occupational Risks (SENSOR), the aim of which is to identify and characterize new case reports of targeted occupational diseases. OA has been included since 1988. Ten states have instituted SENSOR programs, the first four of which started in 1988. The objectives of SENSOR are to identify potentially dangerous sentinel cases in the work environment and consequently to initiate investigations and to implement interventions. The criteria for a case to be classified as OA are: (*i*) a physician diagnosis of asthma, (*ii*) an association between symptoms and work, and (*iii*) exposure to an agent previously associated with asthma or evidence of an association between work exposure and either a significant obstructive decrease in lung function or increase in airways responsiveness (80–82). A summary of SENSOR findings in the states of New Jersey and Michigan for the period 1988–1993 identified 535 cases that met the case definition. Diisocyanates were the most frequent causal agents. The aim of the SENSOR program is not to measure distribution of disease, which renders the incidence figures less comparable to other programs. Thus, using a capture–recapture technique, Henneberger and coworkers arrived at an average annual incidence of OA in Michigan of $58-207/10^6/yr$ for the period 1988–1995 rather than the reported SENSOR figure of $27/10^6/yr$ (83,84). Follow-up industrial sampling detected suspect agents at levels below permissible limits but prompted institution of more comprehensive industrial hygiene measures.

Since 1993, the California SENSOR program has identified all work-related asthma from doctor's first reports (DFRs). A total of 945 cases reported during the first three years (1993–1996) were considered eligible for interview. The case follow-up was planned to gather additional data and to permit identification of new-onset asthma as compared to work-aggravated asthma. The annual reporting rate of work-related asthma was only 25/million, but taking into account the fact that only about one-third of all cases were being captured by DFRs, work-related asthma in California was estimated at 78/million employed workers. However, 35% of the cases were identified as work-aggravated asthma. Interestingly, only 13% of new-onset asthma was associated with exposure to previously known allergens, as compared with a corresponding figure of 53% reported by the Michigan SENSOR project. A remarkable proportion of those agents not designated as allergens were identified as irritants (85).

In the United Kingdom two voluntary reporting schemes have been operating since 1989. The Surveillance of Work-Related and Occupational Respiratory Disease (SWORD) draws on reports on new occupational lung disease reported by specialists in occupational or respiratory medicine throughout the United Kingdom. The other voluntary scheme, Midland Thoracic Society's Rare Respiratory Disease Registry Surveillance Scheme of Occupational Asthma, known as SHIELD, covers only the West Midlands (86). SHIELD focuses on OA. It receives reports from local Medical Boarding Centres in addition to occupational and chest physicians. It has, therefore, a somewhat better coverage than SWORD (87,88). These two voluntary reporting schemes are complementary. SWORD gives the overall national picture, is less vulnerable to temporary variations owing to larger numbers, but is less likely to be complete. SHIELD has the advantage of local contacts facilitating swift investigations of clusters of cases and may be in a better position to assess overlap with the compensation statistics. Results for the 1989–1997 period of SWORD have been reported (89). A summary report of the first 10 years of surveillance under the SWORD surveillance scheme noted that OA remained high with little fluctuations over the last eight years. Chest physicians had classified incident cases according to source and etiology: 87% were attributed to sensitization, 11% to irritant exposure, leaving 2% unspecified. In 1999, diisocyanates were still the most commonly identified sensitizing agents (21% of reported cases), followed by latex (9%), flour and grain (8%), enzymes (8%), laboratory animals and insects (7%), and cobalt (6%). A feature of SWORD is that case descriptions of special interest are circulated among participants. After more than 10 years, the voluntary SWORD surveillance scheme did not experience any decline in reporting (89,90).

In South Africa a voluntary program resembling SWORD was launched in 1996 to monitor occupational respiratory disease. The project, Surveillance of Work-related and Occupational Respiratory Diseases (SORDSA), found that OA was the second most common reported occupational disease with an overall incidence of 13/million in 1996 to 1998. There was an incidence range of 0 to 36/million/yr between the nine participating provinces. The conspicuous differences were likely to reflect availability of health services; 94% of all reports were accounted for by three provinces (91).

In the Province of Quebec, Canada, figures may be obtained from the Quebec Workers' Compensation Board. The comparatively low incidence represents successful claims. Comparing incidence figures with results from surveys in three industries representing snow crab, diisocyanate, and guar gum exposure, the number of diagnosed cases were two to five times the number of claims, the true annual incidence could be some four times higher, i.e., about 100/million. This estimate is close to that of a voluntary scheme reported from British Columbia in 1991 of 92/million (92) and not far off from another voluntary program, PROPULSE, reporting an incidence of 79/million for men and 42/million for women. PROPULSE was a physician-based voluntary system for surveillance resembling SWORD. It was tested for one year only, in 1992 to 1993 (93).

Occupational Disease Registers

Registers on occupational diseases are informative sources. They monitor events longitudinally and are capable of disclosing deviations in incidences, especially in high-risk work environments. Events are reported in a consistent way which make data comparable over the years. As reporting involves national legislation issues and compensation policies, they tend to include data principally on recognized causes of disease, listed substances, and are not likely to be sensitive to discovering new causative agents. Years will pass before new agents, e.g., latex, and diseases, e.g., RADS, turn up in registers. National registers may be on occupational diseases in general, or focusing on specific diseases; however, focus on OA is rare. Consequently they may not hold as detailed and relevant information, for instance, as the voluntary schemes (e.g., SWORD and SHIELD). Registers also vary substantially with respect to ascertainment of cases and physicians' participation. Two very different registers are presented below.

In Finland, a mandatory register on occupational diseases was established in 1964. It is maintained by the Finnish Institute of Occupational Health in Helsinki (FIOH). The Finnish Register on Occupational Diseases (FROD) represents a register based on mandatory reporting by physicians. Since 1974 physicians are obliged by law to report known or suspected occupational diseases to the provincial labor protection authorities. The register receives reports from three sources: (*i*) reports from provincial medical officers to whom physicians are required by law to report all cases of diagnosed occupational disease, (*ii*) claims made of insurance companies, and (*iii*) cases diagnosed at the FIOH. Since 1982 when farmers also became eligible for compensation, there has been relatively good coverage of the working population. The insurance, compulsory for all employed workers, is voluntary for self-employed, roughly half of which have an insurance policy (94). By comparison with most countries, cases are generally ascertained by more reliable objective means. Over 90% of cases are ascertained by serial peak-flow measurements and/or specific inhalation tests (95). Compensation of occupational diseases includes costs of investigations and treatments, retraining, allowances for disablement, and pensions. The rather liberal level of compensation is likely to work as an incentive for workers to come forward with work-related health complaints. The high incidence figures of 150 cases/million working persons reported by the FROD presumably are a result of the diversity of forms of compensation combined with the mandatory reporting structure of this register (94,95).

The Swedish Register of Reported Occupational Diseases (SRROD) is based on self-reporting. Employees complete a form containing information about diagnosis, causes, and the current workplace. The employer countersigns the report. All claims are listed in the SRROD. Information on successful claims is lacking in the register (96). Contrary to what could be expected, the self-reported incidence of OA in Sweden was clearly lower than the Finnish figures.

It seems likely that asthma aggravated by various irritant agents occurring at work will frequently be reported as OA as asthma symptoms certainly will be perceived as causative rather than merely provocative. Consequently, the incidence was high in some occupations not formerly associated with any risk of OA, such as furnace work, foundry and steel-mill work, welding (other than stainless steel welding), and in loggers and cooks. Although these occupations are not known to be associated with sensitizers, they seem to be related to an increased risk of asthma. Based on a recent population study, very similar occupations were reported to have high odd ratios of asthma (96). Self-reporting may have the advantage over mandatory reporting schemes that the latter type may carry an intrinsic risk of overlooking exposures not formerly recognized as compensable inducers.

Voluntary reporting schemes are vulnerable to falling interest among reporting physicians who require continuous active motivation and stimulation of various kinds to keep up the enthusiasm for submitting reports. National registers are, likewise, suffering from an inevitable under-reporting. All workers suffering from work-related asthma symptoms will not be seen by a trained physician, nor will all physicians recognize the causal association with work or even remember to report the event. It is also clear that all workers with such symptoms are not willing to come forward for various reasons, for instance, out of fear of losing the job, especially in countries with a poor compensation policy for occupational diseases. Finally, self-employed people tend to lack an insurance policy, leaving them out of the registers (79,94).

Statutory and Compensation Data

National surveillance programs monitoring occupational diseases and injuries have their own advantages and drawbacks, and they are of comparatively little use with respect to surveillance of specific diseases such as OA. Statutory programs are advantageous in that they involve mandatory reporting, they allow comparisons between occupations and industry distribution figures of various disease groups, and incidence rates can be estimated by occupation or industry type. Drawbacks include under-reporting, especially when insurance policies are involved. With respect to occupational diseases, statutory sources, in general, provide poor information on occupational exposures.

In California, the DFR program has been proven useful (Division of Statistics and Research 1990). It is based on mandatory reporting by physicians by law of all occupational diseases and injuries. Cases have to be reported at the first visit, but not on subsequent visits. It is linked to the workers' compensation scheme. A minority of reported cases are occupational diseases, whereas the vast majority are injuries. The Californian DFR program is an essential part of the Californian SENSOR program (see above) by which index cases are found and subsequently subjected to detailed follow-up employing structured questionnaires.

In the United Kingdom, in addition to the voluntary SWORD and SHIELD schemes, there is a reporting system, the Reporting of Injuries, Diseases, and Dangerous Occurrences Regulations (RIDDOR), to improve the surveillance of occupational disorders. Index cases are supposed to be reported to the Health and Safety Executive by the employer after having been informed in writing by a physician that an employee is suffering from any of a number of listed conditions. An objective of the reporting system is that authorities may institute investigations and hygienic and technical improvements at the workplace. Unfortunately, the RIDDOR is known to receive very few reports annually and is, therefore, not very effective (97). The other official source is provided by the Industrial Injuries Scheme; here all reported OA cases by cause are published annually. The Industrial Injuries Scheme is based on a list of prescribed causes of OA for which the Department of Social Security can accept compensation. In 1990 the list was supplemented by the important category Z which stands for any other sensitizing agent inhaled at work (98). As only those with a disability assessed at 14% or higher are qualified for compensation and the compensation rate is very moderate, it is unlikely that the annual number of applicants reflects true incidence rates of OA (94).

In general, it can be concluded that statutory data and compensation data are vulnerable to deficiencies related to incentives and disincentives during the process of registering and reporting as well as applying for compensation. They are also regulated by national legislation, which hampers comparisons. Still, they may serve as an indication of differences in distribution patterns and causal associations between areas within a country.

Population Studies: Asthma Attributable to Work

From a preventive point of view the fraction of adult-onset asthma that can be attributed to work exposures is interesting. As the *attributable fraction* is the portion of asthma that would not exist were it not for the exposure under scrutiny, a much larger field for preventive strategies opens up. By controlling work environment exposures that are etiologically associated with asthma, alone or, more likely, in combination with other factors, part of adult asthma in general could probably be prevented. The perspectives explain the growing interest in the work-attributable fraction of asthma.

In a review of available population studies Blanc and Toren (1) arrived at a median overall estimate of 9% (range: 2–33%) of the attributable risk of asthma to workplace exposures. This figure rose to 15% when the authors selected only high quality studies, and likewise, Xu and Christiani arrived at an attributable fraction of 15% when studying physician-diagnosed asthma in Beijing residents (99). This prevalence study registered excess asthma in workers exposed to dusts, gas, and chemical fumes, i.e., irritants.

Population-based incidence studies are rare. Milton et al. (100) published a study comprising a cohort of 79,204 health maintenance organization members aged 15 to 55 years. The cohort was followed for three months registering new-onset asthma, re-activation of previous asthma, and exacerbation of asthma. Criteria for onset of clinically significant asthma attributable to work exposures were met by 21% (95% CI, 12–32%).

An exceptionally large study by Karjalainen et al. (101) covered the entire employed Finnish population aged 25 to 59 years. The cohort was followed for 10 years, 1986 to 1998. The unique study was made possible by two registers: one on patients with clinically established, persistent asthma, registered because such patients are entitled to reimbursement of medication costs, and the other was the census data of 1985, 1990, and 1995 classified according to occupation. Combining these registers, relative risks were estimated in jobs associated with exposures and compared with workers employed in administrative work. A total of 49,575 incident cases of asthma were recorded. The attributable fraction of occupation for men was as high as 29% (95% CI, 25–30%) and for women 17% (95% CI, 15–19%). A conservative figure for asthma attributable to work of 5% was previously reported in a study based on the FROD (102).

In a subsequent report on the same population study (103), all known (registered) cases of OA were deleted from the analysis. Interestingly, in typical high-risk occupations such as farming, painting, and baking industry the relative risk of asthma remained significantly high, 1.76 (95% CI, 1.64–1.89), 1.77 (CI, 1.56–2.01), and 2.13 (CI, 1.74–2.83), respectively. Also this study defined an excess risk in various work environments associated with irritants such as dusts, welding and soldering fumes, disinfectants, traffic or other combustion exhaust, and cold air.

From the studies available it is obvious that incidence estimates derived from reporting programs, surveillance schemes, and disease registers invariably are much lower than population-based studies comparing relative risks of asthma attributable to work among exposed and unexposed workers. There may be several reasons for the great differences, one being that population studies are likely to include a much greater part of those individuals ever exposed, reducing survivor effects. The studies may also indicate failure in recognizing association with work exposure or in submitting workers for examinations. It is possible that the higher figures reflect stringent diagnostic criteria, traditionally favoring specific sensitization and overlooking the more complex multifactorial, largely unexplored, etiology of asthma (104).

It may be worth noting that many studies with different designs report increased risks of asthma in work environments associated with irritant exposures (96,99,101,105–108). Increased risks are among construction and textile workers (107) and cleaners (103,105,109), shoemakers and metal plating workers, and electrical machinery workers (103,110). Molds in water damaged buildings, although rarely being IgE mediated, have been suggested as a possible explanation for an increased risk of asthma among educators (111). This receives support from two recent reports on increased risk by mold present at work and at home (112,113).

Studies in High-Risk Work Environments

From a preventive point of view it is necessary to conduct incidence studies in work environments associated with high risk of OA. Such studies identify risk factors including information on host determinants (e.g., atopy, smoking), characterization of exposure, and exposure–response data as well as serially measured effects. An example showing how a prospective study can produce information decisive for preventive strategies is the classical seven-year follow-up study by Juniper et al. (114,115) on detergent industry workers exposed to an enzyme, alcalase, in the late 1960s. By improving engineering controls, reducing exposure by encapsulating the enzyme, and by excluding atopics that had been demonstrated to have an increased risk of sensitization, the incidence of sensitization was reduced from 41% to 11% with a concomitant decrease in the development of respiratory symptoms.

Early prevalence studies in other high-risk occupations, workers exposed to allergy (75) due to laboratory animals and bakeries (116), had demonstrated the importance of atopy as a risk factor for developing respiratory sensitization. Long-lasting discussions, reviewed by Nordman (117), followed on whether atopy should be a reason for exclusion at pre-employment examinations of laboratory animal workers (118,119) as well as bakery workers (116), similar to what had been done in the detergent industry.

A prospective study corroborated the increased risk of atopy for developing symptoms to laboratory animals during the first year, but not during the second and third years, during which nonatopics unexpectedly ran a greater risk of developing symptoms at work than atopics did (120). This seemingly spurious finding may be linked to a more recent prospective study on apprentices exposed to laboratory animals modifying our view on atopy as a risk factor. The study by Gautrin et al. (121) demonstrated that sensitization to domestic pets on entry was a more important determinant than atopy per se (122).

Flour dust exposure in bakeries, pastry making, milling, and animal feeding has attracted the most intensive interest of all high-risk exposures. Cullinan et al. (123) described a nested case–control analysis of the longitudinal phase of a cohort of flour-exposed workers. A total of 300 workers, who had never previously worked in this industry, were included in this analysis. The participants were divided into three exposure categories of inhalable dust exposure: 0.58, 1.17, and 4.37 mg/m^3. Odds ratios derived from logistic regression analysis showed a clear increase in chest, eye/nose, and skin symptoms by increased exposure. Furthermore, SPTs with extracts of wheat flour revealed an increase in positive scores with increasing exposure.

Another important study on dose–response study was conducted by Houba et al. (124) on 393 bakery workers from 21 bakeries (125). Three wheat allergen exposure groups were formed according to job title, with a mean of 0.2, 3.5, and 11.0 µg/m^3, whereas the geometric mean of total inhalable dust exposure levels for the three groups were 0.46, 0.78, and 2.37 mg/m^3. The prevalence of wheat flour sensitization in the three exposure categories increased as follows: 4.4%, 7.8% to 14.1% being somewhat steeper in atopics (4.6%, 11.8%, and 22.9%, respectively). The prevalence of work-related symptoms (rhinitis and/or chest tightness) in relation to wheat allergen exposure increased correspondingly: 15.4%, 23.4%, and 28.7%.

CONCLUSIONS

Primary prevention measures are effective in substantially reducing, but not in eliminating, all new cases of OA within many industries. Medical surveillance for OA among workers at risk appears to be effective, although outcomes of such programs are difficult to ascertain. Public health surveillance is essential in assessing the incidence of OA in general and of OA due to specific causes. Data collected from various sources will guide decisions regarding allocations of effort and resources directed at prevention programs within specific industries.

ACKNOWLEDGMENT

The prevention portion of this chapter has been adapted from a review article prepared by Susan M Tarlo and Gary M Liss, commissioned in 2004 by the journal *Occupational Medicine* (*UK*) and published in 2005.

REFERENCES

1. Blanc PD, Toren K. How much adult asthma can be attributed to occupational factors? Am J Med 1999; 107(6):580–587.
2. American Thoracic Society Statement. Occupational contribution to the burden of airway disease. Am J Respir Crit Care Med 2003; 167:787–797.
3. Brooks SM, Weiss MA, Bernstein IL. Reactive airways dysfunction syndrome (RADS). Persistent asthma syndrome after high level irritant exposures. Chest 1985; 88(3): 376–384.

4. Tarlo SM, Broder I. Irritant-induced occupational asthma. Chest 1989; 96(2):297–300.
5. Bardana EJ Jr. Reactive airways dysfunction syndrome (RADS): guidelines for diagnosis and treatment and insight into likely prognosis. Ann Allergy Asthma Immunol 1999; 83(6 Pt 2):583–586.
6. Prezant DJ, Weiden M, Banauch GI, et al. Cough and bronchial responsiveness in firefighters at the World Trade Center site. N Engl J Med 2002; 347(11):806–815.
7. Banauch GI, Alleyne D, Sanchez R, et al. Persistent hyperreactivity and reactive airway dysfunction in firefighters at the World Trade Center. Am J Respir Crit Care Med 2003; 168(1):54–62.
8. Taylor AN. Role of human leukocyte antigen phenotype and exposure in development of occupational asthma. Curr Opin Allergy Clin Immunol 2001; 1(2):157–161.
9. Niven RM, Pickering CA. Is atopy and smoking important in the workplace? Occup Med (Lond) 1999; 49(3):197–200.
10. Gautrin D, Infante-Rivard C, Ghezzo H, Malo JL. Incidence and host determinants of probable occupational asthma in apprentices exposed to laboratory animals. Am J Respir Crit Care Med 2001; 163(4):899–904.
11. Archambault S, Malo JL, Infante-Rivard C, Ghezzo H, Gautrin D. Incidence of sensitization, symptoms, and probable occupational rhinoconjunctivitis and asthma in apprentices starting exposure to latex. J Allergy Clin Immunol 2001; 107(5):921–923.
12. Venables KM, Upton JL, Hawkins ER, Tee RD, Longbottom JL, Newman Taylor AJ. Smoking, atopy, and laboratory animal allergy. Br J Ind Med 1988; 45(10):667–671.
13. Barker RD, van Tongeren MJ, Harris JM, Gardiner K, Venables KM, Newman Taylor AJ. Risk factors for bronchial hyperresponsiveness in workers exposed to acid anhydrides. Eur Respir J 2000; 15(4):710–715.
14. Cullinan P, Tarlo S, Nemery B. The prevention of occupational asthma. Eur Respir J 2003; 22(5):853–860.
15. Baur X, Huber H, Degens PO, Allmers H, Ammon J. Relation between occupational asthma case history, bronchial methacholine challenge, and specific challenge test in patients with suspected occupational asthma. Am J Ind Med 1998; 33(2):114–122.
16. Bush RK, Stave GM. Laboratory animal allergy: an update. ILAR J 2003; 44(1):28–51.
17. Tarlo SM, Liss GM, Dias C, Banks DE. Assessment of the relationship between isocyanate exposure levels and occupational asthma. Am J Ind Med 1997; 32(5):517–521.
18. Chan-Yeung M, Desjardins A. Bronchial hyperresponsiveness and level of exposure in occupational asthma due to western red cedar (*Thuja plicata*). Serial observations before and after development of symptoms. Am Rev Respir Dis 1992; 146(6):1606–1609.
19. Charous BL, Blanco C, Tarlo S, et al. Natural rubber latex allergy after 12 years: recommendations and perspectives. J Allergy Clin Immunol 2002; 109(1):31–34.
20. Bernstein DI, Karnani R, Biagini RE, et al. Clinical and occupational outcomes in health care workers with natural rubber latex allergy. Ann Allergy Asthma Immunol 2003; 90(2):209–213.
21. Saary MJ, Kanani A, Alghadeer H, Holness DL, Tarlo SM. Changes in rates of natural rubber latex sensitivity among dental school students and staff members after changes in latex gloves. J Allergy Clin Immunol 2002; 109(1):131–135.
22. Tarlo SM, Easty A, Eubanks K, et al. Outcomes of a natural rubber latex control program in an Ontario teaching hospital. J Allergy Clin Immunol 2001; 108(4):628–633.
23. Liss GM, Tarlo SM. Natural rubber latex-related occupational asthma: association with interventions and glove changes over time. Am J Ind Med 2001; 40(4):347–353.
24. Allmers H, Schmengler J, Skudlik C. Primary prevention of natural rubber latex allergy in the German health care system through education and intervention. J Allergy Clin Immunol 2002; 110(2):318–323.
25. Tarlo SM, Wong L, Roos J, Booth N. Occupational asthma caused by latex in a surgical glove manufacturing plant. J Allergy Clin Immunol 1990; 85(3):626–631.
26. Orfan NA, Reed R, Dykewicz MS, Ganz M, Kolski GB. Occupational asthma in a latex doll manufacturing plant. J Allergy Clin Immunol 1994; 94(5):826–830.

27. Valentino M, Pizzichini MA, Monaco F, Governa M. Latex-induced asthma in four healthcare workers in a regional hospital. Occup Med (Lond) 1994; 44(3):161–164.

28. Vandenplas O. Occupational asthma caused by natural rubber latex. Eur Respir J 1995; 8(11):1957–1965.

29. Ho A, Chan H, Tse KS, Chan-Yeung M. Occupational asthma due to latex in health care workers. Thorax 1996; 51(12):1280–1282.

30. Tarlo SM, Sussman GL, Holness DL. Latex sensitivity in dental students and staff: a cross-sectional study. J Allergy Clin Immunol 1997; 99(3):396–401.

31. Liss GM, Sussman GL, Deal K, et al. Latex allergy: epidemiologic study of 1,351 hospital workers. Occup Environ Med 1997; 54:335–342.

32. Sarlo K. Control of occupational asthma and allergy in the detergent industry. Ann Allergy Asthma Immunol 2003; 90(5 suppl 2):32–34.

33. Schweigert MK, Mackenzie DP, Sarlo K. Occupational asthma and allergy associated with the use of enzymes in the detergent industry—a review of the epidemiology, toxicology and methods of prevention. Clin Exp Allergy 2000; 30(11):1511–1518.

34. Cullinan P, Harris JM, Newman Taylor AJ, Hole AM, Jones M, Barnes F, Jolliffe G. An outbreak of asthma in a modern detergent factory. Lancet 2000; 356(9245):1899–1900.

35. Tarlo SM, Liss GM, Yeung KS. Changes in rates and severity of compensation claims for asthma due to diisocyanates: a possible effect of medical surveillance measures. Occup Environ Med 2002; 59(1):58–62.

36. Moussavi A, Dearman RJ, Kimber I, Kemeny DM. Cytokine production by CD4+ and CD8+ T cells in mice following primary exposure to chemical allergens: evidence for functional differentiation of T lymphocytes in vivo. Int Arch Allergy Immunol 1998; 116(2):116–123.

37. Dearman RJ, Kimber I. Cytokine fingerprinting and hazard assessment of chemical respiratory allergy. J Appl Toxicol 2001; 21(2):153–163.

38. Baur X. Are we closer to developing threshold limit values for allergens in the workplace? Ann Allergy Asthma Immunol 2003; 90(5 suppl 2):11–18.

39. Balmes JR. Surveillance for occupational asthma. Occup Med: State Art Rev 1991; 6:101–110.

40. Fabbri LM, Danieli D, Crescioli S, et al. Fatal asthma in a subject sensitized to toluene diisocyanate. Am Rev Respir Dis 1988; 137:1494–1498.

41. Carino M, Aliani M, Licitra C, Sarno N, Ioli F. Death due to asthma at workplace in a diphenylmethane diisocyanate-sensitized subject. Respiration 1997; 64:111–113.

42. Erlich I. Fatal asthma in a baker: a case report. Am J Ind Med 1994; 26:799.

43. Brooks SM. Occupational asthma. Toxicol Lett 1995; 82/83:39–45.

44. National Institute for Occupational Safety and Health. Criteria for a Recommended Standard: Occupational Exposure to Diisocyanates. Cincinnati, Ohio: National Institute for Occupational Safety and Health, 1978 (DHEW Publication no. 78–215).

45. National Institute for Occupational Safety and Health. Preventing Asthma and Death from Diisocyanate Exposure. Cincinnati, Ohio: National Institute for Occupational Safety and Health, 1996 [DHHS (NIOSH) Publication No. 96-111].

46. Ontario Ministry of Labour. Regulation respecting isocyanates made under the Occupational Health and Safety Act, 1980. Revised Statutes of Ontario, 1983; chapter 321, Ontario Regulation 455,80.

47. COSHH. Control of Substances Hazardous to Health Regulations 1988. SI 1657. London: HMO, 1988.

48. Chan-Yeung M, Brooks S, Alberts M, et al. ACCP Consensus Statement: assessment of asthma in the workplace. Chest 1995; 108:1084–1117.

49. Tarlo SM, Banks D, Liss G, Broder I. Outcome determinants for isocyanate induced occupational asthma among compensation claimants. Occup Environ Med 1997; 54(10):756–761.

50. Lozewicz S, Assoufi BK, Hawkins R, Taylor AJ. Outcome of asthma induced by isocyanates. Br J Dis Chest 1987; 81(1):14–22.

51. Gannon PF, Weir DC, Robertson AS, Burge PS. Health, employment, and financial outcomes in workers with occupational asthma. Br J Ind Med 1993; 50(6):491–496.

52. Conner PR. Experience with early detection of toluene diisocyanate-associated occupational asthma. Appl Occup Environ Hyg 2002; 17(12):856–862.

53. Nicholson PJ, Newman Taylor AJ, Oliver P, Cathcart M. Current best practice for the health surveillance of enzyme workers in the soap and detergent industry. Occup Med (Lond) 2001; 51(2):81–92.

54. Merget R, Caspari C, Dierkes-Globisch A, et al. Effectiveness of a medical surveillance program for the prevention of occupational asthma caused by platinum salts: a nested case-control study. J Allergy Clin Immunol 2001; 107(4):707–712.

55. Tee RD, Cullinan P, Welch J, Burge PS, Newman-Taylor AJ. Specific IgE to isocyanates: a useful diagnostic role in occupational asthma. J Allergy Clin Immunol 1998; 101(5):709–715.

56. Liss GM, Tarlo SM, Macfarlane Y, Yeung KS. Hospitalization among workers compensated for occupational asthma. Am J Respir Crit Care Med 2000; 162(1):112–118.

57. Baur X, Stahlkopf J, Merget R. Prevention of occupational asthma including medical surveillance. Am J Ind Med 1998; 34:632–639.

58. Poonai N, van Diepen S, Bharatha A, Manduch M, Deklay T, Tarlo SM. Barriers to diagnosis of occupational asthma in Ontario. Can J Public Health 2005; 96: 230–233.

59. Kraw M, Tarlo SM. Isocyanate medical surveillance: respiratory referrals from a foam manufacturing plant over a five-year period. Am J Ind Med 1999; 35(1):87–91.

60. Bernstein DI, Korbee L, Stauder T, Bernstein JA, Bernstein IL. The low prevalence of occupational asthma and antibody dependent sensitization to diphenylmethane diisocyanate (MDI) in a plant engineered for minimal exposure to diisocyanates. J Allergy Clin Immunol 1993; 92:387–396.

61. Gordon SB, Curran AD, Murphy J, et al. Screening questionnaires for bakers' asthma—are they worth the effort? Occup Med (Lond) 1997; 47(6):361–366.

62. Malo J-L, Ghezzo H, L'Archeveque J, Lagier F, Perrin B, Cartier A. Is the clinical history a satisfactory means for diagnosing occupational asthma? Am Rev Respir Dis 1991; 143:528–532.

63. Meijer E, Grobbee DE, Heederik D. A strategy for health surveillance in laboratory animal workers exposed to high molecular weight allergens. Occup Environ Med 2004; 61:831–837.

64. Bernstein DI, Bernstein IL, Gaines WG, Stauder T, Wilson ER. Characterization of skin prick testing responses for detecting sensitization to detergent enzymes at extreme dilutions. Inability of the RAST to detect lightly sensitized individuals. J Allergy Clin Immunol 1994; 94:498–507.

65. Merget R, Stollfuss J, Wiewrodt R, et al. Diagnostic tests in enzyme allergy. J Allergy Clin Immunol 1993; 92:264–277.

66. Newman Taylor AJ, Nicholson PJ, Cullinan P, Boyle C, Burge PS. Guidelines for the Prevention, Identification & Management of Occupational Asthma: Evidence Review & Recommendations. British Occupational Health Research Foundation, London, www.bohrf.org.uk/downloads/asthevre.pdf, 2004.

67. Malo J-L, Ghezzo H, D'Aquino C, L'Archeveque J, Cartier A, Chan-Yeung M. Natural history of occupational asthma: relevance of type of agent and other factors on the rate of development of symptoms in subjects with disease. J Allergy Clin Immunol 1992; 90:937–943.

68. Chan-Yeung M, Malo J-L. Natural history of occupational asthma. In: Bernstein IL, Chan-Yeung M, Malo J-L, Bernstein DI, eds. Asthma in the Workplace. 2d ed. New York: Marcel Dekker Inc., 1993:129–143 (Chapter 7).

69. Lemiere C, Malo JL, Boulet LP, Boutet M. Reactive airways dysfunction syndrome induced by exposure to a mixture containing isocyanate: functional and histopathologic behaviour. Allergy 1996; 51(4):262–265.

70. Tarlo SM, Boulet LP, Cartier A, et al. Canadian Thoracic Society guidelines for occupational asthma. Can Respir J 1998; 5(4):289–300.

71. Tarlo SM, Liss GM. Occupational asthma: an approach to diagnosis and management. CMAJ 2003; 168(7):867–871.

72. Vandenplas O, Jamart J, Delwiche JP, Evrard G, Larbanois A. Occupational asthma caused by natural rubber latex: outcome according to cessation or reduction of exposure. J Allergy Clin Immunol 2002; 109(1):125–130.

73. Allmers H, Brehler R, Chen Z, Raulf-Heimsoth M, Fels H, Baur X. Reduction of latex allergens and latex-specific IgE antibodies in sensitized workers after removal of powdered natural rubber latex gloves in a hospital. J Allergy Clin Immunol 1998; 102(5):841–846.

74. Baur X, Chen Z, Allmers H. Can a threshold limit value for natural rubber latex airborne allergens be defined? J Allergy Clin Immunol 1998; 101(1 Part 1):24–27.

75. Slovak AJ, Orr RG, Teasdale EL. Efficacy of the helmet respirator in occupational asthma due to laboratory animal allergy (LAA). Am Ind Hyg Assoc J 1985; 46(8):411–415.

76. Taivainen AI, Tukiainen HO, Terho EO, Husman KR. Powered dust respirator helmets in the prevention of occupational asthma among farmers. Scand J Work Environ Health 1998; 24(6):503–507.

77. Cistero Bahima A, Sastre J, Enrique E, et al. Tolerance and effects on skin reactivity to latex of sublingual rush immunotherapy with a latex extract. J Invest Allergol Clin Immunol 2004; 14(1):17–25.

78. Tarlo SM, Sussman G, Contala A, Swanson BA. Control of airborne latex by use of powder-free latex gloves. J Allergy Clin Immunol 1994; 93(6):985–989.

79. Meredith S, Blanc P. Surveillance: clinical and epidemiological perspectives. In: Hendrick DJ, Burge PS, Beckett WS, Churg A, eds. Occupational Disorders of the Lung. W.B. Saunders, 2002:7–23.

80. Baker EL. Sentinel Event Notification System for Occupational Risks (SENSOR): the concept. Am J Public Health 1989; 79(suppl):18–20.

81. Matte T, Hoffman R, Rosenman K, Stanbury M. Surveillance of occupational asthma under the SENSOR model. Chest 1990; 98:173S–178S.

82. Rosenman KD, Reilly MJ, Kalinowski DJ. A state-based surveillance system for work-related asthma. J Occup Environ Med 1997; 39(5):415–425.

83. Henneberger PK, Kreiss K, Rosenman K, Reilly MJ, Chang YF, Geidenberger C. An evaluation of the incidence of work-related asthma in the United States. Int J Occup Environ Health 1999; 5:1–8.

84. Reilly MJ, Rosenman KD, Watt FC, et al. Surveillance for occupational asthma— Michigan and New Jersey, 1988–1992. MMWR CDC Surveill Summ 1994; 43(1):9–17.

85. Reinisch F, Harrison RJ, Cussler S, et al. Physician reports of work-related asthma in California 1993–1996. Am J Ind Med 2001; 39:72–83.

86. DiStefano F, Siriruttanapruk S, McCoach J, Burge PS. The incidence of occupational asthma in the West Midlands (UK) from the Shield surveillance scheme. Eur Respir J 1998; 12(suppl 28):30S.

87. Meredith S. Reported incidence of occupational asthma in the United Kingdom, 1989–1990. J Epidemiol Community Health 1993; 47:459–463.

88. Gannon PFG, Burge PS. A preliminary repot of a surveillance scheme of occupational asthma in the West Midlands. Br J Ind Med 1991; 48:579–582.

89. McDonald JC, Keynes HL, Meredith SK. Reported incidence of occupational asthma in the United Kingdom, 1989–1997. Occup Environ Med 2000; 57:823–829.

90. Meyer JD, Holt DL, Chen Y, Cherry NM, McDonald JC. SWORD "99": surveillance of work-related and occupational respiratory disease in the UK. Occup Med 2001; 51:204–208.

91. Hnizdo E, Esterhuizen TM, Rees D, Lalloo UG. Occupational asthma as identified by the Surveillance of Work-related and occupational respiratory diseases programme in South Africa. Clin Exp Allergy 2001; 31:32–39.

92. Contreras GR, Rousseau R, Chan-Yeng M. Occupational diseases in British Columbia, Canada in 1991. Occup Environ Med 1994; 51:710–712.

93. Provencher S, Labreche FB, Deguire L. Physician based surveillance system for occupational respiratory diseases—the experience of PROPULSE, Quebec, Canada. Occup Environ Med 1997; 54:272–276.

94. Karjalainen A, Kurppa K, Virtanen S, Keskinen H, Nordman H. Incidence of occupational asthma by occupation and industry in Finland. Am J Ind Med 2000; 37:451–458.

95. Torén K. Self-reported rate of occupational asthma in Sweden 1990–1992. Occup Environ Med 1996; 53(11):757–761.

96. Goldman L. RIDDOR revisited. Occup Health (Lond) 1996; 48(4):139–140.

97. Brooks A, Ward FG. Assessment of disability under the Social Security Industrial Injuries Benefit Scheme. Occup Med (Lond) 1997; 47(2):112–116.

98. Xu X, Christiani DC. Occupational exposures and physician diagnosed asthma. Chest 1993; 194:1364–1370.

99. Milton DK, Solomon GM, Rosiello RA, Herrick RP. Risk and incidence of asthma attributable to occupational exposure among HMO members. Am J Ind Med 1998; 33:1–10.

100. Karjalainen A, Kurppa K, Martikainen R, Klaukka T, Karjalainen J. Work is related to a substantial portion of adult-onset asthma incidence in the Finnish population. Am J Respir Crit Care Med 2001; 164:565–568.

101. Reijula K, Haahtela T, Klaukka T, Rantanen J. Incidence of occupational asthma and persistent asthma in young adults has increased in Finland. Chest 1996; 110(1):58–61.

102. Karjalainen A, Kurppa K, Martikainen R, Karjalainen J, Klaukka T. Exploration of asthma risk by occupation—extended analysis of an incidence study of the Finnish population. Scand J Work Environ Health 2002; 28:49–57.

103. Wagner GR, Wegman DH. Occupational asthma: prevention by definition. Am J Ind Med 1998; 33:427–429.

104. Kogevinas M, Anto JM, Sunyer J, Kromhout H, Burney P. Occupational asthma in Europe and other industrialized areas: a population-based study. European Community Respiratory Health Survey Study Group. Lancet 1999; 22(353):1750–1754.

105. Flodin U, Ziegler J, Jonsson P, Axelson O. Bronchial asthma and air pollution at workplaces. Scand J Work Environ Health 1996; 22:451–456.

106. Ng TP, Hong CY, Wong ML, Koh KT, Ling SL. Risks of asthma associated with occupations in a community-based case–control study. Am J Ind Med 1994; 25:709–718.

107. Karjalainen A, Martikainen R, Karjalianen J, Klaukka T, Kurppa K. Excess incidence of asthma among Finnish cleaners employed in different industries. Eur Respir J 2002; 19:90–95.

108. Zock JP, Kogevinas M, Sunyer J, Jarvis D, Torén K, Anto JM. Asthma characteristics in cleaning workers, workers in other risk jobs and office workers. Eur Respir J 2002; 20:679–685.

109. Arif AA, Whitehead LW, Delclos GL, Lee ES. Prevalence and risk factors of work related asthma by industry among United States workers: data from the third national health and nutrition examination survey (1988–1994). Occup Environ Med 2002; 59:505–511.

110. Liss GM, Tarlo SM. Occup Environ Med 2002; 59(8):503–504.

111. Jaakkola M, Nordman H, Piipari R, et al. Indoor dampness and molds and development of adult-onset asthma: a population-based incident case-control study. Environ Health Perspect 2001; 110(5):543–547.

112. Thorn J, Brisman J, Torén K. Adult-onset asthma is associated with self-reported mould or environmental tobacco smoke exposures in the home. Allergy 2001; 56: 287–292.

113. Flindt M. Pulmonary disease due to inhalation of derivatives of *Bacillus subtilis* containing proteolytic enzyme. Lancet 1969; 1:1177–1181.

114. Juniper C, How M, Goodwin B. Bacillus subtilis enzymes: a 7-year clinical, epidemiological and immunological study of an industrial allergen. J Soc Occup Med 1977; 27: 3–12.

115. Järvinen KAJ, Pirilä V, Björksten F, Keskinen H, Lehtinen M, Stubb. Unsuitability of bakery work for a person with atopy: a study on 234 bakery workers. Ann Allergy 1979; 42:192–195.

116. Nordman H. Occupational asthma—time for prevention. Scand J Work Environ Health 1994; 20(special issue):108–115.

117. Cockroft A, Edwards J, McCarthy P. The role of pre-employment allergy screening in animal work. Eur J Respir Dis 1981; 62(suppl 11):42–43.

118. Lutsky I, Ksalbfleish JH, Fink JN. Occupational allergy to laboratory animals: employer practices. J Occup Med 1983; 25:372–376.

119. Botham P, Davies G, Teasdale E. Allergy to laboratory animals: a prospective study of its incidence and of the influence of atopy on its development. Br J Ind Med 1987; 44:627–632.

120. Gautrin D, Ghezzo H, Infante-Rivard C, Malo JL. Natural history of sensitization, symptoms and diseases in apprentices exposed to laboratory animals. Eur Respir J 2001; 17:904–908.

121. Gautrin D, Ghezzo H, Infante-Rivard C, Malo JL. Host determinants for the development of allergy in apprentices exposed to laboratory animals. Eur Respir J 2002; 19: 96–103.

122. Cullinan P, Lowson D, Nieuwenhuijsen MJ, et al. Work related symptoms, sensitization, and estimated exposure in workers not previously exposed to flour. Occup Environ Med 1994; 51:579–583.

123. Houba R, Heederik D, Doekes G. Wheat sensitisation and work related symptoms in the baking industry are preventable: an epidemiological study. Am J Respir Crit Care Med 1998; 158:1499–1503.

124. Houba R, Heederik DJJ, Doekes G, van Run PEM. Exposure–sensitization relationship for a-amylase allergens in the baking industry. Am J Respir Crit Care Med 1996; 154:130–136.

16
Enzymes

Jonathan A. Bernstein
*Division of Allergy–Immunology, Department of Internal Medicine, College of
Medicine, University of Cincinnati, Cincinnati, Ohio, U.S.A.*

Katherine Sarlo
*Central Product Safety Organization, Miami Valley Laboratories, The Procter
and Gamble Company, Cincinnati, Ohio, U.S.A.*

INTRODUCTION

Enzymes are proteins that are used as biocatalysts to reduce or replace the use of
chemicals in a variety of processes (1). As catalysts, enzymes are able to participate
in multiple, repeated processes, making them efficient ingredients in a variety of
industries, including cleaning, food processing, animal feed, fuel alcohol, textile,
paper, and pharmaceuticals. Proteolytic enzymes were first introduced commercially
in Europe in the 1940s as part of an application for soaking and washing soiled linen
(2). In 1967, the first enzyme to be introduced commercially in the United States and
England was Alcalase®. This enzyme, isolated from *Bacillus subtilis* through a
submerged fermentation process, was used in soap detergents. Within three
years, 80% of all soap detergents sold in the United States contained enzymes
(3,4). Shortly thereafter, Flindt and Pepys et al. (5,6) reported the first cases of
respiratory symptoms in detergent workers after inhalation exposure to *Bacillus
subtilis*–derived powdered enzymes, Alcalase and Maxatase®. Out of 25 workers
manifesting respiratory symptoms 20 elicited positive wheal and flare skin test
responses to skin test reagents prepared from the enzymatic material and *Bacillus
subtilis* spore extracts (5). These index cases were strong indicators that enzymes
were highly allergenic materials and that susceptible workers exposed to these
agents were at increased risk of becoming sensitized and developing asthma.

The significance of these initial reports of enzyme sensitization and development of clinical symptoms in and out of the workplace was not fully comprehended
by some of the manufacturers of enzyme-containing products, although it was
recognized that better dust control would reduce potential worker exposures. Thus,
workplace structural and procedural changes were implemented within a short time.
These included manufacturing equipment enclosures, improved work area exhaust
ventilation systems, operational methods for safe handling of enzymes, and novel
enzyme coating methods to reduce enzyme friability and dust generation (7,8).
The American Conference of Governmental Industrial Hygienists implemented

377

a threshold limit value (TLV) for subtilisin of 60 ng/m^3, further driving improvements in exposure control methodologies (9). Despite these preventive measures, plant physicians continued to report enzyme sensitization (e.g., skin-prick test responses) in exposed workers. These findings led to the understanding that all workers exposed to enzymes should be medically monitored at regular intervals for enzyme sensitization in conjunction with strict control of airborne enzyme dust in the workplace (10,11). In fact, manufacturers of enzyme-containing detergent products represent the first industry that voluntarily implemented immunosurveillance programs designed to identify and monitor sensitized enzyme workers. These programs enabled the immediate removal of clinically symptomatic enzyme-sensitized workers from further enzyme exposure in the workplace. Immunosurveillance programs have also been successful in establishing safer operating guidelines for the enzyme industry that has further reduced the risk of enzyme sensitization in exposed workers (12–14).

PREVALENCE AND RISK FACTORS

Epidemiologic surveys conducted in England, the United States, and Canada in the early 1970s demonstrated that detergent workers exposed to *Bacillus*-derived enzymes become sensitized (i.e., developed IgE antibody) at a frequency of 20% to 60% depending on the degree of exposure (15,16). While the frequency of enzyme sensitization and enzyme-induced asthma has been substantially reduced as a result of enzyme dust control measures, the occurrence of occupational asthma (OA) has not been totally eliminated. Identification of risk factors among enzyme-exposed workers for enzyme sensitization and clinical symptoms are not entirely clear. The amount of enzyme exposure and atopy are considered the most important risk factors. The importance of enzyme exposure is based on studies that have demonstrated near total elimination of clinical symptoms and a reduction in sensitization after enzyme exposure was reduced below the current TLV of 60 ng/m^3 in the workplace (9). Nevertheless, OA induced by enzyme sensitizations is still being reported in the medical literature. Recently two cases of OA caused by lipase and one caused by cellulase were reported in workers from two different detergent industries in England, emphasizing the need for continued vigilance and surveillance in this population (17).

The importance of atopy as a risk factor is based on studies which have shown a strong correlation between enzyme-specific IgE-mediated immune responses and clinical disease (18–20). Several studies reported that atopic enzyme detergent–exposed workers were more likely to exhibit enzyme-specific IgE antibodies compared to nonatopic enzyme-exposed workers (21,22). Juniper and Roberts (22) also reported a higher incidence of enzyme-induced asthma in atopic subjects. This association has not been consistently found inasmuch as a recent study of workers in an enzyme production facility failed to show a relationship between atopy and development of enzyme-specific IgE antibodies (23). Although most studies indicate that atopic workers may be more susceptible for becoming sensitized to enzymes, it is still not clear whether or not atopy is predictive of progression to clinical disease (14–21). Flood et al. (21) and Johnsen et al. (23) have reported a higher incidence of enzyme sensitization among smoking workers compared to nonsmoking workers. Other demographic characteristics such as gender, age, and race have not been identified as risk factors for enzyme sensitization (18–23). Recent work by Finn et al. (24) showed that certain major histocompatibility complex (MHC) class II haplotypes were associated with the development of IgE antibody to a protease used in the detergent industry. Because the occurrence of clinical symptoms is currently rare in the detergent industry, it is difficult to assess the relationship between haplotype and symptoms (24).

IMMUNOPATHOGENESIS

Three of the initial symptomatic enzyme-sensitized workers reported by Flindt (5) were studied more extensively by Pepys et al. (6) to define the underlying immunologic mechanism(s) for these reactions. They concluded that the pulmonary symptoms exhibited by these enzyme-sensitized workers involved IgE-mediated immune responses, because all three subjects demonstrated strong immediate skin test reactions to the specific proteolytic enzymes in addition to dual-phase asthmatic responses after specific inhalation challenges (6). Subsequent studies confirmed the central role of enzyme-specific IgE-mediated immune responses in enzyme-induced allergic reactions and asthma (5,10–13,18–21). This conclusion is based on strong correlations between respiratory symptoms, enzyme exposure, positive skin test reactions to enzymes, and specific bronchial inhalation challenges (10,14–18).

The toxicology of enzymes is unique because both proteolytic irritation and IgE-mediated allergy are the major consequences of exposure to enzymes. Animal models have been used to investigate these effects on the respiratory tract. At very high concentrations, proteolytic enzymes can have pronounced toxic effects on airway tissue. Kilburn et al. (25) developed a hamster model for studying morphological changes in the lung induced by the plant-derived enzyme, papain. Papain had previously been reported to produce a lung lesion which resembled centrilobular emphysema in hamster, rabbit, and dog models. Hamsters injected with 1 mg of purified papain in saline developed pulmonary edema and hemorrhage. After four days, there was loss of collagen from alveolar walls but total lung protein, collagen, and elastin did not change (25). Although there was evidence of digestion of alveolar basement membrane connective tissue, cellular repair mechanisms were also observed (25).

Other animal models have been used to study the toxicological effects of enzymes. Guinea pigs exposed to aerosolized solutions and dry powder enzyme at a concentration of 80,000 Gu/m^3 (Gu = glycine units, a measure of enzyme activity) for one hour experienced hypothermia and respiratory distress which was histologically characterized by intraalveolar hemorrhage and infiltration of neutrophils and eosinophils (12). When one-fourth the concentration was administered for half the time, only the inflammatory cell infiltrates were observed. Repeated three to four exposures per week to enzyme aerosols at concentrations which induced only the inflammatory cell infiltrates resulted in systemic sensitization which was demonstrated by immediate percutaneous reactions and passive cutaneous anaphylaxis (12). Sensitized guinea pigs later challenged with enzyme preparations manifested bronchospasm induced by the release of histamine and other bioactive mediators. This observation was confirmed by studies using specific mediator antagonists which blocked this physiologic response (12). In this study, induction of guinea pig sensitization was observed at very high concentrations of enzymes (12). However, other guinea pig studies demonstrated that enzyme sensitization and production of specific IgGla antibodies can also occur after repeated low doses of enzyme exposure (12). Emphysematous histologic changes, reported in the hamster model exposed to papain, were not observed in guinea pig and rat models exposed to other detergent enzymes such as Alcalase and Rapidase® (12). This lack of an effect was postulated to be due to the absence, in detergent enzymes, of elastase which is necessary for the development of emphysema (12).

The toxicologic and immunologic effects of enzymes have also been investigated in Cynomolgus monkeys (26). After these animals were subjected to inhalation exposure of pure enzymes and/or detergents at varying concentrations and combinations for six months, there were no observed histologic, pulmonary function, or biochemical effects at levels of $1 \, mg/m^3$ detergent dust containing $200 \, \mu g/m^3$ enzyme. At higher concentrations there was evidence of bronchiolar constriction, and histology revealed alveolar fibrosis and bronchiolar epithelial hyperplasia. Bronchiolar constriction was reversible over time after cessation of exposure. The monkeys produced precipitating antibodies at all levels of enzyme exposure.

Because IgE-mediated clinical responses were the primary adverse event associated with exposure to enzymes, animal studies focused on understanding allergenic potency of enzymes. Ritz et al. (27) developed a guinea pig intratracheal test to study relative allergenic potencies of enzymes on the respiratory tract of guinea pigs. They found that the initial appearance of respiratory symptoms in guinea pigs after repeated intratracheal enzyme exposure coincided with the initial appearance of enzyme-specific allergic antibodies in the serum. The allergic antibody response increased with the duration and concentration of exposure regardless of whether the enzyme was administered by inhalation or intratracheal instillation (27). They concluded that the guinea pig intratracheal test was a reliable method for studying enzyme-induced respiratory disease (27). Sarlo et al. (28) used the guinea pig intratracheal test to study allergic antibody responses to enzymes at different concentrations and exposure levels. This test has provided useful information for establishing operating guidelines for newer enzyme proteins being developed for use in the detergent industry (28). This model has also been used as a guideline to determine the induction sensitization threshold dose for new enzymes that produced comparable allergic antibody responses previously observed with Alcalase and for which effective plant-operating guidelines already exist. Shifts in threshold doses for sensitization, when nonproteolytic enzymes are mixed with active proteases, have been determined by this technique (29). When the exposure guidelines for new enzymes and new enzyme mixtures were adjusted by extrapolating the guideline for Alcalase, similar rates of enzyme sensitization (skin-prick test reactions) were observed among workers exposed to the new enzymes (29). The guinea pig test has also been used to show that the detergent matrix had an adjuvant effect of allergic antibody production to protease enzyme (29). A mouse intranasal model was also developed to assess allergenic potential of enzymes used in the detergent industry (30). Dose-dependent specific IgG1 and IgE antibodies are produced following three to five intranasal enzyme exposures. In general, the results from the mouse model correlate with those from the guinea pig model (30).

Although animal models provide a valuable tool for studying the toxicologic, histologic, and immunologic effects of specific enzymes, the direct extrapolation of findings in animals, to humans, must be made with caution owing to interspecies differences and variable exposure conditions that occur in the workplace.

SPECIFIC CAUSES OF ENZYME-INDUCED OA

Plant-Derived Enzymes

Papain is the most widely used plant-derived enzyme in industry and research. Papain is a protease enzyme with a molecular weight of 23,000 Da that is produced from the latex of the papaya fruit (*Carica papaya*) (31). Papain is used in hundreds of cosmetic, food, and pharmaceutical consumer products. For example, papain is found in meat tenderizers, fruit juices, beer (as a clarifying agent), digestive aids, medications, and contact lens–cleaning agents (31–33). Papain is an important immunologic reagent used to cleave immunoglobulin molecules into two Fab (antigen-binding) fragments and an Fc (crystallizable) fragment (32). Allergic reactions to papain were reported as early as 1928. However, only a handful of papain-induced asthma cases have been reported (31). Papain is known to induce pulmonary lesions, resembling emphysema, in rat, hamster, rabbit, and dog animal models (34). Because of papain's potent elastolytic activity, there were serious concerns that a similar phenomenon could occur in papain-exposed workers. Tarlo et al. (31) studied 330 papain-exposed workers and found that only seven elicited positive percutaneous reactions to papain. Sensitization was subsequently confirmed by an in vitro radio-allergosorbent test (RAST) assay (31). Baur et al. (32,35) evaluated the clinical effects of papain in a total of 33 exposed workers in two studies. In one study, they observed that seven of 11 papain-exposed workers developed upper and lower respiratory symptoms after variable lengths of exposure. Papain sensitization was confirmed in all seven of these workers by percutaneous testing and papain-specific RAST. Bronchial provocation testing was performed in five of these workers, all of whom demonstrated an immediate asthmatic response (32). One worker also experienced a late asthmatic response four hours after the challenge (32). A subsequent study revealed that the prevalence of papain sensitization was 34.5%. In this study, eight of nine symptomatic workers who underwent specific bronchial provocation testing showed immediate or dual airway responses (35). Novey et al. (33) also reported respiratory symptoms in papain-exposed workers. These correlated with changes in pulmonary function, positive percutaneous reactions, and positive RAST tests to papain. All of these studies confirmed that papain acted as an inhaled allergen which could sensitize exposed workers and cause occupational asthma. Evidence of pulmonary emphysema was not observed by any investigator.

The potential for enzyme exposure and subsequent health effects in the general community has been increasingly recognized. Chymopapain is a proteolytic enzyme, structurally related to papain, which has been used for intradiscal dissolution of herniated lumbar discs (36). This procedure offered a noninvasive alternative approach to surgical laminectomy. Because anaphylaxis and death were reported in 1% of patients undergoing chemonucleolysis, serious concerns about the safety of this procedure were raised (36). Bernstein et al. (36) evaluated 84 patients before they underwent chemonucleolysis by chymopapain percutaneous testing and specific RAST. Three subjects elicited a positive percutaneous reaction which was confirmed by chymopapain IgE-specific RAST in one of these individuals. Thirty-seven percent of subjects who returned for repeat skin testing to chymopapain developed a positive reaction. Atopy was associated with an increased risk for chymopapain sensitization (36). The researchers concluded that skin testing was a more sensitive screening method, compared to RAST for detecting IgE-specific chymopapain antibodies prior to chemonucleolysis. It has been recommended that all subjects being considered for chemonucleolysis be routinely screened for chymopapain sensitization by percutaneous testing (36). Fortunately, this procedure has fallen out of favor. Because chymopapain and papain may cross-react, prior occupational exposure to either papain or chymopapain would constitute an additional risk factor for such patients.

Pepsin is a vegetable-derived enzyme used as an additive in the production of liquors, cheeses, and cereals. Cartier et al. (37) reported an index case of pepsin-induced occupational asthma in an atopic pharmaceutical worker. Pepsin sensitization was confirmed by skin prick testing and IgE RAST. A specific inhalation challenge confirmed the diagnosis of pepsin-induced OA (37).

Bromelain is a purified protease of pineapple (*Ananas comosus*) used in the pharmaceutical industry. A pharmaceutical worker developed OA after 10 years of exposure to bromelain (38). Sensitization was confirmed by skin test reactivity to bromelain extracts and by bromelain-specific RAST. Specific bronchial and oral challenges to bromelain in this subject elicited respiratory and gastrointestinal symptoms, respectively (38). Recent investigations have shown that serological tests can yield false positive IgE responses to bromelain due to cross-reactive carbohydrate determinants from pollens, apple, natural rubber latex, and insect venom (39). These findings indicate that great care must be taken when investigating possible allergy to bromelain.

Gibson et al. (12) performed a cross-sectional survey of a large group of workers in a meat-tenderizing plant where exposure to airborne aerosolized papain, bromelain, and ficin was documented. Good correlation was reported between work-related respiratory symptoms, peak flow variability, and percutaneous reactivity to two or more meat tenderizer–enzyme reagents. They concluded that percutaneous testing was a sensitive method for detecting workers at risk for development of occupational asthma and/or rhinitis (12).

Microbe-Derived Enzymes

The majority of microbe-derived enzymes are commonly produced by bacterial microorganisms belonging to *Bacillus* sp. and *Pseudomonas* sp. and fungal organisms such as *Aspergillus* sp., *Streptomyces* sp., and *Trichoderma* sp. Serine proteases derived from several *Bacillus* organisms (also called subtilisins or subtilopeptidases), were found to be useful in household cleaning agents because of their potent enzymatic activity which was stable over wide ranges of pH and temperature (2). As the enzyme-manufacturing industry rapidly expanded, greater numbers of workers were being continuously exposed to high concentrations of enzyme dusts. As discussed in the Introduction, adverse health effects of enzyme first became apparent in 1967 when 23 of 25 employees of an enzyme-producing plant in England were reported to have developed upper and lower respiratory symptoms (5,6). Shortly thereafter, Newhouse et al. (16) surveyed 271 of 278 workers in a detergent-manufacturing plant in England and found that 21% (57 workers) exhibited skin test reactions to Alcalase. Forty-two of these workers experienced lower respiratory symptoms. Atopy was twice as prevalent among enzyme-sensitized workers as among non-sensitized workers (16). Airway obstruction was demonstrated in 11 of these workers. These workers were reassessed six months later, after modifications to reduce exposure to enzyme dusts were implemented in the workplace. No evidence of deterioration of lung function was observed in the enzyme-sensitized or nonsensitized workers (16). Franz et al. (18) in the United States studied 38 detergent-manufacturing employees, who developed upper and lower respiratory symptoms after exposure to high enzyme dust concentrations. Symptoms ranged from nasal congestion, rhinorrhea, and throat irritation to chest tightness, cough, and shortness of breath. Enzyme sensitization was confirmed by intracutaneous testing to enzymes in 22 of 25 exposed workers manifesting lower respiratory symptoms (18). The prevalence of atopy among these workers was no greater than that found in the normal population. Passive transfer studies using sera from five of the symptomatic workers were positive. Pulmonary function abnormalities were found in 70% of the enzyme-sensitized (skin test positive) workers (18). Subsequent enzyme-specific bronchial challenges revealed a dual airway response in 9 of 10 sensitized workers manifesting lower respiratory symptoms (18). Once enzyme dust control measures were implemented, the frequency of respiratory complaints dramatically decreased (18).

Enzyme-induced sensitization and clinical disease continued to occur in the workplace even though improvements in enzyme dust control were implemented. To further reduce the exposure to enzymes, an encapsulation process called "granulation" was developed to embed the enzyme into a matrix of inorganic salt, resulting in the formation of uniform solid spheres approximately 600 μm in diameter (2,4). Improvements in granulation have decreased the fragility of the encapsulated enzymes. Detergent products were also granulated to reduce the amount of respirable airborne enzyme and detergent dust generated in the detergent-manufacturing process. Additionally, enzyme detergent manufacturers created explicit industry-wide recommendations for the manufacturing industry such as enclosure and exhaust ventilation, worker education, medical monitoring, and work practices for handling enzymes and enzyme containing detergents (10,40). These interventions resulted in significant declines in prevalence of positive enzyme skin test reactions and respiratory illnesses such as asthma (10).

Safety of these modified enzymes among consumers has been studied extensively. In 1985, Pepys et al. (41) investigated the prevalence of enzyme sensitization in the general atopic population by skin testing 136 subjects with preexisting asthma and/or seasonal allergic rhinitis to Alcalase and Maxatase enzymes derived from *Bacillus licheniformis*. They failed to demonstrate cutaneous sensitization in these subjects. It was concluded that consumers who used the newer modified enzyme detergents on a regular basis were at minimal risk for developing enzyme sensitization and clinical symptoms (41). This has been confirmed in a large longitudinal study conducted in the Phillipines where women are known to frequently wash clothes by hand several times a day. Investigators found that none of the 1,980 women (including 655 women who used enzyme-containing detergents for up to a year) enrolled in the study tested positive to enzymes (42).

However, breakdowns in the process and reliance on encapsulation to control exposure can quickly lead to the development of enzyme-induced allergy among the workforce. Liss et al. (10) reported that 25% of workers exposed to encapsulated protease enzyme in the dry bleach industry developed enzyme sensitization confirmed by specific skin testing and RAST.

A recent outbreak of enzyme-induced OA on exposure to amylases and proteases used in detergent manufacturing were reported by Hole et al. (43). Poor adherence to the exposure control methodologies developed by the industry led to 23% sensitization to amylase, 19% sensitization to protease, and six confirmed cases of occupational asthma. OA after exposure to cellulase and lipase enzymes was detected among these workers, demonstrating that sensitization and asthma can also occur following exposure to other classes of microbial enzymes (43).

Mitchell and Gandevia (20) originally addressed the significance of positive skin test responses to enzymes among enzyme-exposed workers by surveying 98 workers who were intermittently exposed to high concentrations of proteolytic enzymes. Fifty percent of these subjects experienced immediate or delayed asthma-like symptoms after enzyme exposure (20). However, there was no significant difference between symptomatic and asymptomatic workers with regard to prevalences of enzyme skin test reactivity to enzymes (20). Subjects with skin test reactivity to three common aeroallergens (*Aspergillus*, dust, and grass pollen) were at significantly greater risk for sensitization to Alcalase. No other risk factors for enzyme sensitization and clinical symptoms were identified (20). It was found that workers could continue to work safely in an enzyme dust–free environment even after they had developed skin sensitization to enzymes. This initial observation was confirmed by numerous other studies; prospective monitoring of the enzyme-detergent workforce for 30 years has shown that individuals with enzyme-specific IgE antibody can continue to work and remain symptom-free as long as exposure to enzyme is controlled (10–12, 14,20,23,44). This has led Sarlo and Kirchner to conclude that the threshold of exposure for elicitation of symptoms is greater than the threshold of exposure needed to induce the production of allergic antibody (44). In addition, some studies have reported that removal of asymptomatic atopic individuals from enzyme exposure was of limited value because enzyme-induced allergic reactions did not differ between atopic and nonatopic individuals (10,20).

Microbial enzymes have been used in the food industry for many years. Alpha-amylase enzymes derived from *Aspergillus oryzae* are commonly added to baking flour to compensate for the low natural content of amylases and carbohydrates fermentable by yeast (45). Alpha-amylase acts to stimulate the growth of *Saccharomyces* which improves the rising of the dough and the quality of the bread (45). Baker's asthma is one of the most common causes of OA in certain parts of the world (45). While flour allergens are a common cause of baker's asthma, the addition of microbial enzymes to facilitate the bread-making process has contributed to this disease. Of the 118 bakery workers surveyed for symptoms, 35 had asthma and/or rhinitis symptoms after contact with flour (45). Skin testing and RAST confirmed IgE-mediated sensitization to wheat flour in all 35 subjects and to rye flour in 33 of them (45). Of the 35 subjects, 12 had positive IgE antibodies by RAST to *Aspergillus*-derived amylase. Specific inhalational challenges to this enzyme reproduced either rhinitis or asthma symptoms in four of these subjects (45). All of the subjects with α-amylase–specific IgE antibodies were atopic (45).

A subsequent study evaluating 140 bakery workers with either upper or lower respiratory symptoms failed to elicit signs of sensitization to wheat or rye flour allergens (46). However, testing of these individuals to the *Aspergillus*-derived enzymes, α-amylase, and glucoamylase, revealed sensitization rates ranging between 5% and 24% (46). Houba et al. (47) showed a clear relationship between exposure and development of enzyme-specific IgE antibody among bakers. The prevalence of IgE sensitization was 1.4%, 12.8%, and 30.4% among workers in low, medium, and high exposure areas, respectively (47). Additional work on enzyme exposure in three large bakeries in the United Kingdom showed that air monitoring for flour antigens or flour dust was a poor means for the identification of fungal amylase (48). These investigators also confirmed the findings of Houba et al. that enzyme-induced sensitization and occupational allergy were highest in workers in areas of the bakery with the highest exposure to enzyme (48). Other investigators have also demonstrated the role of *Aspergillus*-derived enzymes as major allergens in baker's asthma (49). Barber et al. (50) reported that a 14.5 kDa barley salt-soluble protein related to a single protein family of α-amylase/trypsin inhibitors, was a major IgE-binding allergen in patients with baker's asthma.

Documentation of OA has been demonstrated in pharmaceutical workers exposed to enzymes. Losada et al. (51) reported two cases of OA induced by cellulase derived from *Aspergillus niger*. IgE-mediated sensitization to cellulase was confirmed by skin testing and specific IgE immunoassays. Immediate airway responses were induced by bronchial provocation with cellulase dust (51). A cross-sectional survey performed on 94 pharmaceutical workers exposed to *Aspergillus oryzae*–derived β-D-galactoside galactohydrolase revealed that 29% of exposed workers had percutaneous reactivity to this lactase (52). Sensitized lactase workers were nine times more likely to experience upper or lower respiratory symptoms compared to skin test–negative subjects; atopic workers were four times more likely to develop lactase sensitization compared to nonatopic workers (52). Reduction of lactase exposure and restricting atopic workers from working with lactase successfully prevented lactase-induced occupational symptoms (52). Two other groups of investigators have recently reported OA and lactase sensitization in the workplace (53,54). A pharmaceutical worker was reported to have developed OA and rhinitis on exposure to the enzymes, serratial peptidase and lysozyme chloride. Sensitization was confirmed by skin test reactivity and elevated levels of serum-specific IgE to both enzymes (55). The worker experienced a dual asthmatic response after specific bronchoprovocation (55).

Egg-processing workers are known to be at increased risk for developing OA induced by egg proteins such as ovalbumin, ovomucoid, conalbumin, and egg lysozyme (56,57). Bernstein et al. (58) previously reported the first case of OA induced by inhaled egg lysozyme in a worker employed at a plant that manufactured hen egg white–derived lysozyme. IgE-sensitization was confirmed by skin test reactivity and serum-specific IgE antibodies to egg lysozyme (58). Antigen specificity of egg lysozyme–specific IgE was demonstrated by enzyme-linked immunosorbent assay (ELISA) inhibition, and bronchoprovocation was positive to egg lysozyme (58). Since then, a second case of lysozyme-induced OA and sensitization has been reported in the baking industry (59).

Pectinases and other similar enzymes are used in the food industry to clarify fruit juice and aid in the removal of the pith from the fruit prior to processing. OA has been reported to pectinases and gluconase (60). Sen et al. (61) reported OA in 3 of 11 fruit-processing workers exposed to these enzymes. The symptoms developed within three to five months of exposure to the enzymes. All three workers had positive RAST results and positive immunoblot results (using anti-IgE to develop the blots) to the enzymes. The investigators hypothesized that inhalation exposure to enzyme during cleanup procedures and/or from heavily contaminated work clothes were the primary sources of exposure for these individuals (61).

OA from exposure to enzymes used in the animal feed industry has also been described. O'Connor et al. (62) reported OA to phytase and B-gluconase in a 43-year-old man working in an animal feed-manufacturing plant. IgE antibody to both enzymes was detected by skin prick test and by serology (RAST). An immediate and significant drop in lung function forced expiratory volume in one second (FEV_1)/forced vital capacity (FVC) was obtained upon bronchial provocation tests with the enzymes (62).

Symptoms among workers exposed to pancreatic enzymes have been rarely documented. A laboratory technician handling porcine pancreatic amylase developed OA, confirmed by double blind, placebo-controlled inhalation challenge (63). Five parents of children with cystic fibrosis experienced asthma and allergic rhinitis after becoming sensitized following inhalation of pancreatic extracts sprinkled on their children's food (63,64). Avoidance of further exposure to these pancreatic extracts prevented asthma (63). Colten et al. (65) studied 14 workers exposed to airborne hog trypsin in a plant which manufactured plastic polymer resins. Four of these workers were identified based on history to have symptoms consistent with trypsin-induced OA. Hog trypsin sensitization was confirmed by skin test reactivity to trypsin antigens. Three of the workers had immediate asthma responses after specific inhalation challenge (65).

EVALUATION AND TREATMENT

Assessment of enzyme-exposed workers who develop respiratory symptoms should be approached in an algorithmic manner. The initial evaluation should begin with the elicitation of a comprehensive history, which should include information pertaining to the job description, duration of exposure prior to onset of symptoms, temporal relationship between symptoms and the workplace, description of the workplace, length of daily exposure, and use of protective equipment such as clothing, gloves, and masks/respirators. Material safety data sheets and industrial hygiene air sampling data identifying specific exposure(s) should always be reviewed. To assure correct workplace interventions, the evaluating physician should communicate directly with health and safety personnel from the manufacturing site to determine the symptomatic worker's potential source of enzyme exposure. Confirmatory testing should include assessment of atopic status by skin test to common seasonal and perennial aeroallergens and to the specific enzymes encountered in the workplace (63). In preparing enzyme extracts for skin testing, proper preliminary testing of nonexposed control subjects should be performed using serial dilutions of the enzymatic extract to determine the least irritating concentration (8).

Merget et al. (67) compared the sensitivity and specificity of enzyme skin testing, ELISA, and specific bronchial challenge in confirming enzyme-induced sensitization and asthma in 42 workers from the enzyme-manufacturing industry. These workers were exposed to a variety of enzymes including papain, amylase, cellulase, hemicellulase, amyloglycosidase, and bacterial protease. Sensitivity and specificity of the skin prick test and serological test was defined by bronchial challenge. They found 13 workers with positive bronchial challenge tests to different enzymes (67). They found that enzyme skin testing using nondialyzed aqueous enzyme extracts was 100% sensitive and 93% specific compared to serology (ELISA) testing which yielded a sensitivity of only 62% but a specificity of 96% (67). Negative bronchial challenges were observed in only five tests with positive enzyme skin testing. When nonstandard enzyme extracts were used for skin testing, the sensitivity and specificity of the skin test was high, leading the investigators to conclude that the skin test should be the first diagnostic tool to be used in suspected enzyme allergy. They concluded that enzyme skin testing and bronchial provocation testing was essential for confirming enzyme-induced OA (67).

Respiratory status should be assessed by peak flow and/or spirometry at work and away from work and before and after the use of bronchodilators, to document work-related illness and reversible airways disease. A methacholine challenge should be performed to confirm or exclude bronchial hyperresponsiveness when airway obstruction and reversibility cannot be demonstrated. If the diagnosis of enzyme-induced OA remains in question, then enzyme-specific bronchial provocation may be necessary (66). Bronchial provocation should be performed as the last-resort test to diagnose OA to enzymes. Bronchial challenges have been performed using a number of different methods. A standard technique described by Pepys et al. (6) is to have the subject transfer the enzyme powder back and forth between two trays in an enclosed room. The subject's FEV_1 and FVC are measured at different time intervals during this sifting procedure to identify changes in lung function (6). Bronchial provocation has also been performed using capsules of the specific enzyme fitted into a hand-held patient-activated turboinhaler or as an aerosolized solution delivered through a nebulized compressor (35,51). Regardless of the technique used, proper controls should always be included. This involves incorporating a control placebo challenge day. The initial enzyme challenge concentration should typically be two- to threefold lower than the minimal concentration that elicits a positive skin test response. Bronchial challenges should only be performed by experienced personnel in a controlled setting with emergency therapy readily available (66).

MANAGEMENT

Once a diagnosis of enzyme-induced OA has been established, the treatment of choice is to remove the worker from further exposure. Treatment of a worker with enzyme-induced asthma is similar to the treatment of non-OA. This requires regular use of an anti-inflammatory agent to reduce airway inflammation and the potential for airway remodeling and permanent airway obstruction (66). The natural course for clinical improvement among workers with enzyme-induced OA is variable. However, the earlier symptomatic workers are identified in the course of their illness and removed from further exposure, the less likely they will be to suffer irreversible impairment due to airway obstruction. It is not acceptable to treat with medications and allow a symptomatic worker to return to the same job or work area without reducing or eliminating exposure to the causative agent. In the detergent industry, for example, an in-depth analysis of work practices, equipment, formulation, and exposure measurements was done to identify the source of exposure that led to the development of symptoms and to eliminate this source (13).

IMMUNOSURVEILLANCE

A significant problem in correlating enzyme exposure with sensitization has been the lack of reliable enzyme skin test reagents and a standardized approach for skin testing and interpretation of reactions. Studies that reported contradictory findings cited inconsistencies in skin test reagents, skin test methodologies, or in vitro immunoassay sensitivity as reasons for these differences. Early investigations evaluating enzyme-exposed workers were performed using crude enzymatic extracts and may have elicited false positive results in some instances (13).

The standard in vitro immunoassay used to detect specific IgE antibodies in enzyme-exposed workers was the RAST (39). The RAST has been demonstrated to identify 68% of enzyme skin test–positive workers (69). An ELISA has been shown to identify 86% of enzyme skin test–positive workers (69). However, neither of these immunoassays are as sensitive and specific as percutaneous testing (e.g., skin prick test) to determine enzyme sensitization (70).

Dor et al. (68) reported potential problems in performing IgE-specific RAST to various *Bacillus*-derived proteases. For example, they reported that Esperase® derived from *Bacillus licheniformis* undergoes autolysis which can result in the loss of its enzyme reactivity through degradation (68). They found that pretreatment of Esperase with phenylmethylsulfonyl fluoride (PMSF) is required to stabilize the antigen so that it can function as a stable allergen (68). These investigators also found that serum IgE antibodies of sensitized subjects are cross-reactive for Esperase, Alcalase and Savinase, which can limit the specificity of in vitro assays (68). Incomplete inactivation with the PMSF may have contributed to these observations. Using human IgE antibody from workers skin prick test positive to only one of the three enzymes, Esperase, Alcalase, or Savinase, Arlian et al. (71) showed no cross-reactivity among the three enzymes by crossed radioimmunoelectrophoresis.

Sarlo et al. (69) partially addressed the problem with in vitro assays by developing an IgE enzyme–specific ELISA with greater sensitivity and specificity than RAST. Complete agreement between enzyme skin test reactivity and ELISA was demonstrated in 87% of subjects tested, whereas total agreement between skin test reactivity and RAST was present only 77% of the time (69). They concluded that the ELISA was more sensitive for detecting Alcalase-specific IgE antibody in detergent enzyme–exposed workers (69). More recent work with an immunoCAP assay developed to detect IgE antibody to *Bacillus* protease BPN showed 82% sensitivity and 95% specificity, using the skin prick test as the gold standard (72).

Bernstein et al. (70) recently confirmed that skin testing was a more sensitive method for detecting enzyme sensitization in exposed workers. They accomplished this by determining the appropriate skin test dilution which would not elicit a false positive reaction and by showing that the enzymatic extract was not contaminated with other antigens that could cause false positive reactions if the individual had been previously sensitized to antigens that were cross-reactive with the enzyme being tested (70). They found that the range of percutaneous threshold response to enzymes was able to detect "lightly" sensitized subjects whereas the IgE RAST could only detect "highly" sensitized subjects (70). They concluded that skin prick testing was a more sensitive method for longitudinal monitoring of occupational groups that were at risk for enzyme sensitization (70).

Currently, enzyme skin testing is used to screen for sensitization among enzyme-exposed workers. However, workers who demonstrate skin test reactivity to enzymes are not automatically removed from further enzyme exposure because respiratory symptoms do not always immediately follow (12,28,70). Strict control of enzyme dust in the workplace via use of many exposure-control methodologies has been the major determining factor for dramatically reducing enzyme-induced OA and other enzyme-induced allergic reactions (13). Once a sensitized worker clinically manifests upper airway symptoms, such as lacrimation or rhinitis, prompt removal from additional exposure is mandatory to prevent or retard the development of lower airway complications such as asthma. In the detergent industry, the corrective steps taken to eliminate the source of exposure that led to these symptoms allow for these individuals to return to work and work symptom-free.

DIRECTIONS OF FUTURE RESEARCH

Future research is very likely to focus on:

- Long term surveillance protocols of newly hired workers in various enzyme-using or manufacturing facilities to determine genetic susceptibility and risk factors
- Risk factors that might determine clinical asthma in exposed workers
- The presence of differences in sensitization thresholds for different enzymes and whether these thresholds can be used to formulate predictive probability ratios for sensitization and clinical symptoms

- Understanding why enzymes are robust allergens by identification of allergenic T and B cell epitopes, isolating and defining adjuvant loci on various enzyme molecules, and defining the role of enzyme activity in allergy
- Whether sensitization to commercial enzymes precludes allergen immunotherapy with extracts containing protease enzymes
- Genetic modification of enzymes to eliminate allergenicity while retaining their catalytic effects

CONCLUSIONS

Enzymes are widely used in industries to manufacture a number of widely used consumer products. The rapid widespread use of enzymes by a spectrum of industries coupled with the lack of regulatory guidelines for safe enzyme dust exposure levels were two major reasons why enzymes readily surfaced as potent allergens. Many studies have shown that enzyme exposure levels are the key risk factors for enzyme sensitization and disease; atopy, smoking status, and MHC class II haplotype are other risk factors that play a role in sensitization. However, risk factors that determine progression to clinical disease such as asthma remain to be determined. The current paucity of enzyme-induced OA cases makes it difficult to identify these risk factors. Modifications in synthesis of enzymes and improvements in exposure-control techniques in the workplace have been successful in markedly reducing enzyme-induced OA and allergy cases. It is essential that immunosurveillance programs be implemented in the workplace for the early detection and removal of symptomatic enzyme-sensitized workers. Such programs will also provide greater insight into environmental and/or genetic risk factors that contribute to enzyme sensitization and the progression to clinical disease.

REFERENCES

1. Stryer L. Introduction to enzymes. In: Stryer L, ed. Biochemistry. 2nd ed. San Francisco: WH Freeman and Co, 1981:109–131.
2. van Ee J. Historical overview: enzymes in detergency, past to present. In: van Ee J, Misset O, Baas EJ, eds. In Enzymes in Detergency. New York: Marcel Dekker, 1997: 1–9.
3. Zetterstrom O. Challenge and exposure test reactions to enzyme detergents in subjects sensitized to subtilisin. Clin Allergy 1977; 7(4):355–363.
4. Bernstein IL. Enzyme allergy in populations exposed to long term, low level concentrations of household laundry products. J Allergy Clin Immunol 1972; 49:219–237.
5. Flindt ML. Pulmonary disease due to inhalation of derivatives of *Bacillus subtilis* containing proteolytic enzyme. Lancet 1969; 1(7607):1177–1181.
6. Pepys J, Longbottom JL, Hargreave FE, Faux J. Allergic reactions of the lungs to enzymes of *Bacillus subtilis*. Lancet 1969; 1(7607):1181–1184.
7. Bernstein DI, Malo J-L. High molecular weight agents. In: Bernstein IL, Chan-Yeung M, Malo J-L, Bernstein DL, eds. Asthma in the Workplace. New York: Marcel Dekker Inc., 1993:373–398.
8. Belin L, Hoborn J, Falsen E, Andre J. Enzyme sensitization in consumers of enzyme washing powder. Lancet 1970; 2:1153–1157.
9. ACGIH, Threshold limit values and biological exposure indices. Cincinnati: ACGIH, 2004:51.

10. Liss GM, Kominsky JR, Gallagher JS, Melius J, Brooks SM, Bernstein IL. Failure of enzyme encapsulation to prevent sensitization of workers in the dry bleach industry. J Allergy Clin Immunol 1984; 73(3):348–355.
11. Flindt ML. Biological miracles and misadventures: identification of sensitization and asthma in enzyme detergent workers. Am J Ind Med 1996; 29:99–110.
12. Gibson JC, Juniper CP, Martin RB, Weill H. Biological effects of proteolytic enzyme detergents. Thorax 1976; 31:621–634.
13. Schweigert MK, MacKenzie DP, Sarlo K. Occupational asthma and allergy associated with the use of enzymes in the detergent industry – a review of the epidemiology, toxicology and methods of prevention. Clin Exp Allergy 2000; 30:1511–1518.
14. Nicholson PJ, NewmanTaylor AJ, Oliver P, Cathcart M. Current best practice for the health surveillance of enzyme workers in the soap and detergent industry. Occup Med 2001; 51:81–92.
15. Belin LG, Norman PS. Diagnostic tests in the skin and serum of workers sensitized to *Bacillus subtilis* enzymes. Clin Allergy 1977; 7:55–68.
16. Newhouse ML, Tagg B, Pocock SJ. An epidemiological study of workers producing enzyme washing powders. Lancet 1970; 1(7649):689–693.
17. Brandt A, Hole A, Cannon J, et al. Occupational asthma caused by cellulose and lipase in the detergent industry. Occup Environ Med 2004; 61:793–795.
18. Franz T, McMurrain KD, Brooks S, Bernstein IL. Clinical, immunologic, and physiologic observations in factory workers exposed to *Bacillus subtilis* enzyme dust. J Allergy 1971; 47:170–180.
19. Gandevia B, Mitchell C. The dangers of proteolytic enzymes to workers. Med J Aust 1971; 1(19):1032–1033.
20. Mitchell CA, Gandevia B. Respiratory symptoms and skin reactivity in workers exposed to proteolytic enzymes in the detergent industry. Am Rev Respir Dis 1971; 104:1–12.
21. Flood DGS, Blofeld RE, Bruce CF, Hewitt JI, Juniper CP, Roberts DM. Lung function, atopy, specific hypersensitivity, and smoking of workers in the enzyme detergent industry over 11 years. Br J Ind Med 1985; 42:43–50.
22. Juniper CP, Roberts DM. Enzyme asthma: Fourteen years' clinical experience of a recently prescribed disease. J Soc Occup Med 1984; 34:127–132.
23. Johnsen CR, Sorensen TB, Larsen IA, Secher AB, Andreasen E, Kofoed GS, Fredslund, Gyntelberg F. Allergy risk in an enzyme producing plant: a retrospective follow up study. Occup Environ Med 1997; 9:671–675.
24. Finn ES, Pursifull AC, Limardi LC, et al. Complexity of the immune response to a protease and implications for the safety assessment of novel enzyme-containing products. Tox Letters 2003; 144(SL):S33.
25. Kilburn KH, Dowell AB, Pratt PC. Morphological and biochemical assessment of papain-induced emphysema. Arch Intern Med 1971; 127:884–890.
26. Cashner F, Schuyler M, Fletcher ER, Ritz HL, Salvaggio J. Immunological responses of cynomolgus monkeys after repeated inhalation exposures to enzymes and enzyme-detergent mixtures. Toxicol Appl Pharm 1980; 52:62–68.
27. Ritz HL, Evans BLB, Bruce RD, Fletcher ER, Fisher GL, Sarlo K. Respiratory and immunological responses of guinea pigs to enzyme-containing detergents: a comparison of intratracheal and inhalation modes of exposure. Fund Appl Toxicol 1993; 21:31–37.
28. Sarlo K, Fletcher ER, Gaines WG, Ritz HL. Respiratory allergenicity of detergent enzymes in the guinea pig intratracheal test: association with sensitization of occupationally exposed individuals. Fund Appl Toxicol 1997; 39:44–52.
29. Sarlo K, Ritz HL, Fletcher ER, Schrotel KR, Clark ED. Proteolytic detergent enzymes enhance the allergic antibody responses of guinea pigs to non-proteolytic detergent enzymes in a mixture: implication for occupational exposure. J Allergy Clin Immunol 1997; 100(4):480–487.

30. Robinson MK, Horn PA, Kawabata TT, et al. Use of the mouse intranasal test to determine the allergenic potency of detergent enzymes: comparison to the guinea pig intratracheal test. Toxicol Sci 1998; 43:39–46.

31. Tarlo SM, Shaikh W, Bell B, et al. Papain-induced allergic reactions. Clin Allergy 1978; 8:207–215.

32. Baur X, Fruhmann G. Papain induced asthma: diagnosis by skin test, RAST and bronchial provocation test. Clin Allergy 1979; 9:75–81.

33. Novey HS, Keenan WJ, Fairshter RD, Wells ID, Wilson AF, Culver BD. Pulmonary disease in workers exposed to papain: clinico-physiological and immunological studies. Clin Allergy 1980; 10:721–731.

34. Goodman TW, Parslow TG. Immunoglobulin proteins. In: Stites DP, Terr AI, Parslow TG, eds. Basic and Clinical Immunology. Norwalk: Appleton and Lange, 1994: 66–79.

35. Baur X, Konig G, Bencze K, Fruhmann G. Clinical symptoms and results of skin test, RAST and bronchial provocation test in thirty-three papain workers: evidence for strong immunogenic potency and clinically relevant 'proteolytic effects of airborne papain. Clin Allergy 1982; 12:9–17.

36. Bernstein DI, Gallagher JS, Ulmer A, Bernstein IL. Prospective evaluation of chymopapain sensitivity in patients undergoing chemonucleolysis. J Allergy Clin Immunol 1985; 76:458–465.

37. Cartier A, Malo J-L, Pineau L, Dolovich J. Occupational asthma due to pepsin. J Allergy Clin Immunol 1984; 73:574–577.

38. Baur X, Fruhmann G. Allergic reactions, including asthma, to the pineapple protease bromelain following occupational exposure. Clin Allergy 1979; 9:443–450.

39. Ebo DG, Hagendorens MM, Bridts CH, DeClerck LS, Stevens WJ. Sensitization to cross-reactive carbohydrate determinants and the ubiquitous protein profiling: mimickers of allergy. Clin Exp All 2004; 34:137–144.

40. Work Practices for Handling Enzymes in the Detergent Industry. New York, N.Y.:Soap and Detergent Association, 1995.

41. Pepys J, Mitchell J, Hawkins R, Malo J-L. A longitudinal study of possible allergy to enzyme detergents. Clin Allergy 1985; 15:101–115.

42. Cormier EM, Sarlo K, Scott LA, et al. Lack of type I sensitization to laundry detergent enzymes among consumers in the Philippines: results of a 2-year study in atopic subjects. Ann Allergy Asthma Immunol 2004; 92:549–557.

43. Hole AM, Draper A, Jolliffe G, Cullinan P, Jones M, Taylor AJ. Occupational asthma caused by bacillary amylase used in the detergent industry. Occup Environ Med 2000; 57(12):840–842.

44. Sarlo K, Kirchner DB. Occupational asthma and allergy in the detergent industry: new developments. Curr Opin Allergy Clin Immunol 2002; 2:97–101.

45. Bauer X, Fruhmann G, Haug B, Rasche B, Reiher W, Weiss W. Role of *Aspergillus amylase* in baker's asthma. Lancet 1986; 1(8471):43.

46. Baur X, Sauer W, Weiss W. Baking additives as new allergens in baker's asthma. Respiration 1988; 54:70–72.

47. Houba R, van Run P, Doekes G. Airborne levels of alpha-amylase allergens in bakeries. J Allergy Clin Immunol 1997; 99:286–292.

48. Nieuwenhuijsen MJ, Heederik D, Doekes G, Venabvles KM, Newman Taylor AJ. Exposure-response relations of alpha-amylase sensitization in British bakeries and flour mills. Occup Environ Med 1999; 56:197–201.

49. Quirce S, Cuevas M, Diez-Gomez M, et al. Respiratory allergy to Aspergillus-derived enzymes in baker's asthma. J Allergy Clin Immunol 1992; 90:970–978.

50. Barber D, Sanchez-Monge R, Gomez L, et al. A barley flour inhibitor of insect α-amylase is a major allergen associated with baker's asthma disease. FEBS Lett 1989; 248:119–122.

51. Losada E, Hinojosa M, Moneo I, Dominguez J, Gomez MLD, Ibanez MD. Occupational asthma caused by cellulase. J Allergy Clin Immunol 1986; 77:635–639.

52. Bernstein JA, Bernstein DI, Stauder T, Herd Z, Bernstein IL. Allergic sensitization to *Aspergillus oryzae* derived lactase in pharmaceutical workers. J Allergy Clin Immunol 1993; 93:265.

53. Julian JA, Millman JM, Beaudin MA, Dolovich J. Occupational sensitization to lactase. Am J fad Med 1997; 31:570–571.

54. Craig TJ. Lactase induced occupational asthma. J Allergy Clin Immunol 1998; 101:S23.

55. Nahm DH. New occupational allergen in a pharmaceutical industry: serratial peptidase and lysozyme chloride. Ann Allergy, Asthma, Immunol 1997; 78:225–229.

56. Bernstein DI, Smith AB, Moller DR, et al. Clinical and immunologic studies among egg-processing workers with occupational asthma. J Allergy Clin Immunol 1987; 80: 791–797.

57. Smith AB, Bernstein DI, Aw T-C, et al. Occupational asthma from inhaled egg protein. Am J Ind Med 1987; 12:205–218.

58. Bernstein JA, Kraut A, Bernstein DI, et al. Occupational asthma induced by inhaled egg lysozyme. Chest 1993; 103:532–535.

59. Escudero, C, Quirce S, Fernandez-Nieto M, Cuesta J, de las Heras M, Sastre J. Occupational asthma caused by lysozyme in bakers. Allergy(Copen) 2001; 56(suppl 68):237.

60. Hartmann AL. Occupational allergic asthma to the pectolytic enzyme pectinase. Schweirzerische Med Wochen 1987; 113:265–267.

61. Sen D, Wiley K, Williams JG. Occupational asthma in fruit salad processing. Clin Exp All 1998; 28:363–367.

62. O'Connor TM, Bourke JF, Jones M, Brennan N. Report of occupational asthma, due to phytase and beta-glucanase. Occup Environ Med 2001; 58:417–419.

63. Dolan TF Jr, Meyers A. Bronchial asthma and allergic rhinitis associated with inhalation of pancreatic extracts. Am Rev Respir Dis 1974; 110:812–813.

64. Aiken TC, Ward R, Peel ET, Hendrick DJ. Occupational asthma due to porcine pancreatic amylase. Occup Environ Med 1997; 54:762–764.

65. Colten HR, Polakoff PL, Weinstein SF, Strieder DJ. Immediate hypersensitivity to hog trypsin resulting from industrial exposure. N Engl J Med 1973; 292:1050–1053.

66. Bernstein JA, Bernstein DI, Bernstein IL. Occupational asthma. In: Bierman CW, Pearlman DS, Shapiro GG, Busse WW, eds. Allergy, Asthma and Immunology from Infancy to Adulthood. Philadelphia: WB Saunders Company, 1996:529–548.

67. Merget R, Stollfuss J, Wiewrodt R, et al. Diagnostic tests in enzyme allergy. J Allergy Clin Immunol 1993; 92:264–277.

68. Dor PJ, Agarwal MK, Gleich MC, et al. Detection of antibodies to proteases used in laundry detergents by the radioallergosorbent test. J Allergy Clin Immunol 1986; 78: 877–886.

69. Sarlo K, Clark ED, Ryan CA, Bernstein DI. ELISA for human IgE antibody to Subtilisin A (Alcalase): correlation with RAST and skin test results with occupationally exposed individuals. J Allergy Clin Immunol 1990; 86:393–399.

70. Bernstein DI, Bernstein IL, Gaines WG Jr, Stauder T, Wilson ER. Characterization of skin prick testing responses for detecting sensitization to detergent enzymes at extreme dilutions: inability of the RAST to detect lightly sensitized individuals. J Allergy Clin Immunol 1994; 94:498–507.

71. Arlian LG, Vyszenski-Moher DL, Merski JA, Ritz·HL, Nusair TL, Wilson ER. Antigenic and allergenic characterization of the enzymes Alcalase and Savinase by crossed immunoelectrophoresis and crossed radioimmunoelectrophoresis. Int Arch Allergy App Immunol 1990; 91:278–284.

72. Sarlo K, Schnell B, Harbeck RJ, Leto D, Finn EE, Kirchner DB. Sensitivity and specificity of a serological test that detects human IgE antibody to the *bacillus* enzyme Y217L BPN'. The Toxicologist 2004; 78:1262(a).

17

Occupational Asthma in the Baking Industry

Dick Heederik
Division of Environmental and Occupational Health, Institute for Risk Assessment Sciences, University of Utrecht, Utrecht, The Netherlands

Anthony J. Newman-Taylor
Department of Occupational and Environmental Medicine, National Heart and Lung Institute, Royal Brompton and Harefield NHS Trust, London, U.K.

INTRODUCTION

One of the first descriptions of asthma in bakers was given by Ramazzinni in 1700 in *De Morbis artificum diatriba*. However, until the beginning of this century the etiology of this disease was unknown. De Besche (1) suggested for the first time that asthma in bakery workers is an allergic disease. The first systematic investigation in the baking industry was made by Baagöe in 1933 (2). Since then, numerous surveys have been undertaken with the aim of unraveling the etiology of allergic rhinitis and asthma in bakery workers and estimating the risk of developing these diseases. Asthma in bakers and bakery workers is often referred to as "bakers' asthma." This terminology is better avoided because asthma caused by the same agents occurs in workers in other occupations such as flour milling, and in other food producing and processing industries and related industries such as the enzyme-producing and baking ingredient industries; asthma can also be caused by several completely different allergens.

Asthma in bakery workers is one of the most frequently occurring forms of occupational asthma. The annual incidence of asthma in bakery workers has been estimated to be 29 to 41 cases per 100,000 workers, using data from the U.K. SWORD surveillance scheme (3–6), which puts bakery workers among the high-risk group for developing occupational asthma. Data from disease registries in other countries are in agreement with the British data, and according to some occupational disease registries, the number of asthma cases among bakery workers has risen over the last decades (6–10). Cohort studies in bakery workers suggest incidence rates of sensitization and allergy (sensitization and symptoms) that range from 1 to 10 cases per 1000 workers (11–14), considerably higher than what is suggested by registry data. A small study in the United States on the death certificates of 184 individuals who died between 1980 and 1990, with asthma listed as cause or contributing cause of death, revealed an increased age and race-adjusted mortality rate in bakery workers compared to local and national mortality rates (15).

Asthma is the most important manifestation of occupational allergy in bakery workers. Work-related asthmatic symptoms are in most cases preceded by rhinitis and conjunctivitis. Allergens from cereal flours have long been regarded as the major cause of bakers' asthma. But other ingredients of the dough, such as enzymes used as dough improvers or contaminants such as mite allergens and possibly microorganisms, are known to cause allergies in bakers as well. Many cases of bakers' allergy, especially those with asthma and rhinitis, demonstrate the presence of specific IgE to the responsible proteins. Specific inhalation challenges with flour extracts in sensitized workers provoke predominantly immediate asthmatic reactions. Late and dual reactions are also reported (16,17). However, several studies suggest that a considerable number of bakery workers without positive skin-prick tests (SPTs) or specific IgE to flour extracts and other allergens from the bakery environment (enzymes) have work-related asthma symptoms (18–24). This might to some extent be explained by other allergens. Nevertheless, it seems plausible that nonspecific irritation or aggravation of preexisting asthma plays at least some role in explaining the occurrence of respiratory symptoms. Brisman et al. (25) showed, in a small study among 12 mostly symptomatic bakers and 16 controls, that nasal mucosal inflammation occurred related to nasal symptoms. The inflammation may be nonallergic, characterized by activation of neutrophils and fibroblasts. Some studies show that workers without positive SPTs or specific IgE to the most important allergens from the work environment are atopic (22,24).

Important information on the epidemiology of asthma in bakery workers and other flour- and enzyme-exposed workers comes from studies which included clinical evaluations as well as a considerable quantitative exposure assessment component. The development and use of immunoassays, which use the specificity of the immunoglobulin response to measure allergens in dust samples has led to a recent breakthrough in the study of the epidemiology of asthma in bakery workers since the early 1990s. Wheat and α-amylase allergen levels could since then be measured across the baking industry in several countries. Exposure–response relationships have been established for wheat flour allergens and fungal α-amylase used in the flour milling and baking industry, facilitating risk-assessment approaches. Criteria documents from various national and international organizations describe the first attempts to derive exposure standards below which sensitization is less likely. These developments facilitate science-based preventive strategies. There is still a need for prospective studies, and preventive strategies based on recent evidence should be validated and optimized in intervention studies.

ALLERGENS: NATURE AND SOURCES

Cereal Flours

Most reports implicate cereal flours such as wheat flour (*Triticum* sp.), rye flour (*Secale cereale*), and barley flour (*Hordeum vulgare*) as responsible agents causing allergic diseases in bakery workers. Specific IgE antibodies against extracts from these cereal flours have been demonstrated in affected workers by in vivo and in vitro tests (26–28). Although cereal flours are the most common flours bakers work with, flours from other sources may be involved as well. Buckwheat (*Fagopyrum schulentum*), a polygonaceae belonging to the weed group and taxonomically not related to cereal grains, has been mentioned as a cause of IgE-mediated asthma in bakers involved in crepe and health food production (29). Changes in consumer demands over the last decades require production of a greater variety of products, and this ongoing development in its turn leads to the introduction of other flours that contain allergens, such as soy flour.

Strong cross-antigenicity exists between allergens from different cereals. This reflects the taxonomic relationships between at least some of the grain species (26,30,31). Some of the cereal allergens are closely related enzymes or enzyme inhibitors (31–34). The strongest in vitro reactivity had been observed with water-soluble proteins, particularly albumins (35,36). IgE against water-insoluble proteins contained in gliadin, globulin, and glutenin fractions had also been reported (37). The number of potentially relevant allergens is large. A total of 40 different antigens in wheat flour have been identified, of which 20 cross-reacted with rye flour (38). Sera of a majority of sensitized bakers show IgE reactions with many of these proteins, but reaction profiles often differ markedly between individual sera (39). An illustration of the number of proteins involved is presented in Figure 1. Water- or salt-soluble wheat flour proteins from the Bussard cultivar were separated by using two-dimensional gel electrophoresis with immobilized pH gradients. Altogether, more than 100 IgE-binding protein spots were detected. The IgE immunoblots obtained with 10 different sera exhibited a remarkable heterogeneity. Each patient showed an individual IgE-binding pattern with 4 to 50 different allergen spots (40). Reactions to some components in the 12- to 17-kDa range are found most commonly (39–43). One of the major components of the 12- to 15-kDa bands

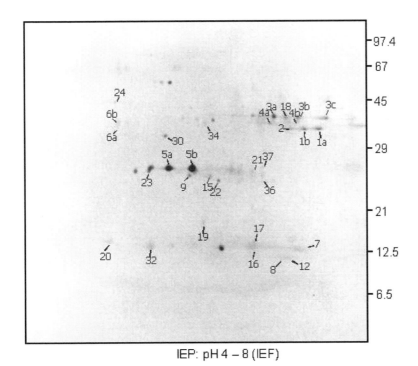

Figure 1 Two-dimensional immunoblot of wheat with serum of one particular wheat-sensitized baker. *Source*: From Ref. 40.

belongs to the α-amylase/trypsin inhibitor family (32,44–46). The allergenicity of purified members of this enzyme-inhibitor family has been shown in vitro (32,47) and in vivo (48), and is found in other cereal species as well (49–52). A 14.5 kDa protein from barley belonging to this family has been associated with bakers' asthma (53). Allergens of 26 to 28 and 35 kDa are homologous to cereal enzymes such as acyl-CoA oxidase and fructose-bisphosphate adolase (45,46) (Fig. 2). However, new allergens are still being identified. Sander et al. (40) recently found four new wheat allergens: two different isoforms of glycerinaldehyde-3-phosphate dehydrogenase, triosephosphate isomerase from *H. vulgare*, and serpin, a serine proteinase inhibitor from *Triticum aestivum*.

Addition of cereal malt flours as dough improvers decreased because of the introduction of fungal amylases. However, malt flours are still being used and contain potent allergens that are probably related to the cereal amylases mentioned earlier (54–56).

Enzymes

A relatively new source of occupational allergies and asthma in the baking industry are enzymes such as fungal α-amylases, proteases, and cellulases. Use of enzymes provides better control of the rising and baking processes. They modify the viscosity of the dough, volume, and coloring of the baked product and lengthen shelf life. The baking industry started using enzymes in the 1970s with rapid increases in the 1980s and 1990s. First reports of enzyme-related respiratory morbidity in bakers come from the early 1980s. Since then, several case reports have been reported of bakers' asthma caused by this enzyme, often in the absence of specific IgE to cereal allergens (54,56–63). The baking industry is probably one of the first intermediary industries, after the primary production industries, where a large-scale use of enzymes occurs and results in an occupational hazard.

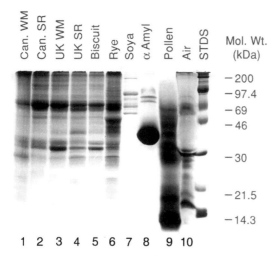

Figure 2   SDS-PAGE of 10 samples + standards. (1) Canadian wholemeal flour; (2) Canadian self-rising flour; (3) U.K. wholemeal flour; (4) U.K. self-rising flour; (5) biscuit flour; (6) rye flour; (7) soya flour; (8) fungal alpha-amylase; (9) rye grass pollen; and (10) air sample eluate.

The most commonly used dough improver, fungal α-amylase (1,4-α-D-glucan glucanohydrolase), usually derived from *Aspergillus oryzae*, is a glycoprotein which catalyses the hydrolysis of internal 1,4-α-glycosidic linkages in polysaccharides. α-Amylase is routinely added in small amounts (mg/kg flour) to baking flour in the flour mills before shipment. Alternatively, commercially available mixtures of dough improvers containing enzymes, fats and sugar, can be added to unenriched flour in the bakery. Several IgE-binding proteins have been detected in crude amylase preparations with a dominating IgE-binding band for a protein with a molecular weight between 51 and 54 kDa (57,62,64–68) (Fig. 3). This band represents the active α-amylase enzyme (65). Commercially available extracts of fungal α-amylase contain several other allergenic proteins with molecular weights of 25 to 27 and 40 kDa (64,65,68,69). Case studies suggest that oral provocation with fungal α-amylase enzyme (70) and bread (71,72) may cause allergic respiratory symptoms in individuals sensitized through airborne amylase. In other studies it was not possible to provoke allergic reactions on consuming bread in individuals with skin test reactions to *Aspergillus fumigatus*, *A. oryzae*, and α-amylase (73). Some studies have shown a loss of allergenicity of heated α-amylase, suggesting that α-amylase in baked food products would indeed not be an important cause of allergic sensitization (74,75). Three other studies suggest, however, that fungal α-amylase partially retains its allergenicity and is still capable of binding IgE antibodies after being heated (72,76,77). Amylases are also present in cereal flour in its native form. IgE antibodies, which bind cereal α-amylases or β-amylases from barley flour, have been demonstrated. Molecular weights of these cereal amylases appeared to be 54, 59, and 64 kDa (66,75). However, cereal and fungal amylases show only minimal immunologic cross-reactivity (66,75), and different allergenic behavior exists between homologous allergens such as α-amylase inhibitor allergens from rye, barley, and wheat (52).

Other allergens are being used in the baking industry and could form a respiratory hazard but seemed less important compared to α-amylase until recently.

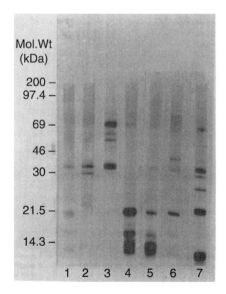

Figure 3   Western blot of Canadian Western Red Spring flour probed with sera of seven patients allergic to flour (1–7). IgE in different sera bind to different flour proteins.

Baur et al. (64,78) studied asthmatic bakers and showed that 5% to 10% were sensitized to fungal glucoamylase and (hemi) cellulase, while sensitization to proteolytic enzymes (protease and papain) was rare. A Finnish study in 365 workers from bakeries, a flour mill, and a crisp bread factory showed that most workers sensitized to enzymes had a positive SPT to fungal α-amylase and very few workers had a positive SPT to fungal proteases, cellulase, or glucose oxidase (79). New surveys are needed to provide reliable information about the sensitization rates to enzymes other than fungal α-amylase.

Storage Mites

Wheat flour in bakeries can be contaminated with storage mites (80), and allergens from storage mites have been suggested as a cause of allergic symptoms in bakery workers (80,81). Epidemiologic studies have shown high prevalence rates of sensitization to storage mites (*Acarus siro*, *Glycophagus domesticus*, *Lepidoglyphus destructor*, *Tyrophagus longior*, *T. putrescentiae*) in bakery workers varying from 11% to 33% (20,21,24,25). However, no difference in sensitization to storage mites could be found in two studies between bakery workers and controls (24,82,83). Others have also reported high prevalence rates of storage mite sensitization in nonoccupationally exposed subjects (82,84,85). This suggests that storage mites are widespread in the environment and that positive skin responses to storage mites among bakers are more an indicator of atopy, rather than a response to an occupational allergen specific to bakers. Moreover, part of the apparent anti–storage mite IgE reactions may be due to cross-reactivity with house dust mites (82,85,86), although according to some studies storage mites also possess storage mite–specific allergenic epitopes (82,85).

Other Allergens

Moulds have also been suggested as causing asthma in some bakers, but their role as a cause of asthma in bakery workers remains controversial (87,88). The prevalence of sensitization in symptomatic bakers significantly differed from that in groups of symptomatic controls (89,90). However, the study by Brisman et al. (25) showed that sensitization rates were low in randomly selected bakery workers. The prevalence of positive SPT to bakers yeast seems low as well (22,25). For most other allergens mentioned in the literature, such as egg yolk and egg white, sesame seeds, nuts (hazelnuts and almonds), etc., only sporadic case reports have been reported, and these allergens present only a marginal contribution to the high prevalence of respiratory allergy in bakers.

MEASUREMENT OF DUST EXPOSURE AND AIRBORNE ALLERGENS

Until recently, dust sampling has been the only tool for exposure assessment in the baking industry. A known volume of air is drawn through a sampling head with a filter and the dust particles are retained on the filter and weighed. The design of the sampling head determines the size of the particulates sampled. For studies in occupational asthma, it is now common to sample the inhalable dust fraction. This is the fraction that is able to penetrate and deposit into the airways. However, despite the widespread availability of dust measurement techniques, reliable exposure data results from large dust measurement series across the bakery industry have only become available since the 1990s (91–95).

Most studies involve large bakeries with distinctly different job categories. Only some data are available for small bakeries, often family-based enterprises. Job rotation is common in small bakeries, and family members are often involved in part of the process. Small bakeries form an important segment of the bread- and pastry-producing industry, especially in some European countries. Results of the available exposure studies show that workers at the front-end of the process of larger industries had the highest eight-hour average dust exposures (dough makers and bread formers average inhalable dust exposures of 3–9 /m^3). Oven workers had intermediate dust exposures (eight-hour average inhalable dust exposures of 1–3 mg/m^3), and workers involved in packing and slicing had the lowest exposures (below 1 /m^3). Some of these studies suggest the presence of small differences in dust exposure between bakeries that produce different products (93,95). High average dust exposure levels were found in Canadian bakeries for workers involved in the production of puff pastry ($N=14$, AM 23 /m^3), bread and buns ($N=17$, AM 18 /m^3), croissants ($N=8$, AM 5.3 /m^3), and cinnamon buns ($N=6$, AM 3.6 /m^3) (95). Data from small bakeries show geometric mean inhalable dust levels of 3.3 /m^3 in bread bakers ($N=36$), 2.0 /m^3 in mixed (bread and confectionary) bakers, and 0.7 /m^3 in confectioners with considerable variability between bakeries (93).

Recently, several assays have become available which allow measurement of allergen levels in personal dust samples. The development of these immunoassays forms an important step forward in quantifying allergen exposure in the bakery industry. These methods are valid, specific, and produce reasonably reproducible results. The sensitivity is sufficient to detect allergens quantitatively in personal samples in the μg/m^3 or even pg/m^3 range. Several different assays have been described for the whole specter of airborne wheat allergens (93,96) by using polyclonal rabbit IgG antibodies and IgG$_4$ antibodies from a pool of IgG$_4$ positive bakery workers in radioallergosorbent test (RAST) and enzyme-linked immunosorbent assays (ELISA), respectively. Similar assays, using affinity-purified polyclonal rabbit IgG or monoclonal antibodies, are available to measure airborne α-amylase allergens (67,68). Some semiquantitative assays have been developed to measure cellulase and xylanase in the air (78). A large-scale European project (MOCALEX) started in 2000 aimed at optimizing and standardizing assays. The results will become available in the coming years.

In two studies, personal dust exposure levels were compared with wheat allergen exposure levels. In the first study, the wheat content of the inhalable dust varied strongly depending on the use of products other than wheat flour (91,93). In the second study, the relationship between dust levels and wheat allergen levels depended on the type of bakery (93). The correlation was strongest in bread bakeries, weakest in pastry bakeries, and intermediate in mixed bakeries. Allergen content of the dust (expressed as the ratio of wheat antigen/dust) varied from 2850 ng/mg for dough makers, 1150 ng/mg for oven staff to 350 ng/mg for slicers, packers, and transport workers in large bakeries. In small family-based bakeries, ratios between 1950 ng/mg (bread bakeries) and 1550 ng/mg (confectioneries) were observed. There were also considerable differences in the ratios of wheat allergen and dust between industries, depending on the end product. For instance, within the group of dough makers, the ratio varied from 4750 ng/mg (wheat bread production) and 1900 ng/mg (crisp bake production) to 550 ng/mg (rye bread production).

For fungal α-amylase, the correlation with dust exposure was only 0.19 in a sample of 357 dust measurements taken in one industry (22,68). This study illustrated that dust concentration is a poor approximation of the allergen exposure level in bakeries, and that misclassification of exposure may occur in epidemiological surveys when bakery workers are classified based on dust exposure levels only. A major drawback of the use of immunoassays is that assay characteristics differ between laboratories. The use of different standard allergen preparations and antibody sources hampers the comparison of allergen levels reported by different research groups. This requires rigid standardization and harmonization in the near future.

Occasionally, particle size distribution of flour dust has been determined, showing that particles larger than $10\,\mu m$ predominate (91,97). Only a small fraction of the dust (approximately 20%) belongs to the respirable fraction (roughly less than $5\,\mu m$). Both the wheat and α-amylase allergens are predominantly present in particulates larger than $5\,\mu m$ (93,98). Exposure to mainly larger particulates has a few important implications. The dust that is generated is airborne for only a short period because sedimentation occurs soon after emission of the dust, and sedimentation of particulates larger than $10\,\mu m$ is only a matter of minutes. Bystander exposures will rarely occur and background exposure levels will be extremely low. As a result, bakery workers will mainly be exposed to a series of short peaks that occur during dusty tasks. A small field study in which the dust exposure was monitored continuously showed that the eight-hour dust exposure could almost entirely be explained by the number of dust peaks that occurred during the day (99).

Little is known about exposure to airborne fungi in bakeries. A large variety of fungal species has been found in bakeries (88,100–103). The dominating mould species varied from study to study, suggesting that local circumstances in each bakery may be very important. Reliable quantitative exposure data for airborne fungi in bakeries have not been published.

EPIDEMIOLOGY

Prevalence and Incidence Data

Sensitization to wheat flour or fungal amylase has been evaluated in a large number of cross-sectional studies, either by skin testing or by measuring specific IgE antibodies in sera. Sensitization rates vary from 5% to 25% for wheat flour and from 2% to 15% for α-amylase (14,15,20–25,83,104,105). Sensitization rates for other allergens from bakeries, such as baker's yeast (*Saccharomyces cerevisiae*), and for enzymes such as xylanase are considerably lower, and in most cases below 1% to 2% (22,25,61,106). Sensitization to other allergens has been reported in case studies, but has not been studied routinely in epidemiological studies. A detailed comparison of the studies is not possible because these tests have been performed with different methods, extracts, and cut-off points. Moreover, little data are available about background levels of sensitization while some occupationally unexposed individuals have specific IgE to allergens possibly due to an increased propensity to develop IgE-mediated sensitization in atopic individuals or because of cosensitization or cross-reactivity to other allergens, for instance pollens (104,107).

A large number of cross-sectional studies have shown that prevalence rates of respiratory symptoms are high. Rhinitis and asthma-like symptoms can be found in 5% to 25% of the workers (14,15,20–25,83,104,105,107). However, several of these studies have important methodological shortcomings. The participation rate is not known, methods have not been described, and information exposure or risk modifiers (atopy, gender, smoking, etc.) are not given.

Apart from information from registry-based studies, information is available on the incidence of bakers' asthma from studies across the industry. Herxheimer (13) studied 1555 Danish bakers in the 1950s in Copenhagen, Denmark. The incidence rate for wheat flour sensitization was in the order of magnitude of 10 per 1000 workers per year, and for respiratory wheat allergy, it was of 3 to 4 per 1000 workers per year. A German cohort study in 880 bakers' apprentices with a five-year follow-up and annual skin-prick testing showed cumulative incidence figures for the number of positive tests of 12% in the second year, 19% in the third, 27% in the fourth, and 30% in the fifth year (14,108). Symptom rates "compatible of allergic rhinitis or asthma" rose as well from 0.2% to 7% in year three and dropped to 4.8% after five years. A major problem of the study was the enormous loss to follow-up, particularly in the later years of the study. The follow-up rates after the second year were below 33% (baseline 100%; first year 74%, second 48%, third 33%, fourth 11%, and fifth 4.2%), which could have biased the prevalence and cumulative incidence rates considerably. In a Swedish study, between 1959 and 1989, the asthma incidence rates were estimated in a retrospective cohort study comprising 2226 workers trained as bakers and two reference categories (109). Males employed as bakers had an incidence rate of 3.0 cases per 1000 person-years, versus 0.9 to 1.9 for the referents. For female bakers, no increased risk was observed. In a more detailed exposure–response analysis, the incidence rate of asthma for the bakers with highest exposure (dough makers) was 7.3 per 1000 person-years in men and 6.5 in women, and for rhinitis 43.4 and 38.5, respectively. There was a significant association between the dust concentration at onset of disease and the risk for asthma or rhinitis. Incidence rates of approximately 2 and 19 per 1000 person-months, respectively, were found for chest and eye/nose symptoms in a British study among newly employed bakers (15). The incidence of positive SPTs to α-amylase was more common (6 per 1000 person-months) than to flour (0.6 per 1000 person-months).

Determinants and Exposure–Response Studies

Two early studies were able to show exposure–sensitization relationships using dust exposure data. A cross-sectional study among 314 bakery workers (110,111) showed that dust exposure, measured in two- to four-hour personal dust samples, was positively associated to wheat flour sensitization in symptom-free workers. In a U.K. study, sensitization to allergens in the work environment was more common among highly exposed workers compared to low-exposed workers (OR = 3.0), when workers were ranked by dust exposure using information on perceived dustiness (25).

More recent studies have included quantitative exposure data on both inhalable dust and airborne allergens. Houba et al. (21) divided 264 workers from bakeries and flour mills, without a previous flour exposure, into three exposure categories: dust (<1, $1–5$, >5 mg/m^3) and wheat (<101, $101–225$, >225 µg/m^3) (Fig 4). The sensitization rate to wheat flour and α-amylase tended to increase with intensity of dust exposure and wheat allergen exposure. Work-related sensitization was more often observed in atopics than in nonatopics. Interestingly, flour and α-amylase sensitization in nonatopics occurred only in those with a high exposure. Work-related sensitization occurred in low-exposed atopics, but more frequently in high-exposed atopics. The authors did not test for statistical significance, but a multiple regression analysis (correcting for age, gender, smoking, and atopic status) did not

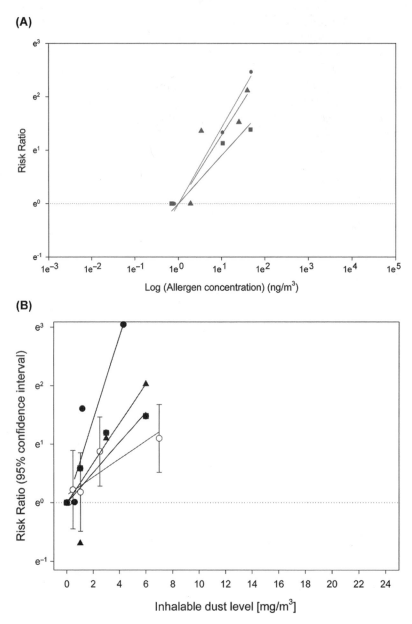

Figure 4 (**A**) Exposure–response relationships for fungal α-amylase [*triangles*: Houba et al. (21); *dots*: Nieuwenhuijsen et al. (117); *squares*: Brisman et al. (118)]. (**B**) Exposure–response relationships for wheat flour allergens. Inhalable dust levels have been taken as a proxy for wheat allergen exposure to facilitate a comparison between studies [*dots*: Cullinan et al. (113) SPT against wheat allergens; *open circles*: Heederik and Houba (112) reanalysis with five exposure categories, specific IgE against wheat allergens; *squares*: Brisman et al. (119) self-reported doctor-diagnosed rhinitis; *triangles*: self-reported doctor-diagnosed asthma]. *Abbreviation*: SPT, skin-prick test.

reveal an independent effect of aeroallergen exposure probably because of lack of sufficient power. Respiratory symptoms were related to wheat allergen levels in atopics, but not in nonatopics.

In a Dutch study, 393 bakery workers were divided into three exposure groups with mean wheat flour allergen exposure levels of 0.2, 3.5, and $11.0\,\mu g/m^3$ (mean dust exposure levels in these groups were 0.5, 0.8, and $2.4\,mg/m^3$, respectively) (23). A strong, statistically significant positive association was found between wheat flour allergen exposure and wheat flour–specific sensitization (Table 1).

These associations were found both in atopic and nonatopic workers, but the relationship was much steeper in the atopics. This study showed that exposure levels have to be reduced at least up to the levels of the lowest exposure category ($0.2\,\mu g/m^3$ wheat allergen exposure or $0.5\,/m^3$ dust exposure during a work shift), to achieve a considerable reduction in risk-sensitization to wheat flour. The same group reported exposure–sensitization relationships for α-amylase allergens in a population of 169 workers from a rusk-producing industry (22). A strong and positive relationship was shown between α-amylase allergen exposure levels and α-amylase–specific sensitization. As for wheat allergens, this relationship differed between atopic and nonatopic bakery workers. A reanalysis of the study on wheat allergen exposure and sensitization has shown that no indications exist for the presence of an exposure threshold. The risk of sensitization increases with increasing exposure and flattens off at higher exposure levels. Interestingly, a similar analysis for symptomatic allergy, defined as sensitization in combination with either upper respiratory work-related symptoms (rhinitis) or asthma, also results in a more sharply increasing exposure–response relationship, and a flattening-off of the relationship, but a reduction of the risk at higher exposure levels (Fig. 5). The shape can be explained by a combination of factors; the prevalence of symptomatic allergy at the very low exposure levels is lower than for sensitization alone, while at higher levels almost all sensitized workers are symptomatic, resulting in a steeper slope than for sensitization only. Flattening-off and reduction in risk at higher exposure levels are probably due to the healthy worker effect, but this needs to be established in longitudinal studies (112).

Several cohort studies have now shown that exposure–response relationships exist, and the results of cross-sectional and cohort studies are consistent. Cohort studies have also shown that those who are sensitized to wheat or amylase have an elevated risk for developing work-related allergy (rhinitis, asthma) symptoms

Table 1   Prevalence of Wheat Flour Sensitization (Specific IgE) by Wheat Allergen Exposure Category and Atopy Defined as Total Serum IgE $\geq 100\,kU/L$ ($N = 346$)

	Positive IgE for wheat flour	
Whole population (N = 346)		
Low wheat allergen exposure	4/90	4.4%
Intermediate wheat allergen exposure	5/64	7.8%
High wheat allergen exposure	27/192	14.1%
Atopic workers (N = 87)		
Low wheat allergen exposure	1/22	4.6%
Intermediate wheat allergen exposure	2/17	11.8%
High wheat allergen exposure	11/48	22.9%
Nonatopic workers (N = 259)		
Low wheat allergen exposure	3/68	4.4%
Intermediate wheat allergen exposure	3/47	6.4%
High wheat allergen exposure	16/144	11.1%

Source: From Ref. 22.

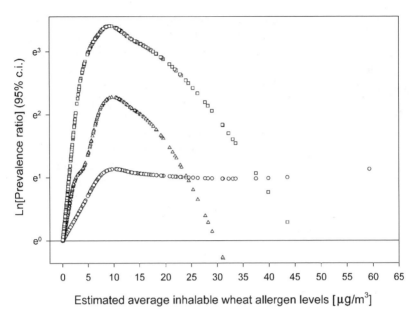

Figure 5 Exposure–response relationship for wheat sensitization, wheat sensitization and work-related rhinitis symptoms, and wheat sensitization and work-related asthma symptoms. *Source*: From Ref. 112.

within a few years, indicating that work-related sensitization is an important risk factor for symptoms (113). Some of these studies also suggest that the sensitization risk flattens off after a few years of follow-up and fewer sensitization cases occur after the first years of exposure; however, the length of follow-up of most studies does not allow firm conclusions on changes in sensitization risk over time.

Atopy is the most important risk modifier of work-related sensitization. In most studies, atopy was defined as a positive SPT to one or more common allergens (grasses, trees, house dust mites, etc.). The risk of work-related sensitization was 5 to 20 times higher in atopics compared to nonatopics. One should be aware that especially cross-sectional studies may overestimate the importance of atopy, because sensitization to grasses and pollens is included in the definition of the atopic status, and cross-reactivity exists between grasses and pollens and wheat sensitization. Only one study identified (24) smoking of cigarettes as a risk factor of work-related sensitization.

DIAGNOSIS

The diagnosis of allergy in bakery and flour mill workers is based on an appropriate history of respiratory symptoms—particularly of the nose and airways—in an individual with relevant exposure at work. Symptoms develop only after an initial symptom-free period of exposure, which can range from months to several years. Rhinitis often accompanies asthma and may have developed before the onset of asthma, but asthma in the absence of rhinitis is not uncommon. The majority of cases identify a clear relationship between periods at work and the development or worsening of their symptoms. Nasal and asthmatic symptoms can develop within minutes of exposure but asthmatic symptoms may develop after several hours. Asthmatic symptoms may resolve within a few hours of leaving work but can persist for 24 hours or more, causing nocturnal waking with asthma. In these circumstances, symptomatic improvement may not be sufficient to be appreciated during a weekend away from work and only recognized during a one- or two-week holiday. Studies have shown that when workers are sensitized, work-related sensitization can be predicted on the basis of a limited set of respiratory symptoms (114,115). This type of information makes it possible to apply short and focused questionnaires on a large scale in exposed populations, and select those with a high sensitization risk for further evaluation.

Objective evidence in support of the diagnosis of occupational asthma can be obtained from *specific IgE* response, series peak flow measurements, or inhalation tests. Specific IgE can be identified either by an immediate "weal and flare" response to a SPT with the relevant allergen or in serum by methods such as RAST. A recent study found that considerable variation exists in SPT reagents from different suppliers (116). The sensitivity of SPT extracts versus a specific challenge was moderate to low (40% and 67%), while the specificity was somewhat better (86% and 100%). In general, specific IgE is a sensitive but not specific test for occupational asthma caused by protein allergens. However, in asthma in bakery and flour mill workers, the large number of potentially relevant allergens—grain, flour, additives (particularly enzymes), and possibly mites and molds—limit the diagnostic value of specific IgE if absent in a patient with an appropriate history. In the majority of cases, in bakery and flour mill workers, allergy is to grain or flour proteins or to the enzyme α-amylase. Because the frequency of specific IgE to these allergens is greater than asthma caused by them, when present, they only have diagnostic value in those occupationally exposed with a history of work-related nasal or asthmatic symptoms. *Serial peak flow measurements*, ideally made at two to three hourly intervals from waking to sleep during a four-week period, which includes periods at and away from work, can identify work-related asthma, with deterioration during periods at work and improvement during absence from work, but do not identify its cause.

The diagnosis of occupational asthma in bakery and flour mill workers can usually be made on the basis of (i) relevant occupation and exposure, (ii) history of work-related respiratory symptoms which have developed since initial occupational exposure, (iii) serial peak flow measurements which show work-related asthma, and (iv) specific IgE to extracts of relevant allergens, usually flour or grain proteins or the enzyme α-amylase. In a few patients, the diagnosis remains unclear even after these investigations. As mentioned, medical decision-making procedures that facilitate combination of information from different diagnostic tests in decision trees may be helpful when surveillance data have to be interpreted (114,115). Because of the important social and financial implications of a diagnosis of occupational asthma—in particular the need to avoid further exposure and change work if asthma is caused by allergy to an agent encountered at work—inhalation testing with relevant allergens may be indicated, although this is now uncommon. Inhalation testing with the responsible allergen can provoke an immediate asthmatic response, which develops within minutes and can last for one to two hours; a late asthmatic response, which develops after one to two hours, is maximal at six to eight hours and has usually resolved by 24 hours, or both—a dual asthmatic response. The late asthmatic reaction is often accompanied by an increase in nonspecific airway responsiveness.

MANAGEMENT

Management of cases of occupational asthma in bakery and flour mill workers is based on the avoidance of further exposure to the cause of their asthma. This can in theory be achieved by (i) reduction in dust exposure at work, (ii) use of respiratory protection, and (iii) change of work. In practice, because once sensitized, individuals react to very low concentrations of inhaled allergen, reduction in dust exposure at work is impractical under the usual work circumstances in bakeries and flour mills. The use of respiratory protection is also usually impractical as a long-term solution in the majority of cases, but can allow an individual to continue in employment and provide time to consider and obtain alternative employment. Avoidance of tasks with high exposure usually requires a change of work. In many cases—particularly, small family-based bakeries—an alternative site of work in the bakery, where exposure to flour can be avoided, cannot be found and exposure is adequately avoided only by leaving work. In large bakeries, relocation at work is a more feasible solution, but even here, because of the dustiness of bakeries and flour mills, avoidance of exposure sufficient to prevent the provocation of asthmatic symptoms can be difficult to ensure. The important social and financial implications of a diagnosis of occupational asthma make it essential that the diagnosis is made only on the basis of sufficient evidence. In the United Kingdom, one-third of cases of occupational asthma were without employment three to five years after the diagnosis had been made (120). Loss of employment consequent upon an incorrect diagnosis can be disastrous. The consequences of misdiagnosis can be as serious as missing the diagnosis. Because of the adverse financial consequences of leaving work in economies with relatively high levels of unemployment, some bakery and flour mill workers with occupational asthma choose to remain in employment, despite being made aware that their asthma is likely to become increasingly severe and may become irreversible. In these circumstances, steps should, where possible in conjunction with their employers, be taken to minimize their exposure to flour dust at work and to wear respiratory protection when exposed to the dust. It is unlikely that these measures alone will be sufficient to control their asthma which should be treated in the same way as asthma not caused by work, with anti-inflammatory and symptomatic treatment taken primarily by inhalation.

PREVENTION

Exposure Standards

Reviews of the literature in the early 1990s made clear that the available evidence on exposure–response studies, if available, was not sufficient to draw conclusions on levels that might protect against the development of sensitization or symptoms (121). The Nordic expert group concluded in 1996 that "... existing data on exposure-response relationships do not allow the identification of a NOAEL for flour dust. Due to the nature of allergy it is unlikely that the setting of a NOAEL for flour dust will be practicable even in the near future." This concept completely shifted following the results from epidemiological studies which incorporated detailed exposure assessment that allowed exposure–response modeling. However, some organizations still do not incorporate the more recent evidence in their proposals for standards, like the HSE in the United Kingdom, which adapted a maximum exposure limit of $10 /m^3$ over eight hours and $30 /m^3$ over 15 minutes (122). Such levels can be met by most modern industries, apart from specific activities, which involve large quantities of flour dust during specific tasks (123). However, results from the epidemiological studies performed in the early 1990s have changed the picture and found an application in risk assessment and several exposure standards have been suggested. In the United States, the ACGIH has adopted a threshold limit value for inhalable flour dust of $0.5/m^3$ averaged over an eight-hour work shift (124). In Sweden, a standard has been adopted of $3/m^3$ over eight hours (125). All these values are either based on no observed adverse effect levels (NOAELs) that have been obtained from the literature or are values that took these NOAELs as starting point, with changes made on the basis of technical feasibility. An entirely different approach has been followed by the DECOS (126). They concluded that on the basis of a reanalysis of a Dutch epidemiological study, no NOAEL can be defined, because the risk increases with increasing exposure and no exposure threshold is observable (112). They therefore calculated the excess risk at a range of exposure levels, using the exposure–response relationship observed, assuming a baseline sensitization rate of 4% to wheat allergens in the general population. An uncertainty factor of two was applied for variation of the allergen content of wheat flour. Excess sensitization risk of 1% and 10% occur at exposure levels of 0.12 and $1.2/m^3$. The socio-economic council will now have to propose a standard on the basis of this information on the excess risk for sensitization in balance with feasibility issues. Application of this approach to the exposure–sensitization studies available for fungal α-amylase leads to excess risk of 1% and 10% against a baseline sensitization risk of 2% for amylase sensitization at exposure levels between 1 and $10\,ng/m^3$, illustrating that exposure levels need to be reduced considerably in this industry to minimize the sensitization risk.

Reduction of Dust and Allergen Exposure

Little quantitative information is available on the contribution of different determinants of exposure in the baking industry (equipment, technology, production lay out, etc.). However, it is clear that several dusty tasks contribute to the high exposures of dough makers and other workers in this industry. Studies using real time aerosol monitors showed that tasks such as emptying bags, compressing empty (paper) bags containing flour or dough improvers, and dusting dough during forming to prevent dough adhesion to surfaces are among the dustiest tasks. Cleaning with brooms or the use of pressurized air lead to high exposures as well. Silo- and bin-cleaning tasks resulted in the highest dust exposure according to one study (123). Some dough makers are involved in weighing of ingredients on simple scales and this activity can lead to high-peak exposures. A recent Canadian study assessed several potential determinants of dust exposure. The study shows that use of horizontal mixers is associated with higher dust exposures than the use of vertical mixers (geometric mean exposure $13.0/m^3$ vs. $3.8/m^3$; $p < 0.001$) (95). Use of divider oil to prevent dough adhesion was associated with considerably lower exposures (geometric mean) than dusting with flour (geometric mean $0.43/m^3$ vs. $12.0/m^3$; $p < 0.001$) (95). Dough brakes lead to exposures that were of the orders of magnitudes higher than in use of other forming methods such as automated forming (95,123). The use of reversible sheeters lead to increased exposures as well, probably because rapid changes in direction of the machine's belt-like surface can result in emissions of dust particles.

The high exposures that occur during the performance of these tasks can be eliminated by fundamental modifications to the baking process and effective use of ventilation technology. The use of flour silos in combination with compressed air to transport flour instead of bags is potentially an effective but fundamental change to the process. Use of exhaust ventilation in a ring around the dough mixer can reduce exposure levels considerably. General room ventilation is seldom effective. Covering dough mixers can further reduce exposure of dough makers when the flour is mixed. Automation of parts of the process is a long-term option that can lead to considerably lower exposure levels (127); however, maintenance of automated equipment seems crucial (95). A major source of wheat exposure occurs when the dough is covered with some flour, often by hand, to prevent sticking. For certain products, the use of divider oil seems possible to reduce exposures. When the use of flour to dust dough is inevitable, these tasks could be performed using flow tables. This requires considerable investments. An unnecessary exposure to amylase occurs if enriched flour is used for this purpose. Exposure to enzymes could be reduced by the use of encapsulated or micropalletized or dissolved enzyme formulations. However, there seems to exist some reluctance to use these alternative enzyme formulations, probably because this might also involve changes in mixing and rising times. Compliance with good house keeping and optimal work practices does lead to lower exposure (128).

SUMMARY

Occupational asthma and rhinitis caused by allergens encountered in bakeries and flour mills is an important occupational health problem, which may be increasing in prevalence. The nature of the responsible allergens and in particular the importance of fungal α-amylase as a cause of asthma in bakers has become clear in recent years. The identification of the responsible allergens and the development of methods to measure their concentration in air have allowed the study of exposure–response relationships. These studies have shown that the frequency of sensitization and respiratory symptoms, both nasal and asthmatic, increases with increasing exposure and implies that the disease incidence can be reduced by improved control of allergen exposure in the workplace. The physiological as well as financial and social consequences, faced by those bakery and flour mill workers who develop occupational asthma, makes application of the scientific findings now available an important priority. Recently obtained information about exposure–risk relationships is now being translated in risk management and exposure control strategies.

ACKNOWLEDGMENTS

We would like to thank Gert Doekes, Remko Houba, and Mark Nieuwenhuijsen for their useful comments and suggestions.

REFERENCES

1. De Besche A. Serologische Untersuchungen über 'allergische Krankheiten' beim Menchen. Acta Pathol Microbiol Scand 1929; 6:115–144.
2. Baagöe KH. Mehlidiosynkrasie als Ursache vasomotorischer Rhinitis und Asthma. Acta Med Scand 1933; 80:310–322.
3. Meredith SK, Taylor VM, McDonald JC. Occupational respiratory disease in the United Kingdom 1989: a report to the British Thoracic Society and the Society of Occupational Medicine by the SWORD project group. Br J Ind Med 1991; 48:292–298.

4. Meredith S. Reported incidence of occupational asthma in the United Kingdom, 1989–1990. J Epidemiol Commun Health 1993; 47:459–463.

5. Meredith SK, McDonald JC. Work-related respiratory disease in the United Kingdom, 1989–1992: report on the SWORD project. Occup Med 1994; 44:183–189.

6. Sallie BA, Ross DJ, Meredith SK, McDonald JC. SWORD'93. Surveillance of work-related and occupational disease in the UK. Occup Med 1994; 44:177–182.

7. Thiel H. Inhalationsallergien bei Bäckern – Aktuelle probleme des Mehlbe rufsasthmas. Lebensversicherungsmedizin 1984; 4:82–87.

8. Bauer X. Allergien inm Backgewerbe. Allergologie 1993; 16:245.

9. Nordman H. Occupational asthma – time for prevention. Scan J Work Environ Health 1994(20 special issue):108–115.

10. Grieshaber R, Rothe R. Obstruktive Atemwegserkrankungen in Bäckereien. Staub 1995; 55:403–407.

11. Mastrangelo G, Bombana S, Priante E, Gallo A, Saia B. Repeated case-control studies as a method of surveillance for asthma in occupations. J Occup Environ Med 1997; 39:51–57.

12. Gadborg E. Allergy to flour. Thesis. Copenhagen, 1956 (as quoted by Bonnevie P. Occupational allergy in bakery, 1958; and In: Thiel H, Kallweit C. Das Bäckerasthma—eine klassische allergische Berufskrankheit, 1984).

13. Herxheimer H. Skin sensitivity to flour in bakers' apprentices. Lancet 1967; 1:83–84.

14. Cullinan P, Lowson D, Nieuwenhuijsen M, et al. Work-related symptoms, specific sensitization and exposure in a cohort of flour workers. Eur Resp J 1995; 19(suppl 8):272s.

15. DeMers MP, Orris P. Occupational exposure and asthma mortality. JAMA 1994; 272:1575.

16. Hendrick DJ, Davies RJ, Pepys J. Bakers' asthma. Clin Allergy 1976; 6:241–250.

17. Nakamura S. On occupational allergic asthma of different kinds newly found in our allergy clinic. J Asthma Res 1972; 10:37–47.

18. Zuskin E, Mustajbegovic J, Schachter EN, Kern J. Respiratory symptoms and ventilatory function in confectionery workers. Occup Environ Med 1994; 51:435–439.

19. Zuskin E, Kanceljak B, Mustajbegovic J, Schachter EN. Immunologic findings in confectionary workers. Ann Allergy 1994; 73:521–526.

20. Cullinan P, Lowson D, Nieuwenhuijsen MJ, et al. Work related symptoms, sensitisation, and estimated exposure in workers not previously exposed to flour. Occup Environ Med 1994; 51:579–583.

21. Houba R, Heederik DJJ, Doekes G, van Run PEM. Exposure-sensitization relationship for α-amylase allergens in the baking industry. Am J Respir Crit Care Med 1996; 154:130–136.

22. Houba R, Heederik D, Doekes G. Wheat sensitization and work related respiratory symptoms are preventable: an epidemiological study. Am J Respir Crit Care Med 1998; 158:1499–1503.

23. De Zotti R, Larese F, Bovenzi M, Negro C, Molinari S. Allergic airway disease in Italian bakers and pastry makers. Occup Environ Med 1994; 51:548–552.

24. Musk AW, Venables KM, Crook B, et al. Respiratory symptoms, lung function, and sensitisation to flour in a British bakery. Br J Ind Med 1989; 46:636–642.

25. Brisman J, Toren K, Lillienberg L, Karlsson G, Ahlstedt S. Nasal symptoms and indices of nasal inflammation in flour-dust-exposed bakers. Int Arch Occup Environ Health 1998; 7:525–532.

26. Block G, Tse KS, Kijek K, Chan H, Chan-Yeung M. Baker's asthma—studies of the cross-antigenicity between different cereal grains. Clin Allergy 1984; 14:177–185.

27. Prichard MG, Ryan G, Musk AW. Wheat flour sensitisation and airways disease in urban bakers. Br J Ind Med 1984; 41:450–454.

28. Sutton R, Skerritt JH, Baldo BA, Wrigley CW. The diversity of allergens involved in bakers' asthma. Clin Allergy 1984; 14:93–107.

29. Valdivieso R, Moneo I, Pola J, et al. Occupational asthma and contact urticaria caused by buckwheat flour. Ann Allergy 1989; 63: 149–152.

30. Baldo BA, Krilis S, Wrigley CW. Hypersensitivity to inhaled flour allergens-comparison between cereals. Allergy 1980; 35:45–56.
31. Sandiford CP, Tee RD, Newman Taylor AJ. Identification of crossreacting wheat, rye, barley and soya flour allergens using sera from individuals with wheat-induced asthma. Clin Exp Allergy 1995; 25:340–349.
32. Fränken J, Stephan U, Meyer HE, König W. Identification of alpha-amylase inhibitor as a major allergen of wheat flour. Int Arch Allergy Immunol 1994; 104:171–174.
33. Nakamura R, Matsuda T. Rice allergenic protein and molecular-genetic approach for hypoallergenic rice. Biosci Biotech Biochem 1996; 60:1215–1221.
34. García-Casado G, Armentia A, Sánchez-Monge R, Sánchez LM, Lopez-Otín C, Salcedo G. A major baker's asthma allergen from rye flour is considerably more active than its barley counterpart. FEBS Lett 1995; 364:36–40.
35. Baldo BA, Wrigley CW. IgE antibodies to wheat flour components. Clin Allergy 1978; 8:109–124.
36. Prichard MG, Ryan G, Walsh BJ, Musk AW. Skin test and RAST responses to wheat and common allergens and respiratory disease in bakers. Clin Allergy 1985; 15:203–210.
37. Walsh BJ, Wrigley CW, Musk AW, Baldo BA. A comparison of the binding of IgE in the sera of patients with bakers' asthma to soluble and insoluble wheat-grain proteins. J Allergy Clin Immunol 1985; 76:23–28.
38. Blands J, Diamant B, Kallós P, Kallós-Deffner L, Løwenstein H. Flour allergy in bakers – identification of allergenic fractions in flour and comparison of diagnostic methods. Int Arch Allergy Appl Immun 1976; 52:392–406.
39. Gómez L, Martin E, Hernández D, et al. Members of the α-amylase inhibitors family from wheat endosperm are major allergens associated with baker's asthma. FEBS Lett 1990; 261:85–88.
40. Sander I, Flagge A, Merget R, Halder TM, Meyer HE, Baur X. Identification of wheat flour allergens by means of 2-dimensional immunoblotting. J Allergy Clin Immunol 2001; 107:907–913.
41. Pfeil T, Schwabl U, Ulmer WT, König W. Western Blot Analysis of Water-Soluble Wheat Flour (*Triticum vulgaris*) Allergens. Int Arch Allergy Appl Immunol 1990; 91: 224–231.
42. Sandiford CP, Tee RD, Newman Taylor AJ. Identification of major allergenic flour proteins in order to develop assays to measure flour aeroallergen. Clin Exp Allergy 1990; 20(suppl 1):3.
43. Sandiford CP, Tee RD, Newman Taylor AJ. Comparison of allergens detected by rabbit and human sera by western blotting of wheat flour. 1991:132.
44. Boisen S. Comparative physico-chemical studies on purified trypsin inhibitors from the endosperm of barley, rye, and wheat. Z Lebensm Unters Forsch 1983; 176:434–439.
45. Posch A, Weiss W, Wheeler C, Dunn MJ, Görg A. Sequence analysis of wheat grain allergens separated by two-dimensional electrophoresis with immobilized pH gradients. Electrophoresis 1995; 16:1115–1119.
46. Weiss W, Huber G, Engel KH, et al. Identification and characterization of wheat grain albumine/globulin allergens. Electrophoresis 1997; 18:826–833.
47. Sanchez-Monge R, Gomez L, Barber D, Lopez-Otin C, Armentia A, Salcedo G. Wheat and barley allergens associated with baker's asthma—glycosylated subunits of the α-amylase-inhibitor family have enhanced IgE-binding capacity. Biochem J 1992; 281: 401–405.
48. Armentia A, Sanchez-Monge R, Gomez L, Barber D, Salcedo G. In vivo allergenic activities of eleven purified members of a major allergen family from wheat and barley flour. Clin Exp Allergy 1993; 23:410–415.
49. Garcia-Olmedo F, Salcedo G, Sanchez-Monge R, Gomez L, Royo J, Carbonero P. Plant proteinaceous inhibitors of proteinases and α-amylases. Oxford Surveys Plant Mol Cell Biol 1987; 4:275–334.
50. Mena M, Sanchez-Monge R, Gomez L, Salcedo G, Carbonero P. A major barley allergen associated with baker's asthma disease is a glycosylated monomeric inhibitor of

insect α-amylase: cDNA cloning and chromosomal location of the gene. Plant Mol Biol 1992; 20:451–458.

51. Adachi T, Alvarez AM, Aoki N, Nakamura R, Garcia VV, Matsuda T. Screening of rice strains deficient in 16-kDa allergenic protein. Biosci Biotech Biochem 1995; 59:1377–1378.

52. García-Casado G, Armentia A, Sánchez-Monge R, Malpica JM, Salcedo G. Rye flour allergens associated with baker's asthma. Correlation between in vivo and in vitro activities and comparison with their wheat and barley homologues. Clin Exp Allergy 1996; 26:428–435.

53. Barber D, Sánchez-Monge R, Gómez L, et al. A barley flour inhibitor of insect α-amylase is a major allergen associated with baker's asthma disease. FEBS letters 1989; 248:119–122.

54. Heyer N. Backmittel als berufsbedingte Inhalationsallergene bei mehlverarbeitenden Berufen. Allergologie 1983; 6:389–392.

55. Jorde W, Heyer N, Schata M. Bäckereirohstoffe als berufsspezifische Allergene. Allergologie 1986:s552–s524.

56. Wüthrich B, Baur X. Backmittel, insbesondere α-Amylase, als berufliche Inhalationsallergene in der Backwarenindustrie. Schweiz med Wschr 1990; 120:446–450.

57. Baur X, Fruhmann G, Haug B, Rasche B, Reiher W, Weiss W. Role of aspergillus amylase in baker's asthma. Lancet 1986; 1:43.

58. Birnbaum J, Latil F, Vervloet D, Senft M, Charpin J. Rôle de l'alpha-amylase dans l'asthme du boulanger. Rev Mal Resp 1988; 5:519–521.

59. Bermejo N, Maria Y, Gueant JL, Moneret-Vautrin DA. Allergie professionnelle du boulanger à l'alpha-amylase fongique. Rev Fr Allergol 1991; 31:56–58.

60. Blanco Carmona JG, Juste Picón S, Garcés Sotillos M. Occupational asthma in bakeries caused by sensitivity to α-amylase. Allergy 1991; 46:274–276.

61. Tarvainen K, Kanerva L, Tupasela O, et al. Allergy from cellulase and xylanase enzymes. Clin Exp Allergy 1991; 21:609–615.

62. Quirce S, Cuevas M, Díez-Gómez ML, et al. Respiratory allergy to *Aspergillus*-derived enzymes in bakers' asthma. J Allergy Clin Immunol 1992; 90:970–978.

63. Valdivieso R, Subiza J, Subiza JL, Hinojosa M, Carlos de E, Subiza E. Bakers' asthma caused by alpha amylase. Ann Allergy 1994; 73:337–342.

64. Baur X, Sauer W, Weiss W. Baking additives as new allergens in baker's asthma. Respiration 1988; 54:70–72.

65. Baur X, Chen Z, Sander I. Isolation and denomination of an important allergen in baking additives: α-amylase from *Aspergillus oryzae* (*Asp o* II). Clin Exp Allergy 1994; 24:465–470.

66. Sandiford CP, Tee RD, Newman Taylor AJ. The role of cereal and fungal amylases in cereal flour hypersensitivity. Clin Exp Allergy 1994; 24:549–557.

67. Sander I, Newhaus-Schroder C, Borowitzki G, Baur X, Raulf-Heimsoth M. Development of a two-site enzyme-linked immunosorbent assay for alpha-amylase from *Aspergillus oryzae* based on monoclonal antibodies. J Immunol Meth 1997; 210:93–101.

68. Houba R, van Run P, Doekes G, Heederik D, Spithoven J. Airborne levels of α-amylase allergens in bakeries. J Allergy Clin Immunol 1997; 99:286–292.

69. Moneo I, Alday E, Sanchez-Agudo L, Curiel G, Lucena R, Calatrava JM. Skin-prick tests for hypersensitivity to α-amylase preparations. Occup Med 1995; 45:151–155.

70. Losada E, Hinojosa M, Quirce S, Sánchez-Cano M, Moneo I. Occupational asthma caused by α-amylase inhalation: clinical and immunological findings and bronchial response patterns. J Allergy Clin Immunol 1992; 89:118–125.

71. Baur X, Czuppon AB. Allergic reaction after eating α-amylase (*Asp o* 2)-containing bread. Allergy 1995; 50:85–87.

72. Kanny G, Moneret-Vautrin DA. α-Amylase contained in bread can induce food allergy. J Allergy Clin Immunol 1995; 95:132–133.

73. Cullinan P, Cook A, Jones M, Cannon J, Fitzgerald B, Taylor AJ. Clinical responses to ingested fungal alpha-amylase and hemicellulose in persons sensitized to *Aspergillus fumigatus*? Allergy 1997; 52:346–349.

74. Alday E, Moneo I, Lucena R, Curiel G. Alpha-amylase hypersensitivity: diagnostic methods. Allergy 1995; 50(suppl 26):88.

75. Baur X, Sander I, Jansen A, Czuppon AB. Sind Amylasen von Backmitteln und Backmehl relevante Nahrungsmittelallergene? Schweiz med Wschr 1994; 124:846–851.

76. Baur X, Czuppon AB, Sander I. Heating inactivates the enzymatic activity and partially inactivates the allergenic activity of Asp o 2. Clin Exp Allergy 1996; 26:232–234.

77. Sander I, Baur X. Evidence for continuous B-cell epitopes on α-amylase of *Aspergillus oryzae* (*Asp o* II). J Allergy Clin Immunol 1994; 93(nr.1 part 2):265.

78. Baur X, Sauer W, Weiss W, Fruhmann G. Inhalant allergens in modern baking industry. Immunol Allergy Pract 1989; 11:13–15.

79. Vanhanen M, Tuomi T, Hokkanen H, et al. Occup Environ Med 1996; 53:670–676.

80. Armentia A, Tapias J, Barber D, et al. Sensitization to the storage mite *Lepidoglyphus destructor* in wheat flour respiratory allergy. Ann Allergy 1992; 68:398–403.

81. Revsbech P, Dueholm M. Storage mite allergy among bakers. Allergy 1990; 45:204–208.

82. Tee RD. Allergy to storage mites – review. Clin Exp Allergy 1994; 24:636–640.

83. De Zotti R, Molinari S, Larese F, Bovenzi M. Pre-employment screening among trainee bakers. Occup Environ Med 1995; 52:279–283.

84. Korsgaard J, Dahl R, Iversen M, Hallas T. Storage mites as a cause of bronchial asthma in Denmark. Allergol Immunopathol 1985; 13:143–149.

85. Müsken H, Bergmann Kch. Vorratsmilben: Biologie, Sensibilisierung, klinische Bedeutung. Allergologie 1992; 15:s189–s196.

86. Johansson E, Johansson SGO, Hage-Hamsten van M. Allergenic characterization of *Acarus siro* and *Tyrophagus putrescentiae* and their crossreactivity with *Lepidoglyphus destructor* and *Dermatophagoides pteronyssinus*. Clin Exp Allergy 1994; 24:743–751.

87. Weiner A. Occupational bronchial asthma in a baker due to *Aspergillus* – a case report. Ann Allergy 1960; 18:1004–1007.

88. Klaustermeyer WB, Bardana EJ, Hale FC. Pulmonary hypersensitivity to *Alternaria* and *Aspergillus* in baker's asthma. Clin Allergy 1977; 7:227–233.

89. Bergmann I, Rebohle E, Wallenstein G, Gemeinhardt H, Thürmer H. Häufigkeit und Bedeutung von Schimmelpilzsensibilisierungen bei Werktätigen in der Backwarenindustrie. Allergie Immunol 1976; 22:297–301.

90. Wallenstein G, Bergmann I, Rebohle E, Gemeinhardt H, Thürmer H. Berufliche Atemtrakterkrankungen durch Schimmelpilze bei Getreidemüllern und Bäckern. Z Erkrank Atm Org 1980; 154:229–233.

91. Nieuwenhuijsen MJ, Sandiford CP, Lowson D, et al. Dust and flour aeroallergen exposure in flour mills and bakeries. Occup Environ Med 1994; 51:584–588.

92. Nieuwenhuijsen MJ, Lowson D, Venables KM, Newman Taylor AJ. Flour dust exposure variability in flour mills and bakeries. Ann Occup Hyg 1995; 39:299–305.

93. Houba R, van Run P, Heederik D, Doekes G. Wheat antigen exposure assessment for epidemiologic studies in bakeries using personal dust sampling and inhibition ELISA. Clin Exp Allergy 1996; 26:154–163.

94. Houba R, Heederik D, Kromhout K. Grouping strategies for exposure to inhalable dust, wheat allergens and α-amylase allergens in bakeries. Ann occup Hyg 1997; 41:287–296.

95. Burstyn I, Teschke K, Kennedy SM. Exposure levels and determinants of inhalable dust exposure in bakeries. Ann Occup Hyg 1997; 41:609–624.

96. Sandiford CP, Nieuwenhuijsen MJ, Tee RD, Newman Taylor AJ. Measurement of airborne proteins involved in Bakers' asthma. Clin Exp Allergy 1994 ; 24:450–456.

97. Burdorf A, Lillienberg L, Brisman J. Characterization of exposure to inhalable flour dust in Swedish bakeries. Ann occup Hyg 1994; 38:67–78.

98. Sandiford CP, Nieuwenhuijsen MJ, Tee RD, Newman Taylor AJ. Determination of the size of airborne flour particles. Allergy 1994; 49:891–893.

99. Jongedijk T, Meijler M, Houba R, Heederik D. Tijdstudies en vergelijkende piekblootstellingsmetingen in ambachtelijke bakkerijen. Tijdschrift voor toegepaste Arbowetenschap 1995; 8:1–8.

100. Charpin J, Lauriol-Mallea M, Renard M, Charpin H. Étude de la pollution fungique dans les boulangeries. Acad Natl Med 1971; 19:52–55.

101. Singh A, Singh AB. Airborne fungi in a bakery and the prevalence of respiratory dysfunction among workers. Grana 1994; 33:349–358.

102. Gemeinhardt H, Bergmann I. Zum Vorkommen von Schimmelpilzen in Bäckereistäuben. Zbl Bakt Abt II 1977; 132:44–54.

103. Wüthrich B. Enzyme: potente inhalative und ingestive Allergene–fehlende Deklarationspflicht von Backmitteln und Backmehl. Schweiz med Wschr 1994; 124:1361–1363.

104. Gautrin D, Infante-Rivard C, Dao TV, Magnan-Larose M, Desjardins D, Malo JM. Specific IgE-dependent sensitization, atopy, and bronchial hyperresponsiveness in apprentices starting exposure to protein-derived agents. Am J Respir Crit Care Med 1997; 155:1841–1847.

105. Smith TA, Lumley KPS, Hui EHK. Allergy to flour and fungal amylase in bakery workers. Occup Med 1997; 47:21–24.

106. Belchi-Hernandez J, Mora-Gonzalez A, Iniesta-Perez J. Baker's asthma caused by *Saccharomyces cerevisiae* in dry powder form. J Allergy Clin Immunol 1996; 97:131–134.

107. Bohadana AB, Massin N, Wild P, Kolopp MN, Toamain JP. Respiratory symptoms and airway responsiveness in apparently healthy workers exposed to flour dust. Eur Respir J 1994; 7:1070–1076.

108. Herxheimer H. The skin sensitivity fo flour of bakers' apprentices. Acta Allergol 1973; 28:42–49.

109. Brisman J, Järvholm BG. Occurrence of self-reported asthma among Swedish bakers. Scand J Work Environ Health 1995; 21:487–493.

110. Hartmann AL, Wüthrich B, Deflorin-Stolz R, Helfenstein U, Hewitt B, Guérin B. Atopie-Screening: Prick-Multitest, Gesamt-IgE oder RAST? Schweiz med Wschr 1985; 115:466–475.

111. Hartmann AL. Berufsallergien bei Bäckern – Epidemiologie; Diagnose, Therapie und Prophylaxe; Versicherungsrecht. München-Deisenhofen, Germany: Dustri-Verlag Dr. Karl Feistle, 1986.

112. Heederik D, Houba R. An exploratory quantitative risk assessment for high molecular weight sensitizers: wheat flour. Ann Occup Hyg 2001; 45:175–185.

113. Cullinan P, Cook A, Nieuwenhuijsen MJ, et al. Allergen and dust exposure as determinants of work-related symptoms and sensitization in a cohort of flour-exposed workers; a case-control analysis. Ann Occup Hyg 2001; 45:97–103.

114. Post WK, Venables KM, Ross D, Cullinan P, Heederik D, Burdorf A. Stepwise health surveillance for bronchial irritability syndrome in workers atrisk of occupational respiratory disease. Occup Environ Med 1998; 55:119–125.

115. Meijer E, Grobbee DE, Heederik D. A strategy for health surveillance in laboratory animal workers exposed to high molecular weight allergens. Occup Environ Med 2004; 61:831–837.

116. Sander I, Merget R, Degens PO, Goldscheid N, Bruning T, Raulf-Heimsoth M. Comparison of wheat and rye flour skin prick test solutions for diagnosis of baker's asthma. Allergy 2004; 59:95–98.

117. Nieuwenhuijsen MJ, Heederik D, Doekes G, Venables KM, Newman Taylor AJ. Exposure-response relations of alpha-amylase sensitisation in British bakeries and flour mills. Occup Environ Med 1999; 56:197–201.

118. Brisman J, Nieuwenhuijsen MJ, Venables KM, Putcha V, Gordon S, Taylor AJ. Exposure-response relations for work related respiratory symptoms and sensitisation in a cohort exposed to alpha-amylase. Occup Environ Med. 2004; 61:551–553.

119. Brisman J, Jarvholm B, Lillienberg L. Exposure-response relations for self reported asthma and rhinitis in bakers. Occup Environ Med 2000; 57(5):335–340.

120. Cannon J, Cullinan P, Newman Taylor A. Consequences of occupational asthma. BMJ 1995; 311:602–603.

121. Tikkainen. Nordic council report of wheat flour, 1996.

122. HSE. Health and Safety Executive. Occupational exposure limits 2002. HSE Caerphilly, UK, EH40/2002.

123. Nieuwenhuijsen MJ, Sandiford CP, Lowson D, Tee RD, Venables KM, Newman Taylor AJ. Peak exposure concentrations of dust and flour aeroallergen in flour mills and bakeries. Ann Occup Hyg 1995; 39:193–201.

124. ACGIH. American Conference of Governmental Industrial Hygienists. Documentation on flour dust. ACGIH, Cincinnati, USA, 1999.

125. Arbetarskyddsstryrelsen Hygiensiska gränsvärden och åtgärder mot luftföroreningar. Stockholm, Sweden, 2000 (in Swedish).

126. DECOS. Wheat and other cereal flour dusts: an approach for evaluating health effects from occupational exposure. Gezondheidsraad, Den Haag, The Netherlands, 2004 (downloadable from www.gr.nl).

127. Jauhiainen A, Louhelainen K, Linnainmaa M. Exposure to dust and α-amylase in bakeries. Appl Occup Environ Hyg 1993; 8:721–725.

128. Elms J, Robinson E, Rahman S, Garrod A. Exposure to flour dust in UK bakeries: current use of control measures. Ann Occup Hyg 2005; 49:85–91.

18

Laboratory Animal, Insect, Fish, and Shellfish Allergy

Susan Gordon
Institute of Occupational Medicine, Riccarton, Edinburgh, Scotland, U.K.

Robert K. Bush
Allergy Section, William S. Middle Veterans Affairs Hospital, Madison, Wisconsin, U.S.A.

Anthony J. Newman-Taylor
Department of Occupational and Environmental Medicine, National Heart and Lung Institute, Royal Brompton and Harefield NHS Trust, London, U.K.

INTRODUCTION

Occupational allergy is an important health problem for those exposed to animals, insects, and shellfish in their place of work. The major source of allergens is the excreta and secreta of the animals and insects, which may be airborne and are inhaled by those working with them. The most usual manifestations of allergy are rhinitis, conjunctivitis, contact urticaria, and asthma; asthma is less common but more important, as those with severe symptoms may be unable to continue in their work. Many exhibiting such allergy, particularly those with asthma, have specific immunoglobulin E (IgE) antibody to the responsible proteins. The presence of specific IgE, identified by skin or serological testing, is helpful in diagnosis. The specificity of the immunological response has been exploited to identify the allergenic proteins in different potential sources and to measure the concentration of airborne allergens in the workplace.

ANIMALS

The importance of laboratory animal allergy (LAA) as an occupational disease was recognized in the early 1970s. In 1976, the British Society for Allergy and Clinical Immunology published preliminary survey results indicating that approximately 23% of the participating animal workers experienced one or more symptoms consistent with LAA (1). Contemporary reports from the United States at that time suggested a lower prevalence rate of 15% (2,3). Subsequent studies, which will be discussed in detail below, have shown that the etiology and high prevalence rate of LAA are remarkably consistent throughout the Western world. Current estimates indicate that 40,000 to 125,000 individuals are exposed to laboratory animals in the United States (4) and 15,000 individuals in the United Kingdom (5).

There is now general recognition of LAA as an occupational disease and an awareness of the factors that contribute to its development. In recent years, formal advice about the prevention of LAA has been published in some countries to complement and support broader health and safety legislation, such as the National Institute for Occupational Safety and Health hazard alert notice in the United States (6) and the Health and Safety Executive (HSE) guidance note EH76 in the United Kingdom (7). However, despite this, there remains no definite evidence that the incidence of the disease is falling. In the United Kingdom, there continues to be approximately 20 to 30 new cases per year of asthma attributable to laboratory animals reported to the surveillance scheme Surveillance of Work and Occupational Respiratory Disease (SWORD). This incidence rate for British workers [200 cases of occupational asthma (OA) per million laboratory and technical assistants] is approximately half that for bakers and one-third for spray painters (8). If contemporary data from Draper et al. (5) for those definitely exposed to small animals is used as the denominator, the incidence rate for asthma and rhinitis may be as high as $1500/10^6$ and $2500/10^6$, respectively—which may still be an underestimate.

Heederik et al. (9) has estimated that there is a wide range in the sensitization potency between various allergens and that for rat urine this can occur at pg/m^3 as compared to ng/m^3 for amylase and $\mu g/m^3$ for flour. Because of the potency of the allergens involved and the importance of allergen exposure as a risk factor for the development of LAA, rigorous control measures are required in the workplace. The emphasis on managing this disease therefore continues to be via effective health and safety management that should incorporate measures for reducing exposure to animal allergens, health surveillance, and effective education and training of staff.

Epidemiology

Although the incidence of OA will reflect the local patterns of occupation, those involving close contact with animals typically report high rates of asthma.

Laboratory Animals

Laboratory animals are a common cause of asthma in countries where medical and veterinary research is undertaken (Western Europe, United States, Japan, and the Antipodes). Observations made about disease frequency from epidemiological studies can be influenced by the study design. While cross-sectional studies are often the simplest to perform, they may be subject to survivor bias. Similarly, the definition and means of determining the endpoint (such as OA) may profoundly affect the estimate of prevalence or incidence of disease. The influence of these factors on the epidemiology of OA has been discussed recently (10). Despite this, there is now a substantial body of data from many investigators that reveals a remarkably consistent disease pattern for allergy to laboratory animals.

Hunskaar and Fosse (11) have reviewed the data from cross-sectional studies reported prior to 1990. Where no special allergen avoidance steps are taken, the prevalence of symptoms of LAA (such as rhinoconjunctivitis, contact urticaria and asthma) among exposed workers varies between approximately 20% and 40%.

The most common symptom is rhinoconjunctivitis occurring in approximately three quarters of the cases. Rhinoconjunctivitis and/or skin symptoms often precede the onset of asthma. Asthma is the least frequently reported but most serious symptom, occurring in approximately one-third of cases. Fortunately, case reports suggest that systemic anaphylaxis after rodent bites or needle-stick injuries is rare (12–14).

This pattern of disease has been supported by the findings of longitudinal studies of up to four years duration. There have been two cohorts of note involving 300 to 400 participants; a British study of newly employed staff at pharmaceutical companies (15) and a Canadian study of apprentices undertaking an animal health technology and veterinary program for three years or more (16–22). The U.K. subjects were observed at six-month intervals, whereas the Canadian subjects were observed at eight months and then annually thereafter. Both studies demonstrate that the majority of cases of LAA develop their symptoms within two years of their exposure. The pattern of disease development confirms the pattern observed with cross-sectional studies in that skin symptoms or rhinoconjunctivitis are experienced before the onset of asthma. The reported incidence rates (per 100 person years) from the United Kingdom were 7.3 for eye/nose symptoms, 4.8 for skin symptoms, 4.1 for sensitization (positive skin-prick test), and 3.5 for respiratory symptoms. Substantially higher incidence rates (per 100 person years) were found among the Canadian apprentices: 12.0 for rhinoconjunctivitis, 7.7 for work-related skin symptoms, 7.9 for antigen skin reactivity, and 2.0 for work-related asthma. Possible reasons cited for these differences are the possibility of "survivor bias" in the U.K. cohort (the initial participants could have had up to four years of exposure before the start of the study) and the fact that the apprentices had exposure to additional animal species. The possibility that the intensity or pattern of exposure to animal allergens differed between the studies was not addressed.

Another measure of the number of cases of OA attributable to laboratory animals can be gained from surveillance schemes. The following data has been provided courtesy of SWORD and Occupational Physicians Reporting Activity (OPRA) as part of The Health and Occupation Reporting network (23). Since the SWORD scheme began in 1989, an estimated 588 cases have been reported (compared to 217 via the OPRA scheme). The breakdown of these cases by year is shown in Table 1.

These results show that despite an apparent decline in the number of cases reported towards the end of the 1990s, the inclusion of cases reported by occupational physicians in the OPRA reports, as well as chest physicians in the SWORD reports, suggest this might not be real. As working practices with laboratory animals continue to improve throughout the United Kingdom, it is possible that this increase is at least in part the result of the HSE inspection and an increased identification of existing cases by occupational health professionals.

Atopy has been consistently identified as a risk factor for the development of allergy to laboratory animals and in particular for asthma. There is some evidence that atopy may shorten the latency period of the disease from initial exposure (24). On the other hand, both cross-sectional (25) and prospective studies have shown that a positive skin-prick test or nasal symptoms associated with exposure to pets are the risk factors for allergy to laboratory animals (16–22). Nguyen et al. (21) have shown that the development of new sensitization to common environmental allergens may occur concomitant with or subsequent to the development of new occupational allergies. Evidence to suggest that smoking might be a risk factor for LAA has been found only when data from three cross-sectional studies were pooled (26).

Table 1 Incidence of Reports of Cases of Occupational
Asthma in the United Kingdom According to SWORD and
OPRA Sentinel-Based Programs

Year	SWORD	OPRA
1989	23	–
1990	26	–
1991	42	–
1992	44	–
1993	35	–
1994	62	–
1995	78	–
1996	58	–
1997	52	–
1998	35	–
1999	18	48
2000	15	60
2001	27	12
2002	24	24
2003	31	73

Note: Cases of LAA reported to SWORD by chest physicians and to
OPRA by occupational physicians, both voluntary reporting schemes with
high participation rates, in the United Kingdom between 1989 and 2004.
Abbreviations: SWORD, surveillance of work and occupational respiratory disease; OPRA, occupational physicians reporting activity; LAA,
laboratory animal allergy.

Recently, the initial reports of the immunological mechanisms involved in the
initiation of the human immune response to Rat n1 that consider genetic susceptibility have been published (27). In a cross-sectional study of U.K. pharmaceutical
workers, Jeal et al. investigated the human leukocyte antigen (HLA) class II
molecules of 109 rat-sensitized individuals and 397 controls. HLA class II molecules
present antigen fragments (epitopes) to T helper cells via T-cell receptor processing;
the more efficiently an antigenic fragment or peptide can bind to these molecules, the
more probable is an effective immune response. Because these molecules are highly
polymorphic, it is plausible that they may contribute to variation in the allergic
response to Rat n1. Jeal et al. have shown that when exposed to rats under similar
conditions, those who developed symptomatic exposure to rat urine were nearly four
times more likely to be HLA-DRβ1*07 positive than those who remained non-
sensitized and asymptomatic. Interestingly, another molecule (HLA-DRβ1*03) was
shown to have a protective effect, and sequencing of both these HLA class II
molecules suggest that the HLA-DRβ1*07 molecule would effectively bind the hydrophobic Rat n1 molecule while HLA-DRβ1*03 would not. However, when considering the factors that contribute most significantly to the development of allergy to
rats, the effect of such markers of individual susceptibility is less than that of exposure.

There is now consistent evidence that the most important risk factor for the
development of sensitization and allergy to rats is exposure to rat urinary proteins
and that the risk increases as allergen exposure increases. The data from three
European studies examining the exposure–response relationship for rat workers
have been pooled (28). These results show that the effect of exposure was particularly
prominent amongst nonatopic workers. Atopic workers were three times more likely

to become sensitized than control subjects, but there was a less clear dose–response relationship. One interpretation of the findings is that the lowest possible exposures measured were sufficient to sensitize atopics whereas the risk for nonatopics was only significant at higher concentrations. A direct positive relationship between exposure intensity and development of symptoms (including chest symptoms) has also been observed (28–30).

There is evidence, direct and indirect, that sensitization to allergens can occur at lower exposure levels than those that provoke symptoms. While no formal exposure measurements were conducted, the prospective study by Botham et al. demonstrated that measures designed to reduce exposure to animal allergens succeeded in reducing the incidence of reported symptoms, but did not reduce the incidence of development of specific IgE (31). This phenomenon has also been observed in those working in the detergent industry (32). Low exposure to rodent allergens has also been found to be associated with the development of specific IgE in a Swedish cohort (33).

The contribution of endotoxin to the development and expression of respiratory symptoms in animal workers is now receiving attention. Although the effect of endotoxin is complex and may depend on the timing and dose (34), endotoxin exposure can cause symptoms in non-sensitized individuals who work with mice (35) and rats (35,36). Endotoxin levels in animal facilities range from 10 to 1500 pg/m^3 (36) with the main reservoirs being the rodent rooms, food, and litter, rather than the animals themselves. The level of endotoxin exposure associated with nasal and chest symptoms was approximately 1 ng/m^3. Endotoxin exposure may contribute to symptoms reported by personnel working with animals who do not have specific IgE antibodies to rodent allergens.

Farm Animals

Exposure to farm animals such as cows and reindeer is an important cause of asthma (37) and contact urticaria in Scandinavia (38). While dairy farming is common in other countries, two factors are considered to be of particular importance in contributing to the high prevalence of the disease in Finland. Because of its northern location, cows are kept in cowsheds (which may form part of the farmhouse) for most of the year, grazing only during the summer months (May to September). It is also a common practice for dairy farmers to brush their animals, which can result in intense exposure to cow dander allergens. Hinze and Bergmann have examined the development of asthma in 67 subjects diagnosed as having asthma because of exposure to cows (39). In common with the progression of hypersensitivity to other animal species, those affected usually experience rhinoconjunctivitis and urticaria prior to developing lower respiratory symptoms. Those with preexisting atopy also tended to develop more severe symptoms. However, in France, respiratory symptoms (chronic bronchitis, moderate bronchial obstruction, and mild decrease in oxygen saturation) observed in dairy farmers ($n = 215$), compared to controls ($n = 110$), were not attributed to allergy to cow or to other occupational allergens (40).

Reindeer herding is another frequent occupation in Scandinavia where its meat is widely used as food. High exposure to reindeer epithelium only occurs in the autumn, when the animals are collected from the forest, marked, and kept in fenced areas over the winter. In a random study of 211 reindeer herders from Northern Finland, only one person had a positive skin-prick test and respiratory symptoms were attributed to extreme weather conditions and/or smoking (41). Allergic reactions to wild animals such as deer and elk can also be an occupational disease of professional hunting guides (42,43). Sensitized individuals may experience asthmatic symptoms when skinning and dressing skins, or washing contaminated clothing. In a study of 15 subjects with exposure to deer and elk, all were highly atopic. Those with pre-existing allergy to domestic animals may be at increased risk of developing IgE-mediated reactions to deer after professional or recreational contact with these animals.

A random study of 125 grooms (and 92 nonexposed controls) who worked with horses in Istanbul has shown that approximately 12% were sensitized to horse-hair as compared to 5% of the controls (44). The pattern of symptoms in the grooms was similar to that seen among other occupational groups. Of those sensitized, 42% reported rhinitis, 35% conjunctivitis, 33% skin symptoms, and 15% asthma. The prevalence of respiratory symptoms among pig and sheep farmers is thought to be probably owing to exposure to other agents such as endotoxin and chemicals rather than allergens (45–48).

Allergens

Rat (*Rattus norvegicus*) and Mouse (*Mus musculus*)

Urine is the major source of allergenic proteins in rats and mice and the low-molecular-weight constituents have been identified as major allergens (49,50). Rat n1 and Mus m1 are synthesized in the liver and belong to the lipocalin family of proteins (51). The complex hormonal control of the production of these molecules, together with detailed structural information and their biological role as phero-mones, have been recently reviewed (52,53). Both Rat n1 and Mus m1 appear in the urine, particularly of male animals after puberty, and disappear after castration or with senility. It has been estimated that the urine of male mice contains approximately four times the amount of Mus m1 than that in the urine of female mice.

All male rats develop chronic renal disease spontaneously owing to the production of Rat n1 and its ability to bind toxic chemicals. Male rats therefore secrete increasing amounts of serum proteins in their urine as they mature. The serum proteins albumin and transferrin, found in rat urine, are allergenic for nearly 30% of rat-sensitive subjects (54). Most common strains of rats and mice produce urine with very similar allergenic composition (55,56). However, strains of rats developed as animal models for diseases such as diabetes, which develop renal disease as a consequence of this, secrete greater amounts of serum proteins in their urine.

The hair and saliva of rats and mice are also important sources of allergens. Extracts of saliva and hair obtained from male rats were subject to immunoblotting studies with serum from 25 or more rat allergic subjects (57). Both extracts contained many IgE-binding components. Fur contained five major IgE-binding bands with relatively high molecular weights (>22 kDa). The most important salivary allergens have molecular weights of less than 22 kDa.

Other Laboratory Animals

Fur, saliva, and urine are allergenic in most guinea pig (*Cavia porcellus*)–sensitized subjects (58,59). The major allergens in pelt and urine were investigated using serum from 40 guinea pig–allergic subjects. Three major allergens were found in both sources with molecular weights of 8, 17, and 20 kDa. N-terminal sequence analysis of the 20 kDa allergen (Cav p1) and 17 kDa allergen (Cav p2) has shown that they are lipocalins that share approximately 60% sequence homology with Mus m1 and Bos d2, respectively (60). Approximately half of subjects had IgE specific for guinea pig serum and albumin. Analysis of dust from guinea pig holding rooms by crossed immunoelectrophoresis has shown that the dust antigens are common to guinea pig dander, fur, saliva, and urine (61).

For rabbits (*Oryctolagus cuniculus*), the urine, fur, saliva, and dander/pelt are all sources of allergens as shown by crossed immunoelectrophoresis (62). Immuno-blotting studies have shown that the molecular weight range of fur allergens (>250–4.4 kDa) was wider than that for saliva (majority <34 kDa). Major salivary allergens with molecular weights of 18 and 21 kDa were identified as lipocalins (63).

There have been few descriptions of allergy to gerbils (14,64), monkeys, and marmosets. Allergy to ferrets has also been reported (65). In an unpublished study on two research workers who presented with symptoms of asthma and rhinitis, specific IgE to two urinary proteins with molecular weights of 22.5 and 17 kDa was observed, the latter only present in the urine of male animals (Scott, Gordon, personal communication).

Other Allergens in the Animal Facility

When managing the risks of occupational allergy in biomedical facilities, attention should also be paid to other sources of allergen. These include natural rubber latex (gloves and medical devices), enzymes (present in animal feed), fish feed (including live bait, chironomids, mealworms), anesthetic gases, chemicals (glutaraldehyde and formaldehyde), and pharmaceutical agents (antibiotics, insulin, etc.).

Other Animals

Hair and dander are considered the most important allergen sources in allergy induced by cows (*Bos domesticus*). Two major allergens have been detected in dander with molecular weights of 20 (Bos d2, a lipocalin) and 22 kDa (66–68). Bos d2 is a weak immunogen (69) and several isoforms exist (70).

Diagnosis and Management of Affected Workers

The diagnosis is based on a history of work-related symptoms (nasal, eye, skin, and chest) in a person who encounters these allergens in their work. Symptoms develop after an initial asymptomatic period of exposure, commonly within the first two or three years of exposure. The typical scenario is the development of sensitization accompanied by nasal and conjunctival symptoms preceding respiratory symptoms, like in the case of other high-molecular-weight allergens (19,71) (Table 2). The major-ity of patients identify a clear relationship between working with animals and the provocation of their symptoms. In sensitized individuals, rhinoconjunctivitis may be provoked within minutes of exposure. Asthma, at least initially, may only be manifest as increased airway responsiveness or may develop only several hours after allergen contact, making identification of the provoking agent more difficult (71). Nasal and eye symptoms can resolve in hours, whereas asthma may persist for several days and cause nocturnal respiratory symptoms with sleep disturbance. Urticaria usually develops at the site of direct skin contact with the allergens. Objective evidence to support a diagnosis can be obtained from a specific immunological response (usually IgE), work-related changes in peak flow rate, and inhalation tests. Specific IgE in serum or identified by a skin-prick test to a specific allergen in general is more sensitive (few false negatives) than a specific test (few false positives) in allergic asthma. The absence of specific IgE is therefore more useful in excluding a specific allergen as

Table 2 Time Course of Work-Related Symptoms and Occupational Diseases in
Apprentices Exposed to Laboratory Animals

	Years in the program				Incidence density[a]
	1	2	3	4	
Number present at visit	136	345	355	98	
Skin reactivity to a	14	37	29	5	85/1075
program-related antigen	(10.3%)	(10.7%)	(8.2%)	(5.1%)	(7.9%)
Work-related symptoms					
Skin	4	33	39	5	81/1051
	(2.9%)	(9.6%)	(11.0%)	(5.1%)	(7.7%)
Rhinoconjunctivitis	17	48	30	4	99/961
	(12.5%)	(13.9%)	(8.5%)	(4.1%)	(10.3%)
Respiratory	1	11	9	1	22/1115
	(0.7%)	(3.2%)	(2.5%)	(1.0%)	(2.0%)
Occupational					
Rhinoconjunctivitis[b]	9	24	29	0	62/1096
	(6.6%)	(7.0%)	(8.2%)	(0%)	(5.7%)
Asthma[c]	5	9	13	1	28/1043
	(3.7%)	(2.6%)	(3.7%)	(1.0%)	(2.7%)

Note: Incident immunological sensitization and rhinoconjunctivitis occur sooner than respiratory symptoms after starting the exposure in the apprenticeship program.
Total number of participants $= 417$ except for the assessment of occupational asthma ($n = 373$) because 44 subjects refused the methacholine test.
[a]Number of cases/person-years in the program.
[b]Defined as incident rhinoconjunctivitis symptoms and skin reactivity to a program-related antigen.
[c]Defined as incident onset of bronchial hyperresponsiveness and skin reactivity to a program-related antigen.
Source: From Ref. 19.

the cause of asthma than its presence is in attributing to it. As for other high-molecular-weight allergens, a combination of IgE-sensitization by skin-prick testing or assessment of specific IgE and the presence of bronchial hyperresponsiveness results in an 80% likelihood of OA.

It is important to distinguish cases of allergy with asthma from those without. The prognosis of those with asthma, who remain exposed to the allergen provoking their symptoms, is probably less good; the longer they remain exposed, the more likely are their symptoms to persist and chronic asthma develops as a result (see Chapter 3). Early diagnosis and the instigation of allergen avoidance measures are therefore of paramount importance. For some, immediate avoidance of animal contact is impossible and time may be required to complete a course of study, retrain and find an alternative employment. In such circumstances, providing the possible consequences to their health are fully explained, support and symptomatic treatment for a short period may be appropriate as long as animal contact has not provoked a life-threatening reaction (acute, severe asthma or anaphylaxis), there is a firm intention to make a job change within an agreed time frame, and allergen exposure can be minimized. This usually requires the conscientious use of good quality respiratory protective equipment whose effectiveness should be monitored by lung function tests. Allergy without asthma is generally easier to manage with respiratory and skin protection and adequate washing and changing facilities on site. The majority of such cases are able to continue to work with animals.

The major occupational health goal for those responsible for the health of persons working with animals, insects, and shellfish must be the progressive reduction in disease incidence. The prevention of disease is most appropriately based on controlling environmental exposure to allergen rather than the identification and exclusion of "susceptible" individuals; the latter is poorly discriminating and identifies the individual rather than the environment as responsible for the problem. The prevention of allergy to animals, insects, and shellfish should therefore be achieved primarily by preventing allergens from becoming airborne and being inhaled, or entering the body via any other route (skin absorption, ingestion, or via mucosal surfaces) and this is discussed in detail elsewhere. It seems that airborne exposure to potent allergens must be virtually eliminated for sensitization to be prevented in most people (9,24,32). However, exposure control measures may be insufficient to prevent sensitization and symptoms in all workers and therefore health surveillance is required.

Measurement of Exposure

While exposure standards have been set in some countries for respiratory sensitizers, there is currently no occupational exposure standard for laboratory animal allergens. Because of the serious health effects and variability in the susceptibility of individuals, it is most likely to be set "as low as reasonably practicable." One serious obstacle at present is the lack of a standardized method to quantify rodent allergens. Recent studies have shown that the type of assay employed may influence the results obtained by up to three orders of magnitude (71,72). Assays that utilize monoclonal antibodies to measure major rodent allergens (such as Rat n1) offer excellent sensitivity and standardization (73,74). An alternative strategy has been adopted for mouse allergens with assays developed using polyclonal antibodies raised to recombinant Mus m1 (74). However, animal room dust is a complex mixture of allergens, and exposure to other allergens (e.g., albumin) that can be important in some circumstances will not be measured with these assays. The number of workplaces performing exposure measurements has grown. The data generated have proved to be useful in the validation of risk assessments, the objective assessment of control measures, and the education of staff.

Control of Exposure

Because of the potency of animal allergens and the nature of scientific work, increasing local ventilation remains the most effective way of controlling exposure. The use of individually ventilated cage (IVC) systems has been shown by several authors to contain rat and mouse allergen, especially when operated at negative pressure to the environment (75–77). When used in conjunction with mobile ventilated cabinets to undertake the transfer of animals to clean cages (78), and the removal of soiled litter via robotic or vacuum means (79), it is possible to minimize exposure to rodent allergens among animal husbandry staff. It has been reported that the IVC systems operated at negative pressure can be used without compromising animal health and that the cost can be recouped (albeit at a large institution) in less than five years (78). Ideally, areas such as holding rooms and cage wash areas, where high levels of allergen may collect, should be maintained at negative pressure to other areas. If exposure to animal allergens is controlled at source, and rooms are kept at negative pressure relative to other communal areas, respiratory protection equipment (RPE) need not be used unless one is in direct contact with animals or their waste.

It is more difficult to reduce exposure when the animals are being employed in procedures. Except in cases where few anaesthetized animals are being used, exposure when performing experiments should be minimized by the use of local exhaust ventilation means, such as class I cabinets and down draft tables. Where this is not possible (as for example in behavioral studies), the possibility of monitoring the experiment by closed circuit television cameras should be explored. Significant exposure to allergen may occur even if there is no direct contact with rodents, such as when changing filters in ventilation systems or during handling of soiled laundry. The studies by Tovey et al. with cat allergen suggests that personal clothing may be an important source and means of distribution of animal allergens (80) but laundering at 60°C with detergent can effectively remove the allergens (81).

The use of good quality respiratory protective equipment (which has been fit tested) is still of fundamental importance. Renstrom et al. have used intranasal sampling to show that disposable P2-masks and air stream helmets reduce exposure to rat and mouse allergens by 90% or more (82).

Inspection Programs

In the United Kingdom, the Health and Safety Executive (HSE) has been undertaking an inspection program of all premises licensed for experimentation on living animals. The aim is to improve the management of health risks in this sector by assessing compliance with current legislation and is also part of a wider national strategy to reduce OA by 30%.

The inspection program commenced in 2002 and coincided with the release of the HSE guidance note EH76 "Control of Laboratory Animal Allergy." The inspection visits were by prior appointment and were made by an Occupational Health Inspector and an Occupational Hygiene Inspector. Sixty-six inspections were carried out between April 2002 and March 2004, primarily of universities. In general, the majority of premises exhibited a "reasonable standard of legal compliance." However, during that period 16 improvement notices were issued to 11 duty holders, the majority ($n = 13$) in the first year of the program. Improvement notices were issued at 20% of the premises inspected and were for poor management of health and safety, inadequate assessment of the risks, insufficiencies in the testing and thorough examination of local exhaust ventilation systems, inadequate training of staff, and failure to undertake fit testing for RPE. However, most were issued for lack of appropriate control measures and health surveillance. The program will be completed in March 2006 with the inspection of a further 50 premises from the commercial sector.

It is evident from this program that even in a sector with a responsible attitude to the risks of occupational allergy, failure of basic health and safety provision was serious enough in a small proportion of facilities to require formal improvement notices to be served. It is also noteworthy that standards of compliance improved as the program progressed. Therefore, continued periodic inspections (by an organization with authority to initiate litigation if required) may be of benefit to maintain the necessary high standards required for preventing LAA.

INSECTS

The presence of specific IgE in cases of sensitivity to an increasing number of insect species has been demonstrated by skin testing and radioallergosorbent allergy testing

(RAST). Various types of occupations can lead to exposures to allergens. The species of insects identified as causing occupational hypersensitivity include flies (83–91), locusts (92,93), grasshoppers (94), bumblebees (95,96), mites (97–102), spiders (103), cockroaches (104), and chironimid midges (105,106).

Entomologists and laboratory workers have developed sensitivity to locusts, crickets, houseflies, blowflies, and screwworm flies. Grain mill workers, dock loaders, and longshoreman may be exposed to beetles, storage mites, and grain weevils. Electrical power plant workers and sewer workers may come in contact with sewer flies and caddis flies at times. Loggers and lumber mill workers have developed sensitivity to the tussock moth. Fish and bait handlers are at risk from exposures to mealworms and blue blowfly and other larvae. Individuals working in the honey industry are exposed to honeybee body dust and venom. Pet food manufactures may be sensitized to chironomids and small animal handlers may become sensitized to fleas.

Epidemiology

The epidemiology of occupational insect allergy has been less well studied than for LAA, primarily because the size of the problem is less than that of LAA.

Individual case reports of occupational allergy to fly species include those of an atopic scientific worker who developed rhinitis when exposed to *Musca domestica* (84), a sewage plant worker who developed rhinoconjunctivitis and then asthma when exposed to sewer flies, *Psychoda alternata* (85), and a doctoral student who experienced anaphylactic symptoms after being bitten by tsetse flies, *Glossina morsitans* (89). A cross-sectional study of 22 research workers who worked with the fruit fly, *Drosophila melanogaster*, demonstrates the potency of insect allergens (86). Seven of the subjects (32%) experienced nasal symptoms; of these four also had lower respiratory tract symptoms and three also had eye symptoms. Similarly 28% of Australian research workers involved in the breeding of the sheep blowfly (*Lucilia cuprina*) used in genetic studies and biological control programs were found to be symptomatic: 24% had upper respiratory tract symptoms, 20% had eye symptoms, 17% had skin symptoms, and 11% either had asthma or experienced tightness of the chest (91). Workers exposed to large numbers of insects in outdoor locations may also be at risk of occupational allergy. At least 25% of the 57 workers employed at a hydroelectric power plant in Canada described work-related symptoms associated with exposure to caddis flies (*Hydropsyche recurvata*) (88). Of the 28 subjects tested, 17 had a positive skin-prick test to caddis fly allergen. Workers were 3.7 times more likely to be sensitized if they worked in areas of high exposure to the caddis fly. Subjects with specific IgE to caddis fly were more likely to report an increased number of work-related symptoms and 10 reported "wheeze" (compared to three who were skin-prick test negative).

Occupational allergy to cockroaches (104), locusts (93), and grasshoppers (*Melanoplus sanguinipes*) (94) has been observed in laboratory workers. Owing to the similarity in observations and the small number of subjects studied [6 (104), 15 (93), and 17 (94) respectively], the findings will be summarized. The prevalence of a positive skin-prick test in these exposed subjects is high (67%, 67%, and 41%, respectively) with over half of the exposed subjects experiencing work-related allergic symptoms. Asthma was seen in 33% of the locust workforce and 24% of the grasshopper workers. All of those experiencing OA had specific IgE to the relevant antigen and had other related symptoms (typically rhinoconjunctivitis in the locust workers and skin sensitivity in the grasshopper workers). Atopy was not necessarily associated with symptomatic or immunological allergy in occupational sensitivity to orthopterans; two out of four skin-prick test positive to cockroach, four out of 10 skin-prick test positive to locust, and five out of seven skin-prick test positive to grasshopper were considered nonatopic.

Case reports of occupational insect allergy include a nonatopic subject who developed severe asthma coincident with the seasonal honey-packing process (95), seven subjects (five nonatopic) who experienced anaphylactic symptoms when stung by bees (96), three female subjects sensitized to spider mites (98,101), nine female subjects with occupational skin and upper respiratory tract symptoms attributed to the urticating hair from the Brazilian spider (103), and a male researcher who developed severe rhinoconjunctivitis after 10 years of collecting live adult chironomid midges (106).

Chironomids are an important environmental inhalant allergen in Japan and have been identified as a source of allergy in those occupationally or recreationally involved in the running of aquariums and in fish-food factory workers (107). As subjects for the study were recruited by advertisement, the prevalence of reported symptoms for the whole group was high (63% prevalence of rhinoconjunctivitis, 45% asthma, etc.). Out of the 32 subjects employed in the fish-food factory, 15 had very high exposure to Chi t1 and of these, five presented with symptoms and specific IgE to Chi t1.

Allergens

There have been attempts to identify and characterize insect allergens. Many of the early studies used immunoblotting techniques to analyze molecular weights of the various allergens. More recent use of molecular biology techniques has identified a number of important allergens from insects, particularly in cockroaches (108–110). Important allergens from cockroaches include Bla g2 (an inactive aspartic proteinase), Bla g4 (calycin), and Bla g5 (glutathione S-transferase). The group 1 cockroach allergens from the German and American cockroaches include the cross-reactive tropomyosin. It is hypothesized that sensitivity to tropomyosins from both house dust mites and cockroaches may confer cross-sensitivity and may also be important in the pathogenesis of sensitivity to shrimp (110–112). An insect hemoglobin (Chi t1) has been identified as the major allergen in midge sensitivity (105,107,113).

There have been a few other studies using data from biochemical studies on insect allergens. Epidemiological studies of workers exposed to a species of flies have generally utilized extracts from whole adult flies (84,86,88). Immunoblotting analysis from the housefly and blowfly showed that most of the allergens had molecular weights between 40 and 60 kDa (87,90). A major allergen from about 70% of blowfly allergic subjects was found at 67 kDa, and a 20 kDa allergen, making a shift to extensive cross-reactivity, was found between different species of flies (84,85,87).

The feces and the peritrophic membrane, a mid-gut secretion that encloses ingested food as it passes through the intestines and encases the feces, when excreted may be important sources of allergens for Othoptera (93,94). Tee et al. (93) identified multiple protein bands by sodium dodecyl sulfate polyacrylamide gel electrophoresis and soluble extracts diluted from whole locust. The protein bands most strongly bound by IgE and identified by immunoblotting of serum from patients allergic to locusts have molecular weights of 18, 29, 37, 42, 54, 66, and 68 kDa. Locust wings have also recently been identified as a novel source of allergen (114). While the cockroach is more likely to be a domestic indoor allergen, there is extensive literature on the allergens as reviewed (108). Honeybee body dust is a major source of allergen for those employed in the honeybee production industry as a means of pollinating plants

(95,96). Venom may also be a source of allergen as well. The role of the pollens originating from plants that feed the insects should not be overlooked as a sensitizing agent either.

As cited above, an important source of allergen for many insect species may be the feces. Therefore, it is not unusual that there may be cross-reactivity between insect feces and feces from the arachnids of the house dust mite family. Further, studies with recombinant and native tropomyosins have demonstrated a cross-reactivity between house dust mite allergens, insects, and shrimp as discussed above.

Several species of insects have been linked to occupational allergy, and in some cases investigation of the aeroallergens has been undertaken primarily to demonstrate the relevant allergen in the air. Tee et al., in their study of the housefly (*Musca domesticus*), demonstrated that the airborne fly allergen(s) originated in part from the dust collecting in the fly-rearing cage were probably of fecal origin (84). Dust from filters collected in a fly-rearing room had a steeper slope than self-inhibition (fly extract), suggesting the presence of additional, but unidentified, allergens in the air. Similarly, feces and the peritrophic membrane are the most likely sources of airborne locust allergens in the species *Schistocerca gregaria* and *Locusta migratoria* (93).

FISHES AND SHELLFISHES

It is well established that occupational exposure and sensitivity to a variety of fish and shellfish in the processing industry are causes of OA. Several species of shellfish have been reported to cause OA including snow crab (*Chinocetes opilis*) (115), Alaska king crab (116–118), lobster (119), shrimp (*Metapenaeus ensis*) (120–122), and scallop (123) and clam (121). Several other fish-derived allergens have been incriminated in case reports and in surveys as reviewed (124). A variety of fishes including salmon (125), trout (126), pilchard, anchovy, and hake (124) also have been described as causes of allergies. Occupational sensitivity to a parasite of fish, *Anisakis simplex*, has also been identified as a cause of asthma (127) and allergic reactions (128). Occupational exposures to seafood allergens can occur both in processing plants and in restaurant workers (119,120). Among the crustacea and mollusk family, tropomyosins appears to be the major sensitizer, and there is extensive cross-reactivity across species. However, in the case of oysters, the oyster itself may not be responsible but a parasite, protochordate, seems to be the principal agent (129,130).

Epidemiology

The first cross-sectional study to examine the prevalence of occupational allergies and asthma in workers processing snow crab (*Chinoecetes* opilis) was published in 1984 by Cartier et al. (115). A total of 313 subjects were employed at two industrial sites in Canada. The freshly caught crabs were boiled and cooled, and the cooked meat was separated from the legs and claws before being canned. The prevalence of work-related symptoms was high in both the plants, with work-related asthma being confirmed in approximately 46 of the 303 workers studied (15% of the total workforce, which corresponds to nearly 97% of the exposed workers). Approximately two-thirds of the workers with asthma had rhinoconjunctivitis and one-third had urticaria. No relationship was found between OA and the presence of atopy. Skin-prick testing with crab antigens found specific IgE in just over half of the asthmatics suggesting that other immunological mechanisms might also be important. Smoking was a risk factor for the development of OA. Further immunological studies reported in 1986 (131) showed that specific IgE to crab antigens could be detected in the serum of the workers by RAST. An improved extract of snow crab cooking water demonstrated that 84% of the 37 asthmatics tested had specific IgE to the extract.

The same group has also reported on clam and shrimp as causes of OA (121). In this study population, the food-processing workers handled lyophilized clam and shrimp and packed the powder into bags. Of the 61 workers employed, 25 worked on the bag production line. Less than 10% of workers reported symptoms associated with exposure to clam and shrimp. Asthma was present in two atopic subjects (4%) who demonstrated specific IgE to both clam and shrimp. The prevalence of sensitization to clam and shrimp was approximately 6% and 15%, respectively. Subjects with specific IgE to clam and/or shrimp often had specific IgE to other seafood species. Additional case reports of OA attributed to lobster and shrimp have been reported in atopic, nonsmoking women working at a fishmongers (120) and in an atopic chef (119). Both had been employed for at least two years before the onset of increasingly severe skin and respiratory symptoms, and both experienced gastrointestinal symptoms after the ingestion of shellfish.

Other epidemiological surveys in which the diagnosis of OA has not been confirmed have been carried out in Alaska king crab processors (132), prawn workers (133), mussel openers (134), and salmon (125), trout (126), and fish meal workers (135) as reviewed (136). A large cross-sectional study has been initiated in South Africa in workers exposed to pilchard, hake, and anchovy. According to preliminary results, skin rashes are highly prevalent (more than 75%) and the prevalence of asthma is estimated as 7% (137).

Allergens

RAST inhibition has been used to detect aerosolized shrimp and clam proteins in the workplace (121). The concentration of snow crab aeroallergen has been found to be highest (1.7 μg allergen on filter equivalent to an airborne concentration of approximately $10 \, \mu g/m^3$) in an area adjacent to the sorting and boiling of crabs, but is virtually undetectable in other areas of the factory where cooked meat is handled (138,139). Allergen concentrations as high as $1000 \, ng/m^3$ have been detected in salmon processing (125).

RESEARCH NEEDS

More complete identification of the allergenic constituents of animals, insects, fishes, and shellfishes is needed, to reduce the concentrations of the most highly allergenic components by efficient environmental means. Prospective studies in apprentices and newly employed personnel are needed to better characterize the natural history of the disease.

REFERENCES

1. Taylor G, Davies GE, Altounyan REC, et al. Allergic reactions to laboratory animals. Nature 1976; 260:280.

2. Lincoln TA, Bolton NE, Garrett AS. Occupational allergy to animal dander and serum. J Occup Med 1974; 16:465–469.
3. Lutsky I, Neuman I. Laboratory animal dander allergy. I. An occupational disease. Ann Allergy 1975; 35:201–205.
4. Seward JP. Occupational allergy to animals. Occup Med 1999; 14:285–302.
5. Draper A, Newman Taylor AJ, Cullinan PC. Estimating the incidence of occupational asthma and rhinitis from laboratory animal allergens in the UK, 1999–2000. Occup Environ Med 2003; 60:604–605.
6. National Institute for Occupational Safety and Health. NIOSH alert: preventing asthma in animal handlers. Publication no. 97-116. NIOSH, 1998.
7. Health and Safety Executive. Control of laboratory animal allergy. Guidance Note EH76. London: HSE Books, 2002.
8. Meredith SK, Taylor V, McDonald JC. Occupational respiratory disease in the United Kingdom: a report to the British Thoracic Society and the Society of Occupational Medicine by the SWORD project group. Br J Ind Med 1991; 48:292–298.
9. Heederik D, Doekes G, Nieuwenhuijsen MJ. Exposure assessment of high molecular weight sensitisers: contribution to occupational epidemiology and disease prevention. Occup Environ Med 1999; 56:735–741.
10. Gautrin D, Newman Taylor AJ, Nordman H, Malo JL. Controversies in epidemiology of occupational asthma. Eur Respir J 2003; 22:551–559.
11. Hunskaar S, Fosse RT. Allergy to laboratory mice and rats: a review of the pathophysiology, epidemiology and clinical aspects. Lab Anim 1990; 24:358–374.
12. Hesford JD, Platts-Mills TAE, Edlich RF. Anaphylaxis after laboratory rat bite: an occupational hazard. J Emerg Med 1995; 13:765–768.
13. Watt AD, McSharry CP. Laboratory animal allergy: anaphylaxis from a needle injury. Occup Environ Med 1996; 53:573–574.
14. Trummer M, Komericki P, Kranke B, Aberer W. Anaphylaxis after a Mongolian gerbil bite. J Eur Acad Dermatol Venereol 2004; 18:634–635.
15. Cullinan P, Cook AD, Gordon S, et al. Allergen exposure, atopy and smoking as determinants of allergy to rats in a cohort of laboratory employees. Eur Respir J 1999; 13:1139–1143.
16. Gautrin D, Infante-Rivard C, Dao TV, Magnan-Larose M, Desjardins D, Malo JL. Specific IgE-dependent sensitization, atopy and bronchial hyperresponsiveness in apprentices starting exposure to protein-derived agents. Am J Respir Crit Care Med 1997; 155:1841–1847.
17. Gautrin D, Ghezzo H, Infante-Rivard C, Malo JL. Incidence and determinants of IgE-mediated sensitization in apprentices: a prospective study. Am J Respir Crit Care Med 2000; 162:1222–1228.
18. Gautrin D, Infante-Rivard C, Ghezzo H, Malo JL. Incidence and host determinants of probable occupational asthma in apprentices exposed to laboratory animals. Am J Respir Crit Care Med 2001; 163:899–904.
19. Gautrin D, Ghezzo H, Infante-Rivard C, Malo JL. Natural history of sensitization, symptoms and diseases in apprentices exposed to laboratory animals. Eur Respir J 2001; 17:904–908.
20. Gautrin D, Ghezzo H, Infante-Rivard C, Malo JL. Host determinants for the development of allergy in apprentices exposed to laboratory animals. Eur Respir J 2002; 19: 96–103.
21. Nguyen B, Ghezzo H, Malo JL, Gautrin D. Time course of onset of sensitization to common and occupational inhalants in apprentices. J Allergy Clin Immunol 2003; 111: 807–812.
22. Rodier F, Gautrin D, Ghezzo H, Malo JL. Incidence of occupational rhinoconjunctivitis and risk factors in animal-health apprentices. J Allergy Clin Immunol 2003; 112: 1105–1111.
23. www.coeh.man.ac.uk/thor.

24. Botham PA, Davies GE, Teasdale EL. Allergy to laboratory animals: a prospective study of its incidence and of the influence of atopy on its development. Br J Ind Med 1987; 44:627–632.

25. Hollander A, Doekes G, Heederik D. Cat and dog allergy and total IgE as risk factors of laboratory animal allergy. J Allergy Clin Immunol 1996; 98:545–554.

26. Venables KM, Upton JL, Hawkins ER, Tee RD, Longbottom JL, Newman Taylor AJ. Smoking, atopy and laboratory animal allergy. Br J Ind Med 1988; 45:667–671.

27. Jeal H, Draper A, Jones M, et al. HLA associations with occupational sensitization to rat lipocalin allergens: a model for other animal allergies? J Allergy Clin Immunol 2003; 111:795–799.

28. Heederik D, Venables KM, Malmberg P, et al. Exposure-response relationships for work-related sensitization in workers exposed to rat urinary allergens: results from a pooled study. J Allergy Clin Immunol 1999; 103:678–684.

29. Nieuwenhuijsen MJ, Putcha V, Gordon S, et al. Exposure-response relations among laboratory animal workers exposed to rats. Occup Environ Med 2003; 60:104–108.

30. Cullinan P, Lowson D, Nieuwenhuijsen MJ, et al. Work-related symptoms, sensitisation and estimated exposure in workers not previously exposed to laboratory rats. Occup Environ Med 1994; 51:589–592.

31. Botham PA, Lamb CT, Teasdale EL, Bonner SM, Tomenson JA. Allergy to laboratory animals: a follow up study of its incidence and of the influence of atopy and pre-existing sensitisation on its development. Occup Env Med 1995; 52:129–133.

32. Sarlo K, Kirchner DB. Occupational asthma and allergy in the detergent industry: new developments. Curr Opin Allergy Clin Immunol 2002; 2:97–101.

33. Renström A, Karlsson AS, Malmberg P, Larsson PH, Hage-Hamsten van M. Working with male rodents may increase risk of allergy to laboratory animals. Allergy 2001; 56:964–970.

34. Singh J, Schwartz DA. Endotoxin and the lung: insight into the host-environment interaction. J Allergy Clin Immunol 2005; 115:330–333.

35. Pacheco KA, McCammon C, Liu AH, et al. Airborne endotoxin predicts symptoms in non-mouse sensitized technicians and research scientists exposed to laboratory mice. Am J Respir Crit Care Med 2003; 167:983–990.

36. Lieutier-Colas F, Meyer P, Pons F, et al. Prevalence of symptoms, sensitization to rats, and airborne exposure to major rat allergen (Rat n 1) and to endotoxin in rat-exposed workers: a cross-sectional study. Clin Exper Allergy 2002; 32:1424–1429.

37. Karjalainen A, Kurppa K, Virtanen S, Keskinen H, Nordman H. Incidence of occupational asthma by occupation and industry in Finland. Am J Ind Med 2000; 37: 451–458.

38. Kanerva L, Susitaival P. Cow dander: the most common cause of occupational contact urticaria in Finland. Contact Dermatitis 1996; 35:309–310.

39. Hinze S, Bergmann K-Chr. Cow hair asthma: symptoms and clinical course. Allergol J 1995; 4:97–101.

40. Chaudemanche H, Monnet E, Westeel V, et al. Respiratory status in dairy farmers in France; cross-sectional and longitudinal analyses. Occup Environ Med 2003; 60: 858–863.

41. Reijula K, Halmepuro L, Hannuksela M, Larmi E, Hassi J. Specific IgE to reindeer epithelium in Finnish reindeer herders. Allergy 1991; 46:577–581.

42. Gillespie DN, Dahlberg MJE, Yunginger JW. Inhalant allergy to wild animals (deer and elk). Ann Allergy 1985; 55:122–125.

43. Spiewak R, Dutkiewicz J. Allergic contact urticaria and rhinitis to roe deer (*Capreolus capreolus*) in a hunter. Ann Agric Environ Med 2002; 9:115–116.

44. Tutluoglu B, Atis S, Anakkaya AN, Altug E, Tosun GA, Yaman M. Sensitization to horse hair, symptoms and lung function in grooms. Clin Exper Allergy 2002; 32:1170–1173.

45. Crook B, Robertson JF, Travers SA Glass, Botheroyd EM, Lacey J, Topping MD. Airborne dust, ammonia, microorganisms, and antigens in pig confinement houses and the respiratory helath of exposed farm workers. Am Ind Hyg Assoc J 1991; 52:271–279.

46. Zuskin E, Kanceljak B, Schachter EN, et al. Immunological and respiratory findings in swine farmers. Environ Res 1991; 56:120–130.

47. Preller L, Heederik D, Boleij JS, Vogelzang PF, Tielen MJ. Lung function and chronic respiratory symptoms of pig farmers: focus on exposure to endotoxins and ammonia and use of disinfectants. Occup Environ Med 1995; 52:654–660.

48. Radon K, Winter C. Prevalence of respiratory symptoms in sheep breeders. Occup Environ Med 2003; 60:770–773.

49. Newman Taylor AJ, Longbottom JL, Pepys J. Respiratory allergy to urine proteins of rats and mice. Lancet 1977:847–849.

50. Gordon S, Tee RD, Newman, Taylor AJ. Analysis of rat urine proteins and allergens by sodium dodecyl sulfate-polyacrylamide gel electrophoresis and immunoblotting. J Allergy Clin Immunol 1993; 92:298–305.

51. Bayard C, Holmquist L, Vesterberg O. Purification and identificaiton of allergenic 2μ-globulin species of rat urine. Biochem Biophys Acta 1996; 1290:129–134.

52. Cavaggioni A, Mucignat-Caretta C. Major urinary proteins, alpha 2μglobulins and aphrodisin. Biochim Biophys Acta 2000; 1482:218–228.

53. Benyon RJ, Hurst JL. Urinary proteins and the modulation of chemical scents in mice and rats. Peptides 2004; 25:1553–1563.

54. Gordon S, Tee RD, Newman Taylor AJ. Analysis of rat serum allergens. J Allergy Clin Immunol 1997; 99:716–717.

55. Finlayson JS, Potter M, Shinnick CS, Smithies O. Components of the major urinary protein complex of inbred mice; determination of NH_2-terminal sequences and comparison with homologous components from wild mice. Biochem Gene 1974; 11:325–335.

56. Schumacher MJ, Tait BD, Holmes MC. Allergy to murine antigens in a biological research institute. J Allergy Clin Immunol 1981; 68:310–318.

57. Gordon S, Tee RD, Stuart MC, Newman Taylor AJ. Analysis of allergens in rat fur and saliva. Allergy 2001; 56:563–567.

58. Swanson MC, Agarwal MK, Yuninger JW, Reed CE. Guinea pig derived allergens. Clinicoimmunologic studies, characterisation, airborne quantitation and size distribution. Am Rev Respir Dis 1984; 129:844–849.

59. Hanada T, Shima T, Ohyama M. Allergic rhinitis in laboratory workers caused by occupational exposure to guinea pigs: an immunological and clinical study. Eur Arch Otorhinolaryngol 1995; 252:304–307.

60. Fahlbusch B, Rudeschko O, Schlott B, et al. Further characterisation of IgE-binding antigens from guinea-pig as new members of the lipocalin family. Allergy 2003; 58:629–634.

61. Walls AF, Newman Taylor AJ, Longbottom JL. Allergy to guinea pigs: II Identification of specific allergens in guinea pig dust by crossed radio-immunoelectrophoresis and investigation of the possible origin. Clin Allergy 1985; 15:535–546.

62. Price JA, Longbottom JL. Allergy to rabbits. II. Identification and characterization of a major rabbit allergen. Allergy 1988; 43:39–48.

63. Baker J, Berry A, Boscato LM, Gordon S, Walsh B, Stuart MC. Identification of some rabbit allergens as lipocalins. Clin Exper Allergy 2001; 31:303–312.

64. McGivern D, Longbottom J, Davies D. Allergy to gerbils. Clin Allergy 1985; 15:163–165.

65. Codina R, Reichmuth D, Lockey RF, Jaen C. Ferret allergy. J Allergy Clin Immunol 2001; 107:927.

66. Ylonen J, Mantyjarvi R, Taivainen A, Virtanen T. Comparison of the antigenic and allergenic properties of three types of bovine epithelial material. Int Arch Allergy Immunol 1992; 99:112–117.

67. Ylonen J, Virtanen T, Hoshmanheimo L, Parkkinen S, Pelkonen J, Mantyjarvi R. Affinity purification of the major bovine allergen by a novel monoclonal antibody. J Allergy Clin Immunol 1994; 93:851–858.

68. Mäntyjärvi R, Parkkinen S, Rythonen M, et al. Complementary DNA cloning of the predominant allergen of bovine dander: a new member of the lipocalin family. J Allergy Clin Immunol 1996; 97:1297–1303.

69. Saarelainen S, Zeiler T, Rautiainen J, et al. Lipocalin allergen Bos d2 is a weak immunogen. Inter Immunol 2002; 14:401–409.

70. Rautiainen J, Auriola S, Konttinen A, et al. Two new variants of the lipocalin allergen bos d2. J Chromatogr B Biomed Sci Appl 2001; 763:91–98.

71. Renström A, Malmberg P, Larsson K, Larsson PH, Sundblad BM. Allergic sensitization is associated with increased bronchial responsiveness: a prospective study of allergy to laboratory animals. Eur Respir J 1995; 8:1514–1519.

72. Hollander A, Gordon S, Renstrom A, et al. Comparison of methods to assess airbrone rat or mouse allergen levels. I. Analysis of air samples. Allergy 1999; 54:142–149.

73. Renstrom A, Gordon S, Hollander A, et al. Comparison of methods to assess rat or mouse allergen levels. II. Factors influencing antigen detection. Allergy 1999; 54:150–157.

74. Renstrom A, Larsson PH, Malmberg P, Bayard C. A new amplified monoclonal rat allergen assay used for evaluation of ventilation improvements in animal rooms. J Allergy Clin Immunol 1997; 100:649–655.

75. Korpi A, Mantyjarvi R, Rautiainen J, et al. Detection of mouse and rat urinary allergens with an improved ELISA. J Allergy Clin Immunol 2004; 113:677–682.

76. Gordon S, Wallace J, Cook A, Tee RD, Newman Taylor AJ. Reduction of exposure to laboratory animal allergens in the workplace. Clin Exp Allergy 1997; 27:744–751.

77. Gordon S, Fisher SW, Raymond RH. Elimination of mouse allergens in the working environment: assessment of individually ventilated cage systems and ventilated cabinets in the containment of mouse allergens. J Allergy Clin Immunol 2001; 108:288–294.

78. Renstrom A, Bjoring G, Hoglund AU. Evaluation of individually ventilated cage systems for laboratory animals: occupational health aspects. Lab Animals 2001; 35:42–50.

79. Schweitzer IB, Smith E, Harrison DJ, et al. Reducing exposure to laboratory animal allergens. Comparative Med 2003; 53:487–492.

80. DeLucca SD, O'Meara TJ, Tovey ER. Exposure to mite and cat allergens as a range of clothing items at home and the transfer of cat allergen to the workplace. J Allergy Clin Immunol 2000; 106:874–879.

81. Tovey ER, Taylor DJ, Mitakakis TZ, DeLucca SD. Effectiveness of laudry washing agents and conditions in the removal of cat and dust mite allergen from bedding dust. J Allergy Clin Immunol 2001; 108:369–374.

82. Renstrom A, Karlsson AS, Tovey E. Nasal sampling used for the assessment of occupational allergen exposure and the efficacy of respiratory protection. Clin Exp Allergy 2002; 32:1769–1775.

83. Gibbons HL, Dille JR, Cowley RG. Inhalant allergy to the screwworm fly. Arch Environ Health 1965; 10:424–430.

84. Tee RD, Gordon DJ, Lacey J, Nunn AJ, Brown M, Newman Taylor AJ. Occupational allergy to the common house fly (*Musca domestica*): Use of immunologic response to identify atmospheric allergen. J Allergy Clin Immunol 1985; 76:826–830.

85. Gold BL, Matthews KP, Burge HA. Occupational asthma caused by sewer flies. Am Rev Respir Dis 1985; 131:949–952.

86. Spieksma FTM, Vooren PH, Kramps JA, Dijkman JH. Respiratory allergy to laboratory fruit flies (*Drosophila melanogaster*). J Allergy Clin Immunol 1986; 77:108–113.

87. Baldo BA, Bellas TE, Tovey ER, Kaufman GL. Occupational allergy in an entomological research centre. II. Identification of IgE-binding proteins from developmental stages of the blowfly *Lucilia cuprina* and other species of adult flies. Clin Allergy 1989; 19:411–417.

88. Kraut A, Sloan J, Silviu-Dan F, Peng Z, Gagnon D, Warrington R. Occupational allergy after exposure to caddis flies at a hydroelectric power plant. Occup Environ Med 1994; 51:408–413.

89. Stevens WJ, Van den Abbeele J, Bridts CH. Anaphylactic reaction after bites by *Glossina morsitans* (tsetse fly) in a laboratory worker. J Allergy Clin Immunol 1996; 98: 700–701.

90. Frigerio C, Aubry M, Gomez F, et al. Occupational allergy to the housefly (*Musca domestica*). Allergy 1997; 52:238–239.

91. Kaufman GL, Gandevia BH, Bellas TE, Tovey ER, Baldo BA. Occupational allergy in an entomological research centre. I Clinical aspects of reactions to the sheep blowfly *Lucilia cuprina*. Br J Indust Med 1989; 46:473–478.

92. Burge PS, Edge G, O'Brien IM, Harries MG, Hawkins R, Pepys J. Occupational asthma in a research centre breeding locusts. Clin Allergy 1980; 10:355–363.

93. Tee RD, Gordon DJ, Hawkins ER, et al. Occupational allergy to locusts: an investigation of the sources of the allergen. J Allergy Clin Immunol 1988; 81:517–525.

94. Soparkar GR, Patel PC, Cockcroft DW. Inhalant atopic sensitivity to grasshoppers in research laboratories. J Allergy Clin Immunol 1993; 92:61–65.

95. Ostrom NK, Swanson MC, Agarwal MK, Yuninger JW. Occupational allergy to honeybee-body dust in a honey-processing plant. J Allergy Clin Immunol 1986; 77: 736–740.

96. Kochuyt AM, Hoeyveld E Van, Stevens EAM. Occupational allergy to bumble bee venom. Clin Exp Allergy 1993; 23:190–195.

97. Michel FB, Guin JJ, Seignalet C, et al. Allergie à Panonychus ulmi (Koch). Rev Franç Allergol 1977; 17:93–97.

98. Reunala T, Bjorksten F, Forstrom L, Kanerva L. IgE-mediated occupational allergy to a spider mite. Clin Allergy 1983; 13:383–388.

99. Cuthbert OD, Jeffrey IG, McNeill HB, Wood J, Topping MD. Barn allergy among Scottish farmers. Clin Allergy 1984; 14:197–206.

100. Kroidl R, Maasch HJ, Wahl R. Respiratory allergies (bronchial asthma and rhinitis) due to sensitization of type I allergy to red spider mite (*Panonychus ulmi KOCH*). Clin Exper Allergy 1992; 22:958–962.

101. Erlam AR, Johnson AJ, Wiley KN. Occupational asthma in greehouse tomato growing. Occup Med 1996; 46:163–164.

102. Kim YK, Son JW, Kim HY, et al. New occupational allergen in citrus farmers: citrus red mite (*Panonychus citri*). Ann Allergy Asthma Immunol 1999; 82:223–228.

103. Castro FF, Antila MA, Croce J. Occupational allergy caused by urticating hair of Brazilian spider. J Allergy Clin Immunol 1995; 95:1282–1285.

104. Steinberg DR, Bernstein DI, Gallagher JS, Arlian L, Bernstein IL. Cockroach sensitization in laboratory workers. J Allergy Clin Immunol 1987; 80:586–590.

105. Baur X. Chironomid midge allergy. Jpn J Allergol 1992; 41:81–85.

106. Teranishi H, Kawai K, Murakami G, Miyao M, Kasuya M. Occupational allergy to adult chironomid midges among environmental research workers. Int Arch Allergy Immunol 1995; 106:271–277.

107. Liebers V, Hoernstein M, Baur X. Humoral immune response to the insect allergen Chi t I in aquarists and fish-food factory workers. Allergy 1993; 48:236–239.

108. Chapman MD. Dissecting cockroach allergens. Clin Exp Allergy 1993; 23:459–461.

109. Helm RM, Pomes A. Cockroach and other inhalant insect allergens. Clin Allergy Immunol 2004; 18:271–296.

110. Arruda LK, Vailes LD, Ferriani VP, Santos AB, Pomes A, Chapman M. Cockroach allergens and asthma. J Allergy Clin Immunol 2001; 107:419–428.

111. Ayuso R, Reese G, Leong-Kee S, Plante M, Lehrer SB. Molecular basis of cross-reactivity: IgE-binding cross-reactive epitopes of shrimp, house dust mite and cockroach tropomyosins. Int Arch Allergy Immunol 2002; 129:38–48.

112. Reese G, Jeong BJ, Daul CB, Lehrer SB. Characterization of recombinant shrimp allergen Pen a1 (tropomyosin). Inter Arch Allergy Immunol 1997; 113:240–242.
113. Tee RD, Cranston PS, Kay AB. Further characterisation of allergens associated with hypersensitivity to the "green nimitti" midge (*Cladotanytarsus lewisi*, Diptera: Chironomidae). Allergy 1987; 42:12–19.
114. Lopata AL, Fenemore B, Jeebhay MF, Gade G, Potter PC. Occupational allergy in laboratory workers caused by the African migratory grasshopper *Locusta migratoria*. Allergy 2005; 60:200–205.
115. Cartier A, Malo JL, Forest F, et al. Occupational asthma in snow crab-processing workers. J Allergy Clin Immunol 1984; 74:261–269.
116. Orford RR, Wilson JT. Epidemiologic and immunologic studies in processors of the King crab. Am J Ind Med 1985; 7:155–169.
117. Beaudet N. OSHA Compliance Issues. Development of asthma in crab processing workers. Appl Occup Environ Hyg 1994; 9:597–598.
118. Ortega HG, Daroowalla F, Petsonk EL, et al. Respiratory symptoms among crab processing workers in Alaska: Epidemiological and environmental assessment. Am J Ind Med 2001; 39:598–607.
119. Patel PC, Cockcroft DW. Occupational asthma caused by exposure to cooking lobster in the work environment: a case report. Ann Allergy 1992; 68:360–361.
120. Lemière C, Desjardins A, Lehrer S, Malo JL. Occupational asthma to lobster and shrimp. Allergy 1996; 51:272–273.
121. Desjardins A, Malo JL, L'Archevêque J, Cartier A, McCants M, Lehrer SB. Occupational IgE-mediated sensitization and asthma due to clam and shrimp. J Allergy Clin Immunol 1995; 96:608–617.
122. Baur X, Huber H, Chen Z. Asthma to Gammarus shrimp. Allergy 2000; 55:96–97.
123. Goetz DW, Whisman BA. Occupational asthma in a seafood restaurant worker: cross-reactivity of shrimp and scallops. Ann Allergy Asthma Immunol 2000; 85:461–466.
124. Jeebhay MF, Robins TG, Lopata AL. World at work: fish processing workers. Occup Environ Med 2004; 61:471–474.
125. Douglas JDM, McSharry C, Blaikie L, Morrow T, Miles S, Franklin D. Occupational asthma caused by automated salmon processing. Lancet 1995; 346:737–740.
126. Sherson D, Hansen I, Sigsgaard T. Occupationally related respiratory symptoms in trout-processing workers. Allergy 1989; 44:336–341.
127. Armentia A, Lombardero M, Callejo A, et al. Occupational asthma by Anisakis simplex. J Allergy Clin Immunol 1998; 102:831–834.
128. Scala E, Giani M, Pirrotta L, et al. Occupational generalised urticaria and allergic airborne asthma due to anisakis simplex. Eur J Dermatol 2001; 11:249–250.
129. Jyo T, Kohmoto K, Katsutani T, Otsuka T, Oka SD, Mitsui S. Hoya (Sea-squirt) asthma. Occup Asthma 1980; 209–228.
130. Gaddie J, Legge JS, Friend JAR, Reid TMS. Pulmonary hypersensitivity in prawn workers. Lancet 1980; 2:1350–1353.
131. Cartier A, Malo JL, Ghezzo H, McCants M, Lehrer SB. IgE sensitization in snow crab-processing workers. J Allergy Clin Immunol 1986; 78:344–348.
132. NIOSH. Asthma-like illness among crab processing workers: Alaska. MMWR 1982; 31:95–96.
133. McSharry C, Anderson K, McKay IC, et al. The IgE and IgG antibody responses to aerosols of Nephrops norvegicus (prawn) antigens: the association with clinical hypersensitivity and with cigarette smoking. Clin Exp Immunol 1994; 97:499–504.
134. Glass WI, Power P, Burt R, Fishwick D, Bradshaw LM, Pearce NE. Work-related respiratory symptoms and lung function in New Zealand mussel openers. Am J Ind Med 1998; 34:163–168.
135. Droszscz W, Kowalski J, Piotrowska B, Pawlowicz A, Pietruszewska E. Allergy to fish in fish meal factory workers. Int Arch Occup Environ Health 1981; 49:13–19.

136. Jeebhay MF, Robins TG, Lehrer SB, Lopata AL. Occupational seafood allergy: a review. Occup Environ Med 2001; 58:553–562.
137. Jeebhay MF, Lopata AL, Robins TG. Seafood processing in South Africa: a study of working practices, occupational health services and allergic health problems in the industry. Occup Med 2000; 50:406–413.
138. Malo JL, Chrétien P, McCants M, Lehrer S. Detection of snow-crab antigens by air sampling of a snow-crab production plant. Clin Exp Allergy 1997; 27:75–78.
139. Weytjens K, Cartier A, Malo JL, et al. Aerosolized snow-crab allergens in a processing facility. Allergy 1999; 54:892–893.

19
Latex Allergy

Olivier Vandenplas
Department of Chest Medicine, Mont-Godinne Hospital, Catholic University of Louvain, Yvoir, Belgium

Donald Beezhold
Analytical Services Branch, NIOSH, Morgantown, West Virginia, U.S.A.

Susan M. Tarlo
Gage Occupational and Environmental Health Unit, Departments of Medicine and Public Health Sciences, University of Toronto, and The Asthma Centre, Toronto Western Hospital, University Health Network, Toronto, Ontario, Canada

INTRODUCTION

Natural rubber latex (NRL) allergy was clearly identified in 1979 in Europe (1) and in 1989 in North America (2,3), although adverse reactions to natural rubber materials had occasionally been described earlier (4). Over the past 15 years, NRL has been increasingly acknowledged as a major cause of IgE-mediated allergy in occupational and nonoccupational environments (5,6). NRL materials can cause a wide spectrum of immediate hypersensitivity reactions, ranging from mild urticaria to extensive angioedema and life-threatening anaphylaxis after cutaneous, mucosal, or visceral exposure. In addition, it has been shown that NRL proteins can bind onto glove powder and can then act as airborne allergens causing rhinitis and asthma (7).

NATURAL RUBBER LATEX

Composition

In the chemical industry, the term latex applies to any emulsion of polymers, including synthetic rubbers and plastics. NRL refers specifically to products derived from the milky fluid, or latex, produced by the laticifers of the tropical rubber tree *Hevea braziliensis* (botanical family of Euphorbiaceae). Laticifers are specialized structures that consist of anastamosed latex-producing cells. Upon wounding, the cytoplasmic content of these cells is expelled and coagulates in order to seal and protect the wounded sites.

Using high-speed centrifugation, NRL can be separated into three components: the "rubber cream" containing the rubber particles, the latex serum (C-serum), and the "bottom fraction" which consists mainly of vacuolar structures called *lutoids*. Rubber particles are spherical droplets containing polymers of *cis*-1,4 poly-isoprene coated with a layer of hydrophilic colloid (proteins, lipids, and phospholipids). Lutoids are vacuoles with an acidic content that are involved in the coagulation of latex through the release of proteins interacting with rubber particles. Fresh NRL consists of about 30% to 40% rubber hydrocarbon and 2% to 3% protein. A number of NRL proteins have been purified and sequenced. Prenyltransferase (38 kDa) is found in the cytosol as well as in association with rubber particles. Rubber elongation factor (14.6 kDa) is bound to the surface of rubber particles. These two enzymes are thought to play a role in the elongation of polyisoprene chains (8). The lutoid bodies contain defense-related proteins. Hevein (4.7 kDa), a major protein of the lutoid bodies, is synthesized as a preproprotein (or prohevein, 20 kDa) that is post-translationally processed into an amino-terminal fragment, hevein, and a carboxyl-terminal domain (14 kDa). Hevein is a lectin-like protein that may be involved in the coagulation of latex by bridging rubber particles (9). Hevein inhibits the growth of chitin-containing fungi through chitin-binding properties (10). Hevein shows structural homology to wheat germ agglutinin and other chitin-binding proteins, while the carboxyl-terminal domain demonstrates homology to wound-inducible proteins in various plants, such as WIN 1 and WIN 2 (11). Hevamine (29 kDa), an enzyme with lysozyme and chitinase properties, has been isolated from the lutoids (12). The lutoid bodies contain glycoproteins that can form complex microfibrils and microhelices.

Processing

Ammonia is added to the fresh latex obtained during tapping of the rubber tree to prevent premature coagulation and bacterial growth. The resulting emulsion is concentrated to obtain a 60% rubber content by centrifuging. Further processing of concentrated NRL varies considerably according to the desired properties of the finished product, but usually includes the following three steps: compounding, coagulation, and vulcanization. Compounding involves the addition of a variety of chemicals including sulfur compounds, antioxidants (e.g., paraphenylenediamine), accelerators (e.g., zinc oxide, thiurams, dithiocarbamates, mercaptobenzothiazole, etc.), fillers, pigments, emulsifiers, and other ingredients. Some of these compounding agents, particularly the accelerators, can cause delayed type-IV hypersensitivity (13). The concentrated liquid NRL is converted to a solid form during the coagulation, or curing, process by dehydration and/or addition of acids, metal ions, or surface-active agents. Vulcanization consists of a heat-catalyzed cross-linking of the *cis*-1,4 polyisoprene chains by sulfur bridges; this process imparts the characteristic property of rubber elasticity. NRL articles are produced either by dipping or by extrusion/compression molding. Typically, gloves are manufactured by dipping porcelain formers, pretreated with a coagulant (e.g., calcium nitrate) and a releasing agent (cornstarch powder), into the compounded liquid NRL. The gloves are then passed through ovens to complete coagulation of NRL and through water baths to extract water-soluble proteins and processing chemicals. Finally they undergo vulcanization and addition of donning powder. For powder-free gloves, the residual releasing agent can be subsequently removed from the gloves through a chlorination wash process.

PATHOGENESIS

There is convincing evidence from both in vitro and in vivo experiments that immediate hypersensitivity reactions caused by NRL materials are mediated through specific IgE antibodies directed against NRL proteins that persist in manufactured products (5,6). Exposure to the NRL proteins occurs by direct contact with the latex product and by inhalation of NRL-contaminated powder aerosolized from powdered gloves. Significant amounts of rapidly elutable endotoxin can contaminate NRL gloves and are also present in glove-generated aerosols (14). Animal models have shown mixed results regarding the role of glove-associated endotoxin. In presence of high dose endotoxin (250,000 EU), the production of Hev b 5 specific IgE was augmented (15). Coexposure to nonammoniated latex (NAL) and low levels of endotoxin (up to 25,000 EU) decreased NRL-specific IgE but enhanced nonspecific airway hyperreactivity (16). Given the nature of these findings, further research to investigate the effects of endotoxins on IgE responses to NRL is necessary.

NRL Allergens

Immunoblotting studies conducted by numerous investigators have identified IgE-binding proteins with molecular weights ranging from 2 to 200 kDa in raw NRL and eluates from NRL-manufactured products (17–27). Antigens with molecular weights of 14, 20, 24, 27, 30, 36, and 46 kDa have been consistently identified. Variations in specific antigen reactivity may be due to differences in source materials, including fresh latex or NAL, ammoniated latex, and finished products. Ammonia treatment and other manufacturing procedures can cause aggregation and/or precipitation of NRL peptides (27–30). Antigenic variability may also result from the methods used for extracting and identifying antigens from NRL products as these methods can lead to conformational alteration and degradation of NRL proteins (30–32). Furthermore, significant differences can be detected in the pattern of IgE reactivity between subjects with NRL allergy (24,26,27,32,33), possibly as a result of differences in the patients' mode of sensitization. Although most studies have failed to demonstrate a correlation between the pattern of IgE reactivity to NRL proteins and clinical manifestations of NRL allergy, some investigations suggest that spina bifida is often associated with the development of IgE antibodies against 24-kDa and 27-kDa proteins (29,34).

Substantial progress has been made in the purification and molecular characterization of NRL allergens. To date, 13 allergens have been officially named by the International Union of Immunological Societies Allergen Nomenclature Committee (35), and several of these exist in multiple isotypes (Table 1) (26,29,30,36–47). Using a proteomic approach, 47 IgE binding proteins were analyzed, resulting in the identification of several known allergen (Hev b 6, 7, 9, and 11) and five new allergen candidates (UDP-glucose pyrophosphorylase, isoflavone reductase, rotamase, thioredoxin, and citrate binding protein) (48). Except for Hev b 4, the named NRL allergens have been cloned and produced by recombinant technologies. The recombinant proteins have been characterized, and for several of the allergens, the T and B cell epitopes have been identified (49–52). Detailed information regarding these allergens can be found in recent reviews (53–55). The use of recombinant or highly purified natural proteins in both laboratory and clinical studies has lead to information on the relative importance of the various individual allergens. By skin-prick testing

Table 1 Natural Rubber Latex (NRL) Allergens

Allergen	Common name	Molecular weight (kDa)	Plant allergen family	Potential cross-reacting allergens	Accession no.	References
Hev b 1	Rubber elongation factor	58/14.6		Papain, fig	AY120685	29,30,36
Hev b 2	β 1-3-glucane	34/36	PR-2		AF311749	37,38
Hev b 3	Small rubber particle protein	24			O82803	29
Hev b 4	Cyanogenic glucosamide	100–115			BI729486	38
Hev b 5	Acidic protein	16		Kiwi	U42640	30,39
Hev b 6.01	Hevein preprotein	20			M36986	11
Hev b 6.02	Hevein	5	PR-3	Banana, avocado Kiwi	P02877	37
Hev b 6.03	C-terminal domain	14	PR-4	Potato	P02877	26,37,40
Hev b 7.01	Patatin homolog (B-serum)	42			U80598	41
Hev b 7.02	Patatin homolog (C-serum)	44		Potato	AJ223038	26
Hev b 8	Profilin	14	Profilin	Pollen, celery	AJ243325	42
Hev b 9	Enolase	51		Molds	AJ132580	43
Hev b 10	Mn-superoxide dismutase	26		Molds	L11707	44
Hev b 11	Class I chitinase	33	PR-3	Banana, avocado	AJ238579	45
Hev b 12	Lipid transfer protein	9.4	PR-14	Stone fruits, peach	AY057860	46
Hev b 13	Early nodule-specific protein	42		Patatin	P83269	47

Note: Allergens are named according to the International Union of Immunological Societies nomenclature. Representative accession numbers are given. Additional information can be obtained at www.allergen.org. *Abbreviation*: PR, pathogenesis-related proteins.

the NR-allergic health care workers with recombinant Hev b 2, 3, 5, 6, 7, and 8, it was found that Hev b 5 (62%), Hev b 6 (66%), and Hev b 7 (41%) were the most common allergens for health care workers (56). More recently, health care workers were skin tested with purified native NRL proteins Hev b 1, 2, 3, 4, 6, 7, and 13 and with recombinant Hev b 5 (57). In this study, Hev b 2 (63%), 5 (65%), 6 (63%), 7 (45%), and 13 (63%) were found to be the most reactive. Interestingly, reactivity of native Hev b 2 (63%) and rHev b 2 (7%) differed significantly between these studies suggesting that the glycosylation on the native protein (compared to the nonglycosylated recombinant form) may play an important role in reactivity to individual Hev b allergens. The contribution of glycosylation to the reactivity/potency of specific NRL allergens has not been well studied.

Assessment of Exposure to NRL Allergens

NRL is widely used in the manufacturing of medical devices (gloves, catheters, drainage tubes, anesthetic masks, tourniquets, dental dams, etc.) as well as in the production of a variety of everyday articles, including household gloves, toys, balloons, condoms, baby pacifiers, sports equipment, elastic straps, mattresses, tires, and adhesives. Various in vitro methods have been used to estimate the allergenic content of NRL materials, including total protein measurements and ELISA and RAST inhibition methods. Total protein assays are easy to perform, but they lack sensitivity and specificity. The results of these assays are strongly influenced by the presence of various chemicals in NRL products that can interfere with these tests (58). Unless precipitation techniques are used to remove interfering substances (59), the results of these tests are unreliable. A modified Lowry test was standardized by the American Society for Testing and Materials (ASTM, D5712) with a protein precipitation step using trichloroacetic acid and phosphotungstic acid to eliminate the interfering substances. This method results in a reasonable estimate of the total protein in the NRL product. ASTM standards recommend that all examination and surgical gloves should contain less than $200 \mu g/dm^2$ of total protein when assessed by this standard test (60).

Many studies have found a marked discordance between the total amount of protein eluting from NRL devices and their allergenic potential, as assessed by skin-prick testing (61–64). For some studies this was due to the failure in removing interfering chemicals, but the lack of correlation may also be due to the nonallergenic nature of some proteins found in NRL products. Immunochemical assays provide a more sensitive and biologically relevant method for determining allergen levels in NRL products (58). ELISA and RAST inhibition methods have been used to estimate the antigen content in NRL products (58,63,65). These methods have shown considerable variations in the allergen content between different brands of gloves and even between different batches of the same brand of gloves (58,63,65). The ASTM has developed a standardized method for quantifying the allergenic potential of latex materials using an inhibition ELISA (ASTM D6499 assay). This test uses a well-characterized rabbit–antilatex reference antisera and an ammoniated NRL protein reference standard, prepared as industry reference materials, to measure antigen levels. The ASTM recommends the presence of less than $10 \mu g/dm^2$ of antigenic protein on examination and surgical gloves when assessed by this standard method. IgE inhibition assays (RAST inhibition) commonly used by individual laboratories are affected by the source of specific IgE and the quality of allergen reference standard. Current work at the ASTM is focused on standardizing monoclonal antibody assays that measure specific allergens. A commercial kit using monoclonal antibodies is available to measure Hev b 1, 2, 5, and 6 as individual ELISA determinations and then combine the results as an indicator of allergenicity. A recent report suggests that measuring only Hev b 5 and Hev b 13 produces a reliable estimate of the allergenic potential (66). While additional work is necessary to standardize an allergen assay, in vivo and in vitro methods have shown that the total protein and allergen content of NRL gloves can be significantly reduced by washing the gloves during the manufacturing process (62,67).

Exposure to NRL allergens can occur from direct contact of NRL materials with the skin, and mucosal and serosal membranes. It has also been demonstrated that NRL protein allergens can bind to powder particles on gloves (or on any powdered rubber product, such as toy balloons) and can become potent airborne allergens (20,60,68–70). Using an inhibition assay, Swanson et al. (71) quantified airborne NRL allergens collected using personal and area samplers at various work sites in a hospital. The amount of airborne NRL allergens correlated with the frequency of glove use, although considerable variation was found among subjects with the same type of job. Substantial amounts of allergens were recovered from coats and surgical scrub suits, suggesting that resuspension from clothing and settled dust may lead to secondary or even remote inhalation exposure. Twenty percent of airborne powder particles were in a respirable size and therefore capable of causing asthma. In a prospective study, NRL aeroallergen levels were strongly correlated with the use of powdered NRL gloves in the operating room and were similar to that found in nonsurgical days when low-allergen gloves were used (72). Another study found that powdered surgical gloves generated lower levels of airborne allergens than did examination gloves, and the allergen was primarily associated with larger particles of size more than $10 \mu m$ (73). In contrast, powdered examination gloves produced a higher proportion of allergenparticles in the respirable range (73).

EPIDEMIOLOGY

Incidence and Prevalence

The incidence of NRL allergy has changed significantly in many occupational settings since the previous edition of this book in 1999. From 1989 to 1999 a number of studies had documented a high incidence of NRL allergy in individuals with occupational exposure to NRL. Most affected were glove wearers and manufacturers (74–81), and patients undergoing multiple surgical procedures (82), particularly in early infancy, such as children with spina bifida and urogenital abnormalities (83–87). Epidemiological studies documented NRL allergy in about 10% of workers manufacturing medical gloves (74) and NRL toys (88). Prevalence figures for NRL allergy had ranged from 2.8% to 17% among health-care workers, including physicians, nurses, laboratory technicians, hospital housekeepers, and dental-care providers (75–80). The highest prevalence rates, ranging from 29% to 65%, were found in children with spina bifida (83–87). In addition, NRL allergy due to gloves was increasingly described in workers in nonmedical environments, including those exposed to chemicals (89), hairdressers (90), and greenhouse workers (81). Few reports have assessed the incidence of NRL allergy. In dental hygiene apprentices reported by Gautrin et al. (91), 110 students were followed after entering the program between 1993 and 1995. On follow-up up to 32 months after entry, seven developed skin sensitization to NRL (6%), while the cumulative incidence of probable occupational rhinoconjunctivitis was 1.8% and probable occupational asthma was 4.5%.

The increasing incidence and prevalence of NRL allergy during that 10-year period were attributed in part to the advent of Standard Precautions in the last half of the 1980s, which resulted in increased use of NRL devices as a protective barrier against viral infections. The increased demand for, and production of, NRL gloves may also have played a role, with the potential for saturation of NRL proteins in the leeching fluid during production and other changes in manufacturing processes (92).

The increased need for tapping of rubber trees and, in some cases, the treatment of Hevea trees with phytohormones to stimulate the production of latex could have enhanced the biosynthesis of some proteins by laticifers, especially defense-related proteins (9,93). Increased recognition of NRL allergy by exposed workers and physicians is also likely to have contributed to the apparent increase in the prevalence of the disease during that time.

Because exposure appears to be the most significant risk factor for developing NRL allergy, it is not surprising that with recognition and intervention measures, the incidence has fallen. Work-related allergic responses from NRL carried by glove powder should no longer be a problem in most occupational settings. As noted, the most reported occupational sensitization was in health-care workers, primarily from the use of high-protein, powdered NRL gloves (6). With this understanding, the protein content of NRL gloves has been significantly reduced by many manufacturers (94), and low-powdered or nonpowdered gloves are available. Several recent studies suggest that when instituted, such changes are very effective in reducing the risk of occupational sensitization in health care workers (95–101). Despite the reductions in incidence of NRL allergy reported from health care facilities where glove changes have been made, it is likely that a significant proportion of facilities have not made specific changes in glove usage. Efforts have been made by NRL glove producers to reduce powder and NRL protein content of NRL gloves used for health care (94). However there is no clear published report to suggest overall effectiveness of this in facilities that have not specifically purchased low-protein, powder-free gloves. Recent reports from various areas of the world indicate that prevalence rates of latex sensitization range from 5.4% to 9.7% among hospital employees with daily NRL contact (102–104). Similarly, it may be expected that improvements in powdered gloves may be slower in non–health care occupations (105,106).

Risk Factors

Although exposure to NRL is intuitively the most relevant risk factor for the initiation of NRL allergy, a clear dose–response relationship between occupational exposure to NRL and IgE-mediated sensitization has not been consistently demonstrated in prevalence surveys. This is because assessment of exposure based on self-reported use of NRL gloves does not reflect the actual level of exposure, as colleagues working in the same environment represent a significant source of airborne allergen (107,108). In addition, cross-sectional studies may be affected by survival bias, because workers with NRL sensitization may tend to use fewer NRL gloves (109). Two epidemiological surveys have provided direct evidence supporting a causal role of exposure to NRL gloves. In a cross-sectional survey of dental students and staff, Tarlo et al. (80) documented a progressive increase in risk of sensitization to NRL by years of exposure as shown by skin-prick test responses to a low-ammoniated raw NRL solution. None of the year 1 or 2 students tested were sensitized (before significant clinical use of NRL gloves), whereas 6% of year 3 students, 10% of year 4 students, and 25% of the staff were sensitized. Symptoms of asthma, rhinoconjunctivitis, and contact urticaria associated with NRL glove exposure were significantly more frequent among those with positive skin tests to NRL. In a prospective cohort study of apprentices, Gautrin et al. (110) found that the cumulative incidence rate of skin reactivity to NRL was significantly higher among dental hygiene students using NRL gloves on a regular basis (6.3%) than among animal health technologists (1%) or pastry makers (1.6%).

The prevalence of sensitization among workers exposed to NRL has never been compared adequately with the figures observed in the general adult population. Prevalence rates of skin reactivity to NRL extracts varied from 0.6% to 4.9% in apprentices assessed before starting occupational exposure (111) and in individuals attending a health-screening visit (112), a preoperative visit (82), or an allergy clinic (113). The figures for clinical allergy to NRL were usually lower, ranging from 1.2% to 3.1% (82,112,113). Higher prevalence rates of NRL sensitization have generally been reported in studies that assessed the levels of NRL-specific IgE antibodies among blood donors (from 3.6% to 7.6%) (114–117). In a population-based survey derived from the Third National Health and Nutrition Examination Survey (1988–1991), Garabrant et al. (118) found that the prevalence of NRL-specific IgE antibodies was not higher among health care workers than among the general population. The reported prevalence rate of NRL sensitization in the general population was, however, much higher (18.4%) than the figures reported in other unexposed populations, raising concern about the specificity of the method used for measuring specific IgE antibodies.

In addition to repeated exposure to NRL products, atopy seems to be the principal determinant for the development of NRL sensitization. Atopy (defined either by immunological tests to common inhalant allergens or by the history) is two- to five-fold more frequent in health care personnel with NRL allergy than in their coworkers without NRL allergy (75,76,78–80,119,120). However, the predictive value of atopy with regard to the development of immunological sensitization and occupational asthma due to NRL is low (79). In a recent study, sensitization to hevein (Hev b 6.02) was associated with the HLA class II alleles DQB1*0302 (DQ8) alone and DQB1*0302(DQ8)-DRB1*04 (DR4) haplotype among health-care workers with NRL allergy (121). Pre-existing dermatitis of the hands is thought to enhance the risk of NRL allergy by facilitating the transcutaneous passage of NRL proteins (122). Hand eczema has been found more frequently in subjects with NRL allergy than in their nonallergic coworkers (75,78–80). In spina bifida children, the development of NRL allergy is associated with atopy and the number of surgical procedures (84,87). Exposure to NRL in infancy is likely to be the crucial factor leading to the high prevalence of NRL sensitization in spina bifida children as compared with adults affected by similar neurological disorders and NRL exposure (123). Reports suggest that allergy to foods can develop before the onset of clinical allergy to NRL products (124), although the role of food allergy as an independent risk factor for the initiation of NRL allergy remains uncertain.

CLINICAL MANIFESTATIONS

Skin and Systemic Reactions

The severity of clinical manifestations of NRL allergy varies according to the route of exposure. Cutaneous exposure to NRL causes local urticaria usually restricted to the site of NRL contact, although systemic reactions have been occasionally reported (3,125,126). In glove wearers, skin symptoms take the form of pruritus, erythema, and hives beginning 20 to 30 minutes after donning NRL gloves. Symptoms of glove-induced itching and redness of the hands have, however, a low predictive value with regard to the presence of NRL allergy, because questionnaire surveys have shown that a high proportion (up to 50%) of health care workers experience glove-related skin symptoms consistent with contact dermatitis in the absence of any demonstrable allergic sensitization to NRL (75,77–79,91). In addition to immediate skin reactions, NRL-exposed workers can also present with persistent dermatitis related to irritant contact dermatitis or delayed hypersensitivity reaction to rubber additives, disinfectants, or drugs (13). Delayed skin reactions to patch tests with NRL suggest that allergic contact eczema to NRL proteins can develop in subjects with or without concomitant urticaria (105,122,127).

Mucosal, visceral, and parenteral exposures to NRL are associated with the greatest risk for developing severe systemic reactions. Anaphylactic reactions have been documented during surgical procedures (2,85,128), deliveries (129), gynecological examinations (130), dental treatment (128), barium enema using balloon-tipped catheters (131,132), and condom-protected sexual intercourse (133). NRL has become the second most common cause of perioperative anaphylactic reactions, accounting for 16% of such adverse events (134). NRL-induced reactions during surgery are characterized by a delayed onset after induction of anesthesia (2). There is also some suggestion that intravenous exposure to NRL allergens can result from injection ports in intravenous lines, plungers on syringes, and stoppers on medication vials (135). Systemic reactions have also been described after ingestion of foods contaminated by NRL allergens when handled by personnel wearing gloves (136). Finally, it should be kept in mind that urticaria and anaphylaxis can occur after remote exposure to NRL allergens transferred from the workplace on hands and clothes (137). Fatal anaphylactic reactions induced by NRL seem, however, to be a rare consequence of NRL allergy (132,138), although a recent survey of U.K. theatre managers found that 18 major anaphylactic reactions and four deaths had occurred among about 500 NRL-allergic patients after they had undergone surgery (139).

Respiratory Symptoms

In the early 1990s, it was demonstrated that exposure to airborne NRL allergens bound to powder particles of gloves (or to any dusted rubber products, such as toy balloons) could result in allergic respiratory reactions, including rhinoconjunctivitis and asthma (7,20,140). These respiratory symptoms have been described primarily among workers manufacturing or using NRL gloves (74,79). A survey of hospital employees showed that asthma is a common manifestation of NRL allergy, and this has been documented through specific inhalation challenges in approximately half of the participants who demonstrated skin sensitization to NRL (i.e., 2.5% of all employees) (79). Surveillance programs and medicolegal statistics indicate that NRL has become one of the leading causes of occupational asthma in the 1990s (141,142). However, only 39% to 68% of subjects with NRL-induced occupational asthma identify NRL gloves as the cause of their asthma, since the work relatedness of respiratory symptoms can be obscured by several factors (143,144). Thus, exposure to airborne NRL allergens is most often intermittent and indirect, resulting from inhalation of NRL allergens disseminated in the air by coworkers handling NRL gloves (107). As a result, subjects who do not use NRL gloves but who experience asthma at work tend to ascribe their asthma to substances other than NRL.

The possibility of respiratory allergy to NRL should be also considered in nonmedical occupations. Rhinoconjunctivitis and asthma caused by NRL gloves have been reported in greenhouse workers (81), hairdressers (105), food processors (145), laboratory workers (146), and pharmaceutical industry workers (89). Although powdered NRL gloves are the most frequent source of exposure to airborne NRL, respiratory reactions have occasionally been described in workers exposed to NRL dust generated by grinding dolls (88) and by processing elasticized fabrics (147). In nonoccupational environments, respiratory symptoms can result from exposure to deflating or bursting toy balloons. One report has suggested that NRL can cause eosinophilic bronchitis, which is characterized by NRL-related cough and sputum eosinophilia in the absence of demonstrable airflow obstruction or nonspecific bronchial hyperresponsiveness (148). At present, it remains unknown whether this syndrome progresses to typical asthma.

Food Allergy

It was recognized early on that individuals with NRL allergy experience allergic reactions after ingestion of banana, kiwi, avocado, and chestnut with an unusually high frequency. In recent years, the list of plant-derived foods causing allergic reactions in NRL-allergic subjects has been extended to include potato, tomato, passion fruit, melon, fig, pineapple, mango, peach, plum, almond, and pepper (124,149–151). Approximately 30% to 50% of individuals with NRL allergy show clinical hypersensitivity to some plant-derived foods, while an even higher proportion (about 70%) demonstrates IgE antibodies against these allergens (124,149,150). The association between allergy to NRL and to plant-derived foods is usually referred to as the "latex-fruit syndrome." The symptoms that are experienced by individuals with the latex-fruit syndrome range from itching of the throat to oral and facial swelling, rhinoconjunctivitis, and anaphylactic shock. It is noteworthy that these hypersensitivity reactions to foods may develop after cessation of occupational exposure to NRL (151). In addition, several reports have described an association between NRL allergy and sensitization to latex from the weeping fig (*Ficus benjamina*) (152), to enzymes extracted from the latex of papaya (*Carica papaya*) (124,153,154), and to pollen (150,155,156). Conversely, a substantial proportion of subjects with fruit allergy show IgE-mediated sensitization to NRL, although only a minority of them will develop clinical hypersensitivity reactions to NRL products (157,158). Several proteins have been identified to be involved in this immunological cross-reactivity between NRL and phylogenetically distant plants, including class I chitinases containing an N-terminal hevein-like domain (Hev b 6.02), a beta-1,3-glucanase (Hev b 2), a patatin-like protein (Hev b 7), and the pan-allergen profilin (Hev b 8) (50,149,155,156,159–161).

DIAGNOSTIC PROCEDURES

Immunological Tests

Most studies have shown that in vitro measurement of NRL-specific IgE using RAST or ELISA methods is less reliable than skin testing (20,122,162–164). There are three FDA-cleared commercial in vitro assays whose diagnostic performance has been carefully compared with skin testing (165). The CAP system (Pharmacia Inc.) and the Alastat microtiter plate assay (Diagnostics Products Corp.), the most commonly used tests, perform comparably, with sensitivities around 75% and specificities of about 97%. The Hy-Tech assay (Hycor) has a greater sensitivity (92%) but a lower (73%) specificity (166). Although anaphylactic events have been reported after skin tests with NRL extracts (162), most investigators agree that skin testing can be performed safely and should be, for the time being, the recommended procedure for demonstrating IgE sensitization to NRL. The use of homemade extracts of NRL materials is not recommended for routine testing, because these extracts are of variable allergenic activity (167). Standardized and validated extracts of NRL are becoming commercially available (168). Further characterization of relevant NRL allergens will make it possible to achieve proper allergen standardization.

Inhalation Challenges

Recent studies have provided evidence that clinical history and immunological testing are sensitive but not specific tools for diagnosing NRL-induced occupational asthma (Table 2) (143,144,169). Among workers investigated for possible occupational asthma caused by NRL gloves, the nature of reported symptoms, including the presence of work-related urticaria and rhinitis, and their timing in relation to workplace exposure do not discriminate between subjects with and without NRL-induced asthma. Awareness of a specific temporal relationship between exposure to NRL gloves and the development of asthma symptoms is more frequently reported by subjects with NRL-induced asthma (143,144). Skin-prick tests to NRL are positive in almost all subjects who demonstrate an asthmatic response to inhalation challenge with NRL gloves, providing a high negative predictive value for the presence of NRL-induced occupational asthma. Conversely, positive immunological tests do not necessarily indicate that NRL is involved in the development of asthmatic reactions. The combination of skin-prick tests with the clinical history increases the sensitivity from 87% to 94% and the negative predictive value from 50%

Table 2 Validity of Procedures for Diagnosing NRL-Induced Occupational Asthma as Compared with Specific Inhalation Challenges

	Sensitivity (%)	Specificity (%)	PPV (%)	NPV (%)	References
Clinical history	92	32	24	94	169
	87	14	75	50	143
	89	50	77	71	144
NSBH	90	7	68	25	143
	90	10	65	33	144
Skin-prick tests to NRL	100	21	74	100	143
	100	20	70	100	144
Specific IgE to NRL	95	40	75	80	144
Clinical history + skin test to NRL	94	36	76	71	143
NSBH[a] + skin test to NRL	84	70	84	70	144

Note: The prevalence rates of NRL-induced occupational asthma, as ascertained by specific inhalation challenges in the studies by Baur et al., Vandenplas et al., and Quirce et al. were 19% (12/62), 69% (31/45), and 63% (19/30), respectively.
[a]Methacholine PC_{20} value less than 4 mg/mL.
Abbreviations: PPV, positive predictive value; NPV, negative predictive value; NSBH, baseline nonspecific bronchial hyperresponsiveness; NRL, natural rubber latex.
Source: From Refs. 143, 144, 169.

to 71%, while the positive predictive value remains unchanged (from 75% to 76%). According to the study by Quirce et al. (143,144) the best specificity (70%) and positive predictive value (84%) are provided by a positive skin-prick test response and an airway hyperresponsiveness. These findings indicate that a diagnostic approach combining the clinical history with immunological testing remains less reliable than the specific inhalation challenges. On the other hand, monitoring of peak expiratory flow rates does not allow for precise identification of the agent causing occupational asthma, because workers may be exposed to multiple asthmogenic agents. Thus, inhalation challenges with NRL should be recommended when the highest level of accuracy is required to establish or exclude a diagnosis of occupational asthma in workers exposed to airborne NRL.

Specific inhalation challenges with NRL should be performed only in specialized centers with facilities to treat severe asthmatic reactions and anaphylactic responses (170–172). However, these tests have proved to be a simple and safe technique, provided that safety requirements and stringent protocols of exposure and monitoring are carefully observed. It has recently been shown that repeated challenge exposures to glove powder do not provoke an increase in immunological sensitization to NRL allergens (173). SIC can be performed either by handling NRL gloves (140,143,144,169,174), by inhaling NRL-loaded cornstarch particles collected from powdered latex gloves (172,173), or by administering aqueous extracts of gloves (175). At present, however, no standardized methodology exists for performing SIC with NRL, because standardization of these tests would require quantification of the amount of NRL allergen delivered and comparison of these levels with those measured at work. The "handling" method is more likely to mimic the mode of exposure encountered at the workplace (i.e., airborne particles) than is the inhalation of nebulized glove extracts. It has been shown that this "realistic" method allows for generating steady concentrations of airborne NRL allergens after a few minutes (144). These findings indicate that the cumulative dose of NRL administered to the patients is mainly determined by the duration of challenge exposure. The dose of NRL allergens required to induce an asthmatic response varies widely from one subject to another, ranging from 25 to 1500 ng (144,174).

MANAGEMENT AND OUTCOME

Pharmacotherapy with antihistamines and corticosteroids does not completely remove the risk of life-threatening anaphylactic reactions to NRL (176). There is some suggestion, from case reports (177–179) and a limited number of placebo-controlled studies (180,181), that immunotherapy with NRL extracts could lead to a reduction in NRL-related symptoms (cutaneous, nasal, and ocular), medication score, and skin and conjunctival reactivity to NRL. Immunotherapy is, however, associated with a high risk of severe local and systemic adverse effects and should be considered unacceptable in its current form. Modified recombinant allergens (182,183), T cell epitope peptides (184), or DNA vaccines (185) could be promising tools for delivering safe and effective NRL allergen immunotherapy (186). A preliminary report suggests that omalizumab, a recombinant and humanized anti-IgE monoclonal antibody, induces an improvement in conjunctival and skin reactivity to NRL (187). At present, avoidance of exposure to NRL-containing products still remains the primary method for management of NRL allergy. Once the diagnosis has been firmly established, NRL-allergic patients should receive complete information about the potential sources of exposure to NRL and the possibility of cross-reactivity with plant-derived foods. All surgical procedures, diagnostic investigations, and dental treatments should be performed strictly in NRL-free environments, regardless of the severity of reactions induced by skin exposure (5,6,188). NRL-allergic individuals should wear a MedicAlert® bracelet or another "allergy identification" device. Those patients who report a history of anaphylactic reaction should be prescribed an autoinjectable epinephrine kit and carefully instructed on how to use it.

In occupational settings, management options include relocation of the worker to an NRL-free work area or conversion of the worker's current area to an NRL safe area. Complete avoidance of exposure to NRL is difficult in health-care environments, as it implies both personal and institutional policy changes. NRL-allergic health-care workers should be instructed to use only NRL-free gloves. However, personal avoidance of NRL gloves is not sufficient to prevent exposure to airborne NRL allergens, because the continued use of powdered NRL gloves by coworkers may disseminate significant amounts of NRL-contaminated powder particles, which are capable of triggering respiratory reactions in allergic workers (71,72,108,189). Thus, every effort should be made to avoid or to minimize indirect airborne exposure to NRL. Nonpowdered gloves with low protein content are effective in reducing the concentration of airborne NRL allergens (71,72,174,190,191) and the level of NRL-specific IgE (191,192), and in preventing the development of asthmatic reactions in health-care workers with NRL-induced asthma (64,174,190). However, the safety of low-protein NRL glove used by coworkers should be properly evaluated on an individual basis, as highly sensitive subjects may still develop asthmatic reactions after prolonged exposure to low-protein gloves (64,174).

There is limited information pertaining to the health and economic outcomes of NRL allergy. A few reports indicate that occupational NRL allergy is associated with a substantial adverse impact on work ability and career options in health-care workers (193,194), particularly in those with NRL-induced asthma (195). A recent follow-up study of workers with NRL-induced occupational asthma found a similar degree of improvement in NRL-related symptoms and nonspecific bronchial hyper-responsiveness in workers who avoided exposure to NRL as compared with those who only reduced exposure (151). These findings indicate that reduction of exposure to NRL can be considered a reasonably safe alternative in those subjects for whom complete NRL avoidance is not feasible. In addition, reduction of exposure to NRL was associated with fewer adverse socioeconomic consequences than complete avoidance. Further investigation is required to determine whether subjects with urticaria and/or rhinitis will develop asthma if they remain exposed to low levels of airborne NRL. It remains unknown whether asymptomatic subjects who demonstrate skin or serological evidence of NRL sensitization will progress to clinical allergy on exposure to NRL products. Nevertheless, it is wise to recommend NRL-free environments during surgical procedures in these individuals with subclinical sensitization to NRL allergens.

PREVENTION

The use of NRL-free materials is undoubtedly the most effective means of preventing sensitization to NRL, as has been reviewed (5). Most NRL devices for medical or consumer purposes can be easily replaced by latex-free materials with similar properties, with the notable exception of medical gloves. At present, the widespread use of NRL-free medical gloves does not appear to be feasible, because synthetic elastomer gloves with satisfactory mechanical and tactile properties are much more expensive than NRL gloves. Vinyl gloves are not as strong as latex gloves, nor do they provide a satisfactory tactile feel. Nevertheless, vinyl or other synthetic gloves should be used where possible for nonsterile procedures, as examination gloves are a significant source of exposure to airborne NRL allergens outside operating rooms. Unless mandated by accepted Standard Precautions, the routine use of NRL gloves by workers and other individuals, such as food handlers and housekeeping personnel, should be discouraged (188).

Because the NRL allergens are closely associated with the donning cornstarch powder (189,196), airborne exposure can be reduced by powder-free or low-powdered gloves or by reducing NRL-allergen content of gloves. Although manufacturers of NRL gloves for health care use have generally reduced the protein and powder content of such gloves to varying degrees (94), widespread switching to NRL gloves with a low allergen and powder content in all exposed health care workers is the logical intervention to reduce exposure to NRL allergens. This approach has been demonstrated to be effective in preventing the development of NRL allergy among health care workers (95–101). In a school of dentistry in Ontario, powdered NRL gloves were substituted with low-protein, powder-free NRL gloves as a result of a cross-sectional survey conducted in 1995 (80). In a repeat survey of the same school in 2000 (97), none of the 57 participating third- and fourth-year students had a positive skin test to NRL, and the only positive skin test responses were in three dental assistants who had not participated in the earlier study. The frequency of contact urticaria and/or pruritus associated with glove use was significantly reduced, and there was a trend toward reduced rates of asthma and rhinoconjunctivitis associated with NRL gloves among all participants. Similarly, in a large Ontario hospital, after changing from powdered NRL gloves to low-protein, low-powdered examination gloves in 1995 and to sterile NRL gloves in 1997 (95), there was a marked fall in the annual rates of "incident reports" and newly diagnosed NRL allergy. Incident reports, which had peaked at 45 in 1994, fell to 0 in 1999, and in that year, only one hospital worker (whose symptoms began in 1997) was newly diagnosed with NRL allergy. Therefore glove changes effectively eliminated the problem of new NRL allergy in this hospital and dental school. Of note, the overall cost of gloves in this hospital did not increase as a result of these changes. Instead of each hospital department ordering gloves individually, glove orders were for the most part consolidated through one supplier, and the bulk ordering led to similar overall costs despite the generally higher costs of safer gloves (95).

Very similar findings in relation to NRL allergy in health-care workers have been reported from the Mayo Clinic by Hunt et al. (98) after changing over to NRL gloves with low or undetectable allergen content. That hospital did not place a restriction on powdered NRL gloves, but it was found that the reduction in glove allergen content was sufficient to reduce airborne NRL allergens carried by the glove cornstarch. Hunt et al. (98) found that NRL-induced symptoms of rhinoconjunctivitis and asthma rarely occurred at sites where the airborne concentration of NRL allergen was below $10 \, ng/m^3$. They reported that measured concentrations of NRL allergens in the Mayo Clinic after the glove changes were usually below $1 \, ng/m^3$ and consistently below $10 \, ng/m^3$ (98), in contrast with previous reports of concentrations 10 to $500 \, ng/m^3$ in settings where high-allergen gloves were used (190,197). They also reported that since the glove changes, there were no new reports to the Employee Health Department of change in work area due to NRL allergy (98). As in the previously cited study (95), costs did not significantly increase with glove changes. More generalized population studies also support the effectiveness of glove changes in reducing occupational NRL allergy. Allmers (99,100) has reported a dramatic reduction in NRL allergy in Germany concurrent with glove changes, and in Ontario, Canada, reductions in compensation claims for NRL-induced occupational asthma have coincided with glove control measures (96), consistent with current recommendations (5). There is less information published as to the implementation of preventive measures for non–health care workers and any impact on sensitization and clinical allergy incidence. Levels of NRL allergen have been reported to be very high in glove-making facilities as recently as in 2000 (198), but current understanding of the risks of sensitization should allow better occupational hygiene measures to reduce skin and airborne exposure of workers to NRL allergen.

Although the total protein content of gloves may not accurately reflect their allergen content (62–64), this does not appear to have been a practical concern in ameliorating the problem of sensitization. Regulatory agencies should establish international standards for the labeling of NRL-containing devices and for measurement of their protein and allergen content. Published data regarding allergen and protein levels in gloves may also prove to be a valuable tool to guide procurement decisions (67,94). Although cost considerations are frequently cited as an objection to converting to non-NRL or low-allergen NRL gloves, reports from North American medical centers have documented no increase in glove costs (95,98). Furthermore, indirect costs such as workers' compensation, disability, loss of work, and medical treatment resulting from NRL exposure must be added into any strict accounting of costs incurred to reduce NRL exposure (199).

The continuing high prevalence of NRL allergy among exposed workers in centers where the use of high-protein NRL gloves is still continued justifies regular medical surveillance by questionnaire and immunological assessment in such settings until the recommendations to change the gloves to low-allergen gloves are implemented. There is also a need for ongoing vigilance and screening for a history of possible NRL allergy in high-risk patients who are undergoing relevant procedures. A positive screening history should be followed up with formal allergy assessment, and when positive or in doubt, NRL-free protocols should be implemented. Children requiring early frequent surgical and medical procedures due to spina bifida or other congenital abnormalities are at such high risk for developing NRL allergy that complete avoidance of exposure to NRL products is needed from birth (200,201).

CONCLUSION, RESEARCH NEEDS, AND PERSPECTIVES

Over the last two decades NRL allergy has become a major cause of medical concern among individuals exposed to NRL-containing materials in medical and nonmedical environments. Intense research efforts have led to the identification of NRL allergens and characterization of pathophysiological mechanisms of the disease. Translation of research findings into workplace practice has significantly altered the course of the NRL allergy outbreak. NRL allergy should be regarded as one of the few conditions where control of exposure is feasible and seems to be effective in reducing the burden of the disease. Further characterization of relevant NRL allergens should allow for developing quantitative assessment of clinically relevant allergens in NRL products and implementing more precise quality standards.

REFERENCES

1. Nutter AF. Contact urticaria to rubber. Br J Dermatol 1979; 101:597–598.
2. Slater JE. Rubber anaphylaxis. N Engl J Med 1989; 320:1126–1130.
3. Spaner D, Dolovich J, Tarlo S, Sussman G, Buttoo K. Hypersensitivity to natural latex. J Allergy Clin Immunol 1989; 83:1135–1137.
4. Fuchs T. Latex allergy. J Allergy Clin Immunol 1994; 93:951–952.
5. Charous BL, Blanco C, Tarlo S, et al. Natural rubber latex allergy after 12 years: recommendations and perspectives. J Allergy Clin Immunol 2002; 109:31–34.
6. Cullinan P, Brown R, Field A, et al. Latex allergy. A position paper of the British Society of Allergy and Clinical Immunology. Clin Exp Allergy 2003; 33:1484–1499.
7. Vandenplas O. Occupational asthma caused by natural rubber latex. Eur Respir J 1995; 8:1957–1965.
8. Dennis MS, Light DR. Rubber elongation factor from *Hevea brasiliensis*. Identification, characterization, and role in rubber biosynthesis. J Biol Chem 1989; 264: 18,608–18,617.
9. Gidrol X, Chrestin H, Tan HL, Kush A. Hevein, a lectin-like protein from *Hevea brasiliensis* (rubber tree) is involved in the coagulation of latex. J Biol Chem 1994; 269:9278–9283.
10. Lee HI, Broekaert WF, Raikhel NV, Lee H. Co- and post-translational processing of the hevein preproprotein of latex of the rubber tree (*Hevea brasiliensis*). J Biol Chem 1991; 266:15,944–15,948.
11. Beezhold DH, Kostyal DA, Sussman GL. IgE epitope analysis of the hevein preprotein: a major latex allergen. Clin Exp Immunol 1997; 108:114–121.
12. Jekel PA, Hartmann BH, Beintema JJ. The primary structure of hevamine, an enzyme with lysozyme/chitinase activity from *Hevea brasiliensis* latex. Eur J Biochem 1991; 200:123–130.
13. Fisher AA. Allergic contact reactions in health personnel. J Allergy Clin Immunol 1992; 90:729–738.
14. Williams PB, Halsey JF. Endotoxin as a factor in adverse reactions to latex gloves. Ann Allergy Asthma Immunol 1997; 79:303–310.
15. Slater JE, Paupore EJ, Elwell MR, Truscott W. Lipopolysaccharide augments IgG and IgE responses of mice to the latex allergen Hev b 5. J Allergy Clin Immunol 1998; 102:977–983.
16. Howell MD, Tomazic VJ, Leakakos T, Truscott W, Meade BJ. Immunomodulatory effect of endotoxin on the development of latex allergy. J Allergy Clin Immunol 2004; 113:916–924.
17. Carrillo T, Cuevas M, Munoz T, Hinojosa M, Moneo I. Contact urticaria and rhinitis from latex surgical gloves. Contact Dermatitis 1986; 15:69–72.
18. Morales C, Basomba A, Carreira J, Sastre A. Anaphylaxis produced by rubber glove contact. Case reports and immunological identification of the antigens involved. Clin Exp Allergy 1989; 19:425–430.
19. Alenius H, Turjanmaa K, Palosuo T, Makinen-Kiljunen S, Reunala T. Surgical latex glove allergy: characterization of rubber protein allergens by immunoblotting. Int Arch Allergy Appl Immunol 1991; 96:376–380.
20. Jaeger D, Kleinhans D, Czuppon AB, Baur X. Latex-specific proteins causing immediate-type cutaneous, nasal, bronchial, and systemic reactions. J Allergy Clin Immunol 1992; 89:759–768.
21. Chambeyron C, Dry J, Leynadier F, Pecquet C, Tran Xaan T. Study of the allergenic fractions of latex. Allergy 1992; 47:92–97.
22. Makinen-Kiljunen S, Turjanmaa K, Palosuo T, Reunala T. Characterization of latex antigens and allergens in surgical gloves and natural rubber by immunoelectrophoretic methods. J Allergy Clin Immunol 1992; 90:230–235.
23. Slater JE, Chhabra SK. Latex antigens. J Allergy Clin Immunol 1992; 89:673–678.

24. Kurup VP, Kelly KJ, Turjanmaa K, et al. Immunoglobulin E reactivity to latex antigens in the sera of patients from Finland and the United States. J Allergy Clin Immunol 1993; 91:1128–1134.

25. Alenius H, Turjanmaa K, Makinen-Kiljunen S, Reunala T, Palosuo T. IgE immune response to rubber proteins in adult patients with latex allergy. J Allergy Clin Immunol 1994; 93:859–863.

26. Beezhold DH, Sussman GL, Kostyal DA, Chang NS. Identification of a 46-kD latex protein allergen in health care workers. Clin Exp Immunol 1994; 98:408–413.

27. Tomazic VJ, Withrow TJ, Hamilton RG. Characterization of the allergen(s) in latex protein extracts. J Allergy Clin Immunol 1995; 96:635–642.

28. Lu LJ, Kurup VP, Fink JN, Kelly KJ. Comparison of latex antigens from surgical gloves, ammoniated and nonammoniated latex: effect of ammonia treatment on natural rubber latex proteins. J Lab Clin Med 1995; 126:161–168.

29. Yeang HY, Cheong KF, Sunderasan E, et al. The 14.6 kd rubber elongation factor (Hev b 1) and 24 kd (Hev b 3) rubber particle proteins are recognized by IgE from patients with spina bifida and latex allergy. J Allergy Clin Immunol 1996; 98: 628–639.

30. Akasawa A, Hsieh LS, Lin Y. Serum reactivities to latex proteins (*Hevea brasiliensis*). J Allergy Clin Immunol 1995; 95:1196–1205.

31. La Grutta S, Mistrello G, Varin E, Pajno GB, Passalacqua G. Comparison of ammoniated and nonammoniated extracts in children with latex allergy. Allergy 2003; 58:814–818.

32. Akasawa A, Hsieh LS, Lin Y. Comparison of latex-specific IgE binding among nonammoniated latex, ammoniated latex, and latex glove allergenic extracts by ELISA and immunoblot inhibition. J Allergy Clin Immunol 1996; 97:1116–1120.

33. Kurup VP, Alenius H, Kelly KJ, Castillo L, Fink JN. A two-dimensional electrophoretic analysis of latex peptides reacting with IgE and IgG antibodies from patients with latex allergy. Int Arch Allergy Immunol 1996; 109:58–67.

34. Alenius H, Palosuo T, Kelly K, et al. IgE reactivity to 14-kDa and 27-kDa natural rubber proteins in latex-allergic children with spina bifida and other congenital anomalies. Int Arch Allergy Immunol 1993; 102:61–66.

35. http://www.allergen.org.

36. Czuppon AB, Chen Z, Rennert S, et al. The rubber elongation factor of rubber trees (*Hevea brasiliensis*) is the major allergen in latex. J Allergy Clin Immunol 1993; 92:690–697.

37. Alenius H, Kalkkinen N, Lukka M, et al. Prohevein from the rubber tree (*Hevea brasiliensis*) is a major latex allergen. Clin Exp Allergy 1995; 25:659–665.

38. Sunderasan E, Hamzah S, Hamid S, Ward MA, Yeang HY, Cardosa MJ. Latex B-serum β-1,3-glucanase (Hev b 2) and a component of the microhelix (Hev b 4) are major allergens. J Nat Rubber Res 1995; 10:82–89.

39. Akasawa A, Hsieh LS, Martin BM, Liu T, Lin Y. A novel acidic allergen, Hev b 5, in latex. Purification, cloning and characterization. J Biol Chem 1996; 271: 25,389–25,393.

40. Alenius H, Kalkkinen N, Reunala T, Turjanmaa K, Palosuo T. The main IgE-binding epitope of a major latex allergen, prohevein, is present in its N-terminal 43-amino acid fragment, hevein. J Immunol 1996; 156:1618–1625.

41. Yeang HY. Natural rubber latex allergens: new developments. Curr Opin Allergy Clin Immunol 2004; 4:99–104.

42. Rihs HP, Chen Z, Rozynek P, Baur X, Lundberg M, Cremer R. PCR-based cloning, isolation, and IgE-binding properties of recombinant latex profilin (rHev b 8). Allergy 2000; 55:712–717.

43. Wagner S, Breiteneder H, Simon-Nobbe B, et al. Hev b 9, an enolase and a new cross-reactive allergen from *Hevea* latex and molds. Purification, characterization, cloning and expression. Eur J Biochem 2000; 267:7006–7014.

44. Wagner S, Sowka S, Mayer C, et al. Identification of a *Hevea brasiliensis* latex manganese superoxide dismutase (Hev b 10) as a cross-reactive allergen. Int Arch Allergy Immunol 2001; 125:120–127.

45. Posch A, Wheeler CH, Chen Z, et al. Class I endochitinase containing a hevein domain is the causative allergen in latex-associated avocado allergy. Clin Exp Allergy 1999; 29:667–672.

46. Beezhold DH, Hickey VL, Kostyal DA, et al. Lipid transfer protein from *Hevea brasiliensis* (Hev b 12), a cross-reactive latex protein. Ann Allergy Asthma Immunol 2003; 90:439–445.

47. Arif SA, Hamilton RG, Yusof F, et al. Isolation and characterization of the early nodule-specific protein homologue (Hev b 13), an allergenic lipolytic esterase from *Hevea brasiliensis* latex. J Biol Chem 2004; 279:23,933–23,941.

48. Yagami T, Haishima Y, Tsuchiya T, Tomitaka-Yagami A, Kano H, Matsunaga K. Proteomic analysis of putative latex allergens. Int Arch Allergy Immunol 2004; 135: 3–11.

49. Chen Z, Van Kampen V, Raulf-Heimsoth M, Baur X. Allergenic and antigenic determinants of latex allergen Hev b 1: peptide mapping of epitopes recognized by human, murine and rabbit antibodies. Clin Exp Allergy 1996; 26:406–415.

50. Raulf-Heimsoth M, Chen Z, Rihs HP, Kalbacher H, Liebers V, Baur X. Analysis of T-cell reactive regions and HLA-DR4 binding motifs on the latex allergen Hev b 1 (rubber elongation factor). Clin Exp Allergy 1998; 28:339–348.

51. Mikkola JH, Alenius H, Kalkkinen N, Turjanmaa K, Palosuo T, Reunala T. Hevein-like protein domains as a possible cause for allergen cross-reactivity between latex and banana. J Allergy Clin Immunol 1998; 102:1005–1012.

52. Beezhold DH, Hickey VL, Slater JE, Sussman GL. Human IgE-binding epitopes of the latex allergen Hev b 5. J Allergy Clin Immunol 1999; 103:1166–1172.

53. Meade BJ, Weissman DN, Beezhold DH. Latex allergy: past and present. Int Immunopharmacol 2002; 2:225–238.

54. Sussman GL, Beezhold DH, Kurup VP. Allergens and natural rubber proteins. J Allergy Clin Immunol 2002; 110:S33–S39.

55. Slater JE. Latex allergens. Clin Allergy Immunol 2004; 18:369–386.

56. Yip L, Hickey V, Wagner B, et al. Skin prick test reactivity to recombinant latex allergens. Int Arch Allergy Immunol 2000; 121:292–299.

57. Bernstein DI, Biagini RE, Karnani R, et al. In vivo sensitization to purified *Hevea brasiliensis* proteins in health care workers sensitized to natural rubber latex. J Allergy Clin Immunol 2003; 111:610–616.

58. Beezhold D, Swanson M, Zehr BD, Kostyal D. Measurement of natural rubber proteins in latex glove extracts: comparison of the methods. Ann Allergy Asthma Immunol 1996; 76:520–526.

59. Yeang HY, Yusof F, Abdullah L. Precipitation of *Hevea brasiliensis* latex proteins with trichloroacetic acid and phosphotungstic acid in preparation for the Lowry protein assay. Anal Biochem 1995; 226:35–43.

60. Beezhold D, Horton K, Hickey V, Daddona J, Kostyal D. Glove powders carrying capacity for latex proteins: analysis using the ASTM ELISA test. J Long Term Effects Med Implants 2003; 13:21–31.

61. Turjanmaa K, Laurila K, Makinen-Kiljunen S, Reunala T. Rubber contact urticaria. Allergenic properties of 19 brands of latex gloves. Contact Dermatitis 1988; 19:362–367.

62. Leynadier F, Tran Xuan T, Dry J. Allergenicity suppression in natural latex surgical gloves. Allergy 1991; 46:619–625.

63. Alenius H, Makinen-Kiljunen S, Turjanmaa K, Palosuo T, Reunala T. Allergen and protein content of latex gloves. Ann Allergy 1994; 73:315–320.

64. Vandenplas O, Delwiche JP, Depelchin S, Sibille Y, Vande Weyer R, Delaunois L. Latex gloves with a lower protein content reduce bronchial reactions in subjects with occupational asthma caused by latex. Am J Respir Crit Care Med 1995; 151:887–891.

65. Jones RT, Scheppmann DL, Heilman DK, Yunginger JW. Prospective study of extractable latex allergen contents of disposable medical gloves. Ann Allergy 1994; 73: 321–325.

66. Yeang HY, Arif SA, Raulf-Heimsoth M, et al. Hev b 5 and Hev b 13 as allergen markers to estimate the allergenic potency of latex gloves. J Allergy Clin Immunol 2004; 114:593–598.

67. Yunginger JW, Jones RT, Fransway AF, Kelso JM, Warner MA, Hunt LW. Extractable latex allergens and proteins in disposable medical gloves and other rubber products. J Allergy Clin Immunol 1994; 93:836–842.

68. Turjanmaa K, Reunala T, Alenius H, Brummer-Korvenkontio H, Palosuo T. Allergens in latex surgical gloves and glove powder. Lancet 1990; 336:1588.

69. Beezhold D, Beck WC. Surgical glove powders bind latex antigens. Arch Surg 1992; 127:1354–1357.

70. Tomazic VJ, Shampaine EL, Lamanna A, Withrow TJ, Adkinson NF Jr, Hamilton RG. Cornstarch powder on latex products is an allergen carrier. J Allergy Clin Immunol 1994; 93:751–758.

71. Swanson MC, Bubak ME, Hunt LW, Yunginger JW, Warner MA, Reed CE. Quantification of occupational latex aeroallergens in a medical center. J Allergy Clin Immunol 1994; 94:445–451.

72. Heilman DK, Jones RT, Swanson MC, Yunginger JW. A prospective, controlled study showing that rubber gloves are the major contributor to latex aeroallergen levels in the operating room. J Allergy Clin Immunol 1996; 98:325–330.

73. Brown RH, Taenkhum K, Buckley TJ, Hamilton RG. Different latex aeroallergen size distributions between powdered surgical and examination gloves: significance for environmental avoidance. J Allergy Clin Immunol 2004; 114:358–363.

74. Tarlo SM, Wong L, Roos J, Booth N. Occupational asthma caused by latex in a surgical glove manufacturing plant. J Allergy Clin Immunol 1990; 85:626–631.

75. Turjanmaa K. Incidence of immediate allergy to latex gloves in hospital personnel. Contact Dermatitis 1987; 17:270–275.

76. Lagier F, Vervloet D, Lhermet I, Poyen D, Charpin D. Prevalence of latex allergy in operating room nurses. J Allergy Clin Immunol 1992; 90:319–322.

77. Salkie ML. The prevalence of atopy and hypersensitivity to latex in medical laboratory technologists. Arch Pathol Lab Med 1993; 117:897–899.

78. Yassin MS, Lierl MB, Fischer TJ, O'Brien K, Cross J, Steinmetz C. Latex allergy in hospital employees. Ann Allergy 1994; 72:245–249.

79. Vandenplas O, Delwiche JP, Evrard G, et al. Prevalence of occupational asthma due to latex among hospital personnel. Am J Respir Crit Care Med 1995; 151:54–60.

80. Tarlo SM, Sussman GL, Holness DL. Latex sensitivity in dental students and staff: a cross-sectional study. J Allergy Clin Immunol 1997; 99:396–401.

81. Carrillo T, Blanco C, Quiralte J, Castillo R, Cuevas M, Rodriguez de Castro F. Prevalence of latex allergy among greenhouse workers. J Allergy Clin Immunol 1995; 96: 699–701.

82. Rueff F, Kienitz A, Schopf P, et al. Frequency of natural rubber latex allergy in adults is increased after multiple operative procedures. Allergy 2001; 56:889–894.

83. Slater JE, Mostello LA, Shaer C. Rubber-specific IgE in children with spina bifida. J Urol 1991; 146:578–579.

84. Yassin MS, Sanyurah S, Lierl MB, et al. Evaluation of latex allergy in patients with meningomyelocele. Ann Allergy 1992; 69:207–211.

85. Kelly KJ, Pearson ML, Kurup VP, et al. A cluster of anaphylactic reactions in children with spina bifida during general anesthesia: epidemiologic features, risk factors, and latex hypersensitivity. J Allergy Clin Immunol 1994; 94:53–61.

86. Mazon A, Nieto A, Estornell F, Reig C, Garcia-Ibarra F. Factors that influence the presence of symptoms caused by latex allergy in children with spina bifida. J Allergy Clin Immunol 1997; 99:600–604.

87. Cremer R, Hoppe A, Korsch E, Kleine-Diepenbruck U, Blaker F. Natural rubber latex allergy: prevalence and risk factors in patients with spina bifida compared with atopic children and controls. Eur J Pediatr 1998; 157:13–16.
88. Orfan NA, Reed R, Dykewicz MS, Ganz M, Kolski GB. Occupational asthma in a latex doll manufacturing plant. J Allergy Clin Immunol 1994; 94:826–830.
89. Vandenplas O, Delwiche JP, De Jonghe M. Asthma to latex and amoxicillin. Allergy 1997; 52:1147–1149.
90. van der Walle HB, Brunsveld VM. Latex allergy among hairdressers. Contact Dermatitis 1995; 32:177–178.
91. Archambault S, Malo JL, Infante-Rivard C, Ghezzo H, Gautrin D. Incidence of sensitization, symptoms, and probable occupational rhinoconjunctivitis and asthma in apprentices starting exposure to latex. J Allergy Clin Immunol 2001; 107:921–923.
92. Truscott W. The industry perspective on latex. Immunol Allergy Clin N Am 1995; 15:89–122.
93. Sanchez-Monge R, Blanco C, Perales AD, et al. Class I chitinases, the panallergens responsible for the latex-fruit syndrome, are induced by ethylene treatment and inactivated by heating. J Allergy Clin Immunol 2000; 106:190–195.
94. Palosuo T, Alenius H, Turjanmaa K. Quantitation of latex allergens. Methods 2002; 27:52–58.
95. Tarlo SM, Easty A, Eubanks K, et al. Outcomes of a natural rubber latex control program in an Ontario teaching hospital. J Allergy Clin Immunol 2001; 108:628–633.
96. Liss GM, Tarlo SM. Natural rubber latex-related occupational asthma: association with interventions and glove changes over time. Am J Ind Med 2001; 40:347–353.
97. Saary MJ, Kanani A, Alghadeer H, Holness DL, Tarlo SM. Changes in rates of natural rubber latex sensitivity among dental school students and staff members after changes in latex gloves. J Allergy Clin Immunol 2002; 109:131–135.
98. Hunt LW, Kelkar P, Reed CE, Yunginger JW. Management of occupational allergy to natural rubber latex in a medical center: the importance of quantitative latex allergen measurement and objective follow-up. J Allergy Clin Immunol 2002; 110: S96–S106.
99. Allmers H, Schmengler J, Skudlik C. Primary prevention of natural rubber latex allergy in the German health care system through education and intervention. J Allergy Clin Immunol 2002; 110:318–323.
100. Allmers H, Schmengler J, John SM. Decreasing incidence of occupational contact urticaria caused by natural rubber latex allergy in German health care workers. J Allergy Clin Immunol 2004; 114:347–351.
101. Jones KP, Rolf S, Stingl C, Edmunds D, Davies BH. Longitudinal study of sensitization to natural rubber latex among dental school students using powder-free gloves. Ann Occup Hyg 2004; 48:455–457.
102. Chen YH, Lan JL. Latex allergy and latex-fruit syndrome among medical workers in Taiwan. J Formos Med Assoc 2002; 101:622–626.
103. Nolte H, Babakhin A, Babanin A, et al. Prevalence of skin test reactions to natural rubber latex in hospital personnel in Russia and eastern Europe. Ann Allergy Asthma Immunol 2002; 89:452–456.
104. Di Lorenzo G, Vitale F, Pacor ML, et al. Prevalence of latex sensitization in health care workers of a general hospital in Palermo, Sicily. J Invest Allergol Clin Immunol 2002; 12:114–119.
105. Nettis E, Dambra P, Soccio AL, Ferrannini A, Tursi A. Latex hypersensitivity: relationship with positive prick test and patch test responses among hairdressers. Allergy 2003; 58:57–61.
106. Conde-Salazar L, Gatica ME, Barco L, Iglesias C, Cuevas M, Valks R. Latex allergy among construction workers. Contact Dermatitis 2002; 47:154–156.
107. Vandenplas O, Delwiche JP, Sibille Y. Occupational asthma due to latex in a hospital administrative employee. Thorax 1996; 51:452–453.

108. Charous BL, Schuenemann PJ, Swanson MC. Passive dispersion of latex aeroallergen in a healthcare facility. Ann Allergy Asthma Immunol 2000; 85:285–290.

109. Grzybowski M, Ownby DR, Peyser PA, Johnson CC, Schork MA. The prevalence of anti-latex IgE antibodies among registered nurses. J Allergy Clin Immunol 1996; 98:535–544.

110. Gautrin D, Ghezzo H, Infante-Rivard C, Malo JL. Incidence and determinants of IgE-mediated sensitization in apprentices. A prospective study. Am J Respir Crit Care Med 2000; 162:1222–1228.

111. Gautrin D, Infante-Rivard C, Dao TV, Magnan-Larose M, Desjardins D, Malo JL. Specific IgE-dependent sensitization, atopy, and bronchial hyperresponsiveness in apprentices starting exposure to protein-derived agents. Am J Respir Crit Care Med 1997; 155:1841–1847.

112. Porri F, Lemière C, Birnbaum J, et al. Prevalence of latex sensitization in subjects attending health screening: implications for a perioperative screening. Clin Exp Allergy 1997; 27:413–417.

113. Hadjiliadis D, Khan K, Tarlo SM. Skin test responses to latex in an allergy and asthma clinic. J Allergy Clin Immunol 1995; 96:431–432.

114. Ownby DR, Ownby HE, McCullough J, Shafer AW. The prevalence of anti-latex IgE antibodies in 1000 volunteer blood donors. J Allergy Clin Immunol 1996; 97:1188–1192.

115. Merrett TG, Merrett J, Kekwick R. The prevalence of immunoglobulin E antibodies to the proteins of rubber (*Hevea brasiliensis*) latex and grass (*Phleum pratense*) pollen in sera of British blood donors. Clin Exp Allergy 1999; 29:1572–1578.

116. Saxon A, Ownby D, Huard T, Parsad R, Roth HD. Prevalence of IgE to natural rubber latex in unselected blood donors and performance characteristics of AlaSTAT testing. Ann Allergy Asthma Immunol 2000; 84:199–206.

117. Senna GE, Crocco I, Roata C, et al. Prevalence of latex-specific IgE in blood donors: an Italian survey. Allergy 1999; 54:80–81.

118. Garabrant DH, Roth HD, Parsad R, Ying GS, Weiss J. Latex sensitization in health care workers and in the US general population. Am J Epidemiol 2001; 153:515–522.

119. Arellano R, Bradley J, Sussman G. Prevalence of latex sensitization among hospital physicians occupationally exposed to latex gloves. Anesthesiology 1992; 77:905–908.

120. Wrangsjo K, Osterman K, van Hage-Hamsten M. Glove-related skin symptoms among operating theatre and dental care unit personnel (II). Clinical examination, tests and laboratory findings indicating latex allergy. Contact Dermatitis 1994; 30:139–143.

121. Rihs HP, Chen Z, Rueff F, et al. HLA-DQ8 and the HLA-DQ8-DR4 haplotype are positively associated with the hevein-specific IgE immune response in health care workers with latex allergy. J Allergy Clin Immunol 2002; 110:507–514.

122. Charous BL, Hamilton RG, Yunginger JW. Occupational latex exposure: characteristics of contact and systemic reactions in 47 workers. J Allergy Clin Immunol 1994; 94:12–18.

123. Konz KR, Chia JK, Kurup VP, Resnick A, Kelly KJ, Fink JN. Comparison of latex hypersensitivity among patients with neurologic defects. J Allergy Clin Immunol 1995; 95:950–954.

124. Blanco C, Carrillo T, Castillo R, Quiralte J, Cuevas M. Latex allergy: clinical features and cross-reactivity with fruits. Ann Allergy 1994; 73:309–314.

125. Beuers U, Baur X, Schraudolph M, Richter WO. Anaphylactic shock after game of squash in atopic woman with latex allergy. Lancet 1990; 335:1095.

126. Fiocchi A, Restani P, Ballabio C, et al. Severe anaphylaxis induced by latex as a contaminant of plastic balls in play pits. J Allergy Clin Immunol 2001; 108:298–300.

127. Sommer S, Wilkinson SM, Beck MH, English JS, Gawkrodger DJ, Green C. Type IV hypersensitivity reactions to natural rubber latex: results of a multicentre study. Br J Dermatol 2002; 146:114–117.

128. Sussman GL, Tarlo S, Dolovich J. The spectrum of IgE-mediated responses to latex. JAMA 1991; 265:2844–2847.

129. Turjanmaa K, Reunala T, Tuimala R, Karkkainen T. Allergy to latex gloves: unusual complication during delivery. BMJ 1988; 297:1029.
130. Mansell PI, Reckless JP, Lovell CR. Severe anaphylactic reaction to latex rubber surgical gloves. BMJ 1994; 308:246–247.
131. Lozynsky OA, Dupuis L, Shandling B, Gilmour RF, Zimmerman B. Anaphylactoid and systemic reactions following saline enema administration. Six case reports. Ann Allergy 1986; 56:62–66.
132. Ownby DR, Tomlanovich M, Sammons N, McCullough J. Anaphylaxis associated with latex allergy during barium enema examinations. Am J Roentgenol 1991; 156:903–908.
133. Turjanmaa K, Reunala T. Condoms as a source of latex allergen and cause of contact urticaria. Contact Dermatitis 1989; 20:360–364.
134. Mertes PM, Laxenaire MC, Alla F. Anaphylactic and anaphylactoid reactions occurring during anesthesia in France in 1999–2000. Anesthesiology 2003; 99:536–545.
135. Primeau MN, Adkinson NF Jr, Hamilton RG. Natural rubber pharmaceutical vial closures release latex allergens that produce skin reactions. J Allergy Clin Immunol 2001; 107:958–962.
136. Beezhold DH, Reschke JE, Allen JH, Kostyal DA, Sussman GL. Latex protein: a hidden "food" allergen? Allergy Asthma Proc 2000; 21:301–306.
137. Karathanasis P, Cooper A, Zhou K, Mayer L, Kang BC. Indirect latex contact causes urticaria/anaphylaxis. Ann Allergy 1993; 71:526–528.
138. Pumphrey RS, Duddridge M, Norton J. Fatal latex allergy. J Allergy Clin Immunol 2001; 107:558.
139. Keh C, Soon Y, Wong LS. Latex allergy: an emerging problem in theatres. Int J Clin Pract 2000; 54:582–584.
140. Lagier F, Badier M, Martigny J, Charpin D, Vervloet D. Latex as aeroallergen. Lancet 1990; 336:516–517.
141. Ross DJ, Keynes HL, McDonald JC. SWORD '97: surveillance of work-related and occupational respiratory disease in the UK. Occup Med (Lond) 1998; 48:481–485.
142. Ameille J, Pauli G, Calastreng-Crinquand A, et al. Reported incidence of occupational asthma in France, 1996–99: the ONAP programme. Occup Environ Med 2003; 60:136–141.
143. Vandenplas O, Binard-Van Cangh F, Brumagne A, et al. Occupational asthma in symptomatic workers exposed to natural rubber latex: evaluation of diagnostic procedures. J Allergy Clin Immunol 2001; 107:542–547.
144. Quirce S, Swanson MC, Fernandez-Nieto M, de las Heras M, Cuesta J, Sastre J. Quantified environmental challenge with absorbable dusting powder aerosol from natural rubber latex gloves. J Allergy Clin Immunol 2003; 111:788–794.
145. Lee A, Nixon R, Frowen K. Reduction of use of latex gloves in food handlers: an intervention study. Contact Dermatitis 2001; 44:75–79.
146. de Groot H, de Jong NW, Duijster E, et al. Prevalence of natural rubber latex allergy (type I and type IV) in laboratory workers in The Netherlands. Contact Dermatitis 1998; 38:159–163.
147. Pisati G, Baruffini A, Bernabeo F, Falagiani P. Environmental and clinical study of latex allergy in a textile factory. J Allergy Clin Immunol 1998; 101:327–329.
148. Quirce S, Fernandez-Nieto M, de Miguel J, Sastre J. Chronic cough due to latex-induced eosinophilic bronchitis. J Allergy Clin Immunol 2001; 108:143.
149. Beezhold DH, Sussman GL, Liss GM, Chang NS. Latex allergy can induce clinical reactions to specific foods. Clin Exp Allergy 1996; 26:416–422.
150. Levy DA, Mounedji N, Noirot C, Leynadier F. Allergic sensitization and clinical reactions to latex, food and pollen in adult patients. Clin Exp Allergy 2000; 30:270–275.
151. Vandenplas O, Jamart J, Delwiche JP, Evrard G, Larbanois A. Occupational asthma caused by natural rubber latex: outcome according to cessation or reduction of exposure. J Allergy Clin Immunol 2002; 109:125–130.

152. Delbourg MF, Moneret-Vautrin DA, Guilloux L, Ville G. Hypersensitivity to latex and *Ficus benjamina* allergens. Ann Allergy Asthma Immunol 1995; 75:496–500.

153. Baur X, Chen Z, Rozynek P, Duser M, Raulf-Heimsoth M. Cross-reacting IgE antibodies recognizing latex allergens, including Hev b 1, as well as papain. Allergy 1995; 50:604–609.

154. Vandenplas O, Vandezande LM, Halloy JL, Delwiche JP, Jamart J, Looze Y. Association between sensitization to natural rubber latex and papain. J Allergy Clin Immunol 1996; 97:1421–1424.

155. Fuchs T, Spitzauer S, Vente C, et al. Natural latex, grass pollen, and weed pollen share IgE epitopes. J Allergy Clin Immunol 1997; 100:356–364.

156. Ganglberger E, Radauer C, Wagner S, et al. Hev b 8, the *Hevea brasiliensis* latex profilin, is a cross-reactive allergen of latex, plant foods and pollen. Int Arch Allergy Immunol 2001; 125:216–227.

157. Garcia Ortiz JC, Moyano JC, Alvarez M, Bellido J. Latex allergy in fruit-allergic patients. Allergy 1998; 53:532–536.

158. Quirce S, Bombin C, Aleman A, Sastre J. Allergy to latex, fruit, and pollen. Allergy 2000; 55:896–898.

159. Chen Z, Posch A, Cremer R, Raulf-Heimsoth M, Baur X. Identification of hevein (Hev b 6.02) in *Hevea* latex as a major cross-reacting allergen with avocado fruit in patients with latex allergy. J Allergy Clin Immunol 1998; 102:476–481.

160. Blanco C, Diaz-Perales A, Collada C, et al. Class I chitinases as potential panallergens involved in the latex-fruit syndrome. J Allergy Clin Immunol 1999; 103:507–513.

161. Seppala U, Palosuo T, Kalkkinen N, Ylitalo L, Reunala T, Turjanmaa K. IgE reactivity to patatin-like latex allergen, Hev b 7, and to patatin of potato tuber, Sol t 1, in adults and children allergic to natural rubber latex. Allergy 2000; 55:266–273.

162. Kelly KJ, Kurup V, Zacharisen M, Resnick A, Fink JN. Skin and serologic testing in the diagnosis of latex allergy. J Allergy Clin Immunol 1993; 91:1140–1145.

163. Turjanmaa K, Reunala T, Rasanen L. Comparison of diagnostic methods in latex surgical glove contact urticaria. Contact Dermatitis 1988; 19:241–247.

164. Hamilton RG, Adkinson NF Jr. Natural rubber latex skin testing reagents: safety and diagnostic accuracy of nonammoniated latex, ammoniated latex, and latex rubber glove extracts. J Allergy Clin Immunol 1996; 98:872–883.

165. Hamilton RG, Peterson EL, Ownby DR. Clinical and laboratory-based methods in the diagnosis of natural rubber latex allergy. J Allergy Clin Immunol 2002; 110:S47–S56.

166. Hamilton RG, Biagini RE, Krieg EF. Diagnostic performance of Food and Drug Administration-cleared serologic assays for natural rubber latex-specific IgE antibody. The Multi-Center Latex Skin Testing Study Task Force. J Allergy Clin Immunol 1999; 103:925–930.

167. Fink JN, Kelly KJ, Elms N, Kurup VP. Comparative studies of latex extracts used in skin testing. Ann Allergy Asthma Immunol 1996; 76:149–152.

168. Turjanmaa K, Palosuo T, Alenius H, et al. Latex allergy diagnosis: in vivo and in vitro standardization of a natural rubber latex extract. Allergy 1997; 52:41–50.

169. Baur X, Huber H, Degens PO, Allmers H, Ammon J. Relation between occupational asthma case history, bronchial methacholine challenge, and specific challenge test in patients with suspected occupational asthma. Am J Ind Med 1998; 33:114–122.

170. Sterk P, Fabbri L, Quanjer P, et al. Airways responsiveness. Standardized challenge testing with pharmacological, physical and sensitizing stimuli in adults. Official statement of the European respiratory Society. Eur Respir J 1993; 6(suppl) 16:53–83.

171. Vandenplas O, Malo JL. Inhalation challenges with agents causing occupational asthma. Eur Respir J 1997; 10:2612–2629.

172. Kurtz KM, Hamilton RG, Schaefer JA, Adkinson NF Jr. A hooded exposure chamber method for semiquantitative latex aeroallergen challenge. J Allergy Clin Immunol 2001; 107:178–184.

173. Kurtz KM, Hamilton RG, Schaefer JA, Primeau MN, Adkinson NF Jr. Repeated latex aeroallergen challenges employing a hooded exposure chamber: safety and reproducibility. Allergy 2001; 56:857–861.

174. Laoprasert N, Swanson MC, Jones RT, Schroeder DR, Yunginger JW. Inhalation challenge testing of latex-sensitive health care workers and the effectiveness of laminar flow HEPA-filtered helmets in reducing rhinoconjunctival and asthmatic reactions. J Allergy Clin Immunol 1998; 102:998–1004.

175. Pisati G, Baruffini A, Bernabeo F, Stanizzi R. Bronchial provocation testing in the diagnosis of occupational asthma due to latex surgical gloves. Eur Respir J 1994; 7:332–336.

176. Kwittken PL, Becker J, Oyefara B, Danziger R, Pawlowski NA, Sweinberg S. Latex hypersensitivity reactions despite prophylaxis. Allergy Proc 1992; 13:123–127.

177. Pereira C, Rico P, Lourenco M, Lombardero M, Pinto-Mendes J, Chieira C. Specific immunotherapy for occupational latex allergy. Allergy 1999; 54:291–293.

178. Nucera E, Schiavino D, Buonomo A, et al. Latex rush desensitization. Allergy 2001; 56:86–87.

179. Pereira C, Pedro E, Tavares B, et al. Specific immunotherapy for severe latex allergy. Allerg Immunol (Paris) 2003; 35:217–225.

180. Leynadier F, Herman D, Vervloet D, Andre C. Specific immunotherapy with a standardized latex extract versus placebo in allergic healthcare workers. J Allergy Clin Immunol 2000; 106:585–590.

181. Sastre J, Fernandez-Nieto M, Rico P, et al. Specific immunotherapy with a standardized latex extract in allergic workers: a double-blind, placebo-controlled study. J Allergy Clin Immunol 2003; 111:985–994.

182. Beezhold DH, Hickey VL, Sussman GL. Mutational analysis of the IgE epitopes in the latex allergen Hev b 5. J Allergy Clin Immunol 2001; 107:1069–1076.

183. Karisola P, Mikkola J, Kalkkinen N, et al. Construction of hevein (Hev b 6.02) with reduced allergenicity for immunotherapy of latex allergy by comutation of six amino acid residues on the conformational IgE epitopes. J Immunol 2004; 172:2621–2628.

184. de Silva HD, Sutherland MF, Suphioglu C, et al. Human T-cell epitopes of the latex allergen Hev b 5 in health care workers. J Allergy Clin Immunol 2000; 105:1017–1024.

185. Slater JE, Paupore E, Zhang YT, Colberg-Poley AM. The latex allergen Hev b 5 transcript is widely distributed after subcutaneous injection in BALB/c mice of its DNA vaccine. J Allergy Clin Immunol 1998; 102:469–475.

186. Sutherland MF, Suphioglu C, Rolland JM, O'Hehir RE. Latex allergy: towards immunotherapy for health care workers. Clin Exp Allergy 2002; 32:667–673.

187. Leynadier F, Doudou O, Gaouar H, et al. Effect of omalizumab in health care workers with occupational latex allergy. J Allergy Clin Immunol 2004; 113:360–361.

188. Task force on allergic reactions to latex. American Academy of Allergy and Immunology. Committee report. J Allergy Clin Immunol 1993; 92:16–18.

189. Mitakakis TZ, Tovey ER, Yates DH, et al. Particulate masks and non-powdered gloves reduce latex allergen inhaled by healthcare workers. Clin Exp Allergy 2002; 32: 1166–1169.

190. Tarlo SM, Sussman G, Contala A, Swanson MC. Control of airborne latex by use of powder-free latex gloves. J Allergy Clin Immunol 1994; 93:985–989.

191. Allmers H, Brehler R, Chen Z, Raulf-Heimsoth M, Fels H, Baur X. Reduction of latex aeroallergens and latex-specific IgE antibodies in sensitized workers after removal of powdered natural rubber latex gloves in a hospital. J Allergy Clin Immunol 1998; 102:841–846.

192. Hamilton RG, Brown RH. Impact of personal avoidance practices on health care workers sensitized to natural rubber latex. J Allergy Clin Immunol 2000; 105:839–841.

193. Kujala VM, Karvonen J, Laara E, Kanerva L, Estlander T, Reijula KE. Postal questionnaire study of disability associated with latex allergy among health care workers in Finland. Am J Ind Med 1997; 32:197–204.

194. Potter PC, Crombie I, Marian A, Kosheva O, Maqula B, Schinkel M. Latex allergy at Groote Schuur Hospital—prevalence, clinical features and outcome. S Afr Med J 2001; 91:760–765.
195. Bernstein DI, Karnani R, Biagini RE, et al. Clinical and occupational outcomes in health care workers with natural rubber latex allergy. Ann Allergy Asthma Immunol 2003; 90:209–213.
196. Poulos LM, O'Meara TJ, Hamilton RG, Tovey ER. Inhaled latex allergen (Hev b 1). J Allergy Clin Immunol 2002; 109:701–706.
197. Baur X, Ammon J, Chen Z, Beckmann U, Czuppon AB. Health risk in hospitals through airborne allergens for patients presensitised to latex. Lancet 1993; 342:1148–1149.
198. Chaiear N, Sadhra S, Jones M, Cullinan P, Foulds IS, Burge PS. Sensitisation to natural rubber latex: an epidemiological study of workers exposed during tapping and glove manufacture in Thailand. Occup Environ Med 2001; 58:386–391.
199. Phillips VL, Goodrich MA, Sullivan TJ. Health care worker disability due to latex allergy and asthma: a cost analysis. Am J Public Health 1999; 89:1024–1028.
200. Ylitalo L, Alenius H, Turjanmaa K, Palosuo T, Reunala T. Natural rubber latex allergy in children: a follow-up study. Clin Exp Allergy 2000; 30:1611–1617.
201. Reider N, Kretz B, Menardi G, Ulmer H, Fritsch P. Outcome of a latex avoidance program in a high-risk population for latex allergy—a five-year follow-up study. Clin Exp Allergy 2002; 32:708–713.

20

High-Molecular-Weight Protein Agents

Santiago Quirce
Department of Allergy, Fundación Jiménez Díaz, Madrid, Spain

David I. Bernstein
Division of Allergy–Immunology, Department of Internal Medicine, College of Medicine, University of Cincinnati, Cincinnati, Ohio, U.S.A.

Jean-Luc Malo
Department of Chest Medicine, Université de Montréal and Sacré-Cœur Hospital, Montreal, Quebec, Canada

INTRODUCTION

High-molecular-weight (HMW) agents are protein-derived antigens that cause sensitization through an immunoglobulin E (IgE)–mediated mechanism. This represents an interesting and useful model of common atopic asthma. Some of the HMW agents are covered in the specific chapters: enzymes (Chapter 16), flour and baking additives (Chapter 17), and laboratory animal allergens, including insect and shellfish emanations (Chapter 18). Here, other proteinaceous agents causing occupational asthma (OA) are described.

ANIMAL-DERIVED ALLERGENS

Mammalian proteins are important sources of occupational allergens that can cause OA. The most important of these is laboratory animal allergens, which are reviewed extensively in Chapter 18.

Allergens in cow dust are important causes of OA in farmers in Finland and are estimated to account for 40% of all new cases of OA in that country; the major purified allergen is designated Bos d 2. Specific IgE to the purified cow allergen, Bos d 2, is a sensitive and specific diagnostic marker of OA (1). Cow-asthmatic dairy farmers show immune reactivity to the major allergen of cow (Bos d 2) and to other cow-derived proteins. The use of purified Bos d 2 marginally increases the performance of diagnostic tests in respiratory cow allergy (1). Specific immunoglobulin G (IgG), on the other hand, is unable to distinguish healthy farm workers from those with OA. Farmers who develop cow hair–specific IgE improve following complete avoidance of exposure to cows (2). Severe asthma during milking of sheep has been described in a worker sensitized to sheep milk proteins, lactoglobulin and casein (3). OA and rhinoconjunctivitis have been reported in a candy worker exposed to dried cow's milk proteins and was confirmed by percutaneous sensitivity to lactalbumin and a positive bronchial challenge test to the same antigen (4).

A farmer raising deer was reported to be sensitized to deer dander and to have OA confirmed by bronchoprovocation testing with deer dander extract. Multiple allergens were identified (size range: 21–110 kDa) (5).

Exposure to raw poultry has recently been reported as a cause of occupational dermatitis, rhinitis, and asthma (6). Eggs were first reported to cause OA in 8 out of 13 bakers spraying egg protein, although sensitization to egg protein was not confirmed (7). In 1987, a survey of 25 egg-processing workers was conducted in an egg-processing plant where high exposures to egg white and egg yolk aerosols were generated (8). Five workers had definite OA confirmed by symptoms and work-related decrements in peak expiratory flow rates (9). Four of the workers exhibited skin-prick test reactions to purified egg proteins, including ovalbumin, conalbumin, lysozyme, and ovomucoid. Specific IgG responses to the aforementioned purified egg white proteins did not discriminate between symptomatic and asymptomatic workers. In a cross-industry survey of egg-processing workers, Smith et al. (10) reported a 34% prevalence of cutaneous sensitization to egg white proteins. Fourteen of the combined workforce of 188 subjects (7%) employed at two plants showed evidence of OA as assessed by a questionnaire, a physician diagnosis of OA, and IgE-mediated sensitization to at least one egg protein. A higher prevalence of egg asthma was found in the "transfer" and "breaking" areas where liquid protein aerosols were generated (12% and 10%, respectively), compared to the drying areas where there was exposure principally to egg powder (5%). Boeniger et al. (11) reported extremely high exposure to ambient egg protein (as high as mean concentration of $644\,\mu g/m^3$) and particulates were of respirable size but particularly increased in areas of a plant where egg protein aerosols were generated (egg breaking and transfer rooms). In this study, atopic egg-processing factory workers were at significantly increased risk for cutaneous sensitization to egg protein allergens, a finding which was not duplicated in similar surveys of egg workers (11). It is possible that the lack of an association in previous cross-sectional surveys of egg sensitivity with atopic status could reflect survivor effects; atopic workers may be more likely to become clinically sensitized and quit their jobs than nonatopic workers. Purified hen egg white lysozyme has been reported as a cause of allergic OA in a worker of the pharmaceutical industry exposed to lysozyme powder (12) and likewise in a cheese worker (13).

Bakery and confectionery workers may also develop OA owing to sensitization to egg proteins (14). Although considered rare, bakery and confectionery workers have been reported to develop the "egg-egg syndrome" or food allergy to eggs subsequent to development of OA, presumably, as a result of IgE-mediated sensitization to ambient egg proteins generated in the workplace (15). The causative role of egg white proteins (lysozyme, ovalbumin, and ovomucoid) in the respiratory symptoms induced by inhalation of egg aerosols among bakers or confectioners has been demonstrated by immunologic and specific inhalation challenge tests (16). The egg white protein that has been most commonly implicated in respiratory allergy among bakery workers is lysozyme, as confirmed by bronchial challenge (16).

A relationship between respiratory type I hypersensitivity to bird antigens and food allergy to egg yolk has been described (the so-called "bird-egg syndrome"). One of the first case reports of this syndrome was a woman with occupational exposure to birds who developed asthma because of bird feathers and serum proteins, followed by severe food allergy to egg yolk (17). In patients with this syndrome, sensitization to airborne bird allergens usually precedes allergy to egg yolk antigens. Egg yolk α-livetin, also known as chicken serum albumin or Gal d 5, has been reported to be the cross-reacting allergen responsible for this association (18,19). Specific inhalation challenge with purified Gal d 5 induced early asthmatic responses as well as allergic manifestations in patients with the bird-egg syndrome (20). Moreover, by using air sampling and immunoblotting, it has been shown that bird serum albumin can be traced in the air of residences with pet birds, demonstrating that Gal d 5 (or other serum albumins from birds) may act as aeroallergens, capable of eliciting respiratory symptoms. Concentrations of Gal d 5 between 3 and 34 µg/mL were sufficient to induce asthmatic responses in sensitized patients during bronchial provocation tests (20).

Although hypersensitivity pneumonitis is the most commonly reported presentation following sensitization to bird antigens, asthmatic responses confirmed by specific inhalation challenges have also been described, particularly among bird fanciers (21,22). Tauer-Reich et al. (23) identified several allergenic components in feather extracts as well as in serum proteins of budgerigar, parrot, pigeon, canary, and hen with molecular weights of 20 to 30 and 67 kDa, the latter allergen very likely corresponding to serum albumin. These investigators showed that inhalable feather dust contains several allergenic components, which cross-react with serum allergens of the same as well as other bird species. IgE antibodies against canary and budgerigar feathers are present in about 20% of canary and budgerigar fanciers with symptoms of atopic disease (24).

A study on 16 poultry workers with work-related rhinitis and asthma showed positive skin tests or radioallergosorbent tests (RAST) to several poultry allergens, including chicken serum, droppings, feathers, or northern fowl mites (*Ornithonyssus sylviarum*) (25). Perfetti et al. (26) reported four poultry-slaughterhouse workers who developed OA confirmed by serial monitoring of spirometry at and away from work. The four subjects showed positive skin-prick tests to chicken feathers and to house dust mites. However, no inhalation challenges were conducted to confirm the implication of chicken feathers as the causative agent of asthma. OA owing to poultry mites has been objectively documented (27), but these mites have been almost eradicated in the modern poultry industry.

MOLD

There are rare reports of mold or yeasts as causes of OA. A case of baker's asthma was proven to be caused by respiratory sensitization to powdered baker's yeast, *Saccharomyces cerevisiae*. Immediate onset of asthma was reported during mixing of yeast with additives and flour (28). Occupational rhinoconjunctivitis and asthma occurred in a research microbiologist working with a slime mold that produced allergenic lysozymal enzymes (29). *Aspergillus* and *Alternaria* mold spores have been isolated from the room air of bakeries. Klaustermeyer et al. (30) reported two bakers with work-related asthma in whom inhalation challenges with either wheat or rye antigens were negative, whereas intracutaneous and bronchial sensitivity were demonstrable to *Aspergillus* and *Alternaria* antigens. In another case report of baker's asthma attributed to respiratory sensitization to *Aspergillus*, a favorable response was observed to allergen immunotherapy with *Aspergillus* antigens (31).

In recent years, putative health effects of indoor mold exposure have been investigated. Some reports have appeared from investigating workers in work environments with obvious mold contamination. Many of the reports in nonoccupational settings have documented a relationship between living in homes with obvious mold growth and respiratory symptoms and generalized manifestations including fatigue, headache, and vague neurological symptoms. However, the exact causal relationship between mold exposure and asthma is obscure.

An outbreak of respiratory disorders was reported by Seuri et al. (32) that was associated with exposure of workers in a military hospital building with substantial chronic water damage. A variety of syndromes were described among 14 employees at the building; the most common was cough, present in nine subjects. Four new cases of asthma were attributed to *Sporobolomyces salmonicolor* exposure and a causal relationship was confirmed by specific inhalation testing, although skin tests with this mold antigen were in the negative. A single case of allergic alveolitis was confirmed and symptoms consistent with occupational rhinitis were also reported. Jaakkola et al. (33) reported in a population-based case–control study that an increased risk for development of asthma was attributable to a workplace where there was visible or olfactory evidence of mold exposure (OR = 1.545; 95% CI, 1.01–2.32). However, the authors did not attempt to confirm a causal link between mold sensitization or exposure and asthma in affected cases.

Santilli and Rockwell (34) evaluated the health effects in two mold-contaminated schools. Environmental sampling for ambient mold counts in one school ranged between 6000 and 50,000 spores/m^3 and was associated with respiratory symptoms, leading to a recommendation to demolish the building. Mold contamination is defined as ambient mold spore counts exceeding 1000 spores/m^3. Among the 85 individuals who reported various work-related symptoms that included nasal congestion, sneezing, cough, wheezing, burning eyes, and fatigue, nine employees were included. Skin testing revealed sensitization to molds in all eight workers who agreed to the testing. The prevalence of asthma in this population was not defined. It is also uncertain if this emerging problem is representative of de novo OA or merely serves as an example of work-aggravated asthma among atopic workers with preexisting mold allergy. Thus, gross contamination of buildings with mold spores has been associated with health effects, manifested by self-reported upper and lower respiratory symptoms that will require more objective characterization in future studies.

PLANTS

Grain dust as well as flour from different sources (wheat, rye, soya, buckwheat, etc.) can cause OA in bakers (Chapter 17). *S. cerevisiae* (28), a yeast, and gluten (35) can also be responsible for OA in bakers. Chlorella algae have caused OA in a pharmacist (36).

Coffee beans have been reported repeatedly to cause OA, as was thoroughly reviewed by Zuskin et al. (37). These authors found a 9% prevalence of asthma and a 25% prevalence of skin reactivity among 45 coffee workers. In the largest epidemiological survey to date, 10% of a group of workers had skin reactions to green coffee beans and 14% of them to the dust that was collected (38). Those subjects who had been employed for a longer period and, therefore, exposed to the dust of green (unroasted) coffee for an equivalent period and with increased specific serum IgE values, had lower forced expiratory volume in one second (FEV)$_1$ results. The extraction of allergens from coffee beans used for bronchoprovocation tests has been described (39,40). Water-soluble extracts from the dust of coffee beans have been used to elicit the causal relationship of symptoms in 22 coffee roastery workers, eight of who had positive bronchial provocation tests and 18 of who had positive prick tests (41). Zuskin et al. (42) studied nine coffee workers who complained of job-related respiratory symptoms. Four had immediate bronchospastic reactions and six had skin reactivity on exposure to green coffee allergens. Roasted coffee can cause OA (43). This case report illustrates that the allergens of green coffee can also be found in roasted coffee albeit at a lesser concentration.

Other beans and seeds from oleaginous plants are also incriminated in the genesis of OA. Several such cases have been reported in the harbor of Marseille (44,45). In Romania, the prevalence of asthma caused by handling the fruit from which castor oil is extracted, by agricultural workers who harvest it has been estimated at 15% of 3000 workers (46) The prevalence of skin reactivity was much higher among symptomatic workers than among asymptomatic workers and reached 80% in those with asthma (46). Castor oil is derived from castor beans (*Ricinus communis*) and is principally used in the production of cosmetics, nylon, explosives, paints, and inks. It was recognized to cause allergic symptoms early in the 20th century, as reviewed by Davison et al. (47). Five cases of asthma caused by castor oil were described by these authors in seamen and laboratory workers (47). IgE antibodies specific to castor bean extracts have been identified (48,49). Seeds of onion (50), sesame (51), fennel (52), sunflower (53), and cacoon (54) can act as sensitizers.

FLOWERS

Although occupational respiratory allergy caused by decorative or horticultural flowers was considered uncommon, over the last years different flowers have been shown to induce occupational rhinitis and asthma, mostly through an IgE-dependent mechanism. Occupational allergy to flowers can be seen among florists, growers, floriculturists, greenhouse workers, gardeners, and flower arrangers. These workers can be exposed to various fresh or dried flowers or nonflowering green plants, which can cause sensitization. These include *Lathyrus odoratus* (55) and baby's breath (*Gypsophila paniculata*) (56), whose allergens have been identified (57), freesia (*Freesia hybride*) and paprika (*Fructus capsici*) (58), amaryllis (*Amaryllis hippeastrum*) (59), spathe flowers (*Spathiphyllum wallisii*) (60), hyacinth (*Hyacinthus orientalis*) (61), narcissus (*Narcissus pseudonarcissus*) (62), and various decorative flowers (63).

A recent cross-sectional survey among 128 florists in Turkey revealed prevalence of work-related asthma symptoms in 14.1% of florists (64). Symptomatic florists were 5.9 times more likely to have a positive skin test response to a flower mix extract. The most prominent risk factors for developing asthma symptoms were work intensity, work duration, small workplace size ($<50\,m^2$), and sensitization to flower mix allergens. Rhinitis and conjunctivitis were also significant risk factors for asthma symptoms (64).

Ornamental dried plants are becoming very popular, however, OA caused by exposure to dried flowers has been reported only with *Limonium tataricum* (65), *G. paniculata* (66), *Carthamus tinctorius*, and *Achillea millefolium* (67).

Weeping fig (*Ficus benjamina*) is a green plant from the genus ficus belonging to the mulberry family. It is used as a decorative houseplant. After reporting two cases of OA (68), Axelsson et al. (69) found that 18 out of 84 plant keepers (21%) had immunological sensitization to the latex from this plant. Allergenic cross-reactivity among *F. benjamina* latex, fig, and other tropical fruits (so called "Ficus-fruit syndrome"), and papain has been reported (70,71). Another nonflowering green plant reported to cause occupational allergic rhinoconjunctivitis is albifloxia (*Tradescantia albifloxia*) (72). A florist suffered from occupational allergic rhinitis and contact urticaria caused by bishop's weed (*Ammi majus*) with demonstration of IgE sensitization (73). A grower of "Bells of Ireland" flowers (*Molucella laevis*) developed seasonal OA owing to IgE-mediated allergy to this flower, which was confirmed by serial measurements of lung function. A specific inhalation challenge elicited a dual asthmatic reaction (74). Recently, the widespread decorative plant "Christmas flower" (*Euphorbia pulcherima*) has been reported to have induced asthma in a sensitized child (75).

Carnation (*Dianthus caryophillus*) is a popular ornamental flower that belongs to the Caryophillacea family, together with *G. paniculata* and *Saponaria officinalis*. This flower was incriminated as the causative agent of occupational rhinitis and asthma in a group of 16 subjects with work-related respiratory symptoms. Specific IgE to allergens from carnation was demonstrated in 15 of these subjects and nasal provocation test with carnation extract was positive in most of them. Immunoblotting showed two major IgE-binding fractions of 34 and 35 kDa in the carnation extract (76). OA owing to simultaneous sensitization to carnation and its common parasite, the red spider mite (*Tetranychus urticae*), has been reported in a greenhouse worker (77) and in a flower supplier (78).

Occupational and environmental IgE-mediated allergy to rose (*Rosa rugosa*) petals and its pollen has been described, affecting mainly the upper airways. Rose handlers, florists, and workers of the rose industry may be at risk of developing rose allergy (79).

Easter lily (*Lilium longiflorum*), belonging to the Liliaceae family, is often used in funeral and bridal decorations and for floral arrangements. Occupational rhinitis and asthma following exposure to Easter lily have been observed in two floral shop workers, as confirmed by positive skin tests, peak flow monitoring, and specific inhalation challenge (80,81). Patients with occupational respiratory allergy to Easter lily usually present concomitant contact urticaria (82) or allergic contact dermatitis (81) to this flower. The prevalence of sensitization to mimosa pollen (*Acacia floribunda*) was 31% in an "at risk" population of floriculturists, whereas it was only 1.2% among atopic subjects. It seems, therefore, that the pollen of *A. floribunda* is potentially allergenic for subjects who are in close proximity (83).

Several cases of occupational respiratory allergy have been reported among workers handling flowers of the Compositae family. In a case series of 14 patients from the Netherlands who had experienced respiratory symptoms (rhinoconjunctivitis, asthma, or both) during their work as florists, growers, or gardeners, the most commonly implicated flowers were chamomile (*Matricaria chamomilla*), Chrysanthemum spp., and *Solidago virgaurea* (84). Out of 14 patients, a positive skin test was seen in 11 patients with exposure to homemade flower extracts of chamomile, in 12 with exposure to solidago, and in seven with exposure to ageratum, all from the Compositae family. The intracutaneous test with mugwort (*Artemisia vulgaris*) extract was positive in all patients, and nearly all subjects had positive IgE (RAST) against mugwort, chrysanthemum, and solidago, suggesting strong allergenic cross-reactivity among different members of the Compositae family. However, the diagnosis of OA was not confirmed by pulmonary function tests in these patients. Sensitization to mugwort pollen was suggested to have positive predictive value in the diagnosis of occupational allergy to Compositae flowers. A florist developed immunological contact urticaria, rhinoconjunctivitis, and late-phase bronchial asthma caused by several Compositae pollen (85).

Sunflower (*Helianthus annus*) is another Compositae flower that may also give rise to occupational allergy. Bousquet et al. (86) reported on a worker who developed occupational rhinoconjunctivitis followed by asthma after exposure to sunflower pollen. This patient had an allergic reaction upon eating honey containing 30% sunflower pollen. Atis et al. (87) reported a 23.5% prevalence of sensitization to sunflower pollen among workers in sunflower processing factories in Turkey. Workers exposed to this pollen had a higher rate of allergic rhinitis and conjunctivitis and showed a significant impairment in lung function as compared to a control group of workers who are not directly exposed to this pollen. The main allergens from sunflower pollen, Hel a 1 (88) and Hel a 2 (89) have been identified and characterized.

Chamomile (*M. chamomilla*) induced occupational contact urticaria, rhinitis, and asthma in a cosmetician who also had allergy to lime flower (90). The globe artichoke (*Cynara scolymus*), a perennial horticultural plant that belongs to the Compositae family, has been reported to induce occupational contact urticaria, rhinitis, and asthma in vegetable warehouse workers through an IgE-mediated mechanism (91,92). Skin-prick tests and IgE determinations to artichoke were positive, and serial peak expiratory flow monitoring confirmed OA in a worker (92).

Immunologic IgE sensitization to the flower of saffron (*Crocus sativus*), a plant commonly grown in Spain for the pistils of its flowers, which yields the species saffron, has been documented among saffron workers (93). Out of 50 saffron handlers, three (6%) were sensitized to saffron pollen and stamen proteins. One worker presented asthma, showing a positive bronchial provocation test, and two patients presented rhinoconjunctivitis, showing positive conjunctival provocation tests. A relevant allergen of 15.5 kDa (profilin) from saffron pollen and stamens was identified by immunoblotting (93). Wall rocket (*Diplotaxis erucoides*) is a common Cruciferae plant that grows in European and American vineyards and olive groves. Its pollen has been shown to elicit IgE-mediated occupational rhinoconjunctivitis and asthma among viticulturists (94,95). Vine (*Vitis vinifera*) pollen has also been reported to cause allergic rhinoconjunctivitis and asthma (96).

GREENHOUSE WORKERS

Cultivation of greenhouse flowers or ornamental plants has emerged as a significant risk factor for asthma (97), with a prevalence of sensitization among exposed workers to workplace allergens greater than 30%. Pollens, molds, and mites, such as the red spider mite *T. urticae*, are the main allergens causing sensitization in this occupational environment. Specific inhalation challenge in the workplace has demonstrated OA in about 20% of the sensitized greenhouse workers (98). The high indoor temperature and humidity facilitates mold growing, particularly of *Cladosporium*, *Penicillium*, *Aspergillus*, and *Alternaria*. Monsó et al. (99) evaluated 39 flower or ornamental plant growers working inside greenhouses in Spain. Sensitization to one or more workplace allergens was found in 13 growers (34.2%), to flowers in eight cases (21%), predominantly to the Compositae such as *Chrysanthemum leucanthemum*, *Solidago canadiensis*, and *H. annus*, and to mold in seven cases (18.4%). Workplace inhalation challenge confirmed OA in three out of five workers with asthma symptoms (prevalence of current OA was 7.7%). These workers were sensitized to several molds in one case, to *Gladiolus* spp. in the second, and to *Aspergillus* and various flowers in the third. However, the specific causative agent inducing OA could not be ascertained. Goldberg et al. (100) have also found a high prevalence (52%) of sensitization to flower allergens in a cross-sectional study of 75 flower growers in Israel. Almost half of the flower growers described ocular or respiratory symptoms associated with occupational exposure to the tested plants.

Sensitization and respiratory symptoms are also very high among greenhouse workers growing bell pepper, with 53.8% of the employees reporting work-related respiratory symptoms (101). In two-thirds of the employees, symptoms at work were associated with an IgE-mediated allergy owing to the high and chronic exposure to bell pepper pollen.

The prevalence of sensitization to chrysanthemum pollen among 104 greenhouse workers was 20.2%, and work-related symptoms, mainly rhinitis, were reported by 56.7% of the employees. Sensitization to chrysanthemum pollen was found to be an important risk factor for the occurrence of work-related symptoms of the upper airways (102).

Three statice (*Limonium sinuatum*) growers, complaining of rhinoconjunctivitis and urticaria induced by harvesting statice in a plastic greenhouse, were shown to have positive reactions following intradermal testing and nasal and eye provocation testing with statice extracts (103). Occupational rhinoconjunctivitis and asthma owing to eggplant (*Solanum melongena*) exposure have been reported in a greenhouse worker, with demonstration of IgE reactivity to eggplant flower petals and pollen (104).

Navarro et al. (105) reported a 25% prevalence of sensitization to *T. urticae* among 246 greenhouse workers. Forty-five of these workers (19%) were allergic to this mite, occurring more often in atopic greenhouse workers. A similar prevalence of sensitization (23%) to the predatory mite *Amblyseius cucumeris* has been reported among exposed horticulturists working in greenhouses (106). Other predatory mites that have been shown to induce IgE-mediated sensitization among greenhouse workers are *Phytoseiulus persimilis* and *Hypoaspis miles* (107).

VEGETABLE GUMS

Several gums have been incriminated as causes of OA. Gums are derived from plants and contain carbohydrates that produce mucilages when they react with water. The various types of gums can be distinguished in the following way (i) gums obtained from exudates, which include (a) acacia or arabic gum derived from *Acacia senegal*, a vegetable grown in Africa, and used in food, pharmaceuticals, and printing; (b) tragacanth, derived from *Astragalus gummifer*, a vegetable grown in Asia and widely used in the printing industry; (c) karaya, derived from *Sterculea urens* (Sterculiacae family), which grows in India and can be used instead of tragacanth; and (ii) gums obtained from seeds, which include (a) carob gum derived from the carob that grows in the Mediterranean region; and (b) guar gum, derived from *Cyamopsis tetragonolobus*, a vegetable grown in India and used in numerous pharmaceutical and food products as well as by carpet manufacturers. Natural gums are high-polymer carbohydrates, which are used as protective colloids and emulsifying agents in food products and pharmaceuticals. In 1933, Spielman and Baldwin (108) described a case of asthma caused by acacia gum. Later, cases of OA among printers exposed to acacia gum were documented. Bohner et al. (109) described 10 such cases, all of who had positive skin tests. Similar cases were also found later (110,111). In 1934, Bullen (112) described a case of asthma in a hairdresser exposed to karaya. In 1943, Gelfand (113) described a case of asthma caused by exposure to tragacanth in a subject working for an import firm. In 1952, Fowler (114) described 32 subjects, all of them printers, who had OA caused by exposure to acacia gum. More recently, guar gum, which is widely used, has been incriminated as causing occupational rhinitis

(115) and asthma (116). The prevalence of sensitization to guar gum among 162 carpet manufacturers has been estimated to vary between 5% (skin testing) and 8% (specific-IgE assessments) (117). In the same survey, it was found that the prevalence of OA as confirmed by specific inhalation challenges was 2%.

Psyllium is a high-molecular-weight gum widely used as a laxative that has been associated with OA, rhinitis, and urticaria associated with sensitization to allergens in the psyllium seed embryo and endospore (118). Allergens are not found in the husk of the psyllium seeds (119). Work-related exposure to psyllium products occurs in several ways—in processing plants that produce psyllium and in nurses chronically handling psyllium when distributing it to patients. Nasal, ocular, and chest symptoms in subjects handling this product have been documented in several case reports (120–129). IgE immunologic sensitization can usually be demonstrated. A self-administered questionnaire showed that 18% of 743 nurses had allergic episodes while handling psyllium, of whom 5% reported respiratory symptoms or hives (127). The prevalence in pharmaceutical workers has been estimated to vary between 28% and 44% (120). A survey of 193 nurses employed by four chronic-care hospitals showed that the prevalence of immunologic sensitization to psyllium varied between 5% (skin testing) and 12% (increased specific IgE levels), whereas 4% had OA as confirmed by specific inhalation challenges (121).

OTHER ALLERGENS

Tea dust can cause respiratory symptoms among workers involved in the primary processing of tea in countries where it is grown (130).The prevalence of OA has been estimated at 6% in 125 workers (131). Shirai et al. (132,133) identified 11 cases of OA owing to exposure to green tea, which is popular in Japan and found evidence that epigallocatechin gallate is the causative agent. The secondary process, tea packing, can be responsible for OA as demonstrated by objective means in four case reports (134,135). Herbal teas made of sage, chamomile, dog rose, and mint can also cause OA as documented in a subject who underwent specific inhalation challenges (136). Various molds that grow on tobacco leaves can be responsible for asthmatic symptoms. These symptoms were reported by a subject, who had a positive inhalation challenge to a fungal extract of *S. brevicaulis* (137). Lander and Gravesen described 16 tobacco workers, including 11 workers who reported asthma symptoms; sensitization was thought to be caused by mircrofungi and/or mites (138).

Garlic dust has been reported to cause OA (139,140). Specific IgE antibodies have been found. Aniseed powder, used as a spice, caused OA confirmed by inhalation challenge (141). Concurrent sensitization and development of IgE-mediated asthma owing to multiple spices (paprika, coriander, and mace) have been documented in a single worker (142). Spices and aromatic herbs have also been reported to cause IgE-mediated sensitization and asthma (143). Although hypersensitivity pneumonitis has been described in cheese workers, OA and bronchitis also seems to represent a significant respiratory ailment (144).

Mushroom powder caused occupational rhinoconjunctivitis and asthma among eight food manufacturing workers who had an immediate skin reaction to a dried mushroom extract, a finding also documented by others (145,146).

Various vegetal products can cause OA: onion (147), potato (148), carrot (149), asparagus (150), chicory (151), sarsaparilla root (152), rose hips (153), ginseng (154), peach leaves (155), fenugreek (156), and kapok (157). Lycopodium powder derived from the herbaceous plant *Lycopodium clavatum* L. has been reported to cause OA in two workers employed by a firm making contraceptive sheaths for men (158). "Maiko" is a dust derived from the tuberous root of devil's tongue (*Amorphophalus konjac*), which is used in the production of a Japanese food product. It has been demonstrated that this agent causes OA through an IgE-mediated mechanism (159). Freeze-dried raspberry used in coating chewing gum can be a cause of OA (160). Pectin powder used in fruit jams causes OA (161). Newmark reported an interesting case of OA owing to hops, presumed to be caused by terpene (162). Various pharmaceutical products can cause OA. Some of these are proteins. Ipecacuanha is a protein product derived from the roots of *Cephaelis ipecacuanha*. It is used as an expectorant or emetic. A survey of 42 employees at a pharmaceutical company was carried out by Luczynska et al. (163). Out of 42 subjects, 19 (45%) had work-related symptoms (rhinitis, conjunctivitis, and/or chest tightness); of these, 10 had skin reactions to ipecacuanha. Three subjects without symptoms also had skin reactions. Specific IgE assessments revealed a similar significant relationship between the presence of symptoms and increased immunological sensitization. Herbs, often prepared by pharmacists and herbalists, are common causes of asthma. Among those, Banha (*Pinella ternata*) (164) and sanyak (165), as well as licorice roots, (166) have been incriminated.

PERSPECTIVES AND RESEARCH NEEDS

HMW agents have been the first agents to be described as responsible for OA. New agents are regularly identified as causing the disease. For many of these agents, the responsible proteins have to be elicited. Also, means to assess IgE-mediated sensitization (validated extracts for skin testing, specific IgE assays, etc.) have to be made available. Reducing exposure, if feasible, to threshold levels that are less likely to induce sensitization and asthma, should be aimed at.

REFERENCES

1. Virtanen T, Zeiler T, Rautiainen J, et al. Immune reactivity of cow-asthmatic dairy farmers to the major allergen of cow (BDA20) and to other cow-derived proteins. The use of purified BDA20 increases the performance of diagnostic tests in respiratory cow allergy. Clin Exp Allergy 1996; 26:188–196.
2. Hinze S, Bergmann KC, Lowenstein H, Hansen GN. Cow hair allergen (Bos d 2) content in house dust: correlation with sensitization in farmers with cow hair asthma. Int Arch Allergy Immunol 1997; 112:231–237.
3. Vargiu A, Vargiu G, Locci F, Giacco S, Del Giacco GS. Hypersensitivity reactions from inhalation of milk proteins. Allergy 1994; 49:386–387.
4. Bernaola G, Echechipia S, Urrutia I, Fernandez E, Audicana M, Fernandez de Corres L. Occupational asthma and rhinoconjunctivitis from inhalation of dried cow's milk caused by sensitization to alpha-lactalbumin. Allergy 1994; 49:189–191.
5. Nahm DH, Park JW, Hong CS. Occupational asthma due to deer dander. Ann Allergy Asthma Immunol 1996; 76:423–426.
6. Schwartz HJ. Raw poultry as a cause of occupational dermatitis, rhinitis and asthma. J Asthma 1994; 31:485–486.
7. Edwards JH, McConnochie K, Trotman DM, Collins G, Saunders MJ, Latham SM. Allergy to inhaled egg material. Clin Allergy 1983; 13:427–432.

8. Bernstein DI, Smith AB, Moller DR, et al. Clinical and immunologic studies among egg-processing workers with occupational asthma. J Allergy Clin Immunol 1987; 80:791–797.

9. Smith AB, Bernstein DI, Aw Tar-Ching, et al. Occupational asthma from inhaled egg protein. Am J Ind Med 1987; 12:205–218.

10. Smith AB, Bernstein DI, London MA, et al. Evaluation of occupational asthma from airborne egg protein exposure in multiple settings. Chest 1990; 98:398–404.

11. Boeniger MF, Lummus ZL, Biagini RE, et al. Exposure to protein aeroallergens in egg processing facilities. Appl Occup Environ Hyg 2001; 16:660–670.

12. Bernstein JA, Kraut A, Bernstein DI, et al. Occupational asthma induced by inhaled egg lysozyme. Chest 1993; 103:532–535.

13. Añibarro B, Fontela JL. Occupational asthma in a cheese worker. Allergy 1996; 51: 960–961.

14. Blanco Carmona JG, Juste Picon S, Garces Sotillos M, Rodriguez Gaston P. Occupational asthma in the confectionary industry caused by sensitivity to egg. Allergy 1992; 47:190–191.

15. Leser C, Hartmann AL, Praml G, Wüthrich B. The egg-egg syndrome: Occupational respiratory allergy to airborne egg proteins with consecutive ingestive egg allergy in the bakery and confectionery industry. J Invest Allergol Clin Immunol 2001; 11:89–93.

16. Escudero C, Quirce S, Fernandez-Nieto M, Miguel J, Cuesta J, Sastre J. Egg white proteins as inhalant allergens associated with baker's asthma. Allergy 2003; 58:616–620.

17. Hoffman DR, Guenther DM. Occupational allergy to avian proteins presenting as allergy to ingestion of egg yolk. J Allergy Clin Immunol 1988; 81:484–488.

18. Szépfalusi Z, Ebner C, Pandjaitan R, et al. Egg yolk alpha-livetin (chicken serum albumin) is a cross-reactive allergen in the bird-egg syndrome. J Allergy Clin Immunol 1994; 93:932–942.

19. Quirce S, Díez-Gómez ML, Eiras P, Cuevas M, Baz G, Losada E. Inhalant allergy to egg yolk and egg white proteins. Clin Exp Allergy 1998; 28:478–485.

20. Quirce S, Marañon F, Umpierrez A, de las Heras M, Fernandez-Caldas E, Sastre J. Chicken serum albumin (Gal d 5) is a partially heat-labile inhalant and food allergen implicated in the bird-egg syndrome. Allergy 2001; 56:754–762.

21. Barr S, Sherman W. Asthma due to parakeet and canary feathers. J Allergy 1961; 32: 17–26.

22. Hargreave FE, Pepys J. Allergic respiratory reactions in bird fanciers provoked by allergen inhalation provocation tests. J Allergy Clin Immunol 1972; 50:157–173.

23. Tauer-Reich I, Fruhmann G, Czuppon AB, Baur X. Allergens causing bird fancier's asthma. Allergy 1994; 49:448–453.

24. van Toorenenbergen AW, Gerth van Wijk R, van Dooremalen G, Dieges PH. Immunoglobulin E antibodies against budgerigar and canary feathers. Int Arch Allergy Appl Immunol 1985; 77:433–437.

25. Bar-Sela S, Teichtahl H, Lutsky I. Occupational asthma in poultry workers. J Allergy Clin Immunol 1984; 73:271–275.

26. Perfetti L, Cartier A, Malo JL. Occupational asthma in poultry-slaughterhouse workers. Allergy 1997; 52:594–595.

27. Lutsky I, Bar-Sela S. Northern fowl mite (*Ornithonyssus sylviarum*) in occupational asthma of poultry workers. Lancet 1982; 2:874–875.

28. Belchi-Hernandez J, Mora-Gonzalez A, Iniesta-Perez J. Baker's asthma caused by *Saccharomyces cerevisiae* in dry powder form. J Allergy Clin Immul 1996; 97:131–134.

29. Gottlieb SJ, Garibaldi E, Hutcheson PS, Slavin RG. Occupational asthma to the slime mold *Dictyostelium discoideum*. J Occup Med 1993; 35:1231–1235.

30. Klaustermeyer WB, Bardana EJ, Hale FC. Pulmonary hypersensitivity to alternaria and aspergillus in baker's asthma. Clin Allergy 1977; 7:227–233.

31. Weiner A. Occupational bronchial asthma in a baker due to Aspergillus. Ann Allergy 1960; 18:1004–1007.

32. Seuri M, Husman K, Kinnunen H, et al. An outbreak of respiratory diseases among workers at a water-damaged building—a case report. Indoor Air 2000; 10:138–145.
33. Jaakkola MS, Nordman H, Piipari R, et al. Indoor dampness and molds and development of adult-onset asthma: a population-based incident case-control study. Environ Health Perspect 2002; 110:543–547.
34. Santilli J, Rockwell W. Fungal contamination of elementary schools: a new environmental hazard. Ann Allergy Asthma Immunol 2003; 90:203–208.
35. Lachance P, Cartier A, Dolovich J, Malo JL. Occupational asthma from reactivity to an alkaline hydrolysis derivative of gluten. J Allergy Clin Immunol 1988; 81:385–390.
36. Ng TP, Tan WC, Lee YK. Occupational asthma in a pharmacist induced by Chlorella, a unicellular algae preparation. Respir Med 1994; 88:555–557.
37. Zuskin E, Valic F, Kanceljak B. Immunological and respiratory changes in coffee workers. Thorax 1981; 36:9–13.
38. Jones RN, Hughes JM, Lehrer SB, et al. Lung function consequences of exposure and hypersensitivity in workers who process green coffee beans. Am Rev Respir Dis 1982; 125:199–202.
39. Karr RM. Bronchoprovocation studies in coffee worker's asthma. J Allergy Clin Immunol 1979; 64:650–654.
40. Lehrer SB, Karr RM, Salvaggio JE. Extraction and analysis of coffee bean allergens. Clin Allergy 1978; 8:217–226.
41. Osterman K, Johansson SGO, Zetterstrom O. Diagnostic tests in allergy to green coffee. Allergy 1985; 40:336–343.
42. Zuskin E, Kanceljak B, Mataija M, Tonkovic-Lojovic M. Specific bronchial reactivity in coffee workers. Arh Hig Rada Toksikol 1989; 40:3–8.
43. Lemière C, Malo JL, McCants M, Lehrer S. Occupational asthma caused by roasted coffee: Immunologic evidence that roasted coffee contains the same antigens as green coffee, but at a lower concentration. J Allergy Clin Immunol 1996; 98:464–466.
44. Charpin J, Zafiropoulo A, Simon L. Asthmes professionnels dus aux oléagineux. J Franç Méd Chir Thor 1961; 15:47–50.
45. Charpin J, Zafiropoulo A, Luccioni R. Asthmes professionnels dans l'industrie des corps gras. Poumon Coeur 1966; 22:513–521.
46. Lupu NG, Dinischiotu GT, Paun R, et al. L'asthme professionnel des cultivateurs de ricin. Concours Méd 1962; 84:5843–5846.
47. Davison AG, Britton MG, Forrester JA, Davies RJ, Hughes DTD. Asthma in merchant seamen and laboratory workers caused by allergy to castor beans: analysis of allergens. Clin Allergy 1983; 13:553–561.
48. Lehrer SB, Karr RM, Muller DJG, Salvaggio JE. Detection of castor allergens in castor wax. Clin Allergy 1980; 10:33–41.
49. Panzani R, Johansson SGO. Results of skin test and RAST in allergy to a clinically potent allergen (castor bean). Clin Allergy 1986; 16:259–266.
50. Navarro JA, del Pozo MD, Gastaminza G, Moneo I, Audicana MT, Fernandez de Corres L. *Allium cepa* seeds: a new occupational allergen. J Allergy Clin Immunol 1995; 96:690–693.
51. Alday E, Curiel G, Lopez-Gil MJ, Carreno D, Moneo I. Occupational hypersensitivity to sesame seeds. Allergy 1996; 51:69–70.
52. Schwartz HJ, Jones RT, Rojas AR, Squillace DL, Yunginger JW. Occupational allergic rhinoconjunctivitis and asthma due to fennel seed. Ann Allergy Asthma Immunol 1997; 78:37–40.
53. Vandenplas O, Vander Borght T, Delwiche JP. Occupational asthma caused by sunflower-seed dust. Allergy 1998; 53:907–908.
54. Rubin JM, Duke MB. Unusual cause of bronchial asthma. Cacoon seed used for decorative purposes. NY State J Med 1974; 74:538–539.

55. Jansen A, Vermeulen A, vanToorenenbergen AW, Dieges PH. Occupational asthma in horticulture caused by *Lathyrus odoratus*. Allergy Proc 1995; 16:135–139.

56. Antepara I, Jauregui I, Urrutia I, Gamboa PM, Gonzalez G, Barber D. Occupational asthma related to fresh *Gypsophila paniculata*. Allergy 1994; 49:478–480.

57. Schroeckenstein DC, Meier-Davis S, Yunginger JW, Bush RK. Allergens involved in occupational asthma caused by baby's breath (*Gypsophila paniculata*). J Allergy Clin Immunol 1990; 86:189–193.

58. vanToorenenbergen AW, Dieges PH. Occupational allergy in horticulture: demonstration of immediate-type allergic reactivity to freesia and praprika plants. Int Archs Allergy Appl Immun 1984; 75:44–47.

59. Jansen APH, Visser FJ, Nierop G, et al. Occupational asthma to amaryllis. Allergy 1996; 51:847–849.

60. Kanerva L, Makinen-Kijunen S, Kiistala R, Granlund H. Occupational allergy caused by spathe flower (*Spathiphyllum wallisii*). Allergy 1995; 50:174–178.

61. Piirila P, Hannu T, Keskinen H, Tuppurainen M. Occupational asthma to hyacinth. Allergy 1998; 53:328–329.

62. Concalo S, Freitas JD, Sousa I. Contact dermatitis and respiratory symptoms from *Narcissus pseudonarcissus*. Contact Dermatitis 1987; 16:115–116.

63. Piirila P, Keskinen H, Leino T, Tupasela O, Tuppurainen M. Occupational asthma caused by decorative flowers: review and case reports. Int Arch Occup Environ Health 1994; 66:131–136.

64. Akpinar-Elci M, Elci OC, Odabasi A. Work-related asthma-like symptoms among florists. Chest 2004; 125:2336–2339.

65. Quirce S, Garcia-Figueroa B, Olaguibel JM, Muro MD, Tabar AI. Occupational asthma and contact urticaria from dried flowers of *Limonium tataricum*. Allergy 1993; 48:285–290.

66. Twiggs JT, Yunginger JW, Agarwal MK, Reed CE. Occupational asthma in a florist caused by the dried plant, baby's breath. J Allergy Clin Immunol 1982; 69:474–477.

67. Compés E, Cuesta J, Fernández-Nieto M, de Miguel J, Quirce S, de las Heras M. Occupational asthma from dried flowers of *Carthamus tinctorius* and *Achillea millefolium*. Allergy 2002; 57:S113.

68. Axelsson G, Skedinger M, Zetterström O. Allergy to weeping fig-a new occupational disease. Allergy 1985; 40:461–464.

69. Axelsson IG, Johansson SG, Zetterström O. Occupational allergy to weeping fig in plant keepers. Allergy 1987; 42:161–167.

70. Diez-Gomez ML, Quirce S, Aragoneses E, Cuevas M. Asthma caused by *Ficus benjamina* latex: evidence of cross-reactivity with fig fruit and papain. Ann Allergy Asthma Immunol 1998; 80:24–30.

71. Hemmer W, Focke M, Gotz M, Jarisch R. Sensitization to *Ficus benjamina*: relationship to natural rubber latex allergy and identification of foods implicated in the Ficus-fruit syndrome. Clin Exp Allergy 2004; 34:1251–1258.

72. Wuthrich B, Johansson SG. Allergy to the ornamental indoor green plant Tradescantia (Albifloxia). Allergy 1997; 52:556–559.

73. Kiistala R, Mäkinen-kiljunen S, Heikkinen K, Rinne J, Haahtela T. Occupational allergic rhinitis and contact urticaria caused by bishop's weed (*Ammi majus*). Allergy 1999; 54:635–639.

74. Miesen WM, van der Heide S, Kerstjens HA, Dubois AE, de Monchy JG. Occupational asthma due to IgE mediated allergy to the flower (Bells of Ireland). Occup Environ Med 2003; 60:701–703.

75. Ibañez MD, Fernandez-Nieto M, Martinez J, et al. Asthma induced by latex from 'Christmas flower' (*Euphorbia pulcherrima*). Allergy 2004; 59:1127–1128.

76. Sanchez-Guerrero IM, Escudero AI, Bartolomé B, Palacios R. Occupational allergy caused by carnation (*Dianthus caryophillus*). J Allergy Clin Immunol 1999; 104:181–185.

77. Cistero-Bahima A, Enrique E, Alonso R, del Mar San Miguel M, Bartolome B. Simultaneous occupational allergy to a carnation and its parasite in a greenhouse worker. J Allergy Clin Immunol 2000; 106:780.

78. Sanchez-Fernandez C, Gonzalez-Gutierrez ML, Esteban-Lopez MI, Martinez A, Lombardero M. Occupational asthma caused by carnation (*Dianthus caryophyllus*) with simultaneous IgE-mediated sensitization to *Tetranychus urticae*. Allergy 2004; 59:114–115.

79. Demir AU, Karakaya G, Kalyoncu AF. Allergy symptoms and IgE immune response to rose: an occupational and an environmental disease. Allergy 2002; 57:936–939.

80. Piirila P, Kanerva L, Alanko K, et al. Occupational IgE-mediated asthma, rhinoconjunctivitis, and contact urticaria caused by Easter lily (*Lilium longiflorum*) and tulip. Allergy 1999; 54:273–277.

81. Vidal C, Polo F. Occupational allergy caused by *Dianthus caryophillus*, *Gypsophila paniculata*, and *Lilium longiflorum*. Allergy 1998; 53:995–998.

82. Piirila P, Lathi A. Contact urticaria and respiratory symptoms from tulips and lilies. Contact Dermatitis 1986; 14:317–319.

83. Ariano R, Panzani RC, Amedeo J. Pollen allergy to mimosa (*Acacia floribunda*) in a Mediterranean area: an occupational disease. Ann Allergy 1991; 66:253–256.

84. de Jong NW, Vermeulen AM, Gerth van Wijk R, de Groot H. Occupational allergy caused by flowers. Allergy 1998; 53:204–209.

85. Uter W, Nohle M, Randerath B, Schwanitz HJ. Occupational contact urticaria and late-phase bronchial asthma caused by compositae pollen in a florist. Am J Contact Dermat 2001; 12:182–184.

86. Bousquet J, Dhivert H, Clauzel AM, Hewitt B, Michel FB. Occupational allergy to sunflower pollen. J Allergy Clin Immunol 1985; 75:70–74.

87. Atis S, Tutluoglu B, Sahin K, Yaman M, Kucukusta AR, Oktay I. Sensitization to sunflower pollen and lung functions in sunflower processing workers. Allergy 2002; 57:35–39.

88. Jimenez A, Moreno C, Martinez J, et al. Sensitization to sunflower pollen: only an occupational allergy? Int Arch Allergy Immunol 1994; 105:297–307.

89. Asturias JA, Arilla MC, Gomez-Bayon N, et al. Cloning and immunological characterization of the allergen Hel a 2 (profilin) from sunflower pollen. Mol Immunol 1998; 35:469–478.

90. Rudzki E, Rapiejko P, Rebandel P. Occupational contact dermatitis, with asthma and rhinitis, from chamomile in a cosmetician also with contact urticaria from both chamomile and lime flowers. Contact Dermatitis 2003; 49:162.

91. Quirce S, Tabar AI, Olaguibel JM, Cuevas M. Occupational contact urticaria syndrome caused by globe artichoke (*Cynara scolymus*). J Allergy Clin Immunol 1996; 97:710–711.

92. Miralles JC, Garcia-Sells J, Bartolome B, Negro JM. Occupational rhinitis and bronchial asthma due to artichoke. Ann Allergy Asthma Immunol 2003; 91:92–95.

93. Feo F, Martinez J, Martinez A, et al. Occupational allergy in saffron workers. Allergy 1997; 52:633–641.

94. Garcia-Ortega P, Bartolome B, Enrique E, Gaig P, Richart C. Allergy to *Diplotaxis erucoides* pollen: occupational sensitization and cross-reactivity with other common pollens. Allergy 2001; 56:679–683.

95. Brito FF, Mur P, Bartolome B, et al. Rhinoconjunctivitis and occupational asthma caused by *Diplotaxis erucoides* (wall rocket). J Allergy Clin Immunol 2001; 108:125–127.

96. Feo Brito F, Martinez A, Palacios R, et al. Rhinoconjunctivitis and asthma caused by vine pollen: a case report. J Allergy Clin Immunol 1999; 103:262–266.

97. Monsó E, Magarolas R, Radon K, et al. Respiratory symptoms of obstructive lung disease in European crop farmers. Am J Respir Crit Care Med 2000; 162:1246–1250.

98. Monsó E. Occupational asthma in greenhouse workers. Curr Opin Pulm Med 2004; 10:147–150.

99.   Monsó E, Magarolas R, Badorrey I, Radon K, Nowak D, Morera J. Occupational asthma in greenhouse flower and ornamental plant growers. Am J Respir Crit Care Med 2002; 165:954–960.
100. Goldberg A, Confino-Cohen R, Waisel Y. Allergic responses to pollen of ornamental plants: high incidence in the general atopic population and especially among flower growers. J Allergy Clin Immunol 1998; 102:210–214.
101. Groenewoud GC, de Jong NW, van Oorschot-van Nes AJ, et al. Prevalence of occupational allergy to bell pepper pollen in greenhouses in the Netherlands. Clin Exp Allergy 2002; 32:434–440.
102. Groenewoud GC, de Jong NW, Burdorf A, de Groot H, van Wyk RG. Prevalence of occupational allergy to Chrysanthemum pollen in greenhouses in the Netherlands. Allergy 2002; 57:835–840.
103. Ueda A, Tochigi T, Ueda T, Aoyama K, Manda F. Immediate type of allergy in statice growers. J Allergy Clin Immunol 1992; 90:742–748.
104. Gil M, Hogendijk S, Hauser C. Allergy to eggplant flower pollen. Allergy 2002; 57:652.
105. Navarro AM, Delgado J, Sanchez MC, et al. Prevalence of sensitization to *Tetranychus urticae* in greenhouse workers. Clin Exp Allergy 2000; 30:863–866.
106. Groenewoud GC, de Graaf in 't Veld C, vVan Oorschot-van Nes AJ, et al. Prevalence of sensitization to the predatory mite *Amblyseius cucumeris* as a new occupational allergen in horticulture. Allergy 2002; 57:614–619.
107. Johansson E, Kolmodin-Hedman B, Kallstrom E, Kaiser L, van Hage-Hamsten M. IgE-mediated sensitization to predatory mites in Swedish greenhouse workers. Allergy 2003; 58:337–341.
108. Spielman AD, Baldwin HS. Atopy to acacia (gum arabic). JAMA 1933; 101:444–445.
109. Bohner CB, Sheldon JM, Trenis JW. Sensitivity to gum acacia, with a report of ten cases of asthma in printers. J Allergy 1941; 12:290–294.
110. Hinault G, Blacque-Bélair A, Buffe D. L'asthme à la gomme arabique dans un grand atelier de typographie. J Franç Méd Chir Thor 1961; 15:51–61.
111. Gaultier M, Fournier E, Gervais P, Vignolet. Un cas d'asthme à la gomme arabique. Histoire clinique, tests cutanés, épreuves fonctionnelles respiratoires. Arch Mal Prof 1960; 21:55–56.
112. Bullen SS. Perennial hay fever from indian gum (Karaya gum). J Allergy 1934; 5: 484–487.
113. Gelfand HH. The allergenic properties of vegetable gums: a case of asthma due to tragacanth. J Allergy 1943; 14:203–219.
114. Fowler PBS. Printers' asthma. Lancet 1952; 2:755–757.
115. Kanerva L, Tupasela O, Jolanki R, Vaheri E, Estlander T, Keskinen H. Occupational allergic rhinitis from guar gum. Clin Allergy 1988; 18:245–252.
116. Lagier F, Cartier A, Somer J, Dolovich J, Malo JL. Occupational asthma caused by guar gum. J Allergy Clin Immunol 1990; 85:785–790.
117. Malo JL, Cartier A, L'Archevêque J, et al. Prevalence of occupational asthma and immunologic sensitization to guar gum among employees at a carpet-manufacturing plant. J Allergy Clin Immunol 1990; 86:562–569.
118. Morgan MS, Arlian LG, Vyszenski-Moher DL, Deyo J, Kawabata T, Fernandez-Caldas E. English plantain and psyllium: lack of cross-allergenicity by crossed immunoelectrophoresis. Ann Allergy Asthma Immunol 1995; 75:351–359.
119. Freeman GL. Psyllium hypersensitivity. Ann Allergy 1994; 73:490–492.
120. Bardy JD, Malo JL, Séguin P, et al. Occupational asthma and IgE sensitization in a pharmaceutical company processing psyllium. Am Rev Respir Dis 1987; 135:1033–1038.
121. Malo JL, Cartier A, L'Archevêque J, et al. Prevalence of occupational asthma and immunologic sensitization to psyllium among health personnel in chronic care hospitals. Am Rev Respir Dis 1990; 142:1359–1366.
122. Gauss WF, Alarie JP, Karol MH. Workplace allergenicity of a psyllium-containing bulk laxative. Allergy 1985; 40:73–76.

123. Scott D. Psyllium-induced asthma. Postgrad Med 1987; 82:160–167.
124. Terho EO, Torkko M. Occupational asthma from psyllium laxatives. Duodecim 1980; 96:1213–1216.
125. Schwartz HJ, Arnold JL, Strohl KP. Occupational allergic rhinitis reaction to psyllium. J Occup Med 1989; 31:624–626.
126. Bernton HS. The allergenicity of psyllium seed. Med Ann Dist Columbia 1970; 39: 313–317.
127. Nelson WL. Allergic events among health care workers exposed to psyllium laxatives in the workplace. J Occup Med 1987; 29:497–499.
128. Breton JL, Leneutre F, Esculpavit G, Abourjaili M. Une nouvelle cause d'asthme professionnel chez un préparateur en pharmacie. Presse Méd 1989; 18:433.
129. Busse WW, Schoenwetter WF. Asthma from psyllium in laxative manufacture. Ann Int Med 1975; 83:361–362.
130. Uragoda CG. Tea maker's asthma. Br J Ind Med 1970; 27:181–182.
131. Uragoda CG. Respiratory disease in tea workers in Sri Lanka. Thorax 1980; 35: 114–117.
132. Shirai T, Reshad K, Yoshitomi A, Chida K, Nakamura H, Taniguchi M. Green tea-induced asthma: relationship between immunological reactivity, specific and non-specific bronchial responsiveness. Clin Exp Allergy 2003; 33:1252–1255.
133. Shirai T, Sato A, Hara Y. Epigallocatechin gallate. The major causative agent of green tea-induced asthma. Chest 1994; 106:1801–1805.
134. Roberts JA, Thomson NC. Tea-dust induced asthma. Eur Respir J 1988; 1:769–770.
135. Cartier A, Malo JL. Occupational asthma due to tea dust. Thorax 1990; 45:203–206.
136. Blanc PD, Trainor WD, Lim DT. Herbal tea asthma. Br J Ind Med 1986; 43:137–138.
137. Lander F, Jepsen JR, Gravesen S. Allergic alveolitis and late asthmatic reaction due to molds in the tobacco industry. Allergy 1988; 43:74–76.
138. Lander F, Gravesen S. Respiratory disorders among tobacco workers. Br J Ind Med 1988; 45:500–502.
139. Lybarger JA, Gallagher JS, Pulver DW, Litwin A, Brooks S, Bernstein IL. Occupational asthma induced by inhalation and ingestion of garlic. J Allergy Clin Immunol 1982; 69:448–454.
140. Anibarro B, Fontela JL, De La Hoz F. Occupational asthma induced by garlic dust. J Allergy Clin Immunol 1997; 100:734–738.
141. Fraj J, Lezaun A, Colas C, Duce F, Dominguez MA, Alonso MD. Occupational asthma induced by aniseed. Allergy 1996; 51:337–339.
142. Sastre J, Olmo M, Novalvos A, Ibanez D, Lahoz C. Occupational asthma due to different spices. Allergy 1996; 51:117–120.
143. Lemière C, Cartier A, Lehrer SB, Malo JL. Occupational asthma caused by aromatic herbs. Allergy 1996; 51:647–649.
144. Dalphin JC, Illig S, Pernet D, Dubiez A, Debieuvre D, Teyssier-Cotte C, Depierre A. Symptômes et fonction respiratoires dans un groupe d'affineurs de gruyère de Comté. Rev Mal Respir 1990; 7:31–37.
145. Symington IS, Kerr JW, McLean DA. Type I allergy in mushroom soup processors. Clin Allergy 1981; 11:43–47.
146. Michils A, Vuyst P De, Nolard N, Servais G, Duchateau J, Yernault JC. Occupational asthma to spores of Pleurotus cornucopiae. Eur Respir J 1991; 1:1143–1147.
147. Valdivieso R, Subiza J, Varela-Losada S, et al. Bronchial asthma, rhinoconjunctivitis, and contact dermatitis caused by onion. J Allergy Clin Immunol 1994; 94:928–930.
148. Quirce S, Gomez ML Diez, et al. Housewives with raw potato-induced bronchial asthma. Allergy 1989; 44:532–536.
149. Quirce S, Blanco R, Diez-Gomez ML, Cuevas M, Eiras P, Losada E. Carrot-induced asthma: immunodetection of allergens. J Allergy Clin Immunol 1997; 99:718–719.
150. Tabar AI, Alvarez-Puebla MJ, Gomez B, et al. Diversity of asparagus allergy: clinical and immunological features. Clin Exp Allergy 2004; 34:131–136.

151. Cadot P, Kochuyt AM, Deman R, Stevens EAM. Inhalative occupational and ingestive immediate-type allergy caused by chicory (*Cichorium intybus*). Clin Exp Allergy 1996; 26:940–944.

152. Vandenplas O, Depelchin S, Toussaint G, Delwiche JP, Weyer R Vande, Saint-Remy JM. Occupational asthma caused by sarsaparilla root dust. J Allergy Clin Immunol 1996; 97:1416–1418.

153. Kwaselow A, Rowe M, Sears-Ewald D, Ownby D. Rose hips: a new occupational allergen. J Allergy Clin Immunol 1990; 85:704–708.

154. Subiza J, Subiza JL, Escribano PM, et al. Occupational asthma caused by Brazil ginseng dust. J Allergy Clin Immunol 1991; 88:731–736.

155. Garcia BE, Lombardero M, Echechipia S, et al. Respiratory allergy to peach leaves and lipid-transfer proteins. Clin Exp Allergy 2004; 34:291–295.

156. Dugue J, Bel J, Figueredo M. Le fenugrec responsable d'un nouvel asthme professionnel. Presse Med 1993; 22:922.

157. Kern DG, Kohn R. Occupational asthma following kapok exposure. J Asthma 1994; 31:243–250.

158. Catilina P, Chamoux A, Gabrillargues D, Catilina MJ, Royfe MH, Wahl D. Contribution à l'étude des asthmes d'origine professionnelle: l'asthme à la poudre de lycopode. Arch Mal Prof 1988; 49:143–148.

159. Kobayashi S. Different aspects of occupational asthma in Japan. In: Frazier CA, ed. Occupational Asthma. New York: Van Nostrand Reinhold Company, 1980:229–244.

160. Sherson D, Andersen B, Hansen I, Kjoller H. Occupational asthma due to freeze-dried raspberry. Ann Allergy Asthma Immunol 2003; 90:660–663.

161. Cohen AJ, Forse MS, Tarlo SM. Occupational asthma caused by pectin inhalation during the manufacture of jam. Chest 1993; 103:309–311.

162. Newmark FM. Hops allergy and terpene sensitivity: an occupational disease. Ann Allergy 1978; 41:311–312.

163. Luczynska CM, Marshall PE, Scarisbrick DA, Topping MD. Occupational allergy due to inhalation of ipecacuanha dust. Clin Allergy 1984; 14:169–175.

164. Kim SH, Jeong H, Kim YK, Cho SH, Min KU, Kim YY. IgE-mediated occupational asthma induced by herbal medicine, Banha (*Pinellia ternata*). Clin Exp Allergy 2001; 31:779–781.

165. Park HS, Kim MJ, Moons HB. Occupational asthma caused by two herb materials, *Dioscorea batatas* and *Pinellia ternata*. Clin Exp Allergy 1994; 24:575–581.

166. Cartier A, Malo JL, Labrecque M. Occupational asthma due to liquorice roots. Allergy 2002; 57:863.

21
Polyisocyanates and Their Prepolymers

Adam V. Wisnewski and Carrie A. Redlich
Department of Internal Medicine, Yale University, New Haven, Connecticut, U.S.A.

Cristina E. Mapp
Section of Hygiene and Occupational Medicine, Department of Clinical and Experimental Medicine, University of Ferrara, Ferrara, Italy

David I. Bernstein
Division of Allergy–Immunology, Department of Internal Medicine, College of Medicine, University of Cincinnati, Cincinnati, Ohio, U.S.A.

INTRODUCTION

Polyisocyanates, a group of low-molecular-weight cross-linking agents, are the most commonly identified cause of occupational asthma (OA) worldwide (1–3). Polyisocyanates are generally synthesized by the reaction of amines or their hydrochlorides with phosgene, and are unique in their ability to catalyze the production of polyurethane—a product of great cultural and commercial importance.

The common feature of all polyisocyanates is the presence of more than one $N=C=O$ group. Diisocyanate monomers (Fig. 1), the forerunners of all polyisocyanates, were first discovered in the late 1840s (4). One prototype, toluene diisocyanate (TDI) was developed by Farben in Germany during World War II for the manufacture of polyurethane, while another, hexamethylene diisocyanate (HDI), was developed by Reinke to create a melt spinnable fiber that would circumvent DuPont's nylon patents (2,4). A number of related compounds have subsequently been developed and utilized commercially, with methylene diphenyl diisocyanate (MDI), naphthalene diisocyanate (NDI), and isophorone diisocyanate (IPDI) being the other major diisocyanates. Diisocyanate dimers, trimers, and polymers based on HDI and MDI are now increasingly being used (Fig. 2). Although these polyisocyanates have inherently lower vapor pressures and volatility in comparison with their corresponding diisocyanate, they can still cause diisocyanate asthma (DA).

Polyisocyanates are used worldwide in a number of important industries. Aliphatic isocyanates such as HDI polymers are used primarily in external coatings and paints (3,5–8). Aromatic isocyanates such as MDI and TDI are used to produce a number of products such as flexible and rigid foams, adhesives, and sealants. For example, they are used extensively in the automobile industry for production of foam rubber cushions,

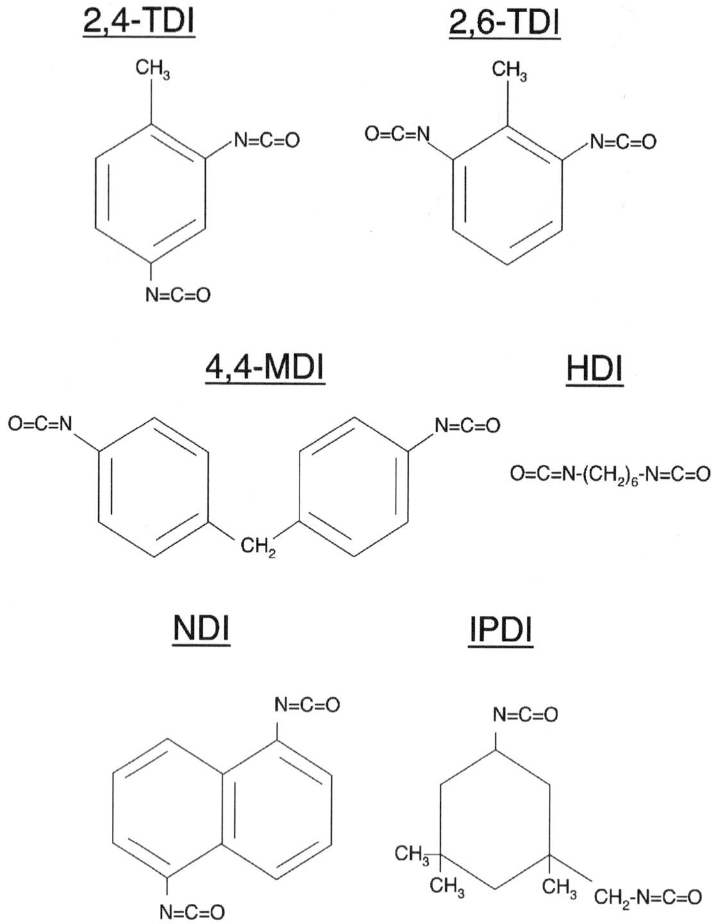

Figure 1 Diisocyanate chemicals.

dashboards, other body parts, and for finished coatings (5–7,9–14). Almost all mold and core processes in modern steel foundries require MDI (12,15–17). MDI also has growing applications such as an insulating material in the building industry, foam mattresses, and footwear, and new uses continue to evolve. MDI is now used to manufacture truck bed liners, synthetic leather, and laminated wood products (8,18).

Environmental exposures of diisocyanates can potentially occur with the use of polyurethane products such as certain glues, insulation products, medical devices, and foam mattresses, in homes, schools, and hospitals. Whether products such as foam mattresses contain free isocyanate groups remains open for debate, but even if present, such diisocyanate exposures will be way below workplace exposures (19).

Worldwide production and consumption of polyisocyanates, mainly MDI and TDI, continues to increase. Production of diisocyanate chemicals has and will continue to increase dramatically in China, where a large corporation has built diisocyanate-manufacturing facilities that produce 11,000 t/yr, and other facilities planned for the future will produce up to 230,000 t annually. Together these ventures will greatly expand the Asian-Pacific market, while the polyisocyanates production rates of United States and Europe are expected to remain steady (20).

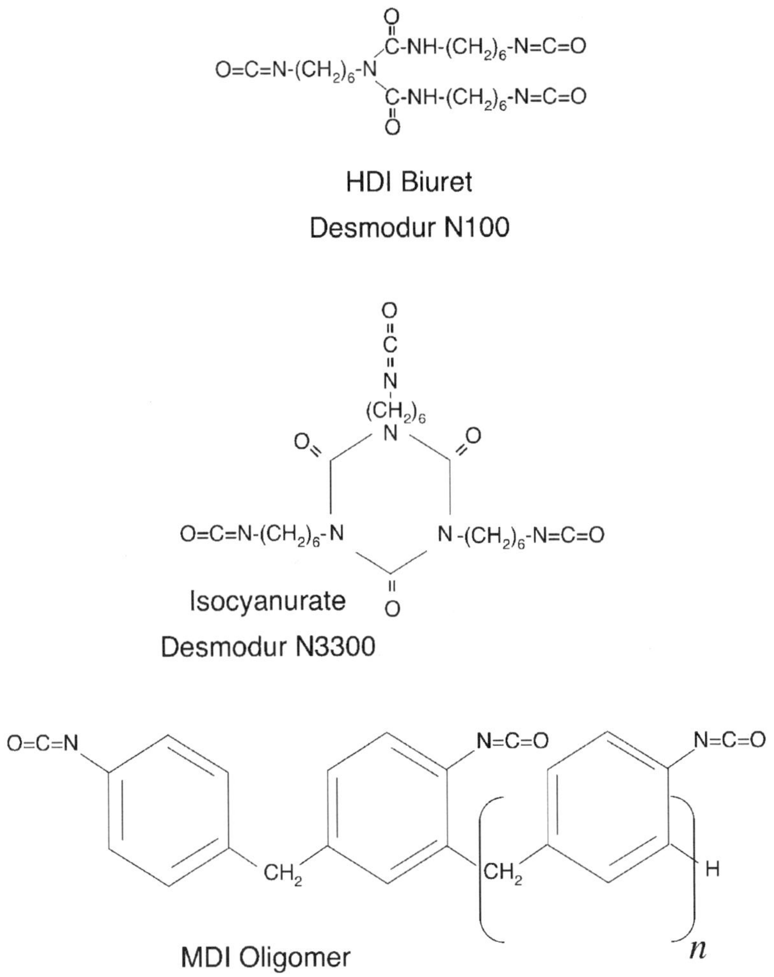

Figure 2 Common polyisocyanate compounds.

BACKGROUND

Almost immediately following the first commercial production of TDI, medical problems arising in associated workers were described. The first report, by Fuchs and Valade in 1951, described the development of asthma in seven of the nine workers exposed to TDI (21). Later reports documented lower respiratory symptoms associated with exposure to other major diisocyanates, even in areas of lower exposure; rare fatal reactions have been documented (9,14,17,22–32). Today, exposure to diisocyanates is recognized as a leading cause of OA; these chemicals are widely produced and consumed in industrialized nations (3,33). Although incidences vary widely depending on the form and type of diisocyanate, and the magnitude, nature, and timing of exposure, it is generally reported that approximately 5% of TDI production workers develop OA on chronic exposure to TDI (34,36). With other polyisocyanates, especially in end-use settings with potentially higher exposures such as spray painting or heat curing foams, asthma prevalences as high as 30% have been estimated (37–39). The structure of the moiety attached to the

N=C=O group (aliphatic or aromatic) and the number of N=C=O groups can alter the vapor pressure and reactivity (7). For example, TDI and HDI are highly volatile at room temperature, whereas MDI is a solid at room temperature and must be heated before considerable vapors are released. Newer polyisocyanates, mainly oligomers of HDI and MDI (Fig. 2) that have vapor pressures much lower than their parent diisocyanate, are being used increasingly (5,7,40). Animal studies suggest some toxicity differences between different diisocyanate monomers and polyisocyanates, but comparative data from human studies are very limited (40).

One of the worst industrial hygiene disasters ever recorded was caused by an accidental release of an isocyanate, monofunctional methyl isocyanate. In 1984, an explosion in a manufacturing plant in Bhopal, India resulted in the release of a cloud of vapor that killed thousands of people living nearby (41). The effects of acute exposure to high levels of methyl isocyanate vapors ranged from irritant symptoms of the upper respiratory tract to lethal lung injury manifested by pulmonary edema and inflammation.

Hypersensitivity pneumonitis (HP), reactive airways dysfunction syndrome (RADS) or irritant-induced asthma, and persistent nonspecific airways hyperresponsiveness are also potential consequences of isocyanate exposure (42). The mechanisms by which isocyanates cause this spectrum of diseases, including asthma and acute toxicity, remain unclear. Because growing numbers of people are occupationally exposed worldwide, better insight into the pathogenesis of isocyanate-induced disorders is needed to improve strategies for diagnosis, prevention, and treatment interventions.

CLINICAL MANIFESTATIONS OF POLYISOCYANATE HYPERSENSITIVITY

The spectrum of disease induced by diisocyanates is broad and includes asthma, RADS or irritant-induced asthma, HP, chemical bronchitis, rhinitis, dermatitis, and pulmonary edema. Asthma is the most common syndrome linked to diisocyanate exposure. Symptoms include rhinorrhea, cough, chest tightness, wheeze, and dyspnea. In many respects, the clinical presentation of isocyanate asthma resembles that of allergic asthma because:

1. only a small proportion of exposed subjects develop asthma,
2. there is a latency period between the onset of exposure and the onset of asthma, and
3. exposure to low levels of the sensitizing agent can induce an attack of asthma. Once an individual has developed asthma, low exposure levels of diisocyanate, as low as 1 ppb for short intervals, may initiate a response (43). Thus, even exposures below those limits mandated by regulatory agencies or those attainable by industrial hygiene methods are often sufficient to stimulate a reaction in a presensitized worker.

In contrast to subjects suffering from asthma induced by aeroallergens, the majority of subjects affected by isocyanate asthma are nonatopic and nonsmokers (44). Although less common than with high-molecular-weight allergens, rhinitis can predate, or coexist with isocyanate asthma (45,46). Onset of asthma is most common in the initial years of exposure to isocyanate. Asthmatic responses following inhalation exposure fall into three categories: (*i*) an early response, usually occurring within minutes following the exposure; (*ii*) a delayed or isolated late asthmatic response occurring 4 to 12 hours after the exposure; or (*iii*) a dual response characterized by both early- and late-phase asthmatic reactions. There have been reports of diurnal association of responses and instances of recurrent late responses over a period of days. An increase in nonspecific airway hyperresponsiveness (NSBH) is usually seen in conjunction with late-phase asthmatic responses. In workers with early responses, NSBH may return to the normal ranges within 24 hours after removal of the worker from the isocyanate environment (47). There have been reports of DA without NSBH; such cases can be explained if airway responsiveness was not tested until after the worker had been removed from work exposure to isocyanates for days or months (48,49). For this reason, methacholine testing, if being used to exclude OA, should be conducted either at work or no later than one to two hours after the last diisocyanate exposure at work (Chapter 7).

The clinical course of isocyanate asthma can be variable. In some workers, asthma resolves following removal of the workers from the isocyanate environment, but in others, asthma persists (50–54). If exposure continues after diagnosis, isocyanate-induced asthma usually persists or often worsens (54,55). The majority of such patients may not recover even years after cessation of diisocyanate exposure (56). The prognosis of OA is better in subjects who, at the time of diagnosis, have better lung function, milder degree of NSBH, shorter duration of exposure and symptoms, and who develop an early (as compared to a late or dual) asthmatic reaction after inhalation challenge with the specific agent. A favorable prognosis is more likely in diisocyanate workers with serum diisocyanate antigen–specific IgE compared to those lacking IgE antibody (56). Prognosis is not influenced by race, sex, or atopy, and it is not improved by relocation to working areas with lower exposure (54,55). Interestingly, persistence of asthma after cessation of exposure is associated with persistent eosinophilic airway inflammation (54,55). In addition to persistent asthmatic symptoms, patients with DA can suffer substantial socioeconomic consequences, including unemployment, decreased wages, and chronic disability (57,58).

High acute irritant-level exposure to diisocyanates has been reported to cause RADS, with the subsequent development of isocyanate sensitization and recurrent asthmatic symptoms at low nonirritant levels documented in a few case reports (59).

EPIDEMIOLOGY

A limited number of longitudinal studies of isocyanate-exposed workers have investigated the incidence and prevalence of isocyanate asthma, primarily in TDI production workers and TDI foam workers (60–62). An annual incidence of isocyanate asthma of 1.8% was seen in a TDI production facility, which declined to less than 1% in a follow-up study, with 6.4% prevalence over a 30-year observation period (62). As noted above, quite variable prevalences of isocyanate asthma have been reported in cross-sectional studies (up to 30%), which are likely related to several factors, including differing exposure conditions, polyisocyanates, coexposures, diagnostic criteria, and possible healthy worker effect (1,40,50,63–65).

Longitudinal studies have also investigated lung function in diisocyanate-exposed workers. Accelerated loss of FEV_1, in diisocyantes polyurethane production workers over a four-year period, and in mold production workers exposed to isocyanates and solvents, has been reported (66,67). However, several recent studies in settings with ongoing medical surveillance have not demonstrated any isocyanate-associated loss in lung function (60,62).

Cross-sectional studies of isocyanate-exposed workers have provided information on the prevalence of isocyanate asthma and risk factors. Generally, greater exposure is associated with a higher prevalence of sensitization and asthma (11,50,69). However, dose–response relationships remain unclear. The impact of factors such as the route of exposure (respiratory, skin), duration of peak exposures, and chemical composition remain poorly defined. Atopy and smoking are not significant risk factors (1,38,44).

UPTAKE, DISTRIBUTION, AND EXCRETION OF POLYISOCYANATES

A number of studies have measured the uptake, distribution, and excretion of polyisocyanates, both in animal models, and in humans exposed under occupational settings. Animal radioisotopic tracing studies with ^{14}C-labeled vapors demonstrate that both MDI and TDI bind to the epithelial linings of the airway in animals, and become broadly distributed throughout the circulatory system, primarily conjugated with albumin (70,71). In clinical studies, HDI has been shown to bind to keratin-18 in the bronchial epithelium and to albumin in the fluid that lines the airway epithelium (72). The total retention rate of isocyanate during human respiratory exposure is estimated to be between 60% and 91%, based on a clinical study by Monso et al. (73). The majority of inhaled isocyanate is excreted in the urine within hours after the exposure (74). However, a pool of isocyanate-conjugated albumin persists in the circulatory system and appears to reach a steady-state level that is dependent upon exposure (75,76). The persistence of isocyanates in vivo in the airways in humans following occupational exposure remains uncertain. In vitro, isocyanate-conjugated proteins can be found in human airway epithelial cells for more than 18 hours post exposure, and may accumulate in phagocytic type cells (77,78).

Together, the published literature from animal and clinical studies clearly demonstrates the uptake of isocyanates via the respiratory tract and excretion via the urine. Other sites, such as the skin, may also take up isocyanates, but this process has not been well quantitated. The persistence of low levels of chemical within the respiratory tract and circulatory system may contribute to immune activation and airways inflammation in exposed workers.

PATHOGENESIS: AIRWAY INFLAMMATION AND CELLULAR RESPONSES

The pathogenesis of isocyanate asthma remains unclear largely due to uncertainties regarding the unique reactivity of the chemical once it is in contact with the human respiratory tract. Like other types of asthma, isocyanate-induced asthma is associated with an inflammatory response in the airways in response to exposure. Increases in the number of CD45$^+$ T cells and eosinophils in airway submucosal tissue have been detected using a diverse array of methods, including broncho-alveolar lavage, endobronchial biopsy, and induced sputum techniques (1,79,80). The increased numbers of CD45$^+$ T cells and eosinophils observed in isocyanate asthma is similar to that observed in nonoccupational types of asthma (81).

Inflammatory changes in the airways of patients with isocyanate asthma differ slightly from that seen in cases of non-OA. An increase in neutrophils and interleukin (IL)-8, a cytokine that induces neutrophils, has been documented in airway secretions of TDI, HDI, and HDI oligomer-exposed individuals (79,82–85). Such findings could relate to irritant effects of isocyanates in susceptible individuals, or to different mechanisms of T-cell (i.e., TH_1) activation in response to exposure.

Immune markers have been investigated in immunocytochemical studies of endobronchial biopsies obtained from workers with DA. In a bronchial biopsy study of workers with DA, Bentley et al. (86) observed an increase in the number of $CD25^+$ T cells and total activated eosinophils. Initially these authors had proposed that the $CD25^+$ T cells represented activated effector T-cell types, because CD25 comprises part of the IL-2 receptor. However, it has recently been appreciated that CD25 is also highly expressed by regulatory T cells (T_{reg}), with the capacity to modulate dendritic cell activity (87). T_{reg} cell responses in isocyanate asthma are yet to be studied.

Two related studies have characterized human T-cell lines derived from endobronchial biopsies of workers with TDI asthma in comparison to that derived from nonoccupational asthmatics (88,89). These studies suggest that $CD8^+$ T cells that secrete interferon (IFN)-γ may predominate in workers with TDI asthma, while $CD4^+$ T cells that make TH_2-type cytokines predominate in nonoccupational "atopic" asthma (88,89). However, more direct in situ characterization of endobronchial biopsies have yielded somewhat conflicting results, demonstrating that TH_2-type $CD4^+$ T cells are found in airway of workers with DA, which may be indistinguishable from that reported in non-OA (9,15,55,80,81,86,90). In situ measurements of cytokines in the airways of individuals with DA have demonstrated the presence of TH_2-type cytokines or chemokines, as well as TH_1 associated cytokines, in both animal models and clinical studies (1,82,90–93).

Analyses of bronchial biopsies have been used to demonstrate polyisocyanate binding to macromolecules in the airway epithelium, with keratin-18 being a predominant in vivo target (72,94). The role of isocyanate–epithelial cell protein conjugates in isocyanate asthma remains unclear, but they may act as antigens that drive airway inflammation following exposure, possibly in an "autoimmune"-like manner. Supportive of this concept are recent studies by Choi et al. (95) demonstrating increased levels of antikeratin antibodies in isocyanate asthmatics as well as individuals with so-called "intrinsic" asthma compared with "atopic" nonoccupational asthmatics.

Reflections of the localized cellular inflammatory response in the lungs of individuals with respiratory disease may also be identified in the peripheral circulation. In isocyanate asthmatics, increases in peripheral blood levels of $CD8^+$ T cells have been reported following exposure in vivo, while in vitro, skewing of the T-cell repertoire in response to isocyanate antigen has been noted (96,97). In one report by Bernstein et al. (97) isocyanate induced preferential usage of particular T-cell antigen receptor genes variable region (V)$_{\beta1}$ and $V_{\beta5}$, while a recent study by Wisnewski et al. (93) demonstrated a strong preferential induction of $V_{\gamma9}V_{\delta2}$ T cells, a subset of which express an unusual $CD8\alpha\alpha^+$ variant. In vitro studies by Lummus et al. (98) document a unique profile of cellular responses to isocyanate antigens, which includes specific increases in monocyte chemoattractant protein (MCP)-1 (originally named histamine-releasing factor) in isocyanate asthmatics, compared to controls. Initial studies indicate that diisocyanate antigen–induced MCP-1 production in vitro may be the best diagnostic indicator of isocyanate asthma, short of specific inhalation challenge (SIC) (99).

To date, studies on isocyanate asthma pathogenesis have yielded somewhat conflicting data, suggesting both differences and similarities with other nonoccupational types of asthma. While TH_2-type airway inflammation is often identifiable in situ, some studies have documented exposure-induced changes that might reflect a more TH_1-like response. In vitro studies also support the concept that isocyanate exposure and asthma may involve cellular responses unlike the typical TH_2 response induced by common environmental allergens.

GENETICS

Further information regarding genetics of OA due to reactive chemicals and isocyanates can be found in Chapter 4. Genetic studies of isocyanate asthma have been limited to date to (*i*) human leukocyte antigen (HLA) genes, which may be directly related to T-cell activation, and (*ii*) genes potentially involved in the metabolism of isocyanates.

HLA class II polymorphisms associated with isocyanate asthma have been identified and upheld in several studies. The data from those studies indicate an association of asthma with HLA DQB1∗0503, but not DQB1∗0501, which differs by a single amino acid (Asp vs. Val) at amino acid 57 (100). These results support the hypothesis of an underlying immunological synapse involving major histocompatibility complex molecule-II (i.e., MHC-II), peptide, and T-cell receptors being central to the development of isocyanate asthma (101,102).

More recent studies on genetic associations between polymorphisms in metabolic enzymes and isocyanate asthma support a different concept, that isocyanate toxicity may be linked to the development of isocyanate asthma. Two studies have suggested an association between common polymorphisms in certain phase I detoxifying enzymes, glutathione S-transferases (GST) M1 and P1, and isocyanate asthma, while others have found associations between phase II detoxifying enzymes, *N*-acetyl transferase 1, phenotype or genotypes and the disease (103–107).

Together, such recent studies have begun to identify specific loci that may be associated with isocyanate asthma. It is likely that isocyanate sensitivity is a multifactorial condition, controlled by a combination of polymorphisms in multiple genes. One long-term goal of future genetic studies is to identify particular genetic haplotypes that might define "at risk" individuals and thus help target disease prevention strategies.

TOXICITY OF ISOCYANATES

Until recently, isocyanate toxicity and sensitization were often studied independently, assuming that the two characteristics were unrelated. However, a number of recent studies have begun to suggest a possible link between the "toxic" properties of isocyanates and the development of allergy. Three parameters that may interconnect toxicity and allergy are (*i*) glutathione, (*ii*) protein conjugation, and (*iii*) oxidative stress.

In 1997, Day et al. (108) showed that isocyanates react rapidly with the reduced form of glutathione (GSH), one of the major antioxidants of the fluid lining the airways, and that GSH–TDI conjugates could be found inside cells that line the airways of exposed animals (109). Furthermore, occupational levels of TDI vapors cause dramatic decreases in GSH levels in primary cultures of human airway epithelial cells in vitro (110). These findings fit with in vivo toxicology studies in rats where one of the first observed effects of acute exposure is decreased levels of GSH inside the airway epithelium, with increased levels of GSH in the fluid lining the airways (111). In animals, drugs that reduce systemic levels of GSH also increase toxicity of isocyanates (112). These findings fit together with the concept that GSH may play a protective role against exposure, based on its ability to "quench" reactive chemicals functionally similar to isocyanates. In light of the recent genetic associations found between GSTs and isocyanate asthma, these findings provide an intriguing link between isocyanate detoxification via GSH and the development of clinical sensitization.

Hints as to how GSH interactions with isocyanates might help protect against isocyanate sensitization have recently emerged. Physiological levels of GSH prevent two processes thought to be central to isocyanate sensitization; isocyanate conjugation to human proteins, and toxicity towards airway epithelial cells (113). While the chemical mechanisms by which GSH is able to impart these protective effects remain undetermined, GSH may be a focal point of future strategies for prevention of isocyanate exposure–induced disease.

GSH-mediated protection from isocyanates may also be important in the context of oxidative stress, given that GSH is a major contributor to thiol–redox homeostasis, which is well known to modulate expression of proinflammatory genes (114–116). The ability of isocyanates to alter thiol–redox homeostasis has been recently shown by three independent studies. In one study by Lantz et al. (110) occupational levels of TDI exposure were shown to decrease intracellular levels of GSH in cultured normal human airway epithelial cells. A second study by Wisnewski et al. (117) used microarray analysis of human airway epithelial cell lines and determined that thioredoxin reductase is upregulated in a dose-dependent manner by subcytotoxic concentrations of isocyanate. Interestingly, the substrate for thioredoxin reductase, thioredoxin, has well-described growth properties for human T cells and, due to early sequencing errors in human thioredoxin, was originally named adult T-cell leukemia–derived factor (118–120). Another study by Elms et al. (121) demonstrated the capacity of isocyanates to modulate redox homeostasis in human monocyte cell lines, with increased intracellular peroxide levels and extracellular adhesion markers on the surface, following in vitro exposure to HDI. Together these studies indicate a link between isocyanate-induced modulation of cellular thiol–redox homeostasis and inflammation, given the intimate link between the two.

ANIMAL STUDIES

Animals have been used to study the direct, acute, and chronic toxic effects of isocyanate exposure, as well as the asthmatic pathophysiology these chemicals are capable of inducing. Animal models have been developed in several different species, each with unique advantages and disadvantages. Experimental models of OA, including those relevant to DA models in rats, guinea pig, and mice, are reviewed in detail in Chapter 6. Novel aspects of experimental models relevant to isocyanates will be discussed here.

Rats: Most of the toxicology studies on the effects of di- and polyisocyanates have been performed in rats. In Wistar rats, the lowest "no-observable-adverse-effects" concentration of different diisocyanates have been determined in acute and chronic exposure settings by focusing on markers of alveolar–capillary barrier permeability, pneumocyte type II activity, release of enzymes from activated phago-cytes, lactate dehydrogenase leakage from injured cells, damaged or increased clara cell activity, surfactant phospholipids, and thiol–redox homeostasis. For aerosols of commonly used HDI and MDI polyisocyanates, the extrapolated lowest no-observed-effects concentrations are roughly similar (0.5–$3 \, mg/m^3$), a concentration roughly one to two orders of magnitude higher than ceiling limits fixed by regulatory agencies for the corresponding diisocyanate. Another report suggests that for poly-meric MDI, concentrations as low as $0.7 \, mg/m^3$ cause transient dysfunction of the pulmonary epithelial barrier, the potential significance of which remains to be deter-mined. Interestingly, depletion of total GSH levels in rats in vivo increases acute respiratory tract polymeric MDI toxicity, consistent with the hypothesis that GSH plays a protective role against exposure, as suggested by in vitro studies (112).

Mice: The advances of transgenic technology for producing overexpressing and gene knockout (KO) mice have provided important new tools for studying human diseases. In the last few years, several investigators have exploited the murine model of isocyanate sensitization first described in 1979 by Tse et al. (122) with several minor modifications and improvements.

Herrick et al. developed an HDI asthma model that involves skin sensitization followed by respiratory tract challenge with HDI–mouse albumin conjugates deliv-ered intranasally. The studies demonstrated a strong dependence of the sensitizing dose on the outcome of exposure as well as a strong genetic susceptibility factor for the development of isocyanate-induced airway inflammatory responses (91,93). Experiments using CD4, CD8, IL-4, and IL-13 KO mice demonstrate that $CD8^+$ T cells mediated contact hypersensitivity responses to HDI in this model, while TH_2-type $CD4^+$ T cells are crucial for isocyanate-induced airway inflammation (91,93). Of note in these studies are the remarkable airway eosinophilia observed and the usage of an HDI albumin conjugates (autologous murine) as the challenge "antigen."

A murine TDI asthma model has recently been described by Lee et al. (123,124) with a slightly different sensitizing regime in which mice are exposed to nebulized TDI (3%) for sensitization and challenge (1%). In this system, vascular endothelial factor (VEGF), matrix metalloproteinase-9 (MMP9), and tissue inhibitor of proteolysis-1 are specifically induced by TDI exposure in sensitized but not unsen-sitized mice. Furthermore, drugs that block VEGF and MMP9 decrease typical TDI-induced pathophysiological changes in the lung, possibly through phosphatidy-linositol 3-kinase–dependent pathways.

Studies by Matheson et al. (78) described a murine TDI asthma model in which mice are exposed to very low sensitizing doses of TDI vapors (0.02 ppm) repeatedly for five days a week for six weeks, in order to mimic occupational exposure (125,126). In this murine model, the effect of the sensitizing dose is well-defined and is consistent with studies by Herrick et al., where acute high-dose exposure led to different responses than lower sensitizing doses. Studies using KO mice show that TH_2-type $CD4^+$ T cells are crucial for sensitization, airway inflammation, and airway hyperreactivity, but also suggest a role for TH_1-type $CD8^+$ T cells and IFN-γ.

A recent study by Vanoirbeek et al. has also established conditions for a TDI murine asthma model and reported dependence of sensitization upon the route and sensitizing dose as mentioned above. The model is similar to the HDI model developed by Herrick et al., in that it involves skin sensitization, and also demonstrates the poten-tially important role for neutrophils in response to exposure (127). This model also further highlights the potential effectiveness of the dermal route of sensitization in inducing respiratory tract hypersensitivity, an observation hinted at by prior clinical studies (18).

Thus, recent years have seen significant utilization of new transgenic mouse strains for studying the pathogenesis of isocyanate asthma. While significant insights have been made, lingering questions remain in translating this research cross-species to humans.

DIAGNOSIS

Diagnosis of DA is often difficult, especially when the asthma is of the delayed type that occurs hours after exposure. Special testing such as a SIC test can provide greater diagnostic certainty but can only be undertaken by a limited number of specialized centers (128). Under certain conditions, workplace challenges may facilitate diagnosis.

During the diagnostic medical evaluation, the dictum of Ramazzini—"ask the patient about his occupation"—is still valid (129). Much essential information can be derived from the history to determine possible contributory host factors, types of agents in the work environment, and the potential for and level of exposure. History should include length and type of present and past employment, including military service, and duration of exposure to diisocyanate agents. Knowledge of past and current hobbies is worth evaluating, because asthma has been reported in individuals exposed to diisocyanates used in these pursuits (130). Development of diisocyanate-induced asthma has been suggested to occur in office workers in a building whose atmosphere was contaminated by diisocyanate discharges from a nearby factory (131). A worker with DA can usually associate his or her asthma with a particular process and can sometimes relate onset of symptoms to exposure to high levels of diisocyanates during an accident or spill (34,35).

On physical examination, chest auscultation reveals wheezing only if the worker has continuous symptoms. Chest X rays are usually negative. If interstitial or patchy infiltrates are observed, hypersensitivity pneumonitis should be suspected (132–135). This complication may rarely be associated with concomitant OA. Rhinitis and conjunctivitis are not infrequent and may be exposure related. The prevalence of upper airway symptoms or signs induced by diisocyanates has not been systematically investigated, but a surprisingly high prevalence was found in one longitudinal study (50). Urticaria, anaphylaxis, eczema, and contact dermatitis have occasionally been reported, but such findings are not useful in diagnosis of DA (50). The use of spirometry, tests of nonspecific airway hyperresponsiveness (i.e., methacholine challenge), as well as workplace challenges and SIC testing, in evaluating DA and OA, are described in detail in Chapters 7, 9, and 10.

LABORATORY TESTING

Immunological tests are of limited clinical value. The few tests available from research laboratories include serological (isocyanate-specific antibody measurements) or cellular measurements of isocyanate-specific proliferative or cytokine responses. Radio-immunoassay testing for isocyanate-specific IgE, has been investigated, but it is well recognized that test sensitivity is too low to serve as a reliable diagnostic marker, and may become undetectable after an undetermined period the worker is away from exposure (136–138). Enzyme-linked immunosorbent assays or western blots for isocyanate-specific IgG are often helpful in confirming prior immunological exposure to isocyanates, and isocyanate-specific IgG may be highly elevated in cases of isocyanate-induced HP. However, such antibodies can be found in nonsymptomatic exposed workers, and this finding appears more relevant to exposure than disease (135,139,140).

In detecting polyisocyanate immunologic reactions, the role of the polyisocyanate–protein conjugate used as the "antigen" is extremely important. Most clinical studies to date have used albumin as the carrier—a good choice based on current in vivo studies in animals and clinical studies. However, methods to avoid under- or oversubstitution of protein carrier moieties remain relatively nonstandardized between laboratories, and new methods for producing "polyisocyanate antigens" continue to evolve (141–148). Mimicking the in vivo microenvironment may be crucial in the production of biologically relevant isocyanate antigens as shown by recent studies using mixed phase (vapor/liquid) exposure systems. A three dimensional model of HDI–albumin conjugates recognized by human immunoglobulins has recently been proposed, based on mass spectrometry analysis and binding studies with these antigens (148). Preliminary studies suggest that "lightly" substituted isocyanate–protein conjugates may be more like those that occur naturally in the airways of exposed workers (148). The possibility that other, nonalbumin carrier proteins exist for isocyanates has not been exhausted and may help explain some of the apparent differences between polyisocyanates and other allergens, if isocyanate conjugates with these proteins also serve as antigens.

Aside from serologic tests, newer tests are being developed to aid in the diagnosis of isocyanate sensitization. In reports to date, one test that has shown only limited promise is the lymphocyte proliferation test, akin to that which has been developed to detect beryllium sensitization (77,149,150). Another cell-based assay recently reported by Bernstein et al. (99) demonstrates the possibility of using isocyanate antigen–induced in vitro expression of MCP-1 as a biomarker for disease (98). Further tests evaluating the repertoire of isocyanate antigens' effects on human immune cells using modern approaches such as microarray, proteomics, or metabolomics, hold promise for the future development of laboratory tests.

BRONCHOPROVOCATION TESTING

A review of SIC testing is presented in detail in Chapter 10. Inhalation challenges may cause early (10–20%), dual (30–50%), or late (30–50%) asthmatic reactions in individuals with a history of asthma induced by TDI (44). The challenge is highly specific because no reaction is induced in normal subjects or in asthmatics not sensitized to TDI. Dual and late, but not early, TDI-induced asthmatic reactions are associated with transient increase of NSBH to methacholine, which lasts for at least 24 hours, and such increase of NSBH is specific because it does not occur in normal subjects or in non-TDI–exposed asthmatics (48,151–153).

Inhalation challenge remains the gold standard for confirming a diagnosis of DA in an individual worker; it is also an important research tool for confirming the diagnosis and monitoring the disease (151–154). Such testing is not without risk to the patient and should not be lightly undertaken, because transient increases in NSBH may persist as long as 30 days after a diisocyanate challenge (155). It is advisable to obtain informed consent from the subject before the test is undertaken.

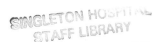
Testing should be performed in specialized centers and conducted by experienced personnel, with all safety measures as recommended by international guidelines (156,157). Although challenges with diisocyanates are highly specific if the test is positive, they may not be sufficiently sensitive, especially if they are performed with subthreshold concentrations. It can also be difficult to generate and monitor the appropriate polyisocyanate, especially aerosols of products such as HDI biuret. Thus, a negative inhalation challenge does not exclude the presence of OA. To determine if a negative test is truly negative, guidelines suggest that workers be reintroduced into the workplace for further monitoring of lung function during exposure to diisocyanates (156).

If moderate or severe respiratory impairment is present, challenge should not be performed. Published guidelines have been issued which formulate standard approaches to performing SIC tests with chemicals (156). A review of evidence to support these recommendations has recently been published (158). Because there is currently no standardized method of provocation testing, it is difficult to interpret and compare results from different centers. Generation and monitoring of the challenge atmosphere must be undertaken only by environmental experts, and in facilities designed especially for challenge procedures that depend on the type of diisocyanate being tested. For some isocyanates, it is very difficult to deliver the agent in an aerosol or vapor phase, and special delivery systems have been devised (157). Sometimes, such as with paint spraying, it has been possible to reproduce the conditions of occupational exposure in the laboratory but, as with all bronchoprovocation tests, it is vital that diisocyanate levels be measured. In all environmental challenges, the importance of appropriate control exposures cannot be overemphasized.

Since SIC testing is usually not available, a workplace challenge study in which a worker is trained to record serial peak expiratory flow rates (PEFR) at intervals of two to four hours before and during the workshift, and at periods away from work including weekends, should be attempted. Burge et al. (159) have shown that occupational exposure studies, in which worksite pulmonary function testing has been performed, can be of value. However, PEFR studies that have shown a high sensitivity in diagnosing OA have typically been performed with the worker being at least two weeks away from work—conditions that can be difficult to achieve (160). However, because it is not possible to always monitor self-recorded peak flow rates, prevarication of data can occur (161). Results should be evaluated with care, because testing is effort dependent and results may be less than ideal in a patient seeking to prove disability. The use of serial peak flow rates in evaluation of OA is reviewed in Chapter 9.

INDUSTRIAL HYGIENE

Quantifying polyisocyanates is complex. The exposures frequently contain mixtures of different polymeric products, and can occur in both vapor and aerosol phase. In addition, there are several different exposure metrics or units used to express isocyanate exposures, making it difficult to compare findings (40). Typically the $N=C=O$ content of an air sample is measured and then expressed as total $N=C=O$ count or mass (40). Methods to measure dermal exposure are limited.

Current isocyanate occupational exposure limits (OELs) are predominantly for diisocyanate monomers, with few for polyisocyanates, even though exposure to polyisocyanates is increasingly predominant. In the United States, the Occupational

Safety and Health Administration has a ceiling permissible exposure limits for TDI and MDI monomers (20 ppb) but no time-weighted average standard for other monomers or polyisocyanates. The American Conference of Governmental Industrial Hygienists and National Institute for Occupational Safety and Health have monomer threshold limit value (TLV) of 5 ppb, but no TLV for polyisocyanates. Thus polyisocyanates remain largely unregulated. European countries are commencing to use the same metric (total reactive isocyanate group) for all isocyanate species, including monomers and polyisocyanates, which should greatly facilitate exposure assessment and control. As mentioned, many workers can relate onset of OA to short-term, high-level exposure in an industrial accident or spill where levels far exceed the TLV. In addition, dermal exposure may also be an important route of sensitization, especially with less volatile polyisocyanates. While levels below the TLV may be appropriate to prevent chronic decrements in lung function, once a worker is sensitized, exposure to levels below the TLV can elicit asthmatic responses (151–153,156).

SURVEILLANCE AND PREVENTION

Surveillance is recommended for DA, based upon the finding that prolonged symptomatic exposure correlates with worse clinical outcomes. However, data on the efficacy and costs of surveillance is more limited. Retrospective studies using Canadian workers' compensation data have demonstrated improved clinical outcomes and fewer cases of asthma associated with the institution of medical surveillance programs, although other factors such as improved hygiene or increased awareness of hazards could also be involved (69,162). A recent model-based approach found a favorable cost effectiveness ratio for screening for isocyanates (39).

Nevertheless, implementation of surveillance programs and improvement in industrial hygiene technology promise to be means of reducing diisocyanate-induced lung diseases. Better controlled methods of avoiding exposure, such as more efficient extractor hoods, dermal protection, and use of positive pressure hoods, may decrease incidence of asthma.

TREATMENT

In workers with confirmed DA, pharmacotherapy should never be considered as an alternative to cessation of exposure. Avoidance and elimination of further ambient diisocyanate exposure is the most essential treatment modality. Once isocyanate exposure has been modified, drug treatment of chronic OA is identical to that of non-OA (163–166).

It is noteworthy that several studies have been performed to examine the effects of pretreatment with pharmacologic agents on isocyanate asthmatic responses elicited by SIC. Oral and inhaled glucocorticoids have been shown to mitigate TDI-induced late asthmatic reactions and associated increases in airway responsiveness, whereas sustained-release of theophylline partially inhibits the early and late asthmatic reactions and has no effect on the increased airway responsiveness (167–170). Atropine, salbutamol alone, cromolyn, verapamil, and ketotifen do not prevent TDI-induced asthmatic reactions and the associated increase of NSBH (169,170).

FUTURE DIRECTIONS IN RESEARCH

Isocyanate asthma is an enigmatic condition and there are unanswered questions regarding disease pathogenesis, susceptibility, and diagnosis. Future studies that may address outstanding issues are listed below:

- *Define possible immunologic mechanisms*: It is unlikely that IgE-mediated immune mechanisms alone explain DA. Further investigation of alternative immune responses, especially those that are cell mediated, may yield new insights. As mentioned, utilization of novel diisocyanate–protein conjugates, prepared in vapor phase as well as liquid phase and at different molar substitution ratios, may help to define immune mechanisms, if they exist. Newly developed murine models, which are able to induce sensitization via chronic inhalational or dermal exposure, are also likely to provide new insights into the immunopathogenesis of DA.
- *Genetic studies*: It is likely that multiple and diverse genes contribute to the pathogenesis of OA. Immune response genes as well as detoxifying enzyme genes have already been linked to DA. Data generated in candidate gene case–control studies in Italy and Finland indicate that genotypic markers (HLA Class II alleles, GST) may partially define susceptibility for DA. Clearly, there may be heretofore-undefined disease-associated gene polymorphisms. Genotypes or genotype combinations associated with DA will need to be investigated in different background populations, but these studies must be controlled for background ethnicity, which would require appropriate genome control markers.
- *Diagnosis*: The SIC test is the most definitive diagnostic method, but is expensive, not widely available, and false negative results can occur. Development of an alternative standardized protocol for performing workplace challenge testing would fill an unmet need. This aim could be achieved in a multicenter study and would likely include assessment of biomarkers of inflammation (i.e., induced sputum inflammatory cells and cytokines), serial testing of lung function, as well as careful workplace exposure assessment and appropriate exposed control groups. It would be necessary to validate results in comparison to those of the SIC test.

REFERENCES

1. Redlich CA, Karol MH. Diisocyanate asthma: clinical aspects and immunopathogenesis. Int Immunopharmacol 2002; 2(2–3):213–224.
2. Mapp C, Butcher BT, Fabbri LM. In: Bernstein D, ed. Polyisocyanates and their prepolymers 1st ed. 2001.
3. Chan-Yeung M, Malo JL, Tarlo SM, et al. Proceedings of the first Jack Pepys Occupational Asthma Symposium. Am J Respir Crit Care Med 2003; 167(3):450–471.
4. Urlich H. Chemistry and Technology of Isocyanates. England: John Wiley & Sons Ltd., 1996.
5. Stowe M, Winewski AV, Holm CT, et al. Cross-sectional study of auto body workers exposed to isocyanates: immunologic responses. Am J Resp Crit Care Med 2005; 171(A).
6. Woskie SR, Sparer J, Gore RJ, et al. Determinants of isocyanate exposures in auto body repair and refinishing shops. Ann Occup Hyg 2004; 48(5):393–403.

7. Sparer J, Stowe MH, Bello D, et al. Isocyanate exposures in autobody shop work: the SPRAY study. J Occup Environ Hyg 2004; 1(9):570–581.
8. Lofgren DJ, Walley TL, Peters PM, Weis ML. MDI exposure for spray-on truck bed lining. Appl Occup Environ Hyg 2003; 18(10):772–779.
9. Fabbri LM, Danieli D, Crescioli S, et al. Fatal asthma in a subject sensitized to toluene diisocyanate. Am Rev Respir Dis 1988; 137(6):1494–1498.
10. Redlich CA, Stowe MH, Coren BA, Wisnewski AV, Holm CT, Cullen MR. Diisocyanate-exposed auto body shop workers: a one-year follow-up. Am J Ind Med 2002; 42(6): 511–518.
11. Redlich CA, Stowe MH, Wisnewski AV, et al. Subclinical immunologic and physiologic responses in hexamethylene diisocyanate-exposed auto body shop workers. Am J Ind Med 2001; 39(6):587–597.
12. Tse KS, Johnson A, Chan H, Chan-Yeung M. A study of serum antibody activity in workers with occupational exposure to diphenylmethane diisocyanate. Allergy 1985; 40(5):314–320.
13. Welinder H, Nielsen J, Bensryd I, Skerfving S. IgG antibodies against polyisocyanates in car painters. Clin Allergy 1988; 18(1):85–93.
14. White WG, Morris MJ, Sugden E, Zapata E. Isocyanate-induced asthma in a car factory. Lancet 1980; 1(8171):756–760.
15. Carino M, Aliani M, Licitra C, Sarno N, Ioli F. Death due to asthma at workplace in a diphenylmethane diisocyanate-sensitized subject. Respiration 1997; 64(1):111–113.
16. Liss GM, Bernstein DI, Moller DR, Gallagher JS, Stephenson RL, Bernstein IL. Pulmonary and immunologic evaluation of foundry workers exposed to methylene diphenyldiisocyanate (MDI). J Allergy Clin Immunol 1988; 82(1):55–61.
17. Zammit-Tabona M, Sherkin M, Kijek K, Chan H, Chan-Yeung M. Asthma caused by diphenylmethane diisocyanate in foundry workers. Clinical, bronchial provocation, and immunologic studies. Am Rev Respir Dis 1983; 128(2):226–230.
18. Petsonk EL, Wang ML, Lewis DM, Siegel PD, Husberg BJ. Asthma-like symptoms in wood product plant workers exposed to methylene diphenyl diisocyanate. Chest 2000; 118(4):1183–1193.
19. Krone CA, Klingner TD, Ely JT. Polyurethanes and childhood asthma. Med Sci Monit 2003; 9(12):HY39–HY43.
20. http://www.bayer.com.
21. Fuchs S, Valade P. Clinical and experimental study of some cases of poisoning by desmodur T (1-2-4 and 1–2-6 di-isocyanates of toluene). Arch Mal Prof 1951; 12(2): 191–196.
22. Friebel H, Luchtrath H. Effects of toluylene diisocyanate (desmodur T) on the respiratory tract. Naunyn Schmiedebergs Arch Exp Pathol Pharmakol 1955; 227(2):93–110.
23. Swensson A, Holmquist CE, Lundgren KD. Injury to the respiratory tract by isocyanates used in making lacquers. Br J Ind Med 1955; 12(1):50–53.
24. Woodbury JW. Asthmatic syndrome following exposure to tolylene diisocyanate. Ind Med Surg 1956; 25(11):540–543.
25. Hama GM. Symptoms in workers exposed to isocyanates; suggested exposure concentrations. AMA Arch Ind Health 1957; 16(3):232–233.
26. Johnstone RT. Toluene-2, 4-diisocyanate; clinical features. Ind Med Surg 1957; 26(1): 33–34.
27. Zapp JA Jr. Hazards of isocyanates in polyurethane foam plastic production. AMA Arch Ind Health 1957; 15(4):324–330.
28. Walworth HT, Virchow WE. Industrial hygiene experiences with toluene diisocyanate. Am Ind Hyg Assoc J 1959; 20(3):205–210.
29. Kessler RC. Pulmonary sensitization to toluene diisocyanate. J Occup Med 1960; 2: 143–147.
30. Elkins HB, McCarl GW, Brugsch HG, Fahy JP. Massachusetts experience with toluene di-isocyanate. Am Ind Hyg Assoc J 1962; 23:265–272.

31. Brugsch HG, Elkins HB. Toluene di-isocyanate (TDI) toxicity. N Engl J Med 1963; 268:353–357.

32. Konzen RB, Craft BF, Scheel LD, Gorski CH. Human response to low concentrations of p,p-diphenylmethane diisocyanate (MDI). Am Ind Hyg Assoc J 1966; 27(2): 121–127.

33. Baur X, Chen Z, Marczynski B. Respiratory diseases caused by occupational exposure to 1,5-naphthalene-diisocyanate (NDI): results of workplace-related challenge tests and antibody analyses. Am J Ind Med 2001; 39(4):369–372.

34. Diem JE, Jones RN, Hendrick DJ, et al. Five-year longitudinal study of workers employed in a new toluene diisocyanate manufacturing plant. Am Rev Respir Dis 1982; 126(3):420–428.

35. Butcher BT, Jones RN, O'Neil CE, et al. Longitudinal study of workers employed in the manufacture of toluene-diisocyanate. Am Rev Respir Dis 1977; 116(3):411–421.

36. Peters JM, Wegman DH. Epidemiology of toluene diisocyanate (TDI)-induced respiratory disease. Environ Health Perspect 1975; 11:97–100.

37. Seguin P, Allard A, Cartier A, Malo JL. Prevalence of occupational asthma in spray painters exposed to several types of isocyanates, including polymethylene polyphenylisocyanate. J Occup Med 1987; 29(4):340–344.

38. Vandenplas O, Malo JL, Saetta M, Mapp CE, Fabbri LM. Occupational asthma and extrinsic alveolitis due to isocyanates: current status and perspectives. Br J Ind Med 1993; 50(3):213–228.

39. Wild DM, Redlich CA, Paltiel AD. Surveillance for isocyanate asthma: a model based cost effectiveness analysis. Occup Environ Med 2005; 62(11):743–749.

40. Bello D, Woskie SR, Streicher RP, et al. Polyisocyanates in occupational environments: a critical review of exposure limits and metrics. Am J Ind Med 2004; 46(5):480–491.

41. Weill H. Disaster at Bhopal: the accident, early findings and respiratory health outlook in those injured. Bull Eur Physiopathol Respir 1987; 23(6):587–590.

42. Luo JC, Nelsen KG, Fischbein A. Persistent reactive airway dysfunction syndrome after exposure to toluene diisocyanate. Br J Ind Med 1990; 47(4):239–241.

43. Butcher BT, Karr RM, O'Neil CE, et al. Inhalation challenge and pharmacologic studies of toluene diisocyanate (TDI)-sensitive workers. J Allergy Clin Immunol 1979; 64(2):146–152.

44. Mapp CE, Boschetto P, Dal Vecchio L, Maestrelli P, Fabbri LM. Occupational asthma due to isocyanates. Eur Respir J 1988; 1(3):273–279.

45. Littorin M, Welinder H, Skarping G, Dalene M, Skerfving S. Exposure and nasal inflammation in workers heating polyurethane. Int Arch Occup Environ Health 2002; 75(7):468–474.

46. Sari-Minodier I, Charpin D, Signouret M, Poyen D, Vervloet D. Prevalence of self-reported respiratory symptoms in workers exposed to isocyanates. J Occup Environ Med 1999; 41(7):582–588.

47. Durham SR, Graneek BJ, Hawkins R, Taylor AJ. The temporal relationship between increases in airway responsiveness to histamine and late asthmatic responses induced by occupational agents. J Allergy Clin Immunol 1987; 79(2):398–406.

48. Mapp CE, Dal Vecchio L, Boschetto P, De Marzo N, Fabbri LM. Toluene diisocyanate-induced asthma without airway hyperresponsiveness. Eur J Respir Dis 1986; 68(2): 89–95.

49. Karol MH, Tollerud DJ, Campbell TP, et al. Predictive value of airways hyperresponsiveness and circulating IgE for identifying types of responses to toluene diisocyanate inhalation challenge. Am J Respir Crit Care Med 1994; 149(3 Pt 1):611–615.

50. Bernstein DI, Korbee L, Stauder T, et al. The low prevalence of occupational asthma and antibody-dependent sensitization to diphenylmethane diisocyanate in a plant engineered for minimal exposure to diisocyanates. J Allergy Clin Immunol 1993; 92(3): 387–396.

51. Banks DE, Rando RJ, Barkman HW Jr. Persistence of toluene diisocyanate-induced asthma despite negligible workplace exposures. Chest 1990; 97(1):121–125.

52. Allard C, Cartier A, Ghezzo H, Malo JL. Occupational asthma due to various agents. Absence of clinical and functional improvement at an interval of four or more years after cessation of exposure. Chest 1989; 96(5):1046–1049.

53. Moller DR, McKay RT, Bernstein IL, Brooks SM. Persistent airways disease caused by toluene diisocyanate. Am Rev Respir Dis 1986; 134(1):175–176.

54. Mapp CE, Corona PC, De Marzo N, Fabbri L. Persistent asthma due to isocyanates. A follow-up study of subjects with occupational asthma due to toluene diisocyanate (TDI). Am Rev Respir Dis 1988; 137(6):1326–1329.

55. Paggiaro P, Bacci E, Paoletti P, et al. Bronchoalveolar lavage and morphology of the airways after cessation of exposure in asthmatic subjects sensitized to toluene diisocyanate. Chest 1990; 98(3):536–542.

56. Piirila PL, Nordman H, Keskinen HM, et al. Long-term follow-up of hexamethylene diisocyanate-, diphenylmethane diisocyanate-, and toluene diisocyanate-induced asthma. Am J Respir Crit Care Med 2000; 162(2 Pt 1):516–522.

57. Vandenplas O, Toren K, Blanc PD. Health and socioeconomic impact of work-related asthma. Eur Respir J 2003; 22(4):689–697.

58. Moscato G, Dellabianca A, Perfetti L, et al. Occupational asthma: a longitudinal study on the clinical and socioeconomic outcome after diagnosis. Chest 1999; 115(1):249–256.

59. Leroyer C, Perfetti L, Cartier A, Malo JL. Can reactive airways dysfunction syndrome (RADS) transform into occupational asthma due to "sensitisation" to isocyanates? Thorax 1998; 53(2):152–153.

60. Clark RL, Bugler J, Paddle GM, Chamberlain JD, Allport DC. A 17-year epidemiological study on changes in lung function in toluene diisocyanate foam workers. Int Arch Occup Environ Health 2003; 76(4):295–301.

61. Clark RL, Bugler J, McDermott M, Hill ID, Allport DC, Chamberlain JD. An epidemiology study of lung function changes of toluene diisocyanate foam workers in the United Kingdom. Int Arch Occup Environ Health 1998; 71(3):169–179.

62. Ott MG, Klees JE, Poche SL. Respiratory health surveillance in a toluene di-isocyanate production unit 1967–97: clinical observations and lung function analyses. Occup Environ Med 2000; 57(1):43–52.

63. Woellner RC, Hall S, Greaves I, Schoenwetter WF. Epidemic of asthma in a wood products plant using methylene diphenyl diisocyanate. Am J Ind Med 1997; 31(1):56–63.

64. Musk AW, Peters JM, Wegman DH. Isocyanates and respiratory disease: current status. Am J Ind Med 1988; 13(3):331–349.

65. Simpson C, Garabrant D, Torrey S, Robins T, Franzblau A. Hypersensitivity pneumonitis-like reaction and occupational asthma associated with 1,3-bis(isocyanatomethyl) cyclohexane pre-polymer. Am J Ind Med 1996; 30(1):48–55.

66. Wegman DH, Musk AW, Main DM, Pagnotto LD. Accelerated loss of FEV- in polyurethane production workers: a four-year prospective study. Am J Ind Med 1982; 3(2):209–215.

67. Akbar-Khanzadeh F, Rivas RD. Exposure to isocyanates and organic solvents, and pulmonary-function changes in workers in a polyurethane molding process. J Occup Environ Med 1996; 38(12):1205–1212.

68. Diller WF. Frequency and trends of occupational asthma due to toluene diisocyanate: a critical review. Appl Occup Environ Hyg 2002; 17(12):872–877.

69. Tarlo SM, Liss GM, Yeung KS. Changes in rates and severity of compensation claims for asthma due to diisocyanates: a possible effect of medical surveillance measures. Occup Environ Med 2002; 59(1):58–62.

70. Kennedy AL, Wilson TR, Stock MF, Alarie Y, Brown WE. Distribution and reactivity of inhaled 14C-labeled toluene diisocyanate (TDI) in rats. Arch Toxicol 1994; 68(7):434–443.

71. Kennedy AL, Stock MF, Alarie Y, Brown WE. Uptake and distribution of 14C during and following inhalation exposure to radioactive toluene diisocyanate. Toxicol Appl Pharmacol 1989; 100(2):280–292.

72. Wisnewski AV, Srivastava R, Herick C, et al. Identification of human lung and skin proteins conjugated with hexamethylene diisocyanate in vitro and in vivo. Am J Respir Crit Care Med 2000; 162(6):2330–2336.

73. Monso E, Cloutier Y, Lesage J, Perreault G, Malo JL. What is the respiratory retention of inhaled hexamethylene di-isocyanate? Eur Respir J 2000; 16(4):729–730.

74. Liu Y, Berode M, Stowe MH, et al. Urinary hexane diamine to assess respiratory exposure to hexamethylene diisocyanate aerosol: a human inhalation study. Int J Occup Environ Health 2004; 10(3):262–271.

75. Johannesson G, Sennbro CJ, Willix P, Lindh CH, Jonsson BA. Identification and characterisation of adducts between serum albumin and 4,4'-methylenediphenyl diisocyanate (MDI) in human plasma. Arch Toxicol 2004; 78(7):378–383.

76. Sennbro CJ, Lindh CH, Tinnerberg H, et al. Development, validation and characterization of an analytical method for the quantification of hydrolysable urinary metabolites and plasma protein adducts of 2,4- and 2,6-toluene diisocyanate, 1,5-naphthalene diisocyanate and 4,4'-methylenediphenyl diisocyanate. Biomarkers 2003; 8(3–4):204–217.

77. Wisnewski AV, Lemus R, Karol MH, Redlich CA. Isocyanate-conjugated human lung epithelial cell proteins: a link between exposure and asthma? J Allergy Clin Immunol 1999; 104(2 Pt 1):341–347.

78. Matheson JM, Lemus R, Lange RW, Karol MH, Luster MI. Role of tumor necrosis factor in toluene diisocyanate asthma. Am J Respir Cell Mol Biol 2002; 27(4):396–405.

79. Lemiere C, Pelissier S, Tremblay C, et al. Leukotrienes and isocyanate-induced asthma: a pilot study. Clin Exp Allergy 2004; 34(11):1684–1689.

80. Maestrelli P, Calcagni PG, Saetta M, et al. Sputum eosinophilia after asthmatic responses induced by isocyanates in sensitized subjects. Clin Exp Allergy 1994; 24(1):29–34.

81. Robinson DS, Hamid Q, Ying S, et al. Predominant TH2-like bronchoalveolar T-lymphocyte population in atopic asthma. N Engl J Med 1992; 326(5):298–304.

82. Park H, Jung K, Kim H, Nahm D, Kang K. Neutrophil activation following TDI bronchial challenges to the airway secretion from subjects with TDI-induced asthma. Clin Exp Allergy 1999; 29(10):1395–1401.

83. Sastre J, Banks DE, Lopez M, Barkman HW, Salvaggio JE. Neutrophil chemotactic activity in toluene diisocyanate (TDI)-induced asthma. J Allergy Clin Immunol 1990; 85(3):567–572.

84. Valentino M, Governa M, Fiorini R. Increased neutrophil leukocyte chemotaxis induced by release of a serum factor in toluene-diisocyanate (TDI) asthma. Lung 1988; 166(6):317–325.

85. Fabbri LM, Boschetto P, Zocca E, et al. Bronchoalveolar neutrophilia during late asthmatic reactions induced by toluene diisocyanate. Am Rev Respir Dis 1987; 136(1): 36–42.

86. Bentley AM, Maestrelli P, Saetta M, et al. Activated T-lymphocytes and eosinophils in the bronchial mucosa in isocyanate-induced asthma. J Allergy Clin Immunol 1992; 89(4):821–829.

87. Shi HZ, Li S, Xie ZF, Qin XJ, Qin X, Zhong XN. Regulatory CD4+CD25+ T lymphocytes in peripheral blood from patients with atopic asthma. Clin Immunol 2004; 113(2):172–178.

88. Del Prete GF, De Carli M, D'Elios MM, et al. Allergen exposure induces the activation of allergen-specific Th2 cells in the airway mucosa of patients with allergic respiratory disorders. Eur J Immunol 1993; 23(7):1445–1449.

89. Maestrelli P, Del Prete GF, De Carli M, et al. CD8 T-cell clones producing interleukin-5 and interferon-gamma in bronchial mucosa of patients with asthma induced by toluene diisocyanate. Scand J Work Environ Health 1994; 20(5):376–381.

90. Maestrelli P, Occari P, Turato G, et al. Expression of interleukin (IL)-4 and IL-5 proteins in asthma induced by toluene diisocyanate. Clin Exp Allergy 1997; 27(11): 1292–1298.

91. Herrick CA, Xu L, Wisnewski AV, Das J, Redlich CA, Bottomly K. A novel mouse model of diisocyanate-induced asthma showing allergic-type inflammation in the lung after inhaled antigen challenge. J Allergy Clin Immunol 2002; 109(5):873–878.

92. Liu Q, Wisnewski AV. Recent developments in diisocyanate asthma. Ann Allergy Asthma Immunol 2003; 90(5 suppl 2):35–41.

93. Wisnewski AV, Herrick CA, Liu Q, Chen L, Bottomly K, Redlich CA. Human gamma/delta T-cell proliferation and IFN-gamma production induced by hexamethylene diisocyanate. J Allergy Clin Immunol 2003; 112(3):538–546.

94. Redlich CA, Karol MH, Graham C, et al. Airway isocyanate-adducts in asthma induced by exposure to hexamethylene diisocyanate. Scand J Work Environ Health 1997; 23(3):227–231.

95. Choi JH, Nahm DH, Kim SH, et al. Increased levels of IgG to cytokeratin 19 in sera of patients with toluene diisocyanate-induced asthma. Ann Allergy Asthma Immunol 2004; 93(3):293–298.

96. Finotto S, Fabbri LM, Rado V, Mapp CE, Maestrelli P. Increase in numbers of CD8 positive lymphocytes and eosinophils in peripheral blood of subjects with late asthmatic reactions induced by toluene diisocyanate. Br J Ind Med 1991; 48(2):116–121.

97. Bernstein JA, Munson J, Lummus ZL, Balakrishnan K, Leikauf G. T-cell receptor V beta gene segment expression in diisocyanate-induced occupational asthma. J Allergy Clin Immunol 1997; 99(2):245–250.

98. Lummus ZL, Alam R, Bernstein JA, Bernstein DI. Diisocyanate antigen-enhanced production of monocyte chemoattractant protein-1, IL-8, and tumor necrosis factor-alpha by peripheral mononuclear cells of workers with occupational asthma. J Allergy Clin Immunol 1998; 102(2):265–274.

99. Bernstein DI, Cartier A, Cote J, et al. Diisocyanate antigen-stimulated monocyte chemoattractant protein-1 synthesis has greater test efficiency than specific antibodies for identification of diisocyanate asthma. Am J Respir Crit Care Med 2002; 166(4): 445–450.

100. Mapp CE, Beghe B, Balboni A, et al. Association between HLA genes and susceptibility to toluene diisocyanate-induced asthma. Clin Exp Allergy 2000; 30(5):651–656.

101. Nel AE, Slaughter N. T-cell activation through the antigen receptor. Part 2: role of signaling cascades in T-cell differentiation, anergy, immune senescence, and development of immunotherapy. J Allergy Clin Immunol 2002; 109(6):901–915.

102. Nel AE. T-cell activation through the antigen receptor. Part 1: signaling components, signaling pathways, and signal integration at the T-cell antigen receptor synapse. J Allergy Clin Immunol 2002; 109(5):758–770.

103. Mapp CE. The role of genetic factors in occupational asthma. Eur Respir J 2003; 22(1):173–178.

104. Piirila P, Wikman H, Luukkonen R, et al. Glutathione S-transferase genotypes and allergic responses to diisocyanate exposure. Pharmacogenetics 2001; 11(5):437–445.

105. Mapp CE, Fryer AA, De Marzo N, et al. Glutathione S-transferase GSTP1 is a susceptibility gene for occupational asthma induced by isocyanates. J Allergy Clin Immunol 2002; 109(5):867–872.

106. Wikman H, Piirila P, Rosenberg C, et al. N-Acetyltransferase genotypes as modifiers of diisocyanate exposure-associated asthma risk. Pharmacogenetics 2002; 12(3):227–233.

107. Berode M, Jost M, Ruegger M, Savolainen H. Host factors in occupational diisocyanate asthma: a Swiss longitudinal study. Int Arch Occup Environ Health 2005; 78(2): 158–163.

108. Day BW, Jin R, Basalyga DM, Kramarik JA, Karol MH. Formation, solvolysis, and transcarbamoylation reactions of bis(S-glutathionyl) adducts of 2,4- and 2,6-diisocyanatotoluene. Chem Res Toxicol 1997; 10(4):424–431.

109. Lange RW, Day BW, Lemus R, Tyurin VA, Kagan VE, Karol MH. Intracellular S-glutathionyl adducts in murine lung and human bronchoepithelial cells after exposure to diisocyanatotoluene. Chem Res Toxicol 1999; 12(10):931–936.

110. Lantz RC, Lemus R, Lange RW, Karol MH. Rapid reduction of intracellular glutathione in human bronchial epithelial cells exposed to occupational levels of toluene diisocyanate. Toxicol Sci 2001; 60(2):348–355.

111. Pauluhn J. Inhalation toxicity of 1,6-hexamethylene diisocyanate homopolymer (HDI-IC) aerosol: results of single inhalation exposure studies. Toxicol Sci 2000; 58(1):173–181.

112. Pauluhn J. Acute inhalation toxicity of polymeric diphenyl-methane 4,4′-diisocyanate in rats: time course of changes in bronchoalveolar lavage. Arch Toxicol 2000; 74(4–5):257–269.

113. Wisnewski AV, Liu Q, Liu J, Redlich CA. Glutathione protects human airway proteins and epithelial cells from isocyanates. Clin Exp Allergy 2005; 35(3):325–327.

114. Rahman I, Gilmour PS, Jimenez LA, MacNee W. Oxidative stress and TNF-alpha induce histone acetylation and NF-kappaB/AP-1 activation in alveolar epithelial cells: potential mechanism in gene transcription in lung inflammation. Mol Cell Biochem 2002; 234–235(1–2):239–248.

115. Rahman I, Mulier B, Gilmour PS, et al. Oxidant-mediated lung epithelial cell tolerance: the role of intracellular glutathione and nuclear factor-kappaB. Biochem Pharmacol 2001; 62(6):787–794.

116. Rahman I, MacNee W. Oxidative stress and regulation of glutathione in lung inflammation. Eur Respir J 2000; 16(3):534–554.

117. Wisnewski AV, Liu Q, Miller JJ, Magoski N, Redlich CA. Effects of hexamethylene diisocyanate exposure on human airway epithelial cells: in vitro cellular and molecular studies. Environ Health Perspect 2002; 110(9):901–907.

118. Iwata S, Hori T, Sato N, et al. Adult T cell leukemia (ATL)-derived factor/human thioredoxin prevents apoptosis of lymphoid cells induced by L-cystine and glutathione depletion: possible involvement of thiol-mediated redox regulation in apoptosis caused by pro-oxidant state. J Immunol 1997; 158(7):3108–3117.

119. Wakasugi N, Tagaya Y, Wakasugi H, et al. Adult T-cell leukemia-derived factor/ thioredoxin, produced by both human T-lymphotropic virus type I- and Epstein-Barr virus-transformed lymphocytes, acts as an autocrine growth factor and synergizes with interleukin 1 and interleukin 2. Proc Natl Acad Sci USA 1990; 87(21):8282–8286.

120. Gasdaska PY, Oblong JE, Cotgreave IA, Powis G. The predicted amino acid sequence of human thioredoxin is identical to that of the autocrine growth factor human adult T-cell derived factor (ADF): thioredoxin mRNA is elevated in some human tumors. Biochim Biophys Acta 1994; 1218(3):292–296.

121. Elms J, Beckett PN, Griffin P, Curran AD. Mechanisms of isocyanate sensitisation. An in vitro approach. Toxicol In Vitro 2001; 15(6):631–634.

122. Tse CS, Pesce AJ. Chemical characterization of isocyanate-protein conjugates. Toxicol Appl Pharmacol 1979; 51:39–46.

123. Lee KS, Jin SM, Kim SS, Lee YC. Doxycycline reduces airway inflammation and hyperresponsiveness in a murine model of toluene diisocyanate-induced asthma. J Allergy Clin Immunol 2004; 113(5):902–909.

124. Lee YC, Song CH, Lee HB, et al. A murine model of toluene diisocyanate-induced asthma can be treated with matrix metalloproteinase inhibitor. J Allergy Clin Immunol 2001; 108(6):1021–1026.

125. Matheson JM, Johnson VJ, Luster MI. Immune mediators in a murine model for occupational asthma: studies with toluene diisocyanate. Toxicol Sci 2005; 84(1):99–109.

126. Matheson JM, Lange RW, Lemus R, Karol MH, Luster MI. Importance of inflammatory and immune components in a mouse model of airway reactivity to toluene diisocyanate (TDI). Clin Exp Allergy 2001; 31(7):1067–1076.

127. Vanoirbeek JA, Tarkowski M, Ceuppens JL, Verbeken EK, Nemery B, Hoet PH. Respiratory response to toluene diisocyanate depends on prior frequency and concentration of dermal sensitization in mice. Toxicol Sci 2004; 80(2):310–321.

128. Bernstein DI, Jolly A. Current diagnostic methods for diisocyanate induced occupational asthma. Am J Ind Med 1999; 36(4):459–468.

129. Rammazzini B. De Morbis Artifictum Diatriba. In: Wright WC, ed. Translated from Latin Text. New York: Hafner, 1964.

130. Pepys J, Hutchcroft BJ. Bronchial provocation tests in etiologic diagnosis and analysis of asthma. Am Rev Res Dis 1975; 112(6):829–859.

131. Darcey D, Lipscomb HJ, Epling C, Pate W, Cherry LP, Bernstein J. Clinical findings for residents near a polyurethane foam manufacturing plant. Arch Environ Health 2002; 57(3):239–246.

132. Merget R, Marczynski B, Chen Z, et al. Haemorrhagic hypersensitivity pneumonitis due to naphthylene-1,5-diisocyanate. Eur Respir J 2002; 19(2):377–380.

133. Yoshizawa Y, Ohtani Y, Hayakawa H, Sato A, Suga M, Ando M. Chronic hypersensitivity pneumonitis in Japan: a nationwide epidemiologic survey. J Allergy Clin Immunol 1999; 103(2 Pt 1):315–320.

134. Buick JB, Todd GR. Concomitant alveolitis and asthma following exposure to triphenylmethane triisocyanate. Occup Med (Lond) 1997; 47(8):504–506.

135. Baur X. Hypersensitivity pneumonitis (extrinsic allergic alveolitis) induced by isocyanates. J Allergy Clin Immunol 1995; 95(5 Pt 1):1004–1010.

136. Baur X, Chen Z, Flagge A, Posch A, Raulf-Heimsoth M. EAST and CAP specificity for the evaluation of IgE and IgG antibodies to diisocyanate-HSA conjugates. Int Arch Allergy Immunol 1996; 110(4):332–338.

137. Baur X, Dewair M, Fruhmann G. Detection of immunologically sensitized isocyanate workers by RAST and intracutaneous skin tests. J Allergy Clin Immunol 1984; 73(5 Pt 1):610–618.

138. Tee RD, Cullinan P, Welch J, Burge PS, Newman-Taylor AJ. Specific IgE to isocyanates: a useful diagnostic role in occupational asthma. J Allergy Clin Immunol 1998; 101(5):709–715.

139. Lushniak BD, Reh CM, Bernstein DI, Gallagher JS. Indirect assessment of 4,4'-diphenylmethane diisocyanate (MDI) exposure by evaluation of specific humoral immune responses to MDI conjugated to human serum albumin. Am J Ind Med 1998; 33(5):471–477.

140. Lemus R, Lukinskeine L, Bier ME, Wisnewski AV, Redlich CA, Karol MH. Development of immunoassays for biomonitoring of hexamethylene diisocyanate exposure. Environ Health Perspect 2001; 109(11):1103–1108.

141. Karol MH, Alarie Y. Antigens which detect IgE antibodies in workers sensitive to toluene diisocyanate. Clin Allergy 1980; 10(1):101–109.

142. Karol MH, Hauth BA. Use of hexyl isocyanate antigen to detect antibodies to hexamethylene diisocyanate (HDI) in sensitized guinea pigs and in a sensitized worker. Fundam Appl Toxicol 1982; 2(3):108–113.

143. Karol MH, Alarie YC. Serologic test for toluene diisocyanate (TDI) antibodies (letter). J Occup Med 1978; 20(6):383.

144. Karol MH, Ioset HH, Alarie YC. Tolyl-specific IgE antibodies in workers with hypersensitivity to toluene diisocyanate. Am Ind Hyg Assoc J 1978; 39(6):454–458.

145. Karol MH, Riley EJ, Alarie Y. Presence of tolyl-specific IgE and absence of IgG antibodies in workers exposed to toluene diisocyanate. J Environ Sci Health C: Environ Health Sci 1979; 13(3):221–232.

146. Karol MH, Sandberg T, Riley EJ, Alarie Y. Longitudinal study of tolyl-reactive IgE antibodies in workers hypersensitive to TDI. J Occup Med 1979; 21(5):354–358.

147. Scheel LD, Killens R, Josephson A. Immunochemical aspects of toluene diisocyanate (TDI) toxicity. Am Ind Hyg Assoc J 1964; 25:179–184.

148. Wisnewski AV, Stowe MH, Cartier A, et al. Isocyanate vapor-induced antigenicity of human albumin. J Allergy Clin Immunol 2004; 113(6):1178–1184.

149. Avery SB, Stetson DM, Pan PM, Mathews KP. Immunological investigation of individuals with toluene diisocyanate asthma. Clin Exp Immunol 1969; 4(5):585–596.

150. Newman LS, Mroz MM, Balkissoon R, Maier LA. Beryllium sensitization progresses to chronic beryllium disease: a longitudinal study of disease risk. Am J Respir Crit Care Med 2005; 171(1):54–60.
151. Mapp CE, Polato R, Maestrelli P, Hendrick DJ, Fabbri LM. Time course of the increase in airway responsiveness associated with late asthmatic reactions to toluene diisocyanate in sensitized subjects. J Allergy Clin Immunol 1985; 75(5):568–572.
152. Sterk PJ, Fabbri LM, Quanjer PH, et al. Airway responsiveness. Standardized challenge testing with pharmacological, physical and sensitizing stimuli in adults. Report Working Party Standardization of Lung Function Tests, European Community for Steel and Coal. Official Statement of the European Respiratory Society. Eur Respir J Suppl 1993; 16: 53–83.
153. Vandenplas O, Malo JL. Inhalation challenges with agents causing occupational asthma. Eur Respir J 1997; 10(11):2612–2629.
154. Butcher BT, Hammad YY, Hendrick DJ. Occupational asthma: identification in the agent. In: Gee JBL, ed. Occupational Lung Disease. New York: Churchill Livingstone, 1984:111.
155. Fabbri LM. Occupational Asthma. In: O'Bryne PM, ed. Asthma as an Inflammatory Disease. New York: Marcel Dekker, Inc., 1990.
156. Tarlo SM, Boulet LP, Cartier A, et al. Canadian Thoracic Society guidelines for occupational asthma. Can Respir J 1998; 5(4):289–300.
157. Banks DE, Sastre J, Butcher BT, et al. Role of inhalation challenge testing in the diagnosis of isocyanate-induced asthma. Chest 1989; 95(2):414–423.
158. Nicholson PJ, Cullinan P, Taylor AJ, Burge PS, Boyle C. Evidence based guidelines for the prevention, identification, and management of occupational asthma. Occup Environ Med 2005; 62(5):290–299.
159. Burge PS, O'Brien IM, Harries MG. Peak flow rate records in the diagnosis of occupational asthma due to isocyanates. Thorax 1979; 34(3):317–323.
160. Perrin B, Lagier F, L'Archeveque J, et al. Occupational asthma: validity of monitoring of peak expiratory flow rates and non-allergic bronchial responsiveness as compared to specific inhalation challenge. Eur Respir J 1992; 5(1):40–48.
161. Malo JL, Cartier A, Ghezzo H, Chan-Yeung M. Compliance with peak expiratory flow readings affects the within- and between-reader reproducibility of interpretation of graphs in subjects investigated for occupational asthma. J Allergy Clin Immunol 1996; 98(6 Pt 1):1132–1134.
162. Tarlo SM, Liss GM. Diisocyanate-induced asthma: diagnosis, prognosis, and effects of medical surveillance measures. Appl Occup Environ Hyg 2002; 17(12):902–908.
163. Tarlo SM, Liss GM. Occupational asthma: an approach to diagnosis and management. Cmaj 2003; 168(7):867–871.
164. Sheffer AL, Silverman M, Woolcock AJ, Diaz PV, Lindberg B, Lindmark B. Long-term safety of once-daily budesonide in patients with early-onset mild persistent asthma: results of the Inhaled Steroid Treatment as Regular Therapy in Early Asthma (START) study. Ann Allergy Asthma Immunol 2005; 94(1):48–54.
165. Rodrigo GJ, Rodrigo C. Triple inhaled drug protocol for the treatment of acute severe asthma. Chest 2003; 123(6):1908–1915.
166. Blake KV. Drug treatment of airway inflammation in asthma. Pharmacotherapy 2001; 21(3 Pt 2):3S–20S.
167. Fabbri LM, Chiesura-Corona P, Dal Vecchio L, et al. Prednisone inhibits late asthmatic reactions and the associated increase in airway responsiveness induced by toluene-diisocyanate in sensitized subjects. Am Rev Respir Dis 1985; 132(5): 1010–1014.
168. Fabbri LM, Di Giacomo R, Dal Vecchio L, et al. Prednisone, indomethacin and airway responsiveness in toluene diisocyanate sensitized subjects. Bull Eur Physiopathol Respir 1985; 21(5):421–426.

169. Mapp C, Boschetto P, dal Vecchio L, et al. Protective effect of antiasthma drugs on late asthmatic reactions and increased airway responsiveness induced by toluene diisocyanate in sensitized subjects. Am Rev Respir Dis 1987; 136(6):1403–1407.

170. Tossin L, Chiesura-Corona P, Fabbri LM, et al. Ketotifen does not inhibit asthmatic reactions induced by toluene di-isocyanate in sensitized subjects. Clin Exp Allergy 1989; 19(2):177–182.

22
Western Red Cedar (*Thuja plicata*) and Other Wood Dusts

Moira Chan-Yeung
Occupational and Environmental Lung Disease Unit, Respiratory Division, Department of Medicine, University of British Columbia and Vancouver General Hospital, Vancouver, British Columbia, Canada

Jean-Luc Malo
Department of Chest Medicine, Université de Montréal and Sacré-Cœur Hospital, Montreal, Quebec, Canada

INTRODUCTION

Exposure to wood dust is a common occurrence in all countries because of its traditional use as fuel and in constructions for human habitation. Exposure to wood dusts can cause contact dermatitis and cancer of the nasopharynx. Respiratory illnesses associated with exposure to wood dust include asthma, hypersensitivity pneumonitis, organic dust toxic syndrome, chronic bronchitis, and mucous membrane irritation syndrome (1,2). In most instances respiratory illness is caused by exposure to chemical compounds in the wood dust. For many types of wood dust, the nature of the responsible chemical compound remains unknown; in others, the disease is caused by exposure to the molds or bacteria growing on the wood chips, bark, or bonding materials used in the wood strips or boards. By far, the most common respiratory illness reported from wood dust exposure is asthma. The disease usually arises as a result of occupational exposure, although in some individuals it may result from exposure in their hobby.

Many different species of wood have been identified as being associated with occupational asthma. They are often highly prized for durability and quality of appearance. The extent to which they are used in construction and furniture industries is not known. Most cases of occupational asthma caused by wood dusts were published as case reports, except that caused by western red cedar (WRC) (*Thuja plicata*). Occupational asthma caused by WRC has been studied extensively because it affects a vast number of workers in the primary industries of the West coast of North America and in countries where red cedar is exported. For this reason, western red cedar asthma (WRCA) will be discussed in detail first.

OCCUPATIONAL ASTHMA DUE TO WRC (*THUJA PLICATA*)

WRC is an important species of wood in the Pacific Northwest region, particularly in the coastal areas. In these areas, cedar accounts for approximately 20% of the total volume of sound wood, the other principal species being Douglas fir and hemlock. It has been used extensively for poles, shakes, shingles, and lumber for exterior construction because of its well-known high durability. WRCA affects sawmill workers, shingle and shake mill workers, workers in remanufacturing plants, carpenters, construction workers, and cabinet makers.

Chemical Composition of WRC

The structural constituents of wood substances, namely cellulose, hemicellulose, and lignan, occur in cedar in roughly the same proportion as they do in other coniferous woods. WRC is different from other species because of its unusually high content of chemical extractives. These extractives of wood are minor nonstructural components that can be extracted from the wood without impairing its structure or strength and include a variety of materials, such as tannin, dyes, pitch, resins, and gums. They are responsible for the smell, taste, and color of the wood (3,4).

Cedar wood extractive may be separated by steam distillation into volatile and nonvolatile fractions (Table 1). The volatile fractions account for only 1% to 1.5% of the heartwood (without bark) while the nonvolatile fractions account for 5% to 15%. The volatile fractions contain at least nine compounds. Some of them

Table 1 Composition of Western Red Cedar Extract

Volatile components
Methyl thujate
Thujic acid
Tropolones
β-Thujaplicinol
γ-Thujaplicin
β-Thujaplicin
α-Thujaplicin
β-Dolabrin
Nazukone
Carvacrol methyl ether
Nonvolatile components (*water soluble*)
Phenolic fraction
Plicatic acid
Plicatin
Thujaplicatin
Thujaplicatin methyl ether
Other lignans
Nonphenolic fraction
Pectic acid
Starch
Hemicellulose
Arabinase
Simple sugars

Source: Adapted from Ref. 4.

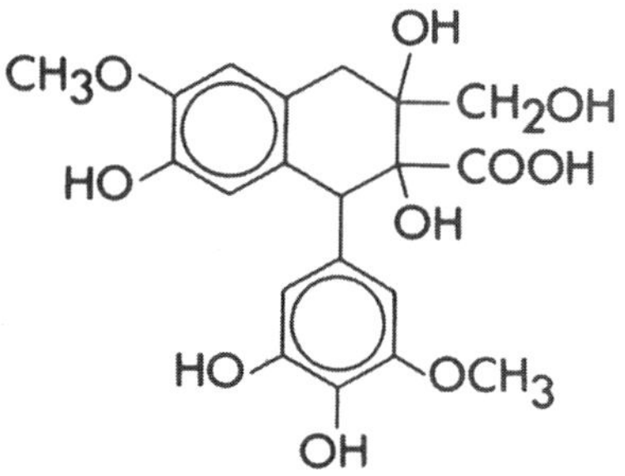

Figure 1 Structural formula of plicatic acid.

have interesting chemical properties. The tropolones, for example, are excellent natural fungicides and are likely to be responsible for the resistance of the wood against decay. They were found to have beta-adrenergic receptor blocking properties (5). Nezucone, an aromatic compound in red cedar, was found to give an asthmatic reaction on inhalation challenge testing in a patient (6). The significance of the tropolones and nezucone in the pathogenesis of WRCA is yet to be determined with careful clinical studies. On the other hand, plicatic acid (PA), a nonvolatile compound, constitutes about 90% of the nonvolatile components by weight. It has a molecular weight of 440 Da; the structural formula is shown in Figure 1. Inhalation challenge test with PA induced an asthmatic reaction similar to that caused by an aqueous extract of the WRC dust, in patients with the disease (7). The asthmatic reaction was found to be specific because patients with asthma and chronic bronchitis without history of exposure did not react on inhalation challenge test (7). PA is, therefore, the most important chemical compound present in the extract of WRC, causing asthma.

Clinical Features

The clinical picture of patients with WRCA is characteristic. Many patients have worked with other wood dusts without any respiratory symptoms. After a period of steady exposure, usually between six weeks and three years (but sometimes as long as 10 years), they develop cough, chest tightness, and wheeze. Some patients experience rhinorrhea several weeks before the onset of respiratory symptoms. In the majority of patients, respiratory symptoms occurred initially after work and at night, waking them up with cough and wheeze. Later, cough, wheeze, and dyspnea occurred during the day and the nocturnal symptoms became more distressing. Symptoms usually improved during weekends and holidays initially; with continued exposure, they became persistent with no remission. At that stage, many patients complained of cough and wheeze immediately on exposure.

The characteristics of the 232 patients included in a study and proven to be suffering from WRCA using inhalation provocation test are shown in Table 2 (8). The proportion of atopic subjects (those with positive prick skin test to one or more common allergens) in this group of patients was 31.4%, not different from those of the general population. This finding suggests that atopic status is not a predisposing factor in WRCA. The other interesting observation is the high proportion of non-smokers and exsmokers (94%) among this patient population (9).

Specific challenge tests can be performed using fine red cedar dust, a crude extract of WRC dust, or PA. The exposure test with fine WRC dust can be performed using the method originally described by Pepys and Hutchcroft (10), by

Table 2 Characteristics of 232 Patients with Documented Western Red Cedar Asthma

Age (yrs)	41.9 ± 11.8
Duration of exposure before onset of symptoms (yrs)	4.1 ± 5.6
Smoking habit (%)	
Nonsmoker	66.8
Exsmokers	28.0
Current smokers	5.2
Atopy[a] (%)	
Positive	31.4
Negative	68.6
Type of asthmatic reaction induced (%)	
Isolated immediate	10.8
Isolated late	42.3
Biphasic or continuous	46.9
Specific IgE antibodies against PA–HSA[b] (%)	20.1

[a]Defined as positive skin-prick test against one or more common allergens.
[b]RAST value greater than 2 was considered as a positive test.
Abbreviations: PA–HSA, plicatic acid–human serum albumin conjugate; RAST, radioallergosorbent test.
Source: Adapted from Refs. 8, 20.

pouring the dust from one container to another, or by a more sophisticated method as described by Vandenplas and Malo (11) in Chapter 10. Specific challenge test can also be performed by aerosolization of the crude WRC extract or with PA (12). PA is however not available commercially. Inhalation challenge tests with an extract of WRC or PA induce three main types of asthmatic reaction: isolated immediate, isolated late, and biphasic or continuous asthmatic reaction (Chapter 10). Systemic or alveolar reaction has not been observed. The proportion of patients with late asthmatic reaction is high (89.2%), either as isolated late or part of biphasic or continuous reaction (Table 2). Recurrent nocturnal asthma over several nights after one single inhalation challenge test has been documented (13).

Patients with a biphasic asthmatic reaction usually have a significantly lower lung function, a greater degree of nonspecific bronchial hyperresponsiveness (NSBH), and the period between the onset of symptoms and diagnosis is longer than in patients with isolated immediate or late asthmatic reaction (14). These findings suggest that the occurrence of biphasic asthmatic reaction at the time of diagnosis is indicative of a greater severity of the disease.

Diagnosis

The diagnosis of WRCA is based on the presence of a compatible taking and objective evidence that exposure to WRC dust causes acute respiratory symptoms and lung function changes. In general, any individual who is exposed to WRC dust in the work place or as a result of their hobby and develops asthma should be suspected of suffering from WRCA.

Skin tests and immunologic tests are not helpful in the confirmation of diagnosis. Both crude WRC extract and PA, or PA conjugated to human serum albumin (PA–HSA), failed to give reactions on skin testing. Specific IgE antibodies to PA–HSA conjugate were detected in only 30% of the red cedar asthma patients, proven by inhalation challenge test (15), and were also detected in 6% of those exposed workers who did not have any respiratory symptom (16).

Prolonged recording of peak expiratory flow (PEF) every two hours during waking hours, for two weeks at work and one week away from work, has been proven by Côté et al. (17) to be both sensitive and specific in the diagnosis of WRCA when compared with the results of specific challenge test with PA. Although serial measurements of NSBH have been used together with prolonged monitoring of PEF effectively in the diagnosis of other types of occupational asthma, Côté et al. (17) did not find that the addition of this measurement improved the sensitivity and specificity of PEF monitoring in this group of patients. This is possibly due to the fact that NSBH persists for a long time in patients with WRCA compared to those due to other agents (18,19).

Outcome

As is the case for occupational asthma, the majority of the patients with WRCA fail to recover several years after the exposure had stopped. A follow-up study of 232 patients about four years after the diagnosis showed that of the 136 patients who left the industry, only 55 (40.4%) recovered completely while the remaining 81 (59.6%) continued to have asthma (8). Early diagnosis and early removal from exposure have been found to be associated with complete recovery in patients with WRCA.

Patients who failed to recover after they left exposure continued to require medications for their asthma. Bronchoalveolar studies of these patients showed a higher total cell count, eosinophil and neutrophil count, and an increase in protein and albumin in the lavage fluid compared to those who recovered (20), therefore suggesting persistent airway inflammation in these patients.

All patients who continued to work with WRC had respiratory symptoms and required medications even though most of them used personal protection. They showed a reduction in forced expiratory flow in one second (FEV_1) and forced vital capacity (FVC) and an increase in NSBH on follow-up examination. Côté et al. (21) found that the use of twin-cartridge respirators offered better protection than airstream helmets. This may be due to the poor compliance to the need of continuous usage of airstream helmets.

A recent follow-up study of 280 patients with WRCA has shown that the longitudinal decline in FEV_1 was significantly greater in those who were still exposed to red cedar compared to those who were exposed but did not have asthma (22). The diagnosis of occupational asthma has considerable socioeconomic implications for the worker and his/her family (23).

Pathogenesis

WRCA is a prototype of asthma caused by exposure to a low-molecular-weight compound. The clinical features and the results of pathogenetic studies are similar to those of diisocyanate-induced asthma. Both nonimmunologic and immunologic mechanisms are likely involved.

Immunologic Mechanisms

The clinical feature of WRCA is one of allergic disease. It affects only a small proportion of exposed workers (prevalence rate of < 2% in sawmills with low dust exposure) (24); reexposure to a small amount of dust may trigger a severe attack of asthma in sensitive subjects. There is a latent period between the onset of exposure and the onset of symptoms. Animals can be sensitized to parenteral administration of PA–HSA conjugate with the production of specific IgG_1 antibodies in guinea pigs and IgE antibodies in rabbits (25). So far, investigations failed to clarify which specific immunologic mechanism(s) is responsible.

The changes in the airway of patients with WRCA are similar to those found in patients with allergic asthma. During late asthmatic reactions induced by PA, increase in eosinophils and albumin and sloughing of bronchial epithelial cells were found in bronchoalveolar lavage fluid (26). Although there was a slight increase in neutrophils 48 hours after challenge, neutrophil infiltration was not a prominent feature earlier. Multiple bronchial biopsies were carried out in three of the patients 24 hours after inhalation challenge. The major findings were denudation of the bronchial epithelium, thickened basement membrane, and infiltration of eosinophils in the bronchial epithelium and submucosa. The occurrence of these inflammatory changes was associated with the development of NSBH. Mediators, predominantly histamine, and LTE_4 were found in the bronchoalveolar lavage fluid during the immediate asthmatic reaction that is induced by PA (27).

When the radioallergosorbent test (RAST) was used, specific IgE antibodies to PA–HSA were found in only 30% of subjects with WRCA proven by specific challenge tests (15); when skin tests were used, the results were negative. Specific IgG antibodies to PA–HSA conjugate were not detected. There was no difference in the frequency of specific IgE antibodies between patients with isolated late reaction and those with biphasic asthmatic reaction (15). The immediate component of the biphasic reaction can be induced on a second challenge in patients who had isolated late reaction alone during the first challenge test, in the absence of specific IgE antibodies (Fig. 2). Although PA was found to release histamine from basophils of most patients with WRCA and not from those of patients with allergic asthma, desensitization of basophils by prior incubation with anti-IgE failed to inhibit histamine release induced by PA (28). Moreover, passive sensitization of human lung fragments with sera from patients with WRCA followed by a challenge with PA failed to release histamine. These findings suggest that specific IgE antibodies to PA–HSA conjugate are unlikely to play a role in the pathogenesis of the disease.

T lymphocytes are important in the pathogenesis of allergic asthma, by participating in the airway inflammatory response, and in the production of specific IgE antibodies. IL-5 produced by CD4 cells is necessary for the maturation of eosinophils, which cause airway damage. In patients with recently diagnosed WRCA, increased numbers of T lymphocytes and activated T lymphocytes were found in the bronchial mucosa (29), similar to the case of patients with diisocyanate-induced asthma (30). When stimulated with PA–HSA conjugate, proliferation of T lymphocyte was found in about 30% of patients (31). The role of T lymphocytes was further defined by the finding that certain HLA types are associated with the predisposition while others with protection against the development of the disease (32).

Nonimmunologic Mechanisms

At high concentrations, PA has several biological activities. It activates the complement system via the classical pathway, leading to the generation of biologically active fragments such as C3a and C5a, both of which can induce histamine release from peripheral human basophils and mast cells, increased vascular permeability, and vasodilatation (33). PA is toxic to bronchial epithelium in high concentrations (34). Crude WRC dust has been shown to release histamine from human and pig lung fragments in vitro (34).

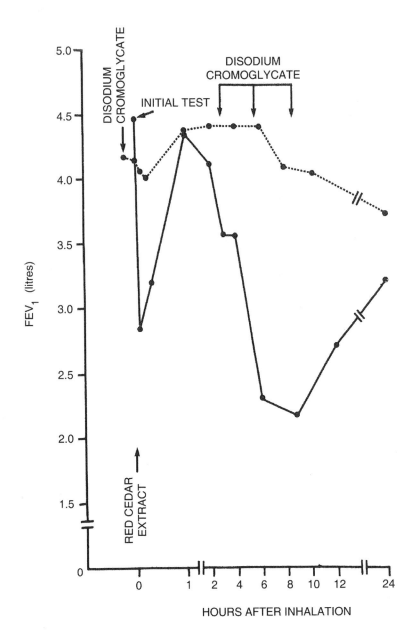

Figure 2   Effect of repeated challenge with plicatic acid on three separate patients with red cedar asthma, showing the occurrence of isolated late reaction after the first challenge and biphasic reaction after the second challenge. PC_{20} decreased after the late asthmatic reaction of the first challenge.

It is likely that both immunologic and nonimmunologic mechanisms are involved in the pathogenesis of WRCA.

Prevalence and Determinants

The prevalence of occupational asthma in workers exposed to WRC dust has been studied by several investigators (Table 3) (36–39). In these studies, a close

Table 3 Epidemiologic Studies of Workers Exposed to Western Red Cedar

Year	Site	Type of industries	Subjects	Age (mean or range)	Smokers (%)	Chronic cough (%)	Chronic phlegm (%)	Wheeze (%)	Work-related asthma (%)	Lung function FEV₁	Lung function FVC	Dust concentration mean–SD or range mg/m³	References
1973	Japan	Furniture	1797	17–60	NA	NA	NA	NA	3.4	NA	NA	NA	(36)
1978	Vancouver, B.C., Canada	Cedar sawmill	405	36.8	53.8	27.4	30.4	13.1	1.1	101%[a]	98.5%[a]	NA	(24)
		Former cedar mill	65	45.9	57.0	23.1	29.7	6.2	4.9				
		Other wood dust	187	42.1	48.7	18.2	17.1	8.6	0	104%[a]	103.4%[a]	NA	(37)
1981	Washington state, U.S.A.	Shake and shingle–cedar	74	NA	NA	20.2[b]			13.5	Cross-shift decrease in FEV₁ greater in WRC workers		4.7±7.45	
		Planer mill–noncedar	58	NA	NA	26.4[b]		5.2				1.3±3.10	
		No wood dust	22	NA	NA	9.0[b]		0					
1984	Vancouver, B.C., Canada	Cedar sawmill	511[c]	44±14	38.2	16.9	16.4	14.7	4.1	−206 mL[d]	−163 mL[d]	NA 0–6	(38)
			394[c]	43±12	30.7	8.9[e]	12.0[e]	12.7	1.6[e]				

[a]Nonsmokers only.
[b]Chronic bronchitis %.
[c]White males only.
[d]Effect of cedar dust exposure versus no exposure adjusted for age, height, and smoking differences.
[e]Differences between cedar sawmill and office workers statistically significant $p < 0.05$.
Abbreviations: FEV₁, forced expiratory volume in one second; FVC, forced vital capacity; NA, not available; WRC, western red cedar.
Source: From Ref. 2.

relationship was found between the prevalence of work-related asthma and the level of dust exposure—the higher the dust concentration, the greater the prevalence of work-related asthma. Brooks et al. (37) studied 74 cedar shake mill workers and 85 personal dust measurements were carried out over a three-day period. Occupational asthma was defined as a positive clinical history and an evidence of 10% drop in FEV_1 was observed, from Monday preshift to any subsequent test during the next three weeks, among 24% of sawyers, 10.5% of packers, 5% of splitters, and in none of deckmen. The average dust exposure concentrations were 6.8, 4.8, 3.6, and 0 mg/m^3, respectively.

Vedal et al. (39) studied 652 cedar sawmill workers (93% participation) and obtained 104 full-shift dust measurements. The dust measurements were used to assign estimates of personal wood dust exposure for 334 workers. Of these, 301 were exposed to less than 1 mg/m^3, 20 to between 1 and 2 mg/m^3, and 13 to levels above 2 mg/m^3. Occupational asthma, defined as the presence of four out of five symptoms consistent with asthma with a temporal relationship with work, and with no asthma prior to employment at the sawmill, was prevalent in 6% and 5% of the low and medium exposure group and in 15% of the high exposure group. After the initial survey in 1982, 26 workers with NSBH and a history of work-related asthma, as defined above, were invited to have a specific challenge test. Eleven workers developed a specific reaction to PA challenge. The prevalence rate of WRCA, defined as specific responsiveness to PA, was 1.7%. During the subsequent six years, six workers developed WRCA at the rate of one per year giving an incidence of 0.3% per year even though the level of exposure in the sawmill was low with very few personal samples above 2.5 mg/m^3. Three of these six workers developed asthma symptoms after they were transferred from low exposure (outside) jobs, with mean exposure levels ranging from 0.01 to 0.27 mg/m^3 (with no samples above 2.5 mg/m^3), to higher exposure (inside) jobs, with mean exposure levels from 0.18 to 0.57 mg/m^3 (with up to 4% of samples over 2.5 mg/m^3) (40).

Given the same degree of exposure, only a small percentage of workers develop asthma. Host susceptibility factors play an important part. As discussed earlier, atopy is not a predisposing host factor in WRCA, since the prevalence of atopy in these patients is not different from that of the general population (18). Smoking is not a predisposing host factor in WRCA as in occupational asthma, due to high-molecular-weight compounds (Chapter 3). On the contrary, the majority of patients with WRCA are life-long nonsmokers. NSBH is unlikely to be a predisposing host factor as workers who developed WRCA did not have NSBH at the onset of a prospective study (18).

A study showed that individuals with HLA Class II antigen, DQB 0302 and DQB 0603 are more susceptible to WRCA while those with DQB 0501 are protected from the disease (35). Similar results were found in patients with diisocyanate-induced asthma; the HLA Class II antigen that confers susceptibility was DQB 0503 (41). These findings further support the importance of T cells in the pathogenesis of occupational asthma due to low-molecular-weight compounds.

Permissible Concentration of Red Cedar Dust

Is there a level of WRC dust that is safe, such that no sensitization can occur below that level? There are very few epidemiologic studies to address this important issue. The Workers' Compensation Board of British Columbia has arbitrarily lowered the permissible concentration of allergenic wood dust such as red cedar dust from 5 to 2.5 mg/m^3. Despite a low dust concentration in a red cedar sawmill with very few samples greater than 2.5 mg/m^3, the incidence of asthma remained at 0.3% per year in a longitudinal study carried out for a period of six years (24). The current permissible concentration has been further lowered to 1 mg/m^3.

OCCUPATIONAL ASTHMA DUE TO OTHER WOOD DUSTS

Eastern white cedar (*Thuja occidentalis*), a "cousin" of WRC that grows in Eastern Canada and Northeastern United States also contains PA, its concentration being approximately half of the one present in WRC. Malo et al. (42) studied 42 (out of 80) employees of a sawmill where eastern white cedar is being processed into shingles. They found three employees with occupational asthma (42) and showed that PA is also present in this wood dust, though at approximately half the concentration as in WRC (43).

Many other types of wood dust have also been shown to cause occupational asthma. The extent to which these types of wood are being used in construction and furniture industry is not known. Most of the cases of occupational asthma due to other wood dusts were published as case reports. The diagnoses were made by inhalation challenge test or by history and positive skin test reaction to the appropriate extracts of wood dust.

The table in the Appendix that contains an extensive list of agents causing occupational asthma with information and key references includes wood dusts. Aqueous extracts of some wood dust such as Iroko (44,45), Palisander (46), Cocobolla (47), Abirucana (48), African maple wood (49), African zebrawood (50), Kejaat wood (51), Quillaja bark (52), and Antiaaris (53) gave immediate wheal and flare reaction on skin testing in sensitive subjects (44–53). In some patients specific IgE antibodies were demonstrated in the sera by using RAST method. In these patients, a type I allergic reaction is likely to be responsible for the asthma reaction. However aqueous extracts of other wood dusts such as Californian red wood (54), Cedar of Lebanon (55), Central American walnut (56), mahogany (57), and oak (57) failed to give positive immediate skin reaction or specific IgE antibodies; precipitating antibodies were not detected in the sera of affected subjects (54–57). The pathogenetic mechanism of asthma induced by these wood dusts is likely to be similar to red cedar asthma. One or several of the chemical compounds present in these trees may be the causative agent(s).

The prevalence of occupational asthma due to various wood dust exposure is not known. Malo et al. (58) described 11 workers with work-related asthma from 10 different sawmills of northwestern and southwestern Quebec and northern Maine, where coniferous trees, spruce, firs, and pines are cut into boards. About 10% of furniture workers exposed to rimu, *Dacrydium cupressinum*, in Wellington, New Zealand, had a history compatible with work-related asthma that was subsequently confirmed by appropriate changes in the PEF recording (59). Several studies have shown that pine wood dust induces respiratory symptoms (60,61). Asthma prevalence related to pine dust exposure was reported by Hessel et al. in 18% of workers exposed to pine dust compared to 12.1% in the general population; those with higher exposure tended to have a higher prevalence of asthma (62). On the other hand, following a very detailed respiratory survey consisting of questionnaire, lung function measurements, skin-prick tests, and measurement of specific-IgE antibodies against molds, among 1205 sawmill workers in Eastern Canada (63), it was found that the workers had normal lung function, and most of their respiratory symptoms could be explained by smoking histories. Workers in pine sawmills had a greater prevalence of skin-prick test to pine than did workers in sawmills where other woods were used. The presence of a positive skin-prick test and/or specific antibodies had no impact on lung function. Nouaigui et al. (57) reported that 5.6% of 197 woodworkers in four plants in Tunisia had asthma. The type of wood the workers were exposed to was not documented in the report. Although the causative agent has not been identified, the results of these studies suggest that many cases of occupational asthma due to wood dust exposure may not be recognized by physicians.

OCCUPATIONAL ASTHMA DUE TO OTHER AGENTS PRESENT IN WOOD DUST

In addition to chemical components of the wood that can cause respiratory sensitization, it is well known that woodworkers can be sensitized to some living organisms, such as molds that grow on wood and develop asthma (64). Côté et al. (65) reported a case of occupational asthma in a plywood factory worker due to a mold of *Neurospora* species growing on the wood under wet conditions (65). This worker had a positive skin reaction and bronchial reaction to challenge with an extract of mold and the wood dust extract.

Formaldehyde and diphenyl-methane diisocyanate (MDI) resins are often used to bond wood fragments for industrial use. Gaseous formaldehyde or MDI can cause irritation of eyes, irritation of the upper respiratory tract, and asthma. A study of plywood mill workers in New Zealand and oriented strand board workers in Alberta, Canada, have shown increased in asthma prevalence compared to controls (66,67).

CHRONIC BRONCHITIS WITH AND WITHOUT AIRFLOW OBSTRUCTION

While it is well known that exposure to a number of wood dusts can induce asthma through sensitization, it is less well recognized that such exposure also gives rise to chronic bronchitis and airflow obstruction. Sawmill workers exposed to WRC dust, known to give rise to occupational asthma, had increased cough and sputum production compared with unexposed office workers with odds ratios of 2.18 and 1.44, respectively ($p > 0.001$ and 0.05, respectively, controlled for age and smoking). These workers had significantly lower lung function compared to office workers after adjusting for differences in age, height, race, and smoking habits and the exclusion of asthmatics from the analysis. The annual decline in lung function in cedar workers was also significantly greater than in the control group in a longitudinal study (68). Noertjojo et al. (68) evaluated exposure–response relationships in a longitudinal study of 243 cedar sawmill workers, by using the office workers as controls and with a follow-up duration of four to 13 years. In this study, 916 dust samples were taken during five separate industrial hygiene surveys for each job title or work area. Cumulative exposure was estimated for each worker, based on the job history, and the average exposure was calculated by dividing cumulative exposure by the duration of employment. Workers were stratified by average exposure level into four groups: control, low, medium, and high. The geometric mean exposure levels were 0.13, 0.30, and 0.61 mg/m^3 in groups with low, medium, and high levels of exposure, respectively. A significant dose–response relationship was found between decline in FVC and cumulative dust exposure; those in the medium and high exposure group had a significantly greater annual decline in FVC compared to the control group. In workers exposed to cedar dust but without asthma, airflow obstruction was associated with average levels of exposure being as low as 0.3 mg/m^3.

There have been several epidemiological studies on the respiratory health effects of exposure to wood dusts other than WRC (Table 4) (Chapter 3). These studies were carried out in either sawmills or furniture factories with workers exposed mostly to softwood. Some studies demonstrated an increase in the prevalence of chronic respiratory symptoms and a dose-dependent relationship between symptoms and lung function and the exposure in sawmill workers, when compared with the unexposed controls (61,62,69–74). Others failed to do so (75–77).

Whitehead et al. (61) conducted an epidemiological study on 354 workers exposed to hardwood dust (mostly maple) and on 220 workers exposed to varying levels of soft wood dust (pine). These workers did not have exposure to other industrial agents such as adhesives and finishing agents. Although an unexposed group was not studied as controls, workers in the high exposure category to both hard wood and pine dust were associated with two to four times the prevalence of low expiratory flow rates compared to those exposed to lower levels of dust irrespective of their smoking habits. These findings indicated that both hard and soft wood exposure is associated with airflow obstruction. Holness et al. (69) studied 50 cabinet workers exposed to different types of wood dust and 50 controls. Woodworkers reported more cough, phlegm, and wheeze but their mean lung function was not significantly different from the controls. Woodworkers, however, had a significant acute decline in lung function over a workshift. A positive correlation was found between baseline lung function and the degree of exposure. Paggiaro et al. (70) studied respiratory symptoms and lung function of 239 workers exposed to wood dust in a furniture plant (70). Significantly higher prevalence rates of cough, phlegm, and wheeze in nonsmoking workers were found compared to the control group derived from a population sample. Although mean lung function results were within normal limits, a lower FEV$_1$% was found in subjects with more years of employment, suggestive of a dose responsive relationship. Shamssain demonstrated that exposure to pine and fiberboard dust was associated with a higher prevalence of chest symptoms and lower lung function among furniture factory workers in Umtata, Republic of Transkei, compared with a group of unexposed subjects (71). Hessel et al. (62) found lower lung function measurements in sawmill workers in Alberta compared with unexposed controls. Halpin et al. (72) studied Welsh sawmill workers exposed to pine, spruce, and Douglas fir and compared the prevalence of respiratory symptoms and lung function abnormalities with unexposed workers (72). They found that workers in high exposed areas had twice the prevalence of work-related respiratory symptoms compared with workers in areas with low dust exposure, while chronic bronchitis and wheeze were twice as prevalent among exposed workers when compared with controls. The increase in symptoms was not accompanied by a significant difference in lung function between groups.

Chan-Yeung et al. (78) included a group of workers in sawmills exposed to Douglas fir, western hemlock, spruce, and balsam in a study of pulpmill workers. These workers were exposed to a mean dust level of 0.5 mg/m^3 (0.1–2.7 mg/m^3)

Table 4 Exposure to Wood Dust, Respiratory Symptoms, Lung Function, and Dust Concentration

Types of industry	Types of wood	N	Mean age (yrs)	Smoker (%)	Chronic cough (%)	Chronic phlegm (%)	Asthma	FEV_1	FVC	Dust level (mg/m^3)	References
Sawmill	*Dalberia sissoo* *Mangifera indici*	W 105 / C 88	W 26.4 / C 28.7	W 70.6 / C 42.0				W 1.8% / C 2.2%	W 28.4% / C NA		(75)
Furniture manufacture	Pine, Tasmania oak, jarrah, blackwood	W 168 / C 46	W 30 / C 39	W 45 / C 50	W 32 / C 41	W 19 / C 24				Machinists 3.2 Cabinet 5.2 Frame maker 3.5 No dose–response	(76)
Furniture factory	?	W 145 / C 152	W 30 / C 39	W 0 / C 0				FEF 81.3%	PEF 89.4%	PFT abnormality correlated with duration of work	(71)
Sawmill	Pine, spruce	W 194 / C 165	W 33.4 / C 34.9	W 43.6 / C 27.9	Chronic bronchitis; W 26.6 / C 13.3	Chronic bronchitis	W 7.4 / C 3.0	Non-smoker W 4133 mL / C 4211 mL	Smoker W 3923 mL / C 4272 mL	1.35 (0.1–2.2 mg/m^3)	(62)
Sawmill		W 105 / J 63 / C 30	W 38 / J 34 / C 39	W 40 / J 23 / C 30	W 58.6 / J 62.2 / C 23.5	W 46.0 / J 67.1 / C 23.5		W 84.6% / J 84.6% / C 94.9%	W 84.7% / J 84.6% / C 93.1%	Dose relationship between exposure and cross-shift changes	(73)
Furniture	Pine	W 2033 / C 474	Male W 37 / C 36.5; Female W 35.9 / C 34.7	Male W 41.7 / C 44.7; Female W 49.1 / C 42.9	Chronic bronchitis Male-NS W 12.8 / C 14.3; Female-NS W 1.4 / C 3.1	Chronic bronchitis Male-CS W 7.2 / C 5.3; Female-CS W 8.9 / C 9.6	Asthma Male-NS W 5 / C 9.6; Female-NS W 5.5 / C 7.9	Asthma Male-CS W 6.0 / C 4.3; Female-CS W 8.9 / C 6.3		Dose relationship between exposure and asthma symptoms	(77)

(Continued)

Table 4 Exposure to Wood Dust, Respiratory Symptoms, Lung Function, and Dust Concentration (*Continued*)

Types of industry	Types of wood	N	Mean age (yrs)	Smoker (%)	Chronic cough (%)	Chronic phlegm (%)	Asthma	Lung function FEV$_1$	FVC	Dust level (mg/m^3)	References
Small scale wood industries	Hardwood and softwood	W 601 C 600	W 29.6 C 28.0	W 23.6 C 23.2	W 50.7 C 39.5	W 47.0 C 30.3	W 9.4 C 7.3			High exposure group > low exposure group in symptoms	(74)
Furniture	White pine	W 650						Reduced FEV$_1$/FVC and MMF associated with level of pine dust exposure		$N=35$ Total dust = 0.2–14.3 mg/m^3	(61)
Sawmill	Spruce, Douglas fir and pine	W 109 C 58			Chronic bronchitis Low dust: 20.7% High dust: 24.4% Control: 9.6%		Low: 3.5% High: 20% Control: 19.2	FEV$_1$ Low: 4.11 L High: 4.06 L Control: 4.13L	FVC Low: 5.02 L High: 4.90 L Control: 5.01L	$N=62$ Low dust: 0.2–1.1 mg/m^3 High dust: 1.3–6.3 mg/m^3 Control: mean 2.5 mg/m^3	(72)
Sawmill, longitudinal	Western red cedar	W 243 C 140						Greater annual decline in FVC in medium- and high-exposure groups		$N=916$ total dust (geo mean) Low: 0.13 mg/m^3 Medium: 0.30 mg/m^3 High: 0.61 mg/m^3	(68)

Abbreviations: W, workers; C, controls; NA, not assessed.

and they had significantly lower lung function compared with workers in the office and log pond of the same mill with no dust exposure. Based on these findings, the investigators suggested that the regulated exposure limit of $5\,mg/m^3$ for soft wood was not adequate to protect the worker's health.

The results of most of the above studies have shown that exposure to different types of wood dust is associated with chronic respiratory symptoms and some impairment of lung function compared to the unexposed. A dose–response relationship was observed between level of exposure and the level of lung function in some studies to indicate that the relationship was significant. Although asthma is the most disabling lung disease among woodworkers, one should realize that inhalation of wood dusts also gives rise to chronic bronchitis with and without airflow obstruction. More recently, Demers et al. (79) reviewed extensively the chemical components and the respiratory effects of exposure to dust of softwood, sampling methods, and particle size consideration and came to the conclusion that health effects from exposure to soft wood dust are observed even when dust levels are below $2\,mg/m^3$.

HYPERSENSITIVITY PNEUMONITIS ASSOCIATED WITH WOOD DUST EXPOSURE

Hypersensitivity pneumonitis often affects sawmill trimmers and pulp and paper mill workers in the wood room and sometimes farmers who handle wood chips (Chapter 29). The antigens responsible for these diseases are often molds growing in wood dust or the bark of the wood, such as *Cryptostroma corticale* in maple bark disease (80), *Penicillium frequentans* in suberosis (81), *Graphium* and *Pullularia* on redwood bark in sequoisis (82), *Alternaria* in woodmills (83), *Aspergillus* and *Thermoactinomyces vulgaris* in moldy wood chips (84), and *Rhizopus* or *Paecilomyces* in wood-trimmer's disease seen in Sweden (85,86).

Of the different types of hypersensitivity pneumonitis, maple bark disease and wood-trimmer's disease were better investigated compared to the others. Maple bark disease was first described in 1932 by Towey et al. (64) and later by Emanuel et al. (80) as seen in workers in the wood rooms of paper mills. The workers were involved in peeling bark from maple logs infected with fungal spores, which were identified as *C. corticale*. High levels of sprecipitating antibodies were found in the sera of patients with hypersensitivity pneumonitis against extracts of this fungus. Wood-trimmer's disease has been described among sawmill workers in Sweden in the late 1960s when conventional outdoor wood drying during the summer was changed to artificial indoor wood drying in special kilns (85). Spores of molds, Rhizopus and Paecilomyces, growing on the wood when it was wet, were found in high concentrations in the sawmills (85). A survey conducted from 1976 to 1978 revealed that in 10 out of 17 Swedish sawmills that employed about 280 workers, about 50% of the wood trimmers had precipitating antibodies mainly to the Rhizopus antigens while 10% to 20% had suffered symptoms compatible with hypersensitivity pneumonitis (87). Serum IgG antibodies to mold spores (*Rhizopus microsporous* ssp, *Paecilomyces variotii*, and *Aspergillus fumigatus*) in two Norwegian sawmill workers were determined; antibody levels were higher and symptoms of mucous membrane irritation, allergic alveolitis, and organic dust toxic syndrome were more frequently found or reported by wood trimmers than by plane operators (88). In British Columbia, six cases of hypersensitivity pneumonitis have been seen from the inland sawmills where spruce, pine, fir, and hemlock are being processed. In three cases precipitating anti-bodies were found in the sera against *A. fumigatus* and *T. vulgaris* (1).

ORGANIC DUST TOXIC SYNDROME

Organic dust toxic syndrome, a syndrome characterized by fever, sometimes shak-ing chills, dry cough, and fatigue, is common among grain handlers and farmers (Chapter 29) (89). It has also been reported among sawmill workers in Sweden (85). Exposure to high concentrations of fungal spores was thought to be the causative factor in the pathogenesis of this condition (90).

RESEARCH NEEDS

The important questions to be addressed by research should include the following:

1. Are there extractives besides PA of WRC dust that can give rise to asthma?
2. What are the definite pathogenic mechanisms of red cedar asthma?
3. What are the genetic susceptibility factors for red cedar asthma?
4. What is the permissible exposure limit for WRC dust and other wood dusts?
5. Are there interactions between genetic susceptibility and levels of exposure?
6. What are the agents (low-molecular-weight agent?) causing occupational asthma to wood dusts besides red and white cedar dusts?

SUMMARY

In this chapter, the respiratory effects of wood dust exposures were reviewed. Many wood dusts can give rise to asthma by sensitization via Type I allergic reaction or by an undetermined immunologic mechanism. Chronic bronchitis, with or without air-flow obstruction, unrelated to smoking, hypersensitivity pneumonitis, and organic dust toxic syndrome, are also found among woodworkers.

Allergic conjunctivitis and rhinitis are also problems among woodworkers. Contact dermatitis from wood dust exposure, however, is the most common com-pensable disease in British Columbia among woodworkers. In many cases it is not the wood dust itself that is causing the dermatitis but contaminants, e.g., lichens growing on the bark of red cedar trees (91). Adenocarcinoma of the nasopharynx is a known disease among woodworkers (92). These conditions cannot be discussed in this chapter in depth, but have been described in detail by Hausen (93).

REFERENCES

1. Enarson DA, Chan-Yeung M. Characterization of health effects of wood dust exposures. Am J Ind Med 1990; 17:33–38.
2. Chan-Yeung M, Malo JL. Occupational respiratory disease associated with forest products industries. In: Harber P, Schenker M, Balmes J, eds. Occupational and Envir-onmental Respiratory Disease. St.Louis: Mosby, 1996:637–653.
3. Gardner JA. Chemistry and utilization of western red cedar. In: Dept of Forestry Publication No. 1023. Ottawa: Ottawa Department of Forestry, 1963.

4. Barton GM, MacDonald BF. The chemistry of utilization of western red cedar. Dept of Fisheries & Forestry, Publication No. 1023. Ottawa: Ottawa Department of Forestry, 1971.

5. Belleau B, Burba J. Occupancy of adrenergic receptors and inhibition of catechol o-methyl transferase by toropolones. J Med Chem 1963; 6:755–759.

6. Shida T, Mimaki K, Sasaki N, Nakagawa Y, Hattovi O. Western red cedar asthma: Occurrance in Oume City, Tokyo and results of inhalation test using "Nezucone" aromatic substance of western red cedar. Areugi—Jpn J Allergol 1971; 20:915–921.

7. Chan-Yeung M, Barton GM, MacLean L, Grzybowski S. Occupational asthma and rhinitis due to western red cedar (*Thuja plicata*). Am Rev Respir Dis 1973; 108: 1094–1102.

8. Chan-Yeung M, MacLean L, Paggiaro PL. Follow-up study of 232 patients with occupational asthma caused by western red cedar (*Thuja plicata*). J Allergy Clin Immunol 1987; 79:792–796.

9. Chan-Yeung M, Lam S. Occupational asthma. Am Rev Respir Dis 1986; 133:686–703.

10. Pepys J, Hutchcroft BJ. Bronchial provocation tests in etiologic diagnosis and analysis of asthma. Am Rev Respir Dis 1975; 112:829–859.

11. Vandenplas O, Malo JL. Inhalation challenges with agents causing occupational asthma. Eur Respir J 1997; 10:2612–2629.

12. Chan-Yeung M, Barton GM, McLean L, Grzybowski S. Bronchial reactions to western red cedar. CMAJ 1971; 105:56–61.

13. Cockcroft DW, Cotton DJ, Mink JT. Nonspecific bronchial hyperreactivity after exposure to western red cedar. Am Rev Respir Dis 1979; 119:505–510.

14. Paggiaro PL, Chan-Yeung M. Pattern of specific airway response in asthma due to western red cedar (*Thuja plicata*): relationship with length of exposure and lung function measurements. Clin Allergy 1987; 17:333–339.

15. Tse KS, Chan H, Chan-Yeung M. Specific IgE antibodies in workers with occupational asthma due to western red cedar. Clin Allergy 1982; 12:249–258.

16. Vedal S, Chan-Yeung M, Enarson DA, Chan H, Dorken E, Tse KS. Plicatic acid-specific IgE and nonspecific bronchial hyperresponsiveness in western red-cedar workers. J Allergy Clin Immunol 1986; 78:1103–1109.

17. Côté J, Kennedy S, Chan-Yeung M. Sensitivity and specificity of PC 20 and peak expiratory flow rate in cedar asthma. J Allergy Clin Immunol 1990; 85:592–598.

18. Chan-Yeung M, Lam S, Koerner S. Clinical features and natural history of occupational asthma due to western red cedar (*Thuja plicata*). Am J Med 1982; 72:411–415.

19. Cartier A, L'Archeveque J, Malo JL. Exposure to a sensitizing occupational agent can cause a long-lasting increase in bronchial responsiveness to histamine in the absence of significant changes in airway caliber. J Allergy Clin Immunol 1986; 78:1185–1189.

20. Chan-Yeung M, Leriche J, Maclean L, Lam S. Comparison of cellular and protein changes in bronchial lavage fluid of symptomatic and asymptomatic patients with red cedar asthma on follow-up examination. Clin Allergy 1988; 18:359–365.

21. Côté J, Kennedy S, Chan-Yeung M. Outcome of patients with cedar asthma with continuous exposure. Am Rev Respir Dis 1990; 141:373–376.

22. Lin FJ, Dimich-Ward H, Chan-Yeung M. Longitudinal decline in lung function in patients with occupational asthma due to western red cedar. Occup environ med 1996; 53:753–756.

23. Marabini A, Ward H, Kwan S, Kennedy S, Wexler-Morrison N, Chan-Yeung M. Clinical and socioeconomical features of subjects with red cedar asthma—a follow up study. Chest 1993; 104:821–824.

24. Chan-Yeung M, Kennedy S, Vedal S. A longitudinal study of red cedar sawmill workers. Am Rev Respir Dis 1990; 139:A81.

25. Chan H, Tse KS, Oostdam J Van, Moreno R, Pare PD, Chan-Yeung M. A rabbit model of hypersensitivity to plicatic acid, the agent responsible for red cedar asthma. J Allergy Clin Immunol 1987; 79:762–767.

26. Lam S, LeRiche J, Phillips D, Chan-Yeung M. Cellular and protein changes in bronchial lavage fluid after late asthmatic reaction in patients with red cedar asthma. J Allergy Clin Immunol 1987; 80:44–50.

27. Chan-Yeung M, Chan H, Salari H, Lam S. Histamine, leukotrienes and prostaglandins release in bronchial fluid during plicatic acid-induced bronchoconstriction. J Allergy Clin Immunol 1989; 84:762–768.

28. Frew A, Chan H, Dryden P, Salari H, Lam S, Chan-Yeung M. Immunologic studies of the mechanisms of occupational asthma caused by western red cedar. J Allergy Clin Immunol 1993; 92:466–478.

29. Frew A, Chan H, Lam S, Chan-Yeung M. Bronchial inflammation in occupational asthma due to western red cedar. Am J Respir Crit Care Med 1994; 151:340–344.

30. Mapp CE, Saetta M, Maestrelli P, et al. Mechanisms and pathology of occupational asthma. Eur Respir J 1994; 7:544–554.

31. Frew AJ, Chan H, Chan-Yeung M. Specificity of antigen-induced T-cell proliferation in western red cedar asthma (WRCA). J Allergy Clin Immunol 1993; 91(abstract):219.

32. Chan-Yeung M, Giclas PC, Henson PM. Activation of complement by plicatic acid, the chemical compound responsible for asthma due to western red cedar (*Thuja plicata*). J Allergy Clin Immunol 1980; 65:333–337.

33. Ayars GH, Altman LC, Frazier CE, Chi EY. The toxicity of constituents of cedar and pine woods to pulmonary epithelium. J Allergy Clin Immunol 1989; 83:610–618.

34. Evans E, Nicholls PJ. Histamine release by western red cedar (*Thuja plicata*) from lung tissue in vitro. Br J Ind Med 1974; 31:28–30.

35. Horne C, Quintana PJE, Keown PA, Dimich-Ward H, Chan-Yeung M. Distribution of HLA class II DQB1 alleles in patients with occupational asthma due to western red cedar. Eur Respir J 2000; 15:911–914.

36. Ishizaki T, Sluda T, Miyamoto T, Matsumara Y, Mizuno K, Tomaru M. Occupational asthma from western red cedar dust (*Thuja plicata*) in furniture factory workers. JOM 1973; 15:580–585.

37. Brooks SM, Edwards JJ, Apol A, Edwards FH. An epidemiologic study of workers exposed to western red cedar and other wood dust. Chest 1981; 80(suppl):30–32.

38. Chan-Yeung M, Vedal S, Kus J, Maclean L, Enarson D, Tse KS. Symptoms, pulmonary function, and bronchial hyperreactivity in western red cedar workers compared with those in office workers. Am Rev Respir Dis 1984; 130:1038–1041.

39. Vedal S, Chan-Yeung M, Enarson D, et al. Symptoms and pulmonary function in western red cedar workers related to duration of employment and dust exposure. Arch Environ Health 1986; 41:179–183.

40. Chan-Yeung M, Desjardins A. Bronchial hyperresponsiveness and level of exposure in occupationnal ashtma due to western red cedar (*Thuja plicata*): serial observations before and after development of symptoms. Am Rev Respir Dis 1992; 146:1606–1609.

41. Balboni A, Baricordi OR, Fabbri LM, Gandini E, Ciaccia A, Mapp CE. Association between toluene diisocyanate-induced asthma and DQB1 markers: a possible role for aspartic acid at position 57. Eur Respir J 1996; 9:207–210.

42. Malo JL, Cartier A, L'Archevêque J, Trudeau C, Courteau JP, Bhérer L. Prevalence of occupational asthma among workers exposed to eastern white cedar. Am J Respir Crit Care Med 1994; 150:1697–1701.

43. Cartier A, Chan H, Malo JL, Pineau L, Tse KS, Chan-Yeung M. Occupational asthma caused by Eastern white cedar (*Thuja occidentalis*) with demonstration that plicatic acid is present in this wood dust and is the causal agent. J Allergy Clin Immunol 1986; 77: 639–645.

44. Azofra J, Olaguibel JM. Occupational asthma caused by iroko wood. Allergy 1989; 44:156–158.

45. Pickering CAC, Batten JC, Pepys J. Asthma due to inhaled wood dusts—western red cedar and iroko. Clin Allergy 1972; 2:213–218.

46. Godnic-Cvar J, Gomzi M. Case report of occupational asthma due to palisander wood dust and bronchoprovocation challenge by inhalation of pure wood dust from a capsule. Am J Ind Med 1990; 18:541–545.

47. Eaton KK. Respiratory allergy to exotic wood dust. Clin Allergy 1973; 3:307–310.

48. Booth BH, Lefoldt RH, Moffitt EM. Hypersensitivity to wood dust. J Allergy Clin Immunol 1976; 57:352–357.

49. Hinojosa M, Moneo I, Dominguez J, Delgado E, Losada E, Alcover R. Asthma caused by African maple (*Triplochiton scleroxylon*) wood dust. J Allergy Clin Immunol 1984; 74:782–786.

50. Bush RK, Yunginger JW, Reed CE. Asthma due to African zebrawood (microberlinia) dust. Am Rev Respir Dis 1978; 117:601–603.

51. Ordman D. Wood dust as an inhalant allergen. Bronchial asthma caused by kejaat wood (*Pterocarpus angolensis*). S Afr Med 1949; 23:973–975.

52. Raghuprasad PK, Brooks SM, Litwin A, Edwards JJ, Bernstein IL, Gallagher J. Quillaja bark (soapbark)-induced asthma. J Allergy Clin Immunol 1980; 65:285–287.

53. Higuero NC, Zabala BB, Villamuza Y García, Gómez C Mogío, Gregorio A Moral de, Sanchez C Senent. Occupational asthma caused by IgE-mediated reactivity to Antiaris wood dust. J Allergy Clin Immunol 2001; 107:554–555.

54. Chan-Yeung M, Abboud R. Occupational asthma due to california redwood (sequoia sempervirens) dusts. Am Rev Respir Dis 1976; 114:1027–1031.

55. Greenberg M. Respiratory symptoms following brief exposure to cedar of Lebanon (*Cedra libani*) dust. Clin Allergy 1972; 2:219–224.

56. Bush RK, Clayton D. Asthma due to Central American walnut (*Juglans olanchana*) dust. Clin Allergy 1983; 13:389–394.

57. Nouaigui H, Gharbi R, M'Rizak N, Jaafar K, Ghachem A, Nemery B. Etude transversale de la pathologie respiratoire chez les travailleurs du bois en Tunisie. Arch Mal Prof 1998; 49:69–75.

58. Malo JL, Cartier A, Boulet LP. Occupational asthma in sawmills of eastern Canada and United States. J Allergy Clin Immunol 1986; 78:392–398.

59. Norrish AE, Beasley R, Hodgkinson EJ, Pearce N. A study of New Zealand wood workers: exposure to wood dust, respiratory symptoms, and suspected cases of occupational asthma. New Zealand Med Journal 1992; 105(934):185–187.

60. Douwes J, McLean D, Slater T, Pearce N. Asthma and other respiratory symptoms in New Zealand pine processing sawmill workers. Am J Ind Med 2001; 38:608–615.

61. Whitehead LW, Ashikaga T, Vacek P. Pulmonary function status of workers exposed to hardwood or pine dust. Am Ind Hyg Ass J 1981; 42:178–186.

62. Hessel PA, Herbert FA, Melenka LS, Yoshida K, Michaelchuk D, Nakaza M. Lung health in sawmill workers exposed to pine and spruce. Chest 1995; 108:642–646.

63. Cormier Y, Mérlaux A, Duchaine C. Respiratory health impact of working in sawmills in Eastern Canada. Arch Environ Health 2000; 55:424–430.

64. Towey JW, Sweany HC, Huraon WH. Severe bronchial asthma apparently due to fungus spores found in maple bark. JAMA 1932; 99:453–459.

65. Côté J, Chan H, Brochu G, Chan-Yeung M. Occupational asthma caused by exposure to neurospora in a plywood factory worker. Br J Ind Med 1991; 48:279–282.

66. Fransman W, McLean D, Douwes J, Demers PA, Leung V, Pearce N. Respiratory symptoms and occupational exposures in New Zealand plywood mill workers. Ann Occup Hyg 2003; 47:287–295.

67. Herbert FA, Hessel PA, Melena LS, Yoshida K, Nakaza M. Respiratory consequences of exposure to wood dust and formaldehyde of workers manufacturing oriented strand board. Arch Environ Health 1994; 49:465–470.

68. Noertjojo HK, Dimich-Ward H, Peelen S, Dittrick M, Kennedy SM, Chan-Yeung M. Western red cedar dust exposure and lung function: a dose-response relationship. Am J Respir Crit Care Med 1996; 154:968–973.

69. Holness DL, Sass-Kortsak AM, Pilger CW, Nethercott JR. Respiratory function and exposure-effect relationships in wood dust-exposed and control workers. JOM 1985; 27:501–506.
70. Paggiaro P, Vellutini M, Viegi G, et al. A cross sectional epidemiological survey on symptoms and lung function of workers in a furniture plant. G Ital Med Lav 1986; 8:145–148.
71. Shamssain MH. Pulmonary function and symptoms in workers exposed to wood dust. Thorax 1992; 47:84–87.
72. Halpin DMG, Graneek BJ, Lacey J, et al. Respiratory symptoms, immunological responses, and aeroallergen concentrations at a sawmill. Occup Environ Med 1994; 51:165–172.
73. Mandryk J, Alwis KU, Hocking AD. Work-related symptoms and dose-response relationships for personal exposures and pulmonary function among woodworkers. Am J Ind Med 1999; 35:481–490.
74. Rongo LMB, Beselink A, Fouwes J, et al. Respiratory symptoms and dust exposure among male workers in small-scale wood industries in Tanzania. J Occup Environ Med 2002; 44:1153–1160.
75. Rastogi SK, Gupta BN, Husain T, Mathur NAJ. Respiratory health effects from occupational exposure to wood dust in sawmills. Am Ind Hyg Assoc J 1989; 50:574–578.
76. Pisaniello DL, Connell KE, Muriale L. Wood dust exposure during furniture manufacture-results from an Australian survey and considerations for threshold limit value development. Am Ind Hyg Assoc J 1991; 52:485–492.
77. Schlunssen V, Schaumburg I, Taudorf E, Mikkelsen AB, Sigsgaard T. Respiratory symptoms and lung function among Danish woodworkers. J Occup Env Med 2002; 44:82–98.
78. Chan-Yeung M, Wong R, MacLean L, et al. Respiratory survey of workers in a pulp and paper mill in Powell River, British Columbia. Am Rev Respir Dis 1980; 122:249–257.
79. Demers PA, Teschke K, Kennedy SM. What to do about softwood? A review of respiratory effects and recommendations regarding exposure limits. Am J Ind Med 1997; 31:385–398.
80. Emanuel DA, Wenzel FJ, Lawton BR. Pneumonitis due to *Cryptostroma corticale* (Maple-Bark Disease). N Eng J Med 1966; 274:1413–1418.
81. Avila R, Villar TG. Suberosis. Respiratory disease in cork workers. Lancet 1968; 1:620–621.
82. Cohen HI, Merigan TC, Kosek JC, Eldridge F. Sequoiosis. A granulomatous pneumonitis associated with redwood sawdust inhalation. Am J Med 1967; 43:785–794.
83. Schlueter DP, Fink JN, GTHensley. Wood-pulp workers' disease: A hypersensitivity pneumonitis caused by alternaria. Ann Int Med 1972; 77:907–911.
84. Thiede WH, Banaszak EF, Fink JN, Unger GF, Scanlon GT. Hypersensitivity studies in Popple (Aspen tree) peelers. Chest 1975; 67:405–407.
85. Belin S. Clinical and immunological data on "wood trimmer's disease" in Sweden. Europ J Respir Dis 1980; 61(suppl 107):169–176.
86. Wimander K, Belin L. Recognition of allergic alveolitis in the trimming department of a Swedish sawmill. Europ J Respir Dis 1980; 61(suppl 107):163–167.
87. Belin L. Health problems caused by actinomycetes and moulds in the industrial environment. Allergy 1985; 40(suppl 3):24–29.
88. Belin L. Sawmill alveolitis in Sweden. Int Arch Allergy Appl Immunol 1987; 82:440–443.
89. doPico GA, Reddan W, Flaherty D, et al. Respiratory abnormalities among grain handlers: A clinical, physiologic and immunologic study. Am Rev Respir Dis 1977; 115:915–927.
90. Malmberg P, Palmgren U, Rask-Anderson A. Relationship between symptoms and exposure to moldy dust in Swedish farmers. Am J Ind Med 1986; 10:316–317.
91. Mitchell JC, Chan-Yeung M. Contact allergy from frullania and respiratory allergy from thuja. Can Med Ass J 1974; 110:653–657.
92. Acheson ED, Cowdell RH, Hadfield E, Macbeth RG. Nasal cancer in woodworkers in the furniture industry. Br Med J 1968; 2:587–597.
93. Hausen B. Woods injurious to human health—A manual. Walter de Gruyter, 1981.

23
Metals

I. Leonard Bernstein
Division of Allergy–Immunology, Department of Internal Medicine, College of Medicine, University of Cincinnati, Cincinnati, Ohio, U.S.A.

Rolf Merget
Research Institute for Occupational Medicine of the Institutions for Statutory Accident Insurance and Prevention (BGFA), Ruhr-University, Bochum, Germany

INTRODUCTION

Occupational asthma induced by inhalation exposure to metals may have been first described by Georgius Agricola, who published "De Re Metallica" in 1556 (1). The author described the possible harmful effects of metallic dust as follows: "On the other hand, some mines are so dry that they are entirely devoid of water and this dryness causeth the workmen even greater harm, for the dust, which is stirred and beaten up by digging, penetrates into the windpipe and lungs and produces difficulty in breathing and the disease the Greeks call 'asthma.'" Admittedly, this excerpt is more likely to pertain to mineworkers' pneumoconiosis than to what would now be called asthma. Although many forms of pulmonary toxicity have been noted after exposure to metals, metalloids, and their respective oxides, salts, and coordination complexes, the occurrence of occupational asthma induced by these substances has only been recognized as a medical entity in the early part of the twentieth century. While the numerical contribution of metal-induced asthma to the overall prevalence of occupational asthma appears to be relatively small, the number of literature citations of these problems continues to increase each year. In addition, significant numbers of workers are exposed to these agents according to the NIOSH 1981–1983 National Exposure Survey (Table 1).

GENERAL PROPERTIES OF METALS

Workers are rarely exposed to pure metals or metalloids, but usually to oxides, sulfides, halides, hydrides, carbides, or other salts of these elements (2). Transition metals also form coordination complexes with ligands such as ammonia, carbon monoxide, cyanogen, organic nitrogen, or sulfur molecules. Bioavailability is also an important determinant of the possible effects resulting from exposure to these substances. Thus, deposits of insoluble metallic compounds in the airways are more

Table 1 Estimated Number of Workers Exposed to Metals and Metallic Salts in the United States, 1981–1983

	All durations		Full-time	
Agent	Total	Female	Total	Female
Nickel: welding, soldering, brazing	139,771	30,830	31,829	8,960
Chromium				
Metal (Cr III)	395,612	11,800	42,181	639
Welding, soldering, brazing	6,876	162	3,774	153
Cobalt: metal, dust fume	79,659	2,718	9,976	44
Vanadium	54,160	2,657	14,867	717
Zinc oxide	1,305,837	248,087	41,410	2,610
Platinum				
Metal	24,836	4,135	1,964	108
Compounds	37,402	18,286	539	
Aluminum				
Metal	1,104,885	102,130	217,084	27,165
Total dust	20,321	1,643	3,374	1,179

likely to be cleared by the mucociliary apparatus, while soluble metallic salts may readily dissociate and be transported as metal ions into lung tissues. Some metals such as cobalt (Co), zinc (Zn), and chromium (Cr) may act as essential trace elements or coenzymes for important metabolic enzyme pathways (3). Indeed, specific metal-binding sites in enzymatic proteins could possibly play a role in the pathogenesis of some metal-related allergic reactions (e.g., platinum interaction with endogenous malic dehydrogenase enzymes) (4). Interaction of metallic ions with other body transport proteins and macromolecules may lead to the development of antigenicity similar to that caused by other organic low-molecular-weight compounds, which may function as haptens (e.g., platinum, chromium, nickel, and cobalt). The biologic activity and impact of some metals is also predicated on their abilities to change oxidation states by oxidation (loss of electrons) and reduction (gain of electrons) (2). As transition metals are electronically stable in more than one oxidation state, these metals play important roles in the catalysis of biologic oxidation reactions. Moreover, their ability to enhance the production of toxic species of oxygen could also be involved in the pathogenesis of nonimmunologic asthma.

DIFFERENTIAL DIAGNOSIS OF METAL-INDUCED ASTHMA

The spectrum of pulmonary toxicity due to inhalation of metallic compounds encompasses a wide range of acute and chronic obstructive syndromes, which in some instances may mimic asthma (2). Inhalation of fumes or dusts from many metallic salts and hydrides may cause chemical tracheobronchitis or chemical pneumonitis with a picture resembling the adult respiratory distress syndrome (5). Similarly, chronic exposure to cobalt (hard metal), aluminum, manganese, titanium dioxide, beryllium, and cadmium are associated with chronic obstructive lung diseases such as chronic bronchitis and pulmonary emphysema (6). Small airway involvement in these diseases may at times be confused with asthma. In the case of occupational exposure to cobalt, alveolitis and asthma may coexist (7). Although the pathogenesis of metal fume fever occurring in welders is not entirely understood, there have been recent reports of associated or superimposed bronchial asthma with this condition. Specific examples of these concurrent entities will be discussed in separate sections under respective individual metals. Finally, small airway disease may at times be a prominent feature of pneumoconiosis with features of diffuse interstitial pneumonitis, for example, hard-metal lung disease or pneumoconiosis with sarcoid-like granuloma formations such as berylliosis (8,9).

OCCUPATIONAL EXPOSURE VARIABLES

Asthma in workers occupationally exposed to metals may not necessarily be because of the metallic exposure. Prior or current cigarette smoking may obfuscate the diagnosis of occupational asthma in some workers. There are other examples of mixed exposures to metals and nonmetals. For example, workers in foundries are far more likely to develop asthma due to methylenediphenyl diisocyanate (MDI), used in some molding resins, than they are to metal oxides. In certain industries, concurrent exposure to sulfur oxide, ozone, chlorine, or nitrogen dioxide may constitute as much or greater risk than exposure to specific metallic compounds. In the platinum-refining industry, for example, workers are not only exposed to the platinum halide salts but also to significant concentrations of chlorine and sulfur dioxide gases (10).

On the other hand, exposure to metals is not necessarily confined to workers involved in metal mining or metallurgical industries. Thus, cobalt-induced bronchial asthma has been described in diamond polishers who use cobalt-containing polishing discs (11). Metallic compounds are used as pigments in the paint and ceramic industry, as catalysts in the chemical industry, or as additives in the plastic industry (12). Finally, significant exposure to metals is not confined to the work environment. Hobbies and domestic activities may lead to clinical sensitivity in susceptible individuals. It has also been suspected that persistence of platinum-induced asthma could be due to continued contact with former platinum workers who retain small amounts of platinum on their clothing (13).

CLASSIFICATION

Because recognition of occupational asthma induced by a variety of metals and their derivatives is relatively recent, a generally acceptable system of classification has not yet evolved. Thus far, this category of occupational asthma has been identified according to specific etiologic agents and terms such as "transitional" metals, "precious" metals (platinum, palladium, etc.), and "hard" metals (tungsten carbide, cobalt, etc.) have been used to define specific asthmatic problems. Because the vast majority of workplace asthma induced by metallic compounds is caused by metallic elements (and their derivatives) located in specific sections of the periodic table of elements, a new classification based on a specific metallic element's position in the periodic table is proposed as a frame of reference for the following discussion of occupational asthma induced by specific agents (Table 2). The 38 elements between groups IIA and III of the periodic table are "transition metals." Thus far, all metallic elements that cause asthma can be classified within the main transition metal series, in the group III metal series, or as indeterminate metals. In this chapter, this numbered classification will encompass the following occupational asthma entities:

Table 2   The Periodic Table of the Elements

	IA	IIA	TRANSITION METALS										III	IV	V	VI	VII	VIII
1	H																	He
2	Li	Be											B	C	N	O	F	Ne
3	Na	Mg											Al	Si	P	S	Cl	Ar
4	K	Ca	Sc	Ti	V	Cr	Mn	Fe	Co	Ni	Cu	Zn	Ga	Ge	As	Se	Br	Kr
5	Rb	Sr	Y	Zr	Nb	Mo	Tc	Ru	Rh	Pd	Ag	Cd	In	Sn	Sb	Te	I	Xe
6	Cs	Ba	La*	Hf	Ta	W	Re	Os	Ir	Pt	Au	Hg	Tl	Pb	Bi	Po	At	Rn
7	Fr	Ra	Ac**	Rf	Db	Sg	Bh	Hs	Mt	Uun	Uuu	Uub		Uuq		Uuh	Uus	

Lanthanides	*	Ce	Pr	Nd	Pm	Sm	Eu	Gd	Tb	Dy	Ho	Er	Tm	Yb	Lu
Actinides	**	Th	Pa	U	Np	Pu	Am	Cm	Bk	Cf	Es	Fm	Md	No	Lr

The transition metals occur between the Group II and Group III alkaline earth metals. These are elements with partially filled d-orbitals. The relevant metals of interest in the induction of occupational asthma are:

1. First period of transition metals between scandium and zinc;
2. Second period of transition metals between yttrium and cadmium;
3. Third period of transition metals between lanthanum, the rare earth elements (lanthanides) and mercury;
4. Group III alkaline earth metals, of which aluminum is the sole relevant metal for occupational asthma.

The rows in the table labeled 1, 2, 3, 4, 5, 6, and 7 correspond to the principal quantum number.

1. First series of transitional metals (also referred to as the "iron group transition metals" between scandium and zinc). This group includes metals such as vanadium, chromium, cobalt, nickel, and zinc.
2. Second series of transitional metals (also referred to as the "palladium group transition metals" between yttrium and cadmium). This group includes ruthenium, rhodium, palladium, and cadmium.
3. Third series of transitional metals (also referred to as the "platinum group transition metals" between hafnium and mercury). This group includes iridium and platinum.
4. Group III metals (aluminum is the sole relevant agent in this series).
5. Indeterminate metals (due to mixtures of alloys or contaminants in manufactured metallic products).

Table 3 is a compilation of metals classified according to their respective orbital structures in the periodic table, their occupational asthma classification numbers defined above, and their propensity to induce IgE mediated asthma after occupational exposure to these agents. According to this classification, it is apparent that the majority of metal-induced asthmatic problems are associated with metals of the first series of transitional metals. However, it should be emphasized that the absolute number of asthma occurrences after exposure to platinum and aluminum far outnumber those after exposure to other metals (14–16).

FIRST SERIES OF TRANSITIONAL METALS

Nickel

Primary nickel industries include mining, milling, smelting, and refinishing processes whereby nickel ores are removed from the ground and transformed into marketable, unfabricated materials such as nickel metal, nickel oxide, and nickel alloy (17). Workers in electroplating industries are commonly exposed to nickel sulfate. Workers involved in the production of nickel catalysts (used in the food industry for hardening of edible oils by hydrogenation) are exposed to both nickel sulfate and nickel hydroxide–carbonate complex. Nickel workers may also be exposed to vapors of nickel carbonyl. The latter compound is extremely toxic to the central nervous system and lung, and the permitted exposure limit is a time-weighted concentration of $0.12\,mg/m^3$. For soluble nickel salts, the exposure limit is $0.1\,mg/m^3$ as the time-weighted average (TWA) concentration for up to an eight-hour workday, 40-hour workweek (18).

Although it is estimated that 140,000 workers in the United States are potentially exposed to nickel, the occurrence of asthma induced by exposure to these salts is uncommon. Moreover, relatively few cases of nickel-induced asthma have been associated with or preceded by contact dermatitis, a frequent outcome of nickel sensitization (19). However, no conclusions can be drawn about the association of nickel dermatitis and asthma because the number of documented asthma reports is too few. Another possible confounding effect of nickel exposure is that coexposure to other metals such as chromium, cobalt, and cadmium often occurs in electroplating, metal grinding, and nickel-battery worksites, respectively (20–22).

Apart from one case of nickel-related Loeffler's syndrome and asthma caused by exposure to nickel carbonyl, there have been about 13 recorded cases of asthma

Table 3 Metals Known to Induce Occupational Asthma

Classification	Periodic system		Chemical form exposed to	TLV/TWA (mg/m^3)	IgE-mediated
	Atomic number	Classification			
Nickel	28	1	Elemental/metal (inhalable)	*1.5*	No
			Soluble compounds, as Ni (inhalable)	*0.1*	Yes
			Insoluble compounds, as Ni (inhalable)	*0.2*[a]	No
			Nickel subsulfide, as Ni (inhalable)	*0.1*[a]	No
			Nickle carbonyl (inhalable)	*0.12 (0.05 ppm)*	Equivocal
Chromium	24	1	Metal and CrIII compounds, as Cr	0.5	No
			Water-soluble CrVI compounds, as Cr	0.05[a]	Yes
			Insoluble CrVI compounds, as Cr	0.01[a]	No
Cobalt	27	1	Metal and inorganic compounds	0.02	Yes
Vanadium	23	1	As V_2O_5 (respirable dust or fumes)	0.05	No
Zinc oxide	30	1	Fume	5	No
			Dust	10	No
Platinum	78	3	Metal	1	No
			Soluble salts, as Pt	0.002	Yes
Aluminum	13	4	Metal dust	10	No
			Pyro powders, as Al	5	No
			Welding fumes, as Al	5	No
			Alkyl	2	No
			Soluble salts, as Al	2	No

TLV/TWA = threshold limit value/time-weighted average: the time-weighted average concentration for a conventional 8-hr workday and a 40-hr workweek, to which it is believed that nearly all workers may be repeatedly exposed, day after day, without adverse effect. Data in italics concern substances for which a change has been proposed ("notice of intended change").

[a]Human carcinogen.

Source: 1998 update TLV/TWA data were supplied by the ACGIH, Cincinnati, Ohio, U.S.A.

occurring after exposure to nickel sulfate (19,20,23–31). Nine of these were documented by controlled bronchial challenge tests (19,20,24–27,30,31). Four workers demonstrated immediate bronchoprovocation response, four workers experienced an isolated late asthmatic reaction, and one exhibited a dual response. Several of these patients also manifested an increase in bronchial hyperresponsiveness for varying periods after the nickel sulfate challenge. Four of the reported cases demonstrated evidence of immediate skin reactivity. Seven out of eight workers with hard-metal asthma thought to be induced by cobalt had positive nickel-specific bronchoprovocation tests (four immediate; three late). This suggested either cross-reactivity or dual sensitization to nickel and cobalt (32). Nickel-reactive hemagglutinating antibodies were first demonstrated by McConnell et al. (23). Modest levels (twice the negative control) of nickel-specific IgE-associated antibodies were demonstrated by Dolovich et al. (33) who showed specific reactivity to a nickel–human serum albumin conjugate, while Novey et al. (26) obtained significantly higher IgE antibody levels using an ionic-exchange resin as the solid phase for the nickel antigen. Specific IgE antibodies were also demonstrated in three other instances (19,20,30). In the cobalt-sensitive workers discussed above, nickel human albumin conjugates elicited specific antibody responses (32). Detailed investigations of possible cell-mediated immune mechanisms were not undertaken in any of these cases.

Chromium

Chromium is a transition metal that is widely used in electroplating processes, metal alloys, pigments, tanning of leather, and production of chromate salts (34). Moreover, many varieties of cement contain traces of chromium, which are responsible for allergic sensitization and contact dermatitis in construction workers. Although chromium metal is thought to be nonallergic, the prevalence of asthma is increased in the chromate miners of Sudan (35). Chromium salts are unequivocally allergenic and have been investigated extensively as causative agents in occupational contact dermatitis. Chromium salts exist naturally in three valence forms: 2, 3, and 6. Bivalent compounds are unstable and have little commercial value. Hexavalent chromium compounds (e.g., chromium trioxide and mono- and bichromates) may have an increased potential for allergenicity because they are more soluble and presumably have easier access into body tissues. It is estimated that 400,000 workers are potentially exposed to hexavalent chromium (18). Workplace standards distinguish between carcinogenic and noncarcinogenic species of hexavalent chromate. Monochromates and bichromates (dichromates of hydrogen, lithium, sodium, potassium, rubidium, cesium, and ammonium, as well as chromium oxide) are considered non-carcinogenic. The workplace environmental limit for hexavalent chromium is a TWA of 0.05 mg of hexavalent chromium/m^3 for up to an eight-hour workday, 40-hour workweek (18).

Although hexavalent chromium is generally acknowledged to be the most frequent skin sensitizer for male industrial workers, it is an uncommon cause of occupational asthma. Documentation of chromium-induced asthma by controlled laboratory bronchial challenge testing has been published in 20 cases (26,31,32,36–40). Six workers demonstrated immediate type bronchoconstrictive responses after inhaling chromium sulfate aerosols. A transient, reversible asthmatic response after bronchial challenge was observed in a metal plating worker (41). Nine workers experienced dual asthmatic responses while four had isolated late reactions. Methacholine-induced hyperresponsiveness was demonstrated in four of these cases (36). Another worker experienced a unique late wheezing reaction six hours after the challenge (37). This was accompanied by a generalized urticarial eruption, facial edema, and periorbital swelling. Cement asthma has been described in building workers (42). Occupational asthma was also reported in a floorer who had both occupational dermatitis and occupational asthma. In this case, it was proposed that the inhalation exposure to chromates occurred by means of smoking rolled cigarettes contaminated with cement (39). Chromium-specific IgE antibodies were demonstrated in the case showing an immediate bronchoconstrictive response (26). In these studies, the chromium salt was adsorbed to a cationic exchange resin as solid phase. Prick tests with 10 mg/mL solutions of chromate salts were positive in two cases (36). In contrast to nickel-induced asthma, a prior history of contact dermatitis and positive patch tests (using 0.5% solution of potassium dichromate) were noted in five cases (38). Evidence of cell-mediated mechanisms was also present in a patient who exhibited an isolated delayed response after chromate challenge (37). In this instance, significant leukocyte inhibitory factor activity to hexavalent chromate was obtained in a dose–responsive fashion.

Cobalt

Cobalt is used in the manufacture of alloys for the electrical, automobile, and aircraft industries (2,6,8). Steel-containing cobalt is used in safety razor blades and surgical instruments. Cobalt is also used in the manufacture of pigments, coloring glass, and enamel. One of the chief uses of cobalt is as a binder for tungsten carbide in sintered hard metals (also called cemented carbides or cermets) and more recently, also in diamond tools. Thus, cobalt incorporated into high-speed polishing discs represents a significant source of exposure for diamond polishers (11). The largest work population exposed to cobalt dust is in the hard-metal industry, because hard metals are used for tools and engine parts that need to sustain high temperatures. Significant exposure to cobalt-containing dust not only occurs during various stages in the manufacturing of hard-metal tools, but also during their maintenance and resharpening. During the latter operations the use of coolants and their continuous recycling has been shown to lead to an enrichment in dissolved cobalt and hence a higher potential for exposure to ionic cobalt in the aerosolized fluids (43).

NIOSH estimates that approximately 80,000 workers are exposed to cobalt materials. Reports of occupational asthma are not infrequent (6,44). In a large industrial survey, Kusaka et al. (45) observed that 5% of hard-metal workers had work-related asthma. This should be distinguished from hard-metal disease. Hard-metal disease is an interstitial pneumonia with clinical presentations resembling hypersensitivity pneumonitis and the potential to evolve to irreversible fibrosis (46). A characteristic pathologic feature of hard-metal lung disease is the presence of "bizarre" multinucleated giant cells in the interstitium and alveoli, and hence in the bronchoalveolar lavage. Hard-metal lung disease has never been reported to occur in subjects exposed to cobalt alone and it is, therefore, likely that the simultaneous presence of cobalt and other particles (such as tungsten carbide or diamond) is required for the development of interstitial pneumonia. However, it is well established by several investigators that cobalt alone can induce asthma in susceptible workers.

Cobalt-induced asthma has been documented in workers involved in the production of cobalt, the manufacture and use of cobalt pigments, the production and maintenance of hard-metal and diamond tools, and the polishing of diamonds (11,41,44,47–50). Provocation tests performed separately with both cobalt and tungsten carbide powder revealed that only cobalt provoked the asthmatic response (51). In addition, investigators have shown that controlled positive challenge to cobalt temporarily increased nonspecific bronchial hyperresponsiveness. It has also been demonstrated that affected workers will react not only to inhaled powder but also to water-soluble cobalt. Delayed bronchial challenge reactions appear to be common (51).

Shirakawa et al. (52) investigated possible immunopathogenesis in 12 cobalt bronchoprovocation-positive patients. None of the patients had positive immediate-type skin tests to cobalt reagents. Six patients demonstrated evidence of cobalt-specific IgE to a cobalt human serum albumin conjugate. One patient showed a borderline significant reaction to cobalt adsorbed to a resin reagent. It was also of interest that five of these workers were considered atopic by virtue of high total IgE titers and positive RAST scores when tested for a battery of common aeroallergens. In a recent cross-sectional survey of 706 workers exposed to hard-metal dust, there was no correlation between cobalt-specific IgE antibodies and cigarette smoking (53). Kusaka et al. (54) observed that two of the patients who had specific IgE antibodies to cobalt also exhibited lymphocyte proliferation responses when their peripheral blood lymphocytes were incubated with either free cobalt or a cobalt human serum albumin conjugate. In a few cases, bronchoalveolar lavage revealed an increase in T lymphocytes with an inverted CD4+/CD8+ ratio (55). These results suggested that cobalt-sensitized lymphocytes may play a role in the immunopathogenesis of some hard-metal asthmatics. However, in the combined studies of Shirakawa et al. and Kusaka et al., it should be noted that five hard-metal asthmatic patients demonstrated neither cobalt-specific IgE nor sensitized lymphocytes. The fact that cobalt and metallic carbides interact with oxygen to produce activated toxic oxygen species suggests that some workers with lower antioxidant defensive mechanisms may be more susceptible to hard-metal disease (56). However, it is not clear whether cobalt-induced asthma is related to the interstitial lung disease associated with cobalt. Because workers occasionally exhibit both asthmatic reactions and parenchymal involvement, it is possible that cobalt asthma may be an "airway variant" of hard-metal disease (7,57,58). As discussed in the nickel section, Shirakawa et al. (59) demonstrated that some workers with cobalt-induced asthma also manifested specific sensitization and positive bronchial responses to nickel sulfate. It is known that nickel is sometimes added to hard metal as a matrix in addition to cobalt. Further evaluation of these workers revealed that four showed evidence of specific IgE antibodies to both cobalt and nickel. Although the authors postulated that cross-reactivity between these two metals was a possibility, it is more likely that these workers developed concurrent hypersensitivity reactions after exposure to both metals.

Vanadium

Vanadium pentoxide is the most important chemical derivative of vanadium in commercial use. It is used as a catalyst for a variety of reactions in the chemical and petroleum refinery industries (60). It is particularly prominent in the production of high-strength steel alloys. Occupational exposure to vanadium pentoxide is primarily an inhalation hazard causing irritation of the upper respiratory tract (61). The recommended threshold limit of vanadium pentoxide dust is 0.5 mg/m^3 of air (19). Acute tracheitis and bronchitis with persistent bronchial hyperresponsiveness can be caused by exposure to vanadium pentoxide. Vanadium-induced asthma is associated with the cleaning of oil tanks ("boilermaker's bronchitis") (62). Information about vanadium-induced asthma is available only from case reports (63). It has been established that this asthma develops in workers without prior history of asthma. The majority of affected workers thus far have been nonatopic. Increased bronchial hyperresponsiveness has been demonstrated in at least two cases. Positive skin tests or any other immunopathogenetic mechanism have not been described. In addition, there are no reports of controlled laboratory challenges to vanadium pentoxide. However, subhuman primates exposed to vanadium pentoxide over a period of weeks develop a pattern of increased hyperresponsiveness to the agent (64).

Zinc

A major use for zinc is in galvanizing, which consists of depositing a fine layer of zinc onto a metal surface (steel sheet, structural sections, and nails) to protect it from corrosion. Other important uses of zinc include various alloys (die castings used in automotive parts) and in brass. Further uses of zinc are as pigments and salts in paints, wood preservation, etc. Zinc chloride is a component of smoke bombs. The most significant exposure to zinc occurs as a result of welding or burning (galvanizing) metals, the fumes of which contain various metal oxides including zinc oxide. Exposure to fumes of zinc oxide is most often associated with metal fume fever, which typically begins 4 to 12 hours after exposure. The manifestations of metal fume fever resemble a flu-like illness, but coughing and shortness of breath may also be present. Episodes may persist anywhere from 24 to 48 hours. Several cases of occupational asthma have been described but considering the extensive usage of zinc-containing metals, the overall prevalence of this problem is negligible (65–67). The threshold limit value of zinc is $5 \, mg/m^3$.

Of the cases with suspected wheezing due to zinc oxide fumes, two patients were subjected to controlled bronchial challenge under laboratory conditions (67). Both workers demonstrated objective evidence of bronchial constriction four to nine hours after the exposure. Fever and leukocytosis occurred in one of the patients, indicating that this individual may have had a combination of occupational asthma and metal fume fever. Increased bronchial hyperresponsiveness was also observed in one patient 24 hours after the exposure. Environmental measurements at the workplace of these two individuals revealed significantly elevated concentrations of zinc after a work-simulated episode of soldering on galvanized iron (22 mg/mL). Another recent case report fulfilled the criteria of occupational asthma, as indexed by a postshift fall of forced expiratory volume in one second (FEV_1), bronchial hyperresponsiveness to methacholine, and an immediate asthmatic response after bronchial challenge (68). Although positive immediate skin tests were demonstrated in this case, it is not certain that IgE-mediated mechanisms were involved (68).

SECOND SERIES OF TRANSITIONAL METALS

Palladium and Rhodium

The occurrence of either skin or clinical sensitization after exposure to precious metals in this category (ruthenium, rhodium, palladium, and silver) is rare (69). Several groups of Russian investigators have reported that some salts of these metals—chiefly palladium—may induce both immediate and delayed hypersensitivity skin reactions and may also elicit direct histamine release from human leukocytes (70–73). The immunogenic potential of palladium was partially corroborated by Biagini et al. (13) who demonstrated that sera from some platinum-sensitive, palladium-exposed workers also elicited a positive PCA response to palladium in subhuman primates. However, these investigators did not observe direct evidence that workers exposed to a variety of precious metal salts other than platinum developed allergic symptoms or asthma to these salts. Daenen et al. (74) recently investigated a case of occupational asthma, which was clearly related to fumes of an electrolysis bath containing palladium chloride. This worker exhibited an isolated positive skin test to tetramminepalladium(II) chloride ($1 \mu g/mL$) as well as a positive bronchial provocation test to this salt administered as an aerosol ($10 \mu g/mL$) for a period of 3.5 minutes (74).

Among a group of 130 catalyst production workers with exposure to a broad spectrum of precious metals, four subjects showed a positive prick test reaction to palladium chloride 10^{-3} mol/L (wheal diameters 6, 3, 2, and 1.5 mm), and the subject with the 6-mm wheal reaction to palladium also demonstrated a 5-mm wheal with rhodium chloride (R. Merget, unpublished). All these subjects showed positive skin-prick tests to platinum salts, and the reactions were interpreted as cross-sensitizations. In another study of 306 South African refinery workers, 38 had positive skin-prick test reactions to platinum salts. Of these, one subject was positive to palladium and six positive to rhodium salts (75). A recent study among 153 Italian refinery workers found positive skin-prick test reactions to rhodium chloride in two subjects; both also showed positive skin-prick tests with hexachloroplatinic acid, suggesting cross-sensitization between the two metallic salts in a small number of cases (76).

Cadmium

Asthma has not been reported after exposure to salts or fumes of cadmium, which is one of the metallic elements in the second long series. Acute exposure to cadmium fumes may cause life-threatening chemical pneumonitis. Recent studies suggest that there is an excess of impaired respiratory function and diffusing capacity, as well as radiologic signs of emphysema, in workers with chronic inhalation exposure to cadmium, when compared with appropriate controls (2).

THIRD SERIES OF TRANSITIONAL METALS

Only two metals in this group have been reported to cause asthma. Whereas platinum salts are among the most prominent causes of occupational asthma, there is only one case report about iridium-induced occupational asthma.

Iridium

A nonsmoking and nonatopic male was exposed to iridium chloride in an electrochemical factory manufacturing titanium anodes. The anodes were coated with various metal salts of the platinum group dissolved in hydrochloric acid. The coating solution was sprayed onto the anodes automatically. The subject developed symptoms of the nose, eyes, and lower airways about three years after the beginning of exposure, and contact urticaria developed about five years later. An iridium chloride skin-prick test showed a positive reaction at a concentration of 5×10^{-4} g iridium (as metal)/mL, and scratch tests with an iridium chloride solution of 5.8×10^{-4} g iridium (as metal)/mL and iridium-salt containing solutions from the workplace produced systemic allergic reactions. Platinum salt allergy was excluded by skin-prick and scratch testing with a hexachloroplatinate solution [4.4×10^{-4} g platinum (as metal)/mL]. Fourteen employees at the same factory did not show skin-prick test reactions to either iridium or platinum salts. The results were interpreted as clinical immediate-type hypersensitivity of the airways to iridium salt (77). Recently, three subjects with positive skin-prick test reactions to iridium chloride were found in a cohort of 153 refinery workers. Sensitization to iridium was accompanied in each case by sensitization to hexachloroplatinic acid (76).

Platinum

Exposure and Epidemiology

The chief occupational exposure to platinum salts occurs during the primary and secondary refining of platinum. In the secondary refining processes, precious metals such as platinum, palladium, rhodium, and ruthenium are reclaimed from scrap metal and expended automobile exhaust catalysts. The scrap is burned to remove carbon and other combustible components. The resultant fine powder is dissolved in hydrochloric acid and chlorine followed by separation, sequential solubilization, and precipitation to yield halide platinum salts (Fig. 1). This manufacturing process also involves exposure to chlorine gas, formaldehyde, sulfur dioxide, hydrazine, hydrogen chloride, and nitric acid. It has been shown that concurrent exposure of subhuman primates to irritants such as those commonly used in the secondary platinum-refining industry could potentiate the effects of platinum salt exposure by increasing pulmonary mucosal permeability (78).

Recently, platinum salt allergy has been reported in catalyst production workers (Fig. 2) (79). The work processes in catalyst production are automated to a high degree in industrialized countries; thus, exposure occurs mostly during maintenance and repair. In contrast to Europe, car catalysts are not submitted to a reduction process prior to installation in cars in the United States. Thus, catalysts still contain halogenated platinum salts when they leave the catalyst production. However, platinum salt allergy has not been described in U.S. automobile workers.

It is estimated that only several thousand workers have significant exposure to the specific platinum salts that have been incriminated as causes of occupational asthma. Thus, platinum salt allergy is not found among the leading causes of occupational asthma worldwide by the number of affected workers, but it is a considerable health problem in some chemical plants with cumulative risks for sensitization of up to 51% within five years (80). The threshold limit value for platinum salts is $2\,\mu g/m^3$; it is not known whether this threshold prevents sensitization because this value has been exceeded even in recent studies (79,81).

Recently, air measurements at workplaces compared exposures over short periods with eight-hour TWA exposure levels at three different industrial sites of a refinery, all with recent cases of respiratory sensitization to platinum salts (82). The eight-hour TWA exposure limit for airborne soluble platinum was exceeded in 2 out of 17 workplaces (where respiratory protection was worn) and short-term exposures exceeded $2\,\mu g/m^3$ at six workplaces, but none of the short-term samples from workplaces where respiratory protection was not worn exceeded the 15-minute exposure level that was three times the eight-hour TWA. The authors concluded that either the current exposure limit is not protective or sensitization occurs via dermal exposure.

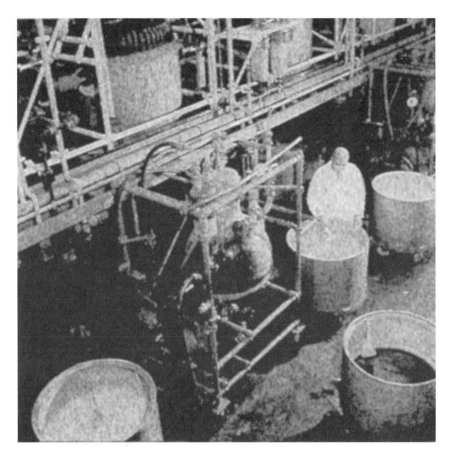

Figure 1 Historical photograph in a precious-metal refinery. The platinum salt is processed in closed reaction tanks; the final product, the yellow platinum salt powder, is obtained after filtration.

Platinum salt–induced occupational asthma has been recognized as early as 1911 in a small number of photographers (82). Further studies were conducted in precious metals refineries, and one study in a catalyst production plant (Table 4). Although two German studies demonstrated workplace air concentrations below 2 $\mu g/m^3$, prevalences of a positive skin-prick test with platinum salts in about 20% of exposed subjects were in the same range as in studies with higher exposure levels. Because few measurements were reported in the German studies, it is likely that exposures were higher than reported. Incidence rates are difficult to compare due to varying durations of follow-up. Interestingly, the three studies of refinery workers gave incidence rates of about 10% per year, whereas this number was much lower in a catalyst plant, possibly because of lower exposure.

Platinum salts induce symptoms in sensitized subjects that are similar to those in IgE-mediated allergies. Symptoms at the time of skin-prick test conversion from negative to positive were reported in 13 out of 14 catalyst production workers in a prospective longitudinal study (28.6% asthma, 64.3% runny nose or sneezing, 35.7% burning or itching eyes, and 35.7% skin rash or itching). The corresponding values for work-related symptoms were 21.4%, 42.9%, 28.6%, and 35.7%, respectively (83). The number of symptoms was considerably higher in a group of 83 workers evaluated

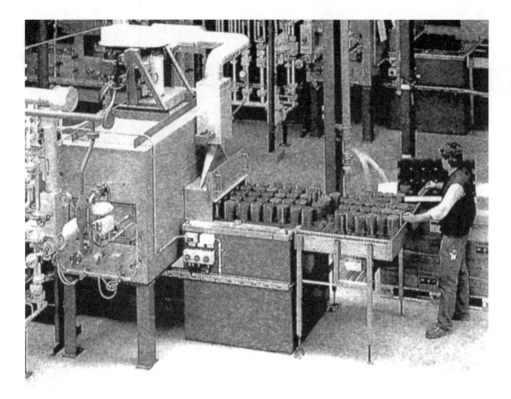

Figure 2 Car catalysts at the end of the production line in a German catalyst production. As the platinum salts were reduced in a reduction furnace, the worker needs no protective equipment.

for compensation (100%, 98%, 63%, and 51%, respectively) (84). These workers had been exposed to platinum salts for longer periods in spite of symptoms. Although this represents a highly selected group, the conclusion can be drawn that symptoms at the beginning of platinum salt allergy may slightly vary, but eventually almost always include rhinitis and asthma. In contrast to baker's rhinitis, rhinitis in platinum salt–allergic subjects without asthma occurs only at the very beginning of the disease.

It has been demonstrated in cross-sectional and longitudinal studies that the prevalence or incidence of platinum salt–skin sensitization correlates closely with occupational asthma. It is the halide moiety, which confers strong allergic properties to platinum salts. Skin-prick test reactions in subjects sensitized to platinum salts are strongly dependent on the halide content of the platinum solution (76,85,86). It has been shown by surveillance data that soluble platinum compounds such as tetramine platinum dichloride have no sensitizing potential (80). This is one of the few instances in which simple and nonconjugated chemicals can be used as reliable reagents for detection of IgE-mediated hypersensitivity responses in the skin. Skin-prick test reactivity has been observed at platinum salt concentrations as low as 10^{-9} g/mL (13). Although it has been reported that symptoms or bronchial hyperresponsiveness may precede skin-prick test positivity (82,88) and skin-prick tests may convert to negative after exposure cessation (Fig. 3), there is general consensus that skin-prick testing is a useful technique for surveillance and early detection of sensitized workers.

Table 4 Prevalence and Incidence Rates of Allergic Symptoms and Positive Skin-Prick Tests with Platinum Salts in Epidemiological Studies of Subjects with Exposure to Platinum Salts

Country	Exposed subjects (n)	Symptoms (%)	SPT+ve (%)	Workplace airborne soluble Pt concentration ($\mu g/m^3$)	Author (year)
Cross-sectional studies					
United Kingdom	16	57	25	0.9–1700	Hunter et al. (1945)
South Africa	306	nd	28	nd	Murdoch et al. (1986)
Germany	20	8	20	<0.08	Merget et al. (1988)
Germany	64	23	19	<0.1	Bolm- Audorff et al. (1992)
United States	107	44	14	>2 in 50–75%	Baker et al. (1990)
Longitudinal studies					
United Kingdom[a]	91	26.9/yr	12.1/yr	nd	Venables et al. (1989)
South Africa[b]	78	20.5/yr	11/yr	>2 in 27%	Calverley et al. (1995)
France[c]	77	13.6/yr	10.4/yr	nd	Niezborala et al. (1996)
Germany[d]	159	0.8/yr	1.8/yr	0.005–3.7 (>2 in 4%)	Merget et al. (2000)

[a]Historical prospective study/2 years (detailed information on incidence is presented only for the first two years of employment), refinery, and preemployment screening for atopy.
[b]Prospective study/2 years, refinery, reemployment screening for atopy.
[c]Historical prospective study/2 years (detailed information on incidence is presented only for the first two years of employment), refinery, and preemployment screening for atopy.
[d]Prospective study/5 years; catalyst plant, and no preemployment screening for atopy, removal from exposure after SPT conversion.
Abbreviations: SPT, skin-prick tests; nd, no data.

A direct comparison between skin-prick and bronchial challenge tests revealed that the skin-prick test has excellent sensitivity and specificity (86). Neither skin-prick tests nor bronchial challenges with platinum salts were positive in nine controls with bronchial hyperresponsiveness. On the other hand, of the 19 subjects with positive skin-prick tests to platinum salts, all subjects had a positive challenge (although one subject had no significant bronchial obstruction, but had coughing and sneezing). Bronchial challenges may be performed by mixing platinum salts with lactose or by direct inhalation of the platinum salt by a nebulizer (86,87,89). Due to the high specificity of skin-prick testing, bronchial challenges, which present as immediate or dual responses, may be avoided if the skin-prick test is positive. According to an international consensus, skin-prick tests (and bronchial challenges) with platinum salts should be performed with sodium hexachloroplatinate at a maximal concentration of 1g/L (90). Positive skin or bronchial reactions with this concentration in controls have not been reported. However, a recent cross-sectional survey found that

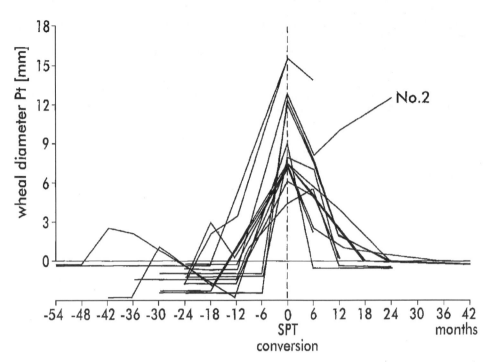

Figure 3 Skin-prick test results with platinum salts of 14 skin-prick test converters in a longitudinal survey. Skin-prick test conversion was set to time "zero." Subjects were removed completely from exposure soon after conversion, with the exception of subject No. 2, who continued to be exposed to small amounts of platinum salts as a workman by contaminated material from the catalyst production. *Source*: From Ref. 83.

skin-prick testing with hexachloroplatinic acid may be more sensitive (23 positive reactions among 153 workers) than testing with sodium hexachloroplatinate (11 positive reactions) (76). This is an unexpected finding and should be examined in the future.

Tenfold dilutions of hexachloroplatinic acid (in a range of 10^{-6} to 10^{-2} mol/L) were used for bronchial challenges (86). However, for safety reasons it is recommended to use doubling doses of sodium hexachloroplatinate in phosphate buffered saline administered using a DeVilbiss 646 dosimeter in a range of about 30 ng to 45 mg (R. Merget, unpublished data). A correlation between bronchial hyperresponsiveness to methacholine and bronchial responsiveness to platinum salts could not be shown; however there was a moderate association between bronchial responsiveness and skin reactivity to platinum salts (16). If bronchial challenges are considered, it is recommended to start with doses in the nanogram range even if methacholine responsiveness is less pronounced.

Due to clearly positive skin test reactions, the immunologic pathogenesis of airway reactions is considered to be an IgE-mediated hypersensitivity reaction. The role of IgE in this disease has been corroborated by both positive passive transfer tests in humans and monkeys with sera from affected workers (91) and IgE radioimmunoassay. Several in vitro procedures with platinum salts conjugated to different proteins or anion exchange resin have been used for the detection of platinum salt sensitivity (13,75,92,93). The sensitivity and specificity of these various in vitro procedures varied between investigators. In all studies, a wide overlap between the amounts of IgE binding to the solid phase occurred between skin-prick test positive and negative subjects. One study found a high correlation between total IgE and in vitro results, but no difference was found for platinum salt "specific" IgE between skin-prick test–positive subjects and nonexposed atopic controls (93). However, others demonstrated by in vitro inhibition experiments that the tests were specific for the respective platinum conjugates (13). Animal experiments showed that platinum salt conjugates with ovalbumin were able to induce specific IgE antibodies in rats (94). In one investigation, the sensitivity of the specific IgE radioimmunoassay was improved by preabsorption of free platinum in serum specimens by polyacrylamide gel (13). It was postulated that small amounts of freely circulating serum platinum competitively competed with the platinum salt conjugate for binding to the test substrate. All studies agreed that the specific radioimmunoassay is less sensitive than skin testing, and there is international consensus that it is not a useful tool in the clinical diagnosis of platinum hypersensitivity (90).

Elevated total IgE levels were reported in subjects with platinum salt allergy (13). Mean total serum IgE was highest in former skin test–positive workers who left the refinery because of platinum salt asthma. Unusually high values (1840 ng/mL or more) were observed in four out of eight of these medically terminated workers. It was suggested that chronic exposure to platinum salts may result in nonspecific immunopotentiation of the isotypic IgE response. This phenomenon had been noted in a rodent experimental model of platinum sensitization (94). However, a recent longitudinal study in a catalyst production plant, where platinum exposure is lower than in refineries, did not show an increase of total IgE in newly hired workers after a follow-up period of up to five years (83). While the presence of heat-stable, short-term sensitizing antibodies to platinum was demonstrated by two independent groups of investigators, the clinical significance of this finding is yet unknown (13,91).

In a cross-sectional refinery study it was shown that platinum salt skin sensitivity generally varied directly with the environmental air concentration of platinum salts in the current employees' production work areas, and the risk of demonstrating platinum salt skin test reactivity increased 1.13 times/1 µg/m^3 increment in work area concentration of platinum salts (10). A recent longitudinal study in a catalyst production plant provided extensive measurements of airborne metallic and soluble platinum concentrations obtained by area sampling for two consecutive years and by personal sampling for one year (79). Area sampling yielded soluble platinum salt air concentrations at the production lines (where cases were detected) within a range of 5 to 549 ng/m^3, while personal sampling showed about one log higher values within a range of 43 to 3697 ng/m^3. Because of the wide variation in the concentrations, a valid threshold for sensitization at the workplace could not be determined (Fig. 4). However, the incidence rate in this study was by far lower than in precious metals refineries with higher workplace exposure (Table 4) indicating a dose–response relationship. This is corroborated by the finding that the degree of exposure was significantly associated with the incidence of platinum salt allergy in a South African refinery (14). Thus, there is sufficient evidence for a dose–response relationship for platinum salt allergy and, to a lesser extent, the effectiveness of primary preventive measures.

Secondary prevention by medical surveillance programs has a long tradition in precious metals refineries. It has been shown in a catalyst production plant that immediate removal from exposure after skin-prick test conversion from negative to positive results in an excellent prognosis (79). It has been recommended that a questionnaire and skin-prick testing with platinum salts be used for surveillance in this study. Earlier results of a U.S. survey in a refinery suggested a role for cold

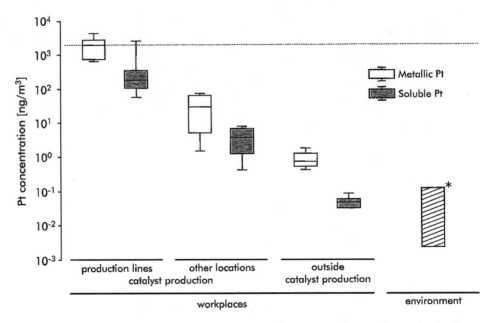

Figure 4 Metallic and soluble platinum workplace air concentrations at the production lines, at other locations in the catalyst production, as well as outside the catalyst production. *As a reference, the concentrations of total platinum in the air at roadsides are presented (literature data). The dotted line represents the TLV for soluble platinum compounds of $2\,\mu g/m^3$.

air challenge in surveillance because there was a strong association between a positive cold air challenge test at baseline measurement and the subsequent conversion to a positive platinum skin test one year later. The follow-up study of the four workers who had a positive cold air challenge and a negative skin test at the initial visit recorded three skin test conversions. In comparison, only 2 out of 63 workers with negative cold air challenge and negative skin tests converted (88).

Several longitudinal studies addressed the question of risk factors for platinum salt allergy. As shown in Table 5, there is a striking agreement that smoking is a strong risk factor for a positive skin-prick test, whereas atopy is not (Table 2) (95). It has not been determined whether smoking cessation programs will result in a decline of cases with sensitization.

In contrast to the U.S. study in a refinery (88), bronchial hyperresponsiveness was not a risk factor in the only prospective longitudinal study of catalyst production workers that included serial testing for bronchial hyperresponsiveness. However, the number of subjects with bronchial hyperresponsiveness in the total cohort was low [8 positive tests out of 115 (7%) in highly exposed subjects at the initial visit] (79).

A recent investigation among refinery workers showed that sensitization to platinum salts was dependent also on genetic factors (97). The human leukocyte-associated antigen (HLA)-DR3 phenotype was significantly associated with skin sensitization to platinum salts (odds ratio, 2.3). Interestingly, this association was modified by the degree of exposure to platinum salts; in that subjects with low exposure showed much higher associations than subjects with high exposure. This study suggests that the importance of genetic susceptibility increases with decreasing degree of occupational exposure.

In a U.S. refinery, it was also found that 10% of workers in the production areas were medically terminated each year because of upper and large airways symptoms (10).

Table 5 Risk Factors for Sensitization Due to Platinum Salts

| Authors (Ref.) | Location | Preemployment screening for atopy | Risk factors (OR) | | |
			Smoking	Atopy	Hyperresponsiveness
Venables et al. (95)	Refinery	Yes	5.1 (1.68–15.2)	2.3 (0.9–6.0)	nd
Calverley et al. (14)	Refinery	Yes	8.0 (2.6–25.0)	nd	nd
Niezborala et al. (96)	Refinery	Yes	5.5 (1.56–19.7)	nd	nd
Merget et al. (79)	Catalyst production	No	3.9 (1.6–9.7)	1.1 (0.9–1.4)	1.1 (0.9–1.3)

Abbreviation: nd, no data.

In this study, a striking persistence of positive platinum skin tests among medically terminated workers was observed. These medically terminated subjects also demonstrated a high prevalence of airway symptoms, abnormal FEV_1/forced vital capacity (FVC) ratios, and positive cold air challenges. This occurred despite the apparent lack of further exposure to platinum salts during an average of five years since respective termination dates. These data were corroborated by a similar study that examined medically terminated refinery workers, all with a positive bronchial challenge to platinum salts (16). Of the 24 workers (71%), 17 still reported asthma symptoms about two years after exposure cessation. Interestingly, skin-prick test converted to negative in three subjects, but this was not accompanied by a reduced responsiveness to methacholine or platinum salt. Also for the total group, bronchial responsiveness to both methacholine and platinum salt were unchanged between initial and final examinations.

GROUP III METAL SERIES

Aluminum

Asthma was first recognized as an occupational health hazard for workers in potrooms of Norwegian aluminum smelters in 1936 (98). Subsequently, the existence of asthma has also been reported in Australian, Dutch, French, Italian, North American, and New Zealand smelters (99–103). The major components of the potroom environment include fluorides in particulate and gaseous forms, dust containing cryolite (Na_3AIF_6), alumina, sulfur dioxide, oxides of carbon, and particulate organic matter (99). Initially, it was thought that an allergic reaction to fluoride in the work environment of the smelter was the cause of potroom asthma, but this widely held belief is yet to be confirmed (98). Whatever the ultimate cause may prove to be, asthma occurring in aluminum smelter workers is now known as "potroom asthma." As the exact etiological agent is unknown, it is customary to use representative TWAs of known pulmonary hazards such as gaseous and particulate fluorides, respirable dust, sulfur dioxide, and coal tar pitch volatiles as an estimate of permissible exposure (99). A recent study suggested that postshift urinary fluoride may be a reasonable exposure index for long-term surveillance, although substantial variation may occur over time and in difficult jobs (100).

There is a large variation in the prevalence and incidence of occupational asthma in the aluminum industry. The estimated incidence of potroom asthma ranged from 0.06% to 4% of exposed workers per year. There is a lower prevalence of potroom asthma reported in North American studies compared to European studies (99). This could be related to different pre-employment medical criteria, prevailing climatic conditions, or the degree of potroom environmental controls. The population at risk also poses problems. This is confounded by high labor turnover in this industry. Forty-four percent of potroom workers in New Zealand left within 12 months, and 71% of Australian smelter workers within three years (99). The results of some cross-sectional analyses are also difficult to interpret because of the healthy survivor effect. Thus, Chan-Yeung et al. (101) were not able to demonstrate any potroom asthma in their study, but this is possibly explained by the fact that five workers left the plant just prior to the study. The relative paucity of documented potroom asthma cases in other Canadian aluminum smelter plants has also been observed by an editor (JLM) of this book. However, his investigative team recently demonstrated a pattern of dual hyperresponsiveness after workplace challenge in a symptomatic, nonsmoking potroom worker six months after he had been removed from further exposure (102).

Several potential risk factors may affect the occurrence of occupational asthma in aluminum potroom workers. At the time of employment, the presence of atopy, particularly hay fever, was a significant risk factor for occupational asthma (103,104). In one of these studies, it was also determined that pre-employment screening for bronchial hyperresponsiveness decreased the incidence of potroom asthma over time, although a few cases continued to occur (103). This study also concluded that atopic history even at lower exposure levels was a risk factor (103). Genotyping for β2 adrenoreceptor, IgE receptor, or TNFα polymorphisms was not predictive of occupational asthma (104). Although in most series the majority of asthmatic cases appeared in smokers, the potential effects of cigarette smoking have not yet been proved because the effect of smoking has not been studied at the same time in matched, unexposed controls.

Symptoms of potroom asthma consist of shortness of breath, wheezing, chest tightness, and cough. While these may occur immediately after exposure, generally the onset of symptoms is delayed. The symptoms become more frequent and severe with repeated exposure. The duration of potroom exposure before the first attack ranges from 1 week to 10 years (106,107). When asthma becomes fully established, it is easy to confirm by objective pulmonary function tests as well as tests measuring bronchial hyperresponsiveness. Positive specific bronchoprovocation results have been demonstrated in two cases. In one of these, an immediate asthma response was observed after challenge with both aluminum powder and aluminum chloride solution. Neutrophil chemotactic activity was increased after an hour and after seven hours following challenges (108). In the other instance, challenge to aluminum welding with or without flux-coated electrodes caused asthma while control exposure to welding on mild steel did not (109). A recent report suggested that exhaled nitric oxide (NO) may be a diagnostic adjunct in nonsmoking potroom workers. Concentrations of NO were not only significantly higher in exposed versus nonexposed workers, but they were also more than doubled in asthmatic compared to nonasthmatic workers (110).

The prognosis of potroom asthma is variable. In some cases, as many as 40% of workers may continue to have asthma after terminating further exposure (105). Bronchial hyperresponsiveness also may persist in many workers (111,112). Some authors have postulated that differences in individual patterns of exposure may account for persistence of asthma. An analogy between this type of persistent asthma and the reactive airways dysfunction syndrome (RADS) has also been suggested (111,112). Several recent reports suggest that early removal from exposure once symptoms are recognized may normalize both FEV_1 and bronchial hyperresponsiveness (113,114). A recent report showing that high plasma fluoride levels in potroom workers are associated with a steeper bronchial hyperresponsiveness dose–response curve and reflects the fact that high airborne fluoride levels are associated with persistent asthma (115). Persistence of asthma after work stoppage has also been reported from industries where smokers have been exposed to other aluminum fluoride compounds ($K_3ALF_6ALF_3$). Apparently, most of these cases occurred when there were high airborne concentrations of total dust up to $53 \, mg/m^3$. Such high peak exposures would certainly be consistent with the onset of RADS.

Although early workers suggested allergy as a possible cause, this association is not convincing. Complete immunological surveys have been conducted in aluminum smelter workers. Mean levels of IgG1, IgA, IgE, recall-delayed hypersensitivity, immune complexes, and antinuclear and/or other autoantibodies were identical in asthmatic and nonasthmatic workers (116). Thus, immune function was normal in both symptomatic and asymptomatic workers in an aluminum smelter. Immediate skin tests to aluminum and fluoride salts were uniformly negative. In one study, six workers showed positive patch tests to 2% NaF (117). The significance of this finding is unknown. A few investigators demonstrated eosinophilia and/or elevated total IgE but such findings are compatible with the presence of atopy, a known risk factor (117,118).

In summary, both cross-sectional and longitudinal studies now indicate that working in aluminum smelters causes occupational asthma. The actual causative agent(s) are unidentified, but it is recognized that dust and fume controls may lessen the overall prevalence of this problem.

INDETERMINATE METALS

Exposure to Steel Products in Welders

In several European population-based studies, the risk of asthma attributable to occupational exposure in welders was among the highest when compared with other occupations (119,120). In the study that explored the risk of asthma among male workers in the construction industry, it was found to be highest among welders and flame cutters with a relative risk of 2.34 (120). The incidence of asthma was compared in welders working with stainless steel or "mild steel". In 127 workers who could be evaluated, 16 had left their jobs because of airway symptoms. This was most likely a "healthy worker" effect because among welders currently working, there was no difference in the incidence of welding-associated asthma (5% for stainless steel; 7% for "mild steel"). It was concluded that welders had a significantly higher prevalence of airway symptoms as compared to a nonwelding control cohort (121). A cross-sectional investigation of asthma in welders concluded that airway responsiveness in regular welders was twice that of workers with negligible exposure after five years of work (122). A recent longitudinal survey of a welding apprenticeship program revealed that the incidence of probable occupational asthma was approximately 3% and that the incidence of bronchial hyperresponsiveness was 11.9% in welders after an average of 15 months of apprenticeship (123). A decline in the pulmonary function among welders has been reported from various parts of the world. In several of these studies, welders who smoked had an increased risk of accelerated decline in pulmonary function (124–127).

Among welders who developed asthma, significant differences have been reported in those who were exposed to solid particles from stainless steel welding fumes as opposed to those engaged in welding of "mild steel". Such differences have been noted throughout the world (128–131). In one of these studies, six workers using a manual metal arc welding technique developed symptoms only after they performed welding operations of stainless steel and not "mild steel" (130). Challenge tests in three of these workers revealed immediate reactions in two of them and dual type reactions in one. Two of these workers had a positive history of exposure to chromates and had undergone patch tests in the past. Inasmuch as stainless steel welding fumes contain significantly higher amounts of chromium and nickel than "mild steel", the investigators of this industrial problem postulated that either the chromium or the nickel in stainless steel welding fumes might be the actual etiologic factor. However, a challenge test to these metallic elements was not performed, so the actual etiologic agent in this group of workers was unknown. A recent cross-shift pulmonary function study demonstrated the influence of duration of stainless welding exposure on the course of lung function during the work shift. After 20 years of stainless steel welding activity, welders had more significant across-shift decreases than "mild steel" welders with a similar duration of welding exposure (131).

Exposure to Steel-Coating Materials

Workers exposed to several processes unique to the steel-manufacturing industry may develop occupational asthma after varying periods of exposure ranging from less than one to eight years. A significant outbreak of industrial asthma occurred in 21 workers exposed to coating materials of rolled steel sheets (132). The coverings were known to contain epoxy resins, acrylics, phenol, formaldehyde, chromates, and polyvinyl chloride. Of great interest, however, was the fact that eight years after the onset of asthmatic symptoms in this plant, it was discovered that toluene diisocyanate (TDI) was liberated during the curing process. Subsequently, two workers in this group demonstrated delayed-onset asthma after a bronchial challenge with TDI. Follow-up survey in this plant after the TDI exposure was eliminated demonstrated that about 40% of the workers still had some work-related asthma, but in the vast majority of cases this was much improved. Although TDI appeared to be the responsible agent in many of these workers, it is possible that employees with residual symptoms of asthma at work could still have increased hyperresponsiveness after exposure to some of the other substances in the coating process.

Welding in General

More than one million workers worldwide perform some type of welding as part of their work duties. A large number of welders experience some type of respiratory illness, which includes entities such as bronchitis, siderosis, asthma, and a possible increase in the instance of lung cancer. In welders' pneumoconiosis, small centrilobular nodules are frequently seen on high-resolution computed tomography (HRCT) scans and there are elevated levels of ferritin that may be of value in diagnosis (133,134). Welders may be exposed to sensitizing anhydrides generated from painted metals (135). There is a single report of a welder who developed RADS after a well-documented acute episode of metal fume fever (136).

DIRECTIONS FOR FUTURE RESEARCH

- Delineation of risk factors for sensitization and/or irritant responses to selected metallic salts
- The specific role of halides versus other ligand complexes in the induction of platinum sensitivity
- Long-term studies comparing platinum workers who continue to be exposed and those removed from exposure to determine factors responsible for persistence of sensitization
- Prospective clinical and laboratory evaluation of potroom asthma
- Genetic predispositions to asthma for both metallic sensitizers and non-sensitizers

CONCLUSION

Occupational asthma occurs after exposure to a variety of metallic compounds. Apart from aluminum, the majority of these agents are salts of elements found in the first, second, and third long series of transitional elements. The prevalence of occupational asthma to various metallic agents varies from rare to as high as 35% in the platinum industry. Both immunological and nonimmunological factors contribute to the pathogenesis of metal-induced occupational asthma. IgE-mediated mechanisms have been demonstrated in nickel-, chromium-, cobalt-, and platinum-induced asthma. The possible contributory role of delayed hypersensitivity is less well understood. Asthma in several metal-fabricating industries has been shown to be due to non-metallic components. Persistence of asthma in several forms of metal-induced asthma may occur if recognition and removal from further exposure are not accomplished as promptly as possible.

REFERENCES

1. Agricola G. de re metalalica. The Mining Magazine (translated by HC Hoover and LH Hoover). London: Mining Journal Ltd, 1912:1556.
2. Nemery B. Metal atoxicity and the respiratory tract. Eur Respir J 1990; 3:202–219.
3. Spivey-Fox MR. Nutritional aspects of metals. In: Lee DHK, ed. Metallic Contaminants and Human Health. New York: Academic Press, 1972:191–208.
4. Friedman ME, Musgrove G, Lee K, Teggins JE. Inhibition of malate dehydrogenase by platinum (II) complexes. Biochem Biophys Acta 1971; 250:286–296.
5. Editorial. Metals and the lung. Lancet 1984; 903:904.
6. Brooks SM. Lung disorders resulting from the inhalation of metals. Clin Chest Med 1981; 2:2235–2254.
7. Van Cutsem EJ, Ceupens JL, Lacquet LM, Demedts M. Combined asthma and alveolitis induced by cobalt in a diamond polisher. Eur J Respir Dis 1987; 70:54–61.
8. Morgan WKC. Other pneumonoconioses. In: Morgan WKC, Seaton A, eds. Occupational Lung Diseases. Philadelphia: WB Saunders, 1975:217–250.
9. Infante PF, Newman LS. Beryllium exposure and chronic beryllium disease. Lancet 2004; 363:415–416.
10. Baker DB, Gann PH, Brooks SM, Gallagher J, Bernstein IL. Cross-sectional study of platinum salts sensitization among precious metals refinery workers. Am J Ind Med 1990; 18:653–664.
11. Gheysens B, Auwerx J, Van den Eeckhout A, Demedts M. Cobalt-induced bronchial asthma in diamond polishers. Chest 1985; 88:740–744.
12. Smith RG. Five metals of potential significance. In: Lee DKH, ed. Metallic Contaminants and Human Health. New York: Academic Press, 1982:139–162.
13. Biagini RE, Bernstein IL, Gallagher JS, Moorman WJ, Brecks S, Gann PH. The diversity of reaginic immune responses to platinum and palladium metallic salts. J Allergy Clin Immunol 1985; 76:794–802.
14. Calverley AE, Rees D, Dowdeswell RJ, Linnett PJ, Kielkowski D. Platinum salt sensitivity in refinery workers: incidence and effects of smoking exposure. Occup Environ Med 1995; 52:661–666.
15. Merget R, Caspari C, Kulzer R, et al. Absence of relationship between degree of nonspecific and specific bronchial responsiveness in occupational asthma due to platinum salts. Eur Respir J 1996; 92:211–216.
16. Merget R, Reineke M, Rückmann A, Bergmann EM, Schultze-Werninghaus G. Nonspecific and specific bronchial responsiveness in occupational asthma due to platinum salts after allergen avoidance. Am J Respir Crit Care Med 1994; 150:1146–1149.
17. Nriagu JO. Nickel in the Environment. New York: Wiley, 1980:1–833.
18. American Conference of Government Industrial Hygienists, 1997 TLFs and BELs, Threshold Limit Values for Chemical Substances and Physical Agents. Biological Exposure Indices, ACHIG, Cincinnati, Ohio, 1998.

19. Eastlander T, Kanerva L, Tupasela O, Keskinen H, Jolanki R. Immediate and delayed allergy to nickel with contact urticaria, rhinitis, asthma and contact dermatitis. Clin Exp Allergy 1993; 23:306–310.

20. Sastre J, Fernandez-Nieto M, Maranon F, Fernandez-Caldas E, Pelta R, Quirce S. Allergenic cross-reactivity between nickel and chromium salts in electroplating-induced asthma. J Allergy Clin Immunol 2001; 108(4):650–651.

21. Kusaka Y, Kumagai S, Kyono H, Kohyama N, Shirakawa T. Determination of exposure to cobalt and nickel in the atmosphere in the hard metal industry. Ann Occp Hyg 1992; 36(5):497–507.

22. Bar-Sela S, Levy M, Westin JB, Laster R, Richter ED. Medical findings in nickel-cadmium battery workers. Isr J Med Sci 1992; 28(8–9):578–583.

23. McConnell LH, Fink JN, Schlueter DP, Schmidt MG Jr. Asthma caused by nickel sensitivity. Ann Intern Med 1973; 78:888–890.

24. Malo J-L, Cartier A, Doepner M, Nieboer E, Evans S, Dolovich J. Occupational asthma caused by nickel sulfate. J Allergy Clin Immunol 1982; 69:55–59.

25. Block GT, Yeung M. Asthma induced by nickel. JAMA 1982; 247:1600–1602.

26. Novey HS, Habib M, Wells ID. Asthma and IgE antibodies induced by chromium and nickel salts. J Allergy Clin Immunol 1983; 72:407–412.

27. Malo J-L, Cartier A, Gagnon G, Evans S, Dolovich J. Isolated late asthmatic reaction due to nickel sulphate without antibodies to nickel. Clin Allergy 1985; 15:95–99.

28. Davies JE. Occupational asthma caused by nickel salts. J Occup Med 1986; 36:29–30.

29. Sunderman FW, Sunderman FW Jr. Loffler's syndrome associated with nickel sensitivity. Arch Intern Med 1961; 107:405–408.

30. Shirakawa T, Morimoto K. Brief reversible bronchospasm resulting from bichromate exposure. Arch Environ Health 1996; 51:221–226.

31. Bright P, Burge PS, O'Hickey SP, Gannon PF, Robertson AS, Boran A. Occupational asthma due to chrome and nickel electroplating. Thorax 1997; 52:28–32.

32. Shirakawa T, Kusaka Y, Fujimura N, Kato M, Heki S, Morimoto K. Hard metal asthma: cross immunological and respiratory reactivity between cobalt and nickel? Thorax 1990; 45:267–271.

33. Dolovich J, Evans SL, Nieboer E. Occupational asthma from nickel sensitivity. I. Human serum albumin in the antigenic determinant. Br J Ind Med 1984; 41:51–55.

34. Burrows D. The dichromate problem. Int J Dermatol 1984; 23:215–220.

35. Ballal SG. Respiratory symptoms and occupational bronchitis in chromate ore miners, Sudan. J Trop Med Hyg 1986; 89(5):223–228.

36. Park HS, Yu HJ, Hung KS. Occupational asthma caused by chromium. Clin Exp Allergy 1994; 24:676–681.

37. Moller DR, Brooks SM, Bernstein DI, Cassedy K, Enrione M, Bernstein IL. Delayed anaphylactoid reaction in a worker exposed to chromium. J Allergy Clin Immunol 1986; 77:451–456.

38. Olaguibel JM, Basomba A. Occupational asthma induced by chromium salts. Allergol Immunopathol 1989; 17:133–136.

39. Nemery B, De Raeve H, Demedts M. Dermal and respiratory sensitization to chromate in a floorer. Eur Respir J 1995; 8(suppl 19):222s.

40. Leroyer C, Dewitte JD, Bassanets A, Boutoux M, Daniel C, Clavier J. Occupational asthma due to chromium. Respiration 1998; 65(5):403–405.

41. Roto P. Asthma, symptoms of chronic bronchitis and ventilatory capacity among cobalt and zinc production workers. Scand J Work Environ Health 1980; 6(suppl): 11–36.

42. Lob M. Allergie respiratoire au ciment. Z Unfallchir Vers Med Berufskr 1985; 78:47–50.

43. Sjogren I, Hillerdal G, Andersson A, Zetterstrom O. Hard metal lung disease: importance of cobalt in coolants. Thorax 1980; 35:653–659.

44. Cirla AM. Cobalt-related asthma: clinical and immunological aspects. Sci Tot Environ 1994; 150:85–94.

45. Kusaka Y, Yokayama K, Sera Y, et al. Respiratory diseases in hard metal workers: An occupational hygiene study in a factory. Br J Ind Med 1986; 43:474–485.

46. Newman LS, Maier LA, Nemery B. Interstitial lung disorders due to beryllium and cobalt. In: Schwartz MI, King TE Jr, eds. Interstitial Lung Disease. 3rd ed. St. Louis: CV Mosby, 1998:367–392.

47. Swennen B, Buchet JP, Stanescu D, Lison D, Lauwerys R. Epidemiological survey of workers exposed to cobalt oxides, cobalt salts, and cobalt metal. Br J Ind Med 1993; 50(9):835–842.

48. Cullen MR. Respiratory diseases from hard metal exposure. A continuing enigma. Chest 1984; 86:513–514.

49. Pillière F, Garnier R, Rousselin X, Dimerman S, Rosenberg N, Efthymiou ML. Asthma aux sels de cobalt. A propos d'un cas dv au resinate de cobalt. Arch Mal Prof 1990; 51:413–417.

50. Bruckner HC. Extrinsic asthma in a tungsten carbide worker. J Occup Med 1967; 9: 518–519.

51. Shirakawa T, Kusaka Y, Fujimura N, et al. Occupational asthma from cobalt sensitivity in workers exposed to hard metal dust. Chest 1989; 95:29–37.

52. Shirakawa T, Kusaka Y, Fujimura N, Goto S, Morimoto K. The existence of specific antibodies to cobalt in hard metal asthma. Clin Allergy 1988; 18:451–460.

53. Shirakawa T, Morimoto K. Interplay of cigarette smoking and occupational exposure on specific immunoglobulin E antibodies to cobalt. Arch Environ Health 1997; 52: 124–128.

54. Kusaka Y, Nakano Y, Shirakawa T, Morimoto K. Lymphocyte transformation with cobalt in hard metal asthma. Ind Health 1989; 27:155–163.

55. Forni A. Bronchoalveolar lavage in the diagnosis of hard metal disease. Sci Tot Environ 1994; 150:69–76.

56. Lison D, Lauwerys R, Demedts M. Nemery B. Experimental research into the pathogenesis of cobalt/hard metal lung disease. Eur Respir J 1996; 9:1024–1028.

57. Davison AG, Haslam PL, Corrin B, Coutts H, Dewar A, Riding WD, Studdy PR, Newman-Taylor AJ. Interstitial lung disease and asthma in hard-metal workers: bronchoalveolar lavage, ultrastructural, and analytical findings and results of bronchial provocation tests. Thorax 1990; 45:267–271.

58. Rivolta G, Nicoli E, Ferretti G, Tomasini M. Hard metal lung disorders: analysis of a group of exposed workers. Sci Tot Environ 1994; 150:161–165.

59. Shirakawa T, Kusaka Y, Fujimura N, Kato M, Heki S, Morimoto K. Hard metal asthma: cross immunological and respiratory reactivity between cobalt and nickel? Thorax 1990; 45:267–271.

60. Hudson TFG. Vanadium: Toxicology and Biological Significance. New York: Elsevier, 1964.

61. Barceloux DG. Vanadium. J Toxicol Clin Toxicol 1993; 37(2):265–278.

62. Kiviluoto M, Rasanen O, Rinne A, Rissanen M. Effects of vanadium on the upper respiratory tract of workers in a vanadium factory. Scand J Work Environ Health 1982; 5:50–58.

63. Musk AW, Tees JG. Asthma caused by occupational exposure to vanadium compounds. Med J Aust 1982; 1:183–184.

64. Knecht EA, Moorman WJ, Clark JC, Lynch DW, Lewis TR. Pulmonary effects of acute vanadium pentoxide inhalation in monkeys. Am Rev Respir Dis 1985; 132:1181–1195.

65. Weir DC, Robertson AS, Jones S, Burge PS. Occupational asthma due to soft corrosive soldering fluxes containing zinc chloride and ammonium chloride. Thorax 1989; 44: 220–223.

66. Malo J-L, Cartier A. Occupational asthma due to fumes of galvanized metal. Chest 1987; 92:375–377.

67. Kawane H, Soejima R, Umeki S, Niki Y. Metal fume and asthma. Chest 1988; 93:1116–1117.

68. Malo J-L, Cartier A, Dolovich J. Occupational asthma due to zinc. Eur Respir J 1993; 6:447–450.

69. Murdoch RD, Pepys J. Platinum group metal sensitivity: reactivity to platinum group metal salts in platinum halide salt-sensitive workers. Ann Allergy 1987; 59:464–469.

70. Bruevich TS, Bogomolets NN, Berezovski B. Sensitizing influence of compounds of noble metals (gold, platinum, ruthenium, rhodium, and silver). Gig Tr Prof Zabol 1980; 5:42–44.

71. Tomilets VA, Dontsov VI, Zakharova IA. Immediate and delayed allergic reactions to group VIII metals in an experiment. Fiziol Zh 1979; 25:653–657 (translation).

72. Tomilets VA, Dontsov VI, Zakharova IA, Kletsov AV. Histamine releasing and histamine binding action of platinum and palladium compounds. Arch Immunol Ther Exp 1980; 28:953–957.

73. Tomilets VA, Zakharova IA. Anaphylactic and anaphylactoid properties of palladium complexes. Farmakol Toksikol 1979; 41:170–173.

74. Daenen M, Rogiers P, Van De Walle C, Rochette F, Demedts M, Nemery B. Occupational asthma caused by palladium. Eur Respir J 1999; 13:213–216.

75. Murdoch RD, Pepys J, Hughes EG. IgE antibody responses to platinum group metals: a large scale refinery survey. Br J Ind Med 1986; 43:37–43.

76. Cristaudo A, Sera F, Severino V, De Rocco M, Di Lella E, Picardo M. Occupational hypersensitivity to metal salts, including platinum, in the secondary industry. Allergy 2005; 60:159–164.

77. Bergman A, Svedberg U, Nilsson E. Contact urticaria with anaphylactic reactions caused by occupational exposure to iridium salt. Contact Dermatitis 1995; 32:14–17.

78. Biagini RE, Moorman WJ, Lewis TR, Bernstein IL. Ozone enhancement of platinum asthma in primate model. Am Rev Respir Dis 1986; 135:719–725.

79. Merget R, Kulzer R, Dierkes-Globisch A, et al. Exposure-effect relationship of platinum salt allergy in a catalyst production plant—conclusions from a five-year prospective cohort study. J Allergy Clin Immunol 2000; 105:364–370.

80. Linnett PJ, Hughes EG. 20 years of medical surveillance on exposure to allergenic and non-allergenic platinum compounds: the importance of chemical speciation. Occup Environ Med 1999; 56:191–196.

81. Maynard AD, Northage C, Hemingway M, Bradley SD. Measurement of short-term exposure to airborne soluble platinum in the platinum industry. Ann Occup Hyg 1997; 41:77–94.

82. Karasek SR, Karasek M. The use of platinum paper. In: Report of the Illinois State Commission of Occupational Diseases to His Excellency Governor Charles S. Deneen, Chicago: Warner Printing Company, 1911:97.

83. Merget R, Caspari C, Dierkes-Globisch A, et al. Effectiveness of a medical surveillance programme for the prevention of occupational asthma due to platinum salts. A nested case-control study. J Allergy Clin Immunol 2001; 107:707–712.

84. Merget R, Schulte A, Gebler A, et al. Outcome of occupational asthma due to platinum salts after transferal to low exposure areas. Int Arch Occup Environ Health 1999; 72:33–39.

85. Cleare MJ, Hughes EG, Jacoby B, Pepys J. Immediate (type I) allergic responses to platinum compounds. Clin Allergy 1976; 6:183–195.

86. Merget R, Schultze-Werninghaus G, Bode F, Bergman EM, Zachgo W, Meier-Syndow J. Quantitative skin prick and bronchial provocation tests with platinum salt. Br J Indust Med 1991; 48:830–837.

87. Hughes EG. Medical surveillance of platinum refinery workers. J Soc Occup Med 1980; 30:27–30.

88. Brooks SM, Baker DB, Gann PH, et al. Cold air challenge and platinum skin reactivity in platinum refinery workers. Chest 1990; 97:1401–1407.

89. Pepys J, Pickering CAC, Hughes EG. Asthma due to inhaled chemical agents—complex salts of platinum. Clin Allergy 1972; 2:391–396.

90. International Platinum Association. Guidance for the medical surveillance of workers exposed to complex salts of platinum. Unpublished draft 1995.

91. Pepys J, Parish WE, Cromwell O, Hughes EG. Passive transfer in man and the monkey of type I allergy due to heat labile and heat stable antibody to complex salts of platinum. Clin Allergy 1979; 9:99–108.

92. Cromwell O, Pepys J, Parish WE, Hughes EG. Specific IgE antibodies to platinum salts in sensitized workers. Clin Allergy 1979; 9:109–117.

93. Merget R, Schultze-Werninghaus G, Muthorst T, Friedrich W, Meier-Sydow J. Asthma due to the complex salts of platinum—a cross sectional survey of workers in a platinum refinery. Clin Allergy 1988; 18:569–580.

94. Murdoch RD, Pepys J. Immunological responses to complex salts of platinum. I. Specific IgE antibody production in the rat. Clin Exp Immunol 1984; 57:107–114.

95. Venables KM, Dally MB, Nunn AJ, et al. Smoking and occupational allergy in workers in a platinum refinery. Br Med J 1989; 299:939–942.

96. Niezborala M, Garnier R. Allergy to complex platinum salts. A historical prospective cohort study. Occup Environ Med 1996; 4:252–257.

97. Newman Taylor AJ, Cullinan P, Lympany PA, Harris JM, Dowdeswell RJ, du Bois RM. Interaction of HLA phenotype and exposure intensity in sensitization to complex platinum salts. Am J Respir Crit Care Med 1999; 160:435–438.

98. Frostad EW. Fluorine intoxication in Norwegian aluminum plant workers. Tidsskr Nor Laegefor 1936; 56:179–182.

99. Abramson MJ, Wlodarczyk JH, Saunders NA, Hemsley MJ. Does aluminum smelting cause lung disease? Am Rev Respir Dis 1989; 139:1042–1057.

100. Seixas NS, Cohen M, Zevenbergen B, Cotey M, Carter S, Kaufman J. Urinary fluoride as an exposure index in aluminum smelting. AIHAJ 2000; 61(1):89–94.

101. Chan-Yeung M, Wong R, MacLean L, et al. Epidemiologic health study of workers in an aluminum smelter in British Columbia—effects on the respiratory system. Am Rev Respir Dis 1989; 127:465–469.

102. Desjardins A, Bergeron JP, Ghezzo H, Cartier A, Malo J-L. Aluminum potroom asthma confirmed by monitoring of forced expiratory volume in one second. Am J Respir Crit Care Med 1994; 150:1714–1717.

103. Sorgdrager B, de Looff AJ, de Monchy JG, Pal TM, Dubois AE, Rijcken B. Occurrence of occupational asthma in aluminum potroom workers in relation to preventive measures. Int Arch Occup Environ Health 1998; 71(1):53–59.

104. Barnard CG, McBride DI, Firth HM, Herbison GP. Assessing individual employee risk factors for occupational asthma in primary aluminum smelting. Occup Environ Med 2004; 61:604–608.

105. Arnaiz NO, Kaufman JD, Daroowalla FM, Quigley S, Farin F, Checkoway H. Genetic factors and asthma in aluminum smelter workers. Arch Environ Health 2003; 58(4):197–200.

106. O'Donnell TV, Welford B, Coleman ED. Potroom asthma: New Zealand experience and follow-up. Am J Ind Med 1989; 15:43–49.

107. Kongerud J, Boe J, Soyseth V, Naalsund A, Magnus P. Aluminum potroom asthma: the Norwegian experience. Eur Respir J 1994; 7:165–172.

108. Park HS, Uh ST, Park CS. Increased neutrophil chemotactic activity is noted in aluminum-induced occupational asthma. Korean J Intern Med 1996; 11(1):69–73.

109. Vandenplas O, Delwiche JP, Vanbilsen ML, Joly J, Roosels D. Occupational asthma caused by aluminum welding. Eur Respir J 1998; 11(5):1182–1184.

110. Lund MB, Oksne PI, Kongerud J. Increased nitric oxide in exhaled air: an early maker of asthma in non-smoking aluminium potroom workers? Occup Environ Med 2000; 57:274–278.

111. Wergeland E, Lund E, Waage JE. Respiratory dysfunction after potroom asthma. Am J Ind Med 1987; 11:627–636.

112. Simonsson BG, Sjoberg A, Rolf C, Haeger-Aronson B. Acute and long-term airway hyperreactivity in aluminum-salt exposed workers with nocturnal asthma. Eur J Respir Dis 1985; 66:105–118.

113. Sorgdrager B, de Looff AJ, Pal TM, van Dijk FJ, de Monchy JG. Factors affecting FEV_1 in workers with potroom asthma after their removal from exposure. Int Arch Occup Environ Health 2001; 74(1):55–58.

114. Soyseth V, Kongerud J, Aalen OO, Botten G, Boe J. Bronchial responsiveness decreases in relocated aluminum potroom workers compared with workers who continue their potroom exposure. Int Arch Occup Environ Health 1995; 67(1):53–57.

115. Hydro Aluminum, Health Department, Ardal Aluminum Plant, Norway. Relation between exposure to fluoride and bronchial responsiveness in aluminum potroom workers with work-related asthma-like symptoms. Thorax 1994; 49:984–989.

116. Mackay IR, Ollihant RC, Laby B, et al. An immunologic and genetic study of asthma in workers in an aluminum smelter. J Occup Med 1990; 32:1022–1026.

117. Saric M, Godnic-Cvar J, Gomzi M, Stilinovic L. The role of atopy in potroom workers' asthma. Am J Ind Med 1986; 9:239–242.

118. Sorgdrager B, Pal TM, de Looff AJ, Dubois AE, de Monchy JG. Occupational asthma in aluminum potroom workers related to pre-employment eosinophil count. Eur Respir J 1995; 8:1520–1524.

119. Kogevinas M, Anto JM, Soriano JB, Tobias A, Burney P. The risk of asthma attributable to occupational exposures. A population-based study in Spain. Spanish Group of the European Asthma Study. Am J Respir Crit Care Med 1996; 154(1):137–143.

120. Karjalainen A, Martikainen R, Oksa P, Saarinen K, Uitti J. Incidence of asthma among Finnish construction workers. J Occup Environ Med 2002; 44(8):752–757.

121. Wang ZP, Larsson K, Malmberg P, Sjogren B, Hallberg BO, Wrangsko K. Asthma, lung function, and bronchial responsiveness in welders. Am J Ind Med 1994; 26(6):741–754.

122. Beach JR, Dennis H, Avery AJ, et al. An epidemiologic investigation of asthma in welders. Am J Respir Crit Care Med 1996; 154(5):1394–1400.

123. El-Zein M, Malo JL, Infante-Rivard C, Gautrin D. Incidence of probable occupational asthma and changes in airway caliber and responsiveness in apprentice welders. Eur Respir J 2003; 22(3):513–518.

124. Erkinjuntti-Pekkanen R, Slater T, Cheng S, et al. Two year follow up of pulmonary function values among welder in New Zealand. Occup Environ Med 1999; 56(5):328–333.

125. Meo SA, Azeem MA, Subhan MM. Lung function in Pakistani welding workers. J Occup Environ Med 2003; 45(10):1068–1073.

126. Wolf C, Pirich C, Valic E, Waldhoer T. Pulmonary function and symptoms of welders. Int Arch Occup Environ Health 1997; 69(5):350–353.

127. Nakadate T, Aizawa Y, Yagami T, Zheg YQ, Kotani M, Ishiwata K. Change in obstructive pulmonary function as a result of cumulative exposure to welding fumes as determined by magnetopneumography in Japanese arc welders. Occup Environ Med 1998; 55(10):673–677.

128. Keskinen H, Kalliomaki P-L, Alanko K. Occupational asthma due to stainless steel welding fumes. Clin Allergy 1980; 10:151–159.

129. Vendenplas O, Dargent F, Auveerdin JJ, et al. Occupational asthma due to gas metal arc welding on mild steel. Thorax 1995; 50:587–588.

130. Sobaszek A, Boulenguez C, Frimat P, Robin H, Haguenoer JM, Edme JL. Acute respiratory effects of exposure to stainless steel and mild steel welding fumes. J Occup Environ Med 2000; 42(9):923–931.

131. Antonini JM, Taylor MD, Zimmer AT, Roberts JR. Pulmonary responses to welding fumes: role of metal constituents. J Toxicol Environ Health A. 2004; 67(3):233–249.

132. Venables KM, Dally MB, Burge PS, Pickering CA, Newman-Taylor AJ. Occupational asthma in a steel coating plant. Br J Ind Med 1985; 42:517–524.

133. Bradshaw LM, Fishwick D, Slater T, Pearce N. Chronic bronchitis, work related respiratory symptoms and pulmonary function in welders in New Zealand. Occup Environ Med 1998; 55(3):150–154.
134. Yoshii C, Matsuyama T, Takazawa A, et al. Welder's pneumoconiosis: diagnostic usefulness of high-resolution computed tomography and ferritin determinations in bronchoalveolar lavage fluid. Intern Med 2002; 41(12):1111–1117.
135. Pfaffli P, Hameila M, Keskinen H, Wirmoila R. Exposure to cyclic anhydrides in welding: a new allergen-chlorendic anhydride. Appl Occup Environ Hyg 2002; 17(11): 765–767.
136. Dube D, Puruckherr M, Byrd RP Jr, Roy TM. Reactive airways dysfunction syndrome following metal fume fever. Tenn Med 2002; 95(6):236–238.

24

Other Chemical Substances Causing Occupational Asthma

Jean-Luc Malo
Department of Chest Medicine, Université de Montréal and Sacré-Cœur Hospital, Montreal, Quebec, Canada

Hae-Sim Park
Department of Allergy and Rheumatology, Ajou University School of Medicine, Youngtongku, Suwon, South Korea

I. Leonard Bernstein
Division of Allergy–Immunology, Department of Internal Medicine, College of Medicine, University of Cincinnati, Cincinnati, Ohio, U.S.A.

INTRODUCTION

Various chemical substances can cause occupational asthma. Chemicals most often implicated as a cause of occupational asthma are the polyisocyanates (Chapter 21). Although the majority of subjects, consulting for possible occupational asthma (OA), are exposed to low-molecular-weight agents (more so than in the case of high-molecular-weight agents), most of the other agents have also been documented in individual case reports. The frequency of occupational asthma caused by these agents has generally not been determined either because the agents are not used extensively or because no sufficient interest was found in carrying out the studies. The mechanism of sensitization has only been determined for some of the agents. Some substances have been found to mediate sensitization through an immunoglobulin (Ig) E–dependent mechanism. Low-molecular-weight agents, which represent the majority of these miscellaneous chemical substances, may cause sensitization by acting as haptens. However, the mechanism of asthma induction remains inconclusive for many other low-molecular-weight agents.

Agents that have been the subject of a larger number of publications are dealt with under specific headings of this chapter. The compendium (Appendix) also provides a list of the chemical agents together with the evidence, which have been reported to cause OA.

AZOBISFORMAMIDE OR AZODICARBONAMIDE

The chemical formula of this compound is $H_2N–CH–O–N=N–O–CH–NH_2$. This product is used in the plastic industry to introduce gas into plastic to make a product that foams when heated. In 1977, Ferris et al. (1) first described that all but one of the 11 workers who were exposed to azodicarbonamide had symptoms characterized by a productive cough. In three of the subjects, forced expiratory volume in one second (FEV_1) recordings on the first day back at work, after a period of four days off work, showed a fall of 21%. In 1981, a survey taken among 151 workers exposed to this product showed that 19% of them had symptoms of late onset asthma (2). No significant changes in spirometry were recorded. Atopy was not a predisposing factor and skin-prick tests with the product were negative. Malo et al. (3) described two subjects who underwent specific inhalation challenges and developed either an isolated late or a dual asthmatic reaction. Case reports, published in 1985 and 2004, documented late asthmatic responses in a worker who was challenged with the product of azodicarbonamide (4). Although blockade of the reaction achieved by administering cromolyn sodium might suggest that mast cells are involved, sensitization has not been proved (4). Four other cases were described, in which one person had a late asthmatic reaction after exposure to the product (5).

AMINES

As reviewed by Hagmar et al. (Table 1) (6), various (approximately 40 different ones) secondary, tertiary, and quarternary amines, which are aliphatic, heterocyclic, or aromatic, have been reported to cause OA.

These products are handled in the primary manufacturing as well as in secondary industries (rubber industry, beauty culture industry, shellac handling industry, color photographs developing industry, antihelminthic drug industry, hair dye manufacturing industry, and fur industry, and industries in which aluminum soldering, acrylate paints, hair dyes, and rubber additives are used). As early as 1951, dermatitis caused by ethelene diamine was diagnosed in 14 subjects involved in the manufacturing of this product (7). Further, Dernehl describes three cases of asthma. In 1963, the same author documented asthma in workers exposed to epoxy resins. Production of epoxy resin is initiated by amines or other materials that act as cross-linking agents, binding the resin molecules together and becoming an intimate part of the polymer molecule (8). In the same year, Gelfand showed that exposure to ethylene diamine, a solvent for shellac, can cause occupational asthma, which was confirmed by specific inhalation challenges (9). Seven other subjects underwent specific inhalation challenges and experienced dual and late asthmatic reactions (10–13). Sargent et al. (14) described lower respiratory tract symptoms and significant changes in bronchial caliber in 25 workers exposed to a mixture of propylamine and triethylenediamine. Environmental controls at the workplace later resulted in the disappearance of significant symptoms and changes in airway caliber in the same workforce (15). Ng found that 3 of the 12 (25%) subjects plus an index case had OA on exposure to various aliphatic polyamines (ethylenediamine, diethylenetriamine, and triethylenetetramine) (16). Savonius et al. (17) described three cases of asthma caused by ethanolamines which are amino alcohols.

McCullagh described a case in whom cutaneous and respiratory sensitivity to piperazine, a heterocyclic amine used as an antihelminthic drug, was observed (18).

Table 1 Occupational Asthma Caused by Amines

Types of amines	Occupational setting	References
Aliphatic amines		
Ethylenediamines		
Ethylenediamine	Manufacturing, rubber industry, cosmetics industry; shellac handling, color photograph development	(7–9,12)
Diethylenetriamine and triethylenetriamine	Manufacturing	(8,14)
Hexamethylenetetramine	Cosmetics	(9)
Ethanolamines		
Monoethanolamine	Cosmetics	(9)
Aminoethylethanolamine	Aluminum soldering	(11,12)
Dimethylethanolamine	Acrylate paints	(13)
Other		
3-Dimethylamino-propylamine	Manufacturing	(15,16)
Heterocyclic amines		
Piperazine	Antihelminthic drug manufacturing	(17–19,22–24)
Aromatic amines		
Benzalkonium chloride	Cleaning agent, disinfectant	(20,21)
p-Phenylenediamine	Fur industry and hair dyes, oil, and rubber additives	(25)

Source: From Ref. 6 (slightly modified).

In another report, two other subjects who underwent specific inhalation challenges in the laboratory developed late asthmatic reactions (19). Benzalkonium chloride, a quaternary amine, also caused a combined cutaneous and respiratory hypersensitivity syndrome (20). Several nurses developed occupational asthma after being exposed to benzalkonium chloride. Under laboratory-controlled conditions, these women developed early or delayed symptoms upon exposure (21).

A survey carried out among 131 subjects exposed to piperazine and ethylenediamine revealed that 8% of them were asthmatic or had experienced asthma associated with exposure to chemicals during their employment (22). Specific IgE antibodies to a piperazine–human serum albumin conjugate were detected in 5 out of 72 exposed workers (7%) (23). In a cohort sample of 602 workers employed in a piperazine producing plant between 1942 and 1979, Hagmar et al. (24) showed a strong exposure–response association between the presence of respiratory symptoms and the degree of exposure. Furthermore, long-term exposure seemed to result in symptoms of chronic bronchitis. Using logistic regressions, the authors showed that age, duration of employment, smoking habits, and previous work-related symptoms all increased the likelihood of developing symptoms. Paraphenylenediamine can also cause asthma in fur workers (25); 37 out of the 80 workers (46%) described by Silberman and Sorrell had symptoms of asthma and 74% of the tested subjects experienced nasal or chest symptoms during specific inhalation challenges.

It is still controversial as to whether amines can cause work-related asthma in employees exposed to isocyanates. In a group of 48 workers exposed to toluene diisocyanate and amines, 13 workers (27%) had respiratory symptoms and 8 (17%) showed increased methacholine reactivity (26). Airborne concentrations of isocyanates were below 0.005 ppm whereas concentrations of amines were 10,000 times greater. Belin et al. (26) therefore concluded that exposure to amines was more likely to have been the cause of the respiratory syndrome than exposure to isocyanates. These results were later contested by Candura and Moscato (27), who documented 12 instances of OA related to toluene diisocyanate and no occurrence of OA to toluene-diamine in workers who underwent inhalation challenges to both products.

The mechanism by which amines cause asthma remains controversial, although evidence of immediate skin reactivity has been seen in some studies.

COLOPHONY AND FLUXES

Colophony is the resin obtained from pine trees, which mainly contains abietic acid and pumaric acid. This product is widely used as a flux in the electronics industry to prevent corrosion. The first report of colophony-induced occupational asthma came from Fawcett et al. (28); they performed specific challenges on four workers who experienced isolated immediate bronchospastic reactions. Burge et al. (29) later described in detail about 21 subjects who had undergone specific inhalation challenges and had developed either isolated immediate (in five subjects), isolated late (in two subjects), or dual (in 12 subjects) asthmatic reactions or an alveolitis type of reaction. The same group of investigators has since thoroughly investigated several aspects of this form of OA (Table 2).

Work-related symptoms were found in 22% of the 446 exposed workers as compared to 6% of a control group of 86 office workers (Fig. 1) (30). In a study of 1339 workers who had left the factory during the previous three years, 4% of solderers had left because of respiratory symptoms as compared to 1% among other shop floor workers and none among the office workers (31). A case–control study comparing 58 affected workers and 48 controls showed that affected workers had a significantly lower preexposure FEV_1 on Monday morning and a more pronounced fall in FEV_1 during shift at work. Atopy was a weak predisposing factor and smoking was not a statistically significant factor (32). In a subsequent article,

Table 2 Colophony Fluxes and Occupational Asthma[a]

Evidence	References
First report: four workers with immediate reactions	(28)
First larger survey in 21 subjects	(29)
Epidemiologic surveys:	
Prevalence of symptoms 22% vs. 4% in controls	(30)
Prevalence of symptoms in those who left is 4% vs. 1% of other shop workers	(31)
Lower Monday morning FEV_1 and more pronounced changes in FEV_1	
During a work shift; atopy is a weak predisposing factor, smoking is not	(32)
Evidence that PEFR monitoring is a useful means of assessment	(33)
Abietic acid as a possible causal agent	(34)
Association between the degree of exposure and work-related symptoms	(35)
Evidence for the persistence of asthma after removal from exposure	(36)

[a]Summary of the original studies, including those by Burge et al. (29).
Abbreviations: FEV_1, forced expiratory volume in one second; PEFR, peak expiratory flow rate.

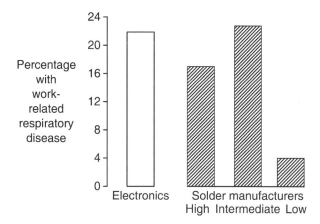

Figure 1 Prevalence of work-related wheeze and breathlessness in electronics workers and manufacturers of colophony fluxes. Significantly lower prevalence is seen in the low-exposure group.

Burge et al. (33) validated the use of serial peak expiratory flow rates in the diagnosis of the condition. Specific bronchial provocation tests were also used by the authors (34). They found that exposure to colophony for 15 minutes or less was sufficient to elicit a reaction in all the 34 workers tested. Reactions were encountered in six workers tested with abietic acid, the principal resin acid in colophony. There was a poor correlation between the level of nonspecific bronchial responsiveness and the response to colophony, but there was an association between the degree of exposure, as assessed by the level of resin acid, and the likelihood of having work-related symptoms. Work-related symptoms were present in 21% of the two higher exposure groups and in only 4% of the lower exposure group (35). Moreover, exposed workers had a significantly lower FEV_1 than unexposed workers (Fig. 2). Follow-up of 39 workers showed that symptoms persisted in half of the affected workers up to four years after the cessation of exposure. Bronchial responsiveness to histamine returned to normal in half of the workers who were no longer exposed ($n = 20$),

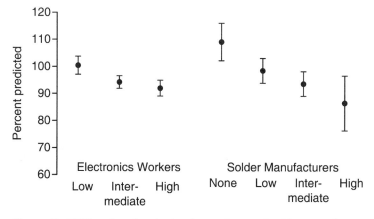

Figure 2 FEV_1 values for electronics workers and solder manufacturers, related to exposure to colophony fumes. Significantly higher FEV_1 values demonstrated in the no-exposure (none) group. *Abbreviation*: FEV_1, forced expiratory volume in one second.

but it returned to normal in only one of the eight workers who were still indirectly exposed to colophony, thus suggesting that a nonspecific bronchial hyperresponsiveness was the result, rather than the cause, of the OA (36). Results of these original works were later summarized by Burge (37). Others have also described cases of occupational asthma caused by colophony (38,39). Colophony-induced asthma was also confirmed in a poultry vender (40). The mechanism of reaction to colophony remains unknown because no specific antibodies have been found.

It was found that unheated colophony can also cause OA (41). The variability of peak expiratory flow rates was assessed using cosinor analysis in workers who were asked to assess their breathing every one to two hours for periods of up to one year (Chapter 9) (42). Several parameters that were calculated from peak expiratory flows data including mesor (24-hour mean), amplitude (24-hour variation), and acrophase (peak time) were different at work and off work.

Weir et al. (43) described two cases of occupational asthma caused by another soldering flux containing zinc chloride and ammonium chloride. The diagnosis was confirmed by serial monitoring of peak expiratory flows and specific inhalation challenges. Another soldering flux containing polyether alcohol–polypropylene glycol has also been reported to cause OA (44).

Elms et al. (45) have recently suggested that colophony first undergoes an oxidation process yielding products that may interact with body proteins to initiate the immune response.

FORMALDEHYDE

Formaldehyde is a chemical used in a wide variety of occupational settings (hospitals, furniture manufacturing, textiles, etc.). Formaldehyde can have irritant effects at higher concentrations, which was described by Harris in 1953 (46) and has been reviewed more recently (47). A level of 3.0 ppm has been proposed as a standard for the onset of toxic effects. Formaldehyde has been used as insulation in many buildings. Acute (48–52) and chronic (53,54) exposure to formaldehyde at concentrations less than 3.0 ppm can cause irritation of the nasal and conjunctival mucosa in normal and asthmatic subjects, but does not generally result in bronchoconstriction. Some normal subjects may develop acute bronchial obstruction after being exposed to 3.0 ppm of formaldehyde during exercise (55). Routine exposure to formaldehyde at concentrations of 2.0 ppm for 40 minutes did not cause significant airway constriction (56) in challenge workers, although other studies have found some effect on airway caliber in carpentry shop workers after a day at work as compared with a control group (57). Gamble et al. (58), found an increase in respiratory symptoms and a decrease in expiratory flow rates at low lung volumes, in rubber workers exposed to a phenol-formaldehyde resin. Schoenberg and Mitchell (59) also found evidence of lower expiratory flow rates in a sample of 63 workers exposed to a phenol-formaldehyde resin. Wallenstein and Rebohle (60) nevertheless concluded that the low percentage of work-related symptoms was evidence of low risk of formaldehyde causing occupational diseases.

Sakula (61) as well as Kerfoot and Mooney (62) initially suspected that formaldehyde can cause occupational asthma, which was reviewed later by others elsewhere (63,64). Hendrick and Lane (65,66) have reported cases where subjects underwent specific inhalation challenges and developed late asthmatic reactions. These were later confirmed by exposing the subjects to low concentrations of formaldehyde, which had not been the case for the subjects initially reported (67). Subsequent to these early reports, the documentation of formaldehyde asthma was a rare occurrence. Frigas et al. (68) were unsuccessful in reproducing bronchial obstruction in 13 subjects with work-related asthma. In a study involving 230 subjects who reported asthma-like symptoms while being exposed to formaldehyde at work, only 12 had significant bronchoconstriction at levels of 1.0 to 2.0 ppm during specific inhalation challenges (69). Urea formaldehyde particles can also cause occupational asthma in subjects exposed to this product incorporated in houses (70), and in carpenters (71), as has been confirmed by specific inhalation challenges. Attempts to detect specific antibodies in the sera of subjects exposed to formaldehyde and to relate it to the symptomatology have so far been unfruitful (72–74) except in two case reports (75). However, exposure to gaseous formaldehyde had induced IgE-mediated sensitization in school children (76). Recently, there are additional sporadic reports of IgE sensitization to formaldehyde, but in none of these cases was specificity proved, and in one of the cases, a very high total IgE may have simply caused a nonspecific reaction (77–79). The physical state of formaldehyde is relevant in causing OA. Cases of OA caused by formaldehyde resin dust, with or without reaction to gaseous formaldehyde, were recently reported (80). Interestingly, Gannon et al. (81) reported seven subjects with OA related to glutaraldehyde; of these, three also experienced an asthmatic reaction on exposure to formaldehyde, which suggests cross-reactivity.

Several recent epidemiologic surveys reported that the prevalence of asthma and work-related respiratory symptoms were higher in formaldehyde-exposed workers than unexposed control cohorts (82). A recent survey of 112 plywood metalworkers in New Zealand also found that asthma symptoms were more common in plywood metalworkers than in the general population and that high exposure to formaldehyde resulted in a much higher prevalence of asthma symptoms (36.4%) than that caused by low exposure (7.9%) (83). The possibility that irritant-induced asthma can be caused by formaldehyde was suggested by a recent case report on persistent asthma in a worker exposed for two hours to formaldehyde that leaked from a malfunctioning reactor gasket. The worker's asthma persisted for at least 13 months (84).

CHLORAMINE T AND OTHER BIOCIDES

Chloramine T is a sterilizing agent used in the food and beverage industry. Chloramine T was reported as a cause of OA in 12 workers of a pharmaceutical company, by Feinberg and Watrous in 1945 (85). Other cases of OA have been observed by different authors (86,87). Late and dual asthmatic reactions to inhalation testing have been documented (88). The mechanism of the reaction is IgE mediated as demonstrated by skin testing (85) and specific IgE assessments. The antigenic determinant is thought to be of the p-toluene sulfonyl group (89), and no evidence of new antigenic determinants related to the carrier could be demonstrated by Wass et al. (90).

Chloramines that are released from the reaction between chlorine releasing agents and pollutants around swimming pools have been incriminated in interesting cases of OA reported in three subjects—two lifeguards and one swimming teacher. These three subjects experienced immediate reactions after laboratory challenge to 0.5 mg/m^3 of nitrogen trichloride (91).

Glutaraldehyde and chlorhexidine are disinfectants commonly used by hospital staff in endoscopy units and radiology departments (92–96). Hexachlorophene is a topical disinfectant, which can cause OA as reported and confirmed through specific inhalation challenges, which caused an immediate reaction that was blocked by the use of sodium cromoglycate (97). Lauryl dimethyl benzyl ammonium chloride is a cleaning agent, which caused OA in a pharmacist who was indirectly exposed to it (98).

Case reports of OA due to three fungicides, tetrachloroisophthalonitrile (99), tributyl tin oxide (100), and captafol (Difolatan) (101), and organic phosphate insecticides (102) have been described.

HAIRDRESSING CHEMICALS

Hairdressers appear to be at increased risk for sensitization and the development of airway symptoms to a number of agents. As early as 1963, paraphenylenediamine was reported to cause occupational asthma among hairdressers (9). Individual case reports of occupational asthma due to persulfate salts were published as early as 1957 (103–109). Blainey et al. (110) found that 4 out of 23 workers (17%) at a hairdressing salon had OA that was confirmed by ammonium persulfate challenges carried out in 22 employees. Several epidemiologic studies on the incidence prevalence of OA in hairdressers revealed a wide range from 0.1 to 88 cases per thousand persons exposed per year (111–113). Recently, serial clinical studies in eight patients revealed a prolonged lapse between symptom onset and diagnosis established by evidence of IgE sensitization and laboratory bronchial provocation tests. In addition, persistence changes and deterioration in FEV_1 was observed in most of these patients despite medical treatment (114). Serum total IgE levels were increased in these workers. This was also found in a larger study of 101 persulfate-exposed workers whose serum levels of total IgE were significantly higher than a matched cohort of unexposed office workers (115). Hairdressers are also exposed to henna, a powder derived from the leaves and roots of a shrub that can cause OA; this has been confirmed by specific inhalation and workplace challenges in two separate reports (116,117). The latter investigators also demonstrated positive skin-prick tests and in vitro IgE-mediated sensitivity to henna. The proximity of exposure to persulfate salts may be significant inasmuch as Merget et al. (118) did not document any case of occupational asthma in 32 employees of a chemical industry where persulfates were used. Paraphenylenediamine is another product handled by hairdressers and has been reported to cause occupational asthma (9).

DIAZONIUM SALTS AND REACTIVE DYES

Diazonium salts are used in photocopying process; an azo-dye results from diazonium salts coupling with light. Armeli originally described four cases of workers with lower respiratory tract symptoms on exposure to diazonium salts (119). Graham et al. (120) described OA in one subject who underwent specific inhalation challenges and developed a late asthmatic reaction with recurrent symptoms over the next two days. The prevalence of work-related respiratory symptoms and increased specific IgE antibodies to diazonium tetrafluoroborate–human serum albumin conjugates was found to be 57% and 20%, respectively, among 45 workers in the polymer industry (121). All workers with increased specific IgE antibodies ($n = 9$) had work-related respiratory symptoms, whereas none of the asymptomatic workers ($n = 10$), and none of those with irritant symptoms only ($n = 10$) had increased specific IgE levels.

Alanko et al. (122) first described and confirmed occupational asthma in four workers exposed to reactive dyes, which are used to create brilliant colors in textile industry. They have shown that the asthma is IgE mediated as demonstrated by immediate skin reactivity and increased specific IgE antibodies in the majority of affected workers (123). Recent surveys were carried out in the dye-producing plant (124) and in textile plants (125) where dyes are used. In a survey of a producing plant employing 309 workers, Park et al. (124) found that 8% of them had skin reactivity to Black GR and 7% of them to Brilliant orange 3R. Seventeen percent of them had increased specific IgE levels to Black GR and 13% to Brilliant orange 3R (124). Specific inhalation challenges were positive in 13 workers. In a survey of 162 textile plant workers exposed to reactive dyes, Nilsson et al. (125) found that 10 had work-related symptoms. Of these, five had evidence of immediate allergic reactivity. Park and Hong (126) found increased levels of specific IgG in 23% and specific IgG_4 in 14% of the 309 workers who were assessed. The presence of increased specific IgG antibodies was associated with increased specific IgE levels and work-related symptoms, although not perfectly so (126).

Carmine E120 is a natural dye extracted from dried females of the arthropod *Dactylopius coccus* (cochineal). It is used in cosmetics, pharmaceutical, and food industries. Tabar-Purroy et al. (127) reported two cases of OA in a natural dye processing industry. The diagnosis was confirmed by specific inhalation challenge testing. Two other cases were reported in butchers who had been exposed during the process of mixing the carmines in sausages (128). In both studies, an IgE-mediated response was suggested.

PHARMACEUTICAL PRODUCTS

The capacity of various pharmaceutical products to induce respiratory sensitization has been studied by several authors (129–131). Chida also found through prospective assessment that the risk of sensitization increases with the degree of exposure (132). Pharmaceutical products derived from proteins or gums (herbs, psyllium, ipecacuanha, pancreatic, and glandular extracts, etc.) are covered in Chapter 20.

Several antibiotics can cause occupational asthma. In 1946, Rosberg (133) described two nurses with occupational asthma due to sulfathiazoles. In 1957, Tara described four subjects who had clinical evidence of asthma after being exposed to penicillin dust (134). Two other cases with evidence of skin and bronchial reactivity to penicillin were reported in 1960 (135). Synthetic penicillin can also be the cause of work-related asthma. Carlesi et al. (136) described six subjects with asthma caused by amoxicillin. Davies et al. (137) confirmed the diagnosis of occupational asthma due to ampicillin in three subjects who underwent specific inhalation challenges and experienced isolated late asthmatic reactions. Cross-reactivity of ampicillin with penicillin was also exhibited by the subjects. Penicillamine, which is a synthetic derivative of penicillin, has also been reported as a cause of occupational asthma as indicated by a late asthmatic reaction after exposure (138). Piperacillin, a semisynthetic penicillin, can also cause OA (139). Cephalosporins induced immediate asthmatic reactions in two pharmaceutical workers (140). The prevalence of occupational asthma due to cephalosporins was found to be 8% (7 out of 91) in 91 workers who were examined by Briatico-Vangosa et al. (141). Third generation cephalosporins, ceftazidine (142), and cefadroxil (143) can also cause occupational asthma. Aminocephalosporanic acid, a derivative, can also induce specific IgE sensitization and asthma (144). Phenylglycine acid chloride makes up the side chains of ampicillin and other antibiotics. An investigation of 24 workers involved in the production of phenylglycine acid chloride was performed by Kammermeyer and Mathews (145). Seven subjects had respiratory symptoms and two underwent specific inhalation challenges, which were both positive. Nine subjects had definite immediate skin reactions to phenylglycine acid chloride. In another study, an immediate skin and bronchospastic reaction was documented in a worker exposed to tetracycline (146). Davies and Pepys described one pharmaceutical worker in whom the diagnosis of OA caused by the macrolide antibiotic spiramycin was confirmed by specific inhalation challenge (147). Evidence of dermatitis and asthma due to spiramycin was also observed in a chick breeder (148). Two other cases were described by Moscato et al. (149) and, in one of them, specific inhalation challenges with adipic acid, an additive used to bind spiramycin, elicited an immediate reaction. Investigation of all 51 employees at a pharmaceutical company processing spiramycin revealed that four (8%) had OA as confirmed by specific inhalation tests (150). The mechanism of the reaction has not been determined. Tylosin tartrate is used in animal food as an antibiotic to prevent dysentery. Tylosin tartrate has been described as causing asthma in a laboratory technician in whom specific inhalation challenges induced a late asthmatic reaction (151).

Alpha-methyldopa can induce late asthmatic reactions, as was shown by Harries et al. (152). A glycyl compound used in the preparation of salbutamol has also been incriminated in causing asthma, confirmed by specific challenges that induced a late reaction (153). Amprolium hydrochloride is used as a food additive in poultries to prevent coccidioidomycosis. It has been reported to cause an immediate bronchoconstriction in subjects on bronchial challenging (154).

Coutts et al. (155) found that 8 out of the 55 subjects (15%) exposed to cimetidine had lower respiratory tract symptoms. In one subject, the diagnosis of occupational asthma was confirmed by specific inhalation challenges, which caused a late asthmatic reaction. Agius described a pharmaceutical worker who was exposed to morphine dust and developed symptoms and spirometric changes similar to that seen with OA (156). Specific IgG and IgG_4 antibodies were also demonstrated in workers exposed to morphine with lowering of this level after the exposure was diminished (157). Two cross-sectional surveys by Moneo et al. (158) and Biagini et al. (159), found a significant association between the presence of immediate skin wheal and flare and symptoms of lung function abnormalities in 28 and 33 opiate workers, respectively. Isonicotinic acid hydrazide, used in the treatment of tuberculosis can cause occupational asthma as was indicated by immediate bronchospasm in a pharmacist for whom evidence of type I sensitization was also confirmed by in vivo and in vitro tests (160,161). Rosenberg et al. (162) described two subjects who developed asthma after handling powdered aminophylline. Delayed reactions to bronchial challenges were observed. Hydralazine, which is an antihypertensive drug, has been shown to cause asthma, eliciting a late reaction after a challenge (163). The mechanism of the reaction is unknown. As discussed in the section on amines in this chapter, piperazine hydrochloride is used as an antihelminthic drug and can cause OA. Hydroxychloroquine was found to cause dermatitis and OA in a pharmaceutical worker (164). Mitoxantrone used as an antineoplastic drug, caused OA in a nurse (165).

POLYVINYLCHLORIDE AND ADHESIVES

Polyvinylchloride (PVC) has been reported to cause OA due to thermal degradation products. Several studies of OA caused by exposure to PVC were published between 1973 and 1977. Sokol et al. (166) published the first evidence of so-called "meat-wrappers asthma" in 1973. They described about three female subjects who developed symptoms after heating PVC with hot wires. Johnson and Anderson (167) described symptoms reported among 15 women employees at a meatpacking plant. Similar symptoms were described in another group of meat wrappers and cutters (168). Identification of the thermal degradation products was later made. Although traces of phthalic anhydride among several other products were identified, none of the exposed workers had specific IgE antibodies to this chemical (169). Andrasch et al. (170) were able to reproduce bronchoconstriction after exposure to PVC and to price label adhesive fumes in some of the workers as observed through serial monitoring of FEV_1. Unheated PVC dust can cause OA (171). Several reports of occupational asthma have appeared since these early investigations. For instance, 20% of the firefighters who were exposed to burning PVC fumes reported physician-diagnosed asthma and/or bronchitis 22 months after exposure (172). Recently, it was determined that the incidence of adult-onset asthma was approximately nine times higher in office workers exposed to degradation products of PVC floor coverings than that of controlled employees in similar work (173). Reports of interstitial lung disease or pneumoconiosis have been described in workers exposed to PVC polymer dust (174). PVC particles have also been shown to exert toxic lung effects in laboratory animals (175).

ACRYLATES

Kopp et al. (176) first described asthma in a subject who used ethylcyanoacrylate-containing instant glue while building model airplanes as a hobby. The subject developed an isolated late asthmatic reaction after bronchial challenges. Pickering et al. (177) and Nakazawa (178) described similar individual cases. The largest series was published by Lozewicz et al (179), who described six subjects who were experiencing either isolated late or dual reactions after exposure to methylmethacrylate and cyanoacrylates. Recent studies demonstrated several cases of OA due to acrylates: one case caused by methacrylate contained in a xerographic toner (180), two cases of asthma and rhinitis in assembly operators handling cyanoacrylate glue (181), and one case of asthma and rhinitis caused by diacrylate in an auto body shop worker (182).

Artificial nail makers and health professionals are exposed to acrylates. The mechanism of sensitization is unknown. A report of six cases of physician-diagnosed OA in cosmetologists working with ethyl methacrylate prompted ventilation modifications, which would significantly control the nail salon technician's exposure to the chemical (183). Ninhydrin, which is used as a laboratory reagent in detection of proteins and peptides, caused occupational asthma in a laboratory technician (184).

ACID ANHYDRIDES

Acid anhydrides were covered in a separate chapter in the previous edition of this book (185). Low-molecular-weight agents, of which trimellitic anhydride, phthalic anhydride, and maleic anhydride are the most common in causing respiratory diseases, are used in resins, plastics, dyes, etc. Recently, it has been reported that cyclic anhydrides can cause asthma (186).

These agents can cause various forms of respiratory diseases (187). First, they can cause direct toxicity to the airways and to the lung with manifestations of epistaxis, hemoptysis, and pulmonary edema. Second, various types of immunologically induced syndromes caused by these agents have been described: (*i*) a cytotoxic syndrome that results in pulmonary hemorrhage with hemoptysis and anemia, (*ii*) a late respiratory systemic syndrome of the hypersensitivity pneumonitis type, (*iii*) an asthmatic reaction associated with the development of an IgE-mediated reaction.

Kern was the first to describe a case of OA and to suggest the IgE-mediated induction of the disease (188). Numerous studies have since convincingly confirmed the IgE process through in vitro and in vivo testing (189–192). Bernstein et al. (193) have shown that the anhydride can act as a hapten or interact with new antigenic determinants.

Several cross-sectional studies in workers exposed to different anhydrides have been published. Zeiss et al. (194) found that 12 out of 474 workers (2.5%) exposed to trimellitic anhydride had asthma or rhinitis symptomatology. A surveillance program of 12 years in a high-risk industry reported by Zeiss identified 17 subjects (3.4%), in approximately 500 workers, with asthma or rhinitis symptoms (185). Barker et al. (195) found that 34 out of the 401 workers (8.8%) exposed to phthalic, maleic, and trimellitic anhydrides had work-related respiratory symptoms. In this study, skin sensitization to anhydrides was found to be present in 3.2% of workers and was significantly associated with smoking, level of exposure, and work-related symptoms. In a study by Grammer et al. (196), rhinitis was present in 22 out of the 25 (88%) subjects who suffered from asthma. Venables et al. (197) found that atopy and smoking were factors significantly associated with the presence of specific IgE to a conjugate of tetrachlorophthalic anhydride. An exposure-symptoms relationship has been found by Venables et al. (198).

A significant association has been found between human leukocyte antigens DR3 and specific IgE to trimellitic anhydride (199). More recently, Jones et al. (200) found a significant association between DQB1*05 gene and sensitization to different types of phthalic anhydrides.

In animal models, injections of anhydrides can cause the development of specific IgE and IgG antibodies (201,202). Antibodies peak three to four weeks after the first injection of anhydrides (202). In workers sensitized to tetrachlorophthalic anhydride and then removed from exposure, the median half-life of specific IgE antibodies was one year (203).

Grammer et al. (204) showed that wearing masks significantly reduced the occurrence of occupational respiratory diseases in 66 workers newly exposed to hexahydrophthalic anhydride and followed up for seven years.

OTHERS

Various chemicals have been incriminated as causes of occupational asthma, primarily in individual case reports or surveys. The list includes:

- freon contained in propellants (205) and hair-sprays, as causing irritation of the airways (206,207); one case of occupational asthma due to heated freon has been described and confirmed by specific inhalation challenges (208);
- furan used in the production of moulds in foundries (209); the diagnosis was confirmed by specific inhalation challenges and serial monitoring of peak expiratory flows;

- paraphenylenediamine in fur workers (25); 37 of 80 workers (46%) had symptoms of asthma; 74% of subjects tested experienced nasal or chest symptoms on specific inhalation challenges performed by inhalation;
- styrene in two plastics manufacturers who had isolated immediate bronchospastic reactions (210);
- enflurane in an anesthesiologist who experienced an asthmatic reaction 11 hours after a specific challenge (211);
- methyl blue contained in electrocardiograph ink (212,213) and terpene contained in rubber gloves (214), in hospital employees;
- exposed workers in a fiberglass plant, in whom the causative agent could not be identified (215), as well as one worker exposed to plexiglas in whom specific inhalation challenges elicited a dual asthmatic reaction (216); plexiglas is a polyacrylic resin that contains methylmethacrylate, which can cause occupational asthma;
- tetrazene, a powder produced by detonator manufacturers; as demonstrated by suggestive peak flows changes and specific inhalation challenges that induced a late asthmatic reaction (217);
- sodium iso-nonanoyl oxybenzene sulphonate in detergent workers; as confirmed by specific inhalation challenges in three workers; the mechanism of the late reaction remains unexplained (218,219);
- polyethylene (220), polypropylene (221), and polyester contained in electrostatic paints (222);
- various machining fluids reported to cause acute pulmonary responses in some (223) but not others (224); oil mists have also been incriminated as a cause of occupational asthma (225,226), although various contaminants present in oil mists can be responsible for their effect as reviewed (227); for at least one subject, the causal agent may be a pine odorant additive (228,229);
- various acids (hydrochloric, hydrofluoric, nitric, perchloric, and sulfuric), although it is not clear whether these reactions are "irritant" or reflect true sensitization (230). In the same way, perfumes can cause asthmatic reactions though it is still debatable if these are of an irritant mechanism (231);
- various chemical agents present in radiology units can cause an excess of asthma in personnel (232), although the frequency has been estimated by some to be probably low (233); an excess of respiratory symptoms has recently been confirmed in more than a thousand medical radiation technologists who were compared to an equivalent number of physiotherapists (82); the authors of the latter study were unable to ascertain if this excess was due to sensitization or irritation reactions to the various agents radiation technologists were exposed to at work (formaldehyde, glutaraldehyde, sulfur dioxide, and acetic acid).

STRUCTURE–ACTIVITY RELATIONSHIPS OF RESPIRATORY SENSITIZATION POTENTIAL

Agius et al. (234) have set various hypothetical mechanisms, based on structure–activity relationship, for the interactions of low-molecular-weight agents, mainly chemical agents, with human molecules. Karol et al. (235) have introduced a model for predicting respiratory sensitization by comparing structure–activity relationships of chemicals as potential sensitizers in a computer-based expert system, Multi Case.

This system enables prediction of sensitizing activity based on structural fragments and physicochemical properties of chemicals whose details are in the database. Approaches to the identification of chemical respiratory sensitizers in a mouse model have been proposed by Kimber et al. (236). Contact allergens, which do not generally cause sensitization of the respiratory tract, provoke a Th-1 type immune response with high levels of interferon-gamma. Exposure of mice to chemical respiratory sensitizers results in the generation of selective Th-2 immune responses with the production of cytokines [interleukin (IL-4 and IL-10)]. This differential response referred to as "cytokine fingerprinting" may provide a clue on the likelihood that a chemical product will cause predominant skin or respiratory sensitization.

MULTIPLE CHEMICAL SENSITIVITY SYNDROME

There are claims that an unusual assortment of symptoms such as headaches, rashes, food intolerance, confusion, chronic vaginal yeast infections, depression, confusion, fatigue, and mental disorientation occur after single or chronic exposures factory workers commonly experience when they come in contact with low levels of organic solvents used in various manufacturing processes (237). A rash of multiple chemical sensitivity (MCS) claims may also occur after exposure to unknown agent(s) associated with the sick building syndrome. Multiple synonyms have been used for MCS. These include total environmental allergy, ecologic illness, environmental illness, 20th-century disease, and the immune dysregulation syndrome. No clear-cut pattern of symptoms has emerged to distinguish a homogeneous group of patients, which would be suitable for epidemiologic investigation. Claims of altered immune responses after exposure to certain chemicals have not been substantiated. One hypothesis that has been proposed is that MCS symptoms represent a chemically triggered syndrome that could alter brain levels of neurotransmitters such as serotonin or acetylcholine. This speculation has not been tested. Several series of typical patients with this syndrome have been evaluated. The common denominator of these clinical reports is a patient presenting with somatoform symptoms as a physical explanation either for unrecognized or self-denied psychiatric disorder. Despite these inconsistencies, patients with this problem claimed to be relieved when they avoid many common environmental agents. Sometimes patients with this disorder have gone to the extremes of building "safe rooms" and wearing charcoal filter or full head respiratory protection. Patients having these symptoms also claim that prior exposure to one or several chemicals were the triggers of current responses to a broad range of unrelated chemicals or odors. None of these multiple chemical reactions have been documented by objective immune or provocative responses (238). It should be emphasized that the atypical and at times bizarre spectrum of nonpulmonary symptoms associated with the MCS syndrome bears no relationship to reactive airways dysfunction syndrome or other chemically induced cases of OA. Therefore, disability compensation of MCS symptoms based on prior occupational exposure alone is not justified by the available facts.

Patients reporting sensitivity to multiple chemicals demonstrate substantial overlap between fibromyalgia and chronic fatigue syndrome. Standardized questionnaires have been used to elucidate symptoms in these patients. A multicenter investigation of both patient- and physician-completed questionnaires revealed that either a four or six domain definition of the MCS syndrome in these questionnaires had reasonable psychometric characteristics (239). Thus far, a variety of mechanisms have been reputed to be involved in this syndrome, but most of these are hypotheses, which have not been proved (240). A recent preliminary study of possible objective indices in the MCS syndrome reported that MCS patients presenting with cough and other airway symptoms demonstrated significantly greater capsaicin-induced cough and higher levels of nerve growth factor in nasal wash samples than control subjects (241).

CONCLUSION AND RESEARCH NEEDS

With the increased use of new chemical products steadily appearing in workplace settings, it is highly probable that the list of agents categorized under the heading of miscellaneous chemical products causing occupational asthma will grow. It is also likely that the increased use of these products will result not only in more documentation of individual cases but also proper surveys of workplaces where the products are used. As for other low-molecular-weight agents, more studies exploring the mechanism of sensitization are needed.

REFERENCES

1. Ferris BG, Peters JM, Burgess WA, Cherry RB. Apparent effect of an azodicarbonamide on the lungs. A preliminary report. J Occup Med 1977; 19:424–425.
2. Slovak AJ. Occupational asthma caused by a plastics blowing agent, azodicarbonamide. Thorax 1981; 36:906–909.
3. Malo JL, Pineau L, Cartier A. Occupational asthma due to azobisformamide. Clin Allergy 1985; 15:261–264.
4. Valentino M, Comai M. Occupational asthma from azodicarbonamide: case report. G Ital Med Lav 1985; 7:97–99.
5. Normand JC, Grange F, Hernandez C, et al. Occupational asthma after exposure to azodicarbonamide: report of four cases. Br J Ind Med 1989; 46:60–62.
6. Hagmar L, Nielsen J, Skerfving S. Clinical features and epidemiology of occupational obstructive respiratory disease caused by small molecular weight organic chemicals. Epidemiol Allergic Diseases Monogr Allergy 1987; 21:42–58.
7. Dernehl CU. Clinical experiences with exposures to ethylene diamines. Ind Med Surg 1951; 20:541–546.
8. Dernehl CU. Hazards to health associated with the use of epoxy resins. J Occup Med 1963; 5:17–21.
9. Gelfand HH. Respiratory allergy due to chemical compounds encountered in the rubber, lacquer, shellac, and beauty culture industries. J Allergy 1963; 34:374–381.
10. Sterling GM. Asthma due to aluminium soldering flux. Thorax 1967; 22:533–537.
11. Pepys J, Pickering CA. Asthma due to inhaled chemical fumes-amino-ethyl ethanolamine in aluminium soldering flux. Clin Allergy 1972; 2:197–204.
12. Lam S, Chan-Yeung M. Ethylenediamine-induced asthma. Am Rev Respir Dis 1980; 121:151–155.
13. Vallières M, Cockcroft DW, Taylor DM, Dolovich J, Hargreave FE. Dimethyl ethanolamine-induced asthma. Am Rev Respir Dis 1977; 115:867–871.
14. Sargent EV, Mitchell CA, Brubaker RE. Respiratory effects of occupational exposure to an epoxy resin system. Arch Environ Health 1976; 31:236–240.
15. Brubaker RE, Muranko HJ, Smith DB, Beck GJ, Scovel G. Evaluation and control of a respiratory exposure to 3-(Dimethylamino)propylamine. J Occup Med 1979; 21: 688–690.

16. Ng TP, Lee HS, Malik MA, Chee CB, Cheong TH, Wang YT. Asthma in chemical workers exposed to aliphatic polyamines. Occup Med 1995; 45:45–48.

17. Savonius B, Keskinen H, Tuppurainen M, Kanerva L. Occupational asthma caused by ethanolamines. Allergy 1994; 49:877–881.

18. McCullagh SF. Allergenicity of piperazine: a study in environmental aetiology. Br J Ind Med 1968; 25:319–325.

19. Pepys J, Pickering CA, Loudon HW. Asthma due to inhaled chemical agents-piperazine dihydrochloride. Clin Allergy 1972; 2:189–196.

20. Bernstein JA, Stauder T, Bernstein DI, Bernstein IL. A combined respiratory and cutaneous hypersensitivity syndrome induced by work exposure to quaternary amines. J Allergy Clin Immunol 1994; 94:257–259.

21. Purohit A, Kopferschmitt-Kubler MC, Moreau C, Popin E, Blaumeiser M, Pauli G. Quaternary ammonium compounds and occupational asthma. Int Arch Occup Environ Health 2000; 73:423–427.

22. Hagmar L, Bellander T, Bergöö B, Simonsson BG. Piperazine-induced occupational asthma. J Occup Med 1982; 24:193–197.

23. Hagmar L, Welinder H. Prevalence of specific IgE antibodies against piperazine in employees of a chemical plant. Int Arch Allergy Appl Immunol 1986; 81:12–16.

24. Hagmar L, Bellander T, Ranstam J, Skerfving S. Piperazine-induced airway symptoms: exposure-response relationships and selection in an occupational setting. Am J Ind Med 1984; 6:347–357.

25. Silberman DE, Sorrell AH. Allergy in fur workers with special reference to paraphenylenediamine. J Allergy 1959; 30:11–18.

26. Belin L, Wass U, Audunsson G, Mathiasson L. Amines: possible causative agents in the development of bronchial hyperreactivity in workers manufacturing polyurethanes from isocyanates. Br J Ind Med 1983; 40:251–257.

27. Candura F, Moscato G. Do amines induce occupational asthma in workers manufacturing polyurethane foams. Br J Ind Med 1984; 41:552–523.

28. Fawcett IW, Newman Taylor AJ, Pepys J. Asthma due to inhaled chemical agents—fumes from "Multicore" soldering flux and colophony resin. Clin Allergy 1976; 6:577–585.

29. Burge PS, Harries MG, O'Brien IM, Pepys J. Respiratory disease in workers exposed to solder flux fumes containing colophony (pine resin). Clin Allergy 1978; 8:1–14.

30. Burge PS, Perks W, O'Brien IM, Hawkins R, Green M. Occupational asthma in an electronics factory. Thorax 1979; 34:13–18.

31. Herks WH, Burge PS, Rehahn M, Green M. Work-related respiratory disease in employees leaving an electronics factory. Thorax 1979; 34:19–22.

32. Burge PS, Perks WH, O'Brien IM, et al. Occupational asthma in an electronics factory: a case control study to evaluate aetiological factors. Thorax 1979; 34:300–307.

33. Burge PS, O'Brien IM, Harries MG. Peak flow rate records in the diagnosis of occupational asthma due to colophony. Thorax 1979; 34:308–316.

34. Burge PS, Harries MG, O'Brien I, Pepys J. Bronchial provocation studies in workers exposed to the fumes of electronic soldering fluxes. Clin Allergy 1980; 10:137–149.

35. Burge PS, Edge G, Hawkins R, White V, Taylor AN. Occupational asthma in a factory making flux-cored solder containing colophony. Thorax 1981; 36:828–834.

36. Burge PS. Occupational asthma in electronics workers caused by colophony fumes: follow-up of affected workers. Thorax 1982; 37:348–353.

37. Burge PS. Occupational asthma due to soft soldering fluxes containing colophony (rosin, pine resin). Eur J Respir Dis 1982; 63(suppl 123):65–67.

38. Innocenti A, Loi F. Occupational allergic asthma due to colophony. Med Lav 1978; 69:720–722.

39. Maestrelli P, Alessandri MV, Dal VL, Bartolucci GB, Cocheo V. Occupational asthma due to colophony. Med Lav 1985; 76:371–378.

40. So SY, Lam WK, Yu D. Colophony-induced asthma in a poultry vender. Clin Allergy 1981; 11:395–399.

41. Burge PS, Wieland A, Robertson AS, Weir D. Occupational asthma due to unheated colophony. Br J Ind Med 1986; 43:559–560.

42. Randem B, Smolensky MH, Hsi B, Albright D, Burge S. Field survey of circadian rhythm in PEF of electronics workers suffering from colophony-induced asthma. Chronobiol Int 1987; 4:263–271.

43. Weir DC, Robertson AS, Jones S, Burge PS. Occupational asthma due to soft corrosive soldering fluxes containing zinc chloride and ammonium chloride. Thorax 1989; 44: 220–223.

44. Stevens JJ. Asthma due to soldering flux: a polyether alcohol-polypropylene glycol mixture. Ann Allergy 1976; 36:419–422.

45. Elms J, Allan LJ, Pengelly I, Fishwick D, Beckett PN, Curran AD. Colophony: an in vitro model for the induction of sensitization. Clin Exp Allergy 2000; 30:209–213.

46. Harris DK. Health problems in the manufacture and use of plastics. Br J Ind Med 1953; 10:255–268.

47. Niemelä R, Vainio H. Formaldehyde exposure in work and the general environment. Occurrence and possibilities for prevention. Scand J Work Environ Health 1981; 7:95–100.

48. Sheppard D, Eschenbacher WL, Epstein J. Lack of bronchomotor response to up to 3 ppm formaldehyde in subjects with asthma. Environ Res 1984; 35:133–139.

49. Witek TJ, Schachter EN, Tosun T, Beck GJ, Leaderer BP. An evaluation of respiratory effects following exposure to 2.0 ppm formaldehyde in asthmatics: lung function, symptoms, and airway reactivity. Arch Environ Health 1987; 42:230–237.

50. Sauder LR, Green DJ, Chatham MD, Kulle TJ. Acute pulmonary response of asthmatics to 3.0 ppm formaldehyde. Toxicol Ind Health 1987; 3:569–578.

51. Harving H, Korsgaard J, Dahl R. Low concentrations of formaldehyde in bronchial asthma: a study of exposure under controlled conditions. Br Med J 1986; 293:310.

52. Harving H, Korsgaard J, Pedersen OF, Molhave L, Dahl R. Pulmonary function and bronchial reactivity in asthmatics during low-level formaldehyde exposure. Lung 1990; 168:15–21.

53. Uba G, Pachorek D, Bernstein J, et al. Prospective study of respiratory effects of formaldehyde among healthy and asthmatic medical students. Am J Ind Med 1989; 15:91–101.

54. Tuthill RW. Woodstoves, formaldehyde, and respiratory disease. Am J Epidemiol 1984; 120:952–955.

55. Green DJ, Sauder LR, Kulle TJ, Bascom R. Acute response to 3.0 ppm formaldehyde in exercising healthy nonsmokers and asthmatics. Am Rev Respir Dis 1987; 135: 1261–1266.

56. Schachter EN, Witek TJ Jr, Brody DJ, Tosun T, Beck GJ, Leaderer BP. A study of respiratory effects from exposure to 2.0 ppm formaldehyde in occupationally exposed workers. Environ Res 1987; 44:188–205.

57. Alexandersson R, Kolmodin-Hedman B, Hedenstierna G. Exposure to formaldehyde: effects on pulmonary function. Arch Environ Health 1982; 37:279–284.

58. Gamble JF, McMichael AJ, Williams T, Battigelli M. Respiratory function and symptoms: an environmental-epidemiological study of rubber workers exposed to a phenol-formaldehyde type resin. Am Ind Hyg Assoc J 1976; 37:499–513.

59. Schoenberg JB, Mitchell CA. Airway disease caused by phenolic (phenol-formaldehyde) resin exposure. Arch Environ Health 1975; 30:574–577.

60. Wallenstein G, Rebohle E. Sensibilisierungen durch formaldehyd bei beruflicher inhalativer exposition. Allerg Immunol 1976; 22:287–295.

61. Sakula A. Formalin asthma in hospital laboratory staff. Lancet 1975; 2:816.

62. Kerfoot EJ, Mooney TF. Formaldehyde and paraformaldehyde study in funeral homes. Am Ind Hyg Assoc J 1975; 36:533–537.

63. Editorial. Formalin asthma. Lancet 1977; 1:790.

64. Editorial. Formaldehyde toxicity. Lancet 1979:620.

65. Hendrick DJ, Lane DJ. Occupational formalin asthma. Br J Ind Med 1977; 34:11–18.
66. Hendrick DJ, Lane DJ. Formalin asthma in hospital staff. Br Med J 1975; 1:607–608.
67. Hendrick DJ, Rando RJ, Lane DJ, Morris MJ. Formaldehyde asthma: challenge exposure levels and fate after five years. J Occup Med 1982; 24:893–897.
68. Frigas E, Filley WV, Reed CE. Bronchial challenge with formaldehyde gas: lack of bronchoconstriction in 13 patients suspected of having formaldehyde-induced asthma. Mayo Clin Proc 1984; 59:295–299.
69. Nordman H, Keskinen H, Tuppurainen M. Formaldehyde asthma-Rare or overlooked? J Allergy Clin Immunol 1985; 75:91–99.
70. Frigas E, Filley WV, Reed CE. Asthma induced by dust from urea-formaldehyde foam insulating material. Chest 1981; 79:706–707.
71. Cockcroft DW, Hoeppner VH, Dolovich J. Occupational asthma caused by cedar urea formaldehyde particle board. Chest 1982; 82:49–53.
72. Patterson R, Pateras V, Grammer LC, Harris KE. Human antibodies against formaldehyde-human serum albumin conjugates or human serum albumin in individuals exposed to formaldehyde. Int Arch Allergy Appl Immunol 1986; 79:53–59.
73. Kramps JA, Peltenburg LT, Kerklaan PR, Spieksma FT, Valentijn RM, Dijkman JG. Measurement of specific IgE antibodies in individuals exposed to formaldehyde. Clin Allergy 1989; 19:509–514.
74. Grammer LC, Harris KE, Shaughnessy MA, et al. Clinical and immunologic evaluation of 37 workers exposed to gaseous formaldehyde. J Allergy Clin Immunol 1990; 86:177–181.
75. Wüthrich EI. Formaldehyd- und phthalisches anydrid-asthma. Schweiz med Wochenschr 1988; 118:1568–1572.
76. Wantke F, Demmer CM, Tappler P, Gotz M, Jarisch R. Exposure to gaseous formaldehyde induces IgE-mediated sensitization to formaldehyde in school-children. Clin Exp Allergy 1996; 26:276–280.
77. Baba K, Yagi T, Niwa S, et al. Measurement of formaldehyde-specific IgE antibodies in adult asthmatics. Arerugi 2000; 49:404–411.
78. Kim CW, Song JS, Ahn YS, et al. Occupational asthma due to formaldehyde. Yonsei Med J 2001; 42:440–445.
79. Doe S, Suzuki S, Morishita M, et al. The prevalence of IgE sensitization to formaldehyde in asthmatic children. Allergy 2003; 58:668–671.
80. Lemière C, Desjardins A, Cloutier Y, et al. Occupational asthma due to formaldehyde resin dust with and without reaction to formaldehyde gas. Eur Respir J 1995; 8:861–865.
81. Gannon PF, Bright P, Campbell M, O'Hickey SP, Burge PS. Occupational asthma due to glutaraldehyde and formaldehyde in endoscopy and x ray departments. Thorax 1995; 50:156–159.
82. Liss GM, Tarlo SM, Doherty J, et al. Physician diagnosed asthma, respiratory symptoms, and associations with workplace tasks among radiographers in Ontario, Canada. Occup Environ Med 2003; 60:254–261.
83. Fransman W, McLean D, Douwes J, Demers PA, Leung V, Pearce N. Respiratory symptoms and occupational exposures in New Zealand plywood mill workers. Ann Occup Hyg 2003; 47:287–295.
84. Vandenplas O, Fievez P, Delwiche JP, Boulanger J, Thimpont J. Persistent asthma following accidental exposure to formaldehyde. Allergy 2004; 59:115–116.
85. Feinberg SM, Watrous RM. Atopy to simple chemical compounds-sulfonechloramides. J Allergy 1945; 16:209–220.
86. Bourne MS, Flindt ML, Walker JM. Asthma due to industrial use of chloramine. Br Med J 1979; 2:10–12.
87. Charles TJ. Asthma due to industrial use of chloramine. Br Med J 1979; 1:334.
88. Dijkman JG, Vooren PH, Kramps JA. Occupational asthma due to inhalation of chloramine-T. I. Clinical observations and inhalation-provocation studies. Int Arch Allergy Appl Immunol 1981; 64:422–427.

89. Kramps JA, van Toorenenbergen AW, Vooren PH, Dijkman JH. Occupational asthma due to inhalation of chloramine-T. II. Demonstration of specific IgE antibodies. Int Arch Allergy Appl Immunol 1981; 64:428–438.

90. Wass U, Belin L, Eriksson NE. Immunological specificity of chloramine-T-induced IgE antibodies in serum from a sensitized worker. Clin Allergy 1989; 19:463–471.

91. Thickett KM, McCoach JS, Gerber JM, Sadhra S, Burge PS. Occupational asthma caused by chloramines in indoor swimming-pool air. Eur Respir J 2002; 19:827–832.

92. Jachuck SJ, Bound PG, Steel J, Blain PG. Occupational hazard in hospital staff exposed to 2 per cent glutaraldehyde in an endoscopy unit. J Soc Occup Med 1989; 39:69–71.

93. Burge PS. Occupational risks of glutaraldehyde. Br Med J 1989; 299:1451.

94. Waclawski ER, McAlpine LG, Thomson NC. Occupational asthma in nurses caused by chlorhexidine and alcohol aerosols. Br Med J 1989; 298:929–930.

95. Cullinan P, Hayes J, Cannon J, Madan L, Heap D, Taylor AN. Occupational asthma in radiographers. Lancet 1992; 340:1477.

96. Pham NH, Weiner JM, Reisner GS, Baldo BA. Anaphylaxis to chlorhexidine. Case Report. Implication of immunoglobulin E antibodies and identification of an allergenic determinant. Clin Exp Allergy 2000; 30:1001–1007.

97. Nagy L, Orosz M. Occupational asthma due to hexachlorophene. Thorax 1984; 39: 630–631.

98. Burge PS, Richardson MN. Occupational asthma due to indirect exposure to lauryl dimethyl benzyl ammonium chloride used in a floor cleaner. Thorax 1994; 49:842–843.

99. Honda I, Kohrogi H, Ando M, et al. Occupational asthma induced by the fungicide tetrachloroisophthalonitrile. Thorax 1992; 47:760–761.

100. Shelton D, Urch B, Tarlo SM. Occupational asthma induced by a carpet fungicide-tributyl tin oxide. J Allergy Clin Immunol 1992; 90:274–275.

101. Royce S, Wald P, Sheppard D, Balmes J. Occupational asthma in a pesticides manufacturing worker. Chest 1993; 103:295–296.

102. Weiner A. Bronchial asthma due to the organic phosphate insecticides. Ann Allergy 1961; 19:397–401.

103. Pichat R, Chatanay R. A propos d'un asthme au persulfate d'ammonium. Arch Mal Prof 1957; 18:280–282.

104. Hardel PJ, Reybet-Degat O, Jeannin L, Paqueron MJ. Asthme des coiffeurs: danger des décolorants capillaires contenant des persulfates alcalins. Nouv Presse Med 1978; 7:4151.

105. Girard JP, Bertrand J. Study of 2% solution of sodium cromoglycate in perennial rhinitis assessed by subjective and objective parameters. Clin Allergy 1975; 5:301–309.

106. Gaultier M, Gervais P, Mellerio F. Deux causes d'asthme professionnel chez les coiffeurs: persulfate et soie. Arch Mal Prof 1966; 27:809–813.

107. Pepys J, Hutchcroft BJ, Breslin AB. Asthma due to inhaled chemical agents-persulphate salts and henna in hairdressers. Clin Allergy 1976; 6:399–404.

108. Baur X, Fruhmann G, Liebe VV. Occupational asthma and dermatitis after exposure to dusts of persulfate salts in two industrial workers. Respiration 1979; 38:144–150.

109. Parra FM, Igea JM, Quirce S, Ferrando MC, Martin JA, Losada E. Occupational asthma in a hairdresser caused by persulphate salts. Allergy 1992; 47(6):656–660.

110. Blainey AD, Ollier S, Cundell D, Smith RE, Davies RJ. Occupational asthma in a hairdressing salon. Thorax 1986; 41:42–50.

111. Leino T, Tammilehto L, Hytönen M, Sala E, Paakkulainen H, Kanerva L. Occupational skin and respiratory diseases among hairdressers. Scand J Work Environ Health 1998; 24:398–406.

112. Cullinan P, Newman Taylor AJ. Aetiology of occupational asthma. Clin Exp Allergy 1997; 27(suppl 1):41–46.

113. Albin M, Rylander L, Mikoczy Z, et al. Incidence of asthma in female Swedish hairdressers. Occup Environ Med 2002; 59:119–123.

114. Munoz X, Cruz MJ, Orriols R, Bravo C, Espuga M, Morell F. Occupational asthma due to persulfate salts: diagnosis and follow-up. Chest 2003; 123:2124–2129.
115. Hollund BE, Moen BE, Lygre SH, Florvaag E, Omenaas E. Prevalence of airway symptoms among hairdressers in Bergen, Norway. Occup Environ Med 2001; 58:780–785.
116. Starr JC, Yunginger J, Brahser GW. Immediate type I asthmatic response to henna following occupational exposure in hairdressers. Ann Allergy 1982; 48:98–99.
117. Bolhaar ST, Mulder M, van Ginkel CJ. IgE-mediated allergy to henna. Allergy 2001; 56:248.
118. Merget R, Buenemann A, Kulzer R, et al. A cross sectional study of chemical industry workers with occupational exposure to persulphates. Occup Environ Med 1996; 53:422–426.
119. Armeli G. Bronchial asthma from diazonium salts. Med Lav 1968; 59:463–466.
120. Graham V, Coe MJ, Davies RJ. Occupational asthma after exposure to a diazonium salt. Thorax 1981; 36:950–951.
121. Luczynska CM, Hutchcroft BJ, Harrison MA, Dornan JD, Topping MD. Occupational asthma and specific IgE to diazonium salt intermediate used in the polymer industry. J Allergy Clin Immunol 1990; 85:1076–1082.
122. Alanko K, Keskinen H, Byorksten F, Ojanen S. Immediate-type hypersensitivity to reactive dyes. Clin Allergy 1978; 8:25–31.
123. Topping MD, Forster HW, Ide CW, Kennedy FM, Leach AM, Sorkin S. Respiratory allergy and specific immunoglobin E and Immunoglobin G antibodies to reactive dyes used in the wool industry. J Occup Med 1989; 31:857–862.
124. Park HS, Lee MK, Kim BO, et al. Clinical and immunologic evaluations of reactive dye-exposed workers. J Allergy Clin Immunol 1991; 87:639–649.
125. Nilsson R, Nordlinder R, Wass U, Meding B, Belin L. Asthma, rhinitis, and dermatitis in workers exposed to reactive dyes. Br J Ind Med 1993; 50:65–70.
126. Park HS, Hong CS. The significance of specific IgG and IgG4 antibodies to a reactive dye in exposed workers. Clin Exp Allergy 1991; 21:357–362.
127. Tabar-Purroy AI, Alvarez-Puebla MJ, Acero-Sainz S, et al. Carmine (E-120)–induced occupational asthma revisited. J Allergy Clin Immunol 2003; 111:415–419.
128. Anibarro B, Seoane J, Vila C, Mugica V, Lombardero M. Occupational asthma induced by inhaled carmine among butchers. Int J Occup Med Environ Health 2003; 16:33–37.
129. Romanski B, Zegarski W. Etiologie de l'asthme et des lésions allergiques de la peau chez les ouvriers d'une usine pharmaceutique. Toulouse Méd 1963; 64:802–804.
130. Kobayashi S, Yamamura Y, Frick OL, Horiuchi Y, Kishimoto S, Miyamoto T. Occupational asthma due to inhalation of pharmacological dusts and other chemical agents with some reference to other occupational asthmas in Japan. Allergology. In: Naranjo P, De Weck A, eds. Proceedings of the VIII International Congress of Allergology, Tokyo, October 1973, 1974; Excerpta Medica, Amsterdam 1974:124–132.
131. Fueki R. Different aspects of occupational asthma in Japan. In: Frazier CA, ed. Occupational asthma. Von Nostrand Reinhold 1980; 229–244.
132. Chida TA. A study on dose-response relationship of occupational allergy in pharmaceutical plant. Jpn J Ind Health 1986; 28:77–86.
133. Rosberg M. Asthma bronchiale caused by sulphathiazole. Acta Med Scand 1946; 126:185–190.
134. Tara S. Asthme à la pénicilline. Arch Mal Prof 1957; 18:274–277.
135. Gaultier M, Fournier E, Gervais P. L'asthme professionnel par allergie à la pénicilline. Arch Mal Prof 1960; 21:13–23.
136. Carlesi G, Ferrea E, Melino C, Messineo A, Pacelli E. Aspects of environmental health and of pathology caused by pollution with amoxicillin in a pharmaceutical industry. Nuovi Ann Ig Microbiol. 1979; 30:185–196.
137. Davies RJ, Hendrick DJ, Pepys J. Asthma due to inhaled chemical agents: ampicillin, bensyl penicillin, 6 amino penicillanic acid and related substances. Clin Allergy 1974; 4:227–247.

138. Lagier F, Cartier A, Dolovich J, Malo JL. Occupational asthma in a pharmaceutical worker exposed to penicillamine. Thorax 1989; 44:157–158.

139. Moscato G, Galdi E, Scibilia J, et al. Occupational asthma, rhinitis and urticaria due to piperacillin sodium in a pharmaceutical worker. Eur Respir J 1995; 8:467–469.

140. Coutts II, Dally MB, Taylor AJ, Pickering CA, Horsfield N. Asthma in workers manufacturing cephalosporins. Br Med J 1981; 283:950.

141. Briatico-Vangosa G, Beretta F, Bianchi S, et al. Bronchial asthma due to 7-aminocephalosporanic acid (7-ACA) in workers employed in cephalosporine production. Med Lav 1981; 72:488–493.

142. Stenton SC, Dennis JH, Hendrick DJ. Occupational asthma due to ceftazidime. Eur Respir J 1995; 8:1421–1423.

143. Sastre J, Quirce S, Novalbos A, Lluch-Bernal M, Bombin C, Umpiérrez A. Occupational asthma induced by cephalosporins. Eur Respir J 1999; 13:1189–1191.

144. Park HS, Kim KU, Lee YM, et al. Occupational asthma and IgE sensitization to 7-aminocephalosporanic acid. J Allergy Clin Immunol 2004; 113:785–787.

145. Kammermeyer JK, Mathews KP. Hypersensitivity to phenylglycine acid chloride. J Allergy Clin Immunol 1973; 52:73–84.

146. Menon MP, Das AK. Tetracycline asthma—a case report. Clin Allergy 1977; 7: 285–290.

147. Davies RJ, Pepys J. Asthma due to inhaled chemical agents—the macrolide antibiotic Spiramycin. Clin Allergy 1975; 1:99–107.

148. Paggiaro PL, Loi AM, Toma G. Bronchial asthma and dermatitis due to spiramycin in a chick breeder. Clin Allergy 1979; 9:571–574.

149. Moscato G, Naldi L, Candura F. Bronchial asthma due to spiramycin and adipic acid. Clin Allergy 1984; 14:355–361.

150. Malo J-L, Cartier A. Occupational asthma in workers of a pharmaceutical company processing spiramycin. Thorax 1988; 43:371–377.

151. Lee HS, Wang YT, Yeo CT, Tan KT, Ratnam KV. Occupational asthma due to tylosin tartrate. Br J Ind Med 1989; 46:498–499.

152. Harries MG, Taylor AN, Wooden J, MacAuslan A. Bronchial asthma due to alphamethyldopa. Br Med J 1979:1461.

153. Fawcett IW, Pepys J, Erooga MA. Asthma due to "glycyl compound" powder—an intermediate in production of salbutamol. Clin Allergy 1976; 6:405–409.

154. Greene SA, Freedman S. Asthma due to inhaled chemical agents—amprolium hydrochloride. Clin Allergy 1976; 6:105–108.

155. Coutts II, Lozewicz S, Dally MB, et al. Respiratory symptoms related to work in a factory manufacturing cimetidine tablets. Br Med J 1984; 288:1418.

156. Agius R. Opiate inhalation and occupational asthma. Br Med J 1989; 298:323.

157. Biagini RE, Klincewicz SL, Henningsen GM, et al. Antibodies to morphine in workers exposed to opiates at a narcotics manufacturing facility and evidence for similar antibodies in heroin abusers. Life Sci 1990; 47:897–908.

158. Moneo I, Alday E, Ramos C, Curiel G. Occupational asthma caused by *Papaver somniferum*. Allergol Immunopathol 1993; 21:145–148.

159. Biagini RE, Bernstein DM, Klincewicz SL, Mittman R, Bernstein IL, Henningsen GM. Evaluation of cutaneous responses and lung function from exposure to opiate compounds among ethical narcotics-manufacturing workers. J Allergy Clin Immunol 1992; 89:108–117.

160. Asai S, Shimoda T, Hara K, Fujiwara K. Occupational asthma caused by isonicotinic acid hydrazide (INH) inhalation. J Allergy Clin Immunol 1987; 80:578–582.

161. Fujiwara K, Saita T, Shimoda T, Asai S, Hara K. Isonicotinic acid hydrazide as an antigen. J Allergy Clin Immunol 1987; 80:582–585.

162. Rosenberg M, Aaronson D, Evans C. Asthmatic responses to inhaled aminophylline: a report of two cases. Ann Allergy 1984; 52:97–98.

163. Perrin B, Malo JL, Cartier A, Evans S, Dolovich J. Occupational asthma in a pharmaceutical worker exposed to hydralazine. Thorax 1990; 45:980–981.

164. Meier H, Elsner P, Wüthrich B. Occupationally-induced contact dermatitis and bronchial asthma in a unusual delayed reaction to hydrochloroquine. Der Hautarzt 1999; 50:665–669.

165. Walusiak J, Wittczak T, Ruta U, Palczynski C. Occupational asthma due to mitoxantrone. Allergy 2002; 57:461.

166. Sokol WN, Aelony Y, Beall GN. Meat-wrapper's asthma. A new syndrome? JAMA 1973; 226:639–641.

167. Johnston CJ, Anderson HW. Meat-wrappers asthma: a case study. J Occup Med 1976; 18:102–104.

168. Brooks SM, Vandervort R. Polyvinyl chloride film thermal decomposition products as an occupational illness. 2. Clinical studies. J Occup Med 1977; 19:192–196.

169. Vandervort R, Brooks SM. Polyvinyl chloride film thermal decomposition products as an occupational illness. 1. Environmental exposures and toxicology. J Occup Med 1977; 19:188–191.

170. Andrasch RH, Bardana EJ, Koster F, Pirofsky B. Clinical and bronchial provocation studies in patients with meatwrapper's asthma. J Allergy Clin Immunol 1976; 58: 291–298.

171. Lee HS, Yap J, Wang YT, Lee CS, Tan KT, Poh SC. Occupational asthma due to unheated polyvinylchloride resin dust. Br J Ind Med 1989; 46:820–822.

172. Markovitz JS. Self reported short- and long-term respiratory effects among PVC-exposed firefighters. Arch Environ Health 1989; 44:30–33.

173. Tuomainen A, Serui M, Sieppi A. Indoor air quality and health problems associated with damp floor coverings. Int Arch Occup Environ Health 2004; 77:222–226.

174. Gong H. Uncommon causes of occupational interstitial lung disease. Curr Opin Pulm Med 1996; 2:405–411.

175. Xu H, Vanhooren HM, Verbeken E, et al. Pulmonary toxicity of polyvinyl chloride particles after repeated intratracheal instillations in rats. Elevated CD4/CD8 lymphocyte ratio in bronchoalveolar lavage. Toxicol Appl Pharmacol 2004; 194:122–131.

176. Kopp SK, McKay RT, Moller DR, Cassedy K, Brooks SM. Asthma and rhinitis due to ethylcyanoacrylate instant glue. Ann Int Med 1985; 102:613–615.

177. Pickering CA, Bainbridge D, Birtwistle IH, Griffiths DL. Occupational asthma due to methyl methacrylate in an orthopaedic theatre sister. Br Med J 1986; 292:1362–1363.

178. Nakazawa T. Occupational asthma due to alkyl cyanoacrylate. J Occup Med 1990; 32:709–710.

179. Lozewicz S, Davison AG, Hopkirk A, et al. Occupational asthma due to methyl methacrylate and cyanoacrylates. Thorax 1985; 40:836–839.

180. Wittczak T, Walusiak J, Ruta U, Palczynski C. Occupational asthma and allergic rhinitis due to xerographic toner. Allergy 2003; 58:957.

181. Quirce S, Baeza ML, Tornero P, Blasco A, Barranco R, Sastre J. Occupational asthma caused by exposure to cyanoacrylate. Allergy 2001; 56:446–449.

182. Weytjens K, Cartier A, Lemière C, Malo JL. Occupational asthma to diacrylate. Allergy 1999; 54:289.

183. Spencer AB, Estill CF, McCammon JB, Mickelsen RL, Johnston OE. Control of ethyl methacrylate exposures during the application of artificial fingernails. Am Ind Hyg J 1997; 58:214–218.

184. Hytonen M, Martimo KP, Estlander T, Tupasela O. Occupational IgE-mediated rhinitis caused by ninhydrin. Allergy 1996; 51:114–116.

185. Zeiss CR, Patterson R, Venables KM. Acid anhydrides. In: Bernstein IL, Chan-Yeung M, Malo JL, Bernstein DI, eds. Asthma in the Workplace. 2nd ed. New York: Marcel Dekker Inc., 1999:479–500.

186. Pfaffli P, Hameila M, Keskinen H, Wirmoila R. Exposure to cyclic anhydrides in welding: a new allergen-chlorendic anhydride. Appl Occup Environ Hyg 2002; 17:765–767.

187. Zeiss CR, Wolkonsky P, Chacon R, et al. Syndromes in workers exposed to trimellitic anhydride. Ann Intern Med 1983; 98:8–12.

188. Kern RA. Asthma and allergic rhinitis due to sensitization to phthalic anhydride: report of a case. J Allergy 1939; 10:164–165.

189. Howe W, Venables KM, Topping MD, et al. Tetrachlorophthalic anhydride asthma: evidence for specific IgE antibody. J Allergy Clin Immunol 1983; 71:5–11.

190. Moller DR, Gallagher JS, Bernstein DI, Wilcox TG, Burroughs HE, Bernstein IL. Detection of IgE-mediated respiratory sensitization in workers exposed to hexahy-drophthalic anhydride. J Allergy Clin Immunol 1985; 75:663–672.

191. Topping MD, Venables KM, Luczynska CM, Howe W, Taylor AJ. Specificity of the human IgE response to inhaled acid anhydrides. J Allergy Clin Immunol 1986; 77:834–842.

192. Nielsen J, Welinder H, Schütz A, Skerfving S. Specific serum antibodies against phthalic anhydride in occupationally exposed subjects. J Allergy Clin Immunol 1988; 82: 126–133.

193. Bernstein DI, Gallagher JS, D'Souza L, Bernstein IL. Heterogeneity of specific-IgE responses in workers sensitized to acid anhydride compounds. J Allergy Clin Immunol 1984; 74:794–801.

194. Zeiss CR, Mitchell JH, Van Peenen PF, et al. A clinical and immunologic study of employees in a facility manufacturing trimellitic anhydride. Allergy Proc 1992; 13:193–198.

195. Barker RD, van Tongeren MJ, Harris JM, Gardiner K, Venables KM, Taylor AJ. Risk factors for sensitisation and respiratory symptoms among workers exposed to acid anhydrides: a cohort study. Occup Environ Med 1998; 55:684–691.

196. Grammer LC, Ditto AM, Tripathi A, Harris KE. Prevalence and onset of rhinitis and conjunctivitis in subjects with occupational asthma caused by trimellitic anhydride. J Occup Environ Med 2002; 44:1179–1181.

197. Venables KM, Topping MD, Howe W, Luczynska CM, Hawkins R, Taylor AJ. Interaction of smoking and atopy in producing specific IgE antibody against a hapten protein conjugate. Br Med J 1985; 290:201–204.

198. Venables KM, Taylor AJ. Exposure-response relationships in asthma caused by tetrachlorophthalic anhydride. J Allergy Clin Immunol 1990; 85:55–58.

199. Young RP, Barker RD, Pile KD, Cookson WO, Taylor AJ. The association of HLA DR3 with specific IgE to inhaled anhydrides. Am J Respir Crit Care Med 1995; 151:219–221.

200. Jones MG, Nielsen J, Welch J, et al. Association of HLA-DQ5 and HLA-DR1 with sensitization to organic acid anhydrides. Clin Exp Allergy 2004; 34:812–816.

201. Larsen CP, Regal RR, Regal JF. Trimellitic anhydride-induced allergic response in the guinea pig lung involves antibody-dependent and -independent complement system activation. J Pharmacol Exp Ther 2001; 296:284–292.

202. Zhang XD, Murray DK, Lewis DM, Siegel PD. Dose-response and time course of specific IgE and IgG after single and repeated topical skin exposure to dry trimellitic anhydride powder in a Brown Norway rat model. Allergy 2002; 57:620–626.

203. Venables KM, Topping MD, Nunn AJ, Howe W, Newman Taylor AJ. Immunologic and functional consequences of chemical (tetrachlorophthalic anhydride)-induced asthma after four years of avoidance of exposure. J Allergy Clin Immunol 1987; 80:212–218.

204. Grammer LC, Harris KE, Yarnold PR. Effect of respiratory protective devices on development of antibody and occupational asthma to an acid anhydride. Chest 2002; 121:1317–1322.

205. Sterling GM, Batten JC. Effect of aerosol propellants and surfactants on airway resistance. Thorax 1969; 24:228–231.

206. Zuskin E, Bouhuys A. Acute airway responses to hair-spray preparations. N Engl J Med 1974; 290:660–663.

207. Schlueter DP, Soto RJ, Baretta ED, Herrmann AA, Ostrander LE, Stewart RD. Airway response to hair spray in normal subjects and subjects with hyperreactive airways. Chest 1979; 75:544–548.

208. Malo JL, Gagnon G, Cartier A. Occupational asthma due to heated freon. Thorax 1984; 39:628–629.

209. Cockcroft DW, Cartier A, Jones G, Tarlo SM, Dolovich J, Hargreave FE. Asthma caused by occupational exposure to a furan-based binder system. J Allergy Clin Immunol 1980; 66:458–463.

210. Moscato G, Biscaldi G, Cottica D, Pugliese F, Candura S, Candura F. Occupational asthma due to styrene: two case reports. J Occup Med 1987; 29:957–960.

211. Schwettmann RS, Casterline CL. Delayed asthmatic response following occupational exposure to enflurane. Anesthesiology 1976; 44:166–169.

212. Keskinen H, Nordman H, Terho EO. ECG ink as a cause of asthma. Allergy 1981; 36:275–276.

213. Rodenstein D, Stanescu DC. Bronchial asthma following exposure to ECG ink. Ann Allergy 1982; 48:351–352.

214. Seaton A, Cherrie B, Turnbull J. Rubber glove asthma. Br Med J 1988; 296:531–532.

215. Finnegan MJ, Pickering CA, Burge PS, Goffe TR, Austwick PK, Davies PS. Occupational asthma in a fibre glass works. J Soc Occup Med 1985; 35:121–127.

216. Kennes B, Garcia-Herreros P, Sierckx P. Asthma from plexiglas powders. Clin Allergy 1981; 11:49–54.

217. Burge PS, Hendy M, Hodgson ES. Occupational asthma, rhinitis, and dermatitis due to tetrazene in a detonator manufacturer. Thorax 1984; 39:470–471.

218. Hendrick DJ, Connolly MJ, Stenton SC, Bird AG, Winterton IS, Walters EH. Occupational asthma due to sodium iso-nonanoyl oxybenzene sulphonate, a newly developed detergent ingredient. Thorax 1988; 43:501–502.

219. Stenton SC, Dennis JH, Walters EH, Hendrick DJ. Asthmagenic properties of a newly developed detergent ingredient: sodium iso-nonanoyl oxybenzene sulphonate. Br J Ind Med 1990; 47:405–410.

220. Gannon PF, Burge PS, Benfield CF. Occupational asthma due to polyethylene shrink wrapping (paper wrapper's asthma). Thorax 1992; 47:759.

221. Malo JL, Cartier A, Pineault L, Dugas M, Desjardins A. Occupational asthma due to heated polypropylene. Eur Respir J 1994; 7:415–417.

222. Cartier A, Vandenplas O, Grammer LC, Shaughnessy MA, Malo JL. Respiratory and systemic reaction following exposure to heated electrostatic polyester paint. Eur Respir J 1994; 7:608–611.

223. Kennedy SM, Greaves IA, Kriebel D, Eisen EA, Smith TJ, Woskie SR. Acute pulmonary responses among automobile workers exposed to aerosols of machining fluids. Am J Ind Med 1989; 15:627–641.

224. Dumas JP, Smolik HJ, Camus P, Jeannin L, Marin A, Klepping J. Réactivité bronchique et exposition professionnelle aux fluides de coupe. Arch Mal Prof 1987; 48: 213–221.

225. Massin N, Bohadana AB, Wild P, Goutet P, Kirstetter H, Toamain JP. Airway responsiveness, respiratory symptoms, and exposures to soluble oil mist in mechanical workers. Occup environ Med 1996; 53:748–752.

226. Rosenman KD, Reilly MJ, Kalinowski D. Work-related asthma and respiratory symptoms among workers exposed to metal-working fluids. Am J Ind Med 1997; 32:325–331.

227. Bukowski JA. Review of respiratory morbidity from occupational exposure to oil mists. Appl Occup Environ Hyg 2003; 18:828–837.

228. Hendy MS, Beattie BE, Burge PS. Occupational asthma due to an emulsified oil mist. Br J Ind Med 1985; 42:51–54.

229. Robertson AS, Weir DC, Burge PS. Occupational asthma due to oil mists. Thorax 1988; 43:200–205.

230. Musk AW, Peach S, Ryan G. Occupational asthma in a mineral analysis laboratory. Br J Ind Med 1988; 45:381–386.
231. Baur X, Schneider EM, Wieners D, Czuppon AB. Occupational asthma to perfume. Allergy 1999; 54:1334–1335.
232. Smedley J, Inskip H, Wield G, Coggon D. Work related respiratory symptoms in radiographers. Occup Environ Med 1996; 53:450–454.
233. Smedley J, Cullinan P, Frew A, Taylor AN, Coggon D. Work related respiratory symptoms in radiographers. Occup Environ Med 1999; 56:646.
234. Agius RM, Nee J, McGovern B, Robertson A. Structure activity hypothesis in occupational asthma caused by low molecular weight substances. Ann Occup Hyg 1991; 35:129–137.
235. Karol MH, Graham C, Gealy R, Macina OT, Sussman N, Rosenkranz HS. Structure-activity relationships and computer-assisted analysis of respiratory sensitization potential. Toxicol Lett 1996; 86:187–191.
236. Kimber I, Bernstein IL, Karol MH, Robinson MK, Sarlo K, Selgrade MK. Identification of respiratory allergens. Fundam Appl Toxicol 1996; 33:1–10.
237. Black DW, Rathe A. Total environmental allergy: 20th century disease or deception. Res Staff Physician 1990; 34:47–54.
238. Barinaga M. Better data needed on sensitivity syndrome. Science 1991; 251:1558.
239. Kutsogiannis DJ, Davidoff AL. A multiple center study of multiple chemical sensitivity syndrome. Arch Environ Health 2001; 56:196–207.
240. Ziem G, McTamney J. Profile of patients with chemical injury and sensitivity. Environ Health Perspect 1997; 105(suppl 2):417–436.
241. Millqvist E, Ternesten-Hasseus E, Stahl A, Bende M. Changes in levels of nerve growth factor in nasal secretions after capsaicin inhalation in patients with airway symptoms from scents and chemicals. Environ Health Perspect 2005; 113:849–852.

25

Reactive Airways Dysfunction Syndrome and Irritant-Induced Asthma

Denyse Gautrin
Université de Montréal, Montreal, Quebec, Canada

I. Leonard Bernstein
Division of Allergy–Immunology, Department of Internal Medicine, College of Medicine, University of Cincinnati, Cincinnati, Ohio, U.S.A.

Stuart M. Brooks
College of Public Health, University of South Florida, Tampa, Florida, U.S.A.

Paul K. Henneberger
Division of Respiratory Disease Studies, NIOSH/CDC, Morgantown, West Virginia, U.S.A.

INTRODUCTION

Although irritant-induced nonimmunological asthma without a latency period had previously been reported, the acronym for this form of occupational asthma (OA) was first derived from the descriptive term "reactive airways dysfunction syndrome" (RADS) in 1985 (1). It was originally defined as asthma occurring after a single exposure to high levels of an irritating vapor, fume, or smoke. Although the term "irritant-induced asthma (IIA) disease" is more consistent with the definitions of OA described in chapter 1, the RADS terminology was retained by the editors because of the high recognition index that it has engendered among the occupational health community as well as the specific diagnostic criteria, which distinguish it from other forms of IIA. Initial symptoms developed within minutes or hours after exposure. In the majority of cases there was continuation of obstructive symptoms and persistent airway hyperresponsiveness for more than one year. The condition is defined here as nonimmunological OA, and, according to this definition, it should be distinguished from other nonimmunological OA entities occurring after longer latent periods of exposure (e.g., meat wrappers' asthma and potroom asthma) and/or fixed obstructive disorders, such as bronchiolitis or bronchiolitis obliterans, resulting from chemical inhalation injury (Chapter 28). As more investigators recognize RADS as a unique form of OA, in future it will be most likely referred as a special phenotype of IIA (2).

CLINICAL DESCRIPTION OF THE SYNDROME

The initial report included 10 individuals who developed a persistent asthma-like illness after a single exposure to high levels of an irritant vapor, fume, gas, or smoke. Respiratory symptomatology and continued presence of nonspecific bronchial hyper-responsiveness (NSBH) were documented in all the subjects for a mean follow-up of three years. In one person, the persistence of disease was documented to have lasted for at least 12 years. Generally, the incremental exposure was short lived, often lasting just a few minutes, but sometimes lasted for 12 hours. Usually, there was a time interval between the exposure and the development of symptoms; this time period was immediate in three subjects, but several hours in the other seven subjects (mean of nine hours). In almost all instances, the exposure was because of an accident or a situation in the work area where there was very poor ventilation and limited air exchange. All the causal etiological agents, although varied in each case, were irritants and included uranium hexafluoride gas, floor sealant, spray paint containing significant concentrations of ammonia, heated acid, 35% hydrazine, fumigating fog, metal coating remover, and smoke inhalation. When tested, all subjects displayed a positive result for methacholine challenge test. There was no identifiable evidence of preexisting respiratory complaints in any of the patients studied. Two subjects were found to be atopic, but in all others no evidence of allergy was identified. Pulmonary function was normal in 3 of 10 subjects and showed airflow limitation in seven.

Typical Courses of Two Sentinel Cases

A previously healthy 41-year-old painter and his partner, a 45-year-old man, worked together spray painting a poorly ventilated apartment during the late fall when the weather was cold. The room was sealed and there was poor fresh air recirculation; the windows were covered with a heavy plastic material, duct tape was placed around the edges to ensure a seal, and the main entrance to the apartment was covered to conserve heat. The painters did not wear approved respiratory protective devices, but only paper masks covering their nose and mouth while they worked. The paint used was a one-stage vinyl latex primer, reported to be rapid-drying, and said to contain 25% ammonia, 16.6% aluminum chlorohydrate, and other additives, many of which were documented irritants.

Both men spray-painted for a total of 12 hours, that is, four hours the first day and eight hours the second. Both of them noted the appearance of an illness beginning at the end of the second day of work, with symptoms of nausea, cough, shortness of breath, paint taste in the mouth, chest tightness, wheezing, and generalized weakness of the limbs. Each worker was subsequently hospitalized for about two weeks with the provisional diagnosis of "chemical bronchitis." A chest roentgenogram of one patient showed "increased bronchovascular markings" consistent with "chemical pneumonitis." After being discharged from the hospital, both painters consulted private physicians and were eventually treated with prednisone, oral theophylline, and aerosol beta2-adrenergic bronchodilators.

On evaluation four months later, there remained persistent symptomatology of wheezing, cough, and exertional dyspnea; in one painter there was also chest discomfort. Separately, each reported newly developed bronchial irritability symptoms, that is, respiratory manifestations after exposure to many and varied nonspecific stimuli such as cold air, dusts, aerosol sprays, smoke, and fumes. The bronchial irritability symptoms were not present before the heavy exposure. Each painter denied a past history of asthma, allergies, rhinitis, frequent colds, dyspnea, or other respiratory symptoms. One of the painters recalled a transient episode of bronchitis 11 years previously without recurrence. Each worker denied a family history of allergy, asthma, or previous respiratory problems. Both had worked only as painters in the past, one for 20 years and the other for 25 years. Both stated that they had never previously spray-painted under the environmental conditions similar to that of the inciting incident. One subject was a cigarette smoker with a 21-year history; the other person was essentially a nonsmoker, having smoked only 20 to 40 cigarettes in his life. A physical examination in one worker disclosed expiratory rhonchi. Laboratory tests of the subjects included normal complete blood counts with 5% eosinophilia in one, normal chest roentgenograms, and negative in vitro battery for common airborne allergens. Pulmonary function testing showed mild airways obstruction; forced expiratory volume in one second (FEV_1)/forced vital capacity (FVC) was 67.7% in one person and 70.3% in the other; forced expiratory flow at the mid-portion of FVC $(FEF)_{25-75}$ was 39.8% and 31.7% of that predicted, respectively.

Over the next year, the two men were followed up with serial clinical evaluations, lung function testing, and methacholine bronchial challenges. The persistence of asthmatic symptoms and airway hyper-responsiveness was noted. Results of methacholine challenges shown in Table 1 demonstrate that NSBH persisted for at least one year in both workers. Because one of the painters reported spray-painting with a polyurethane-based paint several years before, the possibility of isocyanate-induced airway disease was considered. Response to subsequent toluene diisocyanate (TDI) bronchial challenge testing in this person was negative. When last evaluated about 16 to 17 months after the incident, both continued to experience symptoms and had not returned to the painting occupation.

OTHER CASE AND SERIES REPORTS OF RADS

Prior to the 1985 description of RADS, there were a number of reports of workers developing asthma after exposure to high levels of irritants. Although these workers demonstrated evidence of airflow obstruction and symptoms of airway hyper-responsiveness for varying periods after the challenge, they differed from subjects with RADS because the airway hyperresponsiveness was not documented by methacholine or histamine challenge tests. Charan et al. (3) described five victims of accidental inhalation of high levels of SO_2 with three survivors developing severe and others showing mild airway obstruction. Flury et al. (4) described a 50-year-old man who inhaled substantial quantities of concentrated ammonia vapors. Over the next four years serial pulmonary function testing documented the development of

Table 1 Methacholine Reactivity[a]

Date	Subject 1	Subject 2
March 4, 1982	15 inhalation units	29 inhalation units
March 25, 1982	30 inhalation units	28 inhalation units
March 1, 1983	232 µg	52 µg
April 15, 1983	232 µg	–

[a]Positive tests are defined by methacholine doses of <200 inhalation units of 750 µg methacholine.

an obstructive lung disorder. Although methacholine challenges were not performed, the authors indicated that hyperresponsive airways were present and likely the direct result of the inhalation injury. Donham et al. (5) described an acute toxic exposure to high levels of hydrogen sulfide after agitation of liquid manure. One survivor had respiratory symptoms persisting more than two months after the incident. Harkonen et al. (6) followed seven mineworkers who were involved in a pyrite dust explosion and sustained SO_2-induced lung injury. Four years after the accident, an asthma-like condition characterized by reversible airway obstruction was observed in three persons; four workers showed positive histamine challenges, whereas two subjects responded neither to histamine nor to bronchodilators. The authors concluded that NSBH was a frequent sequel of high-level SO_2 exposure and could persist for years.

Subsequent to the original RADS report, other occurrences of RADS were reported. Several of these investigators modified the original criteria of RADS, thereby creating another phenotype of IIA, low-intensity chronic exposure dysfunction syndrome (LICEDS). Tarlo and Broder (2) performed a retrospective review of the files of 154 consecutive workers assessed for OA. Of 59 subjects considered having OA, a subset of 10 persons (and possibly an additional 15) with asthma symptoms for an average of five years were characterized by disease initiated by an exposure to high concentrations of an irritant. The RADS clinical criteria were modified in this study, and exposure was not limited to just a single accident or incident at work. It was concluded that "irritant-induced" OA is not uncommon in a population referred for the assessment of possible OA. The prevalence was estimated to be 6% for definite IIA and 10% for those with a possible diagnosis. Boulet (7) implied that there was prolonged induction of NSBH after the inhalation of high concentrations of irritants in four "normal" subjects and an aggravation of airway hyperresponsiveness in another person with "mild" preexisting asthma. Two of the persons were believed to have developed hyperresponsiveness following an intense short-term exposure alone. Gilbert and Auchincloss (8) reported a case of RADS occurring after a single massive silo dust exposure. In addition to objective evidence of NSBH, flow volume loops revealed a mixed obstructive/restrictive pattern in this worker, presumably on the basis of constriction of bronchioles or alveolar ducts. Other case examples reported as RADS included the following: (i) three Philadelphia police officers exposed to "toxic fumes" from a roadside truck accident (9); (ii) a female computer operator exposed to a floor sealant (10); (iii) workers exposed to TDI (11); (iv) possible exposures to acetic acid (12). Moisan (13) described RADS after smoke inhalation in three subjects. Bernstein et al. (14) evaluated four previously healthy, nonatopic men after acute exposure to toxic levels of anhydrous ammonia fumes. All of these workers exhibited obstructive symptoms, decreases in airway caliber, and persistent NSBH. Many other cases and case series have been reported. By the mid 1990s both the number of case reports and irritant agents have expanded.

Accidental inhalations reported by surveillance of work-related and occupational respiratory disease (SWORD) in the United Kingdom were most commonly caused by chlorine, smoke, and oxides of nitrogen (15). However, an extensive list of agents has been associated with RADS and/or IIA, as shown in Table 2.

RADS cases were identified by the four American states (i.e., California, Massachusetts, Michigan, and New Jersey) that conducted surveillance for work-related asthma (WRA) during the period 1993 to 2003 as part of the Sentinel Event Notification Systems for Occupational Risks (SENSOR). In this sampling period, a total of 445 RADS cases were documented by SENSOR (Chapter 14, Table 1).

Table 2   Agents Associated with RADS and/or Irritant-Induced Asthma

Agent	Type of study	Evidence	References
Acetic acid	Case report	H, S, P	(12)
	Epidemiological	H, S, BHR	(16)
Acids (various)	Case report	H, S, BHR	(2)
	Case report	H, S, BHR, P	(17)
Acid (heated) (+ welding fumes)	Case report	H, S, BHR, P	(1)
Ammonia	Case report	H, S	(4)
		H, S, BHR, P	(14)
		H, S, P	(18)
Bleaching agent	Case report	H, S, BHR	(7)
Calcium oxide	Case report	H, S, BHR	(2)
Chlorine	Case report	H, S, BHR	(2)
	Case report	H, S, BHR, P	(19)
	Epidemiological	H, S, BHR	(20)
Chloropicrin	Experimental	P	(21)
Cleaning agents	Case report	H, S	(22)
Diesel exhaust	Case reports	H, S, BHR	(23)
Diethylaminoethanol	Epidemiological	H, S	(24)
Epichlorohydrin	Experimental	P	(21)
Ethylene oxide	Case report	H, S, BHR, P	(25)
Floor sealant (aromatic hydrocarbons)	Case report	H, S, BHR	(1)
Formalin	Case report	H, S	(26)
Fumigating agent	Case report	H, S, BHR	(1)
Hydrazine	Case report	H, S, BHR	(1)
Hydrochloric acid	Case reports	H, S, BHR	(2,7,9)
Isocyanates	Case report	H, S	(11)
	Case reports	H, S, BHR	(2,27)
	Case report	H, S, BHR, P	(28)
	Experimental	S	(29)
Metal coat remover	Case report	H, S, BHR	(1)
Metam sodium	Epidemiological	H, S, BHR	(30)
Spray paint	Case report	H, S, BHR, P	(1)
Paint (fumes)	Case report	H, S, BHR	(2)
Perchloroethylene	Case report	H, S, BHR	(7)
Phthalic anhydride	Case report	H, S, BHR	(31)
Sulfur dioxide	Case reports	H, S, BHR, P	(6)
	Case report	H, S, BHR	(2)
	Case reports	H, P	(32)
Sulfuric acid	Case report	H, S, BHR	(2,7)
Uranium hexafluoride	Case report	H, S, BHR	(1)
Urea fumes	Case report	H, S, BHR, P	(33)
Fire/smoke (pyrolysis products)	Case report	H, S, BHR	(1)
	Case reports	H, S	(13)
Gases (chlorine, phosgene, mustard, etc.)	Case reports	H, P	(34)
	Case reports	H, S, BHR	(2)

Abbreviations: H, clinical history; S, spirometry; BHR, bronchial hyperresponsiveness; P, pathology.
Source: From Ref. 35.

In Table 3, the most common causal agents of RADS according to the SENSOR data are compared to asthma inducers of new-onset asthma (36). As expected, the two lists differ. Cleaning materials and chemicals not otherwise specified (NOS) lead the RADS list, whereas diisocyanates and lubricants (NOS) are most common for other WRA cases. The authors reported that RADS cases represented 14% of all new-onset WRA cases identified by SENSOR. As shown in Table 4, comparable figures from other studies and surveillance systems ranged from 5% to 18% (36).

PRESENCE OR ABSENCE OF RADS AFTER HIGH-LEVEL IRRITANT EXPOSURES DURING DISASTERS

Exposure to Irritant Gases During War

Thousands of military and civilian personnel experienced high-level exposures to irritants when mustard gas was used as a chemical weapon during the 20th century. On exposure to mustard gas, vesicant, cell damage occurs by the addition of an alkyl group to DNA and the initiation of cytokine-mediated inflammation. Mustard gas was used during World War I and, later by Iraq, during the Iran–Iraq war from 1980 to 1988 (37). One study examined the health of 34,000 Iranians, 13 to 20 years after they had survived exposure to mustard gas in the 1980s. The researchers determined that 42.5% had persistent medical problems of the lungs, defined as FEV_1 or FVC less than 80% of predicted and abnormal lung sounds (37). In another study, researchers identified an elevated prevalence of several lung disorders among 197 Iranian military veterans who had experienced heavy mustard gas exposure 10 years earlier: (*i*) 8.6% diffuse bronchiectasis; (*ii*) 9.6% airway narrowing due to scarring caused by granulation tissue; (*iii*) 10.7% asthma; (*iv*) 12.2% pulmonary fibrosis; and (*v*) 58.9% chronic bronchitis (38). The only respiratory problem among a comparison

Table 3 The Seven Most Frequently Reported Agents for Both Work-Related RADS and Other WRA Cases

RADS		Other WRA	
Agents[a]	No. (%)[b]	Agents[a]	No. (%)[b]
Cleaning materials	18 (15)	Diisocyanates	102 (39)
Chemicals NOS	10 (8)	Lubricants NOS[c]	46 (15)
Chlorine	8 (7)	Formaldehyde	24 (8)
Solvents NOS	8 (7)	Natural rubber latex	22 (7)
Acids, bases, and oxidizers NOS	7 (6)	Glutaraldehyde	19 (6)
Smoke NOS	7 (6)	Epoxy resins	16 (5)
Diesel exhaust	7 (6)	Acrylates NOS	10 (3)

[a]The agent categories are based on a scheme developed by Hunting and McDonald. We created two inclusive agent categories: "cleaning materials" included bleach, cleaning materials NOS, and metal polish; "diisocyanates" included toluene diisocyanate, methylene diisocyanate, naphthalene diisocyanate, hexamethylene diisocyanate, and diisocyanate NOS.
[b]For RADS, the percentages are of the 123 cases. For other WRA, the percentages are of the 301 cases.
[c]This category includes metalworking fluids.
Abbreviations: NOS, not otherwise specified; WRA, work-related asthma.
Sources: From Refs. 36, 40.

Table 4 Percentage of WRA Attributed to RADS or Irritant Asthma, from Surveillance in Four Countries

References	Country (state, province, or region)	Years	Surveillance program (how cases identified)	% RADS or irritant asthma
Henneberger et al. (36)	United States (California, Massachusetts, Michigan, New Jersey)	1993–1995	SENSOR (MD, HDD, WCC)	14% RADS (123/891)
Reilly et al. (41)	United States (Michigan and New Jersey)	1988–1992	SENSOR (MD, HDD, WCC)	8% RADS[a] (42/498)
Rosenman et al. (42)	United States (Michigan)	1988–1994	SENSOR (MD, HDD, WCC)	10% RADS[a] (69/672)
Reinisch et al. (43)	United States (California)	1993–1996	Doctors first reports (MD)	9% RADS (27/290)[b]
Provencher et al. (44)	Canada (Quebec)	1992–1993	PROPULSE (MD)	5% RADS (14/301)[c]
Chatkin et al. (45)	Canada (Ontario)	1984–1988	Ontario Worker Compensation Board (WCC)	5% RADS (12/235)
Tarlo et al. (46) Ross et al. (47)	United Kingdom	1994	SWORD (MD)	9% RADS/irritant asthma (93/1034)[d]
Gannon et al. (48)	United Kingdom (West Midlands Region)	1989–1991	SHIELD (MD)	18% irritant asthma
Hnizdo et al. (49)	South Africa	1996–1998	SORDSA (MD, PR, OHN)	13% irritant asthma (30/225)[e]

[a]The cases from the Michigan SENSOR program are included in Refs. Reilly et al. (38) and Rosenman et al. (39). Some of the cases from Rosenman et al. (39) were included in Henneberger et al. (36).

[b]The 290 cases of WRA were the new-onset cases who were interviewed and could be classified. These cases included 24 RADS and 28 other WRA cases from California that were included in Henneberger et al. (36).

[c]There were 287 cases of OA and 14 cases of inhalation accident/RADS. The combination of these two groups equals 301 cases and 14/301 = 5% RADS.

[d]There were 280 cases of work-related inhalation accidents reported to SWORD in 1994. Based on an earlier study, the researchers estimated that about one-third of the inhalation cases were either asthma or RADS, chiefly because of chemical irritants (215). Thus, about 1/3 × 280 = 93 RADS/irritant asthma cases. With the RADS/irritant asthma cases and other OA cases combined (93 + 941 = 1034), the RADS/irritant asthma cases represented 9% of the total (93/1034 = 9%).

[e]There were 195 cases of OA with latency and 30 cases of asthma induced by irritants. Thus, the percentage of asthma induced by irritants was 30/225 = 13%.

Abbreviations: WRA, work-related asthma; RADS, reactive airways dysfunction syndrome; MD, reports from physicians; HDD, hospital discharge data; WCC, worker compensation claims; PR, reports from provincial representatives; OHN, reports from occupational health nurses; OA, occupational asthma.

Source: From Ref. 36.

group of 86 unexposed veterans was one case of chronic bronchitis. Whether asthma was a direct consequence of RADS in these veterans was not determined.

The Bhopal Industrial Disaster: Chemical Accident

In December 1994, thousands of people were exposed to toxic levels of the irritant methyl isocyanate as the result of an accidental leak at the Union Carbide plant in Bhopal, India. Medical surveys of survivors have identified a variety of adverse respiratory outcomes (50). For example, decrements in FEF_{25-75} were observed at 2 and 10 years after the accident, suggesting persistent small-airways obstruction (51,52). Survivors were not systematically screened with histamine or methacholine challenge to determine whether they were at an increased risk for RADS or other forms of IIA (50,53). However, investigators conducted spirometry before and after administering bronchodilators, which provided some information about whether those tested had fixed or variable obstruction. For example, 11.6% of those tested shortly after the accident responded to a bronchodilator with an improvement of 11% to 20% in FEV_1, and 8.9% had an improvement of over 20% (51). By the third month, these percentages had declined to 7.7% and 8.8%, respectively. The authors concluded that there was no increase in "asthmatic tendency" related to the Bhopal methyl isocyanate exposure (51). Other investigators conducted spirometry before and after inhalation of 200 µg of salbutamol as part of the 10-year follow-up of 74 Bhopal survivors (52). Only 2 of the 74 participants responded to salbutamol. The investigators concluded that IIA was not a common disorder among survivors of the Bhopal accident (52). It would appear that further systematic assessments of the health effects of this industrial accident in larger numbers of survivors are still needed (54,55).

WTC RADS and WTC Cough

On September 11, 2001, terrorist operatives of Osama Bin Laden's Al-Qaida commandeered four U.S. commercial airplanes and initiated an attack on the United States. Two of the planes were flown into the World Trade Center (WTC) towers causing their collapse. The destruction and collapse of the towers generated an intense, short-term exposure to inorganic dust, pyrolysis products, and other respirable materials (56). Nearly 3000 people died and an estimated 250,000 to 400,000 people in the vicinity of the WTC collapse were exposed to the dust, debris, smoke, and chemicals (57). Firefighters and other rescue workers were also exposed to the high levels of the dust and other particulate materials especially during the first few days after the WTC collapse.

WTC Exposures

The specific content of the dust was later measured by the United States Geological Survey (USGS), which collected dust samples from various WTC areas and from steel girder coatings of the WTC debris (58). Most samples were obtained after September 17, 2001, when substantial settling of the dust had already occurred. The composition of the dust was shown to be made up of silicon, aluminum, calcium, magnesium, sodium, and other elements like gypsum; concrete and aggregates (containing calcium and aluminum hydroxides and a variety of silicate minerals containing silicon, calcium, potassium, sodium, and magnesium); particles rich in iron, aluminum, titanium, and other metals that had been used in building construction; and particles of other components, such as computers. Organic carbon in the dusts was most likely from paper, wallboard binder, and other organic materials. The leachate solutions developed alkaline pH values of between 8.2 and 11.8, likely a result of the dissolution of concrete, glass fibers, gypsum, and other material in the dusts. Metals present in relatively high concentrations in the leachate were aluminum, chromium, antimony, molybdenum, barium, manganese, copper, and zinc. The Centers for Disease Control and Prevention (CDC) concluded from an evaluation of environmental data that the level of exposure to most substances did not exceed limits set by the National Institute for Occupational Safety and Health or the Occupational Safety and Health Administration, with concentrations of airborne and respirable particulates ranging up to 2.3 and 0.3 mg/m^3, respectively (59). Fractionations of airborne dust samples revealed that 0.4% to 2% of particulates were respirable (56).

Respiratory Disorders Following WTC Collapse

Following the WTC collapse, several respiratory illnesses were described among rescue workers, including what has been called "WTC cough," persistent hyperresponsiveness/RADS, and acute eosinophilic pneumonia (56,60,61). There were discussions and controversies concerning these conditions (62–65). A high prevalence of rhinitis/sinusitis and gastroesophageal reflux disorders was also noted (56,61).

   WTC Cough.   The WTC cough was defined as a new/worsening persistent cough that developed after the exposure to the WTC site and was accompanied by respiratory symptoms severe enough to require medical leave for at least four weeks (56). The exposure categories were derived retrospectively from the questionnaire data. Although no direct personal exposure profiles were established, there was some confirmation obtained from work records. High exposure was assigned to Fire Department of New York (FDNY) firefighters who reported to the WTC site on the morning of the collapse (<24 hours); a moderate exposure for FDNY workers arriving within two days; low exposure for FDNY workers arriving between three and seven days after the collapse. No exposure was assigned for FDNY officers if they were not at the site for at least two weeks during the rescue operation.

   The specific diagnosis of WTC cough was not formally confirmed until one month after the collapse. In the first medical examination, 332 of 10,116 firefighters (3.3%) met the diagnostic criteria for WTC cough. Within 24 hours after exposure, all 332 FDNY workers with WTC cough reported having a productive cough with black/gray-colored sputum that was "infiltrated with pebbles or particles" (56). WTC cough was more common (8%; 128/1636) in firefighters in the highest exposure category, but cough also developed in 3% (187/6958) with a moderate exposure and 1% (17/1320) with a low exposure. Methacholine challenge testing was performed in about 60% of the WTC cough workers (196/332), and NSBH (as defined by PC$_{20}$ of <16 mg/mL) was present in 24% (47/196); approximately 19% (20/103) of workers without severe cough also showed NSBH (56). Significant numbers of firefighters described dyspnea, chest discomfort, gastroesophageal reflux disease, and upper-airway symptoms. Although the WTC cough cohort had reductions in FVC and FEV$_1$, they were similar in magnitude with no change from the FEV$_1$/FVC% determined before exposure. However, 16% (53/332) showed FEV$_1$/FVC% of <75%. Among those tested, NSBH was noted in about 25% of the firefighters with high levels of exposure, whether or not they had WTC cough.

   Airway Hyperresponsiveness and WTC RADS.   A cohort of firefighters received a follow-up examination six months after the WTC collapse, and the findings were a basis for a second publication describing persistent hyperresponsiveness and RADS (61). RADS was defined as NSBH ($PC_{20} \leq 8$ mg/mL) in conjunction with respiratory symptoms six months post-WTC collapse (61). Subjects designated as having RADS did not include subjects previously identified as suffering from WTC cough reported in the first paper (Prezant, personal communication). However, the authors noted that 13% (19/151) of exposed subjects (mostly in the highly exposed group) subsequently developed "WTC cough" after study enrollment. Of this group, only half (9/18) of the WTC cough group qualified for the diagnosis of RADS (symptoms and NSBH). While it is somewhat difficult to precisely extract numbers from the descriptions provided in the article, at six months there were 16% (20/123) of all exposed study subjects (representing 2% of the population of firefighters) who fulfilled the long-term criteria for the diagnosis of RADS (NSBH).

Significance of WTC Cough, Airway Hyperresponsiveness, and RADS. There were obviously tremendous amounts of dust generated with the fall of the WTC, as most television observers of that fatal day in September can attest. Retrospectively, most firefighters were not exposed to what might be characterized as a massive level of dust exposure by the time they arrived on site or in the days following the collapse of the towers. While not a disqualifying factor, dust exposures have not previously been described for RADS (1). The CDC concluded that the level of WTC dust exposures (0.3–2.3 mg/m^3) when measured several days later did not exceed governmental threshold limit values (15 mg/m^3) or permissible exposure limits (59). Most of the dust consisted of large-sized particles, a small proportion of which (0.4–2%) was respirable (56). Perhaps most of the cough that developed could be attributed to upper airway effects. Sinobronchial disease and rhinitis were prevalent, and these conditions are common causes of cough. In addition, gastroesophageal reflux, another important cause of cough, was also common. One of the features of the dust, which was said to be a characteristic of its irritancy, was its alkalinity (pH > 10) (58,61). However, inhalation of alkaline aerosols does not necessarily cause adverse responses, as determined by Gross et al. (66) who studied 24 asthmatic volunteers exposed to the alkaline aerosols generated during automobile airbag deployment from sodium azide oxidation (67).

The criteria for RADS, as defined by Banauch, were different from the original definition and criteria of RADS described by Brooks et al. (1,68,64). The diagnosis of RADS in the firefighters was established at the six-month evaluation; the subjects were not evaluated within 24 hours of the exposure. In support of the latter point, there was no reporting of inordinate numbers of firefighters visiting emergency rooms within the first 24 hours of the collapse. Of course, firefighters are dedicated professionals who felt an obligation to save as many lives as possible so they chose to work at the site for long hours during the first several days and weeks following the collapse of the towers. Even so, with a severe airway injury of sufficient magnitude to cause classical RADS, emergency medical care is usually necessary (69).

The number of firefighters tested, as compared to the total population at risk, was small with only about 3% of the surveyed firefighters undergoing methacholine challenges. Airway hyperresponsiveness at the six month examination was documented in about 28% of the highly exposed and 8% of the moderately exposed workers, a statistically significant difference. Testing only a fraction of the population may be misleading. As many as one-third of asymptomatic persons in the general population demonstrate a positive methacholine challenge test (70), and approximately 10% of workers with no respiratory symptoms demonstrate methacholine $PC_{20} \leq 8$ mg/mL (71). The sensitivity of methacholine hyperresponsiveness for confirming cases of OA may often be less than 100%, particularly when subjects are no longer exposed to the offending agent (72).

RADS diagnosis requires ruling out preexisting asthma. To qualify for employment as a firefighter, there must be no past history of asthma; this disqualifying fact could possibly have precluded firefighters from mentioning a past history of asthma on their entrance examination (Dorsett Smith, personal communication). Persons with asymptomatic airway hyperresponsiveness are at an increased risk for future development of asthma. On longitudinal follow-up, as many as 45% of asymptomatic persons with bronchial hyperresponsiveness develop asthma during a two- to three-year period (73). The measurements for NSBH show good reproducibility over months to years and may precede the onset of symptomatic clinical asthma by several years (74,75). The finding of a positive methacholine challenge does not necessarily signify disease or asthma. In fact, there is often difficulty in reaching the definitive diagnosis of asthma because of its complex nature and characteristics (76). Although most subjects with active OA show airway hyperresponsiveness (62), this characteristic must be put in context of asthma, which is a dynamic disease, the clinical course of which depends on numerous factors including the lapsed time period since cessation of exposure and treatment (19,77).

Susceptibility (Personal Determinants) for IIA

Even though there were uncertainties about the interpretation of the observed data for firefighters exposed to WTC exposures, the dust does not appear to have the potential for causing lung injury (60). The firefighters with asthma and NSBH presented with new-onset symptoms and findings. How can this observation be interpreted? One explanation may come from the study of Brooks et al. (1) who described two types of IIA that presented as new-onset asthma. The first type was characterized by an intense exposure followed by sudden-onset IIA that corresponded to RADS. The clinical manifestations began within 24 hours. The affected individual was immediately ill and required prompt medical care. In this scenario, RADS was a response to a very excessive (usually brief) accidental exposure to an irritant gas, vapor, or fume. Because of the enormity of the exposure, there was extensive airway damage, which induced bronchial mucosal inflammation; these outcomes led to NSBH and clinical asthma manifestations (78,79). An atopic status was not operative in the pathogenesis of RADS. Likely, the original description of RADS exemplified the extreme end of the spectrum of an irritant effect on the airways (80,81).

In the second phenotype of IIA, a longer onset time (e.g., >24 hours) occurred because the exposure did not involve massive concentrations and the subjects were able to tolerate the exposure for a longer period of time. In this chapter, this form of IIA will be termed LICEDS. Why does an irritant exposure, not considered to be massive or of high level, produce sufficient airway injury to create persistent airway inflammation and airway hyperresponsiveness? Alternative mechanisms other than persistent airway damage caused by massive exposure must be considered. In fact, most acute inhalation injuries clear without residual lung damage.

There may be a susceptibility or risk factor(s) that puts a person at increased risk for developing an acute asthmatic process from this type of exposure. Host susceptibility, such as preexisting asthma or atopy, with its associated inherent biochemical and pathological consequences, is a consideration (82). While subjects with RADS do not show a greater prevalence of allergy/atopy predisposition, a higher percentage (88%) of individuals with the more slowly evolving onset type asthma were atopic (82). Additionally, 40% of persons who presented a new-onset IIA reported a preexisting asthmatic state that was in remission (82); usually, the remission was present for years before the exposure occurred. Persons with asthma in remission may be relatively asymptomatic and do not require medications (70,83–85). Therefore, allergy/atopy status and preexisting asthma may be important risk factors for developing asthma from moderate-level irritant exposures. Whether these or other unknown risk factors for IIA were present in WTC firefighters is unknown, but firefighters might not have mentioned previous atopy or asthma during their childhood or in the distant past, to qualify for employment.

PATHOLOGY

The first descriptions of the pathological features of RADS were mostly those of the chronic stage of the syndrome (1). Brooks and co-workers were the first to perform bronchial biopsies in patients with RADS. Later, bronchial biopsy data reported by Bernstein et al. (14) revealed typical histopathological features of asthma including marked denuded epithelium, submucosal chronic inflammation, and collagen proliferation below the basement membrane. The latter finding had developed in one anhydrous ammonia–exposed patient who had a bronchial biopsy within two weeks after the acute exposure (14).

Deschamps et al. (17,25) performed biopsies on two subjects, the first case three years after exposure to toxic concentrations of ethylene oxide, the second several months after inhalation of a mixture of sodium hypochlorite and hydrochloric acid. They reported severe injury of the epithelial layer as well as inflammatory infiltrates containing lymphocytes. Electron microscopic examination of these biopsy specimens revealed a thickening of connective tissue with collagen fibers. There was no thickening of the basement membrane itself. Histopathological changes in the case of IIA secondary to multiple exposures to an irritant agent have also been described at the chronic stage of the disease. In five workers studied by Gautrin et al. (78) two years after cessation of repeated exposure to high concentrations of chlorine, desquamation of bronchial epithelium and squamous cell metaplasia as well as inflammatory infiltrates consisting of lymphocytes and polynuclear cells with reticulo-collagenic fibrosis in the bronchial wall and thickening of the basement membrane were found. The biopsy specimens of four subjects with IIA and RADS have been examined with immunohistochemical techniques to characterize structural changes further (M. Boulet, personal communication, 1995). Collagen types I, III, IV, and VII, fibronectin, desmin, and laminin beneath the basement membrane, between smooth muscle fibers, and around nerves were observed. These findings indicate marked airway remodeling. Three workers with IIA were investigated by Chan-Yeung et al. (86) five months to one year after exposure to sulfur dioxide, hydrogen peroxide, and acetic acid, respectively; thickening of the basement membrane and cellular infiltration in the mucosa and submucosa were present. In contrast to earlier findings, the inflammatory infiltrates consisted of eosinophils, shown on immunohistology to be activated, and a few T lymphocytes (both CD8+ and CD4+). Two subjects suffering from RADS after a single exposure to toxic fumes were studied by Lemiere et al. (33,28). Bronchial biopsies were performed 46 days and 60 days after the event, respectively.

Immunohistochemical stains revealed that most inflammatory cells were T lymphocytes; no degranulated eosinophils were detected.

Table 5 summarizes the time course of changes in the pathophysiological features in two cases of RADS immediately following the accidental inhalation of chlorine and isocyanates, respectively (Figs. 1 and 2) (19,28). Briefly, there was rapid denudation of the mucosa with fibrinohemorrhagic exudates in the submucosa followed by signs of regeneration of the epithelial layer with proliferation of basal and parabasal cells and subepithelial edema. Five months after the inhalation accident and three months after treatment with inhaled corticosteroids, regeneration of the bronchial epithelium was complete in the first case but only partial in the second case. The time course of the pathological features in these two cases suggests that histological injuries of RADS could be almost completely reversible. Yet, in the specimens described by Brooks et al. (1) from biopsies performed several years after the offending exposure, injuries of the epithelial layer and inflammatory infiltrate were still present. An important difference in the series of cases investigated by Brooks et al. (1) and those by Lemiere et al. (19,28) is the medical management. In the latter series, both subjects were prescribed inhaled corticosteroids after the first bronchoscopy at day 3 and day 45 after exposure to chlorine and isocyanates, respectively. It can be hypothesized that early institution of inhaled corticosteroid treatment may have enhanced the regeneration of bronchial epithelium and reduced the inflammatory reaction (87).

The acute changes of RADS were confirmed in a model in which rats were exposed to high concentrations of chlorine (88). Histological evaluation revealed epithelial flattening, necrosis, and evidence of epithelial regeneration. Bronchoalveolar lavage (BAL) showed an increased number of neutrophils. Maximal abnormality in the appearance of the epithelium occurred between days 1 and 3 and corresponded to the timing of maximal functional changes in lung resistance and NSBH (Fig. 3) (88). Although the functional and pathological abnormalities were resolved in the majority of animals after a variable period, some animals were left with persisting epithelial abnormalities. So, in the animal model of RADS it was shown that institution of parenteral steroids for one week significantly reduced the increased percentage of neutrophils in BAL and had partial beneficial effects on airway wall damage as evidenced by the decrease in the extent of epithelial changes (epithelial flattening, necrosis, and stratification) in goblet cell number and in the amount of smooth muscle (89).

A mouse model (A/J mice) was used recently by Martin et al. (90) to investigate the link between functional changes and the inflammatory response following exposure to chlorine and to explore the possibility that oxidative mechanisms are involved in the injury caused by chlorine. Airway responsiveness to methacholine was measured and inflammation was assessed by lung lavage and histology 24 hours after a five-minute exposure to 100, 200, 400, or 800 ppm chlorine. The presence of tissue oxidation was evaluated by immunostaining with 3-nitrotyrosine (3-NT) in lung lavage cells and pulmonary tissues. Epithelial cells and alveolar macrophages from mice exposed to 800 ppm of chlorine stained for 3-NT residues. Specific inhibition of nitric oxide synthase with an experimental inhibitor (1400 W; 1 mg/kg) suppressed the chlorine-induced changes in responsiveness. These results support the hypothesis that some of the functional and pathological changes in the airways caused by chlorine exposure are associated with oxidative stress and show that inducible NOS is involved in the induction of changes in response to methacholine.

Table 5 Time Course of Histological Lesions After Accidental Inhalation

Interval after accidental inhalation

Case 1: Exposure to toxic concentrations of chlorine (19)

60 hours	15 days	60 days	150 days
Superficial fibrinohemorrhagic layer replacing bronchial epithelium that is sloughed; degeneration of connective tissue	Persistence of superficial hemorrhage; bronchial epithelial sloughing	Regeneration of the epithelial cells (basal, parabasal); collagen degeneration	Complete regeneration of the epithelium layer
	Increased deposition of collagen	Spots of lymphocytes	Numerous basal cells indicating regeneration
		Few polynuclear cells	
		Increase in collagen of basement membrane	

Case 2: Exposure to toxic concentrations of solvents and isocyanates (28)

45 days	98 days
Severe damage of the epithelial layer with few remaining basal cells	Incomplete regeneration of the epithelial layer with few ciliated cells
Subepithelial edema with inflammatory cells underneath the basement membrane	Inflammatory cells persisting in epithelium and connective tissue

Source: From Ref. 87.

(A)   **(B)**

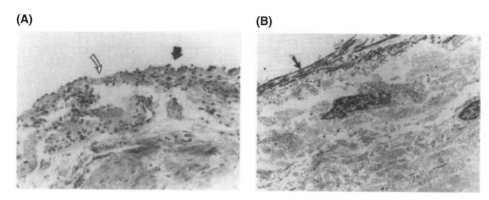

Figure 1 (**A**) Light micrograph of bronchial biopsy 46 days after single massive exposure to isocyanates. Severe loss of epithelial cells (*open arrow*) with few remaining basal cells (*shaded arrow*). Subepithelial edema with inflammatory cells (mainly lymphocytes) underneath basement membrane (hematoxylin-eosin (H-E) stain ×250). (**B**) Electron micrograph of first biopsy. Epithelial cell loss at luminal surface with fibrin deposition and intrafibrillar edema (*arrow*). Epon-embedded material stained with uranyl acetate and lead citrate (×2700). *Source*: From Ref. 28.

HYPOTHESIS OF PATHOGENETIC MECHANISMS

The pathogenesis of RADS is entirely speculative, primarily because the clinical descriptions of the syndrome thus far have been retrospective. Although airway damage in the animal models described earlier appears to confirm the acute changes occurring in RADS, it does not address the diversity of the causative agents and the uncertainties concerning individual susceptibility and risk factors. Moreover, since the initial clinical cases were observed only after high-level irritant exposures, it cannot yet be claimed that the asthma-like reactions caused by low-level respiratory irritants (i.e., LICEDS) are equivalent to RADS. From the currently available meager amount of bronchial biopsy histopathological data, it appears that the

(A)   **(B)**

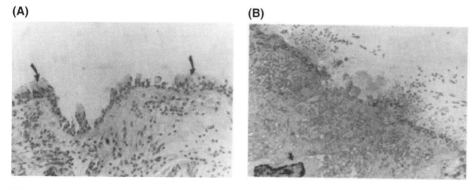

Figure 2 (**A**) Light micrograph of second bronchial biopsy 98 days after isocyanate exposure. Incomplete regeneration of epithelial layer with few ciliated cells (*arrows*). Inflammatory cells (mainly lymphocytes) persist in epithelia and connective tissue (H-E stain ×250). (**B**) Electron micrograph of second biopsy. Epithelial cells with incomplete cilia genesis and dilatation of smooth endoplasmic reticulum. Lymphocytes at bottom (*arrow*) (uranyl acetate and lead citrate staining, ×2700). *Source*: From Ref. 28.

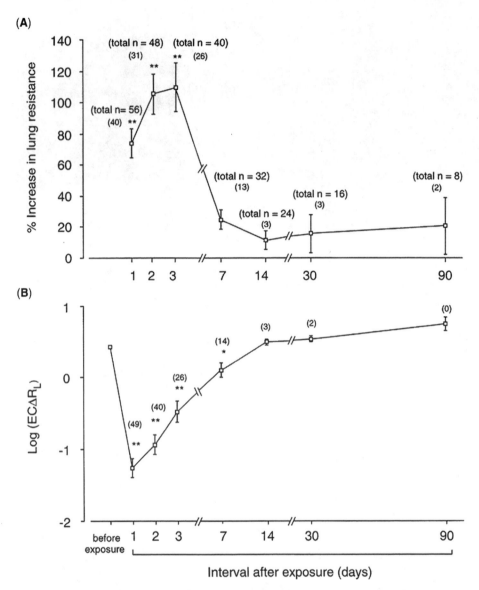

Figure 3 (A) Time course of lung resistance changes after acutre chlorine exposure; (B) time-course of the effective concentration of methacholine required to induce an increase in R_L of 0.20 cmH_2O mL/sec from postsaline inhalation value (EC ΔR_L). Data are expressed as mean - $\pm$ SEM. Statistically significant differences between measured value and baseline value are expressed as **$p < 0.01$, *$p < 0.05$. The total number of rats included and the number of rats with abnormal findings (*in brackets*) are given at each time interval. *Source*: From Ref. 88.

micropathological outcome of RADS is similar to asthma. It may therefore be appropriate to propose a pathogenetic hypothesis commensurate with current knowledge about naturally occurring asthma.

Assuming that RADS is a "big bang" event occurring after a high concentration, and often accidental, single exposure to an irritant gas, vapor, or fume, the high

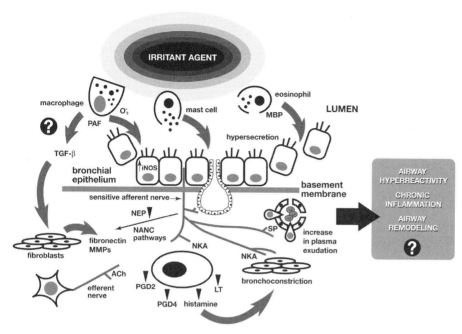

Figure 4 Pathophysiological hypothesis in RADS. *Abbreviations*: Ach, acetylcholine; iNOS, inducible nitric oxide synthase; LT, leukotriene; MBP, major basic protein; MMPs, matrix metalloproteinases; NANC, nonadrenergic, noncholinergic; NEP, neutral endopeptidase; NKA, neurokinin A; PAF, platelet-activating factor; PGD, prostaglandin; SP, substance P; TGF-β, transforming growth factor. *Source*: From Ref. 87.

levels of such irritant exposures will initiate massive airway injury (Fig. 4). The sequelae of the severe epithelial damage may lead to a cascade of changes that include airway inflammation and remodeling. The airway epithelial damage may also lead to direct activation of nonadrenergic, noncholinergic (NANC) pathways via axon reflexes and resultant neurogenic inflammation. Nonspecific macrophage activation and mast cell degranulation may also occur with the release of proinflammatory chemotactic and toxic mediators. Secondary recruitment of inflammatory cells will then enhance the subsequent profound inflammatory response. Subepithelial fibrosis, changes in mucous glands smooth muscle structure, and other changes of remodeling may then ensue.

The important inaugural event involves initiation of bronchial epithelial injury. What exactly transpires is not completely understood, but the injury in some way impairs intrinsic respiratory epithelial function (i.e., loss of ciliary activity, reduced neutral endopeptidase activity, decreased availability of epithelial-derived relaxing factor) and also initiates epithelial cell release of inflammatory mediators with subsequent activation of NANC nerves and transmitter release (neurokinins A and B, substance P, etc.). These combined effects not only induce changes in microvascular permeability but also cause increased mucus cell secretion. The chronic inflammatory process observed in bronchial wall biopsies is probably the end result of secretions from the major effector cells: alveolar macrophages, mast cells, and eosinophils. Many of the inflammatory mediators released by these cells are directly toxic. Others lead to lymphocyte recruitment and subsequent release of a complex cascade of cytokines, which enhance the inflammatory response. It is therefore not surprising that a chronic state of NSBH occurs as an aftermath of RADS.

During the recovery process there may be resolution of inflammation, epithelial cell repair, neural activity inhibition, and improvement of vascular integrity. However, the greater the degree and extent of the initial injury, the more unlikely that a complete recovery will occur. Under the latter conditions there may be deposition of type III collagen under the basement membrane, and such changes may be irreversible. In most cases of RADS due to high-level irritant exposure, the sequelae of the inflammatory response are obviously severe enough to cause chronic persistent asthma with concurrent NSBH.

The importance of airway remodeling in the pathogenesis of RADS (and other types of IIA) is supported by an investigation of workers exposed to repeated accidental inhalations of high and low concentrations of chlorine. Studies were performed to determine if airway obstruction and NSBH were associated with airway remodeling (91). In a prospective cohort of workers from a metal-processing plant, 32 workers were assessed at beginning of employment and five years after. Spirometry and bronchial challenges were performed on both occasions. At follow-up, sputum induction was also performed. Gelatinase (MMP-9) and collagenase (MPP-1) activities were assessed. Increase in bronchial hyperresponsiveness (BHR) (>2 dose decrement in PC_{20}) and/ or decrease in FEV_1 (>11%) were present in 13 subjects (40.7%). These workers had reported more accidental chlorine puffs per year in comparison with the other 19 workers (40.1 + 28.5 vs. 10.6 + 3.8 puffs). Gelatinase activities in activated sputum samples from workers with changes in lung function were significantly higher than in those with no such changes; collagenase activities in nonactivated samples were similar in both groups. These findings suggest that functional decreases associated with repeated exposures to chlorine may be related to airway remodeling. Further studies are needed to identify and quantify the gelatinase subclass involved (MMP-2 or -9).

Several risk or susceptibility factors have been suggested for RADS or LICEDS. Patients with preexistent NSBH (e.g., asthma patients in long-term remission, rhinitis patients with asymptomatic NSBH, and some otherwise normal persons in the general population) might be expected to have underlying pathologic features that would be augmented and worsened by a sudden proinflammatory airway exposure.

What are the possible mechanisms to explain "new-onset" IIA in an individual with an atopy/allergy status? Perhaps atopic persons and possibly individuals with a genetic tendency for allergies (but without overt atopic manifestations) are unique in their responses to irritants. It is known that atopic individuals are at an increased risk for developing asthma, are more likely to show serial accelerated declines in lung function tests, and display exaggerated responses to irritants (39,92–96). Furthermore, IgE, paramount to the atopic state, seems linked to NSBH (97,98).

The roles of bronchial epithelial cells and barrier protection should be considered. Bronchial epithelial cells of atopic subjects react differently to irritant exposures because IgE is bound to their surfaces (99). A further possibility is that a preceding irritant exposure enhances bronchial mucosal permeability which could facilitate sensitization (100,101). The enhanced bronchial mucosal permeability leads to greater penetration of common airborne environmental aeroallergens into the airway mucosa. Previous sensitization to these aeroallergens could then lead to increased allergy/IgE/mast cell interactions and more pronounced mediator release, eventuating into clinically new-onset asthma. An irritant exposure might lead directly to mediator release from various airway cells (e.g., mast cells and bronchial

Table 6 Cardinal Diagnostic Features of RADS

Identification of date, time(s), frequency, and extent of exposure; the latter may be a single
  high exposure, multiple high exposures, or multiple somewhat high exposures (yet still
  higher than either TLV or PEL concentrations)
Symptoms appear within 24 hrs
No latency period between exposure and symptoms
Symptoms less likely to improve away from work
Objective (pulmonary function) tests demonstrate obstruction
Presence and persistence of nonspecific bronchial hyperresponsiveness (as measured by
  methacholine or histamine challenge tests)

Abbreviations: RADS, reactive ariways dysfunction syndrome; TLV threshold limit value; PEL, permissible exposure level.

epithelial cells) and an accentuated airway inflammatory response and NSBH (7). Airway sensitivity to an allergen could be augmented by nonallergic irritant exposure. This has been demonstrated in humans after preexposure to low-levels of ozone and diesel fumes (102,103). In most likelihood, there is also a complex interplay between IIA injury, preexisting airway inflammation, IgE-mediated mechanisms, and genetic factors about which much is not known.

DIAGNOSIS OF RADS

The clinical criteria for confirming the diagnosis of RADS are listed in Table 6. They are determined after a thorough medical and occupational history, abnormal pulmonary function tests, and objective evidence of NSBH.

History and Symptoms

Although there are no rigorous validity data about the predictive value of history, there is no question that it is crucial for the diagnosis of RADS. In contrast to other forms of OA, where the onset of the illness cannot be precisely determined, the onset of RADS usually can be specifically dated. The patient may even be able to identify the exact time of the day that the illness began. The reason for this clear-cut time discrimination is that RADS is a dramatic event, generally following an accident or an unusual precipitous incident. The details remain vividly clear in the subject's mind. The exposure is an irritant and generally a vapor or gas, but on occasion a high-level smoke or dust exposure may be responsible. The original criteria have been modified to encompass both single high-toxic exposures and repetitive exposures to either high toxic or somewhat lower concentrations—yet still above permissible exposure levels of the same irritant. Multiple exposures to low levels of irritants are not included in the original case definition of RADS. Moreover, the terminology of "RADS-consistent symptoms" cannot be rigorously defined and should be discouraged.

A prerequisite of RADS is documenting the onset of a totally new respiratory process. Persons considered to have RADS must not suffer from reactivation of a previously quiescent asthma. RADS is not applicable for the patient with preexisting asthma that worsens with the irritant exposure. Besides preexisting asthma, other entities, such as bronchiolitis obliterans and vocal cord dysfunction, must be considered. In particular, the latter is often falsely considered as RADS. Meticulous review of relevant medical records and careful history taking are imperative to rule out previous respiratory disease.

It is important to document details of the onset with the exact date and time and to distinguish initial severity of disease using objective findings. The documentation may consist of emergency room notes that describe wheezing, reduced arterial oxygen saturation, a reduced FEV_1, a decreased peak flow rate, or a positive methacholine challenge test. The reason for documenting early manifestations (within 24 hours of the exposure) is that individuals with RADS may pursue litigation options. Such patients are examined by several physicians over succeeding months or years. Consequently, reliance solely upon the retrospective description by the patient makes the diagnosis debatable. Acute reported symptomatology could simply be an acute irritant response, and not actual asthma. Therefore, it is essential to document the evolution of serious airway injury in close proximity (e.g., within 24 hours) to the exposure.

The most important historical feature that distinguishes RADS from immunological OA is the presence of a latency period between the initial exposure and disease onset. Therefore, complete knowledge about the suspected etiological agent, the time of exposure, and the subsequent onset of symptoms is essential for an acceptable diagnosis of RADS. Confusion may occur after a single massive exposure to an agent known to cause immunological OA in certain cases (104). For example, although workers with exposures to one or more large spills of TDI are more likely to report asthma symptoms or show changes in lung function tests, an immune mechanism may or may not be demonstrated in such cases (105,106).

Similar to other types of OA, the symptoms of cough, dyspnea, and wheezing may occur. Characteristically, cough is a predominant symptom and may lead to an incorrect diagnosis of "acute bronchitis." Some RADS patients develop an intractable cough, which even interferes with the medical interview and precludes proper spirometric measurements.

The response of symptoms to removal from work may not have the same significance for RADS patients as it does for other types of OA. Workers with RADS are less likely to improve away from work, at least for several months after the first appearance of symptoms. Symptoms usually do not improve over a two-day weekend or an occasional day off, but might gradually taper off within a period of months. Some workers with RADS may note improvement away from work because their newly induced hyperresponsiveness makes them more susceptible to other low-level irritants and physical stimuli in the workplace.

Objective Tests

Changes in airway caliber and airway reversibility are variable in RADS. Abnormalities usually can be demonstrated soon after the initial exposure event. Long-term persistence of airflow limitation depends upon the inciting agent and the initial duration of exposure, both of which determine the degree of epithelial damage and subsequent inflammatory response. Resolution of airways obstruction depends upon the quality and efficiency of the recovery process. Thus, if the recovery is complete, the spirometric tests should become normal. When a RADS patient is well enough to return to work, cross-shift changes in FEV_1 or other obstructive parameters should not be expected to vary, because the industrial event that originally caused RADS is no longer an inciting risk factor for the worker. Thus, in contrast to other forms of OA (both immunological and nonimmunological), pulmonary function tests in RADS workers usually do not vary significantly at or away from work. However, during the active phases of RADS, exaggerated diurnal variation of spirometric values will be present just as in other types of asthma. Therefore, serial peak expiratory flow rate tests are particularly useful in this group of patients for prognosis of the obstructive process (107–109).

Testing for the presence of NSBH in RADS workers is vital for following the course of the disease (110,111). As airway obstruction may resolve within a matter of months, a finding of increased NSBH may be the only objective finding in such patients. In the reported cases that have been followed up, significant NSBH, as measured by methacholine or histamine challenge tests, may be demonstrated for years after the initial inhalation episode (14). The waning or disappearance of NSBH is a good harbinger of recovery (112).

Potentially Novel Diagnostic Techniques for RADS

In recent years, several innovative approaches to the assessment of lower airway inflammation have emerged. These techniques have been evaluated in a number of studies of occupational immunologic asthma but as yet there have been no systemic or prospective investigations of them in IIA.

Total cell and differential counts in sputum samples induced by hypertonic saline have been utilized in several recent OA reports. In general, the presence of increased sputum eosinophils tends to occur more often in immunologic asthma induced by high-molecular-weight compounds, although elevated sputum eosinophils can also be found in asthma due to low-molecular-weight compounds (113). In contrast, Di et al. (114) observed high levels of neutrophil and lower eosinophil counts in the airways of subjects with asthma induced by low-molecular-weight compounds. In the same study, induced sputum results in these subjects were significantly different than in patients with OA due to the action of high-molecular-weight agents which caused increased eosinophils in induced sputum samples. High levels of eosinophils in induced sputum samples may also be found in patients with chronic cough without asthma. Under these conditions, this syndrome is further defined as eosinophilic bronchitis without evidence of variable airflow obstruction or NSBH (115). Since the first report of occupationally induced eosinophilic bronchitis by Maestrelli et al. (116), other case reports have appeared (117–119). OA primarily associated with sputum neutrophils has been reported in workers exposed to metal working fluids and cleaning workers of a swine containment room (120). However, in another report of swine containment workers with a history of asthma, only macrophages were elevated in induced sputum samples (121). It is not clear whether any of the current reports that equate induced sputum measurements as surrogates of airway inflammation can be applied directly to IIA; further research is needed in this area. Of related interest is that several studies have also assayed proinflammatory cytokines, such as IL-6 and IL-8, but no general conclusions can be drawn from such random and uncontrolled studies.

Measurement of exhaled gases, such as hydrogen peroxide and nitric oxide (NO), has been suggested as a surrogate marker for lower airway inflammation. Thus far, most investigators have focused attention primarily on nitric oxide. So far, the chief utility of this test in nonoccupational asthma appears to be its ability to detect changes in mild asthmatic patients and to confirm the ameliorative effects of corticosteroid treatment. In performing the tests, it is essential to exclude nasal NO, which has high concentrations relative to the lower respiratory tract. This can be accomplished by exhalation against resistance which closes the velum during expiration. Because expiratory NO levels are markedly flow dependent, a constant expiratory flow rate is required for reliable measurement. These preconditions may therefore limit the interpretation of the tests in certain subjects. A further possible limiting factor is a recent finding that exhaled NO is increased in patients with chronic obstructive pulmonary disease. This increase was most likely influenced by tobacco-induced lung damage in these patients (122).

The application of exhaled nitric NO as an indicator of airway inflammation secondary to occupational exposure has not been investigated widely, either in immunologic or nonimmunologic asthma. Obata et al. (123) reported that levels of exhaled NO increased 24 hours after challenge with plicatic acid in both responders and nonresponders, and was significant only in nonresponders. Further, no correlations were found between increase in NO and the magnitude of functional changes in the airways. Allmers et al. (124) found no clear relationship between bronchial response and increased NO levels in patients with immunologic asthma. It has been suggested that patients with preexisting atopy may exhibit elevated levels of NO when they have been recently exposed to a relevant allergen (125). Thus, among paper mill workers exposed to bleach, asthmatic workers with preceding atopic problems had higher levels of exhaled NO. In a subsequent report, it was demonstrated that workers exposed to an unusual ozone peak not only developed asthma symptoms but also had higher median concentrations of exhaled NO in comparison with those workers who did not experience such gassing effects (126). Exhaled NO has also been evaluated in patients before and 24 hours after specific bronchial challenge tests to occupational agents (127). In positive challenges which induced bronchoconstriction, a significant increase in exhaled NO was noted. It was particularly accentuated if responding patients had normal or only slightly increased basal NO levels (<14.5 ppb basal NO). On the other hand, patients with both high basal NO levels (>14.5 ppb) and significant bronchoconstriction after challenge did not show significant NO elevations.

Recently, the diagnostic potential of exhaled NO has been assessed in workers exposed to various irritants at work that ultimately cause asthma or asthma-like syndromes. Thus, workers exposed to high concentrations of sulfur dioxide during the process of apricot sulfurization developed asthma-like symptoms with decrements in FEV_1 and FEF_{25-75} (128). Concentrations of serum proinflammatory cytokines, direct nitrite, total nitrite, and nitrate were significantly higher in workers exposed to the sulfurization process than in a normal control cohort (129). These investigators postulated that $TNF\alpha$, IL-1β, IL-6, IL-8, and NO may play a role in the pathogenesis of bronchoconstriction and asthma-like syndromes occurring after the sulfur dioxide exposure. Unfortunately, exhaled NO was not directly evaluated in this study. Swine confinement workers, who reported wheezing, cough, and sinusitis symptoms, were more likely to have small increments in mean exhaled NO than normal controls (121). In a recent study of 218 aluminum smelter workers, 17% of the potroom workers developed asthma-like symptoms. Exhaled NO concentrations in nonsmoking potroom workers were 63% higher than in nonsmoking control subjects evaluated in the same plant. It was interesting that no differences in exhaled NO were found between smoking potroom workers and controls. This most likely was due to known decreases in exhaled NO in chronic cigarette smokers, one of the limitations of the method. Overall, these results are consistent with the notion that increased concentrations of NO in exhaled air in potroom workers may reflect a subclinical degree of airway inflammation caused by exposure to pollutants in the

Table 7 Similarities and Differences Between OA with a Latency Period and RADS

	OA with a latency period	RADS
Latency period	Present	Absent
Diagnosis	Various: PEF monitoring; SIC	History; functional
Pathology	Like asthma	Acute: more epithelial shedding hemorrhage; chronic: more connective tissue
Functional	Better reversibility to BDT	Less reversibility to BDT
Treatment	Steroids useful	Steroids useful

Abbreviations: OA, occupational asthma; BDT, bronchodilator; PEF, peak expiratory flow; SIC, specific inhalation challenge; RADS, reactive airways dysfunction syndrome.
Source: From Ref. 35.

smelting environment (130). Exhaled NO was also studied in synthetic leather workers exposed to organic solvents, such as toluene, xylene, and ketones. Under workplace exposure conditions, the solvent concentrations were high but within permissible exposure levels. Exhaled NO was evaluated at baseline and at the end of the work shift. Exhaled NO increased by 40% in the leather workers at the end of a working day as compared to controls. None of these workers had developed respiratory symptoms. The authors concluded that exhaled NO may be a sensitive tool to monitor possible subclinical effects of occupational proinflammatory substances (131).

Although measurement of exhaled NO may ultimately provide a novel way of estimating lower airway inflammation, it has not yet been investigated on a prospective basis in classical cases of IIA. Such investigations are required before this test can be recommended as part of the current algorithmic approach to IIA.

COMPARISON BETWEEN RADS AND OTHER FORMS OF OA

Common and distinguishing features of RADS and other types of OA are listed in Table 7. From a histopathological point of view, desquamation of the epithelium is found in both conditions. In the acute stage, desquamation is much more extensive in RADS; consequently, regeneration of basal cells is prominent in RADS. The inflammatory exudate, on the other hand, is less intense in RADS. Neutrophils are found in BAL at least in the acute stage of RADS. Lymphocytes are encountered in both types of OA, although they are more numerous in nonoccupational asthma. Eosinophils are commonly found in both natural and OA. However, their presence in RADS has only been reported in two series of cases (78,86). Thickening of the basement membrane is common in both conditions but is more pronounced in RADS. Subepithelial fibrosis is much more pronounced in RADS (78).

From a functional point of view, if airway obstruction is present, it is less responsive to bronchodilators in the case of RADS. Gautrin et al. (78) compared 15 subjects with RADS and 30 subjects with OA with a latency period, all with a FEV_1 of $<80\%$ of predicted normal and with similar intervals from the end of exposure. The mean improvement in FEV_1 after administering a bronchodilator was close to 20% in OA with a latency period, but only 10% in subjects with RADS. As in OA with a latency period, there may be improvement in NSBH for up to two to three years after cessation of exposure (132). Finally, clinical evidence (19) coupled with experimental findings (89) suggests that corticosteroids can improve airway caliber and NSBH in RADS similar to their effects in both OA with a latency period and natural asthma.

EPIDEMIOLOGIC STUDIES

Incidence

It is difficult to estimate the incidence of RADS or a syndrome similar to RADS because of variability in the target populations: i.e., nonoccupational exposure to an accidental spill (133,134) with populations subsequently reporting to a poison control medical center (135) or a worker population (16). In the former instance, a true incidence rate for RADS cannot be calculated because only those self-reporting to a poison or a medical center are evaluated (136). Similarly, in worker populations, NSBH has not been objectively assessed in the entire exposed population but only among subjects consenting to the test (16) or among selected groups of workers at risk of developing RADS (20). Nonetheless, Kern provided an estimate of the incidence of RADS following a single accidental exposure of 56 hospital employees to high concentrations of glacial acetic acid, of whom 51 were assessed within 2.5 hours after the accident (16). Eight workers (16%), with no history of asthma, reported symptoms consistent with RADS within 24 hours after the accident and symptomatic status was related to the degree of exposure. Among the 24 workers who accepted a bronchial challenge test, RADS was confirmed in four subjects and a dose–response relationship was seen corresponding to the degree of acetic acid exposure.

In the United Kingdom, the SWORD data offer a basis for estimating the incidence and outcome of inhalation accidents (137). Between 1990 and 1994, 1180 inhalation accidents were reported; this represented 10% of all work-related lung diseases reported, the fifth most common category. The highest rates were among chemical processors (163.5/million/year), followed by engineers and electricians (32.1/million/year). An investigation of over 700 inhalation accidents (1990–1993) indicated that symptoms lasted for one month or more in 26% of cases, including 9% with asthma or RADS (15). Quantitative SENSOR data for RADS between 1993 and 2003 were discussed above.

Persistence of RADS

Some epidemiological studies addressing the question of the persistence of RADS, or a syndrome with similar features, are summarized in Table 8; for this review, the authors gave preference to studies in which NSBH was assessed. More often than not, there was a lack of information on duration of exposure and concentrations of an irritant agent after an accident. Levels of exposure have been assessed only indirectly through a description of location and employee's movements during the episode (138) or through an analysis of the characteristics of the site (16). In some instances, exposure has been estimated through self-reporting or first-aid reports (139–141). In the absence of estimates of exposure, clinical changes (i.e., dyspnea) associated with accidental inhalations have been used as predictors of lung diseases (138,142).

From the workforce-based studies, there is some evidence that accidental inhalation to high concentrations of irritants leads to persistent symptoms and/or

Table 8 Workforce-Based Surveys of Reactive Airways Dysfunction Syndrome: Long-Term Effects of High-Level Irritant Exposure

No. studied/ population	Type of population	Longest follow-up period	Outcome				Type of irritant exposure; estimated level	Host factors: smoking, personal, asthma	References
			Symptoms	Functional tests	Bronchial responsiveness	Persistence of effects (%)			
59/150 exposed	Longshoremen	2 yrs	Dyspnea: 35% vs. 0%	VC 91% vs. 99.8%; W_{el} 2.7 vs. 1.8; D_{LCO} 94% vs. 109%	No data	Dyspnea: 27%; deficits related to level of exposure	Chlorine; severe vs. minimal	46% smoking, effect not controlled for	(138)
13/20	Construction workers at a pulp mill	12 yrs	Not reported	RV < 80% in 67% (significant change over 12-yr period); FEV_1/FVC <80% in 62% (loss in FEV_1 not greater than the expected 25 mL/yr)	NSBH 38% (5/13) related to initial airway obstruction ($p < 0.05$) and airway trapping ($p < 0.05$)	No initial nonspecific bronchial challenge test	Chlorine	70% smoking	(143)
51/56	Hospital employees	8 mo	No symptoms (70%) vs. transient symptoms (14%) vs. persistent symptoms for at least 3 mos (16%)	Not reported	NSBH 37% (9/24)	RADS in 4/51 (7.8%) approximately 1 yr after accident; relative risk in those w/high exposure: 9.8	Glacial acetic acid; graded by industrial hygienist	No confounding due to preexposure risk factors or smoking	(16)

(Continued)

Table 8 Workforce-Based Surveys of Reactive Airways Dysfunction Syndrome: Long-Term Effects of High-Level Irritant Exposure (*Continued*)

No. studied/population	Type of population	Longest follow-up period	Outcome				Type of irritant exposure; estimated level	Host factors: smoking, personal, asthma	References
			Symptoms	Functional tests	Bronchial responsiveness	Persistence of effects (%)			
90/174	Pulp mill workers	7 yrs	First-aid reports related to work-related chest symptoms (odds ratio=4.4, significant)	FEV$_1$/FVC less in workers with first-aid reports ($p < 0.05$)	No data	Greater decline in FEV$_1$/FVC in gassed group ($p < 0.05$) (95% CI: 0.9–264.6)	Chlorine/ClO$_2$, SO$_2$, welding fumes; first-aid reports/ self-reports of gassing/ nonexposed	Control for age and smoking	(139)
64/71 at risk of developing RADS	Bleach plant workers (survey II)	18–24 mo	Respiratory symptoms: 91%	FEV$_1$ < 80% of predicted: 31% (16/51)	NSBH 57% (29/51)	RADS: 57%, related to severity of initial outcome	Chlorine, ClO$_2$; no. of accidents, severity of initial outcome	53% smokers, no effect of smoking	(20)
20/29 with RADS	Bleach plant workers (survey III)	2–3 yrs	Frequency of dyspnea: 80%	No change in FEV$_1$ after 1 yr	Significant decrease in 6/19 (32%) (PC$_{20}$ ≥ 3.2-fold)	NSBH 74% (14/19)	Chlorine, ClO$_2$; no such exposure during follow-up	No previous history of asthma	(132)

Abbreviations: VC, vital capacity; W_{el}, elastic work of breathing; D$_{LCO}$, diffusing capacity for carbon monoxide; RV, residual volume; FEV$_1$, forced expiratory volume in one second; FVC, forced vital capacity: NSBH, nonspecific bronchial hyperresponsiveness; RADS, reactive airways dysfunction syndrome; PC$_{20}$, provocative concentration causing ≥20% fall in FEV$_1$; CI, confidence intervals.
Source: From Refs. 87, 95.

long-term lung function abnormalities (132,138,139,143,144). By contrast, in the large population-based study, considered to be the most comprehensive follow-up study to date (205 subjects, 145 exposed, and assessed using spirometry initially and at follow-up), no changes were seen in pulmonary function testing over the six-year follow-up period (145). Airway responsiveness, however, was not assessed in this population (145). Comparisons between population- and occupation-based studies are limited owing to differences in exposure characteristics and prevalence of risk factors (143,144). In addition to a single and brief occupational exposure to high concentrations of an irritant, there may be chronic low-level exposure to the same or other agents in the workplace. Under these conditions, it has been hypothesized that the inflammatory reaction occurring in small airways after an accidental exposure to high concentrations of an irritant does not resolve completely because of continuous exposure to the offending stimulus (136).

OTHER FORMS OF IIA OR POSSIBLE VARIANTS OF RADS

Consequences of Low-Level Irritant Exposures

Before the entity of RADS was recognized, repetitive exposure to low concentrations of work-related irritant agents was not thought to give rise to OA. Early epidemiological studies of workers with low-level exposure and subsequent accidental high-level exposure to an irritant were conducted to compare the relative frequency of chest symptoms, increased airway obstruction, and nonspecific airway responsiveness between affected workers and those not exposed to the accidental spill. These studies did not demonstrate major differences between groups (146,147). Later, however, it was suggested that RADS may also include LICEDS, which is defined as a subtype of adult-onset asthma that develops after repeated low-dose exposure to one or more bronchial irritants (148). However, as discussed previously, individuals with this condition should more properly be considered to have a chronic exposure phenotype of IIA.

Variants of RADS

A clinical picture compatible with RADS has been described in several studies following accidental exposures in the community (133,134,149) and in the workplace (142). In a number of studies, the original diagnostic criteria of RADS have been modified to include asthma after repeated exposures to high and somewhat lower concentrations of the same irritant agent (2,20,82,139). When airway responsiveness could not be documented objectively but the other criteria were met, affected individuals were characterized as having symptoms similar to RADS (16) or at risk of developing the syndrome (20). However, the clinical criteria of RADS were not satisfied in such cases.

Activities in Workers Exposed to Chlorine Gas

Several more recent epidemiological surveys that were conducted in workers exposed to both low and high levels of chlorine in pulp mills and paper mills demonstrated adverse outcomes. The main findings are summarized in Table 9. A significantly greater prevalence of persistent wheezing was shown in workers who reported one or more episodes of accidental exposure to chlorine compared to other pulp mill workers with chronic low-level exposure to this irritant, regardless of smoking habits (140). Significantly lower

(*Text continues on page 612*)

Table 9 Workforce-Based Surveys of Reactive Airways Dysfunction Syndrome: Chronic Low-Level Irritant Exposures With or Without (Repeated) High-Level Irritant Exposure(s)

No. studied (exposed vs. nonexposed)	Type of population	Type of study	Outcome — Symptoms	Outcome — Functional tests	Outcome — Airway responsiveness	Prevalence of a syndrome consistent with RADS (%)	Type of irritant exposure and duration	Host factors: smoking, personal asthma	References
147 vs. 124	Pulp mill and papermill workers	Cross-sectional with control group	n.s. difference for chronic nonspecific respiratory disease	n.s. difference between groups for selected measures of lung function	Not assessed	No. of men with obstructive lung disease too small—no rates	Chlorine, ClO_2/SO_2; average Cl exposure duration 20 yrs	Current smokers (69%); control for smoking	(146)
58 with gassing vs. 81 with low exposure	Chlorine plant workers	Cross-sectional	Not related to exposure	Small decrease in MMF related to high exposure plus smoking[a]	Not assessed	Prevalence of ventilatory function impairment (3/139)	Chlorine—background <ppm vs. background + accidental gassing	Ever smokers (73%)	(147)
392 vs. 310	Pulp mill and railyard workers	Cross-sectional with control group	Prevalence of wheezing greater in pulp mill work[a]	FEV_1/FVC and MMF less in young, nonsmoking bleach plant workers[a]	Not assessed	Incidence of asthma in pulp mill workers (2.7/1000) greater than in railyard workers (0.8/1000) n.s.	Chlorine, SO_2, H_2S, CH_2SH; average exposure duration 8.9 yrs	Current smokers (47%), atopy (17%)	(141)

316 vs. 237	Pulp mill and railyard workers	Cross-sectional with control group	Increased prevalence of wheezing in pulp mill with gassing incidents[a]	MMF and FEV_1/FVC less in nonsmoking and ex-smoking pulp mill workers with gassing incidents	Not assessed	Not reported	Chlorine/ClO_2, H_2S, SO_2 and other; average exposure duration 13 yrs	Control for smoking and childhood asthma	(140)
230	Pulp mill and papermill workers	Cross-sectional	Not reported	Changes in FEV_1 and FEV_1/FVC related to gassing[a]	Not assessed	Not reported	Chlorine or SO_2; duration: up to 54 yrs; cumulative exposure index, never vs. accidentally gassed (21%)	Control for smoking and assessment of interaction with cumulative exposure and gassing	(150)
273	Bleach plant workers (survey I)	Cross-sectional	Irritation of the throat (78%), eyes (77%), cough (67%) shortness of breath (54%), headache (63%)	Not performed	Not assessed	Symptoms predictive of irritant-induced chronic lung disease: dyspnea (54%)	Chlorine, ClO_2; most significant exposure episode	Current smokers (53%); asthma or chronic bronchitis (7%), dyspnea not related to smoking or personal asthma	(142)

(Continued)

Table 9 Workforce-Based Surveys of Reactive Airways Dysfunction Syndrome: Chronic Low-Level Irritant Exposures With or Without (Repeated) High-Level Irritant Exposure(s) (*Continued*)

| No. studied (exposed vs. nonexposed) | Type of population | Type of study | Outcome | | | Prevalence of a syndrome consistent with RADS (%) | Type of irritant exposure and duration | Host factors: smoking, personal asthma | References |
			Symptoms	Functional tests	Airway responsiveness				
239/255 grouped according to exposure	Metal processing-plant workers	Cross-sectional	Low prevalence, not related to exposure	FVC less in subjects with mild vs. no symptomatic gassing; FEV_1, FVC, FEV_1/FVC less in workers with frequent gassing with mild symptoms[a]	In 239 workers; proportion with $PC_{20} \leq 32$ mg/mL and dose–response slope related to exposure[a]	No new cases of RADS	Chlorine, HCl; duration ≤ 3 yrs; accidental gassing plus self-evaluation of exposure	Ever smokers (55%), preexistent asthma (3%); control for both	(151)

| 211/239 from above described study (150) | Metal processing-plant workers | Longitudinal (2 yrs) | Persistent symptoms in 8.9%; related to chlorine puffs | In smokers: fall in FEV_1 associated with gassing during follow-up, fall in FEV_1/FVC predicted by number of puffs during follow-up | Increase in BHR (PC_{20} decrease by 1.5-fold) present in 19/211 workers, associated with gassing in the last 2 yrs | No new cases of RADS | Chlorine, HCl; duration ≤ 5 yrs; accidental gassing plus self-evaluation of exposure | Current smokers (22.7%); an interaction was found between gassing and pack-years smoking on lung function changes | (152) |

[a]Significant difference, $p < 0.05$.

Abbreviations: **RADS**, reactive airways dysfunction syndrome; n.s., nonsignificant; MMF, midmaximal flow; FEV_1, forced expiratory volume in one second; FVC, forced vital capacity; PC_{20}, provocative concentration of methacholine inducing a 20% fall in FEV_1; **BHR**, bronchial hyperresponsiveness.

Source: From Ref. 87.

values for maximal mid-expiratory flows and FEV_1/FVC were found among nonsmokers and ex-smokers who reported at least one accidental gassing episode. These findings were confirmed in a longitudinal study in which first-aid reports of symptomatic inhalation accidents were used as estimates of exposure (139). Henneberger et al. (150) found significant changes in FEV_1 and FEV_1/FVC to be associated with high-level irritant gas accidental exposures and cumulative pulp mill exposure and smoking. The changes in lung function appeared to have persisted beyond cessation of exposure to irritant gases. A further study among younger and current workers at the same plant showed that airway obstruction was related to gassing in those with high and moderate pack-year histories of cigarette smoking (153).

Gautrin et al. assessed 239 workers who had experienced repeated exposure to chlorine in a metal-processing plant (151). Data from first-aid records and a detailed occupational history focusing on the occurrence of accidental chlorine puffs made it possible to estimate the degree of exposure. A mild reduction in expiratory flow rates and an increase in airway responsiveness, as assessed through the methacholine dose–response slope, were documented. The changes were significantly greater in workers who experienced mild symptoms than in those who were asymptomatic after exposure to chlorine puffs. In a two-year follow-up study of these workers, a fall in lung function was associated with the number of gassing incidents and the number of chlorine puffs causing mild symptoms among cigarette smokers of 20 pack-years or more. Also, a detectable increase in NSBH (PC_{20} decrease >1.5-fold) was associated with gassing events (152). A surveillance program for workers experiencing gassing incidents was initiated after the first survey to describe the time course of lung function changes. After four years, 13 workers out of the 278 workers at risk had reported a gassing incident at the first-aid unit. Three of those workers whose spirometry and NSBH were within normal range prior to the inhalation accident showed transient but significant changes in lung function (154). Although repetitive exposures to varying concentrations of chlorine gas exhibited irritative effects, it is noteworthy that the appearance of RADS was not uniformly observed.

Asthma Among Cleaners

Professional cleaners have emerged as one of the high-risk groups for WRA in industrialized nations. Based on cases reported by physicians in California during 1993–1996, janitors and cleaners had the highest average annual rate of 625 cases of WRA per 10^6 workers (43). From an analysis of National Health and Nutrition Examination Survey (NHANES) III data collected in the United States, cleaners had the fourth highest odds ratio (OR = 5.44, 95% CI: 2.43–12.18) for work-related wheeze among 28 occupational categories (155). The European Community Respiratory Health Survey (ECRHS) is a population-based study that was conducted in 26 areas in 12 industrialized nations and had over 15,000 participants in the 20 to 44 years age group. Cleaners had the fourth highest odds ratio for asthma (OR = 1.97, 95% CI: 1.33–2.92) among 29 occupational groups, and cleaners and farmers had the most consistent results among the different countries (156). Additional evidence about the association of professional cleaning with asthma comes from Finland (157,158), France (159), Singapore (160), South Africa (161), Spain (162,163), and the United States (164).

Some investigators have implicated the role of sensitizing agents associated with cleaning activities in the development of asthma. For example, a case report from the early 1900s described a pharmacist who developed asthma and was determined to be sensitized to lauryl dimethyl benzyl ammonium chloride, which was a component of the floor cleaner used in his office (165). However, in one study, none of the 334 indoor cleaners tested had IgE specific to detergent enzymes (i.e., protease and amylase) (162). Many studies have implicated irritant agents to be the exposures responsible for WRA among cleaners. Among the 123 cases of work-related RADS that were identified by the SENSOR program during 1993–1995, the most common class of agents was cleaning materials, which were associated with 18 (15%) of the RADS cases (36). Studies conducted in Spain revealed that the risk of asthma was especially elevated among female domestic cleaners (162,163). When the researchers in Spain looked more closely at the work practices among domestic cleaners, which were associated with asthma, they found elevated odds ratios for daily use of bleach (OR = 7.9, 95% CI: 1.6–38) and for use of degreasing sprays at least three times a week (OR = 6.5, 95% CI: 1.1–39) (166). They concluded that asthma among female domestic cleaners was associated with the use of bleach and other irritant cleaning products.

Meat Wrappers' Asthma

This was the term coined for three meat wrappers who were treated in an emergency room for asthma (167). Initial epidemiological investigations recounted a 10% to 57% prevalence of respiratory symptomatology among meat wrappers. The etiological agent was believed to be present in the emissions from the polyvinylchloride meat-wrapping film when it was cut with a hot wire; a fine particulate fume containing di-2-ethylhexyladipate combined with an aerosol or vapor of hydrogen chloride was vaporized (168). Subsequently, a clinical investigation concluded that a component of the emitted fumes from thermally activated price labels was the principal cause of meat wrappers' asthma (169). The major ingredient of the incriminated price label adhesive is dicylohexylphthalate. When heated, it emits irritants, mainly cyclohexyl ether (dicyclohexyl ether) and cyclohexylbenzoate (a cyclohexyl salt of benzoic acid) (144). A potential sensitizer was postulated to be phthalic anhydride, a minor emission product from the heated label (170,171).

Later investigations failed to demonstrate objective evidence of any major airways disease or chronic respiratory hazard among meat wrappers (168,172–174). For instance, in one study, while lower respiratory symptoms were observed in one-third of the meat wrappers, no cross-shift change in FEV_1 was detected, even in the most symptomatic workers (172). Phthalic anhydride was not measurable in the vicinity of the heated price label emissions (168). Thus, it seems unlikely that this emission product is actually present in significant concentrations or that it is present in the air for any reasonable period or even remains stable during heating. Another independent investigation failed to find any evidence of phthalic anhydride–specific IgE and IgG antibodies in exposed workers (172). The paucity of clinical occurrences in the last 25 years relegates this entity to a minor form of IIA.

Formaldehyde

This chemical has myriad applications including use in the chemical and plastics industries, textile processing, disinfectants, the tanning industry, the vulcanization process in the rubber industry, and as a preservative of anatomical and pathological material. A major application was in the production of urea–formaldehyde foam for mobile home insulation and phenol formaldehyde resin for particleboard production. Formaldehyde monomer as well as the degassing of formaldehyde from urea–formaldehyde foam insulation has been reported to cause a variety of symptoms, including asthma (175–178). Asthma caused by low-level exposure is uncommon, but it has been reported in workers with high risk of exposures such as pathologists and nurses working in a dialysis unit (178). There have been very few reported cases of formaldehyde-induced asthma proven by bronchial challenge tests. For example, among 230 exposed workers, positive challenges were obtained in only 12 workers (114). Formaldehyde-specific IgE antibodies have been reported in a case of anaphylactic shock occurring after long-term hemodialysis and in two nurses working in dialysis units (178–180). However, exposure to low levels of indoor formaldehyde does not result in significant levels of specific IgE antibody (181). Low titers of specific IgG antibodies and autoantibodies have been reported in subjects exposed to formaldehyde in various settings (182). The clinical significance of these findings is unclear because no definite correlations can be made between symptoms or other objective findings (180,182). Thus, the current evidence indicates that occupational asthma due to formaldehyde is rare and that most respiratory complaints are the result of the irritant effects of formaldehyde (175,183). The possibility of mixed mechanisms (immunologic and nonimmunologic) excludes this entity from RADS but not entirely from LICEDS.

Potroom Asthma

Although an asthmatic "irritation" syndrome was first observed over 50 years ago in the Norwegian literature, there is still disagreement about how this entity should be classified (184). Pot fume emissions contain particulate and gaseous fluorides, hydrofluoric acid, sulfur dioxide, and cold tar volatiles. Although each of these agents has been suspected as playing a role, there is no convincing evidence that a single agent induces symptoms. The duration of potroom exposure prior to the first attack ranges from one week to 10 years. Thus, those workers who develop symptoms soon after exposure to high peak levels of dust (as high as 54 mg/m^3) could possibly represent a small subset of RADS (185). However, because of the variability of prevalence and prognosis of potroom asthma, the possibility that some workers develop RADS or LICEDS after exposure to aluminum smelter emissions can only be addressed by future prospective epidemiological studies specifically designed to detect and characterize this entity. Potroom asthma is discussed in more detail in Chapter 23.

Machining Fluids

Machine lubricants may have irritant properties because of contamination with trace quantities of metals, additives (i.e., odorants, corrosion inhibitors, antifoam agents, emulsifiers, antioxidants, detergents, viscosity index improvers, antiwear agents, extreme pressure agents), and bactericidal substances. Occupational asthma has been documented in workers exposed to several varieties of machine oil. In one plant where clean suds oil was used, there was a latent period before the workers experienced symptoms (186). Some workers also exhibited asthma after controlled exposures to 1% nebulized aerosols of the clean suds oil. One worker showed a reaction to a pine odorant component in this oil. Other contaminating constituents of the oil were suspected but not proven to induce asthma in some of the other cases (186).

If bacterial substances are not present in sufficient concentrations, oil-in-water machine fluid emulsions will act as good growth media for bacteria and fungi. A study by Kennedy et al. reported significant FEV_1 cross-shift changes in 23.6% of heavily exposed machinists and 9.5% in minimally exposed assembly workers in the same plant (187). The exact etiological agent in machining fluids responsible for the FEV_1 cross-shift changes was not determined, but it was speculated that chemical irritants or endotoxin from contaminating gram-negative bacteria could be potential causes.

Similar to the above discussion of potroom asthma, it is not clear whether this entity should be considered a subtype of RADS, LICEDS, or simply an asthma-like disorder.

Other Workplace Irritants

Many airborne irritants may have the same irritant potential as cigarette smoking. Hypothetically, multiple exposures to such irritants could presumably lead to bronchial mucosal injury and increased permeability to sensitizing agents. Industrial operations utilizing irritant agents are therefore doubly dangerous because of the risk of heavy exposures, and occurrence of accidental spills may lead to nonimmunological and/or immunological asthmatic conditions. Irritant gases (e.g., chlorine and ammonia) are required in the platinum-refining process. Their presence may initiate bronchial epithelial injury.

Researchers in the Netherlands determined that pig farmers who experienced irritant exposures as a result of using disinfectants containing quaternary ammonium compounds (QACs) were at greater risk for sensitization to common allergens (188). Also, they observed an elevated risk for symptoms consistent with asthma among farmers who were both sensitized to common allergens (i.e., atopic) and exposed to QACs, but not among farmers who were only atopic or only exposed to QACs.

Biagini et al. (101) reported that platinum salt immunological sensitization in monkeys required concomitant exposure to ozone before sensitization to platinum salts could be induced. Other animal studies have documented that an antecedent exposure to an airborne irritant enhances the capacity for sensitization to an allergen. Exposure to low levels of SO_2 promotes sensitization in guinea pigs and rats and leads to increased epithelial permeability (189,190). Similar enhancement of allergic sensitization has also been reported to occur after ozone exposure (191). It has also been determined that exposure to low ozone concentrations increases bronchial hyperresponsiveness to allergens in people with atopic asthma (102,103). Other investigations employing prolonged low-level ozone exposure have documented a striking individual variability among normal subjects with a considerable range and response, suggesting that there are subpopulations that are very sensitive to low levels of ozone (192,193). These combined experimental and clinical experiences suggest that the designation of LICEDS in the induction of asthma among susceptible patients in the general population (i.e., atopic patients or "normal subjects" with preexisting but asymptomatic NSBH) is justified.

In a study of young adults with mild atopic asthma, ozone exposure after a late response to an allergen potentiated the eosinophilic inflammatory response that was itself induced by the allergen (194). The severity of allergic responsivity may be a risk factor after mixed allergen/irritant exposures. In a recent study, subjects allergic to ragweed who had rhinitis and/or mild asthma were compared to nonallergic subjects who did not smoke and did not have asthma (195). Both allergic and nonallergic subjects were exposed to ragweed, and then bronchial epithelial cells were harvested and exposed to an acid. The adverse impact of the acid on ciliary activity was less for allergic subjects who had a mild response to the ragweed than for both nonallergic and allergic subjects who had a severe response to the ragweed (195). In a study with rats, coexposure to ozone and endotoxin resulted in greater epithelial and inflammatory responses than observed with exposure to either agent alone (196). The synergistic response was mediated, in part, by neutrophils. It should be emphasized that this possible effect of multiple exposures to low-level irritants has no relationship to the multiple chemical sensitivity syndrome, which involves a variety of nonspecific and nonpulmonary symptoms.

IIA has occurred in several workers who would not be expected to develop this problem. Metal fume fever was initially observed in a worker exposed to heavy metals. This worker experienced symptoms of cough, fever, chills, malaise, and myalgia that were self-limited and of short duration. He also developed wheezing and impaired pulmonary function tests. Contrary to the expected rapid recovery of abnormal respiratory function, he developed prolonged wheezing and pulmonary function abnormalities which was consistent with the RADS syndrome (197). Several workers exposed to the thermal degradation products of chlorofluorocarbons developed acute IIA which persisted. Several other workers exposed to the freon decomposition products developed bronchitis without increase in NSBH. These observations emphasized the variability of exposure outcomes in that workers exposed to the same thermal decomposition accident developed entirely different syndromes (198).

PROGNOSIS

Many individuals with RADS generally continue to report bronchial irritability symptoms and demonstrate evidence of NSBH for years after the inciting incident. These persistent symptoms are analogous to those in TDI, snow-crab processors, or western red cedar workers who have persistent asthma after their exposures have been terminated (199–202). In contrast to immunological asthma in which a more favorable prognostic outcome is associated with a shorter duration of symptoms prior to diagnosis, it is not yet possible to predict which RADS workers will have persistent symptoms and permanent NSBH on the basis of the agent itself or the duration of exposure (203).

The functional sequelae of subjects with RADS or with a suspected syndrome of RADS are due not only to NSBH, but also to persisting airway obstruction (87). Airway obstruction has been documented after inhalation of high levels of irritant agents (17,144). This alteration can persist for several years (1,7,20). Of the ten subjects investigated by Brooks et al. (1), four had a decreased FEV_1 and FVC 4 months to 11 years after the offending exposure. Among three subjects suffering from RADS studied by Boulet, one presented with airway obstruction 6 years after the inhalation accident (7). Bherer et al. demonstrated airway obstruction in 16 of 51 bleach plant workers in a survey that took place 18 to 24 months after these workers had been repeatedly exposed to high concentrations of chlorine and had experienced nasal, conjunctival, and respiratory symptoms within minutes of exposure (20). In these 16 workers, no improvement was found in spirometry 30 to 36 months after the first survey (132).

A restrictive syndrome in association with airway obstruction after exposure to an irritant agent has been described (3,8). Gilbert and Auchincloss hypothesized that the onset of a restrictive pattern could be related to the site of bronchial obstruction (8). Large airway obstruction is more likely to result in an obstructive pattern with a restrictive component if the site of constriction also involves smaller airways. Associated decreases of FEV_1 and FVC have frequently been observed after exposure to high levels of irritant agents (12,86). The concurrent decrease of FVC suggesting a restrictive pattern could be due to hyperinflation with an increased residual volume and therefore not truly restrictive. Thus, it has been demonstrated that 10% of patients with pure obstruction may have a restrictive type of spirogram (204).

Airway responsiveness can either persist for several years after the exposure (1,78) or be reversible within months to years after an inhalation accident (154,205). Bherer et al. studied the time course of clinical and functional behavior of a group of 71 bleach plant workers with suspected RADS, on the basis of the clinical history (20). At 18 to 24 months after these workers were identified and withdrawn from exposure, 22 of 51 (43%) subjects showed normal NSBH. Of the 29 workers with NSBH at the time of the first follow-up, 19 were investigated 30 to 36 months after removal from work; six men had a significantly improved PC_{20} including five for whom the PC_{20} value had returned to a normal range. The six men had normal FEV_1 values on both assessments (132). These subjects had not received either oral or inhaled corticosteroids.

It is still unknown whether treatment with oral or inhaled corticosteroids affects the prognosis of the condition. Randomized studies on RADS are needed to evaluate the efficacy of inhaled corticosteroids. There have been few reports of improvement in pulmonary function with corticosteroid therapy in patients suffering from RADS. Chester et al. reported on two subjects exposed to toxic concentrations of chlorine (206). One was treated with corticosteroids and oxygen therapy while the other received only oxygen therapy. The FEV_1 showed an initial marked improvement in both patients. The first subject continued to improve progressively until her values reached the normal range at the end of the first year while the second subject (although improved at the end of one year) reached a plateau and stabilized at less than 80% of predicted. There is recent evidence that parenteral and/or inhaled steroids may modify the outcome of the condition. In a subject with RADS, treatment with inhaled corticosteroids normalized the heightened NSBH with exacerbation when the treatment was stopped (19).

MANAGEMENT

Because RADS is usually precipitated by an unforeseen industrial accident, removal of the worker is automatic. Emergency treatment of the acute obstructive symptoms might require inhaled or parenteral beta$_2$ agonists, intravenous aminophylline, and/or steroids and oxygen. The specific requirements of each of these agents depends upon the severity of the worker's symptoms.

The use of systemic or inhaled corticosteroids is suggested for managing acute episodes. Similarly, once the acute episode has been managed appropriately, appropriate treatment of the ongoing asthmatic situation is mandatory, using a combination of anti-inflammatory preparations and bronchodilators. Long-term inhaled corticosteroids may be appropriate in reducing the severity of NSBH (19,207,208). It should be stressed that medical therapy is not a substitute for environmental control. This is particularly important for RADS patients who may wish to return to work, because they are particularly susceptible to other, nonspecific irritants in the workplace as a result of the original RADS-induced bronchial hyperresponsiveness (209). In some cases, good protection against the effects of nonspecific irritants may be provided by an airstream helmet (210).

The important long term goals in the management of the worker with IIA asthma are: (*i*) confirm the diagnosis of irritant-induced occupational asthma; (*ii*) gauge the severity of disease; (*iii*) identify aggravants and trigger factors; (*iv*) provide appropriate treatment to curb and reverse the airway inflammation; (*v*) put a high priority on returning the worker back to work, in any capacity, as soon as possible; (*vi*) decide on the best disposition for the worker which may include complete removal from exposure and change to a new job or site; (*vii*) monitor the disease course and ensure patient guidance; and (*viii*) educate patients to develop a partnership in asthma management.

Attempts to return subjects rapidly and efficiently to the workplace are preferable to discontinuation of work. For IIA, removal from exposure may not be required if the risk for recurrent exposure to high levels is not present. However, if the risk for recurrent high levels of exposure is high, removal is the treatment of choice.

RADS is associated with persistent NSBH. Consequently, triggers of NSBH may include workplace irritants, indoor and outdoor air pollutants, changes in environmental temperature or humidity, and physical changes such as exercise, cold air, and high levels of emotional stress. Thus, a strategy of evaluating several exposure environments (including the workplace) at once is preferable. The practitioner should stress efforts to reduce workplace irritant exposures, avoid passive smoking, and limit contacts with vehicle emission and outdoor air pollution. Strategies such as the continued use of respiratory protective devices are not medically ethical for an already sensitized individual.

Education of the workers, their supervisors and coworkers on methods of controlling exposures and on dealing with emergency situations, such as a spill, can be accomplished. Effective control of asthma can be better achieved by educating patients to develop a partnership in asthma management, undergoing regular assessments and monitoring of asthma severity (symptom reports and measurements of lung function), avoiding or controling asthma trigger factors, and establishing an individual medication plan for long-term management.

CONCLUSIONS

IIA represents a spectrum of clinical presentations. In the most extreme case, a single massive exposure leads to the sudden onset of asthma as epitomized by the RADS. The massive exposure causes severe airway injury resulting in persistent airway inflammation and NSBH. Many of these cases resolve or improve over time and especially after treatment with inhaled steroids.

In some cases, the onset of asthma is not so sudden and follows a low level, intense, chronic (LICEDS) exposure to irritants. It is likely that in these individuals, there is a preexisting susceptibility or abnormality responsible for initiation of asthmatic symptoms. Some of these persons suffer from preexisting asthma in remission and the irritant stimulus reactivates (e.g., exacerbates) clinical symptoms. When diagnosing and treating patients with this type of presentation, it is imperative that preexisting history of asthmatic symptoms is carefully identified. The presence of preexisting asthma categorically excludes a diagnosis of RADS. An underlying atopic susceptibility is important because these individuals appear to be primed by showing an exaggerated release of cytokines and other biomediators following certain inhalant stimuli. In this clinical scenario, the irritant exposure causes an exaggerated response and sets up a cascade of biochemical and pathological changes leading to an acute asthma attack.

Even in asthmatic patients controlled by medication, prolonged irritant exposures may aggravate current symptoms and such situations must be clearly distinguished from RADS and LICEDS. Some workplace irritant exposures will pose serious problems for asthmatics and potentially susceptible populations; reducing or eliminating such exposures seems prudent. It is clear that future investigations will better define predisposing risk factors and perhaps uncover new host susceptibilities. Prevention measures for IIA should include the improved recognition of dangerous work, ongoing worker education, and employer commitment to environmental control strategies.

DIRECTIONS OF FUTURE RESEARCH

Major research efforts should encompass many of the following:

- Clinical and or physiologic determinants of RADS compared to LICEDS.
- How can RADS/LICEDS phenotypes of IIA be differentiated from bronchitis, vocal cord dysfunction, postnasal drip, or gastroesophageal reflux?
- Does concurrent exposure to multiple irritants (e.g., ozone, diesel fumes, chlorine, etc.) increase the probability of RADS or LICEDS?
- Can increased cough occurring after irritant exposure be caused by stimulation of unmyelinated C-fibers? How can this be clinically assessed?
- Can the presenting symptom of cough with or without sputum (such as occurred after the WTC disaster) be considered equivalent to RADS or LICEDS?
- Can the diagnosis of RADS ever be made retrospectively when the patient is seen for the first time after a period of time away from the exposure?
- The role of preexistent NSBH in RADS/LICEDS (susceptibility or otherwise) even if the patient is completely unaware of this condition.
- Why does the atopic risk factor differentiate LICEDS from RADS?
- Does RADS/LICEDS increase the severity of allergic symptoms (long or short term or both) in atopic workers who develop these problems?
- Identification of biomarkers for RADS and LICEDS.
- Genetic susceptibility or protective factors for RADS compared to LICEDS.
- What are the basic pathological differences between RADS/LICEDS and diseases of the terminal bronchioles?
- Do diagnostic adjuncts such as exhaled NO and induced sputum for eosinophils/neutrophils aid in the diagnosis either immediately or after a delayed time interval from the original exposure?
- Prospective epidemiologic studies of newly hired workers in industries where both high- and low-intensity exposure to irritants can be expected (e.g., potroom workers, hog farmers).

REFERENCES

1. Brooks SM, Weiss MA, Bernstein IL. Reactive airways dysfunction syndrome (RADS). Persistent asthma syndrome after high level irritant exposures. Chest 1985; 88(3): 376–384.
2. Tarlo SM, Broder I. Irritant-induced occupational asthma. Chest 1989; 96(2):297–300.
3. Charan NB, Myers CG, Lakshminarayan S, Spencer TM. Pulmonary injuries associated with acute sulfur dioxide inhalation. Am Rev Respir Dis 1979; 119(4):555–560.
4. Flury KE, Dines DE, Rodarte JR, Rodgers R. Airway obstruction due to inhalation of ammonia. Mayo Clin Proc 1983; 58(6):389–393.

5. Donham KJ, Knapp LW, Monson R, Gustafson K. Acute toxic exposure to gases from liquid manure. J Occup Med 1982; 24(2):142–145.
6. Harkonen H, Nordman H, Korhonen O, Winblad I. Long-term effects of exposure to sulfur dioxide. Lung function four years after a pyrite dust explosion. Am Rev Respir Dis 1983; 128(5):890–893.
7. Boulet LP. Increases in airway responsiveness following acute exposure to respiratory irritants. Reactive airway dysfunction syndrome or occupational asthma? Chest 1988; 94(3):476–481.
8. Gilbert R, Auchincloss JH Jr. Reactive airways dysfunction syndrome presenting as a reversible restrictive defect. Lung 1989; 167(1):55–61.
9. Promisloff RA, Lenchner GS, Phan A, Cichelli AV. Reactive airway dysfunction syndrome in three police officers following a roadside chemical spill. Chest 1990; 98(4):928–929.
10. Lerman S, Kipen H. Reactive airways dysfunction syndrome. Am Fam Physician 1988; 38(6):135–138.
11. Luo JC, Nelsen KG, Fischbein A. Persistent reactive airway dysfunction syndrome after exposure to toluene diisocyanate. Br J Ind Med 1990; 47(4):239–241.
12. Rajan KG, Davies BH. Reversible airways obstruction and interstitial pneumonitis due to acetic acid. Br J Ind Med 1989; 46(1):67–68.
13. Moisan TC. Prolonged asthma after smoke inhalation: a report of three cases and a review of previous reports. J Occup Med 1991; 33(4):458–461.
14. Bernstein IL, Bernstein DI, Weiss M, Campbell GP. Reactive airways disease syndrome (RADS) after exposure to toxic ammonia fumes. J Allergy Clin Immunol 1989; 83:173.
15. Sallie B, McDonald C. Inhalation accidents reported to the SWORD surveillance project 1990–1993. Ann Occup Hyg 1996; 40(2):211–221.
16. Kern DG. Outbreak of the reactive airways dysfunction syndrome after a spill of glacial acetic acid. Am Rev Respir Dis 1991; 144(5):1058–1064.
17. Deschamps D, Questel F, Baud FJ, Gervais P, Dally S. Persistent asthma after acute inhalation of organophosphate insecticide. Lancet 1994; 344(8938):1712.
18. Leduc D, Gris P, Lheureux P, Gevenois PA, De Vuyst P, Yernault JC. Acute and long term respiratory damage following inhalation of ammonia. Thorax 1992; 47(9):755–757.
19. Lemiere C, Malo JL, Boutet M. Reactive airways dysfunction syndrome due to chlorine: sequential bronchial biopsies and functional assessment. Eur Respir J 1997; 10(1):241–244.
20. Bherer L, Cushman R, Courteau JP, et al. Survey of construction workers repeatedly exposed to chlorine over a three to six month period in a pulpmill: II. Follow up of affected workers by questionnaire, spirometry, and assessment of bronchial responsiveness 18 to 24 months after exposure ended. Occup Environ Med 1994; 51(4):225–228.
21. Buckley LA, Jiang XZ, James RA, Morgan KT, Barrow CS. Respiratory tract lesions induced by sensory irritants at the RD50 concentration. Toxicol Appl Pharmacol 1984; 74(3):417–429.
22. Murphy DM, Fairman RP, Lapp NL, Morgan WK. Severe airway disease due to inhalation of fumes from cleansing agents. Chest 1976; 69(3):372–376.
23. Wade III JF, Newman LS. Diesel asthma. Reactive airways disease following overexposure to locomotive exhaust. J Occup Med 1993; 35(2):149–154.
24. Gadon ME, Melius JM, McDonald GJ, Orgel D. New-onset asthma after exposure to the steam system additive 2-diethylaminoethanol. A descriptive study. J Occup Med 1994; 36(6):623–626.
25. Deschamps D, Rosenberg N, Soler P, et al. Persistent asthma after accidental exposure to ethylene oxide. Br J Ind Med 1992; 49(7):523–525.
26. Porter JA. Letter: acute respiratory distress following formalin inhalation. Lancet 1975; 2(7935):603–604.
27. Berlin L, Hjortsberg L, Wass V. Life-threatening pulmonary reaction to car paint containing a prepolymerized isocyanate. Scand J Work Environ Health 1981; 7:310–312.

28. Lemiere C, Malo JL, Boulet LP, Boutet M. Reactive airways dysfunction syndrome induced by exposure to a mixture containing isocyanate: functional and histopathologic behaviour. Allergy 1996; 51(4):262–265.

29. Ferguson JS, Schaper M, Alarie Y. Pulmonary effects of a polyisocyanate aerosol: hexamethylene diisocyanate trimer (HDIt) or Desmodur-N (DES-N). Toxicol Appl Pharmacol 1987; 89(3):332–346.

30. Cone JE, Wugofski L, Balmes JR, et al. Persistent respiratory health effects after a metam sodium pesticide spill. Chest 1994; 106(2):500–508.

31. Frans A, Pahulycz C. Transient syndrome of acute irritation of the bronchi induced by single and massive inhalation of phthalic anhydride. Rev Pneumol Clin 1993; 49(5): 247–251.

32. Berghoff R. The more common gases; their effect on the respiratory tract. Arch Intern Med 1919; 24:678–684.

33. Lemiere C, Malo JL, Garbe-Galanti L. Bronchial irritation syndrome following inhalation or urea. Histologic and immunohistochemical evaluation. Rev Mal Respir 1996; 13(6):595–597.

34. Black J, Glenny E. Observations on 685 cases of poisoning by noxious gases used by the enemy. Br Med J 1915; 165:165–167.

35. Malo JL, Chan-Yeung M, Lemiere C, et al. Reactive airways dysfunctions syndrome. In: Rose BD, ed. Pulmonary and Critical Care Medicine (CD-Rom version). Wellesley, MA, 1998.

36. Henneberger PK, Derk SJ, Davis L, et al. Work-related reactive airways dysfunction syndrome cases from surveillance in selected US states. J Occup Environ Med 2003; 45(4):360–368.

37. Khateri S, Ghanei M, Keshavarz S, Soroush M, Haines D. Incidence of lung, eye, and skin lesions as late complications in 34,000 Iranians with wartime exposure to mustard agent. J Occup Environ Med 2003; 45(11):1136–1143.

38. Emad A, Rezaian GR. The diversity of the effects of sulfur mustard gas inhalation on respiratory system 10 years after a single, heavy exposure: analysis of 197 cases. Chest 1997; 112(3):734–738.

39. Bascom R, Naclerio RM, Fitzgerald TK, Kagey-Sobotka A, Proud D. Effect of ozone inhalation on the response to nasal challenge with antigen of allergic subjects. Am Rev Respir Dis 1990; 142(3):594–601.

40. Hunting KL, McDonald SM. Development of a hierarchical exposure coding system for clinic-based surveillance of occupational disease and injury. Appl Occup Environ Hyg 1995; 10:317–322.

41. Reilly MJ, Rosenman KD, Watt FC, et al. Surveillance for occupational asthma— Michigan and New Jersey, 1988–1992. MMWR CDC Surveill Summ 1994; 43(1):9–17.

42. Rosenman KD, Reilly MJ, Kalinowski DJ. A state-based surveillance system for work-related asthma. J Occup Environ Med 1997; 39(5):415–425.

43. Reinisch F, Harrison RJ, Cussler S, et al. Physician reports of work-related asthma in California, 1993–1996. Am J Ind Med 2001; 39(1):72–83.

44. Provencher S, Labreche FP, De Guire L. Physician based surveillance system for occupational respiratory diseases: the experience of PROPULSE, Quebec, Canada. Occup Environ Med 1997; 54(4):272–276.

45. Chatkin JM, Tarlo SM, Liss G, Banks D, Broder I. The outcome of asthma related to workplace irritant exposures: a comparison of irritant-induced asthma and irritant aggravation of asthma. Chest 1999; 116(6):1780–1785.

46. Tarlo SM, Liss G, Corey P, Broder I. A workers' compensation claim population for occupational asthma. Comparison of subgroups. Chest 1995; 107(3):634–641.

47. Ross DJ, Sallie BA, McDonald JC. SWORD '1994: surveillance of work-related and occupational respiratory disease in the UK. Occup Med (Lond) 1995; 45(4):175–178.

48. Gannon PF, Burge PS. The SHIELD scheme in the West Midlands Region, United Kingdom. Midland Thoracic Society Research Group. Br J Ind Med 1993; 50(9):791–796.

49. Hnizdo E, Esterhuizen TM, Rees D, Lalloo UG. Occupational asthma as identified by the Surveillance of Work-related and Occupational Respiratory Diseases programme in South Africa. Clin Exp Allergy 2001; 31(1):32–39.

50. Dhara VR, Dhara R. The Union Carbide disaster in Bhopal: a review of health effects. Arch Environ Health 2002; 57(5):391–404.

51. Kamat SR, Patel MH, Pradhan PV, et al. Sequential respiratory, psychologic, and immunologic studies in relation to methyl isocyanate exposure over two years with model development. Environ Health Perspect 1992; 97:241–253.

52. Cullinan P, Acquilla S, Dhara VR. Respiratory morbidity 10 years after the Union Carbide gas leak at Bhopal: a cross sectional survey. The International Medical Commission on Bhopal. BMJ 1997; 314(7077):338–342.

53. Nemery B. Late consequences of accidental exposure to inhaled irritants: RADS and the Bhopal disaster. Eur Respir J 1996; 9(10):1973–1976.

54. Dhara R, Acquilla S, Cullinan P. Has the world forgotten Bhopal? Lancet 2001; 357(9258):809–810.

55. Dhara VR, Cullinan P. Bhopal priorities. Int J Occup Environ Health 2004; 10(1):107.

56. Prezant DJ, Weiden M, Banauch GI, et al. Cough and bronchial responsiveness in firefighters at the World Trade Center site. N Engl J Med 2002; 34711:806–815.

57. Statement of Janet Heinrich Director HCPHI. Representatives: Health Effects in the Aftermath of the World Trade Center Attack. Testimony Before the Subcommittee on National Security, Emerging Threats, and International Relations, 2004.

58. U.S. Geological Survey Web Site. Chemical composition of the WTC dusts and girder coating material. U S Department of the Interior, 2001.

59. CDC. Occupational exposures to air contaminants at the World Trade Center disaster site, New York, September–October, 2001. MMWR Morb Mortal Wkly Rep 2002; 51(21):453–456.

60. Rom WN, Weiden M, Garcia R, et al. Acute eosinophilic pneumonia in a New Yoek City firefighter exposed to World Trade Center. Am J Respir Crit Care Med 2002; 166(6):797–800.

61. Banauch GI, Alleyne D, Sanchez R, et al. Persistent hyperreactivity and reactive airway dysfunction in firefighters at the World Trade Center. Am J Respir Crit Care Med 2003; 168(1):54–62.

62. Nemery B. Reactive fallout of World Trade Center dust. Am J Respir Crit Care Med 2003; 168(1):2–3.

63. Scanlon PD. World Trade Center cough—a lingering legacy and a cautionary tale. N Engl J Med 2002; 347(11):840–842.

64. Truncale T, Brooks S, Prezant DJ, Banauch GI, Nemery B. World Trade Center dust and airway reactivity. Am J Respir Crit Care Med 2004; 169(7):883–884.

65. Beckett WS. A New York City firefighter: overwhelmed by World Trade Center dust. Am J Respir Crit Care Med 2002; 166(6):785–786.

66. Gross KB, Haidar AH, Basha MA, et al. Acute pulmonary response of asthmatics to aerosols and gases generated by airbag deployment. Am J Respir Crit Care Med 1994; 150(2):408–414.

67. Eschenbacher WL, Gross KB, Muench SP, Chan TL. Inhalation of an alkaline aerosol by subjects with mild asthma does not result in bronchoconstriction. Am Rev Respir Dis 1991; 143(2):341–345.

68. Brooks SM, Weiss MA, Bernstein IL. Reactive airways dysfunction syndrome. Case reports of persistent airways hyperreactivity following high-level irritant exposures. J Occup Med 1985; 27(7):473–476.

69. Brooks SM. Occupational asthma. Toxicol Lett 1995; 82–83:39–45.

70. Boulet LP. Asymptomatic airway hyperresponsiveness: a curiosity or an opportunity to prevent asthma? Am J Respir Crit Care Med 2003; 167(3):371–378.

71. Enarson DA, Vedal S, Schulzer M, Dybuncio A, Chan-Yeung M. Asthma, asthmalike symptoms, chronic bronchitis, and the degree of bronchial hyperresponsiveness in epidemiologic surveys. Am Rev Respir Dis 1987; 136(3):613–617.

72. Baur X, Huber H, Degens PO, Allmers H, Ammon J. Relation between occupational asthma case history, bronchial methacholine challenge, and specific challenge test in patients with suspected occupational asthma. Am J Ind Med 1998; 33(2):114–122.

73. Crapo RO, Casaburi R, Coates AL, et al. Guidelines for methacholine and exercise challenge testing-1999. This official statement of the American Thoracic Society was adopted by the ATS Board of Directors, July 1999. Am J Respir Crit Care Med 2000; 161(1):309–329.

74. De Vries K. Clinical significance of bronchial hyperresponsiveness. 1987; 359–371.

75. Hopp RJ, Townley RG, Biven RE, Bewtra AK, Nair NM. The presence of airway reactivity before the development of asthma. Am Rev Respir Dis 1990; 141(1):2–8.

76. National Institute of Health. Guideline for the diagnosis and management of asthma. NHLBI 1997; 1–153.

77. van der HS, De Monchy JG, De Vries K, Dubois AE, Kauffman HF. Seasonal differences in airway hyperresponsiveness in asthmatic patients: relationship with allergen exposure and sensitization to house dust mites. Clin Exp Allergy 1997; 27(6):627–633.

78. Gautrin D, Boulet LP, Boutet M, et al. Is reactive airways dysfunction syndrome a variant of occupational asthma?. J Allergy Clin Immunol 1994; 93(1 Pt 1):12–22.

79. Nagasaka Y, Nakano N, Tohda Y, Nakajima S. Persistent reactive airway dysfunction syndrome after exposure to chromate. Nihon Kyobu Shikkan Gakkai Zasshi 1995; 33(7):759–764.

80. Alberts WM. Reactive airways dysfunction syndrome. Pulm Perspect 1992; 9:1–4.

81. Venables KM. Prevention of occupational asthma. Eur Respir J 1994; 7(4):768–778.

82. Brooks SM, Hammad Y, Richards I, Giovinco-Barbas J, Jenkins K. The spectrum of irritant-induced asthma: sudden and not-so-sudden onset and the role of allergy. Chest 1998; 113(1):42–49.

83. Zhong NS, Chen RC, Yang MO, Wu ZY, Zheng JP, Li YF. Is asymptomatic bronchial hyperresponsiveness an indication of potential asthma? A two-year follow-up of young students with bronchial hyperresponsiveness. Chest 1992; 102(4):1104–1109.

84. Boulet LP, Turcotte H, Brochu A. Persistence of airway obstruction and hyperresponsiveness in subjects with asthma remission. Chest 1994; 105(4):1024–1031.

85. Jones A. Asymptomatic bronchial hyperreactivity and the development of asthma and other respiratory tract illnesses in children. Thorax 1994; 49(8):757–761.

86. Chan-Yeung M, Lam S, Kennedy SM, Frew AJ. Persistent asthma after repeated exposure to high concentrations of gases in pulpmills. Am J Respir Crit Care Med 1994; 149(6):1676–1680.

87. Lemiere C, Malo JL, Gautrin D. Nonsensitizing causes of occupational asthma. Med Clin North Am 1996; 80(4):749–774.

88. Demnati R, Fraser R, Ghezzo H, Martin JG, Plaa G, Malo JL. Time-course of functional and pathological changes after a single high acute inhalation of chlorine in rats. Eur Respir J 1998; 11(4):922–928.

89. Demnati R, Fraser R, Martin JG, Plaa G, Malo JL. Effects of dexamethasone on functional and pathological changes in rat bronchi caused by high acute exposure to chlorine. Toxicol Sci 1998; 45(2):242–246.

90. Martin JG, Campbell HR, Iijima H, et al. Chlorine-induced injury to the airways in mice. Am J Respir Crit Care Med 2003; 168(5):568–574.

91. Gautrin D, Maghni K, Alles M, Lemiere C, Martin JG, Malo JL. Determinants of lung function changes, sputum neutrophilia and metalloproteinases (MMPs) activities in workrers at risk of repeated accidental inhalations of chlorine [abstract]. Eur Respir J 2002; 20(S38):603s.

92. Ackerman V, Marini M, Vittori E, Bellini A, Vassali G, Mattoli S. Detection of cytokines and their cell sources in bronchial biopsy specimens from asthmatic patients.

Relationship to atopic status, symptoms, and level of airway hyperresponsiveness. Chest 1994; 105(3):687–696.

93. Holtzman MJ, Cunningham JH, Sheller JR, Irsigler GB, Nadel JA, Boushey HA. Effect of ozone on bronchial reactivity in atopic and nonatopic subjects. Am Rev Respir Dis 1979; 120(5):1059–1067.

94. Braman SS, Barrows AA, DeCotiis BA, Settipane GA, Corrao WM. Airway hyperresponsiveness in allergic rhinitis. A risk factor for asthma. Chest 1987; 91(5):671–674.

95. Frew AJ, Kennedy SM, Chan-Yeung M. Methacholine responsiveness, smoking, and atopy as risk factors for accelerated FEV1 decline in male working populations. Am Rev Respir Dis 1992; 146(4):878–883.

96. Kagamimori S, Katoh T, Naruse Y, et al. The changing prevalence of respiratory symptoms in atopic children in response to air pollution. Clin Allergy 1986; 16(4):299–308.

97. Gaddy JN, Busse WW. Enhanced IgE-dependent basophil histamine release and airway reactivity in asthma. Am Rev Respir Dis 1986; 134(5):969–974.

98. Doull IJ, Lawrence S, Watson M, et al. Allelic association of gene markers on chromosomes 5q and 11q with atopy and bronchial hyperresponsiveness. Am J Respir Crit Care Med 1996; 153(4 Pt 1):1280–1284.

99. Humbert M, Grant JA, Taborda-Barata L, et al. High-affinity IgE receptor (FcepsilonRI)-bearing cells in bronchial biopsies from atopic and nonatopic asthma. Am J Respir Crit Care Med 1996; 153(6 Pt 1):1931–1937.

100. Van de Graaf EA, Out TA, Roos CM, Jansen HM. Respiratory membrane permeability and bronchial hyperreactivity in patients with stable asthma. Effects of therapy with inhaled steroids. Am Rev Respir Dis 1991; 143(2):362–368.

101. Biagini RE, Moorman WJ, Lewis TR, Bernstein IL. Ozone enhancement of platinum asthma in a primate model. Am Rev Respir Dis 1986; 134(4):719–725.

102. Jorres R, Nowak D, Magnussen H. The effect of ozone exposure on allergen responsiveness in subjects with asthma or rhinitis. Am J Respir Crit Care Med 1996; 153(1):56–64.

103. Molfino NA, Wright SC, Katz I, et al. Effect of low concentrations of ozone on inhaled allergen responses in asthmatic subjects. Lancet 1991; 338(8761):199–203.

104. Moller DR, McKay RT, Bernstein IL, Brooks SM. Persistent airways disease caused by toluene diisocyanate. Am Rev Respir Dis 1986; 134(1):175–176.

105. Brooks SM. Epidemiologic study of workers exposed to isocyanates. NIOSH Health Hazard Evaluation Report, 1980.

106. Karol MH. Survey of industrial workers for antibodies to toluene diisocyanate. J Occup Med 1981; 23(11):741–747.

107. Occupational asthma: recommendations for diagnosis, management and assessment of impairment. Ad Hoc Committee on Occupational Asthma of the Standards Committee, Canadian Thoracic Society. CMAJ 1989; 140(9):1029–1032.

108. Burge PS. Single and serial measurements of lung function in the diagnosis of occupational asthma. Eur J Respir Dis Suppl 1982; 123:47–59.

109. Cartier A, Pineau L, Malo JL. Monitoring of maximum expiratory peak flow rates and histamine inhalation tests in the investigation of occupational asthma. Clin Allergy 1984; 14(2):193–196.

110. Brooks SM. Bronchial asthma of occupational origin. In: Rom W, ed. Environmental and Occupationnal Medicine. Boston: Little Brown, 1992.

111. Cockcroft DW. Bronchial inhalation tests. I. Measurement of nonallergic bronchial responsiveness. Ann Allergy 1985; 55(4):527–534.

112. Lam S, Wong R, Yeung M. Nonspecific bronchial reactivity in occupational asthma. J Allergy Clin Immunol 1979; 63(1):28–34.

113. Lemiere C, Chaboilliez S, Trudeau C, et al. Characterization of airway inflammation after repeated exposures to occupational agents. J Allergy Clin Immunol 2000; 106(6):1163–1170.

114. Di FA, Vagaggini B, Bacci E, et al. Leukocyte counts in hypertonic saline-induced sputum in subjects with occupational asthma. Respir Med 1998; 92(3):550–557.

115. Birring SS, Berry M, Brightling CE, Pavord ID. Eosinophilic bronchitis: clinical features, management and pathogenesis. Am J Respir Med 2003; 2(2):169–173.

116. Maestrelli P, Calcagni PG, Saetta M, et al. Sputum eosinophilia after asthmatic responses induced by isocyanates in sensitized subjects. Clin Exp Allergy 1994; 24(1):29–34.

117. Kobayashi O. A case of eosinophilic bronchitis due to epoxy resin system hardener, methle endo methylene tetrahydro phthalic anhydride. Arerugi 1994; 43(5):660–662.

118. Lemiere C, Efthimiadis A, Hargreave FE. Occupational eosinophilic bronchitis without asthma: an unknown occupational airway disease. J Allergy Clin Immunol 1997; 100(6 Pt 1):852–853.

119. Tanaka H, Saikai T, Sugawara H, et al. Workplace-related chronic cough on a mushroom farm. Chest 2002; 122(3):1080–1085.

120. Larsson BM, Larsson K, Malmberg P, Palmberg L. Airways inflammation after exposure in a swine confinement building during cleaning procedure. Am J Ind Med 2002; 41(4):250–258.

121. Von Essen SG, Scheppers LA, Robbins RA, Donham KJ. Respiratory tract inflammation in swine confinement workers studied using induced sputum and exhaled nitric oxide. J Toxicol Clin Toxicol 1998; 36(6):557–565.

122. Ansarin K, Chatkin JM, Ferreira IM, Gutierrez CA, Zamel N, Chapman KR. Exhaled nitric oxide in chronic obstructive pulmonary disease: relationship to pulmonary function. Eur Respir J 2001; 17(5):934–938.

123. Obata H, Dittrick M, Chan H, Chan-Yeung M. Sputum eosinophils and exhaled nitric oxide during late asthmatic reaction in patients with western red cedar asthma. Eur Respir J 1999; 13(3):489–495.

124. Allmers H, Chen Z, Barbinova L, Marczynski B, Kirschmann V, Baur X. Challenge from methacholine, natural rubber latex, or 4,4-diphenylmethane diisocyanate in workers with suspected sensitization affects exhaled nitric oxide change in exhaled NO levels after allergen challenges. Int Arch Occup Environ Health 2000; 73(3):181–186.

125. Olin AC, Alving K, Toren K. Exhaled nitric oxide: relation to sensitization and respiratory symptoms. Clin Exp Allergy 2004; 34(2):221–226.

126. Olin AC, Andersson E, Andersson M, Granung G, Hagberg S, Toren K. Prevalence of asthma and exhaled nitric oxide are increased in bleachery workers exposed to ozone. Eur Respir J 2004; 23(1):87–92.

127. Piipari R, Piirila P, Keskinen H, Tuppurainen M, Sovijarvi A, Nordman H. Exhaled nitric oxide in specific challenge tests to assess occupational asthma. Eur Respir J 2002; 20(6):1532–1537.

128. Koksal N, Hasanoglu HC, Gokirmak M, Yildirim Z, Gultek A. Apricot sulfurization: an occupation that induces an asthma-like syndrome in agricultural environments. Am J Ind Med 2003; 43(4):447–453.

129. Koksal N, Yildirim Z, Gokirmak M, Hasanoglu HC, Mehmet N, Avci H. The role of nitric oxide and cytokines in asthma-like syndrome induced by sulfur dioxide exposure in agricultural environment. Clin Chim Acta 2003; 336(1–2):115–122.

130. Lund MB, Oksne PI, Hamre R, Kongerud J. Increased nitric oxide in exhaled air: an early marker of asthma in non-smoking aluminium potroom workers? Occup Environ Med 2000; 57(4):274–278.

131. Maniscalco M, Grieco L, Galdi A, Lundberg JO, Sofia M. Increase in exhaled nitric oxide in shoe and leather workers at the end of the work-shift. Occup Med (Lond) 2004; 54(6):404–407.

132. Malo JL, Cartier A, Boulet LP, et al. Bronchial hyperresponsiveness can improve while spirometry plateaus two to three years after repeated exposure to chlorine causing respiratory symptoms. Am J Respir Crit Care Med 1994; 150(4):1142–1145.

133. Hasan FM, Gehshan A, Fuleihan FJ. Resolution of pulmonary dysfunction following acute chlorine exposure. Arch Environ Health 1983; 38(2):76–80.

134. Charan NB, Lakshminarayan S, Myers GC, Smith DD. Effects of accidental chlorine inhalation on pulmonary function. West J Med 1985; 143(3):333–336.

135. Blanc PD, Galbo M, Hiatt P, Olson KR. Morbidity following acute irritant inhalation in a population-based study. JAMA 1991; 266(5):664–669.

136. Kennedy SM. Acquired airway hyperresponsiveness from nonimmunogenic irritant exposure. Occup Med 1992; 7(2):287–300.

137. Sallie BA, Ross DJ, Meredith SK, McDonald JC. SWORD 1993. Surveillance of work-related and occupational respiratory disease in the UK. Occup Med (Lond) 1994; 44(4):177–182.

138. Kowitz TA, Reba RC, Parker RT, Spicer WS, Jr. Effects of chlorine gas upon respiratory function. Arch Environ Health 1967; 14(4):545–558.

139. Salisbury DA, Enarson DA, Chan-Yeung M, Kennedy SM. First-aid reports of acute chlorine gassing among pulpmill workers as predictors of lung health consequences. Am J Ind Med 1991; 20(1):71–81.

140. Kennedy SM, Enarson DA, Janssen RG, Chan-Yeung M. Lung health consequences of reported accidental chlorine gas exposures among pulpmill workers. Am Rev Respir Dis 1991; 143(1):74–79.

141. Enarson DA, Johnson A, Block G, et al. Respiratory health at a pulpmill in British Columbia. Arch Environ Health 1984; 39(5):325–330.

142. Courteau JP, Cushman R, Bouchard F, Quevillon M, Chartrand A, Bherer L. Survey of construction workers repeatedly exposed to chlorine over a three to six month period in a pulpmill: I. Exposure and symptomatology. Occup Environ Med 1994; 51(4):219–224.

143. Schwartz DA, Smith DD, Lakshminarayan S. The pulmonary sequelae associated with accidental inhalation of chlorine gas. Chest 1990; 97(4):820–825.

144. Kaufman J, Burkons D. Clinical, roentgenologic, and physiologic effects of acute chlorine exposure. Arch Environ Health 1971; 23(1):29–34.

145. Jones RN, Hughes JM, Glindmeyer H, Weill H. Lung function after acute chlorine exposure. Am Rev Respir Dis 1986; 134(6):1190–1195.

146. Ferris Jr BG, Burgess WA, Worcester J. Prevalence of chronic respiratory disease in a pulp mill and a paper mill in the United States. Br J Ind Med 1967; 24(1):26–37.

147. Chester EH, Gillespie DG, Krause FD. The prevalence of chronic obstructive pulmonary disease in chlorine gas workers. Am Rev Respir Dis 1969; 99(3):365–373.

148. Kipen HM, Blume R, Hutt D. Asthma experience in an occupational and environmental medicine clinic. Low-dose reactive airways dysfunction syndrome. J Occup Med 1994; 36(10):1133–1137.

149. Chasis H, Zapp J, Bannon J, et al. Chlorine accident in Brooklyn. Occup Med 1947; 4:152–170.

150. Henneberger PK, Ferris Jr BG, Sheehe PR. Accidental gassing incidents and the pulmonary function of pulp mill workers. Am Rev Respir Dis 1993; 148(1):63–67.

151. Gautrin D, Leroyer C, L'Archeveque J, Dufour JG, Girard D, Malo JL. Cross-sectional assessment of workers with repeated exposure to chlorine over a three year period. Eur Respir J 1995; 8(12):2046–2054.

152. Gautrin D, Leroyer C, Infante-Rivard C, et al. Longitudinal assessment of airway caliber and responsiveness in workers exposed to chlorine. Am J Respir Crit Care Med 1999; 160(4):1232–1237.

153. Henneberger PK, Lax MB, Ferris Jr BG. Decrements in spirometry values associated with chlorine gassing events and pulp mill work. Am J Respir Crit Care Med 1996; 153(1):225–231.

154. Leroyer C, Malo JL, Infante-Rivard C, Dufour JG, Gautrin D. Changes in airway function and bronchial responsiveness after acute occupational exposure to chlorine leading to treatment in a first aid unit. Occup Environ Med 1998; 55(5):356–359.

155. Arif AA, Delclos GL, Whitehead LW, Tortolero SR, Lee ES. Occupational exposures associated with work-related asthma and work-related wheezing among U.S. workers. Am J Ind Med 2003; 44(4):368–376.

156. Kogevinas M, Anto JM, Sunyer J, Tobias A, Kromhout H, Burney P. Occupational asthma in Europe and other industrialised areas: a population-based study. European Community Respiratory Health Survey Study Group. Lancet 1999; 353(9166):1750–1754.

157. Jaakkola JJ, Piipari R, Jaakkola MS. Occupation and asthma: a population-based incident case-control study. Am J Epidemiol 2003; 158(10):981–987.

158. Kopferschmitt-Kubler MC, Ameille J, Popin E, et al. Occupational asthma in France: a 1-yr report of the observatoire National de Asthmes Professionnels project. Eur Respir J 2002; 19(1):84–89.

159. Ng TP, Hong CY, Goh LG, Wong ML, Koh KT, Ling SL. Risks of asthma associated with occupations in a community-based case-control study. Am J Ind Med 1994; 25(5):709–718.

160. Buck RG, Miles AJ, Ehrlich RI. Possible occupational asthma among adults presenting with acute asthma. S Afr Med J 2000; 90(9):884–888.

161. Zock JP, Kogevinas M, Sunyer J, et al. Asthma risk, cleaning activities and use of specific cleaning products among Spanish indoor cleaners. Scand J Work Environ Health 2001; 27(1):76–81.

162. Medina-Ramon M, Zock JP, Kogevinas M, Sunyer J, Anto JM. Asthma symptoms in women employed in domestic cleaning: a community based study. Thorax 2003; 58(11):950–954.

163. Rosenman KD, Reilly MJ, Schill DP, et al. Cleaning products and work-related asthma. J Occup Environ Med 2003; 45(5):556–563.

164. Burge PS, Richardson MN. Occupational asthma due to indirect exposure to lauryl dimethyl benzyl ammonium chloride used in a floor cleaner. Thorax 1994; 49(8): 842–843.

165. Zock JP, Medina-Ramon M, Kogevinas M, Sunyer J, Anto JM. Asthma and exposure to irritant agents in domestic cleaning women. Eur Respir J 2004; 24.

166. Sokol WN, Aelony Y, Beall GN. Meat-wrapper's asthma. A new syndrome? JAMA 1973; 226(6):639–641.

167. Vandervort R, Brooks SM. Polyvinyl chloride film thermal decomposition products as an occupational illness: I. Environmental exposures and toxicology. J Occup Med 1977; 19(3):188–191.

168. Andrasch R, Bardana E. Meat wrapper's asthma: an appraisal of a new occupationnal syndrome. J Allergy Clin Immunol 1975; 55:130.

169. Maccia CA, Bernstein IL, Emmett EA, Brooks SM. In vitro demonstration of specific IgE in phthalic anhydride hypersensitivity. Am Rev Respir Dis 1976; 113(5):701–704.

170. Pauli G, Bessot JC, Kopferschmitt MC, et al. Meat wrapper's asthma: identification of the causal agent. Clin Allergy 1980; 10(3):263–269.

171. Brooks SM, Vandervort R. Polyvinyl chloride film thermal decomposition products as an occupational illness. 2. Clinical studies. J Occup Med 1977; 19(3):192–196.

172. Jones RN, Weill H. Respiratory health and polyvinyl chloride fumes. JAMA 1977; 237(17):1826.

173. Krumpe PE, Finley TN, Martinez N. The search for expiratory obstruction in meat wrappers studied on the job. Am Rev Respir Dis 1979; 119(4):611–618.

174. Committee on Aldehydes. Formaldehyde and other aldehydes. Board on Toxicology and Environmental Health Hazards. National Academy of Science, 1981.

175. Day J, Lees R, Clark R. Respiratory effects of formaldehyde and UFFI off-gas following controlled exposure. J Allergy Clin Immunol 1983; 7(suppl):159.

176. Frigas E, Filley WV, Reed CE. Asthma induced by dust from urea-formaldehyde foam insulating material. Chest 1981; 79(6):706–707.

177. Hendrick DJ, Lane DJ. Occupational formalin asthma. Br J Ind Med 1977; 34(1): 11–18.

178. Maurice F, Rivory JP, Larsson PH, Johansson SG, Bousquet J. Anaphylactic shock caused by formaldehyde in a patient undergoing long-term hemodialysis. J Allergy Clin Immunol 1986; 77(4):594–597.

179. Patterson R, Pateras V, Grammer LC, Harris KE. Human antibodies against formaldehyde-human serum albumin conjugates or human serum albumin in individuals exposed to formaldehyde. Int Arch Allergy Appl Immunol 1986; 79(1):53–59.

180. Kramps JA, Peltenburg LT, Kerklaan PR, Spieksma FT, Valentijn RM, Dijkman JH. Measurement of specific IgE antibodies in individuals exposed to formaldehyde. Clin Exp Allergy 1989; 19(5):509–514.

181. Thrasher JD, Wojdani A, Cheung G, Heuser G. Evidence for formaldehyde antibodies and altered cellular immunity in subjects exposed to formaldehyde in mobile homes. Arch Environ Health 1987; 42(6):347–350.

182. Newhouse MT. UFFI dust: nonspecific irritant only?. Chest 1982; 82(4):511–512.

183. Abramson MJ, Wlodarczyk JH, Saunders NA, Hensley MJ. Does aluminum smelting cause lung disease?. Am Rev Respir Dis 1989; 139(4):1042–1057.

184. Wergelund E, Lund E, Waage JE. Respiratory dysfunction after potroom asthma. Am J Ind Med 1987; 11(6):627–636.

185. Robertson AS, Weir DC, Burge PS. Occupational asthma due to oil mists. Thorax 1988; 43(3):200–205.

186. Kennedy SM, Greaves IA, Kriebel D, Eisen EA, Smith TJ, Woskie SR. Acute pulmonary responses among automobile workers exposed to aerosols of machining fluids. Am J Ind Med 1989; 15(6):627–641.

187. Preller L, Doekes G, Heederik D, Vermeulen R, Vogelzang PF, Boleij JS. Disinfectant use as a risk factor for atopic sensitization and symptoms consistent with asthma: an epidemiological study. Eur Respir J 1996; 9(7):1407–1413.

188. Riedel F, Kramer M, Scheibenbogen C, Rieger CH. Effects of SO_2 exposure on allergic sensitization in the guinea pig. J Allergy Clin Immunol 1988; 82(4):527–534.

189. Vai F, Fournier MF, Lafuma JC, Touaty E, Pariente R. SO_2-induced bronchopathy in the rat: abnormal permeability of the bronchial epithelium in vivo and in vitro after anatomic recovery. Am Rev Respir Dis 1980; 121(5):851–858.

190. Osebold J, Gershwin L, Zee Y. Studies on the enhancement of allergic lung sensitization by inhalation of ozone and sulfuric acid aerosol. J Environ Pathol Toxicol Oncol 1990; 3:221–234.

191. Horstman DH, Folinsbee LJ, Ives PJ, Abdul-Salaam S, McDonnell WF. Ozone concentration and pulmonary response relationships for 6.6-hour exposures with five hours of moderate exercise to 0.08, 0.10, and 0.12 ppm. Am Rev Respir Dis 1990; 142(5):1158–1163.

192. Devlin RB, McDonnell WF, Mann R, et al. Exposure of humans to ambient levels of ozone for 6.6 hours causes cellular and biochemical changes in the lung. Am J Respir Cell Mol Biol 1991; 4(1):72–81.

193. Vagaggini B, Taccola M, Cianchetti S, et al. Ozone exposure increases eosinophilic airway response induced by previous allergen challenge. Am J Respir Crit Care Med 2002; 166(8):1073–1077.

194. Hastie AT, Peters SP. Interactions of allergens and irritants in susceptible populations in producing lung dysfunction: implications for future research. Environ Health Perspect 2001; 109(suppl 4):605–607.

195. Wagner JG, Hotchkiss JA, Harkema JR. Effects of ozone and endotoxin coexposure on rat airway epithelium: potentiation of toxicant-induced alterations. Environ Health Perspect 2001; 109(suppl 4):591–598.

196. Dube D, Puruckherr M, Byrd Jr RP, Roy TM. Reactive airways dysfunction syndrome following metal fume fever. Tenn Med 2002; 95(6):236–238.

197. Piirila P, Espo T, Pfaffli P, Riihimaki V, Wolff H, Nordman H. Prolonged respiratory symptoms caused by thermal degradation products of freons. Scand J Work Environ Health 2003; 29(1):71–77.

198. Malo JL, Cartier A, Ghezzo H, Lafrance M, McCants M, Lehrer SB. Patterns of improvement in spirometry, bronchial hyperresponsiveness, and specific IgE antibody

levels after cessation of exposure in occupational asthma caused by snow-crab processing. Am Rev Respir Dis 1988; 138(4):807–812.

199.   Cote J, Kennedy S, Chan-Yeung M. Outcome of patients with cedar asthma with continuous exposure. Am Rev Respir Dis 1990; 141(2):373–376.

200.   Paggiaro PL, Loi AM, Rossi O, et al. Follow-up study of patients with respiratory disease due to toluene diisocyanate (TDI). Clin Allergy 1984; 14(5):463–469.

201.   Chan-Yeung M, MacLean L, Paggiaro PL. Follow-up study of 232 patients with occupational asthma caused by western red cedar (*Thuja plicata*). J Allergy Clin Immunol 1987; 79(5):792–796.

202.   Chan-Yeung M. Immunologic and nonimmunologic mechanisms in asthma due to western red cedar (*Thuja plicata*). J Allergy Clin Immunol 1982; 70(1):32–37.

203.   Gilbert R, Auchincloss Jr JH. The interpretation of the spirogram. How accurate is it for 'obstruction'? Arch Intern Med 1985; 145(9):1635–1639.

204.   Blanc PD, Galbo M, Hiatt P, Olson KR, Balmes JR. Symptoms, lung function, and airway responsiveness following irritant inhalation. Chest 1993; 103(6):1699–1705.

205.   Chester EH, Kaimal J, Payne Jr CB, Kohn PM. Pulmonary injury following exposure to chlorine gas. Possible beneficial effects of steroid treatment. Chest 1977; 72(2):247–250.

206.   Cockcroft DW, Murdock KY. Comparative effects of inhaled salbutamol, sodium cromoglycate, and beclomethasone dipropionate on allergen-induced early asthmatic responses, late asthmatic responses, and increased bronchial responsiveness to histamine. J Allergy Clin Immunol 1987; 79(5):734–740.

207.   Mapp C, Boschetto P, dal Vecchio L, et al. Protective effect of antiasthma drugs on late asthmatic reactions and increased airway responsiveness induced by toluene diisocyanate in sensitized subjects. Am Rev Respir Dis 1987; 136(6):1403–1407.

208.   Smith DD. Medical-legal definition of occupational asthma. Chest 1990; 98(4):1007–1011.

209.   Slovak AJ, Orr RG, Teasdale EL. Efficacy of the helmet respirator in occupational asthma due to laboratory animal allergy (LAA). Am Ind Hyg Assoc J 1985; 46(8):411–415.

210.   Karjalainen A, Martikainen R, Karjalainen J, Klaukka T, Kurppa K. Excess incidence of asthma among Finnish cleaners employed in different industries. Eur Respir J 2002; 19(1):90–95.

26
Asthma Exacerbated at Work

Gregory R. Wagner
Department of Environmental Health, Harvard School of Public Health, Boston, Massachusetts, and NIOSH, Washington, D.C., U.S.A.

Paul K. Henneberger
Division of Respiratory Disease Studies, NIOSH/CDC, Morgantown, West Virginia, U.S.A.

INTRODUCTION

Exacerbation of asthma can result from exposures at home, at work, in the outdoor environment, and in public buildings. There is general agreement in clinical practice that troublesome home environmental exposures should be avoided; physicians often advise asthma patients to rid their homes of carpets, drapes, and other furnishings that might be repositories for allergens. Asthma-related exposures in the work environment are less frequently addressed, because exposures are often beyond the control of the individual patient and an employer may or may not accept their responsibility or have the ability to control exposures. The issue of an affected employee's right to workplace accommodation or compensation further clouds the issue.

Specific studies of asthma exacerbated by workplace exposures are limited in number. In many studies of work-related asthma, work-exacerbated asthma (WEA) is not clearly differentiated from asthma with a work-related onset. For example, the European Community Respiratory Health Survey classifies participants by their current or most recent job, for those who are no longer employed, or by the job they left due to health problems [1,2]. The conditions of that job are then used to determine whether the subject was at risk for exposure to asthma agents; this information is used to determine whether the asthma was work-related. In a population-based study conducted in Norway, the researchers asked participants whether they had ever had respiratory symptoms in relation to work [3]. While these studies are good for identifying the full impact of work on asthma, they do not separate cases characterized by work-related exacerbation of existing asthma from those characterized by work-related onset of asthma. Other investigators have defined and studied WEA as a separate subcategory within the larger category of occupational asthma or work-related asthma.

DEFINITIONS OF WEA

The American College of Chest Physicians published a consensus document on assessment of work-related asthma in 1995 (4). Based on the criteria presented in that document, people were considered to have work-aggravated asthma if they had a diagnosis of asthma and an association between asthma symptoms and work characterized by (i) the presence of asthma symptoms or related medication before entering a new occupational exposure setting and (ii) an increase in symptoms or the need for more or new medication after entering a new occupational exposure setting (4). A similar definition was proposed later in the 1990s as a surveillance case definition for use in the Sentinel Event Notification Systems for Occupational Risks (SENSOR) (5). The SENSOR criteria for work-aggravated asthma are (a) health-care professional's diagnosis consistent with asthma, (b) an association between symptoms and work, (c) asthma symptoms or treatment with asthma medication within the two years before entering a new occupational setting, and (d) increased asthma symptoms or increased asthma medication use upon entering a new occupational setting. There is a longitudinal component to these definitions of work-aggravated asthma. Asthma onset and the presence of asthma symptoms or related medication use must come before entering the new occupational exposure setting, and the condition must worsen after entering. Thus, the clinician or researcher must obtain, either prospectively or retrospectively, knowledge of asthma status before and after subjects enter a new occupational exposure setting.

Medical records may be useful to document an asthma patient's change in status. For example, in a study of recruits who entered the Israel Defense Force at the age of 18 to 21 years, baseline asthma status was established at the time of induction into the military and repeated clinical evaluations documented changes in asthma status over time (6). However, in the absence of medical records, determination of the progression of disease will often depend, at least in part, on subject or patient recall.

Another approach to the definition of WEA is to use self-reported data gathered by questionnaire in clinic- (7,8) or population-based (9–12) studies to determine whether work makes symptoms worse for people with asthma. The definitions for WEA varied to some extent among these studies, as indicated in Table 1. All of the studies were cross-sectional, with the exception of the one by Tarlo et al. (8) which was a retrospective review of data gathered from asthma patients over a 19-year period.

FREQUENCY OF WEA

The frequency of WEA sometimes has been expressed as a percentage of some larger group of work-related asthma cases. From the surveillance of work-related asthma conducted by four states as part of the National Institute for Occupational Safety and Health-sponsored (NIOSH) SENSOR program, 19.1% of the cases registered during 1993–1995 were classified as work-aggravated asthma rather than new-onset asthma (5). From a case series of patients referred for occupational asthma to an occupational and environmental clinic in the United States, 27% were judged to have exacerbation of preexisting asthma (13). Tarlo et al. (14) investigated the status of 469 asthma claims that were accepted by the Ontario Workers' Compensation Board (WCB) during 1984–1988. The WCB group included 234 cases (49.9%) with

Table 1 The Frequency of Work-Exacerbated Asthma

Reference (location of study)	Setting	Definition of work-exacerbated asthma	% with work-exacerbated asthma (n = number with asthma)	
			Among adults with asthma	Among employed adults with asthma
Abramson et al. (9) (Victoria, Australia)	Community based	Self-reported: symptoms exacerbated by workplace conditions	20% (n = 159)	NA[a]
Henneberger et al. (7) (Colorado, U.S.A.)	HMO[b]	Self-reported: current work environment makes asthma worse	25% (n = 1461)	NA
Henneberger et al. (10) (Maine, U.S.A.)	Community based	Self-reported: coughing or wheezing is worse at work	18% (n = 88)	25% (n = 64)
Johnson et al. (11) (6 locations in Canada)	Community based	Self-reported: wheezing or dyspnea at or after work in current job	Wheezing 34% Dyspnea 31% (n = 106)[c]	NA
Saarinen et al. (12) (Finland)	Population based (from those enrolled in national health insurance)	Self-reported: asthma symptoms were caused or made worse by work at least weekly during the past month	NA	21% (n = 969)
Tarlo et al. (8) (Ontario, Canada)	Secondary- and tertiary-referral asthma clinic	Self-reported: worsening of asthma at work and workplace exposure to recognized aggravating factors (including emotional stress), but no likely workplace exposure to sensitizers	3.7% (n = 682)	8.1% (n = 310)

[a]NA, not addressed in publication.
[b]HMO, health maintenance organization.
[c]Limited to those with adult-onset asthma who did not have probable or possible work-related onset of asthma.

aggravation of asthma (AA). In a publication based on the same 469 compensated cases, 68 (14.5% of the 469 total cases and 29.1% of the AA cases) were classified as accident-related AA, which was defined as asthma with worsening of symptoms after an acute accidental exposure to respiratory irritants (15).

Other researchers have identified adults with asthma by clinic records or population-based surveys and then estimated the percentage of the cases having work-exacerbated symptoms. As presented in Table 1, these estimates ranged from approximately 3.7% to 34% among adults with asthma and 8.1% to 25% among employed adults with asthma. This broad range of results may reflect, in part, differences among the studies in subject inclusion criteria and in outcome definition as well as in the source of subjects (Table 1). Some researchers studied asthma patients in a health care setting drawn from the general population, while others looked at people who work and report new symptom patterns associated with their work environment. For example, Tarlo et al. (8) examined the prevalence of work-related asthma among 682 adults (age greater than 17 years) who were diagnosed with asthma in a secondary- and tertiary-referral asthma clinic in Canada (8). Among the 50 cases who reported during their initial clinic visit that their asthma was worse at work, 25 were judged by the investigators to have work-related AA. These 25 cases represented 3.7% of all 682 cases and 8.1% of the 310 cases who had onset of asthma as adults and were employed at the time of the initial clinic visit (8). In a cross-sectional study conducted in a health maintenance organization (HMO) in the United States, 1461 adults with asthma completed a questionnaire (7). This cohort included any adult in the HMO population with a diagnosis of asthma, regardless of whether they were treated by their primary care physician or by a specialist. When asked, 25% of the HMO study participants reported that their asthma was made worse by their current work environment (7).

In a community-based study conducted in Australia, 20% of adults with asthma reported that their symptoms were exacerbated by workplace exposures (9). In a population-based study conducted in the state of Maine in the United States, 16 participants with asthma reported that their coughing or wheezing was worse at work; these participants represented 18.2% of all 88 asthma cases and 25% of the subset of 64 cases who were employed (10). In a study conducted in Finland, the researchers interviewed adults with asthma who had been granted reimbursement for asthma medication by the Finnish Social Insurance Institution (12). During interview, approximately 21% of 969 working adults with asthma reported work-related aggravation of respiratory symptoms at least once a week during the past month (12). The study by Johnson et al. (11) in Canada followed the model of the European Community Respiratory Health Survey. The article was focused on those who fulfilled criteria for probable or possible work-related onset of asthma, but also included findings for others with adult-onset asthma. Wheezing or dyspnea at or after work was reported by 34% and 31%, respectively, of this latter group (12).

EXCESS FREQUENCY OF WEA

One way to address how often work contributes to the exacerbation of asthma is to compare high- to low-risk occupations. In the study of military recruits in Israel, researchers computed the cumulative incidence of asthma onset and worsening over the 30-month study period, which made it possible to compare these figures between different occupational categories (6). Among recruits with a history of rare and mild attacks of dyspnea, normal spirometry, and response to exercise at military induction, worsening of asthma was greater among those in combat units $(78/370 = 21.1\%)$ and maintenance units $(36/236 = 15.3\%)$ than among those who performed clerical tasks $(11/193 = 5.7\%)$. Thus, the excess cumulative incidence, presumably attributable to occupation, was 15.4% for those in combat units and 9.6% for those in maintenance units. Among recruits with mild asthma at induction, characterized by not requiring daily medications and having either mildly impaired spirometry or moderate bronchial hyperresponsiveness, $124/639 = 19.4\%$ of those in the maintenance units had worsening of symptoms compared to $113/606 = 18.6\%$ among those performing clerical tasks.

DISTINCTIVE FEATURES OF ADULTS WITH WEA

A few studies have compared adults with WEA to other adults with asthma or other adults with work-related asthma. Looking first at demographic features (Table 2), the two studies that made comparisons with all other adults with asthma agreed on two findings: The people with WEA were, on average, older but there was little difference by gender (7,12). These two studies did not agree on the impact of cigarette smoking, with one study finding no difference (12) and the other finding that cigarette smoking was more common among asthmatics with WEA (7). One study alone examined race, income, and education as risk factors and found being nonwhite, having lower income, and having less education were associated with work-exacerbation of asthma (7). When Goe et al. (16) used other adults with work-related asthma as the basis for comparison, they found that people with WEA were more likely to be female, young, nonwhite, and nonsmokers.

Table 2 Distinctive Demographic Features of Adults with Work-Exacerbated Asthma

Characteristics of adults with work-exacerbated asthma	Compared to other adults with asthma		Compared to other adults with work-related asthma
	Henneberger et al. (7)	Saarinen et al. (12)	Goe et al. (16)
Gender			
More women	No	No	Yes
Age			
Older	Yes	Yes	No
Younger	No	No	Yes
Race			
More nonwhites	Yes	NA[a]	Yes
Education			
Less	Yes	NA	NA
Annual income			
Lower	Yes	NA	NA
Ever smoked cigarettes			
More likely	Yes	No	No
Less likely	No	No	Yes

[a]NA, not addressed in publication.

Table 3 Distinctive Health and Health Care Features of Adults with
Work-Exacerbated Asthma

Adults with work-exacerbated asthma were more likely to have had:	Compared to other adults with asthma		Compared to other adults with work-related asthma
	Henneberger et al. (7)	Saarinen et al. (12)	Goe et al. (16)
Chronic bronchitis	Yes	NA	NA
Emphysema or COPD	Yes	NA	NA
Allergies	NA	NA	Yes
A family history of allergies or asthma	NA	NA	Yes
Onset of asthma as an adult	NA	Yes	NA
At least one treatment for asthma attack in past year	Yes	NA	NA
A need for asthma medication continuously in past 12 months	NA	Yes	NA
More days with asthma symptoms in past two weeks	Yes	NA	NA
More severe asthma, based on self-report	Yes	NA	NA

Abbreviations: COPD, chronic obstructive pulmonary disease; NA, not addressed in publication.

Distinctive health and health care features of adults with WEA are presented in Table 3. Each item presented is unique to one of the three studies already mentioned (7,12,16). These findings suggest that the people with work-exacerbated symptoms tend to have a more severe form of disease than other adults with asthma.

CLINICAL APPROACH TO A PATIENT WITH WEA

An argument for differentiating between asthma caused by specific sensitizers and WEA is the presumed difference in prognosis with continued workplace exposures. The progression of asthma severity as the result of persistent exposure to sensitizing agents is well recognized, and is the basis for the clinical recommendation to remove someone from exposure, as soon as possible, after diagnosis of occupational asthma (17). Continued exposure to lower levels of the sensitizer and more careful clinical monitoring will often not prevent worsening of the patient's asthma. With irritant-induced or exacerbated work-related asthma, the patient might be able to continue working with lowered exposures and better control of symptoms with medication and not suffer a progression in asthma severity. However, the long-term prognosis for such asthma patients requires additional study (17). Clinical approaches to WEA should include:

- Careful evaluation to ensure that the diagnosis is accurate and is not a misdiagnosis of occupational asthma due to specific sensitizing agents;
- Minimization of exposures triggering exacerbations, preferably through engineering controls;

- Workplace accommodation through job placement away from known triggers in work areas with the least potential exposure to irritants;
- Occasional supplemental use of personal respirators where necessary to protect against unusual conditions. Individuals using respirators must be fit tested and instructed in the use and care of the devices as part of a comprehensive respiratory protection program.
- Referral, as appropriate, to sources of information about relevant social support programs.

CHALLENGES IN STUDYING WEA

Most cross-sectional studies have relied on self reporting to establish WEA status among adults with asthma (7,9–12). With self-reporting goes the opportunity for misclassification due to under- and/or overreporting. Workers with preexisting or quiescent asthma who become sensitized to a new work agent are often erroneously thought to be suffering exacerbations of their preexisting asthma This is not only a challenge in epidemiologic investigations but is also particularly important clinically, as the newly sensitized individuals should be removed from the exposure as quickly as possible.

Some researchers have gone beyond self-reports of WEA. The studies that utilized data from a surveillance program, like SENSOR in the United States (16), or from an asthma clinic, like the study from Ontario, Canada (8), had a more intimate knowledge of the patients, and presumably used that knowledge to judge the veracity of self reports. Another approach was pursued by Milton et al. (18) in a pilot study of new-onset work-related asthma, but it could also be used to investigate WEA. Specifically, the WEA case definition could include both the subject's self report of WEA and the judgment of experts that the subject had experienced occupational exposures that could exacerbate asthma. This would have the advantage of setting a higher standard for WEA case status than has regularly been used in cross-sectional studies.

The need for immediate health care, whether at an emergency department in a hospital, a critical care clinic, or the office of the subject's doctor or increased use of medication are reasonable "objective" indicators of asthma exacerbation. Such visits or medication changes are documented in medical and pharmacy records, eliminating the need to rely on self-reporting alone for the worsening of symptoms. This approach requires access to medical records, which could be monitored prospectively or reviewed retrospectively. There remains the challenge of establishing that conditions at work led to the need for acute care.

Some have suggested that the exacerbation of asthma by workplace exposures might be relatively benign and not contribute to the worsening of the individual's underlying condition (19). One far from benign consequence of WEA is leaving work, either temporarily or permanently. A question about having to leave work due to respiratory health problems has been used in the questionnaires of the European Community Respiratory Health Survey. Moreover, in the province of Ontario in Canada, workers can receive compensation for absences of only a few weeks as the result of WEA. While this endpoint does not directly document an increase in airway inflammation or bronchial hyperresponsiveness, it is easy to collect by questionnaire and is a measure of the impact of occupational exposures on asthma.

With enough clinical data, it would be possible to document that someone with asthma has experienced an increase in airway inflammation or bronchial hyperresponsiveness. This would require repeated clinical follow-up, and also require the determination of whether changes were related to work rather than some other source of harmful exposures. Researchers could also determine the severity level of asthma in patients over time and whether changes were related to workplace exposures.

CLASSIFICATION OF WEA

There have been disagreements within the occupational respiratory research community on how to classify WEA. In an editorial published in 1998, Wagner and Wegman noted that occupational asthma is usually defined "by the specific response to an agent capable of provoking sensitization" (20). They argued that this definition of occupational asthma should be broadened to include "preexisting asthma exacerbated by workplace environmental exposures," noting that this condition can result in significant disability, and that broadening the definition of occupational asthma would motivate prevention. Other researchers, commenting on the editorial, argued that WEA should not be considered as occupational asthma, but should be included in the broader category of work-related asthma (19). The commenting authors justified a more restrictive definition of occupational asthma on the basis of different mechanisms of disease, different medical approaches, and the need to treat the conditions differently in social insurance (workers' compensation) systems. These apparent differences have diminished over time as the diverse mechanisms of asthma initiation and exacerbation are explored. Recognition that WEA is an important source of work disability and a target for prevention is increasing, and the need for social insurance and compensation systems to provide assistance for people with WEA is starting to be addressed.

CONCLUSIONS

Exacerbation of asthma can result from exposures at home, at work, in the outdoor environment, and in public buildings. Asthma-related exposures in the work environment are less frequently addressed, because exposures are often beyond the control of the individual patient and an employer may or may not accept responsibility or have the ability to control exposures. The issue of an affected employee's right to workplace accommodation or compensation further clouds the issue. The incidence of asthma exacerbated at work among employed adults with asthma ranges between 8% and 25%, depending on the epidemiologic criteria utilized. Under specific exposure conditions, an excess cumulative incidence of WEA may be found in certain occupations. Compared to other adults with asthma, workers with WEA on average are older, and in one study this problem was more likely to be found in nonwhites and those with less education and lower incomes. Continued exposure to lower levels of the agents responsible for WEA must be avoided in the same manner as new-onset asthma. However, it is possible that some of these patients may continue working with reduced exposures and adequate use of controller medications without suffering progression of asthma severity, although close monitoring over time is necessary.

Most cross-sectional studies have relied on self-reporting to establish the presence of WEA. However, visits to hospitals, critical care clinics, or the office of the subject's doctor with a need for increased medication are reasonable "objective indicators" of asthma exacerbation. Current research demonstrates that WEA is an important source of work disability and an appropriate target for prevention. Additional outcomes research can help define how to address this problem more effectively.

DIRECTIONS OF FUTURE RESEARCH

- Prospective surveillance of newly hired workers (preferably apprentices) with histories of currently controlled asthma or asthma in remission in workplaces where asthma triggers are likely to be encountered.
- Outcomes in the above studies vis a vis: (i) number and frequency of asthma flares, (ii) the effects of workplace exposure on asthma control or severity— both short term and long term, (iii) the extent of temporary or permanent time lost from work as a result of exposure, (iv) the health consequences of continuing employment at such worksites, (v) the responses to various interventions, and (vi) amount of time required to resolve and reestablish control of asthma.
- Health surveillance programs should fine tune annual incidence data by including a separate category of WEA.
- Further examination of the economic, social (e.g., family), and productivity impact of work-exacerbated and new-onset asthma over time.
- Comparison of the incidence of new onset asthma and WEA in industries before and after introduction of optimal environmental controls.

REFERENCES

1. Fishwick D, Pearce N, D'Souza W, et al. Occupational asthma in New Zealanders: a population based study. Occup Environ Med 1997; 54: 301–306.
2. Kogevinas M, Anto JM, Soriano JB, Tobias A, Burney P. The risk of asthma attributable to occupational exposures: a population-based study in Spain. Am J Respir Crit Care Med 1996; 154:137–143.
3. Bakke PS, Gulsvik A. Work-related asthma: prevalence estimates by sex, age and smoking habits in a community sample. Int J Tuberc Lung Dis 2000; 4:649–656.
4. Chan-Yeung M. Assessment of asthma in the workplace. ACCP consensus statement. Chest 1995; 108:1084–1117.
5. Jajosky RA, Harrison R, Reinisch F, et al. Surveillance of work-related asthma in selected U.S. states using surveillance guidelines for state health departments, California, Massachusetts, Michigan, and New Jersey, 1993–1995. MMWR CDC Surveill Summ 1999; 48(3):1–20.
6. Katz I, Moshe S, Sosna J, Baum GL, Fink G, Shemer J. The occurrence, recrudescence, and worsening of asthma in a population of young adults: impact of varying types of occupation. Chest 1999; 116:614–618.
7. Henneberger PK, Hoffman CD, Magid DJ, Lyons EE. Work-related exacerbation of asthma. Int J Occup Environ Health 2002; 8:291–296.
8. Tarlo SM, Leung K, Broder I, Silverman F, Holness DL. Asthmatic subjects symptomatically worse at work: prevalence and characterization among a general asthma clinic population. Chest 2000; 118:1309–1314.

9. Abramson ML, Kutin JJ, Rosier MJ, Bowes G. Morbidity, medication, and trigger factors in a community sample of adults with asthma. Med J Aust 1995; 162:78–81.
10. Henneberger PK, Deprez RD, Asdigian N, Oliver LC, Derk S, Goe SK. Workplace exacerbation of asthma symptoms: findings from a population-based study in Maine. Arch Environ Health 2003; 58:781–788.
11. Johnson AR, Dimish-Ward HD, Manfreda J, et al. Occupational asthma in adults in six Canadian communities. Am J Respir Crit Care Med 2000; 162:2058–2062.
12. Saarinen K, Karjalainen A, Martikainen R, et al. Prevalence of work-aggravated symptoms in clinically established asthma. Eur Respir J 2003; 22:305–309.
13. Wheeler S, Rosenstock L, Barnhart S. A case series of 71 patients referred to a hospital-based occupational and environmental medicine clinic for occupational asthma. West J Med 1998; 168:98–104.
14. Tarlo SM, Liss G, Corey P, Broder I. A workers' compensation claim population for occupational asthma: comparison of subgroups. Chest 1995; 107:634–641.
15. Chatkin JM, Tarlo SM, Liss G, Banks D, Broder I. The outcome of asthma related to workplace irritant exposures: a comparison of irritant-induced asthma and irritant aggravation of asthma. Chest 1999; 116:1780–1785.
16. Goe SK, Henneberger PK, Reilly MJ, et al. A descriptive study of work-aggravated asthma. Occup Environ Med 2004; 61:512–517.
17. Friedman-Jimenez G, Beckett WS, Szeinuk J, Petsonk EL. Clinical evaluation, management, and prevention of work-related asthma. Am J Ind Med 2000; 37:121–141.
18. Milton DK, Solomon GM, Roseillo RA, Herrick RF. Risk and incidence of asthma attributable to occupational exposure among HMO members. Am J Ind Med 1998; 33:1–10.
19. Malo J-L, Chan-Yeung M. Comment on the editorial. Occupation asthma: prevention by definition. Am J Ind Med 1999; 35:207.
20. Wagner GR, Wegman DH. Occupational asthma: prevention by definition. Am J Ind Med 1998; 33:427–429.

27

Acute Airway Diseases Due to Organic Dust Exposure

Moira Chan-Yeung
Occupational and Environmental Lung Disease Unit, Respiratory Division, Department of Medicine, University of British Columbia and Vancouver General Hospital, Vancouver, British Columbia, Canada

I. Leonard Bernstein
Division of Allergy–Immunology, Department of Internal Medicine, College of Medicine, University of Cincinnati, Cincinnati, Ohio, U.S.A.

Susanna Von Essen
Pulmonary and Critical Care Medicine Section, Department of Internal Medicine, University of Nebraska Medical Center, Omaha, Nebraska, U.S.A.

Jaspal Singh
Department of Medicine, Duke University Medical Center, Durham, North Carolina, U.S.A.

David A. Schwartz
Duke University Medical Center and Durham Department of Veterans Affairs Medical Center, Durham, North Carolina, U.S.A.

INTRODUCTION

A number of agents in agricultural environments have been shown to give rise to asthma-like syndromes. The term "asthma-like syndrome" has been used to describe an acute nonallergic airway response arising from inhalation of various agents in the agricultural environment characterized by symptoms of chest tightness, wheeze, and/or dyspnea, which may or may not be associated with cross-shift decline in forced expiratory volume in one second (FEV_1) (usually less than 10%), which is dose related, and evidence of acute neutrophilic airway inflammation. As symptoms may occur on first exposure and specific antigens and antibodies have not been identified, the syndrome is likely to be an inflammatory response to exposure and not an allergic reaction.

Of the organic dusts, cotton dust, grain dust, and swine confinement exposure have been studied more extensively. Acute respiratory symptoms and cross-shift declines in FEV_1 have also been described among poultry workers (chicken catchers), slaughterhouse workers, garbage handlers, and poultry farmers who are exposed to a number of airborne contaminants, including mixtures of organic poultry dust, skin debris, feathers, insect parts, aerosolized feed, and poultry excreta as well as a variety of viable bacteria and gram-negative bacterial endotoxin.

In this chapter we discuss asthma-like syndromes in workers exposed to cotton dust, grain dust, and swine confinement facilities, and the evidence that endotoxin, an agent common to all these working environments, is at least partially responsible for the syndrome. In both cotton and grain dust exposures, acute airflow obstruction may lead to irreversible airflow obstruction in some workers.

COTTON AND OTHER TEXTILE DUSTS

Byssinosis is a generic term applied to acute and chronic airway disease among those occupationally exposed to vegetable dust arising from the processing of cotton, flax, hemp, jute, and possibly other textile fibers. Observations regarding respiratory disease attributable to these vegetable dusts date to the early 18th century (1).

Today the production of cotton products is equally commercially important to developed and developing countries. Industries pertaining to processing of flax and hemp remain regionally important, which continue to provide traditional textile products. Thus, millions of workers are occupationally exposed to these vegetable dusts worldwide. In the United States more than 300,000 workers are directly exposed to cotton dust, primarily in the textile industry, but also in cotton ginning, cotton warehousing and compressing, cotton classing offices, cottonseed oil and delinting mills, bedding and batting manufacturing, and utilization of waste cotton for a wide variety of products.

Two febrile syndromes characterized by fever, cough, and other constitutional symptoms including headache and malaise are also associated with byssinosis and textile manufacturing. These occur most frequently with exposure to low-grade, spotted cotton. Mattress-maker's fever and weaver's cough may be considered together because of their characteristically high attack rate and probable similar etiology. Mill fever, which is characterized by fever, malaise, myalgia, fatigue, and often cough, was a common complaint among workers first exposed to high levels of these vegetable dusts; with the prevailing cotton dust levels in the western world it now rarely occurs. These febrile syndromes are similar to other febrile syndromes described among agricultural workers exposed to high levels of contaminated vegetable dusts.

It is now clear that symptoms typical of byssinosis are observed among others occupationally exposed to vegetable dusts. Many of those exposed are employed in agriculture, which typically involves daily exposure, rather than the cyclical workweek exposure of textile workers. It is also clear that exposure to organic dusts in textile and nontextile operations will often result in asthma-like symptoms. This often results in self-selection or transfer of the affected worker out of dusty jobs or entirely out of the industry. Now there is also evidence that exposure to textile dusts results in heightened airway reactivity and that atopy is a risk factor for the development of vegetable dust–induced bronchoconstriction (2). These observations are likely to become more relevant with regulation of cotton dust to lower levels. This may allow toleration of lower exposure to cotton dust by many of those who were previously selected out of these industries because of asthma, thereby resulting in increased risk to the development of chronic airway disease.

Epidemiology

The term byssinosis was first used by Proust (3) in 1877 to describe respiratory disease among textile workers. It arises from the Latin word, byssus, which means fine and valuable textile fiber known to the ancients, usually referring to flax, but also cotton, silk, and other natural textile fibers. Although Ramazzini was the first to describe asthma and chronic respiratory disease arising from the processing of textiles, there are abundant important historical descriptions about respiratory disease among textile workers. These were variously described as tracheal phthisis, spinner's phthisis, cotton pneumonia, stripper's asthma, or stripper's and grinder's asthma. The first description of the symptom pattern now associated with byssinosis, that is, respiratory symptoms most severe at the start of the working week, was given in 1845 by Mareska and Heyman:

"All the workers have told us that the dust bothered them much less on the last days of the week than on the Monday and Tuesday. The masters find the cause of this increased sensitivity to be in the excesses of the Sunday, but the workers never fail to attribute it to the interruption of work which, they say, makes them lose, in part, their habituation to the dust" (4).

The British Home Office established a Departmental Committee on Dust in Card Rooms in the Cotton Industry (5), which in its 1932 report described the disease as respiratory in nature with three stages: (i) the stage of irritation, characterized by "a cough and tight feeling in the chest. This is usually temporary, passing off in one or two days, but the susceptibility returns during a short absence from work, such as at the weekend." This stage developed after approximately five years of exposure to cotton dust in the opening and cardroom areas and entirely disappeared on removal from a dusty atmosphere; (ii) the state of temporary disablement or incapacity, which is described as the one that occurs after being "exposed to the dust for some 10 or more years" where the worker "suffers from early bronchitis or asthma, or both, associated with cough and mucous expectoration. This condition may lead in time to partial incapacity"; and (iii) the stage of total disablement or incapacity: In this advanced stage there is chronic bronchitis, with emphysema. Cough is present with mucous or mucopurulent expectoration and shortness of breath on exertion. This condition is incurable, and at this stage work in the dusty atmosphere becomes impossible, but improvement may take place and further progress of the disease may be arrested or retarded by removal from the dusty environment of the cardroom. In the final stage of the malady the continued strain on the right side of the heart is apt to lead ultimately to cardiac failure (5).

Contemporary studies about cotton textile workers' mortality have not revealed consistent excesses in overall mortality. Assessment of respiratory mortality has been difficult to determine because of a lack of adequate work history data and lack of smoking histories. Enterline and Kendrick studied 6281 white male cotton textile workers employed in Georgia mills (6). They found an overall mortality similar to that of asbestos building product and asbestos friction material workers but less than that of asbestos textile workers. There was no evidence of excess respiratory deaths among all cotton workers when cause-specific rates were compared to U.S. white male mortality rates. There was, however, an increase in cardiovascular and all causes of death with increasing duration of exposure. Of interest was a deficit in lung cancer deaths that led Enterline to suggest that there may be a cancer inhibitor, possibly endotoxin, in cotton dust (7). Recent studies of lung cancer in China have confirmed significantly less lung cancer among cotton textile workers after controlling for smoking (8). While methodologic factors were considered, these authors concluded that their findings are consistent with Enterline's hypothesis that some tumor-inhibiting factor(s) may be present in dusts from cotton and other vegetable fibers.

Early morbidity studies of cotton and flax workers found an unusually high prevalence of respiratory disease, particularly among those working in high–dust exposure areas (4,9,10). In Great Britain, byssinosis was made a compensable disease in 1942 and, on the basis of the number of cases compensated, was thought to be a disappearing disease. Schilling and Goodman rediscovered byssinosis when they studied Lancashire mills to investigate an apparent increase in cardiovascular mortality (11,12). In a series of studies extending over a 10-year period, Schilling contributed significantly to our understanding of the epidemiology of respiratory diseases among textile workers. He developed, and tested for reliability and validity, a series of questions that were added to the British Medical Research Council (BMRC) respiratory questionnaire, which provided the basis for his byssinosis grading scheme (Table 1) (13).

Schilling's questionnaire and grading scheme has been the standard for worldwide epidemiologic studies of workers exposed to textile and other vegetable dusts. To validate the grading scheme, he demonstrated that cotton workers with increasing grades of byssinosis have corresponding increases in airway obstruction. Together with Roach, he was the first to quantify a strong linear dose–response relationship between total and respirable cotton dust and the prevalence of byssinosis, which largely explained differences in prevalence in various mill work areas (14). He was also the first to report that smoking was an important risk factor in determining byssinosis prevalence (12,13).

However Schilling's clinical grading does have deficiencies, in that it does not take into account either the irritant effects of dust exposure or the lung function changes which may occur in asymptomatic workers. To address these deficiencies a new classification has been proposed (Table 2) (15).

Since Schilling's publications, similar findings have been reported among textile workers from many countries around the world. Recent studies confirm the presence of byssinosis, but especially nonspecific respiratory symptoms and associated lung function abnormalities among Chinese cotton textile workers (16,17). While byssinosis is now much less prevalent, it is still found among Lancashire cotton textile workers (18) and flax workers in Normandy, France (19). In addition to those exposed in primary textile mill operations, the disease has been reported among cotton ginners (20,21), cottonseed oil and delinting workers (20,22), workers in waste cotton operations (23), those in garneting (bedding and batting operations) (24), and those processing soft hemp (25,26) and flax (27–30). Byssinosis has not been typically found among those processing "hard" fibers of sisal or jute (31,32). However, one study reported typical byssinosis among Tanzanian sisal workers with very high–dust exposure (33) and studies in a few jute mills in India reported objective changes consistent with byssinosis in a considerable number of exposed workers

Table 1 Byssinosis Grading Scheme

Grade 0	No symptoms of chest tightness or breathlessness on Mondays
Grade 1/2	Occasional chest tightness on Mondays, or mild symptoms such as irritation (cough) of the respiratory tract on Mondays
Grade 1	Chest tightness and/or breathlessness on Mondays only
Grade 2	Chest tightness and/or breathlessness on Mondays and other workdays

Table 2 New Grading System of Byssinosis

Classification	Symptoms
Grade 0	No symptoms
Byssinosis	
Grade B1	Chest tightness and/or SOB on most of first day back at work
Grade B2	Chest tightness and/or SOB on the first and other days of the working week
Respiratory tract irritation	
Grade RTI 1	Cough associated with dust exposure
Grade RTI 2	Persistent phlegm (i.e., on most days during three months of the year) initiated or exacerbated by dust exposure
Grade RT1 3	Persistent phlegm initiated or made worse by dust exposure either with exacerbations of chest illness or persisting for 2 yrs or more
Lung function	
Acute changes	
No effect	A consistent[a] decline in FEV_1 of less than 5% or an increase in FEV_1 during the work shift
Mild effect	A consistent[a] decline of between 5% and 10% in FEV_1 during the work shift
Moderate effect	A consistent[a] decline between 10% and 20% in FEV_1 during the work shift
Severe effect	A decline of 20% or more in FEV_1 during the work shift
Chronic changes	
No effect	FEV_1[b] 80% of predicted value[c]
Mild to moderate effect	FEV_1 60–79% of predicted value[c]
Severe effect	FEV_1[b] less than 60% of predicted value[c]

[a]A decline occurring in at least three consecutive tests made after an absence from dust exposure of two days or more.
[b]Predicted values should be based on data obtained from local populations or similar ethnic and social class groups.
[c]By a preshift test after an absence from dust exposure of two days or more.
Abbreviations: FEV_1, forced expiratory volume in one second; SOB, shortness of breath.

(34). In addition, symptoms consistent with byssinosis have been reported among workers exposed to herbal tea processing and among workers engaged in swine confinement housing operations (35,36).

Several investigations (21,29,37–40) have now confirmed, with remarkable uniformity, Schilling's early dose–response findings, despite differences in dose-measurement technique, study population composition, and source of raw product. More recent studies have demonstrated that reliance on total dust measurement may provide a misleading indication of risk, as much of the mass may be composed of cotton lint (41).

In the United States, measurement of inhalable dust (less than 15 u in aerodynamic diameter) has proven to be a reliable and valid dust measurement for assessment of vegetable dust dose–response (42). Most of these studies have concentrated on preparation and on yarn-production workers, with little attention given to weavers and others exposed to cotton dust. One study examined both preparation and yarn processors, who were found to have similar dose–response relationships, and weavers, who were found to have a quantitatively different dose–response

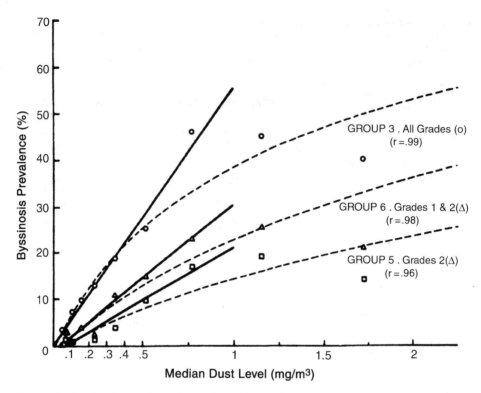

Figure 1 Byssinosis prevalence by grade and by median dust level among cotton preparation and yarn area workers: linear regressions and fitted probit dose-response curves.

relationship (Fig. 1) (42). Studies of changes in lung function over a Monday working shift have provided objective data on dose-related declines in FEV_1, which were consistent with the dose–response relationships based on byssinosis prevalence (42). Based on these data, a permissible exposure limit for exposure to raw cotton dust has been promulgated by the U.S. Department of Labor: for preparation and yarn operations, a time-weighted concentration of $0.2\,mg/m^3$ of air, and for weavers, $0.75\,mg/m^3$ of air (43).

In the United Kingdom a different approach was taken. In a study comparing work area and personal sampling techniques, a 7.8-fold difference in measurement between the two techniques was found in the earliest cotton spinning processes, falling to a ratio of 1.4 in ring spinning. This suggested that work area sampling may underestimate an individual's exposure in the earlier processes where byssinosis is most prevalent. This work has led to the introduction of a new cotton exposure standard in the United Kingdom, based on a personal sampling technique (44).

Dose–response data are less available for cotton dust exposures outside the cotton textile industry, but there is evidence of a dose–response relationship for other cotton operations and for processing of flax and hemp (45,46). Based on all available data, the World Health Organization has recommended limits for several of these exposures (47).

Assessment of chronic cough and phlegm, as defined from the BMRC respiratory questionnaire, has been an integral part of most epidemiologic studies of cotton, hemp, and flax textile workers (48). While not a uniform observation, most surveys have reported increased rates of chronic cough and phlegm among those with heavy cotton dust exposure, especially among those with symptoms of byssinosis (49,50). Similarly, indices of dyspnea, as assessed by the BMRC questionnaire, have been shown to be strongly associated with dustier exposures and have been found to be increased among those with more severe grades of byssinosis (25,26,28,46). As with many other epidemiologic studies of respiratory disease, smoking has been found to be a powerful risk factor for chronic cough and phlegm and for measures of dyspnea (42,51).

Two major effects of vegetable dust on lung function have been reported in epidemiologic studies. The first is a chronic effect characterized by airway obstruction and manifested by reductions in FEV_1, forced vital capacity (FVC), and FEV_1/FVC with increased dust concentration and duration of exposure. The second is an acute effect characterized by measures demonstrating bronchoconstriction over a working shift of exposure to cotton dust, especially after an absence from exposure for two or more days (Fig. 2) (52,53). Spirometric evaluation, typically conducted prior to the Monday shift in Western countries, has confirmed Schilling's observation that those with symptoms of byssinosis, as a group, may be expected to have lower expiratory flow rates than comparable controls. Furthermore, those with chronic cough and phlegm, in addition to symptoms of chest tightness, have been found to have a further decrease in lung function (49–51,54). In large cross-sectional studies, smoking has also been found to exert a significant additive decrease in preshift lung function (41,42,55). Studies by Schacter et al. (56) suggest that smoking may be more related to abnormalities in maximum expiratory flows at 50% and 25%, whereas cotton dust appears to be either more important or as important as the smoking effect on FVC and FEV_1 among cotton textile workers with long exposures.

McKerrow et al. (57) were the first to observe a reduction in expiratory flow rates over a work shift, a reduction that was most marked after an absence from

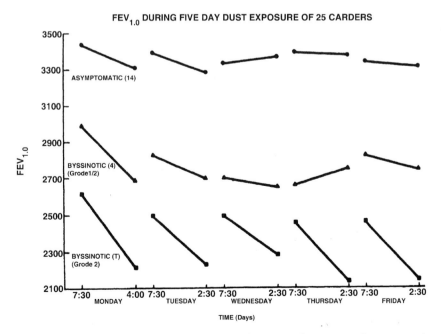

Figure 2 Pattern of response among 25 cardroom workers exposed to cotton dust.

exposure and especially among workers in areas with higher dust levels. From these observations they suggested that symptoms of Monday chest tightness and dyspnea might be explained by the reduction in expiratory flow rate. This hypothesis has been questioned, as many with symptoms of byssinosis do not exhibit work shift decrements and because the degree of reduction, although statistically significant in epidemiologic studies, is typically not considered clinically significant (decrement of 10% or more) (58).

It has been further observed that subjects with bronchitis and byssinosis tend to have greater cross-shift decrements in expiratory flow than those with byssinosis alone (51,54). On the basis of the epidemiologic association between byssinosis grade and mean decrement in expiratory flow, Bouhuys et al. (59) proposed a functional grading scheme. Subsequent reports have shown that the relationship between a Monday decline in FEV_1 of 200 cc, as proposed by Bouhuys, is highly variable. An appreciable proportion of those without symptoms of byssinosis have a Monday decrement of greater than 200 cc or 5%, whereas many with byssinosis symptoms do not show even a modest decline (49,60). Nevertheless, because expiratory flow can be easily measured in untrained subjects and provides an objective indicator of biologic effect to vegetable dusts, spirometry before and following exposure has been widely used in epidemiologic studies. Those exposed to cotton, soft hemp, and flax dusts usually have greater decrements in expiratory flow than those exposed to similar dust levels from "hard fibers" (45,46). Those exposed at higher dust levels have been found to show more marked decrements, and the dose–response relationship between respirable dust and decrement in flow rates approximates that for byssinosis symptoms (21,24,42).

In a series of experimental cardroom studies utilizing volunteer subjects exposed to a wide variety of cottons at different levels of dust exposure, Castellan et al. (61,62) have demonstrated a stronger dose–response relationship between vertically elutriated endotoxin than vertically elutriated dust and have concluded that these observations strongly support the hypothesis that endotoxin plays a causative role in the acute pulmonary response to cotton dust. As the volunteer subjects were not textile workers, these investigators were unable to assess the pattern of symptoms characteristic of byssinosis. Kennedy et al. (63) in a dose–response study in Shanghai, reported a significant association with current endotoxin level and the prevalence of byssinosis and chronic bronchitis, but not with dust alone. While smoking clearly affects baseline spirometric levels, there is conflicting evidence regarding the influence of smoking on acute changes in lung function (49,53,63). Cross-shift decline in FEV_1 remains a very useful epidemiologic tool, and despite its limitations in its application to individual workers, it has been incorporated as one feature of the medical surveillance examinations required by the U.S. Cotton Dust Standard (43).

Several studies have evaluated lung function prospectively (2,39,64–67). In each of these studies, conclusions were necessarily based upon survivor populations and include other selection biases, which usually tend to minimize occupational effects. Prospective assessments of decline in lung function have been carried out on workers exposed to high levels of cotton dust in Yugoslavia, India, and China, all of which demonstrated accelerated mean annual declines in FEV_1, which were associated with higher dust exposures that were several times higher than the U.S. Cotton Dust Standard (68–70). Berry et al. (65) reported roughly twice the annual decline in FEV_1 among cotton textile workers as among synthetic textile workers. The decline attributable to cotton dust was slightly greater, but similar in magnitude, to that attributable to smoking, and was somewhat greater among those working in dustier areas and among those exposed for shorter periods of time than longer periods. Merchant et al. (39), who studied a single cotton textile mill several times over a single year, found that those exposed to high levels of cotton dust (many of whom were new employees) had 10-month declines as high as 280 cc, and that smaller dose-related increased 10-month declines in FEV_1 occurred among workers in three other work areas with less dust exposure and longer tenure. A community study of active and retired older cotton textile workers found cotton textile workers to have a higher prevalence and attack rate of respiratory symptoms than controls, and that both men and women cotton textile workers had greater annual declines than did community controls. This study confirmed the cross-sectional assessment of this community and reported a significantly higher proportion of textile workers than nontextile worker controls to be severely impaired (55,64).

In the first published prospective study of lung function among cotton textile workers exposed at or below the U.S. Cotton Dust Standard, Glindmeyer et al. (66) found no accelerated decline in FEV_1 among slashers and weavers exposed below the cotton dust standard and no accelerated decline among nonsmoking yarn-processing workers exposed at the cotton dust standard. However, smoking yarn-processing workers were found to have accelerated loss in annual FEV_1, even below the cotton dust standard of $0.2 \, mg/m^3$; dose-related increases in decline in annual FEV_1 were observed among men and women smokers and nonsmokers, thereby unambiguously confirming the dose–response findings from the cross-sectional studies of byssinosis prevalence and cross-shift decline in FEV_1 on which the U.S. Cotton Dust Standard was based (37,43). While these aggregate data support the hypothesis that those with increased acute responses are at increased risk for increased declines in lung function over time, as suggested by Bouhuys (26,69,71), this question is not fully resolved.

Clinical Evaluation

Signs and Symptoms

The hallmark of byssinosis is the characteristic symptom of chest tightness that typically occurs following a weekend away from exposure. Chest tightness is described by workers, often accompanied by placing a hand over their chest, as a heaviness on their chest, as chest congestion, as difficulty taking a deep breath, and sometimes as a band-like feeling around their chest. The onset of chest tightness is variable, as noted in the British Home Office report which described the symptoms in 100 cardroom workers, 93% of whom described respiratory symptoms (5). Of these, 59% experienced their most severe symptoms during the first half of the working shift and 41% during the second half of the shift. In all workers, symptoms were most severe on the first day of the working week. This time period is important as it distinguishes byssinosis from occupational asthma, which tends to increase in severity over the working week. Affected workers often compare the feeling of chest tightness to that of a chest cold. Frequently chest tightness is accompanied by a cough, which is more prominent on Monday. Indeed, a Monday cough may be the only symptom. A history of chronic productive cough is frequently obtained. Among older workers who have been exposed to cotton dust for many years, a history of exertional dyspnea is a common finding. Among those severely affected, chest tightness and dyspnea occur on all workdays, with relief coming only on weekends and holidays, if then.

All of these symptoms become more severe if the period away from cotton dust exposure is prolonged, i.e., the affected individual appears to lose exposure tolerance. Conversely, Monday symptoms do not occur if exposure occurs seven days a week, as often occur with cotton ginning. Symptoms are more severe and more frequent among smokers (39,40). Occasionally, a worker with typical byssinosis will report that symptoms of Monday chest tightness disappeared when he or she stopped smoking without an apparent change in dust exposure (51).

There are no typical or characteristic signs found upon physical examination of workers with symptoms of byssinosis. While the symptomatic worker frequently exhibits a productive cough, on examination the chest is usually relatively quiet. Wheezing is not commonly found early in the course of the disease. Among those severely affected, all the physical findings of advanced chronic airflow limitation may be observed.

A number of nonspecific symptoms are observed among those exposed to cotton dust, apart from byssinosis. Work-related ocular and nasal irritation are now the most common symptoms complained of in U.K. textile mills (72). In this study of 1452 textile workers, 17.5% of cotton workers complained of eye irritation and 11% of nasal irritation. There was no relationship between these symptoms and atopy, byssinosis, or dust concentration, suggesting the presence of unidentified agents in textile dusts which are unrelated to the concentration of dust. Chronic bronchitis was first documented in cotton textile workers by Molyneux and Tombleson (60) in 1970. Even at the dust exposure levels currently prevailing in Lancashire textile mills an excess of chronic bronchitis is still demonstrable. A study of 2991 cotton and synthetic textile workers reported a prevalence of chronic bronchitis of 6.9% in cotton workers and 4.5% in synthetic fiber workers (73). After controlling for smoking, cotton workers were significantly more likely to suffer from chronic bronchitis. This was most marked in workers over 45 years of age and was significantly associated with cumulative cotton dust exposure. In the cotton population the presence of chronic bronchitis was associated with a small, significant decrement in lung function when symptomatic workers were compared to age, sex and smoking matched asymptomatic workers. In a recent 15-year follow-up study on Chinese cotton textile workers compared to silk workers, long-term exposure to cotton dust was associated with occurrence of byssinosis manifested by chest tightness, chronic cough, dyspnea, and chronic bronchitis (67).

Febrile syndromes that have been associated with cotton processing include mattress maker's fever and weaver's cough. These conditions occur among experienced workers and are characterized by a high attack rate, a clear-cut febrile episode, severe cough, and dyspnea. Most of these outbreaks have been attributed to mildewed yarn. These febrile syndromes are similar to those common among agricultural workers who are frequently exposed to high concentrations of moldy grain, hay, or silage (74–77). Because the clinical presentation is the same, and because the etiology of all of these febrile syndromes is probably from microorganism toxins, the term organic dust toxic syndrome (ODTS) has recently been suggested in an attempt to codify this condition (see Chapter 29) (78). It is likely that the febrile syndromes arising from high levels of cotton or grain dust are also attributable to endotoxins, which are now well-known constituents of these vegetable dusts.

Newly hired workers, and those who first go into dusty cotton-processing areas for a period of a few hours, may experience mill fever (79), which has also been called cardroom fever, dust chills, dust fever, cotton cold, cotton fever, weaver's fever, and, among flax workers, heckling fever (80). A similar syndrome has been described among those exposed to high concentrations of grain dust (78). Symptoms, which typically occur 8 to 12 hours following heavy dust exposure, consist of chills, headache, thirst, malaise, sweating, nausea, which may be accompanied by vomiting, and a transient fever, followed by fatigue. Without further exposure, these symptoms subside spontaneously within a day or two, but the fatigue may continue for several days. With repeated exposure, such as that experienced by a newly hired textile worker, these symptoms may occur for several days until the worker is "seasoned" or develops a tolerance (79). This "seasoning" is well recognized by workers exposed to high–dust concentrations.

Another common complaint of new workers or visitors to mills with high exposures to cotton dust is tobacco intolerance (51). Also a common finding among mill visitors who have a history of asthma, and who may not have had an asthma attack for years, is immediate onset of clinical asthma, which may be severe and often requires medical intervention (74). With the improved dust control achieved through implementation of the Cotton Dust Standard, mill fever and tobacco intolerance are now infrequent observations. However, it has been suggested that better dust control may allow many more workers with airway hyperresponsiveness to remain in vegetable dust-processing operations and that these workers may constitute a high-risk group for future development of airway obstruction (81).

Treatment

Research on medical treatment for byssinosis has been confined to acute events. Clinical trials have relied almost exclusively on changes in flow rates among active workers as the indicators of effect. While propranolol has been shown to increase bronchoconstriction with hemp dust exposure, antihistamines and ascorbic acid have been found to protect against this effect (82,83). Similarly, inhaled bronchodilators (salbutamol, isoprenaline, and orciprenaline) will prevent or reverse flow rate changes (82–84). Finally, pre-exposure treatment with cromolyn sodium tends to block bronchoconstriction (82–84). Inhaled beclomethasone also appears to reduce the flow rate response to cotton dust exposure (84). It must be emphasized that these beneficial physiologic effects occur without similar documentation in regard to symptoms. Thus, while the bronchoconstricting effect of these organic dusts, which is usually not severe, may be blocked or reversed, there is no evidence that use of these drugs will necessarily suppress byssinosis symptoms or retard the progression of cotton dust–induced obstructive airway disease. Therefore, these drugs cannot be considered as preventive measures. Management of severe cases of byssinosis does not differ from that for chronic bronchitis and emphysema.

Pathology

Schilling and Goodman (11) reviewed pathologic observations on lungs of workers with long cotton dust exposure, as made by several early investigators, and concluded that the pulmonary pathology was that of chronic bronchitis and emphysema. In one report lungs were fixed in inflation from 10 autopsies of workers with over 20 years of cotton dust exposure. Nine of these cases were found to have chronic bronchitis and/or emphysema, which was more marked among those working in high–dust exposure areas. These five and two others had evidence of right ventricular hypertrophy, and four of these cases were judged to have died of cor pulmonale. Gough and Woodcock described lungs of cotton textile workers with histories of byssinosis as having inflammation of the bronchi with squamous metaplasia and generalized emphysema, which was somewhat more prominent in proximity to dust deposits (11).

Three more recent studies of lung pathology in cotton textile workers have been reported (85–87). Edwards et al. (85) studied lungs from 43 patients who had long exposures to cotton dust and had been receiving industrial benefits for byssinosis. The lungs were distended with formalin at necropsy. Gross examination revealed 27 (63%) with no significant emphysema, 10 (23%) with varying degrees of centrilobular emphysema, and 6 (14%) with panacinar emphysema. Most cases showed heavy black dust pigmentation, often associated with centrilobular dilation of distal airspaces. There was, however, significantly more mucous gland hyperplasia and hypertrophy of smooth muscle in the upper and lower lobar bronchi and significantly less connective tissue and cartilage in cases than in controls. While the authors suggested that both smoking (17 cases) and air pollution from living in the Lancashire region could have contributed to these pathologic lesions, this study did not assess these possible risk factors.

Pratt et al. (86) studied lungs fixed in inflation from 44 textile workers and 521 nontextile workers. Their study had the advantage of using lungs properly prepared for evaluation of emphysema and knowledge of smoking status. It was limited, however, by lack of documentation of cotton dust exposure, the extent of that exposure, and the small numbers of nonsmoking textile workers (eight cases). Nevertheless, significantly more mucous gland hyperplasia and goblet cell metaplasia were found among textile workers. Centrilobular emphysema was slightly, but insignificantly, increased among textile workers. Moran, who conducted a study of cotton textile workers over an 18-year period, reported an odds ratio of 2.2 for emphysema among active and highly exposed cotton textile workers compared to a group of noncotton workers (87). The results of this study suggested that there may be a shift to an earlier age of onset of emphysema among certain exposed cotton textile workers, but details regarding specific cotton dust and smoking exposures were not available. Of relevance to the question of emphysema among cotton textile workers is a recent animal model of intratracheally instilled cotton dust endotoxin in hamsters. This revealed both functional and morphologic evidence of mild emphysematous lesions (88).

In summary, the available pathologic data consistently find evidence of considerably more airway disease (both large and small airway lesions of chronic bronchitis), while the data regarding emphysema are incomplete. There appears to be historical evidence for the existence of emphysema and some recent clinical and animal morphologic evidence for an increase in emphysema among those with heavy cotton dust exposure. An autopsy study of a larger number of cotton textile workers with well-documented occupational and smoking histories is needed to resolve this issue.

Etiology

Although there is consensus that some component(s) of the cotton plant, or an associated plant contaminant, is responsible for the acute symptoms of byssinosis, a single causal etiology has not yet been fully established. Etiologic hypotheses have focused on plant-derived materials chiefly in the bract (the fine leaves below the cotton boll) or contaminating microorganisms and/or their constituents (chiefly gram-negative–derived bacterial endotoxin). Both in vivo and in vitro investigations with water-soluble extracts from cotton bracts have revealed their ability to cause both acute airways obstruction and inflammation. Early experiments with water-soluble cotton bract extracts (CBE) suggested that biologic activity induced by such substances were similar to histamine itself or an intermediate substance causing histamine release (89). As research in this area progressed, a number of other pharmacologic smooth muscle agonists were isolated from various types of CBE. These include agonists having properties similar to 5-hydroxytryptamine, prostaglandins, thromboxane, and acetylcholine. Of these substances, the 5-hydroxytryptamine–like agonist had the most potent effects (90). It was found primarily in presenescent cotton extracts as well as standard cotton dust extracts prepared for research purposes. Research about smooth muscle agonist substances in CBE has also raised the possibility that such substances could work as primary releaser agonists on a variety of human cells and therefore indirectly cause release of 5-hydroxytryptamine, thromboxane, histamine, and various leukotrienes. The latter hypothesis has yet to be proven. Several nonwater-soluble substances have also been purported to contract smooth muscle and act as proinflammatory agents. These include tannins, terpenoid aldehydes, and the phytoalexin, lacinilene C methylester (LCME) (91). These lipid-soluble materials stimulate recruitment of polymorphonuclear leukocytes to the airways in experimental animals. In addition, LCME also has been shown to have potent smooth muscle-contracting properties that are slow to develop but result in very strong contractility. β-1,3 Glucan, a component of fungal cell walls, is also found in cotton dust (92) and has been reported to have biological activity on alveolar macrophages (93). However exposure experiments in guinea pigs and mice have failed to show evidence of airway inflammation (94).

The role of endotoxin in the pathogenesis of byssinosis will be discussed in the section on endotoxin.

Prevention

Given our current state of knowledge regarding the etiology of byssinosis and the lack of practical biological assays, risk assessment depends on measurement of dust concentrations, and prevention depends largely on dust control in the workplace (95). Significant improvements in exhaust ventilation and in dust control technology and application have resulted in reduced risk in most areas of textile mills in the United States. A second control technology, which appears promising in experimental studies, is cotton washing (53). Although this preprocessing has been found to reduce symptoms and functional changes among experimentally exposed subjects (largely through removal of fine dust), it is not yet clear whether cotton washing will be technically feasible prior to spinning. It is recognized to be efficacious for certain cotton products (medicinal cotton and cotton batting) that do not require spinning and is so recognized by the U.S. Cotton Dust Standard (43). A recent report that bactericidal treatments of opened cotton capsules with benzododecinium are effective in reducing endotoxin content has not yet been applied in a clinically relevant situation (96).

While dust control is the foundation of a respiratory disease prevention program in the cotton-processing industries, medical surveillance and employee education also play important roles. Smoking and the interaction between smoking and cotton dust exposure are clearly important risk factors in byssinosis and chronic lung disease arising from cotton dust exposure. Therefore, it is essential that information regarding the adverse effects of smoking, and the combined effects of smoking and cotton dust exposure, be made available to workers through employee education and smoking cessation programs. Workers who continue to smoke should be placed in low dust exposure areas (41,65). It is also essential to stress the use of appropriate work practices to reduce dust exposure. Periodic medical examinations designed to detect those acutely affected and those with chronic lung disease are important and can be effective (65). Through the use of a standard questionnaire, it is possible to ascertain a sound occupational and smoking history and to screen for byssinosis, bronchitis, dyspnea, and other common medical conditions. Simple, routine spirometry will identify many of those acutely affected and should detect all with significant impairment.

All of these prevention provisions—allowable dust concentrations, work practices, and medical surveillance—are detailed in the Department of Labor Cotton Dust Standard promulgated in 1978 (42). With the four-year grace period given the industry to implement all provisions, this standard has now been in place for 15 years. Evaluation of the efficacy of the standard has been examined by Glindmeyer et al. (65) who found that the standard provided protection from progressive declines in lung function for all of those working in slashing and weaving areas and for all yarn-processing workers, except for smokers, who still showed progressive losses in lung function below the $0.2 \, mg/m^3$ standard. This finding, which is consistent with previous cross-sectional and prospective studies of smoking cotton textile workers, points up the importance of medical surveillance and appropriate placement of smoking textile workers, but raises the possibility that dust levels may need to be further controlled to protect this sector of the workforce.

GRAIN DUST

It has been known for a long time that exposure to grain dust is harmful to the lungs. Ramazzini (97) in 1713 described a disease among "sifters and measurers of grain" which led to dyspnea and early death. In North America there are several million farmers, about 250,000 grain elevator workers, 50,000 people engaged in grain milling and baking, and an unknown number of workers in feedmills and dockworkers loading and unloading grain. These individuals are at risk of exposure to grain dust and flour dust. Grain is processed in three different types of elevators, country, terminal, and transfer. The process is basically the same in each type of elevator: receiving, grading, weighing, transferring, binning, drying, cleaning, and shipping. Country elevators store and clean grain trucked to them by farmers before being shipped to terminal elevators or local mills. Most country elevators are manned by one or two workers and are not ventilated. Dust levels in these elevators are high (98). Terminal elevators process grain from country elevators, clean, grade, and store grain before shipping to other parts of the country or for export. Transfer elevators do not process grain although they resemble terminal elevators in other respects.

Grain dust is generated by the abrasion of kernels when grain is being handled. It has been estimated that when passing through a typical elevator, each ton of grain handled generates three to four pounds of dust (98). Levels of dust in elevators are influenced by the type of grain handled, the degree of activity, the extent of enclosure at transfer points when grain falls freely from one conveying system to another, the efficiency and upkeep of exhaust ventilation provided at transfer points, and work and housekeeping practices (98).

Characteristics of Grain Dust

The physical and chemical compositions of grain dust vary depending on the geographic site, the type of grain, the wetness of the season, storage temperature, and many other factors. The major components of grain dust include fractured grain kernels, fractured weed seeds, husks, storage mites, insects, bacteria, molds, and chemicals such as pesticides and insecticides and silica.

All types of grain dust contain husk or pericarp fragments in addition to respirable particles. Scanning electron microscopy has shown that each type of dust consists of a distinct assortment of particles. Small husk fragments and "trichome-like" objects are common (99). Many grain workers complain that their respiratory symptoms are worse when they handle barley and oats. These two types of grain dust contain many fine needle-like fragments compared to other types of grain dust.

The microflora of grain dust changes during the process of harvesting and storage. During harvest, many fungi produce spores that become airborne in large quantities. *Cladosporium* and *Alternaria* are found in all samples of harvester dust (100). Once the grain is placed in storage, the microflora changes depending on the water content, the degree of spontaneous heating and the aeration of the grain bulk. The predominant fungus is *Ustilago* but *Cladosporium* and *Alternaria* are also found.

Storage mites of genera *Glycyphagus*, *Tyrophagus*, *Acarus*, and *Goheiria* are found in grain dust (101). The number of mites in grain dust is directly related to the water content of the dust. Particles from weevils, insects, rodents, birds, and their excreta are also found in grain dust. In addition, grain workers are also exposed to herbicides, aluminum phosphide, and other types of pesticides such as malathion. The pathogenic role of these various components of grain dust on respiratory health of grain workers is not known.

Pathogenic Mechanisms of Acute Bronchoconstriction from Grain Dust Exposure

There are two possible mechanisms for grain dust to induce acute airway disease: by sensitization to one of its components or by direct airway injury leading to inflammation from one of the toxins contaminating the dust.

Allergen-Induced Airflow Obstruction or Grain Dust Asthma

Grain dust asthma has been described by several investigators (102–106). These cases were documented by specific challenge tests with either crude grain dust or grain dust extract. Immediate, late, and biphasic asthmatic responses have been described. Systemic responses (fever and leukocytosis) also occurred after challenge testing in some grain workers (102,106). A few control subjects also had fever and leukocytosis after challenge testing when exposure levels were high (106).

The mechanisms these reactions were further evaluated by inhibition studies (103). The immediate asthmatic response was inhibited by pretreatment with disodium cromoglycate, while the late response was partially inhibited by treatment with beclomethasone diproprionate before and at intervals after challenge testing similar to those found in allergic asthma. Those with bronchial reaction had increase in nonspecific bronchial hyperresponsiveness and eosinophils but in those without such a response to challenge testing. These findings are similar to patients with allergic asthma. Most studies were unable to demonstrate positive skin test reaction to grain dust extract or a correlation between an asthmatic response to grain dust, and an immediate skin reaction to grain dust extract (103–106) and specific antibodies have not been found in the sera of patients with an asthmatic response on inhalation challenge (102,103). However, a study of an animal feed facility in Korea has shown that 13/43 (30.2%) workers had high levels of specific IgE antibodies to a grain dust extract; these antibodies were inhibited by the same extract but not by house dust or storage mite and corn dust (107). Immunoblot analysis of this grain dust extract showed eight IgE binding components with two bound to IgE in more than 50% of the sera tested. The same investigators also found specific IgE, IgG, and IgG4 antibodies to corn dust in employees working in animal feed industry (108). These antibodies were found in both symptomatic and asymptomatic employees. The significance of these antibodies in the pathogenesis of grain dust asthma has yet to be elucidated.

Agent(s) Responsible for Grain Dust–Induced Asthma.   The agent in grain dust responsible for grain dust asthma is unknown. Studies to identify the responsible airborne allergens in grain dust have met with little success. doPico et al. (109) studied 11 grain workers, including using extracts of durum wheat, durum wheat airborne dust, and grain insects and mites for specific inhalation challenge tests. Only one subject had a positive bronchial response to durum wheat airborne dust extract and none reacted to mites or insect extracts. Davies et al. (105) reported recurrent nocturnal asthma after inhalation challenge with grain dust in a farmer. Allergy skin testing and serological tests suggested the grain mite, Glycyphagus destructor, to be the allergen likely responsible for recurrent asthma in this patient. Warren et al. (106) reported a grain handler with asthma due to the Canadian storage mite, *Lepidoglyphus destructor*. They tested 100 asthmatics and found that 12% were sensitized to this storage mite while 4% were also sensitized to another storage mite, Acarus siro. Sensitization to a weevil, sitophilus oryzae, which infest granaries, has been reported to cause immediate and late phase reactions after inhalation of grain dust (110,111). No other studies have successfully identified allergen(s) in grain dust responsible for grain dust–induced asthma.

Prevalence of Grain Dust–Induced Asthma.   There is no information on the prevalence of allergic grain dust–induced asthma. It has been suggested that asthmatics are likely to seek other employment and leave the industry shortly after starting employment. The results of a prevalence study for grain dust asthma in 669 male grain workers and 560 controls of male office workers in Vancouver (112) support this notion. The prevalence of atopy (defined as immediate skin reactivity to one or more common allergens) was 17.3% versus 31.3%, respectively, while the prevalence of current asthma was 2.4% versus 2.7%, respectively. Eleven (1.6% of the total) out of 26 asthmatic grain workers claimed that their asthma started after employment to suggest possible relationship between grain dust exposure and asthma. The prevalence of allergic grain dust–induced asthma is likely to be low even though the prevalence of wheeze in grain workers is higher than the controls in many epidemiologic studies (113,114).

Asthma-Like Syndrome or Nonallergen-Induced Airflow Obstruction.   There are a number of studies (115–118) showing that a proportion of grain workers demonstrate cross-shift decline in lung function which may or may not be associated with respiratory symptoms such as cough, sputum production, wheeze, or chest tightness (Table 3). Gandevia and Ritchie (115) were the first to report a mean fall in FEV_1 of -291 mL over a work shift in a group of dockworkers unloading grain. Several investigators subsequently confirmed this finding. The cross-shift decline in lung function in grain workers appears to be directly related to the level of dust exposure (116,117) or to endotoxin (119) and is associated with an increase in peripheral blood leukocyte count but not to age, smoking habit, duration of employment,

Table 3 Cross-Shift or Cross-Week Changes in Lung Function

| Group | Location | n | Change in FEV_1 (mL) | | References |
			Cross-shift	Cross-week	
Dockworkers	Australia	24	−291.0 wheat dust −107.0 rock dust	NA	(115)
Dockworkers	United Kingdom	6	VC decrease by 200–800 mL		(116)
Grain	Wisconsin	248	−8.0	NA	(117)
Civic		192	+36.3	NA	
Grain	Vancouver	485	−22.0	−34.0	(118)
Sawmill		65	+71.0	+100.0	
Grain	Iowa	582	NA	−87.0	(119)
Control		153	NA	+82.0	
Grain	Toronto	47	Significant reduction in V_{50} and V_{75} on Mondays and Wednesday within days Significant reduction in FVC within week		(120)
Civic		15	No similar changes		

Abbreviations: NA, not available; FEV_1, forced expiratory volume in one second.

atopic status, or skin test reactivity to grain dust antigens. Previously unexposed individuals also developed acute decreases in lung function when exposed to high concentrations of grain dust (116,117). These characteristics suggest that, in most individuals, the acute cross-shift decline in lung function is not an IgE-mediated reaction but a nonallergic response to some constituent(s) of grain dust. This syndrome is similar to byssinosis described in workers with cotton dust exposure, but different from "classical" asthma because it is not associated with eosinophilia and persistent nonspecific bronchial hyperresponsiveness (121).

Clapp et al. (119,122) induced airflow obstruction in grain handlers and in healthy volunteers after inhalation challenge with a corn dust extract. The degree of airflow obstruction induced was similar to that observed following challenge with equivalent concentrations of endotoxin (119,123). Deetz (124) showed that among health volunteers, a single inhalation of corn dust extract resulted in significant airflow obstruction within 10 minutes and persisted for 48 hours. Atopic status does not appear to be an important determinant of airflow obstruction following inhalation of corn dust extract (125).

The nonallergic airway disease induced by grain dust exposure is not known but is unlikely to be due to sensitization. Several lines of evidence indicate that the physiologic response to grain dust is primarily mediated by an acute inflammatory response in the respiratory tract. In vitro studies have shown that grain dust activates both the classical and alternative complement pathways (126,127). Human inhalation studies have demonstrated that grain dust induces airflow obstruction in previously unexposed individuals (109,128) and in a dose-dependent manner (109,128) associated with accumulation of neutrophils in the upper and lower respiratory tract following inhalational challenges (122,129). In animals, a study has shown that inhaled grain dust causes a neutrophilic response in the lower respiratory tract (130). Grain dust has also been shown to release neutrophil chemotactic factors (131) and IL-1 (132) from macrophages. In mice, IL-10, given intravenously before challenge with corn dust extract, reduced the degree of airway hyperresponsiveness and the degree of airway inflammation due to corn dust challenge (133). These findings strongly suggest that a specific toxin(s), capable of inducing neutrophil chemotaxis in previously exposed and also unexposed individuals, is responsible for the development of airway inflammation and airflow obstruction in grain handlers. It is now believed that endotoxin is one of the primary agents in grain and other organic dust that causes airway inflammation and airflow obstruction. It will be discussed in detail below.

Febrile Syndrome Associated with Grain Dust Exposure

Grain fever, reported in 6% to 32% of exposed workers in different studies (134–139), is an acute illness occurring during or shortly after exposure to a high concentration of grain dust. The illness is characterized by facial warmth, headache, malaise, myalgia, fever, chilliness, throat and tracheal burning sensation, chest tightness, dyspnea, cough, and expectoration; it is often associated with airflow obstruction without detectable parenchymal abnormalities. Peripheral blood leuko-cytosis and a left shift of the differential count can be found in most subjects during such an episode. Chest radiography is usually normal. doPico et al. (128) exposed six grain workers and six controls to very high levels of grain dust (mean respirable dust concentration, $84 \, mg/m^3$) for 120 minutes. All subjects developed symptoms of grain fever. Because controls also developed similar symptoms as grain workers, immuno-logic mechanisms were thought to be unlikely. Moreover, grain fever is not asso-ciated with alveolitis, as is seen with hypersensitivity pneumonitis, and serum precipitating antibodies are absent. doPico et al. (128) postulated that grain fever is due to bacterial endotoxin in the grain dust releasing chemical mediators directly in the airways.

Grain fever has also been classified as an ODTS, a syndrome which is often associated with exposure to massive concentrations of spores of fungi or thermophi-lic actinomycetes (140).

Chronic Effects of Grain Dust Exposure

There is increasing evidence that exposure to grain dust leads to the development of chronic lung disease and associated respiratory disability. The evidence is found in a num-ber of epidemiologic studies, which can be divided into two categories: cross-sectional studies, and longitudinal studies which focused on exposure response relationships.

Cross-Sectional Studies.   Early cross-sectional prevalence studies (before 1978) were conducted on grain workers mostly without unexposed comparison groups (134–139). They showed a high prevalence of respiratory symptoms in grain workers. Of these studies, two also found significant reductions in pulmonary function in grain workers compared to population prediction equations (122,137). A negative relation-ship was found between duration of exposure and MMF level (139). Although detailed information on exposure was not available, some ambient air measurements indicated that exposure levels were often high, ranging from 10 to $800 \, mg/m^3$ (141).

Most cross-sectional studies carried out after 1978 included external compari-son groups. They demonstrated increased prevalence rates for respiratory symptoms and significantly lower average lung function levels in grain workers compared to external comparison groups (Table 4). Most of these studies were conducted among grain elevator workers or farmers (118,142–149). In one study (143) the combined effect of both smoking and grain dust exposure resulted in lower mean levels of lung function than either exposure alone.

Table 4 Effect of Grain Dust Exposure on Symptoms and Lung Function in Grain Elevator Workers–Cross-Sectional Studies with Control Groups

Site, year (Ref.)	Group and number	Mean age	Current smokers (%)	Symptoms (%)				Grain fever (%)	Lung function		
				Cough	Phlegm	Wheeze	Dyspnea		FEV_1	FVC	
New York, 1968 (136)	G: 55	49.8	60	27	NA	16	29	33	69%p	94%p	Effect of smoking = effect of exposure; no smoking–exposure interaction
	C: 56										
Thunder Bay, Ontario, 1979 (120)	G: 441	49.3	60	40	NA	7	20	NA	78%p	98%p	Effect of smoking > effect of exposure; no smoking–exposure interaction
	C: 180	40.0	52	45	45	5	16	1	93%p	108%p	
Vancouver, British Columbia, 1980 (118)	G: 610	42.0	48	32	32	5	14	0.5	98%p	115%p	Effect of smoking = effect of exposure; no smoking–exposure interaction
	C: 136	37.8	49	35	34	32	30	0	99%p	100%p	
Alberta, 1981 (142)	G: 63	44.3	29	23	22	25	21	NA	102%p	105%p	Effect of smoking > effect of exposure; no smoking–exposure interaction
	C: 63	46.9	38	36	—	24	25	14	87%p	103%p	
Saskatchewan, 1983 (143)	G: 390	46.9	38	32	—	32	11	NA	100%p	104%p	Effect of smoking = effect of exposure; exposure and smoking additive
	C: 63	30.6	50	16	—	27	NA	NA	110%p	NA	
Cape Town, 1985 (144)	G: 582	30.6	50	8	—	20	NA	NA	110%p	NA	
	C: 390	36.9	68	46	35	24	25	NA	2.6 L	3.8 L	

(Continued)

Table 4 Effect of Grain Dust Exposure on Symptoms and Lung Function in Grain Elevator Workers–Cross-Sectional Studies with Control Groups (*Continued*)

Site, year (Ref.)	Group and number	Mean age	Current smokers (%)	Symptoms (%) Cough	Phlegm	Wheeze	Dyspnea	Grain fever (%)	Lung function FEV$_1$	FVC
Eastern France, 1995 (145)	C: 153	36.1	68	30	17	10	20	NA	2.6 L	3.8 L
	G: 118	38	44	30	30	5	17	NA	100%p	100%p
France, 1995 (146)	C: 164	38	51	15	15	4	16	NA	100%p	100%p
	G: 142	42.1	44.4	14.8	13.4	18.3	27.4	NA	99.9%p	101.1%p
Shanghai, 1998 (147)	C: 37	42.4	Pack-yrs	0	0	8.1	10.9	NA	102.6%p	103.6%p
	Male									
	G: 312	35.8	7.3	32.7	28.8	4.8	–	24.3	3.36 L	4.17 L
	C: 138	32.7	5.6	3.6	2.2	2.2	–	0	3.44 L	4.17 L
	Female									
	G: 162	32.5	–	23.5	27.2	3.1	–	27.2	2.54 L	3.06 L
	C: 97	30.1	–	5.2	0	4.1	–	0	2.55 L	2.98 L

Abbreviations: %p, percent predicted; L, liter; NA, not available; G, control; FEV$_1$, forced expiratory volume in one second; FVC, forced vital capacity.

Longitudinal Studies. Follow-up studies were carried out mostly in Canadian grain elevators. Studies of grain elevator workers in British Columbia showed a greater annual decline in airflow rates compared with controls, in both the three-year and the six-year longitudinal study, especially among older workers (150–153). Ontario grain workers also had a slightly more rapid, but not statistically significant, decline in lung function over a period of three years compared with controls (154). As grain workers who left this employment had significantly more cough and breathlessness at the initial study than those who remained (a difference not seen in the comparison population), this suggested a "healthy worker" effect that favors the "fitter" individuals to remain in the exposed workforce.

Two short-term (few months) follow-up studies (155,156) indicated that, among young workers, part of the lung function changes may be reversible with cessation of exposure. However, the results of the longer duration follow-up studies indicated that continuous exposure was accompanied by chronic respiratory symptoms and reductions in lung function. Retired grain elevator workers had significantly lower lung function compared with retired civic workers despite cessation of exposure, even among lifetime nonsmokers (Fig. 2) (157). They also reported significantly greater breathing related impairment in activities of daily living (unrelated to asthma), indicating that grain dust exposure leads to chronic respiratory disability in some workers. A recent study from Saskatchewan grain elevators found that the annual decline in lung function became smaller after dust control program has been in place (158).

Analysis of Exposure–Response Relationships. Several well-designed studies have shown a dose-dependent relationship between the level of exposure and lung function declines. A significant relationship was found between airflow rates and grain dust level in Ontario grain elevator workers (120). Enarson et al. (159) compared exposure levels between workers with the largest FEV_1 decline over a six-year period and those with the smallest FEV_1 decline in a nested case–control study. The group with the largest FEV_1 decline was significantly more likely to be employed in high dust jobs. Using an industry specific job exposure matrix to compute cumulative and average grain dust exposure values for 454 grain elevator workers, Huy et al. (160) found significant exposure response relationships between cumulative dust exposure and increased prevalence of chronic phlegm and dyspnea, and reductions in both FEV_1 and FVC. The retirees from this cohort, who had a 5% acute cross-shift drop in FEV_1 of 5% or greater in 1975, had a significantly greater annual rate of decline in FEV_1 (–60.7 mL/yr) compared to the annual decline of –34.2 mL/yr in those without an acute cross-shift change in 1975 (161). This effect was most pronounced in workers with the highest dust exposure jobs in 1975.

In a Dutch study of 315 animal feed workers, reductions in lung function were found to correlate with dust and endotoxin levels (162) while a follow-up study of this cohort showed a significant correlation between lung function decline and grain dust level (163). Jorna et al. (164) reported significant exposure-related increases in chronic bronchitis and wheezing and decreases in airflow rates among 194 animal feed workers in the Netherlands. Even workers in the lowest exposure group ($0–4\,mg/m^3$, on average) had significant reductions in FEV_1 and MMF compared with the nonexposed group. In a recent collaborative study in which data from the Dutch grain elevator and animal feed workers and Canadian grain elevator and grain loading workers were pooled, exposure–response relationships of similar magnitude were demonstrated for current grain dust exposure and years employed among these diverse populations when exposure sampling methods and analytic approaches were harmonized (165).

In summary, the results of numerous cross-sectional and longitudinal studies and the consistent exposure–response relationship constitute in a strong body of evidence linking grain dust exposure and deleterious chronic effects on the respiratory system.

Nature of Chronic Lung Disease Due to Grain Dust Exposure. The specific nature of the chronic lung disease due to grain dust exposure is unclear. Autopsy carried out on three grain workers who died as a result of the illness showed that the lungs were not only emphysematous, but had diffuse granulomata with fibrosis as well (134). Most of the epidemiologic studies with detailed pulmonary function measurements showed chronic airflow limitation. Because many grain workers are also smokers, the presenting clinical features (i.e., of chronic airflow obstruction) are difficult to distinguish from those caused by smoking. However, some of the recent studies (153,155,156,161,163) indicated that exposure to grain dust–induced changes in FVC as well as FEV_1, suggesting the possibility of parenchymal involvement as well. This needs to be confirmed by more comprehensive clinical and pathological examination of nonsmoking grain workers with chronic pulmonary function abnormalities.

Threshold Limit Value for Grain Dust

As the dysfunction caused by grain dust exposure affects a relatively high proportion of exposed workers and the abnormalities induced are inflammatory and frequently nonallergic, it should be possible to prevent or reduce the severity of the response by controlling the ambient dust levels. Theoretically it is possible to determine the relationship between various levels of exposure and the resulting physiologic changes and thereby provide a guide to the permissible concentration for grain dust. This can be done by determining the levels of grain dust in the air at the same time as the physiologic measurements are undertaken in a workforce. This would not, however, provide measurements of cumulative exposure. For this purpose, a trend in dust exposure, obtained from a monitoring program, would be required.

In 1977, Labour Canada implemented a medical and dust surveillance program in the grain industry. Workers are required to have a medical examination including questionnaire, spirometry, and chest X-ray every three years. Regular dust monitoring of the elevators is also mandatory. At that time, Labour Canada adopted a permissible concentration of $10 \, mg/m^3$ for grain dust, similar to that for nuisance dust at that time, because there were very few epidemiologic studies. A number of epidemiologic studies were conducted as part of the medical surveillance program in Canada (118,150–152,155,156,158). All the studies showed that grain workers had more respiratory symptoms and lower lung function compared to the controls even when the dust levels in the elevators were below $10 \, mg/m^3$.

Enarson et al. (159) showed that workers exposed to levels of dust less than $4 \, mg/m^3$ were not at risk for developing rapid decline in lung function. doPico et al. (128) showed a significantly higher prevalence of work-related respiratory symptoms and decrements in lung function over an eight-hour work shift in grain workers compared to controls when the mean level of total dust exposure was below $5 \, mg/m^3$ $(3.3 + 7.0 \, mg/m^3)$. Furthermore, recent studies in which exposure–response relationships have been investigated in detail (160–165) confirmed that the permissible concentration for grain dust should be lowered to at least $5 \, mg/m^3$. The American Governmental Conference of Industrial Hygienists has recommended $4 \, mg/m^3$ as the permissible concentration of grain dust (166).

EXPOSURE IN SWINE CONFINEMENT BARNS

Increasing numbers of hogs are raised in confinement barns for economic reasons. As hog farms have increased in size, it has become common for workers to spend eight hours or more per day in these barns. The hogs eat feed consisting of ground grain and soybeans. Their waste is usually flushed out with water, and the manure slurry is stored in a pit under the floor of the barn or in an outdoor storage structure. The workers are exposed to dust in the air, which is rich in endotoxin. They also inhale a variety of gases, including ammonia (Fig. 3). It was recognized in the 1970s and 1980s that work in this setting is associated with symptoms consistent with the asthma-like syndrome (167). Other respiratory disorders caused by work in this environment include bronchitis, allergic asthma, mucous membrane irritation, and ODTS (168). It has subsequently been determined that the exposure to dust, endo-toxin, and ammonia together cause airway disease in swine confinement barn work-ers (169,170). Persons affected can include veterinarians as well as individuals responsible for daily care and feeding of the hogs. The problem of airway disease secondary to work in swine confinement barns persists despite innovations in the design and management of these facilities (171).

Clinical Features

Swine confinement workers commonly develop symptoms of airway disease, including cough that may or may not be productive of sputum, chest tightness, wheezing, and dyspnea on exertion (167,172–174). They often report nocturnal cough, wheeze, and chest tightness. Their symptoms commonly are worse after work in the swine confinement barns and may be improved after time spent away from the farm. There is a dose–response relationship between hours worked inside the hog barn and

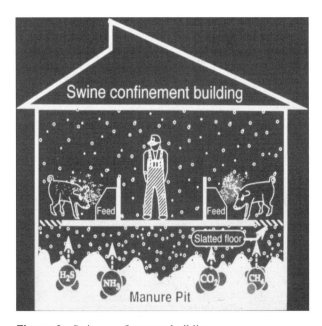

Figure 3 Swine confinement building.

respiratory symptoms (175). Rarely, persons with these complaints are found to suffer from asthma secondary to an allergic response to porcine proteins, with elevated IgE levels (176–178). IgG antibodies to porcine proteins are commonly identified in the serum of workers but are not associated with clinical symptoms (179). Other individuals may have underlying asthma or COPD that is exacerbated by exposure to the swine confinement barn environment. However, many workers who develop airway disease symptoms have no previous history of COPD or allergic asthma. Their clinical picture can be most consistent with the asthma-like syndrome, if cough, wheeze, and chest tightness are the most prominent symptoms. Alternatively, the picture may be more consistent with chronic bronchitis if cough with sputum production is the main complaint (180). Their symptoms can develop within weeks after the start of work in this setting (181). More commonly, the symptoms are reported after several years of work in swine confinement barns.

Spirometry results may be normal or may reveal mild airway obstruction (174). Less often there is evidence of more severe airway obstruction. The presence of severe airway obstruction on spirometry is rarely found in workers who do not smoke cigarettes. The effect of tobacco smoke on lung function is somewhat greater than that of swine confinement barn exposure (173). Certain individuals who work in this setting have an accelerated loss of lung function, which may become apparent in young workers (181,182). A cross-shift drop in FEV_1 is a common finding in swine confinement workers and is predictive of an accelerated loss in lung function (183,184).

Nonspecific bronchial hyperresponsiveness is often demonstrated in the swine confinement workers, including those who have normal spirometry (174,185). The results can be positive in both symptomatic workers and in those without symptoms. Bronchial hyperresponsiveness can be seen after a single exposure in previously unexposed persons (185,186). Interestingly, the response to methacholine inhalation after hog barn exposure is greater in previously unexposed nonfarming subjects than in farmers, suggesting adaptation to this environment (185).

Measurement of exhaled nitric oxide (NO) has been used as a tool for assessing airway inflammation in swine confinement workers as well as in asthmatics. Acutely exposed, naïve subjects have larger elevations in exhaled NO than do workers (186,187). There is evidence that the inflammatory response is downregulated in workers when compared to naïve subjects exposed to this environment, which likely explains the difference in NO values (188). Interestingly, the NO values of workers are also considerably lower than those of asthmatic subjects (189).

Bronchoalveolar lavage (BAL) has been a useful tool for defining the airway disease seen in swine confinement workers. Persons newly exposed to this work environment have a profound neutrophilic inflammation of the airways (190). Lymphocytes and macrophages are also present in increased numbers in the lower respiratory tract of naïve subjects when compared to normal control subjects. In contrast, workers have a much less pronounced elevation in these measures (191). Eosinophils are not increased in the lower respiratory tract of either group.

Pathogenesis

The evidence available from epidemiologic studies indicates that exposure to dust, endotoxin, and ammonia is a risk factor for developing the asthma-like syndrome (169,192,193). Current recommendations include keeping total dust levels below $2.5\,mg/m^3$ and ammonia levels below 7.0 ppm to reduce the risk of airway disease symptoms (168). There is also some evidence that the presence of other microbial products, such as peptidoglycan, contribute to the airway disease seen in the workers (194).

Inhalation of dust from swine confinement barns induces a profound inflammatory response in the upper and lower respiratory tract. Inflammatory changes observed include the presence of increased numbers of neutrophils, lymphocytes, and macrophages. Interestingly, this inflammatory response is much less pronounced in workers than in naive subjects (188). There is evidence that L-selectin shedding may play a role in the downregulation of the inflammatory response (195). The healthy worker effect may also help explain this finding.

The inflammatory response seen after swine confinement barn exposure is systemic in nature. IL-6 and IL-8 are commonly elevated in the blood and airways of persons exposed to this environment, which likely explains the presence of increased numbers of neutrophils in the upper and lower respiratory tract (187,196,197).

Exhaled NO is somewhat elevated in workers exposed to the swine confinement barn environment when compared to normal controls, at levels lower than those seen in naive subjects with this exposure (186,198). Levels of exhaled NO in the workers are also considerably lower than those of asthmatic persons (189). NO levels may affect mucus secretion and the airway microcirculation in exposed workers.

Treatment

Management of airway disease in hog confinement barn workers should begin with reducing exposure to dust, endotoxin, and ammonia inside the barns to levels below those associated with airway disease symptoms. These goals can be reached most easily if levels of dust, endotoxin, and ammonia are monitored on an ongoing basis. Routinely measuring ammonia levels is feasible at this time. Measuring the amount of dust and endotoxin in the air requires greater investment in technology and is usually done only in a research setting. At this time, it is a common practice to adjust ventilation for the purpose of preventing respiratory illness in the hogs, which are more tolerant of high ammonia, dust, and endotoxin levels than are the workers. Ideally, air quality is monitored routinely for the purpose of preserving workers' health. When problems with air quality are identified, ventilation should be increased, and the barns should be cleaned more frequently. Managers may resist increasing ventilation because doing so will increase the need to heat the barns during the cold months of the year in temperate climates, thus raising operating expenses. In most cases, the air quality of the barns is not formally monitored. It must be noted that simple visual inspection for assessment of cleanliness of the barns does not serve as a substitute for industrial hygiene measurements (199).

It has been recommended that swine confinement barn workers wear respirators on a routine basis. Most workers do not find these respirators comfortable. Compliance with this recommendation is generally poor although educational interventions can increase knowledge regarding the importance of respirator use (200). It is estimated that fewer than 30% of workers routinely wear respirators. There is evidence that use of N-95 respirators reduces airway inflammation (201). A study of naive subjects intentionally exposed to the swine confinement barn environment revealed that those who wore respirators had less neutrophilic upper airway inflammation and a smaller fall in FEV_1 than did those who did not use personal protective equipment. Others have found that the increase in bronchial responsiveness and influx of neutrophils seen after swine confinement barn exposure is not abolished by respirator use (186,202).

The potential value of use of medications to control airway disease symptoms after swine confinement barn exposure has been explored in several in vivo and in vitro studies. However, at this time no pharmacologic agent has been identified as being clearly effective for airway disease symptoms in swine confinement barn workers.

Outcomes

A relatively small number of published studies describe outcomes from working in swine confinement barns. It has been shown that young workers lose lung function at an accelerated rate (181). The presence of a cross-shift drop in FEV_1 has been found to be a predictor of a loss of lung function over time (184). Severe airway obstruction in some individuals was reported in a case series from Canada (203). However, this outcome does not appear to be common.

ENDOTOXIN AND AIRWAY DISEASE CAUSED BY ORGANIC DUST EXPOSURE

Endotoxins are lipopolysaccharide (LPS) fragments that coat the outer membrane of gram-negative bacteria. Significant amounts of endotoxin are found in settled dusts and ambient air of occupational and domestic environments, though in highly variable quantities. Common occupational sources of exposure include livestock, grain dust, and textiles, but significant concentrations also occur in the household from pets, carpeting, and indoor ventilation systems (204). Several investigators have also found endotoxin in tobacco smoke (205) and particulate matter in air pollution (206). Although our lungs are constantly exposed to endotoxins in the environment, the host response to inhaled endotoxin varies. The role of endotoxin in airway disease pathogenesis remains to be precisely defined.

Airway Responses to LPS

Inhalation of LPS can cause a host of airway responses including symptoms of chest tightness, myalgias, fevers, chills, and dyspnea. The corresponding physiological responses include airflow obstruction, enhanced airway hyperresponsiveness, and a reduction in alveolar diffusion capacity. At the cellular level, recruitment of resident macrophages and neutrophils has been demonstrated in BAL fluid; likewise, increased concentrations of inflammatory mediators (e.g., IL-1, IL-6, IL-8, and TNF-α) have been recovered from BAL fluid after inhalation or local instillation of LPS (4). With acute exposure to inhaled endotoxin, murine models not only demonstrate histologic inflammation, but also airway hyperresponsiveness and neutrophilic cellular response in the BAL fluid (207). Thus it appears that inhaled endotoxin induces a physiologic and inflammatory airway reaction that phenotypically resembles an acute asthma flare. However, unlike an asthma flare, the pathophysiologic response to inhaled LPS or to dusts containing LPS can be reproduced in nonasthmatic subjects (208).

In patients with mild atopic asthma, exposure to air containing low levels of endotoxin ($250 \, \text{ng/m}^3$) for four hours before bronchial challenge with allergen significantly increased both bronchial reactivity and airway eosinophilia (209). Thus, asthmatic and atopic individuals appear to be more susceptible to the effects of inhaled endotoxin.

Chronic exposure to endotoxin may also be associated with the development of chronic obstructive lung disease. In mice, chronic intratracheal exposure to LPS elicits lung pathologic changes similar to human COPD-associated inflammation (210). In rats, acute exposure to intratracheal LPS alters lung histology even after 16 days beyond the acute exposure with a resulting increase in extracellular matrix, differentiation of myofibroblasts, and altered secretion of surfactant by newly differentiated Type II pneumocytes (211). Subchronic inhalation of LPS in mice results in persistent airway hyperresponsiveness and airway remodeling (212). Textile workers who developed byssinosis (thought now to be mainly due to chronic occupational endotoxin exposure) developed severe obstructive airway disease. Similarly, swine confinement workers developed symptomatic chronic airflow obstruction; corresponding histology revealed thickening of the airway basement that was similar to COPD (213). Understanding such mechanisms of injury will lead to new insight in the pathogenesis of chronic airway diseases.

Endotoxin as an Etiological Factor for Airway Disease in Organic Dust Exposure

Endotoxin was initially suspected as an etiologic agent in byssinosis. Endotoxin is present in all parts of cotton plants, but particularly high concentrations are found in microorganisms on cotton bracts. The airborne concentration of endotoxin in cotton mill dust depends upon the degree of contamination of the cotton (usually lower grade cotton) processed, ventilation, and the textile process. Most of the human studies have been performed in worker populations stratified by current and cumulative dust or endotoxin exposure. Castellan et al. (61) reported that decline in FEV_1 correlated highly with dustborne endotoxin concentration among volunteers selected for reactivity to cotton dust. Similarly Rylander et al. (214) observed respiratory function decreases among cotton workers in experimental card-rooms. However CBE that are purified to remove endotoxin may still cause bronchoconstriction in human volunteers (215). In another study, the level of endotoxin exposure significantly correlated with the prevalence of chronic bronchitis and a decrease in FEV_1 among exposed cotton workers (216). However, this study also found that workers in the highest endotoxin exposure category had less byssinosis, a smaller cross-shift change in FEV_1, and better baseline pulmonary function than other workers. This suggested that this particularly high-exposure group had either become less reactive, as a result of tolerance to repeated high exposures, or that the group represented a healthy survivor population.

The evidence that endotoxin is at least one of the agents responsible for airway disease in organic dust exposure is based on the results of a number of studies. First, the concentration of inhaled endotoxin in the bioaerosol is strongly associated with the development of acute decrements in airflow among cotton (63,217,218), swine confinement (219), and poultry workers (220), and appears to be the most important occupational exposure associated with development (221) and progression (222) of airway disease in agricultural workers. In addition, the concentration of endotoxin in domestic environment adversely affects asthmatics, with higher concentrations of ambient endotoxin associated with greater degrees of airflow obstruction (223,224). Second, inhaled endotoxin (223,225–228), grain dust (122,128), or cotton dust (61,62,217,229) can cause airflow obstruction in naive or previously unexposed subjects. Furthermore, asthmatic individuals develop airflow obstruction at lower concentrations of inhaled endotoxin than normal controls (228). Finally,

exposure–response studies have shown that inhaled grain dust and endotoxin produce similar physiologic and biologic effects (122,123); the concentration of endotoxin appears to play an important role in the acute biological response to grain
dust (123,230,231); a competitive antagonist for LPS (*Rhodobacter spheroides*
diphosporyl lipid A) reduces the inflammatory response to inhaled grain dust
(232); and genetic or acquired hyporesponsiveness to endotoxin substantially reduces
the biological response to grain dust (230). In aggregate, these studies indicate that
endotoxin is an important cause of organic dust–induced airway disease.

Pathogenesis

The pathologic response to inhaled grain dusts involves a complex interaction between the innate and adaptive immune systems, which are modified by host-specific
factors, such as genetic predisposition (Fig. 4). A pivotal role in this response is likely
played by the alveolar and airway macrophage. Animal inhalation studies have
shown that grain dust, such as endotoxin, induces a profound neutrophilic response
in the lower respiratory tract (130,131,230). This does not appear to be dependent on
complement, because inactivation of complement will not affect the influx of neutrophils following exposure to endotoxin (233). Moreover, transfer of macrophages
from endotoxin-sensitive mice to endotoxin-resistant mice will render the resistant
mice sensitive to the toxic effects of endotoxin (234). Animal studies have also shown
that inhalation of endotoxin results in a dose-dependent influx of neutrophils to
the alveoli which can be partially inhibited by prior treatment with TNF-α specific

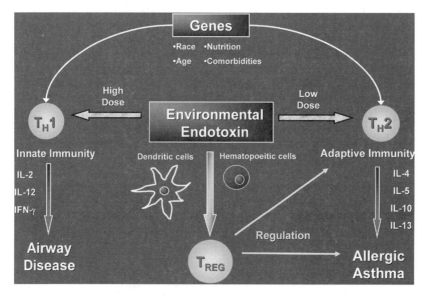

Figure 4 Environmental endotoxin, depending on dose and timing, can result in predominantly either an adaptive or innate immune response. Endotoxin directly and indirectly stimulates lung resident (dendritic) and recruited (hematopoietic) cells, which in turn interact with
Treg cells. The Treg cells modulate the adaptive immune system to develop clinical allergy
and/or asthma. Individual genetic predilection, modified by other factors of host susceptibility,
mediates this complex interaction.

antibodies (235). Grain dust is directly chemotactic for neutrophils, and can induce alveolar macrophages to release factors that have potent chemotactic activity for neutrophils (109). Following inhalation of grain dust, the production and release of specific proinflammatory cytokines (TNF-α, IL-1β, IL-6, and IL-8) have been demonstrated in the lungs of humans (221,223).

Epithelial cells may also be involved in recruitment and modulation of the inflammatory response. Interestingly, epithelial cells respond poorly to endotoxin and appear to require a specific host-derived signal (TNF-α or IL-1) for induction of IL-8 (236). The inability to respond to LPS has been demonstrated in vitro in A549 cells (237) and bronchial epithelial cells (238); however, if these cells are exposed directly to either TNF-α or IL-1 they are able to produce and release IL-8. In a baboon model of sepsis, pretreatment with anti-TNF-α antibody significantly reduced the circulating concentration of IL-8 (239), suggesting that TNF-α and/or IL-1 are needed to stimulate other cells to release IL-8 and promote neutrophil chemotaxis. Interestingly, IL-8 is clearly upregulated in the airway epithelia following inhalation of corn dust extract (221,240) and MIP-2, thought to be the murine homolog of IL-8, is produced and released in the lungs of mice following inhalation of corn dust extract (229). These findings suggest that inhaled grain dust initiates a complex interaction between macrophages and other inflammatory (primarily neutrophils) and structural (bronchial epithelial) cells, and this interaction is mediated by specific proinflammatory cytokines that are initially released by alveolar macrophages.

Hygiene Hypothesis—Can Exposure to Endotoxin Be Beneficial?

Several studies suggest that chronic low levels of exposures to endotoxin during infancy may reduce the risk of developing atopy and even asthma. The controversial "hygiene hypothesis" has been extensively reviewed by Liu (241). Some epidemiologic studies have observed a lower prevalence of allergic rhinitis, asthma, and inhalant allergen sensitization in persons who have grown up around higher concentrations of endotoxin or experienced significant respiratory infections (e.g., measles, tuberculosis). The number of childhood febrile infections in the first year of life by parental self-report was also associated with decreased risk of the development of asthma and atopy (242). Early participation in daycare and older siblings (presumably exposing children to more microbial pathogens) appear to reduce the risk of atopy and asthma (243). Increased endotoxin levels in house dust correlated with lower levels of allergic sensitization in German children (244), and higher levels of endotoxin in a child's mattress was associated with a lesser incidence of hay fever and atopic sensitization (245). In young mice, presensitization with ovalbumin attenuates the hyperresponsiveness to inhaled LPS (207). All of these studies highlight a potential mechanism whereby chronic exposure in early life may be protective from the eventual development of asthma and atopy. As intriguing as these studies are, much of these data are merely associations. Furthermore, other epidemiologic studies do not support this association. In fact, epidemiological findings have been published that suggest that individuals exposed to endotoxin early in life may be at higher risk of developing asthma. For instance, crowding in the home (246) and increased public hygiene are associated with the development of asthma. Moreover, a recent study has shown that higher levels of domestic endotoxin may be a risk factor for the development of asthma in young children (247). Nevertheless, there is sufficient evidence to suggest that environmental exposure to high doses of endotoxin in early life can reduce the risk of developing asthma and atopy.

Genomics of Endotoxin Response

Given our current understanding of the innate immune receptor/signaling pathway (248), a number of potential candidate genes emerge that may play an important role in controlling the response to innate immune stimuli. For instance, a polymorphism of TLR4 (Asp299Gly) is observed in approximately 10% of individuals in the general population and has been associated with a blunted response to LPS in vitro and with diminished airway response to inhaled LPS (249). A recent study found that the TLR4 polymorphism is more prevalent in asthmatic Swedish children, especially those with atopic asthma, suggesting that an inability to respond to endotoxin places one at higher risk of Th2 mediated diseases (250). Though a large family-based cohort study did not find TLR4 polymorphisms to be associated with asthma or atopy (251), another recent study found that individuals with the TLR4 polymorphism appear to have an increased risk of being atopic (252). Concordantly, the presence of CD14 (a ligand for the TLR4 receptor) can modify the response to inhaled LPS (253), whereas a genetic polymorphism for CD14 may determine severity of atopy (254). Polymorphisms of genes involved in the TLR pathway (e.g., IRAK-4, NEMO, Csp-12) that are involved in other human diseases are also being investigated regarding their contribution toward asthma susceptibility (255).

SUMMARY

Exposure to organic dusts, such as cotton and grain, can lead to the development of acute and chronic airflow obstruction. In some individuals, acute bronchoconstriction is the result of sensitization to some components of organic dust (asthma); in others, acute bronchoconstriction is due to direct tissue injury and inflammation (asthma-like syndrome). Chronic exposure to organic dust has also been shown to give rise to chronic airflow obstruction in some individuals. Endotoxin, present in most of the organic dusts, may be the most important etiological factor responsible for acute and chronic airway disease due to organic dust exposure. Further research is necessary to identify other agents responsible for it.

DIRECTIONS FOR FUTURE RESEARCH

- Further understand the role of innate immunity in modulating the adaptive immune response.
- Identify the key genetic variants that modulate the response to inhaled endotoxin.
- Develop biosensors that detect respirable endotoxin.
- Determine whether interventions directed at endotoxin inhalation have an effect on the development and progression of airway disease.
- Do substances other than endotoxin (e.g., β-1,3 d-glucan) contribute to the pathogenesis of byssinosis and other acute airway disease due to organic dust exposure?
- Standardization of techniques for measuring endotoxin levels in dust collected from the air of swine confinement barns, grain elevators, and cotton mills.
- There needs to be a systematic attempt to obtain more histopathologic data on airway disease due to exposure to organic dust such as cotton and

grain and to determine whether emphysema is a true complication of these exposures.

- Animal experiments to determine whether organic dust exposure increases or decreases in animals' ability to develop specific IgE-mediated allergic symptoms.
- Cross-sectional and prospective studies to determine if engineering and industrial hygiene measures designed to improve air quality in swine confinement barns are effective in terms of reducing the risk for airway disease in swine confinement workers.
- Studies to determine the long-term prognosis of persons with airway disease secondary to work in swine confinement barns.
- Studies of gene–environment interactions that might help predict which swine confinement barn workers are at higher risk for developing airway disease from this work.
- Development of monitoring devices for measuring dust and endotoxin levels in swine confinement barns that are suitable for routine use on farms.

REFERENCES

1. Ramazzini B. A Treatise of the Diseases of Tradesmen. London: Bell, 1705.
2. Sepulveda MJ, Castellan RM, Hankinson JL, Cocke JB. Acute lung function response to cotton dust in atopic and non-atopic individuals. Br J Ind Med 1984; 41:487–449.
3. Proust AA. Traite d'Hygiene Publique et Privee. Paris: G. Masson, 1877.
4. O'Grady NP, Praes HL, Pugin J, et al. Local inflammatory responses following bronchial endotoxin installation in humans. Am J Respir Crit Care Med 2001; 163: 1591–1598.
5. Report of the Departmental Committee on Dust in Cardrooms in the Cotton Industry. London: Great Britain Home Office, 1932.
6. Enterline PE, Kendrick MA. Asbestos-dust exposures at various levels and mortality. Arch Environ Health 1967; 15:181–186.
7. Enterline PE, Kykor JE, Keleti O, Lange JH. Endotoxins, cotton dust, and cancer. Lancet 1985; 265:934–935.
8. Levin LI, Gao YT, Blot WJ, Wei Z, Fraumeni JF. Decreased risk of lung cancer in the cotton textile industry in Shanghai. Cancer Res 1987; 47:5777–5781.
9. Hill AB. Sickness amongst operatives in Lancashire cotton spinning mills (with special reference to the cardroom). Rep Ind Hlth Res Bd Rept No. 59, HMSO, London, 1930.
10. Malcolm AG. The influence of factory life on the health of the operative as founded upon the medical statistics of the class in Belfast. JR Statist Soc 1856; 19:170.
11. Schilling RSF, Goodman N. Cardiovascular disease in cotton workers. Part I. Br J Ind Med 1952; 9:146–153.
12. Schilling RSF. Byssinosis in cotton and other textile workers. Lancet 1956; 2:261–265, 319–324.
13. Schilling RSF, Hughes JPW, Dingwall-Fordyce I, Gilson JC. An epidemiological study of byssinosis among Lancashire cotton workers. Br J Ind Med 1995; 12:217–227.
14. Roach SA, Schilling RSF. A clinical and environmental study of byssinosis in the Lancashire cotton industry. Br J Ind Med 1960; 17:1–9.
15. Recommended health-based occupational exposure limits for selected vegetable dusts. Report of a WHO study group, WHO Technical Report Series 684. Geneva: World Health Organization, 1983.
16. Christiani DC, Eisen EA, Wegman DH, et al. Respiratory disease in cotton textile workers in the People's Republic of China. Scand J Work Environ Health 1986; 12:40–45.

17. Christiani DC, Eisen EA, Wegman DH, et al. Respiratory disease in cotton textile workers in the People's Republic of China. II. Pulmonary function result. Scand J Work Environ Health 1986; 12:46–50.

18. Fishwick D, Fletcher AM, Pickering CAC, Niven R, McL R, Faragher EB. Lung function in Lancashire cotton and man made fibre spinning mill operatives. Occup Environ Med 1996; 53:46–50.

19. Cinkotai FF, Emo P, Gibbs ACC, Caillard JF, Jouany JM. Low prevalence of byssinotic symptoms in 12 flax scutching mills in Normandy, France. Br J Ind Med 1988; 45:325–328.

20. El Batawi MA. Byssinosis in the cotton industry in Egypt. Br J Ind Med 1962; 19: 126–130.

21. El Batawi MA, Schilling RSF, Valic F, Wolfod J. Byssinosis in the Egyptian cotton industry: changes in ventilatory capacity during the day. Br J Ind Med 1964; 21:13–19.

22. Noweir MH, El-Sadek Y, El-Dakhakhry AA. Exposure to dust in the cottonseed oil extraction industry. Arch Environ Health 1969; 19:99–102.

23. Engleberg AL, Piacitelli GN, Petersen M, et al. Medical and industrial hygiene characterization of the cotton waste utilization industry. Am J Ind Med 1985; 7:93–108.

24. U.S. Department of Health, Education and Welfare, Public Health Service, National Institute for Occupational Safety and Health, Health Hazard Evaluation Determination. Report No. 76, 73–523. Cincinnati, Ohio: Stearns & Foster Company, 1978.

25. Bouhuys A, Lindell SD, Lundin G. Experimental studies in byssinosis. Br Med J 1960; 1:324–326.

26. Bouhuys A. Experimental studies in byssinosis. Arch Environ Health 1963; 6:56–61.

27. Carey OCR, Elwood PC, McAuley JR, Merrett JD, Pemberton J. Byssinosis in flax workers in Northern Ireland. A Report to the Minister of Labour and National Insurance, The Government of Northern Ireland. Belfast: HMSO, 1965.

28. Elwood PC. Respiratory symptoms in men who had previously worked in a flax mill in Northern Ireland. Br J Ind Med 1965; 22:38–42.

29. Elwood PC, Pemberton J, Merrett JD, Carey JCR, McAuley JR. Byssinosis and other respiratory symptoms in flax workers in Northern Ireland. Br J Ind Med 1965; 19:27–37.

30. Elwood PC, Pemberton J, Merrett JD, Carey OCR, McAuley JR. Prevalence of byssinosis and dust levels in flax preparers in Northern Ireland. Br J Ind Med 1966; 23: 188–193.

31. Mair A, Smith DH, Wilson WA, Lockhart W. Dust diseases in Dundee textile workers. Br J Ind Med 1960; 17:272–276.

32. McKerrow CB, Gilson JC, Schilling RSF, Skidmore JW. Respiratory function and symptoms in rope workers. Br J Ind Med 1965; 22:204–209.

33. Khogoli M, Lakha AS, Milla MH, Dahoma A. Byssinosis, respiratory symptoms and spirometric lung function tests in Tanzanian sisal workers. Br J Ind Med 1976; 35:123–128.

34. Chattopadhyay BP, Saiyed HN, Mukherjee AK. Byssinosis among jute mill workers. Int Health 2003; 41:265–272.

35. Castellan RM, Boehlecke BA, Petersen MR, Merchant JA. Herbal tea workers pulmonary function and symptoms. Proceedings of the International Conference on Byssinosis. Chest 1981; 79:815–855.

36. Merchant JA, Donham KJ. Health risks from animal confinement units. In: Dosman JA, Cockcroft DW, eds. Principles of Health and Safety in Agriculture. Boca Raton, FL: CRC Press, 1989:58–61.

37. Merchant JA, Lumsden JC, Kilburn KH, et al. Dose response studies in cotton textile workers. J Occup Med 1973; 15:222–230.

38. Fox AJ, Tombelson JBL, Watt A, Wilke AO. A survey of respiratory disease among cotton operatives. Part II. Symptoms, dust estimations, and the effect of smoking habit. Br J Ind Med 1973; 30:48–53.

39. Merchant JA, Lumsden JD, Kilburn KH, et al. Intervention studies of cotton steaming to reduce biological effects of cotton dust. Br J Ind Med 1974; 31:261–274.

40. Molyneux MBK, Berry O. The correlation of cotton dust exposure with the prevalence of respiratory symptoms. Proceedings of the International Conference on Respiratory Disease in Textile Workers, Alicante, Spain, 1968:177–183.

41. Merchant JA, Kilburn KH, O'Fallon WM, et al. Byssinosis and chronic bronchitis among cotton textile workers. Ann Int Med 1972; 76:423–433.

42. Merchant JA, Lumsden J, Kilburn KH, et al. An industrial study of the biological effects of cotton dust and cigarette smoke exposure. J Occup Med 1973; 15:212–221.

43. U.S. Department of Labor. National Institute for Occupational Safety and Health, Cotton Dust Title 29: Code of Federal Regulations. Part 1910.1043.

44. Niven R, McL R, Fishwick D, et al. A study of the performance and comparability of the sampling response to cotton dust of work area and personal sampling techniques. Ann Occup Hyg 1992; 36(4):349–362.

45. Gilson JC, Stott H, Hopwood BEC, Roach SA, McKerrow CB, Schilling RSF. Byssinosis: the acute effect on ventilatory capacity of dusts in cotton ginneries, cotton, sisal and jute mills. Br J Ind Med 1962; 18:9–18.

46. Valic F, Zuskin E. Effect of different vegetable dust exposures. Br J Ind Med 1972; 29:293–297.

47. WHO study group. Recommended Health-Based Occupational Exposure Limits for Selected Vegetable Dusts, WHO Technical Report Series 684. Geneva, Switzerland: World Heath Organization, 1983.

48. Medical Research Council Committee on Aetiology of Chronic Bronchitis. Standardized questions on respiratory symptoms. Br Med J 1960; 2:1665.

49. Imbus HR, Suh MH. Byssinosis: a study of 10,133 textile workers. Arch Environ Health 1973; 26:183–191.

50. Lammers B, Schilling RSF, Wolford J. A study of byssinosis, chronic respiratory symptoms, and ventilatory capacity in English and Dutch cotton workers, with special reference to atmospheric pollution. Br J Ind Med 1964; 21:124–134.

51. Merchant JA. Epidemiological studies of respiratory diseases among cotton textile workers, 1970–1973. Dissertation, University of North Carolina, 1973.

52. Merchant JA, Halprin JM, Hanson JR, et al. Evaluation before and after exposure—the pattern of physiological response to cotton dust. Ann NY Acad Sci 1974; 221:38–43.

53. Merchant JA, Lumsden JC, Kilburn KH, et al. Preprocessing cotton to prevent byssinosis. Br J Ind Med 1973; 30:237–247.

54. Valic F, Zuskin E. Pharmacological prevention of acute ventilatory capacity reduction in flax dust exposure. Br J Ind Med 1973; 30:381–384.

55. Bouhuys A, Gilson JC, Schilling RSF. Byssinosis in the textile industry. Arch Environ Health 1970; 21:475–478.

56. Schacter EN, Kapp MC, Maunder LR, Beck G, Witek TJ. Smoking and cotton dust effects on cotton textile workers: an analysis of the shape of the maximum expiratory flow volume curve. Environ Health Perspect 1986; 66:145–148.

57. McKerrow EB, McDermott M, Gilson JC, Schilling RSF. Respiratory function during the day in cotton workers: a study in byssinosis. Br J Ind Med 1958; 15:75–83.

58. Bates DV, Macklem P, Christie RV. Respiratory Function in Disease. 2nd ed. Philadelphia: W.B. Saunders Company, 1971.

59. Bouhuys A, Gilson JC, Schilling RSF, van de Woestijne KP. Chronic respiratory disease in hemp workers. Am J Med 1969; 46:526–537.

60. Molyneux MKB, Tombleson JBL. An epidemiological study of respiratory symptoms in Lancashire mills, 1963–1966. Br J Ind Med 1970; 27:225–234.

61. Castellan RM, Olenchock AA, Hankinson JL, et al. Acute bronchoconstriction induced by cotton dust: dose-related responses to endotoxin and other dust factors. Ann Int Med 1984; 101:157–163.

62. Castellan RM, Olenchock SA, Kinsley KB, Hankinson JL. Inhaled endotoxin and decreased spirometric values. N Engl J Med 1987; 317:605–610.
63. Kennedy SM, Christiani DC, Eisen EA, et al. Cotton dust and endotoxin exposure–response relationships in cotton textile workers. Am Rev Respir Dis 1987; 135:194–210.
64. Beck GJ, Schachter EN, Maunder LR, Bouhuys A. The relation of lung function to subsequent employment status and mortality in cotton textile workers. Chest 1981; 79: 265–305.
65. Berry G, McKerrow CB, Mollyneux MKB, Rossiter CE, Tombleson JBL. A study of the acute and chronic changes in ventilatory capacity of workers in Lancashire cotton mills. Br J Ind Med 1973; 301:25–36.
66. Glindmeyer HW, Lenfante JJ, Jones RN, Rando RJ, Kader HAA, Weill H. Exposure-related declines in the lung function of cotton textile workers. Am Rev Respir Dis 1991; 144:675–683.
67. Wang XR, Wang XR, Eisen EA, et al. Respiratory symptoms and cotton dust exposure; results of a 15 year follow up observation. Occup Environ Med 2003; 60:935–941.
68. Zuskin E, Ivankovic D, Schacter EN, Witek TJ. A ten-year follow-up study of cotton textile workers. Am Rev Respir Dis 1991; 143:301–305.
69. Kamat JR, Kamat GR, Salpekar VY, Lobo E. Distinguishing byssinosis from chronic obstructive pulmonary disease. Am Rev Respir Dis 1981; 124:31–40.
70. Christiani DC, Wegman DH, Eisen EA. Cotton dust exposure and longitudinal change in lung function. Am Rev Respir Dis 1990; 141:A589.
71. Bouhuys A, Schoenberg JB, Beck GJ, Schilling RSF. Epidemiology of chronic lung disease in a cotton mill community. Lung 1977; 154:167–186.
72. Fishwick D, Fletcher AM, Pickering CAC, Niven R, McL R, Faragher B. Ocular and nasal irritation in operatives in Lancashire cotton and synthetic mills. Occup Environ Med 1944; 51:744–748.
73. Niven R, McL R, Fletcher AM, et al. Chronic bronchitis in textile workers. Thorax 1997; 52:22–27.
74. Hamilton JD, Germino VH, Merchant JA, Lumsden JC, Kilborn KH. Byssinosis in a nontextile worker. Am Rev Respir Dis 1973; 107:464–466.
75. Dutkiewicz J. Exposure to dust-borne bacteria in agriculture. I. Environmental studies. Arch Environ Health 1978; 33:250–259.
76. Olenchock AA, Lenhart SW, Mull JC. Occupational exposure to airborne endotoxins during poultry processing. J Toxicol Environ Health 1982; 9:339–349.
77. Pratt DS, May JJ. Feed-associated respiratory illness in farmer. Arch Environ Health 1984; 39:43–48.
78. do Pico GA. Health effects of organic dusts in the farm environment. Report on diseases. Am J Ind Med 1986; 10:261–265.
79. Arlidge JT. The Hygiene Diseases and Mortality of Occupations. London: Percival and Company, 1982.
80. Caminita BH, Baum WF, Neal PA, Schneiter R. A review of the literature relating to affection of the respiratory tract in individuals exposed to cotton dust. Public Health Bulletin No. 297. Washington, D.C., U.S. Government Printing Office, 1949.
81. Rylander R, Schilling RSF, Pickering CAC, Rooke GB, Dempsey AN, Jacobs RR. Effects alter acute and chronic exposure to cotton dust: the Manchester criteria. Br J Ind Med 1987; 44:577–579.
82. Zuskin E, Valic F, Bouhuys A. Byssinosis and airway responses to exposure to textile dust. Lung 1976; 154:17–24.
83. Zuskin E, Bouhuys A. Protective effect of disodium cromoglycate against airway constriction induced by hemp dust extract. J Allergy Clin Immunol 1976; 57(5): 473–479.
84. Fawcett IW, Merchant JA, Simmonds SP, Pepys J. The effect of sodium cromoglycate, beclomethasone diproprionate and salbutamol on the ventilatory response to cotton dust in mill workers. Br J Dis Chest 1978; 29:29–38.

85. Edwards C, MacArtney J, Rooke G, Ward F. The pathology of the lung in byssinotics. Thorax 1975; 30:612–623.

86. Pratt PC, Vollmer RT, Miller JA. Epidemiology of pulmonary lesions in non-textile and cotton textile workers: a retrospective autopsy analysis. Arch Environ Health 1980; 35:133–138.

87. Moran TM. Emphysema and other chronic lung disease in textile workers: an 18-year autopsy study. Arch Environ Health 1983; 38:267–276.

88. Milton DK, Godleski JJ, Feldman HA, Greaves IA. Toxicity of intratracheally instilled cotton dust, cellulose and endotoxin. Am Rev Respir Dis 1990; 142:184–192.

89. Bouhuys A. Byssinosis, Breathing, Physiology, Environmental and Lung Disease. New York: Grune & Stratton, 1976:416–440.

90. Russell JH, Gilberstadt ML, Rolstad RA, Rohrbach MS. Airway smooth muscle and platelet responses to several varieties of cotton bracts. Lung 1984; 162:89–97.

91. Russell JH, McCormick JP. Lacinilene C methyl ether (LCME) constricts tracheal smooth muscle. Environ Res 1988; 45(1):118–126.

92. Rylander R, Bergstrom R, Goto H, Yuasa K, Tanaka S. Studies on endotoxin and beta-1,3 glucan in cotton dust. Proceedings of the 13th Cotton Dust Research Conference, Nashville, Tennessee, 1989:46–47.

93. Di Luzio NR. Lysozyme, glucan-activated macrophages in neoplasia. J Reticuloendothel Soc 1979; 26:67–81.

94. Castronova V, Robinson VA, Frazer DG. Pulmonary reactions to organic dust exposures: development of an animal model. Environ Health Perspect 1996; 104(1):41–53.

95. Merchant JA. Byssinosis: progress in prevention (editorial). Am J Public Health 1983; 73(2):37–138.

96. Hend IM, Milnera M, Milnera SM. Bactericidal treatment of raw cotton as the method of byssinosis prevention. AIHA J 2003; 64:88–94.

97. Ramazzini B. De Morbis Articum. Translated by W.C. Wright. New York: Hafner Publishing, 1964.

98. Farant JP, Moore CF. Dust exposures in the Canadian industries. In: Dosman JA, Cotton DJ, eds. Occupational Pulmonary Disease, Focus on Grain Dust and Health. New York: Academic Press, 1980:477–506.

99. Dashek WV, Olenchock SA, Mayfield JE, Wirtz GH, Wolz DE, Young CA. Carbohydrate and protein contents of grain dusts in relation to dust morphology. Environ Health Perspect 1986; 66:135–143.

100. Lacy J. The microflora of grain dusts. In: Dosman JA, Cotton DJ, eds. Occupational Pulmonary Disease: Focus on Grain Dust and Health. New York: Academic Press, 1980:417–440.

101. Cuthbert OD, Wraith EG, Brostoff J, Brighton ND. The role of mites in hay and grain dust allergy. In: Dosman JA, Cotton DJ, eds. Occupational Pulmonary Disease: Focus on Grain Dust and Health. New York: Academic Press, 1980:469–476.

102. Warren CPW, Cherniak RM, Tse KS. Hypersensitivity reaction to grain dust. J Allergy Clin Immunol 1974; 53:139–149.

103. Chan-Yeung M, Wong R, MacLean L. Respiratory abnormalities among grain elevator workers. Chest 1979; 75:461–467.

104. Broder I, Davies G, Hutcheon M, et al. Variables of pulmonary allergy and inflammation in grain elevator workers. J Occup Med 1983; 25:43–47.

105. Davies RJ, Green M, McSchofield N. Recurrent nocturnal asthma after exposure to grain dust. Am Rev Respir Dis 1976; 14:1011–1015.

106. Warren CPW, Holford-Strevens V, Sinha RN. Sensitization in a grain handler to the storage mite Lepidoglyphus destructor (shrank). Ann Allergy 1983; 50:30–38.

107. Park HS, Nahm DH, Suh CH, et al. Occupational asthma and specific IgE sensitization to grain dust. J Korean Med Sic 1998; 13:275–280.

108. Park HS, Nahm DH, Kim HY, Suh CH, Kim KS. Role of specific IgE, IgG, and IgG4 antibodies to corn dust in exposed workers. Korean J Intern Med 1998; 13:88–94.

109. doPico GA, Jacobs S, Flaherty D, Rankin J. Pulmonary reaction to durum wheat: a constituent of grain dust. Chest 1982; 81:55–61.

110. Lunn JA, Hughes DT. Pulmonary hypersensitivity to the grain weevil. Br J Ind Med 1967; 24:158–161.

111. Kleine-Tebbe J, Jeep S, Josties C, Meysel U, O'Connor A, Kunkel J. IgE-mediated inhalant allergy in inhabitants of a building infested by the rice weevil (*Sitophilus oryzae*). Ann Allergy 1992; 69:497–503.

112. Chan-Yeung M. Grain dust asthma, does it exist? In: Dosman J, Cockcroft D, eds. Principles of Health and Safety in Agriculture. Academic Press, 1990:169–171.

113. Senthilselvan A, Chen Y, Dosman JA. Predictors of asthma and wheezing in adults. Grain farming, sex, and smoking. Am Rev Respir Dis 1993; 148:6676–6680.

114. Senthilselvan A, Pahwa P, Wang P, McDuffie HH, Dosman JA. Persistent wheeze in grain elevator workers should not be ignored. Am J Respir Crit Care Med 1996; 153:701–705.

115. Gandevia B, Ritchie B. Relevance of respiratory symptoms and signs to ventilatory capacity changes after exposure to grain dust and phosphate rock dust. Br J Ind Med 1966; 23:181–187.

116. McCarthy PE, Cockcroft AE, McDermott M. Lung function after exposure to barley dust. Br J Ind Med 1985; 42:106–110.

117. doPico GA, Reddan W, Anderson S, Flaherty D, Smalley E. Acute effects of grain dust exposure during a work shift. Am Rev Respir Dis 1983; 128:399–404.

118. Chan-Yeung M, Schulzer M, MacLean L, Dorken E, Grzybowski S. Epidemiologic health survey of grain elevator workers in British Columbia. Am Rev Respir Dis 1980; 121:329–336.

119. Clapp WD, Thorne PS, Frees KL, Zhang X, Lux CR, Schwartz DA. The effects of inhalation of grain dust extract and endotoxin on upper and lower airways. Chest 1993; 104:825–830.

120. Corey P, Hutcheon M, Broder I, Mintz S. Grain elevator workers show work-related pulmonary function changes and dose-effect relationships with dust exposure. Br J Ind Med 1982; 39:330–337.

121. Enarson DA, Vedal S, Chan-Yeung M. Fate of grainhandlers with bronchial hyperreactivity. Clin Invest Med 1988; 11:193–197.

122. Clapp WD, Becker S, Quay J, et al. Grain dust-induced airflow obstruction and inflammation of the lower respiratory tract. Am J Respir Crit Care Med 1994; 150:611–617.

123. Jagielo PJ, Thorne PS, Watt JL, Frees KL, Quinn TJ, Schwartz DA. Grain dust and endotoxin inhalation produced similar inflammatory responses in normal subjects. Chest 1996; 110:263–270.

124. Deetz DC, Jagielo PJ, Quinn TJ, Thorne PS, Bleuer SA, Schwartz DA. The kinetics of grain dust-induced inflammation of the lower respiratory tract. Am J Respir Crit Care Med 1997; 155:254–259.

125. Blaski CA, Clapp WD, Thorne PS, et al. The role of atopy in grain dust-induced airway disease. Am J Respir Crit Care Med 1996; 154:334–340.

126. Olenchock SA, Mull JC, Major PC, Peach MJ, Gladish ME, Taylor G. In vitro activation of the alternative pathway of complement by settled grain dust. J Allergy Clin Immunol 1978; 62:295–300.

127. Olenchock SA, Mull JC, Major PC. Extracts of airborne grain dusts activate alternative and classical complement pathways. Ann Allergy 1980; 44:23–28.

128. doPico GA, Flaherty D, Bhaansali P, Chavaje N. Grain fever syndrome induced by inhalation of airborne grain dust. J Allergy Clin Immunol 1982; 69:435–443.

129. Von Essen SG, McGranaghan S, Cirian D, O'Neill D, Spurzem JR, Rennard SI. Inhalation of grain sorghum dust extract causes respiratory tract inflammation in human volunteers. Am Rev Respir Dis 1991; 143:A105.

130. Keller GE, Lewis DM, Olenchock SA. Demonstration of inflammatory cell population changes in rat lungs in response to intratracheal instillation of spring wheat dust using

lung enzymatic digestion and centrifugal elutriation. Comp Immun Microbiol Infect Dis 1987; 10:219–226.

131. Von Essen SG, Robbins RA, Thompson AB, Ertl RF, Linder J, Rennard S. Mechanisms of neutrophil recruitment to the lung by grain dust exposure. Am Rev Respir Dis 1988; 138:921–927.
132. Lewis DM, Mentnech MS. Extracts of airborne grain dusts simulate interleukin-1 (IL-1) production by alveolar macrophages. Am Rev Respir Dis 1984; 129:A161.
133. Quinn TJ, Taylor S, Wohlford-Lenane CL, Schwartz D. IL-10 reduces grain induced airway inflammation and airway hyperreactivity. J Appl Physiol 2000; 88:173–179.
134. Smith AR, Greenburg L, Siegel W. Respiratory disease among grain handlers. Ind Bull. (Dept of Labour, New York State) 1941; 20:1.
135. Williams N, Skoulas A, Merriman JE. Exposure to grain dust. I. A survey of the effects. J Occup Med 1964; 6:319–329.
136. Kleinfeld M, Messite J, Swencicki RE, Shapiro J. A clinical and physiological study of grain handlers. Arch Environ Health 1968; 16:380–384.
137. Tse KS, Warren P, Janusz M, McCarthy DS, Cherniack RM. Respiratory abnormalities in workers exposed to grain dust. Arch Environ Health 1973; 27:74–77.
138. doPico GA, Reddan W, Flaherty D, et al. Respiratory abnormalities among grainhandlers: a clinical, physiologic, and immunologic study. Am Rev Respir Dis 1977; 115:915–927.
139. Sheridan D, Deutscher C, Tan L, et al. The relationship between exposure to cereal grain dust and pulmonary function in grain workers. In: Dosman JA, Cotton D, eds. Occupational Pulmonary Disease: Focus on Grain Dust and Health. New York: Academic Press, 1979:229–238.
140. Rask-Andersen A, Malmberg P. Organic dust toxic syndrome in Swedish farmers: symptoms, chemical findings and exposure in 98 cases (Abstract). Am J Ind Med 1989; 17:116–117.
141. Farant JP, Moore CF. Dust exposures in Canadian grain industry. Am Ind Hyg Assoc J 1978; 39:177–193.
142. Herbert FA, Woytowich V, Schram E, Baldwin D. Respiratory profiles of grain handlers and sedentary workers. Can Med Assoc J 1981; 125:46–50.
143. Cotton DJ, Graham BL, Li KYR, Froh F, Barnett GD, Dosman JA. Effects of grain dust exposure and smoking on respiratory symptoms and lung function. J Occup Med 1983; 25:131–141.
144. Yach D, Myers J, Bradshaw D, Benatar SR. A respiratory epidemiologic survey of grain mill workers in Cape Town, South Africa. Am Rev Respir Dis 1985; 131:505–510.
145. Massin N, Bohadana AB, Wild P, Kolopp-Sarda MN, Toamain JP. Airway responsiveness to methacholine, respiratory symptoms, and dust exposure levels in grain and flour mill workers in Eastern France. Am J Ind Med 1995; 27:859–869.
146. Gimenez C, Fouad K, Choudat D. Chronic and acute respiratory effects among grain mill workers. Int Arch Occup Environ Health 1995; 67:311–315.
147. Ye T, Huang J, Shen Y, Lu P, Christiani DC. Respiratory symptoms and pulmonary function among Chinese rice-granary workers. Int J Occup Environ Health 1998; 4:155–159.
148. Broder I, Mintz M, Hutcheon P, et al. Comparison of respiratory variables in grain elevator workers and civic outside workers of Thunder Bay, Canada. Am Rev Respir Dis 1979; 119:193–203.
149. Dosman JA, Cotton DJ, Graham B, Li R, Froh F, Barnett D. Chronic bronchitis and decreased forced expiratory flow rates in life-time nonsmoking grain workers. Am Rev Respir Dis 1980; 121:11–16.
150. Chan-Yeung M, Schulzer M, MacLean L, et al. A follow up study of the grain elevator workers in the Port of Vancouver. Arch Environ Health 1981; 36:75–80.
151. Chan-Yeung M, Enarson DA. Prospective changes in lung function in grain elevator workers in large terminals in Vancouver. In: Dosman J, Cockcroft D, eds. Principles of Health and Safety in Agriculture. Academic Press, 1990:131–134.

152. Schulzer M, Enarson DA, Chan-Yeung M. Analyzing cross-sectional and longitudinal lung function measurements: the effects of age. Can J Statist 1985; 13:7–15.
153. Chan-Yeung M, Ward H, Enarson DA, Kennedy SM. Five cross-sectional studies of grain elevator workers. Am J Epidemiol 1992; 136:1269–1279.
154. Broder I, Corey P, Davies G, et al. Longitudinal study of grain elevator workers and control workers with demonstration of healthy worker effect. J Occup Med 1985; 27:873–880.
155. Broder I, Mintz S, Hutcheon MA, Corey PN, Kuzyk J. Effect of layoff and rehire on respiratory variables on grain elevator workers. Am Rev Respir Dis 1980; 122:601–608.
156. Broder I, Hutcheon MA, Mintz S, et al. Changes in respiratory variables of grain handlers and civic workers during their initial months of employment. Br J Ind Med 1984; 41:94–99.
157. Kennedy SM, Dimich-Ward H, Desjardins A, Kassam A, Vedal S, Chan-Yeung M. Respiratory health among retired grain elevator workers. Am J Respir Crit Care Med 1994; 150:59–65.
158. Pahwa P, Senthilselvan A, McDuffie HH, Dosman JA. Longitudinal decline in lung function measurements among Saskatchewan grain workers. Can Respir J 2003; 10:135–141.
159. Enarson DA, Vedal S, Chan-Yeung M. Rapid decline in FEV1 in grain handlers—relation to level of dust exposure. Am Rev Respir Dis 1985; 132:814–817.
160. Huy T, De Schipper K, Chan-Yeung M, Kennedy SM. Grain dust and lung function: exposure response relationships. Am Rev Respir Dis 1991; 144:1314–1321.
161. Kennedy SM, Dimich-Ward H, Chan-Yeung M. Relationship between grain dust exposure and longitudinal changes in pulmonary function. In: Human Sustainability in Agriculture: Health Safety and Environment. Michigan: Lewis Publishers, 1995: 13–18.
162. Smid T, Heederik D, Houba R, Quanjer PH. Dust- and endotoxin-related respiratory effects in the animal feed industry. Am Rev Respir Dis 1992; 146:1474–1479.
163. Post WK, Heederik D, Houba R. Exposure related lung function decline and selection processes among workers in the animal feed and grain processing industry. Wageningen Agricultural University, Wageningen, 1996.
164. Jorna THJM, Borm PJA, Valds J, Houba R, Wouters EFM. Respiratory symptoms and lung function in animal feed workers. Chest 1994; 106:1050–1055.
165. Peelen SJM, Heederik D, Dimich-Ward H, Chan-Yeung M, Kennedy SM. Comparison of dust related respiratory effects in Dutch and Canadian grain handling industries. A pooled analysis. Occup Environ Med 1996; 53:559–566.
166. American Conference of Governmental Industrial Hygienists (ACGIH). 2000 TLVs and BEIs Threshold Limit Values for Chemical Substances and Physical Agents and Biological Exposure Indices. Cincinnati, Ohio: ACGIH, 2000.
167. Donham KJ, Rubino MJ, Thedell TD, Kammermeyer J. Potential health hazards to agricultural workers in swine confinement buildings. J Occup Med 1977; 19:383–387.
168. Von Essen S, Donham K. Illness and injury in animal confinement workers. Occup Med: State Art Rev 1999; 14(20):337–350.
169. Reynolds SJ, Donham KJ, Whitten P, Merchant JA, Burmeister LF, Popendorf WJ. Longitudinal evaluation of dose-response relationships for environmental exposures and pulmonary function in swine production workers. Am J Ind Med 1996; 29(1):33–40.
170. Vogelzang PFJ, van der Gulden JWJ, Folgering H, et al. Endotoxin exposure as a major determinant of lung function decline in pig farmers. Am J Respir Crit Care Med 1998; 157:15–18.
171. Andersen CI, Von Essen SG, Smith LM, Spencer J, Jolie R, Donham KJ. Respiratory symptoms and airway obstruction in swine veterinarians: a persistent problem. Am J Ind Med 2004; 46(4):386–392.
172. Holness DL, O'blenis EL, Sass-Kortsak A, Pilger C, Nethercott JR. Respiratory effects and dust exposures in hog confinement farming. Am J Ind Med 1987; 11(50):571–580.

173. Iversen M, Pedersen B. Relation between respiratory symptoms, type of farming and lung function disorders. Thorax 1990; 45(12):919–923.

174. Schwartz DA, Donham KJ, Olenchock SA, et al. Determinants of longitudinal changes in spirometric function among swine confinement operators and farmers. Am J Respir Crit Care Med 1995; 151(1):47–53.

175. Radon K, Danuser B, Iversen M, et al. Respiratory symptoms in European animal farmers. Eur Respir J 2001; 17:747–754.

176. Harries MG, Cromwell O. Occupational asthma caused by allergy to pigs' urine. Brit Med J 1982; 284:867.

177. Larsen FO, Roepstort V, Sigsgaard T, Hjort C, Poulsen LK, Norn S. Does inhalation allergy to pig exist? Inflamm Res 1997; 46(suppl 1):S65–S66.

178. Matson SC, Swanson MC, Reed CE, Yunginer JW. IgE and IgG-immune mechanisms do not mediate occupation-related respiratory or systemic symptoms in hog farmers. J Allergy Clin Immunol 1983; 72:299–304.

179. Thorne PS, Donham KJ, Dosman J, Jagielo P, Merchant JA, Von Essen S. Report of the Occupational Health Group: Proceedings from Understanding the Impacts of Large Scale Swine Production: an Interdisciplinary Scientific Workshop; June 29–30, 1995:1–41.

180. Dosman JA, Lawson JA, Kirychuk SP, Cormier Y, Biem J, Koehncke N. Occupational asthma in newly employed workers in intensive swine confinement facilities. Eur Respir J 2004; 24:698–702.

181. Zejda JE, Hurst TS, Rhodes CS, et al. Respiratory health of swine producers: focus on young workers. Chest 1993; 103:702–709.

182. Senthilselvan A, Dosman JA, Kirychuk SP, et al. Accelerated lung function decline in swine confinement workers. Chest 1997; 111(6):1733–1741.

183. Schwartz DA, Landas SK, Lassise DL, Burmeister LF, Hunninghake GW, Merchant JA. Airway injury in swine confinement workers. Ann Int Med 1992; 116:630–635.

184. Kirychuk S, Senthilselvan A, Dosman JA, et al. Predictors of longitudinal changes in pulmonary function among swine confinement workers. Can Respir J 1998; 5(6):472–478.

185. Palmberg L, Larsson B-M, Malmberg P, Larsson K. Airway responses of healthy farmers and nonfarmers to exposure in a swine confinement building. Scand J Work Environ Health 2002; 28(4):256–263.

186. Sundblad B-M, Larsson B-M, Palmberg L, Larsson K. Exhaled NO and bronchial responsiveness in healthy subjects exposed to organic dust. Eur Respir J 2002; 20:426–431.

187. Von Essen SG, Scheppers LA, Robbins RA, Donham KA. Respiratory tract inflammation in swine confinement workers studied using analysis of induced sputum and exhaled nitric oxide. Clin Toxicol 1998; 36:557–565.

188. Von Essen S, Romberger D. The respiratory inflammatory response to the swine confinement building environment: the adaptation to respiratory exposures in the chronically exposed worker. J Agric Safety Health 2003; 9(3):185–196.

189. Robbins RA, Floreani AA, Von Essen SG, et al. Measurement of exhaled nitric oxide by three different techniques. Am J Respir Crit Care Med 1996; 153:1631–1635.

190. Larsson KA, Eklund AG, Hansson LO, Isaakson B-M, Malmberg PO. Swine dust causes intense airways inflammation in healthy subjects. Am J Respir Crit Care Med 1994; 150:973–977.

191. Larsson K, Eklund A, Malmberg P, Belin L. Alterations in bronchoalveolar lavage fluid but not in lung function and bronchial responsiveness in swine confinement workers. Chest 1992; 101:767–774.

192. Zejda JE, Barber E, Dosman JA, et al. Respiratory health status in swine producers relates to endotoxin exposure in the presence of low dust levels. JOM 1994; 36(1):49–56.

193. Vogelzang PF, van der Gulden JW, Folgering H, Heederick D, Tielen MJ, van Schayck CP. Longitudinal changes in bronchial responsiveness associated with swine confinement dust exposure. Chest 2000; 117(5):1488–1495.

194. Zhiping W, Malmberg P, Larsson BM, Larsson L, Saraf A. Exposures to bacteria in swine-house dust and acute inflammatory reactions in humans. Am J Respir Crit Care Med 1996; 154(5):1261–1266.

195. Israel-Assayag E, Cormier Y. Adaptation to organic dust exposure: a potential role of L-selectin shedding? Eur Respir J 2002; 19(5):833–837.

196. Wang Z, Malmberg P, Larsson P, Larsson B-M, Larsson K. Time course of interleukin-6 and tumor necrosis factor-α increase in serum following inhalation of swine dust. Am J Respir Crit Care Med 1996; 153:147–152.

197. Palmberg L, Larsson B-M, Malmberg P, Larsson K. Induction of IL-8 production in human alveolar macrophages and human bronchial epithelial cells in vitro by swine dust. Thorax 1998; 53:260–264.

198. Romberger DJ, Bodlak V, Von Essen SG, Mathisen T, Wyatt TA. Hog barn dust extract stimulates IL-8 and IL-6 release in human bronchial epithelial cells via PKC activation. J Appl Physiol 2002; 93(1):289–296.

199. Cormier Y, Israël-Assayag E, Racine G, Duchaine C. Farming practices and the respiratory health risks of swine confinement buildings. Eur Respir J 2000; 15:560–565.

200. Gjerde C, Ferguson K, Mutel C, Donham K, Merchant J. Results of an educational intervention to improve the health knowledge, attitudes and self-reported behaviors of swine confinement workers. J Rural Health 1991; 7:278–286.

201. Dosman JA, Senthilselvan A, Kirychuk SP, et al. Positive human health effects of wearing a respirator in a swine barn. Chest 2000; 118(3):852–860.

202. Larsson B-M, Larsson K, Malmberg P, Palmberg L. Airways inflammation after exposure in a swine confinement building during the cleaning procedure. Am J Ind Med 2002; 41(4):250–258.

203. Holness DL. What actually happens to the farmers? Clinical results of a follow-up study of hog confinement farmers. In: Dosman JA, Cockcroft DW, eds. Principles of Health and Safety in Agriculture. Boca Raton, FL: CRC Press, 1995:69–71.

204. Reed CE, Milton DK. Endotoxin-stimulated innate immunity: a contributing factor for asthma. J Allergy Clin Immunol 2001; 108:157–166.

205. Hasday JD, Bascom R, Costa JJ, Fitzgerald T, Dubin W. Bacterial endotoxin is an active component of cigarette smoke. Chest 1999; 115:829–835.

206. Mueller-Anneling L, Avol E, Peters JM, Thorne PS. Ambient endotoxin concentrations in PM10 from Southern California. Environ Health Perspect 2004; 112:583–588.

207. Cochran JR, Khan AM, Elidemir O, et al. Influence of LPS exposure on airway function and allergic responses in developing mice. Pediatr Pulmonol 2002; 34:267–277.

208. Rylander R, Bake B, Fisher JJ, Helander IM. Pulmonary function and symptoms after inhalation of endotoxin. Am Rev Respir Dis 1989; 140:981–986.

209. Boehlecke BA, Peden D, Hazucha M. Exposure to low level of endotoxin for four hours increased response to inhaled mite allergen in mild asthmatics. Am J Respir Crit Care Med 1999; 159:A699.

210. Vernoy JHJ, Dentener MA, van Suylen RJ, Buurman Wouters EFM. Long-term intratracheal LPS exposure results in chronic lung inflammation and persistent pathology. Am J Respir Cell Mol Biol 2002; 26:152–159.

211. Domenici L, Pieri L, Galle MB, Romagnoli P, Adembri C. Evolution of endotoxin-induced lung injury in rats beyond the acute phase. Pathobiology 2004; 71:59–69.

212. Brass DM, Savov JD, Gavett SH, Haykal-Coates N, Schwartz DA. Subchronic endotoxin inhalation causes chronic airway disease. Am J Physiol: Lung Cell Mol Physiol 2003; 285:L755–L761.

213. Schwartz DA, Landas SK, Lassise DL, Burmeister LF, Hunninghake GW, Merchant JA. Airway injury in swine confinement workers. Ann Intern Med 1992; 116(8):630–635.

214. Rylander R, Haglind P. Exposure of cotton workers in an experimental cardroom with reference to airborne endotoxins. Environ Health Perspect 1986; 66:83–86.

215. Buck MG, Wall JH, Schachter EN. Airway constrictor response to cotton bract extracts in the absence of endotoxin. Br J Ind Med 1986; 43:220–226.

216. Rylander R, Snella M. Acute inhalation toxicity of cotton plant dusts. Br J Ind Med 1976; 33:175–180.

217. Haglind P, Rylander R. Exposure to cotton dust in an experimental cardroom. Br J Ind Med 1984; 41:340–345.

218. Rylander R, Haglind P, Lundholm M. Endotoxin in cotton dust and respiratory function decrement among cotton workers in an experimental cardroom. Am Rev Respir Dis 1985; 131:209–213.

219. Donham K, Haglind P, Peterson Y, Rylander R, Belin L. Environmental and health studies of farm workers in Swedish swine confinement buildings. Br J Ind Med 1989; 46:31–37.

220. Thelin A, Tegler O, Rylander R. Lung reactions during poultry handling related to dust and bacterial endotoxin levels. Eur J Respir Dis 1984; 65:266–271.

221. Schwartz DA, Thorne PS, Yagla SJ, et al. The role of endotoxin in grain dust-induced lung disease. Am J Respir Crit Care Med 1995; 152:603–608.

222. Schwartz DA, Donham KJ, Olenchock SA, et al. Determinants of longitudinal changes in spirometric functions among swine confinement operators and farmers. Am J Respir Crit Care Med 1995; 151:47–53.

223. Michel O, Ginanni R, Le Bon B, Content J, Duchateau J, Sergysels R. Inflammatory response to acute inhalation of endotoxin in asthmatic patients. Am Rev Respir Dis 1992; 146:352–357.

224. Michel O, Kips J, Duchateua J, et al. Severity of asthma is related to endotoxin in house dust. Am J Respir Crit Care Med 1996; 154:1641–1646.

225. Cavagna G, Foa V, Vigliani EC. Effects in man and rabbits of inhalation of cotton dust or extracts and purified endotoxins. Br J Ind Med 1969; 26:314–321.

226. Herbert A, Carvalheiro M, Rubenowitz E, Bake B, Rylander R. Reduction of alveolar-capillary diffusion after inhalation of endotoxin in normal subjects. Chest 1992; 102:1095–1098.

227. Rylander R, Bake B, Fischer JJ, Helander IM. Pulmonary function and symptoms after inhalation of endotoxin. Am Rev Respir Dis 1989; 140:981–986.

228. Michel O, Duchateau J, Sergysels R. Effect of inhaled endotoxin on bronchial reactivity in asthmatic and normal subjects. J Appl Physiol 1989; 66:1059.

229. Boehlecke B, Cocke J, Bragg K, et al. Pulmonary function response to dust from standard and closed boll harvested cotton. Chest 1981; 79:77S–81S.

230. Schwartz DA, Thorne PS, Jagielo PJ, White GE, Bleuer SA, Frees KL. Endotoxin responsiveness and grain dust-induced inflammation in the lower respiratory tract. Am J Physiol 1984; 267:L609–L617.

231. Jagielo PJ, Thorne PS, Kern JA, Quinn TJ, Schwartz DA. The role of endotoxin in grain dust-induced inflammation in mice. Am J Physiol: Lung Cell Mol Physiol 1996; 270:L1052–L1059.

232. Jagielo PJ, Quinn TJ, Qureshi N, Schwartz DA. Grain dust induced lung inflammation is reduced by Rhodobacter Sphaeroides Disphosphoryl Lipid A. Am J Physiol 1998; 274:L26–L31.

233. Snella M, Rylander R. Lung cell reactions after inhalation of bacterial lipopolysaccharides. Eur J Respir Dis 1982; 63:550–557.

234. Freudenberg MA, Galanos C. Induction of tolerance to lipopolysaccharide (LPS)-D-galactosamine lethality by pretreatment with LPS is mediated by macrophages. Infect Immun 1988; 56:1352–1357.

235. Kips JC, Tavernier J, Pauwels RA. Tumor necrosis factor causes bronchial hyperresponsiveness in rats. Am Rev Respir Dis 1992; 145:332–336.

236. Strieter RM, Standiford TJ, Rolfe MW, Kunkel SL. Interleukin-8. In: Kelley J, ed. Cytokines of the Lung. Marcel Dekker, Inc., 1993:281–306.
237. Standiford TJ, Kunkel SL, Basha MA, et al. Interleukin-8 gene expression by a pulmonary epithelial cell line. J Clin Invest 1990; 86:1945–1953.
238. Nakamura H, Yoshimura K, Jaffe HA, Crystal RG. Interleukin-8 gene expression in human bronchial epithelial cells. J Biol Chem 1991; 266:19611–19617.
239. Redl H, Schlag G, Ceska M, Davies J, Buurman WA. Interleukin-8 release in baboon septicemia is partially dependent on tumor necrosis factor. J Inf Dis 1993; 167: 1464–1466.
240. Schwartz DA. Grain dust, endotoxin, and airflow obstruction. Chest 1996:57s–63s.
241. Liu AH. Endotoxin exposure in allergy and asthma: reconciling a paradox. J Allergy Clin Immunol 2002; 109:379–392.
242. Calvani M Jr, Alessandri C, Bonci E. Fever episodes in early life and the development of atopy in children with asthma. Eur Respir J 2002; 20:391–396.
243. Ball TM, Castro-Rodriguez JA, Griffith KA, Holberg CJ, Martinez FD, Wright AL. Siblings, day-care attendance, and the risk of asthma and wheezing during childhood. N Engl J Med 2000; 343:538–543.
244. Gehring U, Bischof W, Fahlbusch B, Wichmann H, Heinrich J. House dust endotoxin and allergic sensitization in children. Am J Respir Crit Care Med 2002; 166:939–942.
245. Braun-Fahrlander C, Riedler J, Herz U, Eder W, et al. Environmental exposure to endotoxin and its relation to asthma in school-age children. N Engl J Med 2002; 347:869–877.
246. Cardoso MR, Cousens SN, de Goes Siqueira LF, Alves FM, D'Angelo LA. Crowding: risk factor or protective factor for lower respiratory disease in young children? BMC Public Health 2004; 4:19.
247. Park J, Gold DR, Spiegelman DL, Burge HA, Milton DK. House dust endotoxin and wheeze in the first year of life. Am J Respir Crit Care Med 2001; 163:322–328.
248. Akira S, Takeda K. Toll-like receptor signaling. Nat Rev Genet 2004; 4:499–511.
249. Arbour NC, Lorenz E, Schutte BC, et al. TLR4 mutations are associated with endotoxin hyporesponsiveness in humans. Nat Genet 2000; 25:187–191.
250. Fageras Bottcher M, Hmani-Aifa M, Lindstrom A, et al. A TLR4 polymorphism is associated with asthma and reduced LPS-induced IL-12 responses in Swedish children. J Allergy Clin Immunol 2004; 114:561–567.
251. Raby BA, Klimecki WT, Laprise C, et al. Polymorphisms in Toll-like receptor 4 are not associated with asthma or atopy-related phenotypes. Am J Respir Crit Care Med 2002; 166:1449–1456.
252. Yang IA, Barton SJ, Rorke S, et al. Toll-like receptor 4 polymorphism and severity of atopy in asthmatics. Genes Immun 2004; 5:41–45.
253. Alexis N, Eldridge M, Reed W, Bromberg P, Peden DB. CD14-dependent airway neutrophil response to inhaled LPS: role of atopy. J Allergy Clin Immunol 2001; 107:31–35.
254. Koppelman GH, Reijmerink NE, Colin Stine O, et al. Association of a promoter polymorphism of the CD14 gene and atopy. Am J Respir Crit Care Med 2001; 163:965–969.
255. Cook DN, Pisetsky DS, Schwartz DA. Toll-like receptors in the pathogenesis of human disease. Nat Immun 2004; 5:975–979.

28

Chronic Airway Disease Due to Occupational Exposure

Eva Hnizdo[a]
Division of Respiratory Disease Studies, NIOSH, Morgantown, West Virginia, U.S.A.

Susan M. Kennedy
School of Occupational and Environmental Hygiene, University of British Columbia, Vancouver, British Columbia, Canada

Paul D. Blanc
Division of Occupational and Environmental Medicine, Department of Medicine, University of California–San Francisco, San Francisco, California, U.S.A.

Kjell Toren
Departments of Occupational and Environmental Medicine and Allergology, Sahlgrenska University Hospital, Sahlgrenska Academy at Göteborg University, Göteborg, Sweden

I. Leonard Bernstein
Division of Allergy–Immunology, Department of Internal Medicine, College of Medicine, University of Cincinnati, Cincinnati, Ohio, U.S.A.

Moira Chan-Yeung
Occupational and Environmental Lung Disease Unit, Respiratory Division, Department of Medicine, University of British Columbia and Vancouver General Hospital, Vancouver, British Columbia, Canada

INTRODUCTION

Long before personal cigarette smoking was widespread, medical writers recognized that dusty trades were associated with various lung diseases. Much of this, often termed "miner's phthisis," was due to inorganic dusts and is best understood by today's nosology as one of the pneumoconioses (with or without super-imposed tubercular disease). Nonetheless, clinical syndromes consistent with chronic

---

[a] The findings and conclusions in this chapter are those of the author and do not necessarily represent the views of the National Institute for Occupational Safety and Health.

bronchitis or airway obstruction, in particular among persons experiencing heavy organic dust inhalation, were also well described throughout the 19th century (1,2).

By the mid-20th century, occupational exposures, characterized by dusty trades, were generally presumed to be contributors to chronic bronchitis specifically and, by extension, the airway disease generally. A key 1953 analysis of mortality data from the 1930s found that work in dusty trades, even within the same social class, was linked to bronchitis mortality (3). In 1958, Fletcher himself noted that, "men who work in dusty trades, especially coal miners, have a higher prevalence of symptoms of bronchitis and emphysema..." (4). When Fletcher's landmark studies downplayed the role of chronic bronchitis in the progression of airway obstruction, the ascendancy of cigarette smoking as a major independent risk factor for the latter tended to eclipse all other potential associations. This was most especially true of possible links between occupational exposures and chronic obstructive pulmonary disease (COPD), with or without concomitant chronic bronchitis.

Over the ensuing 30 years since 1960, many epidemiological studies investigated the question of COPD in relation to occupational exposures. During this time, a number of industry-based and population-based studies did publish interesting and surprisingly consistent findings indicating that work-related exposures were linked to symptoms of bronchitis or COPD/emphysema, or to airway obstruction by lung function testing. In many of these investigations, occupational risk was not a study focus and often the occupational findings were published as little more than a controlling cofactor in multivariate modeling. At the same time, exposure-specific studies were providing new insights relevant to the biological plausibility of industrial toxins and airway obstruction. For example, research linked occupational cadmium exposure to emphysema in a dose-dependent manner, while other studies delineated the pulmonary function characteristics of fixed obstruction in byssinosis (5,6).

The revival of general biomedical interest in occupational exposures in the causation of chronic bronchitis, COPD, and emphysema has been revived through the seminal work of Dr. Becklake (7). Early on, she had observed the airway obstruction of irritant gas inhalation among miners exposed to explosive blast fumes (7) and had also shown that lung function decline among gold miners need not be linked to the extent of radiographic disease (8,9). Beginning in 1989, she authored a series of reviews and informal meta-analyses systematically compiling together the scattered epidemiological reports that had been appearing in the medical literature. The key analysis from this series included five large population-based studies (two from the United States and one each from Italy, France, and Poland), all showing longitudinal decline in airflow or a greater prevalence of airflow obstruction associated with work-related inhalation of gases and vapors or fumes and dust or both categories of exposure. In the same analysis, Becklake also summarized data from nine industry-specific studies (almost all inorganic dust) indicating an accelerated lung function decline (10–12). Becklake's work was followed by a series of other reviews and commentaries addressing this question anew (13–17).

The spectrum of occupational COPD also encompasses exposure to toxic agents which cause irreversible inflammatory disease in the terminal bronchioles, respiratory bronchioles, and alveolar ducts. The unique histopathology features of bronchiolitis (B) and bronchiolitis obliterans (BO) clearly distinguish these airway diseases from other COPD entities. In recent years, workplace exposure to a variety of toxic agents has been directly associated with these outcomes. Although the total number of reported cases has been modest, future industry-specific epidemiologic studies may be warranted. Because workplace experience with B or BO is limited, relevant clinical data will be discussed in the context of specific causal agents.

In this chapter, we first present the epidemiological evidence of chronic airflow obstruction based on specific occupational or industrial groups relevant to cohorts with specific exposures. Second, after summarizing findings relevant to specific exposures, we will review the population attributable risk percent (PAR%) or attributable fraction of COPD and chronic bronchitis related to workplace exposures across all occupational groups rather than limited to a single industrial cohort.

EXPOSURE TO MINERAL DUST

Occupational exposure to mineral dust occurs in many industrial operations worldwide. Occupational mineral dust exposures can be broadly categorized as strongly fibrogenic dusts (silica, asbestos, and coal) and other mineral dusts (emery, graphite, gypsum, marble, mica, perlite, plaster of Paris, Portland cement, silicon, silicon carbide, soapstone, and talc) that may also be associated with adverse lung effects (18). Mineral dust-induced pneumoconioses [silicosis, asbestosis, and coal workers' pneumoconiosis (CWP)] and associated tuberculosis have been the main causes of morbidity and mortality directly attributable to mineral dust exposure at workplace. Many epidemiological studies of specific industry cohorts, however, have demonstrated that exposure to mineral dusts, primarily the more highly fibrogenic types of dusts, is associated with increased levels of obstructive lung function impairment and increased prevalence of chronic bronchitis (11,13,19–21). Extending this association from highly dust-exposed groups to those with lower mineral dust exposure in the absence of radiological signs of pneumoconiosis is an area of ongoing research (21,22).

In addition to the classic features of COPD whose predominant pathological features are emphysema, small airway disease, and chronic bronchitis (23) in mineral dust–exposed workers, lung fibrosis and pulmonary tuberculosis can also cause airflow limitation (24–26). Epidemiologic investigations of exposure–response relationships between indices of occupational dust exposure and lung function impairment, symptoms of chronic bronchitis, and mortality from COPD, adjusted for the confounding effect of age and tobacco smoking, can provide an evidence on whether a particular occupational exposure has a potential of increasing the risk of COPD in the exposed workers. Given the complexity of COPD etiology, however, to obtain reliable estimates of the exposure–response relationships, a relatively large sample size of exposed workers, and if possible a comparable control group, may be required. In many workplace cohorts the number of exposed workers may be relatively small, causing the estimated effect to have a large error leading to poor study power to detect a relationship. For this reason, epidemiological studies conducted on large mining populations often provide the most reliable estimates of the exposure–response relation between mineral dust exposure and lung function impairment (13). Another generalizable problem is the parallel relationships (collinearity) among age, exposure measured in dust-years, and cigarette exposure measured in pack years. This can also increase error terms in estimating equations or lead to overadjustment that masks a true exposure–effect relationship.

In this section, an overview of the evidence on the effect of mineral dust exposure on airflow obstruction is provided, focusing on the issue of whether the risk of airflow obstruction is increased due to mineral dust exposure independent of radiological signs of pneumoconiosis. The following are discussed in sequence: the potential mechanisms by which mineral dusts can cause airflow obstruction, the epidemiological evidence from mining cohorts, focusing on the exposure–response relation, and the evidence from other mineral dust exposure studies.

Pathophysiology of Chronic Obstructive Lung Disease Due to Mineral Dusts

There are multiple pathophysiological mechanisms by which mineral dusts may potentially initiate lung injury leading to airflow obstruction, chronic bronchitis, and emphysema, all independent of fibrosis. Upon deposition, mineral dust particles reach two critical target cells in the lung: macrophages and epithelial cells (27,28). Ingestion of various mineral dust particles by the macrophage (phagocytosis) has been shown to lead to macrophage activation resulting in an increased release of a wide range of products that may react with various target cells in the lung to cause tissue damage. The potential mechanisms of cell injury include cytotoxicity (28–31) leading to generation of reactive oxygen/nitrogen species (31) and secretion of proinflammatory factors (32), cytokines, chemokines, elastase (31,32) and fibrogenic factors (33,34). Mineral dusts analyzed in terms of these mechanisms and found to be toxic include crystalline silica, coal dust, kaolin, talc, bentonite, and feldspar.

In addition to macrophage mediated effects which include cytokine networking with epithelial cells, epithelial cells may interact directly with deposited particles. This may lead to hyperplasia of mucus-producing glands and increased mucus production in the bronchus as well as inflammatory processes in conducting and peripheral airways and in alveolar tissue leading to bronchitis (28,35) and emphysema (31,32,35–39). Dust particles can also cause epithelial cell injury that facilitates penetration of the particles through the walls of small airways and can cause localized fibrosis (33,34,40).

Mineral dust airway disease defined by focal fibrosis in respiratory bronchioles associated with mineral dust exposure has been reported as a pathological process causing airflow limitation in mineral dust-exposed workers (41–44). Nonetheless the association between small airways impairment and silica dust has been reported in only one study (45) and was not found in another when specifically assessed (46). Although data on direct pathological correlates of airflow obstruction in mineral dust exposure are limited, findings of emphysema have often served as a surrogate marker for the concomitant risk of COPD. In coalminers' lungs, typical centrilobular emphysema is caused by coal dust deposition forming the coal macula (47). In silicosis, studies have shown poor correlations between spirometry and profusion of nodules on the chest radiograph and CT scan, while significant inverse correlations were found between CT emphysema score and forced expiratory volume in one second (FEV_1) and D_{LCO} (48–53). Silica dust exposure appears to be associated with more emphysema than asbestos dust (49). In addition, there is an exposure-response relationship between silica dust exposure and emphysema assessed on paper-mounted whole-lung sections at autopsy (54–56). Nonetheless, the degree of emphysema found in silica dust–exposed miners who were never smokers was not correlated with lung function measured five years prior to death (57). Among gold miners, however, emphysema found at autopsy was found to be the most important predictor of lung function measured five years prior to death (58).

Coal Mining Dust—Epidemiological Evidence

Epidemiological studies of British, U.S., and Italian coal miners have established the existence of an exposure–response relationship between cumulative coal dust exposure and decreased lung function. The association was found in smokers, ex-smokers, and never-smokers, and across all age groups. The studies demonstrated that the severity of the impairment associated with coal mining dust exposure puts coal miners at an increased risk of COPD. Because of this evidence, COPD (i.e., chronic bronchitis and emphysema) are now compensable occupational diseases among coal miners in many countries (e.g., Britain, Germany, South Africa). The issues that are currently debated in scientific literature are whether current permissible concentrations of coal mining dust (2 mg/m^3 in the United States) can increase the risk of COPD, especially in the absence of CWP (21).

Several large studies based on a large industry-wide survey of more than 30,000 British coal miners, initiated during 1953–1958 with follow-up studies up to 1991, have shown excessive losses of FEV$_1$ with cumulative dust exposure with dose-dependent relationship and independent of the presence of CWP; the loss was found to be greatest in younger men and in men with respiratory symptoms (Table 1)

Table 1 Epidemiological Studies of the Effect of Coal Mining Dust Exposure on Airflow Limitation

Country (Reference)	N	Design	Reduction of FEV$_1$ (mL/ghm^{-3}) [mL/(mg/m^3–yrs)][a]	Cumulative exposure mean ghm^{-3} (mg/m^3–yrs)[a]	Comment
United Kingdom (59)	3581	Cross-sectional	0.6	175	Current miners
United Kingdom (60)	4059	Cross-sectional	0.76	174	The effect observed across all ages
United Kingdom (61)	2757	Cross-sectional	1.04	204	South Wales miners
			0.08	148	Yorkshire miners, no effect was observed in N.E. England miners (ghm^{-3} = 103)
United States (62)	7139	Cross-sectional	0.69		
United States (63)	977	Cross-sectional	5.9[a]	15.4[a]	Miners who started work from 1970
United Kingdom (64)	1677	Longitudinal	0.42	117	Loss over 11 yrs in relation to previous exposure
United States (65)	1161	Longitudinal	1.6		Loss over 11 yrs in relation to current exposure
Italy (66)	909	Longitudinal	10.9[a]	1.8–6.1[a]	Sardinian coal miners follow-up 1983–1993

[a]Applies to studied done in U.S. (62) and Italy (66).
Abbreviation: FEV$_1$, forced expiratory volume in one second.

(59,60,64,67). Investigating the severity of the impairment associated with coal dust exposure, one study reported that the risks of having symptoms of chronic bronchitis and FEV_1 less than 80% predicted and FEV_1 less than 65% predicted were almost doubled in men with the highest exposure category of 348 ghm^{-3} (61). The excess loss of FEV_1 persisted even after dust levels were substantially reduced in coal miners employed after 1970 (68,69). Another study found that adjusted FEV_1 was on average 155 mL (95% CI, 74–236 mL) lower in miners than in the controls, the difference being greatest in younger men (62).

The findings of the National Study of CWP in the United States of coal miners were essentially similar (Table 1) (62,63). Coal mining dust was also associated with higher rate of decline in lung function (65). Other important occupational risk factors that were reported to contribute to increased rate of decline in lung function in the U.S. coal miners included work practices such as lack of use of respiratory protection, participation in explosive blasting, roof bolting, and use of dust control sprays that used water that had been stored in holding tanks (70). Furthermore, a rapid decline in FEV_1 of 60 mL/yr or more was associated with early retirement from coal mining, increased risk of respiratory morbidity, and increased mortality from nonmalignant respiratory disease (NMRD) (71). Relationships between exposure to coal mining dust and increased mortality from COPD have also been found in British, U.S., and Dutch studies (72–74).

Exposure–response relationship for airflow obstruction and coal mining dust was also found in a longitudinal study of Italian coal miners (66).

In summary, the epidemiological evidence from coal mining studies shows an exposure–response between various outcomes of COPD and indices of coal mining dust exposure. It has been estimated that 8.0% (95% CI, 3.4% to 13.7%) of nonsmoking coal miners with a cumulative respirable dust exposure of 123 ghm^{-3} (considered equivalent to 35 years of work with a mean respirable dust level at current allowed limits of 2 mg/m^3) could be expected to develop a clinically important (>20%) loss of FEV_1 attributable to dust (13). Among smoking miners, the estimate attributable to dust was 6.6% (95% CI, 4.9% to 8.4%), (13) but the combined effect of dust and smoking can potentially account for a large number of cases of COPD attributable to dust through the combined effect (75).

Silica Dust—Epidemiological Evidence

Despite the dramatic reduction of silica dust exposure levels in most developed countries during the last century (76), airflow limitation and associated COPD remain health issues in workers exposed to silica dust (22). Recent epidemiologic studies show that silica dust exposure can lead to airflow limitation in the absence of radiological signs of silicosis and that airflow limitation associated with silica dust exposure occurs in many different types of industrial operations (77–99).

Epidemiological studies of hard rock miners demonstrated that the FEV_1, forced vital capacity (FVC), and FEV_1/FVC ratio, adjusted for age, height, and tobacco smoking, decreased with increasing cumulative respirable dust exposure both in smokers and nonsmokers (77,78). The average loss in lung function attributable to silica dust exposure, estimated for a 50-year-old white South African gold miner exposed for 24 years to standard exposure levels, was equivalent to an average excess loss of 9.8 mL/yr of FEV_1 and 9.0 mL/yr of FVC (22). Similar results were also observed among black South African gold miners (79), Canadian hard rock miners (80), Western Australian miners (81), and U.S. molybdenum miners (82) (Table 2).

Table 2 Epidemiological Studies of the Effect of Mineral Dust (Silica and Mixed) on Lung Function Loss in Selected Studies

Silica dust exposure (Reference)	N	Age	Years	Mean exposure to silica dust		Loss of lung function associated with mean cumulative dust exposure or duration of exposure		
				Respirable dust (mg/m³); % silica	Cum. respirable dust (mg/m³–yr)	FEV_1 (mL) loss/yr of exposure	FEV_1 %	FVC (mL)
South African gold (77,78)	2260	50	24	0.6[a]; 15	13.4	236; 9.8	2.3	217
South African gold miners (79)	1197	46	25	0.6[a]; 15	NA	200; 8; 447[b]	3.3	NS 351[b]
Canadian hard rock miners (80)	95	39	13	0.5; 8	NA	325	NS	364
U.S. hard rock miners (82)	281	44	9	NA;19	8.3	155	NS	NS
Silica dust exposed subjects (83)	3445	38	7	<0.2[c]; NA	NA	31:4.3	4.5	NS
Swedish granite crushers (84)	45	52	22	0.16[c]; NA	7.2	150	3.2	NS
Norwegian tunnel workers (85)	345	40	19	2; 24	15.3	162	NA	NA
Dutch construction workers (88)	1335	42	19	NA; NA	NA	117	NS	126
Dutch construction workers (87)	144	36	11	0.8; 9	7.0	NS	2.2	NS
Brick-manufacturing workers (88)	382	35	16	2	NA	NS	NS	18.5
Italian ceramic workers (93)	380	35	5	NA	NA	NA; 5.7	NA; 9.2	NA
Stone carvers (94)	97	33	11	0.2–0.9[c]; NA	NA	195; 18	NS	207
Potato sorters (98)	172	45	12	2.2; 12	NA	124; 11	3.8	NS

[a]Respirable dust measured before hydrochloric acid treatment.
[b]Additional loss associated with silicosis ILO category 3/3.
[c]Respirable silica.
Abbreviations: FEV₁, forced expiratory volume in one second; NS, not significant; NA, not available.

Several recent epidemiological studies have shown that silica dust exposure constitutes a hazard for airflow limitation in many nonmining industries (granite crushers, tunnel workers, construction workers, brick-manufacturing workers, slate workers, stone carvers, ceramic workers, refractory ceramic fiber industry, etc.) (Table 2). A dose-dependent relationship between exposure, either in the duration of employment or in the dust level, and lung function level or lung function decline was found in some of these studies. The effect of employment in silica dust–exposed occupations was even detected in a large general population–based cross-sectional study of Norwegian men of 30 to 46 years of age (83). Workers with 15 or more years of silica dust exposure had a statistically significant excess loss of FEV_1 of 4.3 mL (95% CI, 1.1–7.5) with each year of exposure; the exposure–response relationship was similar among nonsmokers, ex-smokers, and smokers. This study is also addressed in the later section on PAR% estimates.

Several mortality studies of cohorts of silica dust–exposed workers reported increased mortality from NMRD (100,101) and from COPD (102,103). Generally, NMRD combines deaths from pneumoconioses and COPD.

In summary, the epidemiological evidence from large studies of hard rock miners demonstrates an exposure–response relation for airflow limitation and silica dust exposure that is not dependent on the presence of silicosis. In addition, several recent industry-based studies show that the silica dust–associated airflow limitation can occur in a variety of industrial settings.

Asbestos Dust—Epidemiological Evidence

Occupational exposure to asbestos dust occurred mainly in the past in mining, in asbestos product manufacturing, and in workplaces where asbestos was used for its heat insulation properties. In the presence of asbestosis, lung function impairment associated with asbestos dust exposure is primarily of restrictive nature (20,104,105). Nonetheless, several epidemiologic studies have shown that exposure to asbestos dust can be associated with obstructive as well as restrictive lung function impairment (106–113). This suggests that asbestosis-related functional changes can be coexistent with dust-related airway disease (20). In a longitudinal study, workers with heavy asbestos exposure had a steeper decline in both FEV_1 and FVC in comparison to workers exposed to cement and polyvinyl chloride; this steeper decline was found in nonsmokers and smokers (112). Other occupational groups potentially exposed to asbestos and investigated for asbestos-related lung function impairment were electricians (114), boilermakers (115), and plumbers and pipe fitters (116) from the construction industry in Edmonton, Canada. All three groups of workers had significantly higher prevalence of respiratory symptoms in comparison with telephone workers, but only the pipe fitters and plumbers combined together had significantly lower FVC in comparison with the telephone workers (115,116).

Portland Cement

Some studies reported significantly lower $FEV_1\%$ values in workers exposed to cement in comparison to unexposed workers, suggesting that exposure to occupational factors in cement plants may lead to obstructive impairment (117–120). One of these studies also reported very high respirable dust exposure ($> 40\,mg/m^3$). However, in two recent studies, no relation between exposure to Portland cement dust and airflow limitation was found (121,122). These results suggest that exposure levels may play an important role in disease causation with Portland cement exposure. It should also be noted that Portland cement manufacture is also associated with irritant gas (sulfur dioxide) exposure; thus this particular exposure may be as relevant to the epidemiology of irritant gas as mineral dust exposure.

Mineral Dust—Summary Comments

Many epidemiological studies show association between occupational mineral dusts and increased lung function impairment in nonsmokers and in smokers after adjustment for smoking. There can be several mechanisms by which mineral dust exposure causes lung function impairment even in the absence of radiological signs of pneumoconiosis or a restrictive pattern of impairment. Depending on the type of dust, exposure pattern, and individual susceptibility, there can be pathologic states with various effects on pulmonary function: chronic bronchitis, bronchiolitis, and emphysema, which cause airflow obstruction. The large epidemiological studies on coal and gold miners show that both coal and silica dust are associated with obstructive impairment due to the effect of dust itself and are independent of the presence of pneumoconiosis radiographically or restriction physiologically. The variability between the smaller studies in the estimated excess loss in lung function and the pattern of impairment may be due to differences in exposure levels, dust toxicity, the prevalence of pneumoconiosis, sample size, and the prevalence of smoking, because smoking usually potentiates the effect of dust on morbidity and mortality from COPD (75). Because of the complexity of the various mechanisms involved in airflow limitation in mineral dust–exposed workers, it is difficult in smaller studies to discern the individual risk factors in the absence of good data on occupational exposure, radiological changes, and smoking history.

EXPOSURE TO ORGANIC DUSTS

There is considerable evidence that agricultural exposures are associated with the development of chronic airway disease. These exposures included dusts from cereal grain, animal feed, soil, and components of microorganisms such as endotoxin and fungi which initiate an inflammatory process in the airways and may ultimately lead to chronic airway disease. We have already presented evidence of development of chronic airflow obstruction due to chronic exposure to cotton dust (Stage IV byssinosis) and grain dust in Chapter 27 and wood dust in Chapter 22. In this section, the effects of chronic exposure to organic dust in crop and dairy farming are discussed. It should be noted that fewer studies have been conducted among crop and dairy farmers compared with other types of organic dust.

Crop Farmers

The prevalence of chronic bronchitis from mailed questionnaire surveys was 7.5% among Finnish farmers (123) and 23% among cattle farmers in Manitoba (124). Dosman et al. (125) reported significantly lower lung function in farmers in Saskatchewan compared with controls. A questionnaire study of crop farmers in Europe found that 12.4% had chronic phlegm, 3.3% asthma, 14.9% wheeze, and 15.2% organic toxic syndrome (126). Another cross-sectional study of European and Californian crop farmers (127) found that rhinitis and asthma were less prevalent in European farmers than in Californian farmers (12.7% vs. 23.9% and 2.8% vs. 4.7%), but chronic bronchitis and toxic pneumonitis were more prevalent in Europe than in California (10% vs. 4.4% and 12.2% vs. 2.7%). The high prevalence of chronic bronchitis and toxic pneumonitis in European farmers was attributable to indoor work (Table 3).

On the other hand, some studies failed to detect differences in the prevalence of symptoms or lung function abnormalities in grain farmers compared with controls as in Manitoba (128) and in England and Wales (131). In addition, low prevalence of symptoms has been reported among Hispanic farm workers in the citrus, tomato, and grape industries (132).

Dairy Farmers

In general, farming involving animals tended to have a higher prevalence of symptoms than farming involving grain or crops (Table 3). Babbott et al. (129) reported chronic bronchitis in 30% of smoking and 16% of nonsmoking dairy farmers in Vermont compared with 21% and 10% in respective controls. Lung function was significantly lower in nonsmokers only. In France, higher prevalence of chronic bronchitis and lower lung function were found among nonsmoking dairy farmers than in nonsmoking controls (130,133). Higher rates of chronic bronchitis were also reported among Yugoslavian cattle breeders compared with other farm workers (134). A study of agricultural workers in a rural area in Tuscany showed that the prevalence of chronic bronchitis was related to jobs in the cowshed (135). Measurements of organic dust were carried out on six different farms in Switzerland by Catbomas et al. (136). The concentration of PM_{10} was found to be 109 to 2207 $\mu g/m^3$ of daily barn activities in winter months and from 76 to 4862 $\mu g/m^3$ for hay storage in summer time; these levels were similar to those found in other dairy farms in Finland and in the United States. Although levels of dust were not measured in other farming facilities, the authors considered that these levels were moderate to high and suggested that long-term exposure to these levels may lead to the development of chronic obstructive lung disease (COLD). Chaudemanche et al. (137) conducted a follow-up study on the cohort of French dairy farmers in Doubs. They demonstrated an accelerated decline in FEV_1/FVC among farmers compared to controls after adjustment for other covariates, again suggesting that farmers were at a higher risk for developing COLD (Table 3).

Organic Dust—Summary Comments

There is considerable evidence that chronic exposure to organic dusts is associated with development of chronic airflow obstruction, especially for cotton and grain dust exposure when studies of relatively large numbers of workers were found to have excessive decline in lung function with a dose–response relationship irrespective of smoking. In cotton dust exposure, there is pathological evidence of airway disease from autopsy findings; in grain workers, pathological findings were scarce. In a study of retired grain workers, significant airflow obstruction was found even in nonsmokers. While endotoxin present in organic dust is likely to be responsible for acute or chronic airflow obstruction, other contaminants such as beta-glucan in molds may also be responsible. Further studies are required to identify the pathogenesis of airflow obstruction arising from exposure to these organic dusts.

Table 3 Studies of Farmers and Farm Workers

References	Type/method	Place/population	N	Prevalence of symptoms (%)	Lung function
(123)	All farmers/postal survey	Finland Farmers Nonfarmers	9699 NA	Chronic cough 2 0.7	NA
(124)	All farmers/mailed questionnaire	Manitoba Farmers	833	Chronic bronchitis Dyspnea 23 14	NA
(128)	All farmers/questionnaire	United Kingdom Farm workers Controls	428 356	Chronic bronchitis: no difference between groups	Dairy farmers and silage workers more likely to have reduced FEV
(125)	All farmers/questionnaire and spirometry	Saskatchewan Farmers Nonfarmers	1824 556	Chronic bronchitis Dyspnea 11 33 7.7 18.2	FEV_1% p FVC% p 96.1 97.7 102.8 106.1
(129)	Dairy farmers/questionnaire and spirometry	Vermont Dairy farmers Controls	198 516	Chronic sputum Smokers Nonsmokers 30 16 21 10	FEV_1/FVC < 70% Smokers Nonsmokers 20% 14% 18% 7%
(130)	Dairy farmers/questionnaire and spirometry	France Dairy farmers Controls	250 250	Chronic bronchitis Men Women 17.7 5.8 9.2 2.5	FEF% p VC% p 78.8 95.2 90.1 98.6

Abbreviations: FEV_1, forced expiratory volume in one second; FVC, forced vital capacity; FEF, forced expiratory flow; p, predicted; NA, not available.

EXPOSURE TO IRRITANT GASES AND FUMES

Studying the pulmonary effects of exposure to irritant gases and fumes alone is complicated by the fact that most workplaces are complex environments where gases and fumes are comingled with dust particles larger than the submicron particles that comprise fumes. For example, in many workplaces, welders are exposed not only to metal fumes and gases, but also to larger inorganic particles (or dusts) generated by other industrial operations nearby in the workplace (138). This is also true of many metal industry and construction workplaces (139,140). Intensive animal confinement (141) and pulp and paper manufacturing (142) operations also expose employees to complex mixtures of irritant gases in addition to organic particulate matter and bioaerosols. Furthermore, in many of these environments there are concomitant exposures to agents that provoke asthma and acute nonspecific airway hyperresponsiveness that may or may not progress to chronic bronchitis symptoms and chronic airflow obstruction (143,144).

Nevertheless, there is a growing body of evidence that exposure to irritant gases and fumes can lead to both acute and chronic airflow limitations. Some evidence also suggests that these exposures in combination with inorganic and organic particulate matter may augment the effect of exposure to dust alone. This has been seen in mining and smelter workers (80,145), workers in rubber manufacturing (146,147), welders (148–150), tunnel and road workers (85,151,152), firefighters (153–155), and, recently, in a general population-based case–control study of risk factors for COPD (156). The remainder of this section will review evidence from occupational groups where exposure to irritant gases and fumes predominate over inorganic and organic particulate matter, and examine population-based studies in which investigators have attempted to separate the effect of gases and fumes from dust.

Welding

Airborne exposures associated with welding include volatilized metal and submicron particles from both the welding rod and the base metal being welded; smoke or fume from burning of metal coatings, shielding gases, fluxes; and, often, dust or other airborne contaminants present in the surrounding workplace. The nature and extent of exposures experienced by welders have been reviewed by many authors (157–160) and, although they have been shown to vary widely, exposure levels are often in excess of regulated occupational exposure limits or guidelines (138–141).

Some welders experience acute airflow obstruction demonstrated by changes in airflow rates over a work shift (161,162) or changes in nonspecific bronchial responsiveness in response to welding exposures (143). Laboratory studies have provided evidence that welding exposure is linked to oxidative stress thus providing mechanistic support for the hypothesis of inflammatory mediated airway obstruction (163–165). Epidemiologic studies have shown welders to experience increased cough and phlegm in association with measures of increased cumulative exposure to welding (150,166); however, one study found that bronchitis symptoms were reversible and not associated with lung function decline over a subsequent three-year period (161). The possibility that the inflammatory response to welding fume components may be lessened by the development of "tolerance" has been suggested (167).

Evidence of chronic airflow obstruction in relation to measures of welding exposure has been seen in most but not all studies designed to investigate this outcome. Several investigations of shipyard welders and burners found dose-related increased chronic bronchitis symptoms and airflow obstruction especially among welders who were current or former smokers (148,149,168); one study also reported functional changes in small airways among nonsmoking welders (169), and in a long-itudinal investigation of the same population of shipyard welders and burners in which welding-related functional abnormalities had been limited to smokers in cross-sectional analysis, Chinn et al. found airflow obstruction in both smokers and nonsmokers that was linked to the nonuse of local exhaust ventilation while welding. Functional changes appeared to be reversible only among those welders who were consistently using local exhaust ventilation (148). An earlier study of welders in the engineering industry found that welders were more likely to be absent from work due to upper respiratory tract infection and that welders who smoked had some evidence of small airway obstruction (reduced mid-maximal flow rates) compared to nonwelders, but no differences were seen when comparing nonsmoking welders and nonwelders (170).

Industries at High Risk for "Gas and Fume" Exposure in Addition to Dust

Other environments in which irritant gases and fumes are commonly encountered include foundries and smelters, rubber production, pulp and paper production, and animal confinement operations. Few studies of foundry and smelter workers report pulmonary effects of gases or fumes separately from the effects of dust (particularly silica and asbestos) or polycyclic aromatic hydrocarbons. In a study of workers at a small iron foundry, Gomes et al. (97) found reduction in measures of airflow among workers in high dust exposure jobs, and in one job with high exposure to gases and fumes but low dust exposure. Similarly, in a study that included underground miners and smelter workers, Manfreda et al. (80) found abnormal airflow rates (compared to expected values) only in smoking smelter workers but not in miners. The main exposure difference between the two work groups was exposure to sulfur dioxide and metal fumes among smelter workers. Among tunnel construction workers, exposure to nitrogen dioxide (from blasting gases and diesel fumes) was associated with increased longitudinal decline in airflow rates (151).

Rubber production workers exposed to high levels of rubber curing fumes have been shown to have increased prevalence of chronic bronchitis symptoms, significantly reduced airflow rates, and a greater longitudinal decline in lung function, compared to internal control groups (147,171,172). A recent study of Dutch rubber workers found no exposure-related symptom differences or acute changes in lung function, but did find an association between cumulative exposure and airflow obstruction (173). Finally, another recent study of Norwegian asphalt workers found a significantly higher prevalence of COPD (defined as FEV_1/FVC ratio less than 0.7 plus chronic bronchitis symptoms) compared to outdoor construction workers (152). None of these studies were able to differentiate the effects of dust from those of "fume" in the populations studied. Rubber "fume" includes a wide variety of cyclohexane soluble chemicals, whose concentrations vary greatly with production associated factors (174).

Pulp and paper workers are also exposed to organic dusts (e.g., wood and paper) and highly irritating gases (such as chlorine, chlorine dioxide, and ozone) especially in bleaching operations. Numerous studies have shown that high exposure peaks to these irritant gases are linked to increased acute airflow obstruction and increased asthma in pulp workers (144,175–177). The relationship of exposures in this industry to chronic airflow obstruction has also been investigated. Increased mortality for obstructive lung disorders was seen among Swedish pulp and paper workers (178), but not in U.S. workers (179). Among the U.S. pulp and paper population, episodes of high exposure to chlorine or sulfur dioxide were associated with chronic changes in spirometric measures of airflow (180). Similar findings have been seen in populations of workers exposed to organic dusts in combination with highly irritating gases such as ammonia, especially in animal confinement agriculture (181–184). An exposure–response relationship between chronic airflow obstruction and duration of exposure in hog barns was even observed recently among swine veterinarians (185), and Donham et al. (183) found a significant synergistic effect of dust and ammonia combined on airflow rates among poultry workers.

Irritants—Summary Comments

A number of studies show that exposures to irritant gases and fumes can work additively or synergistically with exposure to airborne particulate matter (both organic and mineral dust) to enhance the risk of COPD across a broad range of industries and settings. These studies are supported by laboratory evidence of airway inflammation in response to specific metals and metal fume mixtures and irritant gases.

EXPOSURE TO TOXIC AGENTS THAT CAUSE BRONCHITIS AND BRONCHIOLITIS OBLITERANS (BO)

Nature of Obstructive Disease in the Terminal Airways

In recent years, workplace exposure to several toxic agents has been associated with acute bronchiolitis, which often evolves into a chronic bronchiolar inflammatory process termed BO. If the toxic exposure is of specific type and/or of sufficient magnitude, there can be rapid progression to obliterative bronchiolitis (BO), a small airway inflammatory disease involving the terminal bronchioles, respiratory bronchioles, and alveolar ducts to various degrees. Although formerly considered to be rare, it is now more frequently diagnosed in adults as a complication of chronic graft versus host as well as in other conditions, such as in association with connective tissue diseases over and above sporadic toxin-related cases. In addition, the condition is often idiopathic in form. When BO occurs together with an organizing pneumonia, the designation bronchiolitis organizing pneumonia (BOOP) or cryptogenic organizing pneumonia (COP) is used. As opposed to BO, associated with a poorly reversible, obstructive ventilatory deficit, BOOP is associated with restrictive finding on lung function and a decreased D_{LCO}. Although BOOP has also been reported in association with certain occupational triggers, it will not be considered further here.

Occupational Agents Associated with BO

Both acute and chronic exposure to occupational agents may induce BO. Acute exposure to a number of toxic agents may cause acute respiratory distress which initially might resemble irritant-induced asthma. As the disease process evolves, however, the clinical-physiologic-radiologic changes of BO become evident.

Acute injury by toxic gases is a common cause of BO and has been reported after inhalation of high concentrations of nitrogen dioxide, sulfur dioxide, ammonia, hydrogen fluoride, phosgene, hydrogen bromide, and hydrogen chloride (187–194).

It is important to remember that these outcomes appear to be quite uncommon, even in larger series of irritant gas exposed persons. The typical scenario among these affected workers is that they initially develop chemical pneumonitis followed by a silent interval with subsequent development of the severe, irreversible BO syndrome. In 1984, a massive leak of methyl isocyanate in an Indian pesticide plant caused many lethal and sublethal respiratory injuries (195). Long-term chronic lung disability in many exposed workers suggested fibrosing constrictive BO but pathological confirmation is scarce. The chronic nature of some cases of BO was further confirmed by an investigation of 77 Iranian war veterans who were exposed to very low levels of a chemical warfare agent, sulfur mustard, and initially suffered no acute respiratory effects. Serial lung high resolution CAT scans, questionnaire data, and pulmonary function tests in these subjects later revealed significant air trapping in over one-third of them. Septal wall thickening and bronchiectasis were also demonstrated in five and three cases, respectively.

Man-Made Organic Fibers

The role of man-made organic fibers, as a potential cause of BO has received considerable attention in recent years (197). This may have coincided with new industrial developments of producing respirable fine-diameter fibers. In 1998, symptomatic workers with unexplained radiographic and physiologic abnormalities in a nylon flocking plant had open lung biopsies which revealed interstitial pneumonia in six cases and BOOP in one case, respectively (198). All seven biopsies also showed peribronchiolar, vascular, interstitial lymphoid nodules with germinal centers, and most had lymphocytic bronchiolitis and interstitial fibrosis. Review of tissue specimens from workers at a different nylon flock plant demonstrated similar findings. This investigation caused a wild flurry of accusations and counter-accusations between management in the nylon flock company and the investigational team (196). This culminated in a Centers for Disease Control consensus clinical-pathologic workshop which concluded that nylon flock had caused a heretofore undescribed form of lymphocytic bronchiolitis and peribronchiolitis (199,200). Of interest was the fact that six of these cases improved after removal from the workplace, and six others who had improved and decided to return to their original jobs had relapses (200).

Food Flavorings

The most recent outbreak of toxin-related BO occurred in eight workers in a microwave-popcorn production plant (201). These workers developed severe BO and had to be removed from the workplace. This experience led to an expanded study involving the remaining workers in the plant. This was a combined questionnaire and spirometric epidemiologic survey in which 87% of the current workforce participated. Analysis of these results revealed that workers at this plant had 3.3 times the expected rate of clinical obstructive symptoms and twice the expected rate of physician-diagnosed asthmatic/chronic bronchitis. There was also a strong association between the highest exposure quartile of diacetyl, a volatile butter-flavor ingredient, and the extent of airway obstruction found in these workers.

Miscellaneous Causes

Individual instances of BO have occurred after exposure to incinerator fly ash, animal feed, spices, and benzalkonium (202–205).

BO—Summary Comments

Acute and chronic irreversible injury to terminal small airways may at times be confused with asthma or other COPD diseases. For the most part B and BO are caused by known toxic agents, but several epidemics of BO have occurred after previously unrecognized toxic substances. Bronchiolitis and BO should be considered as a possible cause in the differential diagnosis of workplace obstructive syndromes.

DEFINING THE PROBLEM OF COPD FROM AN EPIDEMIOLOGICAL PERSPECTIVE

COPD refers to a single clinical condition, but also serves as an umbrella term or category that subsumes several different and only partially overlapping disease entities. Moreover the conditions that are included or separated from the COPD categorization may vary depending on the nature of the epidemiological investigation involved. COPD is characterized by airflow limitation that is not fully reversible. Two main pathological conditions causing COPD are chronic bronchitis and emphysema. Often the two diseases processes overlap and thus their relative contribution is difficult to discern. In epidemiological research the presence of COPD can be ascertained using pulmonary function testing and using ATS/ERS definitions of COPD or doctor diagnosis of COPD, chronic bronchitis, or emphysema. A related, more overarching category of chronic obstructive lung disease (COLD) further includes asthma, but the COLD categorization will not be considered further in this discussion.

Thus, the term COPD has been applied heterogeneously depending on the setting of its use. Some degree of clinical standardization, including severity gradation, has been attempted through international efforts. For example, the recent promotion of "GOLD" criteria attempts to set guidelines based on postbronchodilator spirometry that can be used to categorize or "stage" persons with COPD according to symptoms and lung function (206). Nonetheless, large gaps remain between COPD defined at the level of the individual person, usually a patient in a clinical setting, with the definition based on subjective and objective medical criteria (such as incorporated in the GOLD guidelines), and COPD defined at a population level, based on epidemiological criteria intended to consistently estimate case incidence and prevalence.

Epidemiological analyses of COPD generally rely upon one of two approaches to case definition. Survey research (including secondary analyses of administrative or other data sets) relies upon "report" of one of the underlying COPD conditions. This can be restricted to COPD and emphysema only or also can include chronic bronchitis, as noted above. When chronic bronchitis is included, stratified analyses with and without this condition subset are often presented. The COPD categorization in epidemiological terms can be based on the subject's responses to a questionnaire affirming that the respondent has received a physician's diagnosis of at least one of the target conditions of interest. It can also be based on diagnostic data (for example, International code of death (ICD)-based conditions, prescribed medication, or medical test results) identified through medical records or insurance claims. Some large epidemiological field studies define cases based on primary data collected as part of the study. For COPD, primary definition in these studies depends on spirometry (although cut-off values defining obstruction may vary), whereas chronic bronchitis is typically defined through a standard battery of questionnaire items establishing the presence of productive cough for three months in two consecutive years.

Both of these epidemiological approaches have advantages and disadvantages. Survey approaches allow larger, less costly sampling, but have less precision due to misdiagnosis and potential biases due to recall and access to care. Field studies are limited by case selection effects and, in particular, by limited ability to assess emphysema (given that diffusing capacity measurements and sensitive radiographic assessment are rarely included in such studies). Importantly, despite differences in methodology, epidemiological investigations of COPD provide important measures of association and risk that cannot be gleaned from individual case reports or even large clinical series.

The most familiar epidemiological measure of risk is the relative risk (RR) and the related estimate, the odds ratio. By comparing exposed to unexposed groups, these measures are used commonly to gage the strength of a link between a suspect risk factor and a specific disease outcome. Attributable risk is a different epidemiological measure that can be even more relevant when analyzing factors linked to COPD. Attributable risk, more specifically the "PAR%," integrates the magnitude of the RR together with the general frequency of the exposure in the population. A putative exposure (Exposure I), for example, may carry with it an exceeding high RR, but this exposure may be experienced only by very few people within the population at large. In that case, the actual number of cases induced may be quite small. If another risk factor for the same disease (Exposure II) could have a much lower RR in absolute terms, but may be more ubiquitous, the number of cases it induces may be far greater. Thus, the proportion of all cases of disease attributable to Exposure II will be higher—it will be associated with a larger PAR%. The calculation of the PAR% from an epidemiologic data set can be performed using different algebraic equations. In some cases a published report may not present actual PAR% values but does provide the data (exposure proportion and RR) that allow a post-hoc calculation. The PAR% can also be estimated with corresponding confidence intervals that take into account the variance in cofactors tested in the predictive model.

Regardless of the method of calculation, a key characteristic shared by all PAR% values is that they provide an estimate of the disease caused, at least in part, by the factor in question. This is often described as the burden of disease that would be removed if this factor were eliminated. The PAR%, by definition, recognizes that two factors may act upon each other to magnify risk and that removing either one would reduce disease causation. Indeed, the combined PAR% values calculated for a series of risk factors may very well add to greater than 100% if the effects of these risk factors are multiplicative rather than solely additive.

The epidemiology of occupational asthma has benefited greatly from insights drawn from attributable risk-based approaches (see Chapter 3). The PAR% is no less relevant to the study of occupational COPD. The first reason is because of key diagnostic differences between COPD and asthma, and the second reason is because of the strong link between cigarette smoking and COPD. In asthma, clinical criteria can provide for the diagnosis of occupational disease at the individual patient level, allowing differentiation between work-related and nonwork-related cases. For example, a clinical case series of adults with new-onset asthma could be stratified between those with occupationally related disease based on predefined diagnostic criteria and those who do not meet a clinical definition of occupationally related asthma. On this basis, the incidence of occupational asthma can be estimated and can be compared to general incidence rates. This is not tantamount to a PAR%, and issues of underdiagnosis and underdetection would temper the interpretation of such estimates. Nonetheless, this can provide a basis for population-based inferences of the occupationally related burden of asthma. Occupational COPD does not lend itself to such an approach. At present, there is no set of generally accepted clinical criteria by which an individual patient is likely to be diagnosed as having "occupational COPD." Furthermore, even the term "chemical bronchitis," which is sometimes used in clinical practice, does not have a standard application; emphysema is rarely, if ever, diagnosed as work related. Occupational disease surveillance programs and registries, although acknowledged to under-report asthma, capture virtually no COPD. In general, workers' compensation insurance schemes have resisted awards for work-related COPD.

The direct and powerful link between cigarette smoking and COPD is the second reason why PAR%-based epidemiological assessments of work-related disease are important in COPD. Although theoretical models of COPD induction have always allowed for other causes beyond cigarette smoking, in clinical practice, smoking is typically considered the sole relevant risk factor for such disease. Adopting a PAR% approach to the question of smoking, occupation, and COPD is particularly illuminating precisely because, based on PAR% analyses, "only" 80% of COPD is attributable to smoking. Therefore, a minimum of one in five cases is related to other factors. Moreover, potential interactions between exposures (for example, occupational exposure and cigarette smoking) could mean that the actual PAR% for non-smoking factors may be even higher. Finally, the epidemiological approach takes into account cigarette smoking exposure on a group level, using appropriate statistical methods to adjust for the impact of this factor, while teasing out occupational risk factors that might otherwise be obscured.

CONTRIBUTION OF OCCUPATION TO THE BURDEN OF COPD

With renewed attention to the question of occupation as a potentially causative factor in COPD, additional studies subsequently appeared that further supplemented the existing literature. In 2001, the American Thoracic Society (ATS) undertook development of a position statement on the "Occupational Contribution of the Burden of Airway Disease." This review was submitted and approved by the ATS in 2002 and published in 2003 (208). The ATS position statement also reviewed the scientific literature in relation to asthma and occupation, but that topic will not be addressed here. The ATS statement findings in relation to COPD and occupation

Table 4 The Occupational Contribution to the Burden of COPD

Disease endpoint	Number of studies	Number of subjects	Countries included	Median PAR%	Range PAR%
Chronic bronchitis	8	> 38,000	8	15	4–24
Breathlessness	6	> 25,000	6	13	6–30
Airflow obstruction	6	> 12,000	5	18	12–55

Note: Based on the analysis presented in the 2002 ATS position statement.
Abbreviations: COPD, chronic obstructive pulmonary disease; PAR%, population attributable risk percent; ATS, American Thoracic Society.
Source: From Ref. 208.

are summarized in Table 4. As with the earlier 1988 review by Becklake, this analysis found a consistent link between occupational exposure and COPD based on PAR% estimates.

It should be noted that although several study endpoints are included in Table 4, many are multiple endpoints derived from the same study (10 independent studies in total). Nonetheless, the consistency and the strength of the associations are impressive. Since the ATS publication, a number of additional analyses have further reinforced the body of evidence linking occupation to COPD. A large study of COPD-related mortality in high and low dust-exposed construction workers in Sweden found a PAR% of 11% overall and 53% among nonsmoking workers (209). A nationwide telephone survey of occupation and COPD in the United States has found a smoking-adjusted occupational PAR% for COPD of 20%, increasing to 28% after excluding those with chronic bronchitis alone without concomitant COPD or emphysema (210). A secondary analysis of the U.S. National Health and Nutrition Examination Survey (NHANES) found that occupationally associated PAR% of airway obstruction was 19% overall and 31% among nonsmokers (211,212). Other reports were also published as the ATS review studies have also indicated the same direction of association between work-related factors and airway obstruction or chronic bronchitis (212–218). Beyond these studies, other analyses of the effects of occupational exposure among persons with alpha-1-antitrypsin deficiency serve to further support the biological plausibility of work-related COPD (219,220). Taken together, these studies support a causal association between occupational exposures to vapor, gas, dust, and fume and COPD.

OVERALL SUMMARY

The body of scientific evidence supports a causal link between occupational exposures broadly defined as gases, vapors, dusts, and fumes and COPD, including airway obstruction, chronic bronchitis, and emphysema. The findings across a number of locations using a variety of analytic methods have been remarkably consistent.

A number of studies have suggested that the strength of the effect of having worked in a "dusty trade" is in a range consistent with the risk associated with light to moderate smoking. We do not yet have strong data delineating the potential interactive effects of noxious workplace exposures combined with smoking, although it is likely that this is more than additive based on the PAR% estimates for both that have been observed.

Even without potential synergism as an issue, on the individual level smoking cessation remains a mainstay for both primary prevention of COPD incidence and secondary prevention of disease progression. This does not mean that ongoing exposure to substantial workplace exposure to gases, dusts, fumes, and vapors should be ignored. To the degree to which nonspecific airway hyperresponsiveness is a comorbid finding in COPD and may be worsened by ongoing workplace exposures, the attribution of this component of disease should parallel the attribution of work-aggravated or work-exacerbated asthma. Retrospective attribution may prove far more challenging, especially in the face of a substantive cigarette smoking history. Each individual case requires a detailed review of all of the salient risk factors. The epidemiological perspective makes clear that simply because a person has been an active smoker does not mean that occupational factors did not play a role in the development of his or her lung disease.

DIRECTIONS FOR FUTURE RESEARCH

- Further studies to determine the pathogenesis of airway disease due to chronic exposure to various dusts, fumes, and vapors in the workplace
- Histopathologic studies on airway disease due to exposure to organic dust such as cotton and grain to determine whether emphysema is a true complication of these exposures
- Studies directed to investigate the independent effects of exposure to various dusts, vapors, and fumes in the workplace and smoking and their interaction
- Studies to determine the effects of exposure to multiple contaminants in the workplace
- Studies to determine the long-term prognosis of persons with airway disease secondary to exposures in the workplace
- Development of animal models with one or more agents that have been shown to induce BO to study the cellular response and various inflammatory indices
- Prospective evaluation of affected workers with BO using physiological tests and proinflammatory markers

REFERENCES

1. Thackrah C. The Effects of Arts, Trades, and Professions, and of Civic States and Habits of Living, on Health and Longevity. 2nd ed. London: Longman, 1832.
2. Greenhow EH. Chronic Bronchitis. Philadelphia, PA: Blakston Son & Co., 1868.
3. Goodman N, Lane RE, Rampling SB. Chronic bronchitis: an introductory examination of existing data. Br Med J 1953; 2(4830):237–243.
4. Fletcher CM. Disability and mortality from chronic bronchitis in relation to dust exposure. AMA Arch Ind Health 1958; 18:368–373.
5. Davison AG, Newman Taylor AJ, Darbyshire J, et al. Cadmium fume inhalation and emphysema. Lancet 1988; 1(8587):663–667.
6. Honeybourne D, Pickering CA. Physiological evidence that emphysema is not a feature of byssinosis. Thorax 1986; 41:6–11.
7. Becklake MR, Goldman HI, Bosman AR, Freed CC. The long-term effects of exposure of nitrous fumes. Am Rev Tuber 1957; 76:398–409.
8. Becklake MR, Du Preez L, Lutz W. Lung function in silicosis of the Witwatersrand gold miner. Am Rev Tuber Lung Dis 1958; 77:400–412.
9. Becklake MR. When the chest x-ray does not tell the whole story. Am J Respir Crit Care Med 2001; 164(10):1761–1762.
10. Becklake MR. Occupational pollution. Chest 1989; 96(4):S372–S378.
11. Becklake MR. Occupational exposures: evidence for a causal association with chronic obstructive pulmonary disease. Am Rev Respir Dis 1989; 140:S85–S91.
12. Becklake MR. The work relatedness of airways dysfunction. In: Proceedings of the 9th International Symposium on Epidemiology in Occupational Health [DHHS (NIOSH) Publication No. 94–112]. Cincinnati, OH: U.S. Department of Health and Human Services, Public Health Service, Centers for Disease Control and Prevention, National Institute for Occupational Safety and Health, 1992:1–28.
13. Oxman AD, Muir DCF, Shannon HS, Stock SR, Hnizdo E, Lange HJ. Occupational dust exposure and chronic obstructive pulmonary disease. Am Rev Respir Dis 1993; 148:38–48.

14. Hendrick DJ. Occupation and chronic obstructive pulmonary disease (COPD). Eur Respir J 1994; 7:1032–1034.
15. Walter R, Gottlieb DJ, O'Connor GT. Environmental and genetic risk factors and gene-environment interactions in the pathogenesis of chronic obstructive lung disease. Environ Health Perspect 2000; 108(suppl 4):733–742.
16. Burge PS. Occupation and COPD. Eur Respir Rev 2002; 12(86/87):293–294.
17. Viegi G, Di Pede C. Chronic obstructive lung diseases and occupational exposure. Curr Opin Clin Immunol 2002; 2:115–121.
18. Lange AM. Characterization and measurements of the industrial environment. In: Merchant JA, ed. Mineralogy Occupational Respiratory Disease. U.S. Dept of Health and Human Services (NIOSH) Publication No. 86–102, 1986.
19. Higgins ITT. The epidemiology of chronic respiratory disease. Prev Med 1973; 2:14–33.
20. Becklake MR. Occupational exposures as causes of chronic airways disease. In: Rom WR, ed. Environmental and Occupational Medicine. 3rd ed. Philadelphia: Lippincott-Raven Publishers, 1998.
21. Coggon D, Taylor AN. Coal mining and chronic obstructive pulmonary disease: a review of the evidence. Thorax 1998; 563:398–407.
22. Hnizdo E, Vallyathan V. Chronic obstructive pulmonary disease due to occupational exposure to silica dust: a review of epidemiological and pathological evidence. Occup Environ Med 2003; 60:237–243.
23. American Thoracic Society. Standard for the diagnosis and care of patients with chronic obstructive pulmonary disease. Am J Respir Crit Care Med 1995; 152:S77–S120.
24. Wang XR, Christiani DC. Respiratory symptoms and functional status in workers exposed to silica, asbestos, and coal mine dust. J Occup Environ Med 2000; 42:1076–1084.
25. Gamble JF, Hessel PA, Nicolich MJ. Relationship between silicosis and lung function. Scand J Work Environ Health 2004; 30:5–20.
26. Hnizdo E, Singh T, Churchyard G. Chronic pulmonary function impairment caused by initial and recurrent pulmonary tuberculosis following treatment. Thorax 2000; 55:32–38.
27. Schins RPF, Borm PJA. Mechanisms and mediators in coal dust induced toxicity: a review. Ann Occup Hyg 1999; 43:7–33.
28. Castranova V. From coal mine dust to quartz: mechanisms of pulmonary pathogenicity. Inhal Toxicol 2000; 12(suppl 3):7–14.
29. Hunter DD, Castranova V, Stanley C, Dey RD. Effects of silica exposure on substance P immunoreactivity and preprotachykinin mRNA expression in trigeminal sensory neurons in Fischer 344 rats. J Toxicol Environ Health 1998; 24:593–605.
30. Bernard AM, Gonzales-Lorenzo JM, Siles E, Trujillano G, Lauwerys R. Early decrease of serum clara cell protein in silica-exposed workers. Eur Respir J 1994; 7:1932–1937.
31. Vallyathan V. Generation of oxygen radicals by minerals and its correlation to cytotoxicity. Environ Health Perspect 1994; 102(suppl 10):111–115.
32. Zay K, Loo S, Xie C, Devine DV, Wright J, Churg A. Role of neutrophils and alpha1-antitrypsin in coal- and silica-induced connective tissue breakdown. Am J Physiol 1999; 276; Lung Cell Mol Physiol 20:L269–L279.
33. Dai J, Gilks B, Price K, Churg A. Mineral dust directly indices epithelial and interstitial fibrogenic mediators and matrix components in the airway wall. Am J Respir Crit Care Med 1998; 158:1907–1913.
34. Rom WN. Relationship of inflammatory cell cytokines to disease severity in individuals with occupational inorganic dust exposure. Am J Ind Med 1991; 19:15–27.
35. Vallyathan V, Shi X. The role of oxygen free radicals in occupational and environmental lung disease. Environ Health Perspect 1997; 105(suppl 1):165–177.
36. Becher R, Hetland RB, Refsnes M, Dahl JE, Dahlman HJ, Schwarze PE. Rat lung inflammatory responses after in vivo and in vitro exposure to various stone particles. Inhal Technol 2002; 13:789–805.

37. Li K, Keeling B, Churg A. Mineral dusts cause collagen and elastin breakdown in the rut lung: a potential mechanism of dust induced emphysema. Am J Respir Crit Care Med 1996; 153:644–649.

38. Li K, Zay K, Churg A. Mineral dusts oxidize methionine residue. Possible mechanism of dust-induced inactivation of α-1-antitrypsin. Ann Occup Hyg 1997; 41(suppl 1): 379–383.

39. Churg A, Zay K, Li K. Mechanisms of mineral dust-induced emphysema. Environ Health Perspect 1997; suppl 5:1215–1218.

40. Churg A. The uptake of mineral particles by pulmonary epithelial cells. State of the Art. Am J Respir Crit Care Med 1996; 154:1124–1140.

41. Wright JL, Harrison N, Wiggs B, Churg A. Quartz but not iron oxide cause air-flow obstruction, emphysema, and small airways lesions in the rat. Am Rev Respir Dis 1988; 138:129–135.

42. Churg A, Wright JL. Small-airway lesions in patients exposed to nonasbestos mineral dusts. Hum Pathol 1983; 14:688–693.

43. Churg A, Wright JL, Wiggs B, Pare PD, Lazar N. Small airways disease and mineral dust exposure. Prevalence, structure, and function. Am Rev Respir Dis 1985; 131: 139–143.

44. Wright JL, Cagle P, Churg A, Colby TV, Myers J. Diseases of the small airways. Am Rev Respir Dis 1992; 146:240–262.

45. Chia KS, Ng TP, Jeyaratnam J. Small airways function of silica-exposed workers. Am J Ind Med 1992:155–162.

46. Gevenois PA, Sergent G, De Maertelaer V, Gouat F, Yernault J-C, De Vuyst P. Micronodules and emphysema in coal mine dust or silica exposure: relation with lung function. Eur Respir J 1998; 12:1020–1024.

47. Ruckley VA, Gauld SJ, Chapman JS, et al. Emphysema and dust exposure in a group of coal workers. Am Rev Respir Dis 1984; 129:528–532.

48. Begin R, Ostiguy G, Cantin A, Bergeron D. Lung function in silica-dust exposed workers. A relationship to disease severity assessed by CT scan. Chest 1998; 94:539–545.

49. Kinsella M, Muller N, Vedal S, Staples C, Abboud RT, Chan-Yeung M. Emphysema in silicosis. A comparison of smokers with nonsmokers using pulmonary function testing and computed tomography. Am Rev Respir Dis 1990; 141:1497–1500.

50. Bergin CJ, Muller NL, Vedal S, Chan-Yeung M. CT in silicosis: correlation with plain films and pulmonary function tests. AJR 1986; 146:477–483.

51. Begin R, Filion R, Ostiguy G. Emphysema in silica- and asbestos-exposed workers seeking compensation. A CT scan study. Chest 1995; 108:647–655.

52. Cowie RL, Hay M, Glyn-Thomas R. Association of silicosis, lung dysfunction, and emphysema in gold miners. Thorax 1993; 48:746–749.

53. Wang X, Yano E. Pulmonary dysfunction in silica-exposed workers: a relationship to radiographic signs of silicosis and emphysema. Am J Ind Med 1999; 36:299–306.

54. Becklake MR, Irwig L, Kielkowski D, Webster I, de Beer M, Landau S. The predictors of emphysema in South African gold miners. Am Rev Respir Dis 1987; 135:1234–1241.

55. de Beer M, Kielkowski D, Yach D, Steinberg M. Selection bias in a case-control study of emphysema. S Afr J Epidemiol Infect 1992; 7:9–13.

56. Hnizdo E, Sluis-Cremer GK, Abramowitz JA. Emphysema type in relation to silica dust exposure in South African gold miners. Am Rev Respir Dis 1991; 143:1241–1247.

57. Hnizdo E, Sluis-Cremer GK, Baskind E, Murray J. Emphysema and airway obstruction in non-smoking South African gold miners with long exposure to silica dust. Occup Environ Med 1994; 51:557–563.

58. Hnizdo E, Murray J, Davison A. Correlation between autopsy findings for chronic obstructive lung disease and in-life disability in South African gold miners. Int Arch Occup Environ Health 2000; 73:235–244.

59. Rogan JM, Attfield MD, Jacobsen M, Rae S, Walker DD, Walton WH. Role of dust in the working environments in development of chronic bronchitis in British coal miners. Br J Ind Med 1973; 30:217–226.

60. Soutar CA, Hurley JF. Relation between dust exposure and lung function in miners and ex-miners. Br J Ind Med 1986; 43:307–320.

61. Marine WM, Gurr D, Jacobsen M. Clinically important respiratory effects of dust exposure and smoking in British coal miners. Am Rev Respir Dis 1988; 137:106–112.

62. Attfield MD, Hodous TK. Pulmonary function of U.S. coal miners related to dust exposure estimates. Am Rev Respir Dis 1992; 145:605–609.

63. Seixas NS, Robins TG, Attfield MD, Moulton LH. Longitudinal and cross sectional analyses of exposure to coal mine dust and pulmonary function in new miners. Br J Ind Med 1993; 50:929–937.

64. Love RG, Miller BG. Longitudinal study of lung function in coal-miners. Thorax 1982; 37:193–197.

65. Attfield MD. Longitudinal decline in FEV_1 in the United States coalminers. Thorax 1985; 40:132–137.

66. Carta P, Aru G, Barbier MT, Avataneo G, Casula D. Dust exposure, respiratory symptoms, and longitudinal decline of lung function in young coalminers. Occup Environ Med 1996; 53:312–319.

67. Hurley JF, Soutar CA. Can exposure to coalmine dust cause a severe impairment of lung function?. Br J Ind Med 1986; 43:150–157.

68. Soutar C, Campbell S, Gurr D, et al. Important deficits of lung function in three modern colliery populations. Am Rev Respir Dis 1993; 147:797–803.

69. Soutar CA, Hurley JF, Miller BG, Cowie HA, Buchanan D. Dust concentration and respiratory risks in coalminers: key risk estimates from British Pneumoconiosis Field Research. Occup Environ Med 2004; 61:477–481.

70. Wang ML, Petsonk EL, Beekman LA, Wagner GR. Clinically important FEV_1 declines among coal miners: an exploration of previously unrecognized determinants. Occup Environ Med 1999; 56:837–844.

71. Beeckman LA, Wang ML, Petsonk EL, Wagner GR. Rapid declines in FEV_1 and subsequent respiratory symptoms, illnesses, and mortality in coal miners in the United States. Am J Respir Crit Care Med 2001; 163:633–639.

72. Miller BG, Jacobsen M. Dust exposure, pneumoconiosis, and mortality of coal miners. Br J Ind Med 1985; 42:723–733.

73. Kuempel ED, Stayner LT, Attfield MD, Buncher CR. Exposure-response analysis of mortality among coal miners in the United States. Am J Ind Med 1995; 28:167–184.

74. Meijers JMM, Swaen GMH, Slangen JJM. Mortality of Dutch coal miners in relation to pneumoconiosis, chronic obstructive pulmonary disease, and lung function. Occup Environ Med 1997; 54:708–713.

75. Hnizdo E, Baskind E, Sluis-Cremer GK. Combined effect of silica dust exposure and tobacco smoking on the prevalence of respiratory impairments among gold miners. Scand J Work Environ Health 1990; 16:411–422.

76. American Thoracic Society. Adverse effects of crystalline silica exposure. Am J Respir Crit Care Med 1997; 155:761–765.

77. Wiles FJ, Faure MH. Chronic obstructive lung disease in gold miners. In: Walton WH, ed. Inhaled Particles IV. Part 2. Oxford: Pergamon Press, 1977:727–735.

78. Hnizdo E. Loss of lung function associated with exposure to silica dust and with smoking and its relation to disability and mortality in South African gold miners. Br J Ind Med 1992; 49:472–479.

79. Cowie RL, Mabena SK. Silicosis, chronic airflow limitation, and chronic bronchitis in South African gold miners. Am Rev Respir Dis 1991; 143:80–84.

80. Manfreda J, Sidwall G, Maini K, West P, Cherniack RM. Respiratory abnormalities in employees of the hard rock mining industry. Am Rev Respir Dis 1982; 126:629–634.

81. Holman CD, Psaila-Savona P, Roberts M, McNulty JC. Determinants of chronic bronchitis and lung dysfunction in Western Australian gold miners. Br J Ind Med 1987; 44:810–818.

82. Kreiss K, Greenberg LM, Kogut SJH, Lezotte DC, Irvin CG, Cherniack RM. Hardrock mining exposure affects smokers and non-smokers differently. Am Rev Respir Dis 1989; 139:1487–1493.

83. Humerfelt S, Eide GE, Gulsvik A. Association of years of occupational quartz exposure with spirometric airflow limitation in Norwegian men aged 30–46 years. Thorax 1998; 53:649–655.

84. Malmberg P, Hedenstrom H, Sundblad B-M. Changes in lung function of granite crushers exposed to moderate highly silica concentrations: a 12 year follow up. Br J Ind Med 1993; 50:726–731.

85. Ulvestad B, Bakke B, Melbostad E, Fuglerud P, Kongerud J, Lund MB. Increased risk of obstructive pulmonary disease in tunnel workers. Thorax 2000; 55:277–282.

86. Ulvestad B, Bakke B, Eduard W, Kongerud J, Lund MB. Cumulative exposure to dust causes accelerated decline in lung function in tunnel workers. Occup Environ Med 2001; 58:663–669.

87. Meijer E, Kromhout H, Heederik A. Respiratory effects of exposure to low levels of concrete dust containing crystalline silica. Am J Ind Med 2001; 40:133–140.

88. Tjoe-Nij E, de Meer G, Smit J, Heederik D. Lung function decrease in relation to pneumoconiosis and exposure to quartz-containing dust in construction workers. Am J Ind Med 2003; 43:574–583.

89. Zuskin E, Mustajbegovic J, Schachter EN, Kern J, Doko-Jelinic J, Godnic-Cvar J. Respiratory findings in workers employed in brick-manufacturing industry. JOEM 1998; 40:814–820.

90. Chen YH, Wu TN, Liou SH. Obstructive pulmonary function defects among Taiwanese firebrick workers in a 2-year follow-up study. J Occup Environ Med 2001; 43:969–975.

91. Liou SH, Chen YP, Shih WY, Lee CC. Pneumoconiosis and pulmonary function defects in silica-exposed fire brick workers. Arch Environ Health 1996; 51:227–233.

92. Cowie HA, Wild P, Beck J, et al. An epidemiological study of the respiratory health of workers in the European refractory ceramic fiber industry. Occup Environ Med 2001; 58:800–810.

93. Forastiere F, Goldsmith DF, Sperati A, et al. Silicosis and lung function decrements among female ceramic workers in Italy. Am J Epidemiol 2002; 156:851–856.

94. Yingratanasuk T, Seixas N, Barnhart S, Brodkin D. Respiratory health and silica exposure of stone carvers in Thailand. Int J Occup Environ Health 2002; 8:301–308.

95. Ng TP, Tsin TW, O'Kelly FJ, Chan SL. A survey of the respiratory health of silica-exposed workers in Hong Kong. Am Rev Respir Dis 1987; 135:1249–1254.

96. Ahman M, Alexandersson R, Ekholm U, Bergstrom B, Dahlqvist M, Ulfvarson U. Impeded lung function in moulders and coremakers handling furan resin sand. Int Arch Occup Environ Health 1991; 63:175–180.

97. Gomes J, Lloyd OL, Norman NJ, Pahwa P. Dust exposure and impairment of lung function at a small iron foundry in a rapidly developing country. Occup Environ Med 2001; 58:656–662.

98. Jorna THJM, Borm PJA, Koiter KD, Slangen JJM, Henderson PT, Wouters EFM. Respiratory effects and serum type II procollagen in potato sorters exposed to diatomaceous earth. Int Arch Occup Environ Health 1994; 66:217–222.

99. Neukirch F, Cooreman J, Korobaeff M, Periente R. Silica exposure and chronic airflow limitation in pottery workers. Arch Environ Health 1994; 49:459–464.

100. Steenland K, Brown D. Mortality study of gold miners exposed to silica and nonasbestiform amphibole minerals: an update with 14 more years of follow-up. Am J Ind Med 1995; 27:217–229.

101. Costello J, Castellan RM, Swecker GS, Kullman GJ. Mortality of a cohort of US Workers employed in crushed stone industry, 1940–1980. Am J Ind Med 1995; 27:625–640.

102. Hnizdo E. Combined effect of silica dust and tobacco smoking on mortality from chronic obstructive lung disease in gold miners. Br J Ind Med 1990; 47:656–664.

103. Reid PJ, Sluis-Cremer GK. Mortality of white South African gold miners. Occup Environ Med 1996; 53:11–16.

104. Wang ML, Lu PL. Lung function studies in asbestos workers. Scand J Work Environ Health 1985; 11:34–42.

105. Becklake MR. Asbestos and other fiber-related diseases of the lungs and pleura: distribution and determinants in populations. Chest 1991; 100:248–254.

106. Harber P, Dahlgren J, Bunn W, Lockey J, Chase G. Radiographic and spirometric in diatomaceous earth workers. JOEM 1998; 40:22–28.

107. Kilburn KH, Warshaw RH, Einstein K, Bernstein J. Airway disease in non-smoking asbestos workers. Arch Environ Health 1985; 40:293–295.

108. Copes R, Thomas D, Becklake MR. Temporal patterns of exposure and non-malignant pulmonary abnormality in Quebec chrysotile workers. Arch Environ Health 1985; 40:80–87.

109. Demers RY, Neale AV, Robins T, Herman SC. Asbestos-related disease in boiler-makers. Am J Ind Med 1990; 17:327–339.

110. Kennedy SM, Vedal S, Muller N, Kassam A, Chan-Yeung M. Lung function and chest radiograph abnormalities among construction insulators. Am J Ind Med 1991; 20: 673–684.

111. Hall SK, Cissi JH. Effects of cigarette smoking on pulmonary function in asymptomatic asbestos workers with normal chest radiographs. Am Ind Hyg Assoc J 1982; 43: 381–386.

112. Siracusa A, Cicioni C, Volpi R, et al. Lung function among asbestos cement factory workers: cross-sectional and longitudinal study. Am J Ind Med 1984; 5:315–325.

113. Algranti E, Mendonca EMC, DeCapitani EM, Freitas JBP, Silva HC, Bussacos MA. Non-malignant asbestos-related diseases in Brazilian asbestos cement workers. Am J Ind Med 2001; 40:240–254.

114. Hessel PA, Melenka LS, Michaelchuk D, Herbert FA, Cowie RL. Lung health among electricians in Edmonton, Alberta, Canada. JOEM 1998; 40:1007–1012.

115. Hessel PA, Melenka LS, Michaelchuk D, Herbert FA, Cowie RL. Lung health among boilermakers in Edmonton, Alberta. Am J Ind Med 1998; 34:381–386.

116. Hessel PA, Melenka LS, Michaelchuk D, Herbert FA, Cowie RL. Lung health among plumbers and pipefitters in Edmonton, Alberta. Occup Environ Med 1998; 55:678–683.

117. Kalacic I. Ventilatory lung function in cement workers. Arch Environ Health 1973; 26:84–85.

118. Saric M, Kalacic I, Holetic A. Follow-up of ventilatory lung function in a group of cement workers. Br J Ind Med 1976; 33:18–24.

119. Shamssain MH, Thompson J. Effect of cement dust on lung function in Libyans. Ergonomics 1988; 31:1299–1303.

120. Mengesha YA, Bekele A. Relative chronic effects of different occupational dusts on respiratory indices and health of workers in three Ethiopian factories. Am J Ind Med 1998; 34:373–380.

121. Siracusa A, Forcina A, Volpi R, Mollichella E, Cicioni C, Fiordi T. An 11-year longitudinal study of the occupational dust exposure and lung function of polyvinyl chloride, cement and asbestos cement factory workers. Scand J Work Environ Health 1988; 14:181–188.

122. Fell AKM, Thomassen TR, Kristensen P, Egeland T, Kongerud J. Respiratory symptoms and ventilatory function in workers exposed to Portland cement dust. JOEM 2003; 45:1008–1014.

123. Terho EO. Work-related respiratory disorders among Finnish farmers. Am J Ind Med 1990; 18:269–272.
124. Warren CPW, Manfreda J. Respiratory symptoms in Manitoba farmers: association with grain and hay handling. CMA J 1980; 122:1259–1264.
125. Dosman JA, Graham BL, Hall D, van Loon, Bhasin P, Froh F. Respiratory symptoms and pulmonary function in farmers. J Occup Med 1987; 29:38–42.
126. Monso E, Magarolas R, Radon K, et al. Respiratory symptoms of obstructive lung disease in European crop farmers. Am J Respir Crit Care Med 2000; 162:1246–1250.
127. Monso E, Schenker M, Radon K, et al. Region-related risk factors for respiratory symptoms in European and Californian farmers. Eur Respir J 2003; 21:323–331.
128. Manfreda J, Cheang M, Warren CPW. Chronic respiratory disorders related to farming and exposure to grain dust in a rural adult community. Am J Ind Med 1989; 15:7–19.
129. Babbott FL, Gump DW, Sylvester DL, Macpherson BV, Holly C. Respiratory symptoms and lung function in a sample of Vermont dairymen and industrial workers. Am J Public Health 1980; 70:241–245.
130. Dalphin JC, Pernet D, Dubiez A, Debieuvre D, Allemand H, Depierre A. Etiologic factors of chronic bronchitis in dairy farmers, case control study in the Doubs region of France. Chest 1993; 103:417–421.
131. Heller FR, Hayward DM, Farebrother MTB. Lung function of farmers in England and Wales. Thorax 1986; 41:117–121.
132. Gamsky TE, Schenker MB, McCurdy SA, Samuels SJ. Smoking, respiratory symptoms, and pulmonary function among a population of Hispanic farmworkers. Chest 1992; 101:1361–1368.
133. Dalphin JC, Dubiez A, Monnet E, et al. Prevalence of asthma and respiratory symptoms in dairy farmers in the French province of the Doubs. Am J Respir Crit Care Med 1998; 158:1293–1498.
134. Milosevic M. The prevalence of chronic bronchitis in agricultural workers of Slavonia. Am J Ind Med 1986; 10:319–322.
135. Talini D, Monteverdi A, Carrara M, Paggiaro PL. Risk factors for chronic respiratory disorders in a sample of farmers in middle Italy. Monaldi Arch Chest Dis 2003; 59: 52–55.
136. Catbomas RL, Bruesch H, Fehr R, Reinbart W, Kubn M. Organic dust exposure in dairy farmers in an alpine region. Swiss Med Weekly 2003; 132:174–178.
137. Chaudemanche H, Monnet E, Westeel V, et al. Respiratory status in dairy farmers in France; cross-sectional and longitudinal analyses. Occup Environ Med 2003; 60: 858–863.
138. Matczak W, Gromiec J. Evaluation of occupational exposure to toxic metals released in the process of aluminum welding. Appl Occup Environ Hyg 2002; 17:296–303.
139. Woskie SR, Kalil A, Bello D, Virji MA. Exposures to quartz, diesel, dust, and welding fumes during heavy and highway construction. AIHA J (Fairfax, Va) 2002; 63:447–457.
140. Rappaport SM, Weaver M, Taylor D, Kupper L, Susi P. Application of mixed models to assess exposures monitored by construction workers during hot processes. Ann Occup Hyg 1999; 43:457–469.
141. Kirychuk S, Senthilselvan A, Dosman JA, et al. Predictors of longitudinal changes in pulmonary function among swine confinement workers. Can Respir J 1998; 5:472–478.
142. Kauppinen T, Teschke K, Astrakianakis G, et al. Assessment of exposure in an international study on cancer risks among pulp, paper, and paper product workers. AIHA J (Fairfax, Va) 2002; 63:254–261.
143. Contreras GR, Chan-Yeung M. Bronchial reactions to exposure to welding fumes. Occup Environ Med 1997; 54:836–839.
144. Olin AC, Granung G, Hagberg S, et al. Respiratory health among bleachery workers exposed to ozone and chlorine dioxide. Scand J Work Environ Health 2002; 28(2): 117–123.

145. Kennedy SM, Wright JL, Mullen JB, Pare PD, Hogg JC. Pulmonary function and peripheral airway disease in patients with mineral dust or fume exposure. Am Rev Respir Dis 1985; 132:1294–1299.

146. Fine LJ, Peters JM. Studies of respiratory morbidity in rubber workers. Part III. Respiratory morbidity in processing workers. Arch Environ Health 1976; 31:136–140.

147. Fine LJ, Peters JM. Respiratory morbidity in rubber workers: II. Pulmonary function in curing workers. Arch Environ Health 1976; 31:10–14.

148. Chinn DJ, Stevenson IC, Cotes JE. Longitudinal respiratory survey of shipyard workers: effects of trade and atopic status. Br J Ind Med 1990; 47:83–90.

149. Cotes JE, Feinmann EL, Male VJ, Rennie FS, Wickham CA. Respiratory symptoms and impairment in shipyard welders and caulker/burners. Br J Ind Med 1989; 46:292–301.

150. Nakadate T, Aizawa Y, Yagami T, Zheg YQ, Kotani M, Ishiwata K. Change in obstructive pulmonary function as a result of cumulative exposure to welding fumes as determined by magnetopneumography in Japanese arc welders. Occup Environ Med 1998; 55:673–677.

151. Bakke B, Ulvestad B, Stewart P, Eduard W. Cumulative exposure to dust and gases as determinants of lung function decline in tunnel construction workers. Occup Environ Med 2004; 61:262–269.

152. Randem BG, Ulvestad B, Burstyn I, Kongerud J. Respiratory symptoms and airflow limitation in asphalt workers. Occup Environ Med 2004; 61:367–369.

153. Betchley C, Koenig JQ, van BG, Checkoway H, Reinhardt T. Pulmonary function and respiratory symptoms in forest firefighters. Am J Ind Med 1997; 31:503–509.

154. Musk AW, Peters JM, Bernstein L, Rubin C, Monroe CB. Pulmonary function in firefighters: a six-year follow-up in the Boston Fire Department. Am J Ind Med 1982; 3:3–9.

155. Mustajbegovic J, Zuskin E, Schachter EN, et al. Respiratory function in active firefighters. Am J Ind Med 2001; 40:55–62.

156. Mastrangelo G, Tartari M, Fedeli U, Fadda E, Saia B. Ascertaining the risk of chronic obstructive pulmonary disease in relation to occupation using a case-control design. Occup Med (Lond) 2003; 53:165–172.

157. Susi P, Goldberg M, Barnes P, Stafford E. The use of a task-based exposure assessment model (T-BEAM) for assessment of metal fume exposures during welding and thermal cutting. Appl Occup Environ Hyg 2000; 15:26–38.

158. Dryson EW, Rogers DA. Exposure to fumes in typical New Zealand welding operations. N Z Med J 1991; 104:365–367.

159. Hewett P. The particle size distribution, density, and specific surface area of welding fumes from SMAW and GMAW mild and stainless steel consumables. Am Ind Hyg Assoc J 1995; 56:128–135.

160. Antonini JM, Lewis AB, Roberts JR, Whaley DA. Pulmonary effects of welding fumes: review of worker and experimental animal studies. Am J Ind Med 2003; 43:350–360.

161. Beckett WS, Pace PE, Sferlazza SJ, Perlman GD, Chen AH, Xu XP. Airway reactivity in welders: a controlled prospective cohort study. J Occup Environ Med 1996; 38:1229–1238.

162. Fishwick D, Bradshaw LM, Slater T, Pearce N. Respiratory symptoms, across-shift lung function changes and lifetime exposures of welders in New Zealand. Scand J Work Environ Health 1997; 23:351–358.

163. Li GJ, Zhang LL, Lu L, Wu P, Zheng W. Occupational exposure to welding fume among welders: alterations of manganese, iron, zinc, copper, and lead in body fluids and the oxidative stress status. J Occup Environ Med 2004; 46:241–248.

164. Antonini JM, Lawryk NJ, Murthy GG, Brain JD. Effect of welding fume solubility on lung macrophage viability and function in vitro. J Toxicol Environ Health A 1999; 58:343–363.

165. Taylor MD, Roberts JR, Leonard SS, Shi X, Antonini JM. Effects of welding fumes of differing composition and solubility on free radical production and acute lung injury and inflammation in rats. Toxicol Sci 2003; 75:181–191.

166. Bradshaw LM, Fishwick D, Slater T, Pearce N. Chronic bronchitis, work related respiratory symptoms, and pulmonary function in welders in New Zealand. Occup Environ Med 1998; 55:150–154.

167. Fine JM, Gordon T, Chen LC, et al. Characterization of clinical tolerance to inhaled zinc oxide in naive subjects and sheet metal workers. J Occup Environ Med 2000; 42:1085–1091.

168. Chinn DJ, Cotes JE, el Gamal FM, Wollaston JF. Respiratory health of young shipyard welders and other tradesmen studied cross sectionally and longitudinally. Occup Environ Med 1995; 52:33–42.

169. Hjortsberg U, Orbaek P, Arborelius M Jr. Small airways dysfunction among non-smoking shipyard arc welders. Br J Ind Med 1992; 49:441–444.

170. Hayden SP, Pincock AC, Hayden J, Tyler LE, Cross KW, Bishop JM. Respiratory symptoms and pulmonary function of welders in the engineering industry. Thorax 1984; 39:442–447.

171. Fine LJ, Peters JM. Respiratory morbidity in rubber workers: I. Prevalence of respiratory symptoms and disease in curing workers. Arch Environ Health 1976; 31:5–9.

172. Zuskin E, Mustajbegovic J, Schachter EN, Doko-Jelinic J, Budak A. Longitudinal study of respiratory findings in rubber workers. Am J Ind Med 1996; 30:171–179.

173. Meijer E, Heederik D, Kromhout H. Pulmonary effects of inhaled dust and fumes: exposure-response study in rubber workers. Am J Ind Med 1998; 33:16–23.

174. Kromhout H, Swuste P, Boleij JS. Empirical modelling of chemical exposure in the rubber-manufacturing industry. Ann Occup Hyg 1994; 38:3–22.

175. Kennedy SM, Enarson DA, Janssen RG, Chan-Yeung M. Lung health consequences of reported accidental chlorine gas exposures among pulpmill workers. Am Rev Respir Dis 1991; 143:74–79.

176. Salisbury DA, Enarson DA, Chan-Yeung M, Kennedy SM. First-aid reports of acute chlorine gassing among pulpmill workers as predictors of lung health consequences. Am J Ind Med 1991; 20:71–81.

177. Olin AC, Ljungkvist G, Bake B, Hagberg S, Henriksson L, Toren K. Exhaled nitric oxide among pulpmill workers reporting gassing incidents involving ozone and chlorine dioxide. Eur Respir J 1999; 14:828–831.

178. Wingren G, Persson B, Thoren K, Axelson O. Mortality pattern among pulp and paper mill workers in Sweden: a case-referent study. Am J Ind Med 1991; 20:769–774.

179. Ferris BG Jr, Puleo S, Chen HY. Mortality and morbidity in a pulp and a paper mill in the United States: a ten-year follow-up. Br J Ind Med 1979; 36:127–134.

180. Henneberger PK, Ferris BG Jr, Sheehe PR. Accidental gassing incidents and the pulmonary function of pulp mill workers. Am Rev Respir Dis 1993; 148:63–67.

181. Schwartz DA, Donham KJ, Olenchock SA, et al. Determinants of longitudinal changes in spirometric function among swine confinement operators and farmers. Am J Respir Crit Care Med 1995; 151:47–53.

182. Donham KJ, Reynolds SJ, Whitten P, Merchant JA, Burmeister L, Popendorf WJ. Respiratory dysfunction in swine production facility workers: dose-response relationships of environmental exposures and pulmonary function. Am J Ind Med 1995; 27:405–418.

183. Donham KJ, Cumro D, Reynolds S. Synergistic effects of dust and ammonia on the occupational health effects of poultry production workers. J Agromed 2002; 8:57–76.

184. Radon K, Monso E, Weber C, et al. Prevalence and risk factors for airway diseases in farmers—summary of results of the European Farmers' Project. Ann Agric Environ Med 2002; 9:207–213.

185. Andersen CI, Von Essen SG, Smith LM, Spencer J, Jolie R, Donham KJ. Respiratory symptoms and airway obstruction in swine veterinarians: a persistent problem. Am J Ind Med 2004; 46:386–392.

186. Vermeulen R, Heederik D, Kromhout H, Smit HA. Respiratory symptoms and occupation: a cross-sectional study of the general population. Environ Health 2002; 1:5.

187. Milne JE. Nitrogen dioxide inhalation and bronchiolitis obliterans. A review of the literature and report of a case. J Occup Med 1969; 11(10):538–547.

188. Woodford DM, Coutu RE, Gaensler EA. Obstructive lung disease from acute sulfur dioxide exposure. Respiration 1979; 38(4):238–245.

189. Horvath EP, doPico GA, Barbee RA, Dickie HA. Nitrogen dioxide-induced pulmonary disease: five new cases and review of the literature. J Occup Med 1978; 29(2):103–110.

190. Ducatman AM, Ducatman BS, Barnes JA. Lithium battery hazard: old-fashioned planning implications of new technology. J Occup Med 1988; 39(4):309–311.

191. Konichezky S, Schattner A, Ezri T, Bokenboim P, Geva D. Thionyl-chloride-induced lung injury and bronchiolitis obliterans. Chest 1993; 104(3):971–973.

192. Kraut A, Lilis R. Chemical pneumonitis due to exposure to bromine compounds. Chest 1988; 94(1):208–210.

193. Lenci G, Wacker G, Schulz V, Muller KM. Bronchiolitis obliterans following nitrogen dioxide (NO_2) inhalation: clinical-roentgenologic-histologic study. Pneumologie 1990; 44(1):32–36.

194. White CS, Templeton PA. Chemical pneumonitis. Radiol Clin North Am 1992; 30(6):1231–1243.

195. Weill H. Disaster at Bhopal: the accident, early findings and respiratory health outlook in those injured. Bull Eur Physiopathol Respir 1987; 23(6):587–590.

196. Merrill WW, Beckett WS, Raymond LW, et al. Flock worker's lung. Ann Intern Med 1999; 130(7):615.

197. Warheit DB, Hart GA, Hesterberg TW, et al. Potential pulmonary effects of man-made organic fiber (MMOF) dusts. Crit Rev Toxicol 2001; 31(6):697–736.

198. Kern DG, Crausman RS, Durand KT, Nayer A, Kuhn C III. Flock worker's lung: chronic interstitial lung disease in the nylon flocking industry. Ann Intern Med 1998; 129(4):261–272.

199. Boag AH, Colby TV, Fraire AE, et al. The pathology of interstitial lung disease in nylon flock workers. Am J Surg Pathol 1999; 23(12):1639–1645.

200. Eschenbacher WL, Kreiss K, Lougheed MD, Pransky GS, Day B, Castellan RM. Nylon flock-associated interstitial lung disease. Am J Respir Crit Care Med 1999; 159(6): 2003–2008.

201. Kreiss K, Gomaa A, Kullman G, Fedan K, Simoes EJ, Enright PL. Clinical bronchiolitis obliterans in workers at a microwave-popcorn plant. N Engl J Med 2002; 347(5): 330–338.

202. Boswell RT, McCunney RJ. Bronchiolitis obliterans from exposure to incinerator fly ash. J Occup Environ Med 1995; 37(7):850–855.

203. Spain BA, Cummings O, Garcia JG. Bronchiolitis obliterans in an animal feed worker. Am J Ind Med 1995; 28(3):437–443.

204. Alleman T, Darcey DJ. Case report: bronchiolitis obliterans organizing pneumonia in a spice process technician. J Occup Environ Med 2002; 44(3):215–216.

205. Di Stefano F, Verna N, Di Giampaolo L, Boscolo P, Di Cioacchino M. Cavitating BOOP associated with myeloperoxidase deficiency in floor cleaner with an incidental heavy exposure to benzalkonium compounds. J Occup Health 2003; 45(3):182–184.

206. Global Initiative for Chronic Obstructive Lung Disease. Global strategy for the diagnosis, management, and prevention of chronic obstructive pulmonary disease. NHLBI/WHO report. NIH, NHLBI Publication Number 2701, April 2001.

207. Xu X, Christiani DC, Dockery DW, Wang L. Exposure-response relationships between occupational exposures and chronic respiratory illness: a community-based study. Am Rev Respir Dis 1992; 146:413–418.

208. Balmes J, Becklake M, Blanc P, et al. American Thoracic Society statement: occupational contribution to the burden of airway disease. Am J Respir Crit Care Med 2003; 167:787–797.
209. Bergdahl IA, Toren K, Erikkson K, et al. Increased mortality in COPD among construction workers exposed to inorganic dust. Eur Respir J 2004; 23:402–406.
210. Trupin L, Earnest G, San Pedro M, et al. The occupational burden of chronic obstructive pulmonary disease. Eur Respir J 2003; 22:1–9.
211. Hnizdo E, Sullivan PA, Bang KM, Wagner G. Association between chronic obstructive pulmonary disease and employment by industry and occupation in the U.S. population: a study of data from the Third National Health and Nutrition Examination Survey. Am J Epidemiol 2002; 156:738–746.
212. Hnizdo E, Sullivan PA, Bang KM, Wagner G. Airflow obstruction attributable to work in industry and occupation among U.S. race/ethnic groups: a study of NHANES III data. Am J Ind Med 2004; 46:126–135.
213. Suadicani P, Hein HO, Meyer HW, Gyntelberg F. Exposure to cold and draught, alcohol consumption, and the NS-phenotype are associated with chronic bronchitis: an epidemiological investigation of 3387 men aged 53–75 years: the Copenhagen male study. Occup Environ Med 2001; 58:160–164.
214. Mak GK, Gould MK, Kuschner WG. Occupational inhalant exposure and respiratory disorders among never-smokers referred to a hospital pulmonary function laboratory. Am J Med Sci 2001; 322(3):121–126.
215. Zock JP, Sunyer J, Kogevinas M, Kromhout H, Burney P, Anto JM. The ECRHS Study Group. Occupation, chronic bronchitis, and lung function in young adults. Am J Respir Crit Care Med 2001; 163:1572–1577.
216. Hertzberg VS, Rosenman KD, Reilly MJ, Rice CH. Occupational and environmental disease: effect of occupational silica exposure on pulmonary function. Chest 2002; 122:721–728.
217. Lange P, Parner J, Prescott E, Vestbo J. Chronic bronchitis in an elderly population. Age Ageing 2003; 32:636–642.
218. de Meer G, Kerkhof M, Kromhout H, Schouten JP, Heederik D. Interaction of atopy and smoking on respiratory effects of occupational dust exposure: a general population-based study. Environ Health: Global Access Sci Source 2004; 3(6):1–7.
219. Piitulainen E, Tornling G, Eriksson S. Effect of age and occupational exposure to airway irritants on lung function in non-smoking individuals with α_1-antitrypsin deficiency (PiZZ). Thorax 1997; 52:244–248.
220. Mayer AS, Stoller JK, Bartelson BB, Ruttenber AJ, Sandhaus RA, Newman LS. Occupational exposure risks in individuals with PI*Z α_1-antitrypsin deficiency. Am J Respir Crit Care Med 2000; 162:553–558.

29

Hypersensitivity Pneumonitis and Organic Dust Toxic Syndromes

Yvon Cormier
Institut Universitaire de Cardiologie et de Pneumologie, Laval University and Hospital, Laval, Quebec, Canada

Mark Schuyler
Department of Internal Medicine, University of New Mexico School of Medicine, Albuquerque, New Mexico, U.S.A.

INTRODUCTION—HYPERSENSITIVITY PNEUMONITIS

Hypersensitivity pneumonitis (HP) is a lung disease caused by an immune response to inhaled antigen to which the subject has previously been sensitized. HP is essentially defined by the clinical presentation, causative agent, and pathophysiology because the disease has no pathognomonic marker. There is a wide spectrum of clinical presentations from the most acute phase characterized by fever, chills, general malaise, cough, and dyspnea to a more insidious progressive dyspnea over several months if not years. This wide spectrum of presentations has led to the separation of HP into three classical phases: acute, subacute, and chronic. These distinctions are poorly defined and therefore have little clinical relevance. What is important is whether the disease is present or not.

Farmer's lung was the first form of HP to be described both clinically and etiologically by Pepys in 1960 (1). Clinical description of farmer's lung went as far back as 1555 when Olaus Magnus, the last Catholic archbishop of Sweden, published a history of the northern people that described respiratory difficulties from the dust produced during threshing in winter (2). Ramazzini in 1713, recognized respiratory problems in sifters and measurers of grain that probably represented both asthma and HP (3). Farmer's lung was described in England in 1932 (4). Since then, the number of settings and etiological agents has continuously grown to a point where there are now some 100 environments known to be at risk. Most forms of HP have been named for the setting or the agent responsible (e.g., bird fancier's disease, humidifier lung, hot tub lung, etc.). Some of these different types of HP are presented in Table 1.

Table 1   Common Occupational Causes of HP

Disease	Antigen source	Probable antigen
Plant products		
FLD	Moldy hay	Thermophilic actinomycetes
		SR (*Micropolyspora faeni*)
		Thermoactinomyces vulgaris
		Aspergillus sp.
		Penicillium sp.
		Candida sp.
		Absidia corymbifera
		Wallemia sebi
		Fusarium sp.
Bagassosis	Moldy pressed sugarcane (bagasse)	Thermophilic actinomycetes
		Thermoactinomyces sacchari
		T. vulgaris
Mushroom worker's disease	Moldy compost and mushrooms	Thermophilic actinomycetes
		SR
		T. vulgaris
		Aspergillus sp.
		Mushroom spores
Suberosis	Moldy cork	*Penicillium* sp.
		Aspergillus sp.
		Cork
Malt worker's lung	Contaminated barley	*Aspergillus clavatus*
Maple bark disease	Contaminated maple logs	*Cryptostroma corticale*
Sequoisis	Contaminated redwood dust	*Graphium* sp.
		Pullularia sp.
Soybean lung	Soybeans in animal feed	Soybean hull antigens
Wood pulp worker's disease	Contaminated wood pulp	*Alternaria* sp.
Wood dust HP	Contaminated wood dust	*Bacillus subtilis*
		Alternaria
		Pine sawdust
Cheese workers' disease	Cheese or cheese casings	*Penicillium* sp.
Wood trimmer's disease	Contaminated wood trimmings, at times in sawmills	*Rhizopus* sp.
		Mucor sp.
Greenhouse lung	Greenhouse soil	*Aspergillus* sp.
		Penicillium sp.
		Cryptostroma corticale
Potato riddler's lung	Moldy hay around potatoes	Thermophilic actinomycetes
		SR
		T. vulgaris
		Aspergillus sp.
Tobacco workers' disease	Mold on tobacco	*Aspergillus* sp.
Wine grower's lung	Mold on grapes	*Botrytis cinerea*
Soy sauce brewers' lung	Fermentation starter for soy sauce	*Aspergillus oryzae*
Tiger nut dust	Tiger nut dust	*Junia avellaneda*
Riding school lung	Hay in horse stall	Thermophilic actinomycetes
		SR
		T. vulgaris

(*Continued*)

Table 1   Common Occupational Causes of HP (*Continued*)

Disease	Antigen source	Probable antigen
Stipatosis	Esparto grass (*Stipa tenacissima*) used to make plaster	Esparto grass antigens Thermophilic actinomycetes *SR* *Aspergillus* sp.
Algarroba lung	Livestock feed	Algarroba (legume) antigens
Salami lung	Mold on salami casings	Fungi *Penicillium camembertii*
Peat moss lung	Mold on peat moss	Fungi *Penicillium* sp. *Monocillium* sp.
Miller's lung	Grain weevils in wheat flour	*Sitophilus granarius* proteins
Fertilizer lung	Contaminated fertilizer	*Streptomyces albus*
Nylon plant lung	Biomass in air-conditioning system	*Cytophaga* (gram-negative bacteria)
Konnyaku lung	Konnyaku manufacturing	*Hujikia fusiforme* (algae)
Animal products		
Pigeon breeder's disease	Pigeon droppings	Altered pigeon serum (probably IgA) Pigeon bloom (derived from feathers) Pigeon intestinal mucin
Turkey handler's disease	Turkey products	Turkey proteins
Chicken breeder's lung	Chicken feathers	Chicken feather proteins
Laboratory worker's HP	Rat fur	Rat urine protein
Shell lung	Oyster or mollusk shell	Shell proteins
Sericulturists' lung	Silk worm larvae	Silk worm larvae proteins
Reactive chemicals		
TDI HP	TDI	Altered proteins (albumin + others)
MDI HP	MDI	Altered proteins
HDI HP	HDI	Altered proteins
TMA HP	TMA	Altered proteins
Other		
Ventilator lung	Contaminated humidifiers, dehumidifiers, air conditioners, and heating systems	Thermophilic actinomycetes *Thermoactinomyces candidus* *T. vulgaris* *Penicillium* sp. *Cephalosporium* sp. *Debaryomyces hansenii* Amoebae *Klebsiella* sp. *Candida* sp.
Tractor lung	Contaminated tractor cab air conditioner	*Rhizopus* sp.
Metal working fluid HP	Contaminated metal-working fluid	*Pseudomonas* sp. *Acinetobacter* sp. *Mycobacterial* sp.
Smut lung	Japanese handicrafts	*Ustilago esculenta*

Abbreviations: FLD, farmer's lung disease; HDI, hexamethylene diisocyanate; HP, hypersensitivity pneumonitis; MDI, diphenylmethane diisocyanate; *SR*, *Saccharopolyspora rectivirgula*; TDI, toluene diisocyanate; TMA, trimetallic anhydride.

Definition

There are no clear definitions of HP. The definition can be approached from an immunopathological angle or from its clinical aspects. However, both of these approaches are difficult because we do not have a clear understanding of all of the immune mechanisms involved or a clinical presentation definable in a single entity. For the acute form, the patient usually presents with fever and chills three to eight hours after an obvious exposure (e.g., handling moldy hay). This suggests a delayed type immune response (type III antigen/antibody). The antigen/antibody implication in the pathogenesis has never been proved and the histology of granuloma formation and lymphocytic infiltrates mitigates against that mechanism. The more insidious presentation of subacute or chronic forms would better fit with a type IV cellular mediated immunity.

We propose a tentative definition as follows: "HP is an inappropriate immune response to inhaled antigens that causes shortness of breath, a restrictive lung defect, interstitial infiltrates seen on lung imaging [chest X ray and high-resolution computed tomography (HRCT)] due to the accumulation of large numbers of activated T lymphocytes in the lungs." The disease is sometimes further characterized by episodic bouts of fever a few hours after exposure.

Clinical Manifestations

Signs and Symptoms

Acute illness typically begins 4 to 12 hours after exposure, with the patient describing a flu-like illness characterized by symptoms of cough, dyspnea, chest tightness, fevers, chills, malaise, and myalgias. Symptoms are usually accompanied by physical findings of fever, tachypnea, tachycardia, and crepitant rales. The acute symptoms of HP typically abate or improve within 24 hours, only to recur hours after repeat antigen exposure. Because of the transient nature of this form of HP, the physical signs, especially fever and tachycardia, are often no longer present when the patient is examined by a physician.

Manifestations of the more insidious presentations are often not specific and are more difficult to diagnose. Exertional dyspnea and cough are the predominant symptoms, with sputum production, fatigue, anorexia, and weight loss also reported. Physical examination may be normal or reveal basilar crackles. Cyanosis and right heart failure may be evident with severe fibrotic disease. Digital clubbing is occasionally found in late stages. Clubbing occurred in approximately half of patients in a case series of pigeon breeder's disease and was associated with a poorer prognostic outcome (5). These patients are often diagnosed as having idiopathic pulmonary fibrosis. For example, Japanese researchers found that a considerable number of patients diagnosed as HP had typical idiopathic interstitial fibrosis on lung biopsy (6).

Diagnostic Criteria

With the ubiquity of potential environmental antigens (often in unsuspected workplace or home environments), the difficulties in identifying and measuring relevant antigenic exposures, the variable disease manifestations, and the often-subtle clinical presentation leading to under-recognition and misdiagnosis of HP continue to plague clinicians. A high degree of clinical suspicion and a careful history remain essential for early disease recognition.

Numerous diagnostic criteria for the disease have been published (7,8). Most of these are opinions of experts and based on the description of the disease. None of these have been validated. Recently, the American Thoracic Society HP study group has published the first validated clinical predictive rules for the diagnosis of HP (9). That study shows that classical cases of HP can sometimes be confirmed or ruled out with a high degree of certainty by simple clinical criteria. These criteria are: (i) exposure to a known offending antigen, (ii) positive specific serum antibodies, (iii) recurrent episodes of symptoms, (iv) inspiratory crackles, (v) symptoms four to eight hours after exposure, and (vi) weight loss. Unfortunately, many, if not most, cases fall outside the diagnostic capacity of this rule. This rule is heavily weighed on known exposure and offending antigen; if these are not obvious, the diagnosis cannot be made without further tests. Additional procedures include HRCT, lung functions, bronchoalveolar lavage (BAL), lung biopsies, and antigen challenge (suspected environment or laboratory).

Clinical Evaluation

Physiology

Pulmonary function abnormalities in HP are classically restrictive, with a decrease in forced vital capacity, one-second forced expiratory volume, and total lung capacity. Lung diffusion capacity is the most consistently altered lung function and the degree of its decrease is usually greater than that of the lung volumes or flows (10,11). These tests are obviously nonspecific, because most interstitial lung diseases show a similar pattern. Arterial blood gas analysis usually shows O_2 desaturation of variable degree. These abnormalities improve or even correct themselves within a month after exposure removal or corticosteroid therapy (12).

The insidious form or repeated bouts of acute episodes can lead to irreversible lung damage in the form of lung fibrosis or emphysema (13,14). Methacholine hyperresponsiveness has been described in 22% to 60% of patients with HP (15–18). The incidence of asthma increased from 1% prior to a diagnosis of farmer's lung disease (FLD) to 7% within five years after the diagnosis of FLD in a Finish study of 1031 farmers with HP (19).

Radiology

In the acute form of disease, the chest radiograph may be normal, but typically shows diffuse interstitial infiltrates [Fig. 1(A)].

HRCT is the most useful imaging tool to clearly evaluate the lung involvement. Widespread diffuse ground-glass opacification, areas of decreased attenuation and mosaic perfusion, and centrilobular micronodules are the most common and characteristic CT manifestations of HP [Fig. 1(B)] (20–23).

Either patchy or diffuse ground-glass attenuation was observed in 52% of subacute and 71% of chronic forms of bird breeder's HP (24). Honeycombing is present in more advanced chronic cases. Emphysematous changes can be seen as an important irreversible sequella of HP. The emphysematous changes can occur in nonsmoking HP patients, but the characteristics of the emphysema are not different from those seen in smokers. Mediastinal lymph nodes may be enlarged, but hilar adenopathy is rare (20). These nodes are usually smaller than those seen in sarcoidosis or cancer (25).

(A)   **(B)**

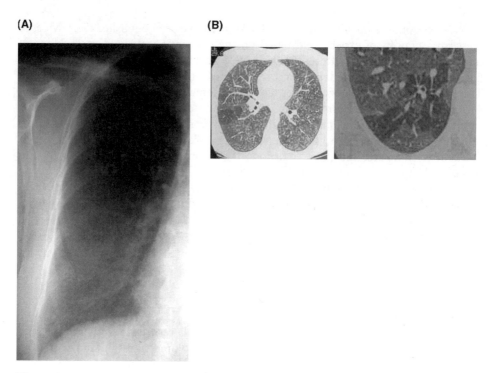

Figure 1 (**A**) Posterioanterior chest film of a patient with acute HP showing typical interstitial infiltrates which predominate in the lower lung fields. (**B**) HRCT image showing patchy alveolar infiltrates characteristic of acute HP. *Abbreviations*: HP, hypersensitivity pneumonitis; HRCT, high-resolution computed tomography.

Specific Antibodies

The finding of specific antibodies against the suspected antigen in the serum of a patient with suspected HP indicates antigen exposure sufficient to generate a humoral immunological response and may be a helpful diagnostic clue (26). These antibodies have classically been called precipitins because they were measured by the double diffusion method of Outcherlony, which uses an antigen containing gel and the addition of positive serum leading to the precipitating of an antigen/antibody complex (27). This test is not sensitive and has been widely replaced by the enzyme-linked immunosorbant assay technique. The finding of specific antibodies signifies that the patient has been exposed to that antigen and has developed an immune response to the antigen. Most individuals with positive antibodies do not have HP. Serum precipitins were found in 3% to 30% of asymptomatic farmers and in up to 50% of asymptomatic pigeon breeders (28–31). The prevalence of positive tests in asymptomatic individuals can fluctuate, with subjects testing variably positive or negative at different times (32). The absence of serum antibodies suggests that the patient does not have HP or that the wrong antigen has been tested. False-negatives may occur because of poorly standardized commercial laboratory antigens, insensitive laboratory techniques, use of underconcentrated sera, or the wrong choice of antigen for testing (33). Serum precipitins may disappear over variable periods of time after exposure ceases, adding to the difficulty of antigen-specific diagnosis (34).

Other Laboratory Studies

In the acute illness, peripheral blood leukocytosis with neutrophilia and lymphopenia is often present. Eosinophilia is unusual. Mild elevation in erythrocyte sedimentation rate, C-reactive protein, and immunoglobulins of IgG, IgM, or IgA isotypes are occasionally evident, reflecting acute or chronic inflammation. Skin tests have not been useful in the diagnosis of HP (35).

Inhalation Challenge

The use of inhalation challenge in the diagnosis of HP is limited by the lack of standardized antigens and techniques. Inhalation of an aerosolized antigen suspected to be causative is helpful only when acute symptoms and clinical abnormalities are part of the disease presentation and likely to occur within hours after exposure (36). Observation of the acute symptoms on exposure to the suspect environment with postexposure monitoring of symptoms, temperature, leukocyte count, spirometry, and chest radiograph may be preferable to laboratory challenge. Interpretation of results is often difficult, and inhalation challenge is not recommended in most patients with suspected HP except in a research context.

Bronchoalveolar Lavage

BAL can be very useful in the evaluation of patients with HP and in excluding other conditions that mimic the illness, though BAL findings are nonspecific and, by themselves, nondiagnostic (37). Typically, a marked lavage lymphocytosis is found. Other diseases such as sarcoidosis, military tuberculosis, berylliosis, and bronchiolitis obliterans organizing pneumonia can also give a lymphocytosis in BAL. The absolute number of BAL lymphocytes is usually higher in HP than in other lymphocytic lung diseases. It was originally believed that the lymphocytes CD4/CD8 ratio could differentiate HP from sarcoidosis, HP having a low ratio and sarcoidosis a high ratio (38). Recent studies, however, show that the CD4/CD8 ratio varies considerably in HP with ratios as high as those seen in sarcoidosis (39). Increased BAL neutrophils are observed shortly after antigen exposure. Total white cell numbers are increased, often up to fivefold of that seen in controls. The absolute number of macrophages is increased, although their percentage in lavage is reduced due to the higher number of lymphocytes. Mast cells are increased in patients with HP, though their pathogenic role remains unclear (40). Concentrations of IgG, IgM, and IgA antibodies are typically increased in BAL in subjects with HP (though smoking may mitigate this effect), as are total protein and albumin (41,42). The BAL lymphocytosis may persist for years following removal from exposure and despite improvement in other clinical parameters, limiting its utility as a tool to follow the course and progression of disease (43). Asymptomatic farmers and pigeon breeders may have BAL lymphocytosis, further limiting the diagnostic utility of lavage (44,45).

Pathology

Lung biopsy may be indicated in patients who do not meet the clinical criteria for a definitive diagnosis or to rule out other diseases requiring different treatment. Transbronchial biopsies are of limited values, and thoracoscopic lung biopsy is occasionally required (46). Special stains and cultures are helpful to distinguish HP from infectious granulomatous conditions such as fungal and mycobacterial diseases.

Histopathology in 60 Wisconsin patients with farmer's lung biopsied during the active phase of their disease showed an interstitial alveolar infiltrate in 100% (consisting of plasma cells, lymphocytes, and occasional eosinophils), granulomata in 70%, unexpectedly mild interstitial fibrosis in 65%, and bronchiolitis to some degree in 50% of the biopsy specimens; no vasculitis was observed in any case (47).

Coleman and Colby studied 27 patients with putative HP and found a "diagnostic triad" of (i) cellular infiltrates of lymphocytes and plasma cells of varying density along airways, (ii) interstitial infiltrates of lymphocytes and plasma cells varying from mild to very dense, and (iii) single, non-necrotizing, randomly scattered granulomata in the parenchyma with some in bronchiolar and alveolar walls, but without mural vascular involvement (48). Eosinophils were scant or absent. About 80% of clinically proven cases were estimated as demonstrating the triad, which may, however, be present in other interstitial diseases.

Sarcoidosis may be particularly difficult to distinguish from HP, but certain histopathologic features may help. In sarcoidosis, but not in HP, granulomata are found in perivascular and intramural areas of blood vessels. Infiltrates of lymphocytes and plasma cells are found only in and around granulomata in sarcoidosis, whereas in HP such infiltrates are also seen involving the parenchyma at sites distant from granulomata. Ultrastructural studies have revealed similar, nonspecific air–blood barrier lesions of alveolar epithelial or endothelial injury and inflammation with type II cell hyperplasia and fibrosis in both HP and sarcoidosis (49).

The pathology of HP is sometimes that of nonspecific interstitial pneumonia and the usual interstitial pneumonia changes can be seen in chronic cases (50). These descriptions may therefore mislead the physician to make an inappropriate diagnosis.

Epidemiology

The epidemiology of occupation-related HP is meaningful only when it relates to specific types of HP. Definitive prevalence studies are difficult for several reasons (51,52). The diagnosis depends on a group of clinical and laboratory findings, none of which are pathognomonic. Symptoms are not specific, and it is impractical in large epidemiological studies to use chest roentgenograms, BAL, lung biopsies, and inhalation challenge studies in either the suspected environment or the laboratory. Serum precipitins and BAL lymphocytosis indicate exposure, not disease. Thus, identification of individuals with clinical HP in any occupational groups is tentative, so the accuracy and value of relevant epidemiological studies are questionable.

Variables complicating prevalence studies in individuals and groups include the extent of environmental exposure, geographic location, rainfall and other local conditions, characteristics and hygiene of facilities and processes, safety and control measures, exposure precautions, awareness of the hazard, and host factors. Despite these built-in problems, many epidemiological studies have been carried out, mainly in farmer's lung, bird fancier's lung, and building-related exposures or contaminated humidification devices (53).

Farmer's lung is primarily a disease of dairy farmers. Early studies that reported high prevalence utilized questionnaires only, but more recent studies with strict criteria for diagnosis indicate an annual incidence of 44 per 100,000 among farming population in Finland and 23 per 100,000 in Sweden (54). An overall prevalence of 0.42%, or 420 per 100,000, was found in 1400 Wisconsin dairy farmers (55). Differences among various studies have been attributed to geographic location, rainfall, and type of farming as well as to epidemiological methods. Bird fancier's or breeder's lung among populations appropriately exposed has ranged from 3% to 15%. Budgerigar (parakeet) fanciers in Britain have a HP prevalence rate of 0.5% to 7.5%. Outbreaks of HP from contaminated humidifiers in office buildings have affected 15% to 52% of exposed individuals. Few useful data are available for other occupation-related HP. Of note is the diminished frequency and even disappearance of a specific HP after the cause is recognized and controlled. Maple bark stripper's lung and bagassosis, for example, have essentially disappeared as occupational diseases.

Pathophysiology

There are multiple immunological markers present in subjects with HP that suggest that immune mediation is important in the pathogenesis of this syndrome (28,56–61). In addition, the necessity for previous sensitization (indicated by the presence of antibody in virtually all patients with HP) suggests immunologic mediation.

The presence of serum antibody in patients with HP and the timing of symptoms after exposure (2–9 hours) led to the hypothesis that HP represents an example of immune complex–mediated lung disease (1). However, the presence of antibody in exposed but not ill subjects, the lack of correlation of the presence of serum antibody and pulmonary function tests, the presence of HP in a patient with hypogammaglobulinemia, the appearance of HP in a HIV-infected patient as the peripheral blood lymphocyte count recovered, the lack of evidence of complement consumption during acute exposure, the pathology which includes granulomatous changes, and the findings from animal models strongly suggest that cell-mediated immune processes are very important in HP (48,62–64).

Exploration of cell-mediated (type IV) hypersensitivity mechanisms in human HP has focused largely on cell phenotypes, functional patterns, and cytokine release in BAL fluids. Alveolar lymphocytosis consists predominantly of CD8+ T cells in HP, varying with the stage of disease and causative agent (65). Analysis of the T cell receptor, β-chain–variable region in HP BAL lymphocytes showed overexpression of a particular β-chain–variable segment reported to belong to the lymphocyte subset that accounts for the alveolitis in HP (CD8+), and resolution of alveolitis was accompanied by normalization of the T cell subsets (66). More recent data reveal that the expansion of the BAL CD8+ cells is clonal, is dependent on continued exposure of the subject to the responsible antigen, and is likely due to antigenic stimulation, rather than the effects of superantigen (67). The presence of serum IgG_4 antibody to pigeon antigens correlates with lack of symptoms in pigeon breeders (60). Because IgG_4 is an immunoglobulin isotype that is induced by interleukin (IL)-4 and suppressed by IFNγ, this suggests that symptomatic HP may be characterized by the predominance of Th1 type immunologic reactivity.

Activated CD8+ cells, macrophages, and resultant cytokines characterize the lymphocyte-rich alveolitis in HP and putatively account for progression to clinical disease. IL-1, tumor necrosis factor (TNF), MIP-1α, and IL-8 are elevated in BAL fluids and synthesized and released by BAL cells (68,69). Other substances increased in HP BAL include fibroblast growth factors, type III procollagen, fibronectin, vibronectin, and hyaluronic acid. Surfactant protein A, associated with macrophage immunomodulatory function, is altered in BAL fluids obtained from HP patients (70). Serine proteinase inhibitors, α1-proteinase inhibitor, secretory leukocyte proteinase inhibitor, and elafin (elastase-specific inhibitor) are present in BAL and may play a role in resolution and control of HP (71). Asymptomatic, exposed individuals may also demonstrate a lymphocyte-rich BAL, and the presence of BAL lymphocytosis does not predict the later development of disease (44,72). The mechanisms of BAL lymphocytosis could include the influence of chemokines and/or a decrease of lymphocyte apoptosis (73–75).

Although increased numbers of CD8+ T lymphocytes in BAL of recently exposed HP patients have been reported by several investigators, others have found no consistent phenotypic preponderance, despite increased T lymphocyte proliferation, activation, and function. Increased populations of CD4+ and CD8+ lymphocytes, mast cells, and various sorts of cytotoxic cells, including natural killer cells and major histocompatibility complex (MHC)-restricted and non-MHC–restricted cytotoxic lymphocytes, have been found in lungs of HP patients (76,77).

Pursuit of antigenic epitopes on the relatively crude extracts of *Saccharopolyspora rectivirgula* (*SR*), the agent responsible for FLD, or avian proteins has shown that the relevant T lymphocytes recognized a wide range of proteins that induce proliferation, but without any clear meaning for pathogenesis (78,79). An adjuvant effort of the etiological agent itself or a concurrent viral infection may initiate or enhance disease in susceptible individuals, and suppressor cells of lymphocyte or macrophage lineage have been postulated to explain the absence or limitation of inflammation in exposed, asymptomatic individuals. Because of necessary limitations in using patients in experimental studies and the inadequacies of in vitro techniques for such a purpose, several species of animals have been utilized to help elucidate pathogenesis (80). Recent studies have included adoptive transfer and genetically manipulated mice in attempts to elucidate the role of T cells.

Many of the agents responsible for HP can act as adjuvants and are particulate (promoting retention of antigen within the lung for prolonged periods of time), persistent, and nondegradable. They can interact with humoral mediators (complement and antibody) and cells in the lung to produce inflammation. The agents can induce injury by causing polymorphonuclear leukocytes and macrophages to release phlogistic substances such as reactive oxygen compounds, proteolytic enzymes, and products of arachidonic acid metabolism, such as prostaglandins and leukotrienes. The agents can also cause the production and release of IL-1, TNFα, IL-12, IL-6, monocyte chemotactic protein (MCP)-1 and MIP1α from macrophages and lymphokines (IL-2, IFNγ, and B cell growth and differentiation factors) from lymphocytes (81,82).

Injury to the lung caused by the above factors could allow enhanced pulmonary exposure to inhaled antigen, which might promote immunologic sensitization and subsequent pulmonary damage. The result of all these processes is pulmonary inflammation.

Cyclosporin A, a potent immunosuppressant of T cell function, has been found to suppress disease in rabbit and murine models of HP. Nude mice did not exhibit pulmonary lesions characteristic of HP following exposure which was able to produce lesions in the thymus-intact littermates' ability to express pulmonary lesions could be transferred with T cells from sensitized mice (83–86).

Most recent work has used *SR*, the agent responsible for FLD, administered into the lungs of mice. The readouts in these experiments were usually pulmonary histologic abnormalities and BAL fluid parameters. In general, the response of the lung to intratracheal *SR* is dependent on IFNγ, perhaps dependent on IL-12, and is associated with upregulation of vascular adhesion molecules such as E-selectin, P-selectin, and VCAM-1 (87–91). The mechanism of decreased influx of lymphocytes into the lungs of IFNγ-deficient mice likely involves decreased production of the IFNγ-dependent chemokines IP-10, Mig, and I-Tac (88). Although most mouse strains respond similarly to *SR*, DBA/2 mice express less pulmonary inflammation, perhaps due to increased IL-4 mRNA stability and subsequent Th2 bias, compared to C57Bl/6 animals (89,92,93). Chemokines (MCP-1, MIP-1α, MIP-2) are increased in BAL fluid, but are not necessary for the expression of experimental HP (94–97). IL-10 appears to downregulate the inflammatory response (98). Viral infection (both recombinant Sendai virus and Sendai) accentuates pulmonary inflammation (95,99). Nicotine exposure decreases the pulmonary inflammatory and systemic immunologic response (100).

A slight modification of the above model is repetitive injection of antigen into mice. This is similar to the events that occur in humans and likely involves immune events, as blockage of costimulatory signals by CTLA4-Ig reduces pulmonary inflammation, specific antibody, and cytokine (IL-4, IL-10, IFNγ) production (101). Concurrent Sendai viral infection has been shown to enhance HP in mice receiving repeated intranasal instillations of *SR* (102). A common phenomenon in animals injected repetitively with i.t. antigen is diminution of pulmonary inflammation despite continuing injections, which might be regulated by IL-10 (103,104).

These models differ from human disease in many important aspects. Human disease occurs after repetitive inhalation of the responsible material and is not associated with the use of adjuvants. Previous exposure is necessary in human HP, and there is evidence of sensitization in patients with HP (antibody and cellular sensitization). Most importantly, only a minority of exposed individuals develops the disease. In general, these models examine the direct effects of the responsible agents on the lung (toxicity, and aspects of the innate immune system), but not the adaptive immunologically mediated effects that are dependent on previous sensitization. Therefore, this approach cannot easily separate the direct effects of the agents on the lung from those induced by adaptive immunity.

Adoptive transfer models of HP allow differentiation between direct lung damage (i.e., toxicity), sensitization (the development of antibody and cellular reactivity), and the results of immunologic reactions (the interaction of antigen with antibody and/or cells). This can be accomplished by transfer of the putatively responsible cells or antibody into a recipient animal, before challenging that animal with an agent that causes HP. Adoptive transfer of HP induced by *SR* in animal models has been successful using the transfers of cultured lymphocytes from sensitized, syngeneic strain II guinea pigs, Lewis rats, and inbred mice to naive recipients subsequently challenged with inhaled or instilled intrapulmonary antigen (105–107).

Adoptive transfer HP in mice is not mediated by serum antibody, but by T cells (92,86). The cells can be from the spleen, peripheral- or lung-associated lymph nodes, or peritoneum. Both in vivo sensitization and in vitro culture with antigen are required. The pulmonary injury is characterized by increased numbers of mononuclear cells in the lungs in both perivascular and peribronchiolar locations. CD4+ cells are responsible for the transfer and interact with recipient CD4+ cells (103,108,109). The bulk of pulmonary inflammatory cells in the recipient animals originate from the host and not from the transferred cells (110). The transferring cells have the characteristics of Th1 cells, and are a mixture of naive and memory (as defined by CD44, CD45RB, and LECAM-1 markers) (107,111) CD4+ cells. Th1 cell lines are capable of transfer and Th2 cells lines are incapable of transfer (112).

Animal studies have led to the conclusions that Th1 CD4+ lymphocytes and cytotoxic cells are major effector cells of experimental HP. So far, none of the cellular humoral, cytokine, mediator, in vitro, or in vivo studies in humans or animals fully explains the pathogenesis of HP. The combinations of cells, cytokines, and other substances that are both necessary and sufficient for the progression to clinical disease or result in downregulation without clinical disease remain uncertain. How these findings relate to human disease with CD8+ lymphocytosis in BAL, what is responsible for and regulates the influx of effector cells, inflammatory cytokines, and other mediators, and what downregulates and modulates the responses of the lung that lead to resolution and control are questions motivating further research.

Natural History and Prognosis

Studies on the natural history and prognosis of recovery from HP have been hampered by variable diagnostic criteria, limited duration of follow-up, failure to characterize or control for ongoing antigen exposure, and probably differences in antigen potencies that may affect recovery. While the clinical course of HP is variable, if illness is recognized early and recurrent attacks are avoided, the prognosis for recovery is usually quite good. Recurrent illness and ongoing antigen exposure can lead to chronic, progressive, and occasionally fatal lung disease (18,34,113,114).

Following acute attacks of HP, there is usually rapid improvement in lung vital capacity and diffusion capacity in the first two weeks. Generally, single acute episodes are self-limited. Continued symptoms and progressive lung impairment have been reported after recurrent acute attacks and even after a single severe attack (115–117).

The chronic form of HP, with insidious symptoms and more subtle clinical abnormalities, is often recognized later in the course of illness and may have a poorer prognosis (118). Symptomatic pigeon breeders followed up for 18 years showed a fourfold average rate of decline in pulmonary function compared to the expected rate (119). In a follow-up study of 33 FLD cases, airflow obstruction with or without emphysema was found in 13, suggesting that asthma and emphysema are more common sequelae of HP than previously recognized (14).

No single functional or biochemical marker exists to predict outcome. The BAL lymphocytosis is of no prognostic value as it may persist for years following removal from exposure and despite clinical recovery (120). Precipitating antibodies also have doubtful prognostic significance for the development of persistence of HP. Age at diagnosis, duration of antigen exposure after onset of symptoms, and total years of exposure before diagnosis seem to have predictive value in the likelihood of recovery from pigeon breeder's lung disease (121). Pigeon breeders with HP were more likely to improve or recover completely, if they had been in contact with birds for less than two years. Neither the form of clinical presentation (acute vs. chronic) nor the degree of lung function abnormality at the time of diagnosis was related to recovery in another study of pigeon breeder's disease (122). Rather, younger age at diagnosis (27 vs. 42 years) and exposure to antigen for less than six months after symptom onset were associated with complete recovery.

Treatment and Prevention

Primary prevention is probably not feasible in most instances. The main reason for this is that only a small fraction of individuals exposed to an environment that can lead to HP ever do get the disease. For example, it is unlikely that all dairy farmers would agree to wear respirators when only 3 per 1000 ever develop farmer's lung. This having been said, preventing the risk of exposure does have its place. All farmers should understand the risk of working with moldy hay and take all possible measures to decrease such exposures. Bird fanciers will not abandon their hobby, but better education of individuals who cohabitate with pigeons could help decrease the incidence of pigeon breeder's disease.

Once the disease is present, contact avoidance is the most effective form of treatment. Contact avoidance is as effective as oral corticosteroids in promoting recovery from HP (12). Contact avoidance is however not always achievable. This is especially true when the contact is in the workplace or in the living environment (e.g., pigeons).

There is increasing evidence that some farmers who develop HP can continue their profession if appropriate measures are taken (113,123). Strategies recommended to reduce both FLD recurrence and incident cases include efficient drying of hay and cereals before storage, use of mechanical feeding systems, and better ventilation of farm buildings (124). The use of lactic-acid producing bacteria as hay additives to minimize mold contamination is of no apparent benefit as it does not decrease the amount of airborne farmer's lung antigen (125). A six-year follow-up study of farmers with HP revealed that 50% to 60% remained on the farm; by 15 years, as many as 70% had returned to farming (34,126). In such cases, regular follow-up of pulmonary function, radiography, and symptoms is essential to detect clinical deterioration and direct efforts to minimize antigen exposure.

Avoidance of exposure by eliminating the offending antigen from the environment may be difficult. Despite animal removal and appropriate cleaning, high levels of bird antigen could still be detected 18 months later (127). The efficacy of various types of respirators in preventing disease progression is largely unknown. Helmet-type, powered air-purifying respirators have been used to prevent episodic exposure in individuals with previous acute episodes of farmer's lung (128). Prolonged wearing of respiratory protection is limited by the fact that most respirators are hot and cumbersome. Dust respirators offer substantial, but in some cases incomplete, protection against organic dusts and are not recommended once sensitization has occurred (129).

Indoor microbial contamination is often related to problems with control of moisture. Source, dilution, and administrative controls are used to reduce these indoor contaminants (130). Source control includes preventing leaking and flooding, removing stagnant water sources, eliminating aerosol humidifiers and vaporizers, and maintaining indoor relative humidity below 70%. Complete elimination of indoor allergens is probably impossible.

Drug Treatment

Oral corticosteroids are the only known drug type currently available for the treatment of HP. Although steroids are active in controlling the disease activity, there is no evidence that such treatment modifies long-term outcome (18). The dose required is also unknown. Small doses (20 mg/day of prednisone) are as effective as contact avoidance in the initial outcome of acute HP (12). Higher doses have been recommended in acute severe disease, but because no studies have looked at dose response, there are no clear dose recommendations. Empirically, it would seem reasonable to give a short-course, high-doses treatment (50 mg/day of prednisone) in acutely ill patients. The steroids could be stopped as soon as the patient has recovered to a stable clinical condition (usually within a few days). When contact can be avoided, there is no justification for prolonged steroid uses. In the case of HP, when the contact cannot be avoided (e.g., dairy farmer) longer courses of low doses of prednisone (20 mg/day) will control the disease activity and is therefore justifiable. Such treatment can be prolonged until the contact can be ceased (e.g., early spring).

In these cases, care should then be taken to add required treatment for potential side effects of the long-term use of prednisone.

Inhaled steroids and β-agonists may be helpful in patients with HP manifested by symptoms of chest tightness and cough with airflow limitation on pulmonary function testing (131). No data exist from controlled clinical trials on the efficacy of inhaled steroids in the treatment of HP.

ORGANIC DUST TOXIC SYNDROME

Definition and Clinical Presentation

The term "organic dust toxic syndrome" (ODTS) was coined in 1985 at the Skokloster, Sweden workshop on the Health Effects of Organic Dust in the farm environment (132). Before that date, the disease was variously known as mycotoxicosis, atypical farmer's lung, silo unloader's syndrome, and inhalation fever (mill fever, humidifier fever, or grain fever) (133,134). Although first described in relation to organic dust exposure on the farm, ODTS can occur wherever abundant organic particles are inhaled. Cases have been reported from exposure to a print shop, wood chip compost, and recycle processing (135–137). Manifestations of ODTS include fever, myalgia, chest tightness, cough, headache, and dyspnea that arise three to eight hours after exposure (134).

Etiology and Mechanisms

ODTS is produced by inhalation of organic dusts or aerosols containing large quantities of microorganisms. What substance or substances are responsible for clinical manifestations is controversial. Immunological mechanisms play no role in the pathogenesis of this condition. Endotoxins and mycotoxins seem to be involved; the inhalation of endotoxin itself is able to induce a response similar to ODTS (138,139). Cases of ODTS have been reported, however, where endotoxin levels in the inhaled air were too low to account for the syndrome, suggesting a combination of factors in pathogenesis (140).

Inhaled "toxins" probably initiate a cascade of mediator release. Cytokines can recruit inflammatory cells to the lung and airways and contribute to systemic manifestations. Inhaled endotoxin (lipopolysaccharide) and exposure to swine confinement buildings induce the release of IL-1, IL-6, and TNFα from lung cells (141,142). Acute exposure to swine confinement buildings, however, induces a transient increase in bronchial responsiveness to inhaled methacholine that is not seen in typical ODTS (134,143,144).

The hypothesis that ODTS is toxic is supported by (*i*) a delay between exposure and the occurrence of symptoms that is too short for infectious process, (*ii*) lack of necessity for prior exposure/sensitization, (*iii*) absence of serum antibodies (precipitins) to the suspected etiological agent or source, (*iv*) incrimination of massive quantity of airborne materials in most cases, (*v*) susceptibility to ODTS by all similarly exposed individuals, and (*vi*) spontaneous recovery within 24 hours or so after withdrawal from exposure (145).

Clinical Evaluation

Except for fever during the acute illness, objective evaluation in most patients with ODTS will include normal physical findings, chest radiograms, and lung function (134). Although some degree of bronchospasm has been described, no persistent increase in airway responsiveness to methacholine is seen (146,147). Peripheral blood neutrophilia is often present (134). Arterial blood gases are unremarkable, although a mild respiratory alkalosis due to hyperventilation may sometimes be found. Bronchoscopy in the acute stage reveals diffusely inflamed bronchial mucosa, and BAL contains abundant neutrophils (146,148). BAL done after resolution of the symptoms retrieves increased numbers of lymphocytes (146).

Treatment and Outcome

The treatment of ODTS is supportive. Analgesics can be given for chest pain and myalgia; antipyretics can be used if needed; cough suppressants may be required if coughing is severe. Antibiotics are not indicated, nor are inhaled or systemic corticosteroids helpful in shortening the duration of symptoms. The best treatment is prevention by educating individuals at risk to avoid unprotected breathing in poorly ventilated, potentially contaminated environments. The usual outcome is spontaneous resolution without sequelae (147). The syndrome will recur with repeated exposure.

Differential Diagnosis

ODTS may be difficult to differentiate from acute HP or an infectious process (Table 1). History of exposure, appropriate constellation of symptoms, and paucity of objective findings will help establish the diagnosis of ODTS. The relationship, if any, between repeated bouts of ODTS and the development of HP remains unclear (149).

Epidemiology

The incidence of ODTS is difficult to establish, as its prevalence in the farming population varies considerably from one country to another and from one type of farming to another (148,149). This syndrome is, however, much more frequent than farmer's lung in a population at risk. A study of Swedish farmers found that the incidence of febrile reactions, the majority of which were considered to be ODTS, was 100 per 10,000 farmers per year, in contrast to a farmer's lung incidence of 2 to 3 per 10,000 farmers per year (54).

OVERALL SUMMARY

HP and ODTS are lung diseases typically associated with farming; although this may still be true for ODTS, HP is now much more frequent in environments other than farming where the prevalence is steadily decreasing as farming practices modernize. The most important challenges in the diagnosis of HP are its variable clinical presentations and the large number of environments contaminated by organic dust that can potentially cause HP. A key in diagnosing HP is to think about it in all patients presenting with recurrent febrile episodes and/or interstitial lung involvement. The pathophysiology of ODTS seems mostly a toxic response to an overwhelming exposure to microbial toxins, while that of HP is only partially understood. We know that HP is a delayed-type immune response to inhaled antigens to which the individual has previously been sensitized. The immune response implicates an enhanced antigen presentation by alveolar macrophages and possibly dendritic cells and a Th1 type of lymphocytic activation.

DIRECTIONS FOR FUTURE RESEARCH

- Meaningful future research will require multicenter international collaborations to have enough cases to answer clinical and immunopathological questions.
- Use of modern assays of cell function such as proteomics and gene array techniques may allow insight into mechanisms of HP.
- Animal models of HP are available and have been very useful in helping us understand some of the immunopathology of the disease.
- A clear definition of HP is required to establish precise epidemiological data. Additional diagnostic criteria will have to be developed for difficult cases, and standardized research facilities using specific antigenic provocation may be needed to advance our knowledge on HP.

REFERENCES

1. Pepys J. Hypersensitivity diseases of the lungs due to fungi and organic dusts. Monogr Allergy 1969; 4:1–147.
2. Rask-Anderson A. Pulmonary reactions to inhalation of mould dust in farmers with special reference to fever and allergic alveolitis. Acta Univ Ups 1988:8–20.
3. Ramazzini B. Latin text of 1713 revised, with translation and notes by WC Wright. In: Wright W, ed. The Classics of Medicine Series. Chicago: University of Chicago Press, 1983:243–248.
4. Campbell J. Acute symptoms following work with hay. Br Med J 1969; 2:1143–1144.
5. Sansores R, Salas J, Chapela R, Barquin N, Selman M. Clubbing in hypersensitivity pneumonitis. Its prevalence and possible prognostic role. Arch Int Med 1990; 150(9):1849–1851.
6. Hayakawa H, Shirai M, Sato A, et al. Clinicopathological features of chronic hypersensitivity pneumonitis. Respirology 2002; 7(4):359–364.
7. Richerson HB, Bernstein IL, Fink JN, et al. Guidelines for the clinical evaluation of hypersensitivity pneumonitis. Report of the Subcommittee on Hypersensitivity Pneumonitis. J Allergy Clin Immunol 1989; 84(5 Pt 2):839–844.
8. Terho E. Diagnostic criteria for farmer's lung disease. Am J Ind Med 1986; 10:329.
9. Lacasse Y, Selman M, Costabel U, et al. Clinical diagnosis of hypersensitivity pneumonitis. Am J Respir Crit Care Med 2003; 168(8):952–958.
10. Dinda P, Chatterjee SS, Riding WD. Pulmonary function studies in bird breeder's lung. Thorax 1969; 24(3):374–378.
11. Sansores R, Perez-Padilla R, Pare PD, Selman M. Exponential analysis of the lung pressure-volume curve in patients with chronic pigeon-breeder's lung. Chest 1992; 101(5):1352–1356.
12. Cormier Y. Treatment of hypersensitivity pneumonitis (HP): comparison between contact avoidance and corticosteroids. Can Respir J 1994; 1:223–228.
13. Perez-Padilla R, Salas J, Chapela R, et al. Mortality in Mexican patients with chronic pigeon breeder's lung compared with those with usual interstitial pneumonia. Am Rev Respir Dis 1993; 148(1):49–53.

14. Lalancette M, Carrier G, Laviolette M, et al. Farmer's lung. Long-term outcome and lack of predictive value of bronchoalveolar lavage fibrosing factors. Am Rev Respir Dis 1993; 148(1):216–221.

15. Warren C, Tse K, Cherniack R. Mechanical properties of the lung in extrinsic allergic alveolitis. Thorax 1978; 33:315–321.

16. Freedman PM, Ault B. Bronchial hyperreactivity to methacholine in farmers' lung disease. J Allergy Clin Immunol 1981; 67(1):59–63.

17. Monkare S. Clinical aspects of farmer's lung: airway reactivity, treatment and prognosis. Eur J Respir Dis Suppl 1984; 137:1–68.

18. Monkare S, Haahtela T. Farmer's lung—a five-year follow-up of eighty-six patients. Clin Allergy 1987; 17(2):143–151.

19. Kokkarinen JI, Tukiainen HO, Terho EO. Asthma in patients with farmer's lung during a five-year follow-up. Scand J Work Environ Health 1997; 23(2):149–151.

20. Hansell DM, Moskovic E. High-resolution computed tomography in extrinsic allergic alveolitis. Clin Radiol 1991; 43(1):8–12.

21. Akira M, Kita N, Higashihara T, Sakatani M, Kozuka T. Summer-type hypersensitivity pneumonitis: comparison of high-resolution CT and plain radiographic findings. Am J Roentgenol 1992; 158:1223–1228.

22. Buschman DL, Gamsu G, Waldron JA Jr, Klein JS, King TE Jr. Chronic hypersensitivity pneumonitis: use of CT in diagnosis. AJR Am J Roentgenol 1992; 159(5):957–960.

23. Hansell DM, Wells AU, Padley SP, Muller NL. Hypersensitivity pneumonitis: correlation of individual CT patterns with functional abnormalities. Radiology 1996; 199(1):123–128.

24. Remy-Jardin M, Remy J, Wallaert B, Muller NL. Subacute and chronic bird breeder hypersensitivity pneumonitis: sequential evaluation with CT and correlation with lung function tests and bronchoalveolar lavage. Radiology 1993; 189(1):111–118.

25. Cormier Y, Brown M, Worthy S, Racine G, Muller NL. High-resolution computed tomographic characteristics in acute farmer's lung and in its follow-up. Eur Respir J 2000; 16(1):56–60.

26. Dalphin JC, Toson B, Monnet E, et al. Farmer's lung precipitins in Doubs (a department of France): prevalence and diagnostic value. Allergy 1994; 49(9):744–750.

27. Ouchterlony O. Antigen-antibody reactions in gels. Acta Pathol Microbiol Scand 1953; 32:231.

28. Banham SW, McSharry C, Lynch PP, Boyd G. Relationships between avian exposure, humoral immune response, and pigeon breeders' disease among Scottish pigeon fanciers. Thorax 1986; 41(4):274–278.

29. Carrillo T, Rodriguez de Castro F, Cuevas M, Diaz F, Cabrera P. Effect of cigarette smoking on the humoral immune response in pigeon fanciers. Allergy 1991; 46(4):241–244.

30. Fink JN, Schlueter DP, Sosman AJ, et al. Clinical survey of pigeon breeders. Chest 1972; 62(3):277–281.

31. Elgerfors B, Belin L, Hanson LA. Pigeon breeder's lung. Clinical and immunological observations. Scand J Respir Dis 1971; 52(3):167–176.

32. Cormier Y, Belanger J. The fluctuant nature of precipitating antibodies in dairy farmers. Thorax 1989; 44(6):469–473.

33. Krasnick J, Meuwissen HJ, Nakao MA, Yeldandi A, Patterson R. Hypersensitivity pneumonitis: problems in diagnosis. J Allergy Clin Immunol 1996; 97(4):1027–1030.

34. Barbee RA, Callies Q, Dickie HA, Rankin J. The long-term prognosis in farmer's lung. Am Rev Respir Dis 1968; 97(2):223–231.

35. Williams J. Inhalation and skin tests with extracts of hay and fungi in patients with farmer's lung. Thorax 1963; 18:182–196.

36. Ramírez A, Pérez-Padilla R, Selman M, Sansores R. Inhalation challenge test with avian antigens for the differential diagnosis of pigeon breeder's disease (PBD). Am J Respir Crit Care Med 1996; 153:A546.

37. Drent M, Mulder PG, Wagenaar SS, Hoogsteden HC, van Velzen-Blad H, van den Bosch JM. Differences in BAL fluid variables in interstitial lung diseases evaluated by discriminant analysis. Eur Respir J 1993; 6(6):803–810.

38. Godard P, Clot J, Jonquet O, Bousquet J, Michel FB. Lymphocyte subpopulations in bronchoalveolar lavages of patients with sarcoidosis and hypersensitivity pneumonitis. Chest 1981; 80(4):447–452.

39. Grubek-Jaworska H, Hoser G, Droszcz P, Chazan R. CD4/CD8 lymphocytes in BALF during the efferent phase of lung delayed-type hypersensitivity reaction induced by single antigen inhalation. Med Sci Monit 2001; 7(5):878–883.

40. Laviolette M, Cormier Y, Loiseau A, Soler P, Leblanc P, Hance AJ. Bronchoalveolar mast cells in normal farmers and subjects with farmer's lung. Diagnostic, prognostic, and physiologic significance. Am Rev Respir Dis 1991; 144(4):855–860.

41. Patterson R, Wang JL, Fink JN, Calvanico NJ, Roberts M. IgA and IgG antibody activities of serum and bronchoalveolar fluid from symptomatic and asymptomatic pigeon breeders. Am Rev Respir Dis 1979; 120(5):1113–1118.

42. Calvanico NJ, Ambegaonkar SP, Schlueter DP, Fink JN. Immunoglobulin levels in bronchoalveolar lavage fluid from pigeon breeders. J Lab Clin Med 1980; 96(1):129–140.

43. Cormier Y, Belanger J, Laviolette M. Prognostic significance of bronchoalveolar lymphocytosis in farmer's lung. Am Rev Respir Dis 1987; 135(3):692–695.

44. Cormier Y, Belanger J, Beaudoin J, Laviolette M, Beaudoin R, Hebert J. Abnormal bronchoalveolar lavage in asymptomatic dairy farmers. Study of lymphocytes. Am Rev Respir Dis 1984; 130(6):1046–1049.

45. Cormier Y, Belanger J, Laviolette M. Persistent bronchoalveolar lymphocytosis in asymptomatic farmers. Am Rev Respir Dis 1986; 133(5):843–847.

46. Lacasse Y, Fraser RS, Fournier M, Cormier Y. Diagnostic accuracy of transbronchial biopsy in acute farmer's lung disease. Chest 1997; 112(6):1459–1465.

47. Reyes N, Wenzel F, Lawton B, Emanuel D. The pulmonary pathology of farmer's lung disease. Chest 1982; 81:142–146.

48. Coleman A, Colby TV. Histologic diagnosis of extrinsic allergic alveolitis. Am J Surg Pathol 1988; 12(7):514–518.

49. Planes C, Valeyre D, Loiseau A, Bernaudin JF, Soler P. Ultrastructural alterations of the air-blood barrier in sarcoidosis and hypersensitivity pneumonitis and their relation to lung histopathology. Am J Respir Crit Care Med 1994; 150(4):1067–1074.

50. Vourlekis JS, Schwarz MI, Cool CD, Tuder RM, King TE, Brown KK. Nonspecific interstitial pneumonitis as the sole histologic expression of hypersensitivity pneumonitis. Am J Med 2002; 112(6):490–493.

51. Lopez M, Salvaggio JE. Epidemiology of hypersensitivity pneumonitis/allergic alveolitis. Monogr Allergy 1987; 21:70–86.

52. Fink JN. Epidemiologic aspects of hypersensitivity pneumonitis. Monogr Allergy 1987; 21:59–69.

53. Johnson C, Bernstein I, Gallegher J, Bonventre P, Brooks S. Familial hypersensitivity pneumonitis induced by Bacillus subtilis. Am Rev Respir Dis 1980; 122:339–348.

54. Malmberg P, Rask-Andersen A, Hoglund S, Kolmodin-Hedman B, Read Guernsey J. Incidence of organic dust toxic syndrome and allergic alveolitis in Swedish farmers. Int Arch Allergy Appl Immunol 1988; 87(1):47–54.

55. Marx JJ, Guernsey J, Emanuel DA, Merchant JA, Morgan DP, Kryda M. Cohort studies of immunologic lung disease among Wisconsin dairy farmers. Am J Ind Med 1990; 18(3):263–268.

56. McSharry C, Banham SW, Boyd G. Effect of cigarette smoking on the antibody response to inhaled antigens and the prevalence of extrinsic allergic alveolitis among pigeon breeders. Clin Allergy 1985; 15(5):487–494.

57. Christensen LT, Schmidt CD, Robbins L. Pigeon breeders' disease–a prevalence study and review. Clin Allergy 1975; 5(4):417–430.

58. Cormier Y, Belanger J, Durand P. Factors influencing the development of serum precipitins to farmer's lung antigen in Quebec dairy farmers. Thorax 1985; 40(2):138–142.

59. Terho EO, Husman K, Vohlonen I. Prevalence and incidence of chronic bronchitis and farmer's lung with respect to age, sex, atopy, and smoking. Eur J Respir Dis Suppl 1987; 152:19–28.

60. Kitt S, Lee CW, Fink JN, Calvanico NJ. Immunoglobulin G4 in pigeon breeder's disease. J Lab Clin Med 1986; 108(5):442–447.

61. Schuyler MR, Thigpen TP, Salvaggio JE. Local pulmonary immunity in pigeon breeder's disease. A case study. Ann Int Med 1978; 88(3):355–358.

62. Lee TH, Wraith DG, Bennett CO, Bentley AP. Budgerigar fancier's lung. The persistence of budgerigar precipitins and the recovery of lung function after cessation of avian exposure. Clin Allergy 1983; 13(3):197–202.

63. Schkade PA, Routes JM. Hypersensitivity pneumonitis in a patient with hypogammaglobulinemia. J Allergy Clin Immunol 1996; 98(3):710–712.

64. Morris AM, Nishimura S, Huang L. Subacute hypersensitivity pneumonitis in an HIV infected patient receiving antiretroviral therapy. Thorax 2000; 55(7):625–627.

65. Ando M, Konishi K, Yoneda R, Tamura M. Difference in the phenotypes of bronchoalveolar lavage lymphocytes in patients with summer-type hypersensitivity pneumonitis, farmer's lung, ventilation pneumonitis, and bird fancier's lung: report of a nationwide epidemiologic study in Japan. J Allergy Clin Immunol 1991; 87(5):1002–1009.

66. Trentin L, Zambello R, Facco M, et al. Selection of T lymphocytes bearing limited TCR-Vbeta regions in the lung of hypersensitivity pneumonitis and sarcoidosis. Am J Respir Crit Care Med 1997; 155(2):587–596.

67. Facco M, Trentin L, Nicolardi L, et al. T cells in the lung of patients with hypersensitivity pneumonitis accumulate in a clonal manner. J Leukoc Biol 2004; 75(5): 798–804.

68. Denis M. Proinflammatory cytokines in hypersensitivity pneumonitis. Am J Respir Crit Care Med 1995; 151(1):164–169.

69. Denis M, Bedard M, Laviolette M, Cormier Y. A study of monokine release and natural killer activity in the bronchoalveolar lavage of subjects with farmer's lung. Am Rev Respir Dis 1993; 147(4):934–939.

70. Cormier Y, Israel-Assayag E, Desmeules M, Lesur O. Effect of contact avoidance or treatment with oral prednisolone on bronchoalveolar lavage surfactant protein A levels in subjects with farmer's lung. Thorax 1996; 51(12):1210–1215.

71. Tremblay GM, Sallenave JM, Israel-Assayag E, Cormier Y, Gauldie J. Elafin/elastase-specific inhibitor in bronchoalveolar lavage of normal subjects and farmer's lung. Am J Respir Crit Care Med 1996; 154(4 Pt 1):1092–1098.

72. Cormier Y, Letourneau L, Racine G. Significance of precipitins and asymptomatic lymphocytic alveolitis: a 20-yr follow-up. Eur Respir J 2004; 23(4):523–525.

73. Oshima M, Maeda A, Ishioka S, Hiyama K, Yamakido M. Expression of C-C chemokines in bronchoalveolar lavage cells from patients with granulomatous lung diseases. Lung 1999; 177(4):229–240.

74. Pardo A, Smith KM, Abrams J, et al. CCL18/DC-CK-1/PARC up-regulation in hypersensitivity pneumonitis. J Leukoc Biol 2001; 70(4):610–616.

75. Laflamme C, Israel-Assayag E, Cormier Y. Apoptosis of bronchoalveolar lavage lymphocytes in hypersensitivity pneumonitis. Eur Respir J 2003; 21(2):225–231.

76. Drent M, Grutters JC, Mulder PG, van Velzen-Blad H, Wouters EF, van den Bosch JM. Is the different T helper cell activity in sarcoidosis and extrinsic allergic alveolitis also reflected by the cellular bronchoalveolar lavage fluid profile? Sarcoidosis Vasc Diffuse Lung Dis 1997; 14:31–38.

77. Semenzato G, Trentin L, Zambello R, Agostini C, Cipriani A, Marcer G. Different types of cytotoxic lymphocytes recovered from the lungs of patients with hypersensitivity pneumonitis. Am Rev Respir Dis 1988; 137(1):70–74.

78. Mendoza F, Melendro EI, Baltazares M, et al. Cellular immune response to fractionated avian antigens by peripheral blood mononuclear cells from patients with pigeon breeder's disease. J Lab Clin Med 1996; 127(1):23–28.
79. Allen JT, Spiteri MA. Pigeon breeder's disease. J Lab Clin Med 1996; 127:10–12.
80. Richerson HB. Hypersensitivity pneumonitis–pathology and pathogenesis. Clin Rev Allergy 1983; 1(4):469–486.
81. Denis M, Ghadirian E. Transforming growth factor-beta is generated in the course of hypersensitivity pneumonitis: contribution to collagen synthesis. Am J Respir Cell Mol Biol 1992; 7(2):156–160.
82. Denis M, Ghadirian E. Murine hypersensitivity pneumonitis: production and importance of colony-stimulating factors in the course of a lung inflammatory reaction. Am J Respir Cell Mol Biol 1992; 7(4):441–446.
83. Kopp WC, Dierks SE, Butler JE, Upadrashta BS, Richerson HB. Cyclosporine immunomodulation in a rabbit model of chronic hypersensitivity pneumonitis. Am Rev Respir Dis 1985; 132(5):1027–1033.
84. Takizawa H, Suko M, Kobayashi N, et al. Experimental hypersensitivity pneumonitis in the mouse: histologic and immunologic features and their modulation with cyclosporin A. J Allergy Clin Immunol 1988; 81(2):391–400.
85. Denis M, Cormier Y, Laviolette M. Murine hypersensitivity pneumonitis: a study of cellular infiltrates and cytokine production and its modulation by cyclosporin A. Am J Respir Cell Mol Biol 1992; 6(1):68–74.
86. Takizawa H, Ohta K, Horiuchi T, et al. Hypersensitivity pneumonitis in athymic nude mice. Additional evidence of T cell dependency. Am Rev Respir Dis 1992; 146(2):479–484.
87. Gudmundsson G, Hunninghake GW. Interferon-gamma is necessary for the expression of hypersensitivity pneumonitis. J Clin Invest 1997; 99(10):2386–2390.
88. Nance S, Cross R, Fitzpatrick E. Chemokine production during hypersensitivity pneumonitis. Eur J Immunol 2004; 34(3):677–685.
89. Gudmundsson G, Monick MM, Hunninghake GW. IL-12 modulates expression of hypersensitivity pneumonitis. J Immunol 1998; 161(2):991–999.
90. Schuyler M, Gott K, Cherne A. Is IL12 necessary in experimental hypersensitivity pneumonitis? Int J Exp Pathol 2002; 83(2):87–98.
91. Pan LH, Yamauchi K, Sawai T, et al. Inhibition of binding of E- and P-selectin to sialyl-Lewis X molecule suppresses the inflammatory response in hypersensitivity pneumonitis in mice. Am J Respir Crit Care Med 2000; 161(5):1689–1697.
92. Schuyler M, Gott K, Haley P. Experimental murine hypersensitivity pneumonitis. Cell Immunol 1991; 136(2):303–317.
93. Butler NS, Monick MM, Yarovinsky TO, Powers LS, Hunninghake GW. Altered IL-4 mRNA stability correlates with Th1 and Th2 bias and susceptibility to hypersensitivity pneumonitis in two inbred strains of mice. J Immunol 2002; 169(7):3700–3709.
94. Schuyler M, Gott K, Cherne A. Mediators of hypersensitivity pneumonitis. J Lab Clin Med 2000; 136(1):29–38.
95. Gudmundsson G, Monick MM, Hunninghake GW. Viral infection modulates expression of hypersensitivity pneumonitis. J Immunol 1999; 162(12):7397–7401.
96. Schuyler M, Gott K, Cherne A. Experimental hypersensitivity pneumonitis: role of MCP-1. J Lab Clin Med 2003; 142(3):187–195.
97. Schuyler M, Gott K, French V. The role of MIP-1a in experimental hypersensitivity pneumonitis. Lung 2004; 182:135–149.
98. Gudmundsson G, Bosch A, Davídson BL, Berg DJ, Hunninghake GW. Interleukin-10 modulates the severity of hypersensitivity pneumonitis in mice. Am J Respir Cell Mol Biol 1998; 19(5):812–818.
99. Cormier Y, Israel-Assayag E, Fournier M, Tremblay GM. Modulation of experimental hypersensitivity pneumonitis by Sendai virus. J Lab Clin Med 1993; 121(5):683–688.

100. Blanchet MR, Israel-Assayag E, Cormier Y. Inhibitory effect of nicotine on experimental hypersensitivity pneumonitis in vivo and in vitro. Am J Respir Crit Care Med 2004; 169(8):903–909.

101. Israel-Assayag E, Fournier M, Cormier Y. Blockade of T cell costimulation by CTLA4-Ig inhibits lung inflammation in murine hypersensitivity pneumonitis. J Immunol 1999; 163(12):6794–6799.

102. Cormier Y, Tremblay GM, Fournier M, Israel-Assayag E. Long-term viral enhancement of lung response to Saccharopolyspora rectivirgula. Am J Respir Crit Care Med 1994; 149(2 Pt 1):490–494.

103. Schuyler M, Gott K, Shopp G, Crooks L. CD3+ and CD4+ cells adoptively transfer experimental hypersensitivity pneumonitis. Am Rev Respir Dis 1992; 146(6):1582–1588.

104. Schuyler M, Gott K, French V. The role of IL-10 in experimental hypersensitivity pneumonitis. Am J Respir Crit Care Med 2004; 169:A83.

105. Schuyler M, Cook C, Listrom M, Fengolio-Preiser C. Blast cells transfer experimental hypersensitivity pneumonitis in guinea pigs. Am Rev Respir Dis 1988; 137(6):1449–1455.

106. Richerson HB, Coon JD, Lubaroff D. Adoptive transfer of experimental hypersensitivity pneumonitis in the LEW rat. Am J Respir Crit Care Med 1995; 151(4):1205–1210.

107. Schuyler M, Gott K, Cherne A, Edwards B. Th1 CD4+ cells adoptively transfer experimental hypersensitivity pneumonitis. Cell Immunol 1997; 177(2):169–175.

108. Schuyler M, Gott K, Edwards B, Nikula KJ. Experimental hypersensitivity pneumonitis. Effect of CD4 cell depletion. Am J Respir Crit Care Med 1994; 149(5):1286–1294.

109. Schuyler M, Gott K, Edwards B, Nikula KJ. Experimental hypersensitivity pneumonitis: effect of Thy1.2+ and CD8+ cell depletion. Am J Respir Crit Care Med 1995; 151(6):1834–1842.

110. Schuyler M, Gott K, Fei R, Edwards B. Experimental hypersensitivity pneumonitis: location of transferring cells. Lung 1998; 176(3):213–225.

111. Schuyler MR, Gott K, Edwards B. Adoptive transfer of experimental hypersensitivity pneumonitis: CD4+ cells are memory and naive cells. J Lab Clin Med 1994; 123(3):378–386.

112. Schuyler M, Gott K, Edwards B. Th1 cells that adoptively transfer experimental hypersensitivity pneumonitis are activated memory cells. Lung 1999; 177(6):377–389.

113. Braun SR, doPico GA, Tsiatis A, Horvath E, Dickie HA, Rankin J. Farmer's lung disease: long-term clinical and physiologic outcome. Am Rev Respir Dis 1979; 119(2):185–191.

114. Kokkarinen J, Tukiainen H, Terho EO. Mortality due to farmer's lung in Finland. Chest 1994; 106(2):509–512.

115. Barrowcliff DF, Arblaster PG. Farmer's lung: a study of an early acute fatal case. Thorax 1968; 23(5):490–500.

116. Chasse M, Blanchette G, Malo J, Malo JL. Farmer's lung presenting as respiratory failure and homogeneous consolidation. Chest 1986; 90(5):783–784.

117. Greenberger PA, Pien LC, Patterson R, Robinson P, Roberts M. End-stage lung and ultimately fatal disease in a bird fancier. Am J Med 1989; 86(1):119–122.

118. Grammer LC, Roberts M, Lerner C, Patterson R. Clinical and serologic follow-up of four children and five adults with bird-fancier's lung. J Allergy Clin Immunol 1990; 85(3):655–660.

119. Schmidt CD, Jensen RL, Christensen LT, Crapo RO, Davis JJ. Longitudinal pulmonary function changes in pigeon breeders. Chest 1988; 93(2):359–363.

120. Leblanc P, Belanger J, Laviolette M, Cormier Y. Relationship among antigen contact, alveolitis, and clinical status in farmer's lung disease. Arch Intern Med 1986; 146(1):153–157.

121. Allen DH, Williams GV, Woolcock AJ. Bird breeder's hypersensitivity pneumonitis: progress studies of lung function after cessation of exposure to the provoking antigen. Am Rev Respir Dis 1976; 114(3):555–566.

122. de Gracia J, Morell F, Bofill JM, Curull V, Orriols R. Time of exposure as a prognostic factor in avian hypersensitivity pneumonitis. Respir Med 1989; 83(2):139–143.

123. Cormier Y, Belanger J. Long-term physiologic outcome after acute farmer's lung. Chest 1985; 87(6):796–800.

124. Zejda JE, McDuffie HH, Dosman JA. Epidemiology of health and safety risks in agriculture and related industries. Practical applications for rural physicians. West J Med 1993; 158(1):56–63.

125. Duchaine C, Meriaux A, Brochu G, Cormier Y. Airborne microflora in Quebec dairy farms: lack of effect of bacterial hay preservatives. Am Ind Hyg Assoc J 1999; 60(1):89–95.

126. Bouchard S, Morin F, Bedard G, Gauthier J, Paradis J, Cormier Y. Farmer's lung and variables related to the decision to quit farming. Am J Respir Crit Care Med 1995; 152(3):997–1002.

127. Craig TJ, Hershey J, Engler RJ, Davis W, Carpenter GB, Salata K. Bird antigen persistence in the home environment after removal of the bird. Ann Allergy 1992; 69(6):510–512.

128. Nuutinen J, Terho EO, Husman K, Kotimaa M, Harkonen R, Nousiainen H. Protective value of powered dust respirator helmet for farmers with farmer's lung. Eur J Respir Dis Suppl 1987; 152:212–220.

129. Hendrick D, Marshall R, Faux J, Krall J. Protective value of dust respirators in extrinsic allergic alveolitis: clinical assessment using inhalation provocation tests. Thorax 1981; 36:917–921.

130. Macher JM. Inquiries received by the California Indoor Air Quality Program on biological contaminants in buildings. Experientia Suppl 1987; 51:275–278.

131. Carlsen KH, Leegaard J, Lund OD, Skjaervik H. Allergic alveolitis in a 12-year-old boy: treatment with budesonide nebulizing solution. Pediatr Pulmonol 1992; 12(4): 257–259.

132. Rylander R. Lung diseases caused by organic dusts in the farm environment. Am J Ind Med 1986; 10(3):221–227.

133. Emanuel DA, Wenzel FJ, Lawton BR. Pulmonary mycotoxicosis. Chest 1975; 67(3):293–297.

134. May JJ, Stallones L, Darrow D, Pratt DS. Organic dust toxicity (pulmonary mycotoxicosis) associated with silo unloading. Thorax 1986; 41(12):919–923.

135. Mamolen M, Lewis DM, Blanchet MA, Satink FJ, Vogt RL. Investigation of an outbreak of "humidifier fever" in a print shop. Am J Ind Med 1993; 23(3):483–490.

136. Weber S, Kullman G, Petsonk E, et al. Organic dust exposures from compost handling: case presentation and respiratory exposure assessment. Am J Ind Med 1993; 24(4): 365–374.

137. Sigsgaard T, Abel A, Donbaek L, Malmros P. Lung function changes among recycling workers exposed to organic dust. Am J Ind Med 1994; 25(1):69–72.

138. Fogelmark B, Sjostrand M, Rylander R. Pulmonary inflammation induced by repeated inhalations of beta(1,3)-D-glucan and endotoxin. Int J Exp Pathol 1994; 75(2):85–90.

139. Rylander R, Bake B, Fischer JJ, Helander IM. Pulmonary function and symptoms after inhalation of endotoxin. Am Rev Respir Dis 1989; 140(4):981–986.

140. Malmberg P, Rask-Andersen A, Lundholm M, Palmgren U. Can spores from molds and actinomycetes cause an organic dust toxic syndrome reaction? Am J Ind Med 1990; 17(1):109–110.

141. Lewis D, Olenchock S. Cellular immune reactions to grain dust and extracts of grain dusts. In: Dosman JA, Cockcroft D, eds. Principles of Health and Safety in Agriculture. Boca Raton, FL: CRC Press, 1989:72–75.

142. Wang Z, Malmberg P, Larsson P, Larsson BM, Larsson K. Time course of interleukin-6 and tumor necrosis factor-alpha increase in serum following inhalation of swine dust. Am J Respir Crit Care Med 1996; 153(1):147–152.

143. Cormier Y, Duchaine C, Israel-Assayag E, Bedard G, Laviolette M, Dosman J. Effects of repeated swine building exposures on normal naive subjects. Eur Respir J 1997; 10(7):1516–1522.

144. Larsson KA, Eklund AG, Hansson LO, Isaksson BM, Malmberg PO. Swine dust causes intense airways inflammation in healthy subjects. Am J Respir Crit Care Med 1994; 150(4):973–977.

145. Brinton WT, Vastbinder EE, Greene JW, Marx JJ Jr, Hutcheson RH, Schaffner W. An outbreak of organic dust toxic syndrome in a college fraternity. JAMA 1987; 258(9): 1210–1212.

146. Lecours R, Laviolette M, Cormier Y. Bronchoalveolar lavage in pulmonary mycotoxicosis (organic dust toxic syndrome). Thorax 1986; 41(12):924–926.

147. May JJ, Marvel LH, Pratt DS, Coppolo DP. Organic dust toxic syndrome: a follow-up study. Am J Ind Med 1990; 17(1):111–113.

148. Emanuel D, Marx J, Ault B, Roberts R, Kryda M. Organic dust toxic syndrome (pulmonary mycotoxicosis)– a review of the experience in central Wisconsin. In: Dosman JA, Cockcroft D, eds. Principles of Health and Safety in Agriculture. Boca Raton, FL: CRC Press, 1989:72–75.

149. Malmberg P, Rask-Andersen A, Palmgren U, Hoglund S, Kolmodin-Hedman B, Stalenheim G. Exposure to microorganisms, febrile and airway-obstructive symptoms, immune status and lung function of Swedish farmers. Scand J Work Environ Health 1985; 11(4):287–293.

30
Building-Related Illnesses

Dick Menzies
Respiratory Epidemiology Unit, Department of Medicine and Epidemiology and Biostatistics, Montreal Chest Institute, McGill University, Montreal, Quebec, Canada

Kathleen Kreiss
Division of Respiratory Disease Studies, NIOSH Field Studies Branch, NIOSH, Morgantown, West Virginia, U.S.A.

INTRODUCTION

Over the past 30 years, a new man-made ecosystem has developed—the controlled environment within the sealed exterior shells of modern office buildings. Air pollution may occur in this indoor environment caused by the occupants, their work activities, equipment, plants, furnishings, building materials, and even the ventilation systems themselves. In the vast majority of office buildings in North America, the major mechanism to remove these pollutants and to provide a healthy, comfortable indoor environment is the heating, ventilation, and air-conditioning (HVAC) system. These highly automated systems are often run by only one or two operators. These operators have very little training in health and, in large buildings, have little contact with building occupants. When the sealed exterior shells of modern office buildings are damaged, water incursion through the building envelope can give rise to damp building materials and furnishings, which often support microbial growth.

It is therefore not surprising that health problems related to this ecosystem—termed "building-related illnesses" (BRI)—have emerged in the past three decades. Although the health effects are usually mild, these illnesses can be severe. And even if mild, the public health impact is major, because more than half of the adult workforce in North America and Western Europe work in this environment (1), and most adults in these countries spend more than 90% of their lives within an indoor environment. It has been estimated that 20% to 30% of the occupants of the one million nonindustrial buildings in the United States, or as many as 30 million workers, have work-related symptoms related to this environment (2), and this may result in economic losses of $22 billion annually in the United States (3,4). As a result, this problem has attracted the attention of research scientists from a variety of domains including architecture, engineering, industrial hygiene, biochemistry, microbiology, and epidemiology. It has also attracted the attention of the media, the public, and increasingly, the legislators, all of whom are demanding a solution to this problem. Finally, given that this work environment is not directly controlled by workers, but

737

usually by the employer or building owner, the work environment should be subject to government regulation. Although such regulation should consider the valid economic interests of building owners, the primary objective of such regulations must be the protection of workers from recognized hazards.

This chapter reviews studies describing the health effects of the nonindustrial, nonresidential indoor environment. The evidence cited—of outbreaks, population-based studies, and experimental manipulations of the nonindustrial building environment—have been used to synthesize a conceptual model of this problem. These evidences have also been used to develop recommendations for prevention or remediation, and to aid health professionals in evaluating workers with health problems potentially related to this work environment.

DEFINITIONS

Ventilation rate: This term means the rate of delivery of outdoor air to the indoor environment. This is usually expressed as a volume of air per unit time per occupant, such as cubic feet per minute per person (CFMpp) or liters per second per person (LSP). This may also be expressed in air changes per hour (ACH), meaning the proportion of indoor air replaced by outdoor air every hour.

Work-related symptom: Symptom that occurs in a work-related pattern is called a work-related symptom. In the simplest form, these are symptoms that occur after arrival at work and resolve upon leaving work. For some immunologically mediated illnesses, symptoms may occur in the evening after work, become progressively worse over the work week, and improve on days off work.

BRI: Illnesses that can be causally linked to indoor environmental exposure within a building are termed BRI (5). The term is restricted here to illnesses that arise in nonindustrial environments such as office buildings, schools, hospitals, or day-care centers.

Specific BRI: Illnesses characterized by reasonably homogeneous clinical pictures in which a causative agent or physiologic mechanism can be identified are termed specific BRI. The most severely affected individuals will have abnormalities on physical, laboratory, or radiographic examinations.

Nonspecific BRI: Here there is occurrence of symptoms—mucous membrane complaints, headache, and difficulty concentrating—which are tightly linked with being inside of a nonindustrial building (5), yet no objective health effects can be found. This term might be taken to imply that the absence of objective health effects makes the symptoms less important. However, in many instances, the absence of objective health effects is not so much because they are truly absent but rather because they are not measured. The cause for the symptoms, formerly known as "sick building syndrome" (SBS), is not known (6), and at present there is no known measurement which predicts the likelihood of either the presence or absence of these symptoms among building occupants. The concept of "sick" or "healthy buildings" arose from early investigations, conducted by industrial hygienists, engineers, and architects, with expertise in the evaluation of buildings rather than in the evaluation of human occupants. These early investigators believed that there were two distinct populations of buildings: "sick" buildings in which many workers had building-related symptoms and "healthy" buildings, in which few workers had symptoms—presumed to be non-work related. This concept has been proved incorrect. Epidemiological surveys in office buildings selected without regard to occupant health status have demonstrated that prevalence of work-related symptoms range in a continuous fashion from low (but not zero) to high (7–16). For example, in a study of 47 buildings in Britain, the average number of symptoms reported by the workers in each building ranged in a continuous fashion from 1.5 in the least symptomatic building population, to 5 in highly symptomatic populations. No single cutoff point or criterion could distinguish problem from non-problem buildings. Although generally non-problem buildings had a lower average number of symptoms reported, there was considerable overlap with problem buildings (8). Regardless of terminology, buildings in which building-related symptoms occur require investigation and remediation, and affected workers should be "treated" by resolving the deficiencies in the building environment.

SPECIFIC BRI

Specific BRI are diverse and include toxic illness from carbon monoxide exposures (17–19); dermatitis due to fibrous glass released from building materials and duct work lining (20,21); and rare reactions to specific materials used in buildings, such as photocopier fumes (22) and carbonless copy paper (23–25). However, from a public health and investigative viewpoint, the building-related diseases of interest are asthma, hypersensitivity pneumonitis, humidifier fever, allergic rhinitis/sinusitis, noncommunicable infections, and communicable infections. This last set of illnesses has microbial causes, even if the specific organism is not always identified in an individual patient or outbreak (Table 1).

Microbial Causes

Microbes that affect human health within the indoor environment originate from two sources—humans and the environment. Microbes from human sources typically cause disease through infectious mechanisms. They include common viruses such as rhinovirus, influenza, adenovirus, and measles. Airborne transmission of viruses within the indoor environment has been well documented. Severe acute respiratory syndrome is caused by a new coronavirus that quickly achieved global recognition as it appears to be highly transmissible within the indoor environment and causes severe manifestations with a high case-fatality rate. Transmission of bacterial disease, such as pneumococcal pneumonia, has been demonstrated within indoor environments. *Mycobacterium tuberculosis*, a pathogen which can remain viable airborne for more than 24 hours within the indoor environment, has been transmitted in a wide range of indoor environments, including office buildings (31).

Noncommunicable infections from environmental sources also occur in buildings and are more readily identified as building related. Examples include *Legionella pneumonia* and fungal infections in immunocompromised persons in hospital settings. Microbes from environmental sources must have conditions conducive to their amplification and must have a means of dissemination in aerosol form. For example, *Legionella pneumophila* has been found in water-cooling towers and in humidification and water supply systems, and aerosols from these reservoirs can cause pneumonia with a case fatality of 10% to 15% (26,39). This organism is also associated with Pontiac fever, a milder flu-like illness (27,28), which may not be an infection.

Dissemination of environmental microbes can be caused by aerosols of non-viable microorganisms, their constituents, or their toxins, which can be inhaled by building occupants. Environmental bacteria, fungi, and protozoa can cause health effects through allergic, cellular immune, toxic, or irritant mechanisms.

Table 1 Major Specific Building-Related Illnesses

Disease	Study[a]	References	Building	Indoor source	Exposure
Infections					
Legionnaires' disease and Pontiac fever	Case reports: sporadic or epidemic	(26–28)	Large buildings (office, hospital, hotel)	Cooling tower, airconditioning, or humidifier	*Legionella pneumophila*
Flu illness and common cold	Cross-sectional Longitudinal	(29)	Office buildings	Human source	Respiratory virus
Tuberculosis	Index case followed by cross-sectional	(30) (31)	Military barracks Office buildings	Human source	*Mycobacterium tuberculosis*
Immunological					
Hypersensitivity pneumonitis and humidifier fever	Case reports	(32)	Office buildings	Humidifier	Multiple bacteria, fungus, actinomycetes
	Index cases followed by cross-sectional	(33–35)	Office buildings Factory	Air, conditioning, humidifier Ventilation unit Cardboard boxes	*Aspergillus, Penicillium* spp. or multiple organisms
Allergy					
Dermatitis, rhinitis, and asthma	Case reports		Office buildings	Surface dust and carpet, clothing	Dust mite, plant product, animal allergen, fungus
	Index cases followed by cross-sectional	(36,37)	Office building and factory	Humidifier; water incursion	Unknown
Rhinitis					
Contact urticaria, laryngeal edema	Case reports	(22–25)	Office buildings	Carbonless copy paper	Alkylphenol novolac resin
Irritant					
Dermatitis	Case reports	(20,38)	Office buildings	Ceiling boards	Fiber glass
Upper and lower respiratory irritation	Case report	(17)	Office buildings	Tobacco smoke, vehicle exhaust, any combustion process	Combustion pollutants: CO, NO_2

[a]Because of space restrictions, references were limited to certain case reports, studies of index cases followed by an epidemiological evaluation, or field studies when available.

Source: Adapted from Ref. 5.

Allergic manifestations are IgE mediated and typically occur soon after exposure to microbial products such as proteins or components of the cell wall. Symptoms range from itchy, watery eyes, nasal stuffiness, congestion, and discharge typical of allergic rhinitis, to chest tightness, wheezing, and difficulty breathing typical of asthma. Persons with a personal or family history of allergy or atopic illnesses are more likely to manifest allergic responses to airborne microbial contaminants.

The other major mechanism of immune reaction is a cell-mediated response to inhaled antigens. This lymphocyte response often manifests only hours after exposure, making the diagnosis of building-related hypersensitivity pneumonitis less obvious than with immediate allergic responses. Manifestations resemble pneumonia with dyspnea, chest tightness, hypoxia in severe cases, and systemic symptoms of fever, chills, and sweats. Hypersensitivity pneumonitis has also been described with several other occupational exposures involving bacterial and fungal aerosols, such as farmer's lung. Interestingly, nonsmokers are at particularly high risk for this type of immune response. Milder reactions involving systemic symptoms only have been termed "humidifier fever." Whether the pathogenic mechanism is the same as that for hypersensitivity pneumonitis is unknown, but these syndromes may coexist and result from similar immunological responses to fungi, bacteria, or protozoa contaminating humidifiers or ventilation systems (33–35). Hypersensitivity pneumonitis outbreaks have been associated with either microbially contaminated ventilation system components or with water-damaged building components.

In hypersensitivity pneumonitis outbreaks, when all exposed workers have been carefully examined, prevalence of illness is often high and a wide spectrum of manifestations has been described (33,35,40). For example, in a group of 14 workers exposed to levels of *Penicillium* of 5000 to 10,000 CFU/m^3, one nonsmoking worker developed hypersensitivity pneumonitis, another with history of atopy and cigarette smoking developed asthma, while six others developed nonspecific respiratory symptoms (35). In an industrial setting, 548 workers were exposed to airborne *Aspergillus* species, of whom 152 had positive serum precipitins (33). Among these 152 workers, 29 were asymptomatic, 8 had symptoms but did not meet the case definition, and 115 could be classified as cases of hypersensitivity pneumonitis. Less than 10% of these cases had any objective abnormalities; i.e., the vast majority were diagnosed on the basis of symptoms alone. In addition, these cases reported increased occurrence of nonspecific symptoms such as fatigue, headache, and mucosal irritation compared to exposed workers without precipitins. In an unusual study in which symptomatic workers without radiographic or restrictive pulmonary function abnormalities underwent transbronchial biopsy and bronchoalveolar lavage, most had mononuclear cell infiltrates or granulomas, consistent with hypersensitivity pneumonitis (41). In such outbreaks, without the "sentinel cases," workers with less severe responses would have been indistinguishable from, and potentially labeled as, workers with nonspecific BRI, or even diagnosed as humidifier fever.

Building-related asthma is recognized less often than building-related hypersensitivity pneumonitis, possibly because asthma is a common disease with many nonoccupational causes. The literature documenting increased risk of asthma and respiratory symptoms in damp residential environments is robust (42–44). Outbreaks of asthma related to exposures in water-damaged or damp commercial and office buildings have been reported rarely and the causative microbial agent(s) are often not identified (36,37,45–47; Cox-Ganser, in preparation). Of interest, many buildings with cases of hypersensitivity pneumonitis also have elevated rates of recent-onset asthma, as well as high rates of nonspecific building-related symptoms

(35,36,45–47). Sarcoidosis and idiopathic pulmonary fibrosis are also sometimes seen in workers in buildings where other workers have asthma and hypersensitivity pneumonitis (35,36,48; Cox-Ganser, in preparation).

It is possible that hypersensitivity pneumonitis, humidifier fever, and asthma result from different pathophysiological responses to the same exposure. Because the pathogenetic mechanisms of humidifier fever and hypersensitivity pneumonitis have not been clearly distinguished, it is possible that they represent different manifestations of the same illness (49). What determines whether the manifestations are mild and self-limited (Pontiac fever, humidifier fever), or severe (legionnaires' pneumonia, or hypersensitivity pneumonitis) may include the interaction of individual susceptibility, and type and level of exposure. Airborne concentrations of the causative agents, when identified, have rarely been measured in building-related outbreaks of immunologic lung disease. Within the industrial environment, epidemiological studies of "farmer's lung" show that higher exposures resulted in a higher proportion affected (50,51), as well as more severe symptoms.

Microorganisms produce a substantial array of toxins, and their health effects are complex. All gram-negative bacteria have endotoxin in their cell walls. Experimental endotoxin exposures, in high concentrations, produce acute reactions with fever, difficulty breathing, and changes in lung function (52–54). In cross-sectional studies, exposure to endotoxin or gram-negative bacteria have been linked to nonspecific building-related symptoms (55–57). Residential endotoxin has been associated with wheezing in infancy (58), childhood asthma (44), and asthma severity in clinical case series (59,60). In several investigations of hypersensitivity pneumonitis, endotoxin levels have been high (41,49,61). However, in cross-sectional studies and clinical series such as these, endotoxin may be a marker of exposure to bioaerosols and is not necessarily the etiologic agent. Other confounding factors may have resulted in the effects seen. In several other studies, no relationship between endotoxin levels and health effects was found.

Fungi have glucans in their cell walls, which like endotoxins, can trigger inflammatory symptoms and induce mediators in cell systems and in animals. Whether glucans and fungal-specific extracellular polysaccharides are etiologic agents of building-related symptoms or markers of etiologic exposures is currently being investigated.

The health effects of mycotoxins produced by certain fungi, such as *Stachybotrys atra*, are more controversial (62). Health effects have been attributed to mycotoxin exposure in the indoor environment, in case reports and case series (63), but measurement methods for airborne mycotoxins are not available. In one case–control study, *Stachybotrys* exposure was linked to pulmonary hemorrhage in infants (64). However, in a subsequent publication by the same agency, the study methods were heavily criticized, findings reversed in reanalysis, and conclusions withdrawn. In summary, although many microbes produce toxins under specific conditions of growth, and intuitively toxins cannot be good, there is inconclusive evidence that they cause health effects in the concentrations found in the indoor environment (42).

Influence of Ventilation in Modifying Communicable Infection

The studies that examined the relationship between ventilation rate and characteristics and transmission, or attack rate, of communicable respiratory infections are summarized in Table 2. A major strength of some of these studies is the measurement of objective health outcomes. A limitation is that the methodology and the

Table 2 Influence of Ventilation Rate on Transmission of Respiratory Infections Within Buildings

Author (References)	Study population		Infection	Ventilation		Rate or RR
	Building type (N)	Worker type (N)		Method of measurement	Vent level compared	
Brundage (30)	Barracks	Recruits (2,633,916)	Febrile respiratory illness	Design	1.2 LSP, 95% recirculated	RR. 1.5
					10 LSP, 60% recirculated	Reference
Warshauer (65)	Residence (N = 3)	Scientists (165)	Rhinovirus	Design	No outdoor air	RR 4-0
					"Considerable"	Reference
Nardell (31)	Office building	Office workers (67)	Tuberculosis (TST conversion)	Worksite CO_2	2.4 LSP	78%
					7.0 LSP	40% (observed)
						27%
Hoge (66)	Prison	Prisoners (46)	Pneumococcal pneumonia	Supply air flow Room CO_2	11.8 LSP	0/1,000
					7.2 LSP	3.1/1,000
					3.8 LSP	4.4/1,000
					3.4 LSP	7.3/1,000
					2.0 LSP	
Drinka (67)	Nursing home	Patients (688)	Influenza A	% recirculation Floor space per resident	0% recirculated, 88 FT^2/resident	3/184 = 2%
					30% recirculated, 57 FT^2/resident	31/196 = 16%
					30% recirculated, 54 FT^2/resident	18/194 = 9%
					70% recirculated, 24 FT^2/resident	16/114 = 14%
Menzies (68)	Hospitals (N=17)	Health workers (1200)	Tuberculosis (TST conversion)	Tracer gas	2 ACPH	Reference
					<2 ACPH	RR 3.4

Abbreviation: LSP, liters per second per person.

units of ventilation measurement varied substantially among studies. In the study of transmission of common colds in an Antarctic station, actual ventilation rates were not measured, but there were large differences in outdoor air supply according to building ventilation design (65). In all these studies the comparison or control populations should have been very similar because selection into the indoor environments with different ventilation rates was independent of characteristics of the exposed subjects. In the study of nursing home residents, potential differences in population characteristics, such as vaccination rates and severity of underlying illnesses, were accounted for in the design and analysis (67). Nevertheless the populations and environments studied were unusual—an Antarctic station, army housing, nursing homes, or prisons. The studies in the office environment evaluated health outcomes of tuberculosis transmission (3), self-reported episodes of colds (29), short-term sick leave thought largely attributable to respiratory infection (31), and sickness absence and consultation with medical specialists such as otorhinolaryngologists (69). These studies consistently demonstrated a relationship between lower ventilation rate and increased attack rate of disease, or other evidence of transmission. It should be noted that standard air filtration systems installed in HVAC systems of nonindustrial buildings are not effective in filtering out microorganisms. This can only be achieved with high-efficiency particulate air (HEPA) filters.

A number of population-based studies have demonstrated a clear link between ventilation levels and infectious disease transmission. These include measles outbreaks, excess occurrence of febrile respiratory disease among military recruits housed in mechanically ventilated barracks compared to naturally ventilated barracks (30), and excess occurrence of *Streptococcal pneumonia* in prison inmates where there was greater crowding and less ventilation. In one study, an office worker with contagious TB infected many of her coworkers, some of whom had no direct contact but worked in offices ventilated with the same recirculated air as the affected worker. The high levels of recirculation acted to disseminate the infection throughout the building (31). A second study detected significantly higher transmission of TB infection in hospital workers caring for TB patients in clinical units with low levels of ventilation (68). Office workers had increased sickness absence owing to respiratory illnesses if they shared an office (29), and military personnel reported more respiratory symptoms if they were housed in air-conditioned barracks (70). These findings imply that economy measures such as greater recirculation of air, open concept offices, or smaller work stations may result in greater transmission of respiratory pathogens with increased human illness and net economic loss.

Other Causative Agents

Damp conditions may lead to degradation of building materials which can result in generation of asthmagens and irritants associated with respiratory, conjunctival, and dermal symptoms. A ninefold increase in asthma incidence among office workers was attributed to degradation of polyvinyl chloride floor coverings which released the markers 2-ethyl-1-hexanol and 1-butanol (71). Dampness-related alkaline degradation of di(ethylhexyl)-phthalate, a plasticizer in polyvinyl chloride floor materials covering concrete, can be detected in indoor air concentrations of 2-ethyl-1-hexanol and has been associated with increased asthma symptoms (72). Phthalates in floor dust are associated with allergic symptoms among children (44).

Exposure to common indoor allergens such as dust mites, plant products, and passively transported allergens may occur in any occupied building, and result in upper or lower respiratory symptoms. Rarely other specific exposures can produce specific immune-mediated illnesses. These include photocopier fumes producing hypersensitivity angiitis (22) and carbonless copy papers producing urticaria, laryngeal edema (23,24), or pharyngitis (25).

Upper and lower respiratory symptoms may also represent irritant responses from exposure to nonallergic agents. Exposure to man-made vitreous fibers can result in sore throat and cough (20) accompanied by itching skin and burning eyes. Release of glass fibers may occur from ceiling boards which are damaged or movement of these boards by building vibrations or room pressure changes when doors are opened or closed (20). Mucosal irritation with respiratory symptoms and increased respiratory tract infections can occur following exposure to nitrogen dioxide (NO_2) indoors. This can be caused by the inhalation of exhaust fumes or simply outdoor air, if the levels are very high (73,74). Formaldehyde is well recognized as a mucosal irritant, but there have not been any well-documented outbreaks of illness related to exposure to formaldehyde in office buildings.

NONSPECIFIC BRI

In cross-sectional surveys in buildings, selected without regard to the occupants' health status, up to 60% of workers reported at least one work-related symptom, and 10% to 25% reported such symptoms occurring twice weekly or more frequently (10,11,14,15,75,76). Therefore nonspecific BRI is much more common and has much greater impact at the population level than specific BRI.

Associations with Demographic, Personal, and Medical Factors

As summarized in Table 3, the reporting of work- or building-related symptoms has been strongly and consistently associated with several personal and work characteristics in cross-sectional studies. History of atopic illness or asthma is consistently associated with symptom reporting in all studies—presumably reflecting a heightened sensitivity to the indoor environment. Female gender and younger age are generally associated with increased symptom reporting in most, although not all, studies. This may be the result of heightened sensitivity to environmental conditions, as has been demonstrated experimentally (85–89), or exposure to worse environmental conditions than their coworkers, as has been documented in some studies (90–92).

Psychosocial factors, such as work stress, have been consistently associated with symptom reporting. On pshychologic testing, symptomatic and asymptomatic office workers have similar test results (93); it is well known that psychosocial factors are associated with other conditions such as cardiovascular disease (94), and there is evidence that increased stress may be the result, rather than the cause, of health problems (95). An important source of stress at work can be conflict with the management. Since the management is also responsible for building operations, conflict between workers and management may lead to mistrust in the management regarding the indoor environment. This may result in the belief by workers that their work environment is harmful, and thereby, lead to substantial reporting bias. Differences in personal, medical and psychosocial characteristics may confound comparison of differences of symptom prevalence in workers in different buildings.

Table 3 Personal, Demographic, and Work Characteristics Associated with Nonspecific BRI

	Studies finding an association		Studies finding no association	
	Subjects (N)	References	Subjects (N)	References
Personal factors				
Female gender	23,764	(7–9,11,15,77–81)	3948	(13)
Younger age	17,166	(8,13,15,77,80)	8450	(7,9)
Cigarette smoking/atopy/allergy/asthma	23,662	(7,9–11,13,15,77,78,82)	–	
Personal	8433	(11,15)	13,944	(7,9,13,86)
Passive	15,017	(8,15,78)	5,338	(11,13)
Psychosocial factors	21,762	(7,9,11,13,15,78,79)	–	
Work-related factors				
Clerical work	9301	(7,8,11)	6489	(9,86)
Work with video display terminals	22,277	(7,9,11,13,15,77)	880	(95)
Work with carbonless paper	16,373	(7,9,15,83,84)	–	
Photocopiers: work with, or nearby	10,720	(7,9,11,83)	3948	(13)
Worksite factors				
Open concept office type	6489	(9,77)	3948	(13)
Crowding	11,430	(7,15,83)	–	

Abbreviation: BRI, building-related illness.

Although these factors can be measured, and therefore controlled for using multi-variate analysis techniques, it is impossible to control for possible reporting bias related to psychosocial factors such as work stress or conflict. Another potential limitation of this approach is overadjustment with multivariate analysis. Certain types of work or office equipment may be markers for exposure. In such circumstances, multivariate adjustment for these factors may obscure potentially important observations.

Thermal Factors

In two cross-sectional studies (77,85) and one experimental study (96), symptoms were significantly associated with relatively small differences in temperatures as shown in Table 4. The temperatures measured were all within the range 22°C to 26°C, traditionally considered acceptable (102). This may be explained by age- and gender-related differences in physiological responses to temperature (86,87). Both low and high humidity have been associated with symptoms (Table 4) (8,96–99,101). This may appear contradictory, but symptoms associated with lower humidity are usually those of mucosal irritation, whereas symptoms associated with high humidity tend to be systemic and/or respiratory; this suggests different mechanisms underlying the associations. This association of symptoms with temperature and humidity contradicts the long-standing belief that these are only "comfort parameters" (97–99,101–103) and suggests that these factors should be more carefully monitored and controlled.

Role of Microbial Contaminants

Most environmental fungi and bacteria require only water and a carbon source for growth. Carbon substrates can be dust, furnishings, or building materials. Many organisms grow well in the absence of light (in fact natural sunlight will often kill them). Given these simple requirements for growth, it should be no surprise that environmental microorganisms are ubiquitous in the indoor environment. Abundant growth, leading to high concentrations, can occur on any surface with sufficient water. This includes building materials that have been damaged by flooding, ground water, or spillage; anywhere that condensation of water occurs, such as in air-conditioning systems; or where there is standing water, such as in water cooling towers and humidification systems. Microbial contamination has been identified within all parts of modern ventilation systems, including filters, air-conditioning chillers, drip pans, and ducts. In one study, low concentrations of *Alternaria* in the filters of some HVAC systems of large office buildings were linked to respiratory symptoms and positive allergy skin tests to *Alternaria*. However this relationship was detected only in 2% of the total study population and only by means of a complex series of investigations (104). In addition, mold and bacterial contamination is common in areas of food preparation or consumption.

Fungi and bacteria have been implicated, because of the association of nonspecific BRI with indicators of potential microbial contamination such as high humidity (8,97,98), surface dust (7,13), carpets (7,13,83), and air conditioning (12,14,75,105). Microorganisms and/or their toxins have been detected in high concentrations at sites of localized water damage (63), and in HVAC systems—on cooling coils (106), filters (107), duct work (108,109), humidifiers (37), drip pans (106), and air-cooling units (32,35,106). Despite this, airborne microbial levels have been low and inconsistently associated with symptoms in field studies, as shown in Table 5 (55,90 97,105,106,111). Microbial indices in dust have correlated more frequently with health

Table 4 Association of Nonspecific BRI with Temperature and Humidity

Observational studies, parameter measured (unit)	Symptoms not associated			Symptoms associated		
	Mean	Range	Reference	Mean	Range	Reference
Temperature (°C)	23.0	22.4–24.0	(97)	23.0	21–26	(77)
				23.3	21–26	(85)
Relative humidity (%)					10–20%	(85)
					>40%	(8,98)

Experimental studies, parameter varied (unit)	No change in symptoms				Reduction in symptoms			
	Subjects (N)	Baseline level	Postinterv level	References	Subjects (N)	Baseline level	Postinterv level	References
Temperature (°C)					339		1.5° lower	(96)
Relative humidity (%)								
Field studies					211	24%	33%	(101)
					339	25%	40%	(96)
Chamber studies	12	50%	80%	(99)	12	18%	50%	(99)
	8	9%	50%	(100)				

Abbreviation: BRI, building-related illnesses.

Table 5 Association of Nonspecific BRI with Airborne Microorganisms

Author (Ref.)	Study design	Population Persons (N)	Buildings (N)	Exposure assessment Type	Microbiological class	Concentration measured Mean (cfu/m^3)	Range (cfu/m^3)	Symptom associated
Skov (97)	Cross-sectional	2369	14	Area	Fungi,	32	0–111	None
					Bacteria,	574	120–2,100	None
					Thermophilic actinimycetes		0	None
Nelson (111)	Cross-sectional	383	3	Personal	Fungi,	10	0–100	None
					Bacteria,	42	5–240	None
					Thermophilic actinomycetes	7	1–140	None
Menzies (110)	Case-control	100	6	Personal	Fungi	27	2–200	None
Harrison (105)	Cross-sectional	4610	15	Area	Total bacteria	342	80–961	None
					Fungi	97	2–978	Nose, skin, throat
Teeuw (55)	Cross-sectional	1355	19	Area	GM (−) bacteria	17	1–33	SBS—all symptoms
					Fungi	45	28–75	None
Menzies (90)	Repeated measures	704	2	Area	Fungi	14	8–17	None

Abbreviations: BRI, building-related illnesses; GM (−), gram-negative; SBS, sick building syndrome.

outcomes than airborne levels (25,43,55,56,58–60,112), although some studies have correlated airborne endotoxin or (1,3)-β-D-glucans with health (113).

Role of Other Contaminants

Approaches and guidelines for contaminant concentrations in the indoor nonindustrial environment have been issued by authoritative agencies such as the World Health Organization (6), American Society for Heating, Refrigerating and Air-Conditioning Engineers (ASHRAE) (114), and others (115). However, there is very little information to indicate the true health effects in the indoor population.

The term "volatile organic compounds" (VOCs) refers to many different compounds produced from a wide variety of sources within office buildings (116). These include new building materials or furnishings (the "new car smell"), cleaning agents, paints, solvents, microbial effluents, and equipment such as laser printers, photocopiers, and carbonless paper. In three single-blind chamber studies (Table 6) of controlled exposures administered to human volunteers, a mix of VOCs commonly found in office environments resulted in mucosal irritation (89,120,126,127). However, the concentrations of VOCs used (5000–50,000 $\mu g/m^3$) were far higher than those detected in most field studies (Table 6) (90,97,117–119). In these field studies, associations of symptoms with concentrations of VOCs are inconsistent, although, associations were detected in studies where concentrations were higher. Studies of controlled exposures to concentrations of VOCs usually found in the office environment would be of great interest.

Airborne dust may arise from indoor activity, particularly if there is inadequate cleaning, or from intake of outdoor air if there is inadequate filtration in the HVAC system. In cross-sectional surveys, airborne dust levels have generally been low, although there have been some associations with symptoms, particularly eye irritation (Table 6). The association between dust levels and systemic symptoms in one study may have resulted from associated, but unmeasured, contaminants (90). In one chamber study, young, healthy, male volunteers were exposed to increasing concentrations of environmental tobacco smoke. Even at the lowest level of exposure, 58 $\mu g/m^3$, subjects reported increased eye and nasal irritation, and their respiratory pattern was altered. Eye blink rate increased at much higher concentrations (125). Surface dust and carpets are reservoirs of fungi (44), endotoxin (112,128), VOCs (44), phthalates (97,116), and house dust mites, which may be released when disturbed, and result in health effects (129). In one experimental study, subjects who were unaware of the change demonstrated reduction of symptoms and increased productivity in the absence of an old carpet pollution source from the office environment, compared to when it was present (130). In another study, replacement of carpet by low-emitting vinyl floor material, along with HVAC renovation, was effective in reducing nonspecific BRI in one part of a building, in comparison with the non-intervention part of the building (126,131). Symptom reduction following intensive cleaning has also been documented (132,133).

Formaldehyde is commonly detected in low concentrations in the indoor office environment. Sources include building materials and furnishings. Exposures in the home environment to concentrations of formaldehyde exceeding 0.3 ppm resulted in symptoms of headache, eye, nose, and skin irritation in 71% of those surveyed. On the other hand, among subjects exposed to concentrations of less than 0.1 ppm, only 7% reported symptoms—no different from an unexposed control population (88). A similar relationship was seen between mucosal irritative symptoms and levels

Table 6 Association of Nonspecific BRI with VOCs and Airborne Dust

Author (Ref.)	Year	Population Persons (N)	Population Buildings (N)	Exposure assessment	VOCs or dust measured Mean (μg/m³)	VOCs or dust measured Range (μg/m³)	Symptoms associated
VOCs–field studies [all cross-sectional except (90)]							
Norback (117)	1990	261	11	Area	380	50–1380	Mucosal + systemic
Skov (97)	1990	215	4	Area	590	70–3190	None
Hodgson (118)	1991	147	3	Personal	1247		Mucosal + systemic
Sundell (119)	1993	1087	29	Area	70	3–740	None
Menzies (90)	1996	702	2	Area	941	160–2353	Acute mucosal
VOCs–chamber studies							
Molhave (120)	1986	150		Direct	5000 25,000		Mucosal ↓ Neurobehavioral performance
Otto (121,122)	1990	62		Direct	25,000		Mucosal, headache, fatigue No change in performance
Kjaergaard (89)	1991	35		Direct	25,000		Mucosal irritation ↓ FEV_1 ↑ Ocular tears/leukocytes ↓ Neurobehavioral performance
Dust–field studies [all cross-sectional except (90)]							
Weber (123)	1984	472	6	Personal	133	10–962	Eye irritation
Norback (124)	1990	129		Area	16	8–24	Eye symptoms
Hodgson (118)	1991	147	5	Personal	52	1–110	None
Harrison (105)	1992	4610	15	Area	30		None
Menzies (90)	1996	704	2	Area	22	13–19	Systemic
Dust–chamber studies							
Weber (123)	1984	33		Direct			Eye irritation at lowest level
Walker (125)	1996	17		Direct	58		Nasal, eye irritation, altered respiration
					217		Increased eye blink rate

Abbreviations: VOCs, volatile organic compounds; BRI, building-related illnesses.

of formaldehyde exposure in an industrial environment (134). In cross-sectional surveys among office workers (Table 7), exposure levels have been generally low and associations with symptoms rarely detected. In chamber studies, the odor detection threshold has been noted to be very low although there is a considerable range. Given the very low threshold for odor detection and the unpleasantness of formaldehyde odor, most investigators have found a strong association between detection of formaldehyde odor and the reporting of symptoms. In an ingenious study using a special apparatus that limited experimental formaldehyde exposure to the corneal surface of one eye, ocular irritation was reported only at significantly higher concentrations when the experimental subjects were not able to detect formaldehyde odors (138).

Sources of carbon monoxide in nonindustrial environments include improperly vented combustion such as the heating system (141) and/or intake of automotive exhaust fumes either from outdoor air or from an enclosed garage that is attached to the building (17). As summarized in Table 7, only one out of four studies detected an association between carbon monoxide levels and central nervous system (CNS) symptoms (139). As mentioned earlier, occult carbon monoxide poisoning may give rise to nonspecific symptoms of fatigue, headache, and difficulty concentrating (19). This has only been described in individuals exposed in the home environment, but could occur in the office environment from exposure to high enough levels.

The effects of exposure to environmental tobacco smoke have recently been reviewed (142), updating the comprehensive information available from nearly 20 years ago that focused largely on residential exposures (143). Workplace exposures to environmental tobacco smoke appear more deleterious than residential exposures and contribute to increased incidence of airway disease and prevalence of respiratory symptoms, asthma, and chronic bronchitis. These findings support continued multifaceted efforts to eliminate smoking from public indoor environments.

Potential Combined Effect of Multiple Agents

Most surveys of the nonindustrial, nonresidential environment have detected many contaminants known to cause health effects, but all at lower concentrations than previously demonstrated to cause these effects. Very few studies have examined the hypothesis that symptoms could result from a combination of two or more of these agents. In one report, an outbreak of illness among office workers was linked to exposure to carbon monoxide, ozone, and pentane, all at concentrations believed safe. Illness was more common among those with lower body weight, making a toxic effect more plausible (139). In a second report, symptoms were found to be more common in workers from two buildings, who were exposed to higher total contaminant load (90). Two experimental studies provide data in support of these observations. Exposure to 0.12 ppm of ozone for one hour increased subsequent bronchial reactivity to inhaled allergens (144), while volunteers exposed to 0.82 ppm of formaldehyde had a four times greater occurrence of mucosal irritation when also exposed to air from a "sick" building (137).

Role of Ventilation in Nonspecific BRI

Type of Ventilation System

Cross-sectional studies conducted in the 1980s identified that mechanically ventilated buildings had a higher prevalence of nonspecific BRI (5). Six of these studies were

Table 7 Association of Nonspecific BRI with Formaldehyde and Carbon Monoxide

Author (Ref.)	Year	Persons (N)	Buildings (N)	Exposure assessment	Mean (µg/m³)	Range (µg/m³)	Symptoms associated
Formaldehyde—field studies [all cross-sectional except (90)]							
Main (135)	1983	21 exposed		Area	0.87 ppm	0.2–1.6	Headache, mucosal, fatigue
		18 not exposed					
Horvath (134)	1988	113		Area		<0.05	4% sore throat
						0.05–0.4	8% sore throat
						0.4–1.0	22% sore throat
						1.0–3.0	33% sore throat
Skov (97)	1990	1018	4	Area	80 µg		None
Norback (117)	1990	261	11	Area	11 µg	0–30	None
DeBortoli (136)	1990	785	10	Area	450 µg	0–139	None
Sundell (119)	1993	1087	29	Area	31 µg	11–59	Mucosal, skin
Menzies (90)	1996	704	2	Area	0.03 ppm	0.01–0.05	None
Formaldehyde—Chamber studies							
Ahlstrom (137)	1986	64		Direct		>60 µg	Odor
Hempel (138)	1996	10		Direct		>0.88 ppm	Eye irritation

Author (Ref.)	Year	Persons (N)	Buildings (N)	Exposure assessment	Mean (ppm)	Range (ppm)	Symptoms associated
Carbon monoxide—field studies [all cross-sectional except (90)]						CO level	
Faust (139)	1981	22	1	Area		5–25	CNS
Robertson (140)	1985	241	2	Area		1–7	None
Hodgson (118)	1991	147	5	Personal	4.5		None
Menzies (90)	1996	704	2	Area	3.9	2–5.5	None

Abbreviations: BRI, building-related illnesses; VOCs, volatile organic compounds.

reanalyzed by Mendell and Smith (14). Using pooled data from these studies, building-related symptoms were most consistently associated with the presence of air conditioning, not simply mechanical ventilation. Subsequent studies, as summarized in Table 8, have confirmed that air conditioning is a consistent risk factor for nonspecific BRI. Recently, more serious morbidity has been suggested by a population-based study of French women, who had higher sickness absence and consulted medical specialists more frequently if they worked in air-conditioned buildings (69). Respiratory, allergic, and mucosal membrane symptoms have been the most consistently associated with air conditioning.

The underlying mechanism for this relationship has not been characterized. As seen in Table 9, the relationship between mechanical ventilation, ventilation rate, and occurrence of BRI is complex. Although it is reasonably certain that certain contaminants will increase in concentration if outdoor air supply is reduced, other contaminants may demonstrate a variable response. The most consistent evidence implicates microbial contamination of central air-conditioning systems. Air-conditioning systems are almost always wet because water condensation is inevitable. The microbes usually detected within HVAC systems have very simple growth requirements: water and carbon sources such as cellulose or dust. As a result, microbial contamination has been detected in all parts of HVAC systems, including filters, cooling coils, drip pans, and supply air ducts, as summarized in Table 9. The majority of outbreaks of specific BRI, where a cause was identified, have been traced to fungal, bacterial, and protozoal contamination of HVAC systems (26,33,35,48,104,106,108,109,160–169). In these outbreaks, symptoms resolved with remediation of microbial contamination. If the ventilation systems themselves are a source of BRI, then differences in ventilation rate (outdoor air supply) will have little relationship with symptom occurrence among workers in those buildings. Similarly, when water damage of the building structure or contents leads to microbial reservoirs, ventilation rates may have little effect in diminishing exposures by dilution.

Cross-Sectional Studies of Levels of Ventilation

Over the past 15 years, as summarized in Table 10, 14 large-scale cross-sectional studies investigated the relationship between ventilation rate and building-related symptoms or illnesses. These studies have involved approximately 30,000 workers in 500 buildings in North America and Europe. Most involved office buildings, but some involved schools, hospitals, and day care centers. The majority of the studies estimated ventilation rate from measures of worksite carbon dioxide (CO_2), although a substantial minority utilized exhaust airflow measurements. Most utilized self-reported work-related symptoms, although a few utilized perceived air quality, or environmental satisfaction or dissatisfaction as the primary outcomes. Very few studies utilized the assessment of objective outcome measures.

Results from these studies were not consistent. Perceived air quality was associated with lower ventilation rates in only one of three studies, where this was the primary outcome. Even in the one positive study, the correlation was relatively weak; air quality ratings were slightly worse only at the lowest ventilation levels. Self-reported work-related symptoms were the most commonly measured outcome. Of all the cited studies, the centers with the lowest levels of ventilation found no association between these low levels and symptoms (172). Yet in the same study, and in others (10,39,76,173), symptoms were lower at higher ventilation rates. In one study, there was no association of CO_2, in levels which ranged from 400 to 2000 with symptoms

Table 8 Cross-Sectional Studies of Type of Ventilation System and Building-Related Symptoms/Illnesses

Author (reference) year	Country	Study population Building-types and (N)	Workers (N)	Comparison (reference = natural)	Symptoms associated
Finnegan (145) 1984	Britain	Office (8)	951	Air conditioning (steam humidifier)	CNS, mucosal
				Air conditioning + water humidifier	CNS, mucosal, skin, resp
Hedge (146) 1984	Britain	Office (3)	1332	Mechanical	Headache
				Air conditioning + water humidifier	CNS, mucosal
Robertsons (140) 1985	Britain	Office (2)	241	Air conditioning	CNS, eye, mucosal
Burge (8) 1987	Britain	Office (42)	4373	Mechanical	None
				Air conditioning + humidifier	CNS, nasal, resp
Skov (147) 1987	Denmark	Office (14)	2778	Mechanical	None
				Air conditioning + water humidifier	CNS, mucosal, skin
Zweers (15) 1992	Netherlands	Office (61)	7043	Mechanical	None
				Air conditioning	Skin, eye, mucosal, CNS, fever
				Humidifier + air conditioning	Skin, eye, mucosal, CNS, fever
Richards (70) 1993	Saudi Arabia	(barracks)	2598	Air conditioning	Sore throat, cough; rhinorrhea less likely
Fisk (83) 1993	United States	Office (12)	880	Mechanical	Fatigue, dry skin
				Air conditioning	Fatigue, dry skin, respiratory
Sundell (10) 1994	Sweden	Office (160)	4943	Mechanical	None
				Air conditioning humidifier	None
Jaakhola (12) 1995	Finland	Office (41)	2678	Mechanical	Only throat
				Air conditioning	Throat, lethargy
				Air conditioning + water humidifier	Nasal, lethargy
				Air conditioning + steam humidifier	Mucosal, allergic
Smedge (148) 1997	Sweden	Schools (40)	1210	Exhaust only	Odds of worse PAQ: 1.8
				Supply + exhaust	Odds of worse PAQ: 0.7

(Continued)

Table 8 Cross-Sectional Studies of Type of Ventilation System and Building-Related Symptoms/Illnesses (*Continued*)

| | | Study population | | Comparison | |
Author (reference) year	Country	Building-types and (N)	Workers (N)	(reference = natural)	Symptoms associated
Vincent (149) 1997	France	Office (3)	1144	Air conditioning Fan coil unit	Headache, nasal, throat None
Walinder (150,151) 1998	Sweden	Schools (12)	234	Mechanical	Lower nasal patency Higher nasal lysozyme
Teculescu (81) 1998	France	Office (2)	776	Air conditioning	Chest tightness Sick absence
Costa (152) 2000	Brazil	Stores (43)	309	Air conditioning	Skin, eye, nasal, throat, respiratory
Preziosi (69) 2004	France	Working professional women	920	Air conditioning	Sickness absence, otorhinolaryngology and dermatology consultations

Note: Data for this table taken from the references listed and additional data from (14)
Abbreviations: CNS, central nervous system; SBS, sick building syndrome; PAQ, perceived air quality.

Table 9 Ventilation System as the Source or Solution to Specific Contaminants

Chemical parameters	
Formaldehyde	Increased ventilation rate will reduce levels (73,77,90)
Carbon monoxide	Improper intake of auto exhaust will increase levels (153)
TVOCs	Ventilation systems may be important source (154,155) Increased ventilation will reduce levels (73,77,90,156)
NO_2	Improper intake of exhaust fumes may increase levels (153) Increased intake of outdoor air will increase levels (153)
Dust	Mechanical ventilation airconditioning reduces dust levels compared to natural (157) Increased intake of outdoor air increases indoor levels (153)
Microbial	
Fungi/bacteria	Contamination has been documented on: HVAC filters (104,158,159) Drip pans (106,159) Humidifiers (37,159) Air cooling towers (32,35,106) Air-conditioning coils (106,159,161) Air washers (160) Dust in ducts (55,108)
Toxins	Endotoxin and mycotoxins have been extracted from HVAC dust (55,108).

Abbreviations: HVAC, heating, ventilation, and air-conditioning; TVOC, total volatile organic compounds.

in four buildings, but there was an association between higher CO_2 levels and lethargy in a single building (176). The findings emphasize that increased outdoor air ventilation rate may be beneficial in certain buildings—maybe because of greater crowding, or other factors. Even more puzzling is that two studies found that higher levels of ventilation were associated with more symptoms of irritation of mucosal membranes and skin (173,177). It has been suggested that (173) because these two studies were conducted in Nordic countries in winter, the excess of symptoms at higher ventilation levels may have been the result of very low indoor humidity resulting from intake of large amounts of cold dry outdoor air. Another possible explanation is that the high ventilation rates in these buildings might have reflected prior indoor air–quality problems for which ventilation rates had already been increased without successfully reducing symptoms.

Studies using objective health measures such as nasal patency or inflammatory markers have detected greater problems at lower ventilation rates, and a single study found greater documented sickness absence associated with lower ventilation rates— an important finding given the economic impact of work absence.

A study conducted in homes in Norway examined ventilation rate, indicators of indoor pollutants, and bronchial obstruction (asthma) in infants. No direct relationship was found between ventilation rate and asthma in this case–control study. However, sources of indoor pollutants such as polyvinyl chlorides, dampness problems,

Table 10 Cross-Sectional Studies of Ventilation Rate and Building-Related Symptoms/Illness, [1 CFMpp = 0.4719 LSP]

Author (reference) year	Study population			Measurement of ventilation	Comparison vent levels	Symptoms associated with ventilation level
	Country	Building-types and (N)	Workers (N)			
Skov (97) 1990	Denmark	Town hall (14)	2369	Worksite CO_2	500–1300 ppm (range of CO_2	No symptoms
Zweers (170) 1990	Denmark	Town hall (4)	855	Air flow	5.9–16 LSP	No symptoms
Jaakhola (78,171) 1991	Finland	Office (1)	1719	Exhaust air flow % of recirculation	7–15 LSP 15–25 LSP >25 LSP	No symptoms No symptoms Reference level
Zweers (15) 1992	Netherlands	Office (61)	7043	Worksite CO_2	485–1239 ppm (range of CO_2)	Inverse relationship (higher CO_2 = lower symptoms)
Hill (80) 1992	United States	Office (5)	206	Worksite CO_2	493–610 ppm (range of CO_2)	No symptoms
Fisk (83) 1993	United States	Office (12)	880	Average worksite CO_2 (40 hrs)	370–580 ppm (range of CO_2)	No symptoms
Ruotsalaiman (172) 1994	Finland	Day care (30)	268	Exhaust air flow	0–2.4 LSP 2.5–4.9 LSP 5.0 LSP	None Lethargy and odors Reference level
Sundell (10) 1994	Sweden	Office (160)	4943	Exhaust air flow or tracer gas	<13.6 LSP 13.6 LSP	Any symptom (weak association—Figure 1) Reference level
Nordstrom (173) 1995	Sweden	Hospitals (8)	225	Exhaust air flow	0.6–17 LSP (range)	Eye, throat, skin with higher ventilation levels
Jaakhola (76) 1995	Finland	Office (14)	399	Exhaust air flow	<5 LSP 5–15 LSP 15–25 LSP >25 LSP	Mucosal, allergic Mucosal, allergic Reference level Mucosal, allergic

Hedge (174) 1995	United States	Office (5)	939	Worksite CO_2	468–664 ppm (Range of CO_2)	No symptoms No environmental ratings
Nelson (175) 1995	United States	Office (4)	646	Worksite CO_2	540–792 ppm (range of CO_2)	No symptoms No environmental ratings
Bluyssen (155) 1996	Europe	Office (56)	6537	CO_2, air flow, tracer gas	0–56 LSP 4–1500 ppm over OA (range of CO_2)	Modest relationship of lower vent (10–20 LSP) with poor perceived air quality (Fig. 2)
Smedge (148) 1997	Sweden	Schools (40)	1410	Worksite CO_2 Tracer gas	425–2800 ppm CO_2 0.1–22 LPS	PAQ—not associated with CO_2 PAQ—not associated with air change
Vincent (149) 1997	France	Office (3)	1144	Worksite CO_2 Indoor/outdoor CO_2 ratio	880 vs. 912 2.0 vs. 2.1	SBS symptoms SBS symptoms
Walinder (150,151) 1998	Sweden	School (12)	234	Tracer Gas	1.1–9.0 LSP	No nasal patency Higher nasal lysozyme
Apte (39) 2000	United States	Office (33)	1579	Worksite CO_2 (average or maximum)	>300 ppm CO_2 over OA	Mucosal/respiratory (NOT a dose–response relationship)
Milton (3) 2000	United States	Office (40)	3720	Worksite CO_2 (end of day or maximum)	12 LSP 24 LSP	1.5 RR Short term sick leave Reference level
Niven (176) 2000	Britain	Office (5)	947	Worksite CO_2	400–2000(overall) 500–1000 (1 building) (range of CO_2 ppm)	None Lethargy

Abbreviations: CFMpp, cubic feet per minute per person; LSP, liters per second per person; PAQ, perceived air quality.

and textile materials, were associated with asthma in infants, and the effect was two to three times greater in homes with low outdoor air–exchange rates (178).

Six experimental field studies are summarized in Table 11. In two, the initial ventilation rates were very low, and ventilation levels were substantially modified in all studies. Despite this, in four studies, no relationship was detected between ventilation level and symptoms or environmental satisfaction. The two field studies finding an association employed a single cross-over design, so seasonal or other temporal changes may have accounted for the modest benefit seen. It is also possible that in the buildings where increased ventilation appeared to result in benefits, there were stronger indoor pollutant sources than in the buildings where no such benefit was detected. The sixth study found a significant difference in certain symptoms and environmental ratings between levels of 3 and 30 LSP. There was greater improvement in all measured outcomes when ventilation was increased from 3 to 10 LSP than when ventilation was increased from 10 to 30 LSP.

In summary, while increased ventilation may be important in some buildings as an intervention, the etiology of building-related symptoms and ventilation effects on diverse sources of contaminants are too complex to expect that all problems in all buildings will be resolved with simple increases in ventilation rates.

Measurement of Ventilation in the Indoor Environment

In the nonindustrial environment, CO_2 measures rarely exceed 1000 ppm or 0.1%, and the maximum concentration reported was 2800 ppm or 0.28%. Direct toxic effects of CO_2 are not expected at these concentrations. The current North American industry standards for minimum outdoor air delivery is expressed in CFMpp or LSP. Since the only source of CO_2 in the vast majority of nonindustrial buildings is the human occupants, measurement of CO_2 is the simplest and most direct method to verify that ventilation per occupant meets the current standard. Calculation of outdoor air delivery is as follows:

$$CFMpp = [(0.75/60) \times (1,000,000 - \text{indoor } CO_2)]/[\text{indoor } CO_2 - \text{outdoor } CO_2]$$

where:

    CFMpp = cubic feet per minute per person
    0.75/60 = amount of pure CO_2 (cubic feet) produced by one sedentary adult
           per minute
    Indoor CO_2 = concentration of CO_2 in the indoor environment
    Outdoor CO_2 = concentration of CO_2 in outdoor air at the same time
    For example: If outdoor $CO_2 = 350$ ppm, and indoor $CO_2 = 1000$ ppm, then
           CFMpp = 19.2

As summarized in Table 12, CO_2 has a number of important advantages when used as a proxy of ventilation. CO_2 concentrations reflect all ventilation entering the indoor space, including air delivered by mechanical ventilation systems, entering through open windows and doors, or infiltrating through the building envelope. In older buildings, the latter can be very substantial. The most important advantage is that CO_2 can be measured rapidly and easily with relatively inexpensive infrared direct reading instruments capable of precision to within 1 ppm. Because of this, as shown in Table 3, CO_2 has already been used in numerous large-scale epidemiologic surveys. This experience provides a growing body of evidence to link different CO_2 concentrations in the indoor environment to health effects. There is no

Table 11 Experimental Studies of Ventilation Rate and Building-Related Symptoms/Illnesses

Author (Ref.) year	Country	Study population		Measurement of ventilation	Comparison vent levels high–low (liters/second/person)	Symptoms associated
		Buildings (N) and type	Workers (N)			
Turiel (73) 1983	United States	2 (office)	593	Design (method not clarified)	20–23 vs. 4–6	Odors (symptoms not analyzed)
Jaakhola (171) 1991	Finland	1 (office)	1719	% Recirculation Exhaust air flow	26 vs. 6.5 26 vs. 10.4	Total number of symptoms (No dose response seen)
Wyon (96) 1992	Sweden	1 (hospital)	222	Supply/exhaust air flow	17 vs. 12 24 vs. 17	None None
Menzies (77) 1993	Canada	4 (office)	1546	CO_2 at worksites	30 vs. 14	None
Jaakhola (179) 1994	Finland	2 (office)	75	% Recirculation	20 vs. 6	None
Wargocki (180) 2000	Denmark	1 (office)	30	Tracer gas Worksite CO_2	3 vs. 30	Odors, PAQ, dryness of mouth, throat, concentration, overall well-being

Abbreviation: PAQ, perceived air quality.

Table 12 Comparison of Ventilation Measurement Methods

Methods	Advantages	Limitations	References
CO_2	Measurement is easy, inexpensive, and rapid. Inexpensive instruments accurate to 1 ppm Can be measured at multiple sites and on multiple occasions. Measures all ventilation Infiltration plus delivered	Only accounts for human source of pollutants Requires equilibrium—of occupants, and CO_2 concentration, hard to obtain. Does not give air change rates Must measure multiple sites and out doors.	(3,15,31,39,66,73,77,80,83,148,149 174–176,181–184)
Air flow	Easy, quick, inexpensive Multiple measures possible Independent of human occupants Does not require equilibrium	Measures only delivered air Does not measure infiltration or entry through windows or doors, nor short-circuting. Does not account for occupant density/crowding	(10,66,76,78,98,96,170–173,179)
Tracer gas	Considered the gold standard Measures all ventilation Independent of other building factors or operations Independent of occupants	Complex, slow, and very expensive Very few research groups able to do this limited number of measures—can not account for spatial or temporal variability.	(68) (10,148,150)
Design parameters	Simplest—need only engineering or architect plans or specifications	Does not meaure actual ventilation nor its effectiveness.	(65,73,185)
% Recirculation	Simple, quick, cheap Multiple measures can be made	Does not measure actual ventilation, nor occupants, nor infiltration	(67,77,78,171,179)

Note: In one study CO_2 was used as a tracer gas.
Source: From Ref. 186.

question that the indoor environment is complex and highly variable between buildings. It is also highly variable within individual buildings because of spatial and temporal variability. Therefore, use of a measure, like CO_2, that can be measured at many sites and at many times allows a more credible estimate of exposure–response relationships in large-scale epidemiologic studies.

Despite these advantages, use of CO_2 has several important limitations. The most important is that it is an indicator only of human sources of pollutants (181), not building sources (187). To illustrate the potential limitations, an extreme example would be a large building with substantial indoor pollutant sources (building materials, furnishings, and carpets), but only one occupant. In this building, CO_2 concentrations would remain low, even at very low ventilation rates, but levels of other pollutants could be high enough to cause significant health effects. A second problem is that the CO_2 concentrations must reach equilibrium, meaning a steady state, to make a valid estimate of air exchange rates.

Measurement of HVAC airflow, usually at supply diffusers or exhaust air intakes within occupied space, can be made quickly, easily, and precisely with inexpensive equipment. This measures only air delivered by the ventilation system, but does not account for reduction in the ventilation system effectiveness, occupant density (crowding), or for building sources of pollutants.

Tracer gas methods are considered the gold standard in the measurement of ventilation rates (188), but their major disadvantage is that these techniques are complex, slow, and expensive. As a result, very few epidemiologic studies have used these techniques. Also they are not practical for use in the investigation of possible building-related symptoms/illnesses.

Use of design parameters of the HVAC system to estimate ventilation is a very problematic approach. This does not either measure actual ventilation or account for such variables as ventilation effectiveness, other building conditions, outdoor conditions, or occupancy. This method is particularly inaccurate in older buildings where the current HVAC system functioning may be very different from that which was initially designed, due to postconstruction changes of the building or in the HVAC system, and normal wear and tear (189,190).

The percentage of recirculation is easy to measure; the only requirement is simultaneous measurement of CO_2 or temperature, in HVAC supply, and in return and outdoor air.

Complex Interrelationship of Indoor Contaminants

There is substantial temporal and spatial variability of CO_2 and other indoor pollutants within large nonindustrial buildings (85). This variability is related to differences in occupancy, local sources of pollutants, and ventilation effectiveness. Accurate assessment of workers' exposure to actual ventilation conditions and related indoor pollutants must account for this temporal and spatial variability, by repeated measurements at the same sites at different times, and also by taking measurements at multiple sites.

Certain pollutants, such as total VOCs and formaldehyde (73,77,90,156,170, 175,180,182), have correlated strongly with measures of outdoor air exchange. These chemicals are produced almost exclusively within buildings and are found in very low concentrations in outdoor air (191). Nevertheless, the correlation with ventilation rate will be weaker if there are strong sources from building materials or furnishings and will be better if the major sources are from humans or from their day-to-day activities (photocopying, printing, etc.). The major source of NO_2 and carbon monoxide in urban environments is automobile exhaust. Therefore, these two pollutants are generally at higher concentrations outdoors than indoors (191). These contaminants have been correlated with ventilation rate in some studies, and greater outdoor air supply (lower CO_2) was associated with higher indoor NO_2 (90).

At higher ventilation rates, indoor levels of dust (124) and bacteria (73,183) may be higher or lower (90,183). The relationships are complex because these parameters are often elevated in outdoor air, but sources of these contaminants may be found within the occupied spaces, or in the HVAC system (157). Local sources for microbial contaminants include carpets, furnishings, humans themselves, and localized areas damp damage (128,192,193). Local sources for particulates are the same plus cigarette smoking and certain work activities (191). The ventilation system may be an important source of microbial contaminants (33,104,106,161) or their toxins (108). Buildings with tightly sealed outer shells, air conditioning, and efficient filter systems may be unaffected by outdoor concentrations of dust and microbes (157). In buildings where the HVAC system itself has heavy microbial contamination, that is, these systems are the sources of fungi and bacteria, then increasing the ventilation rate will not change indoor concentrations of airborne microbial contaminants or their toxins.

Temporal and Spatial Variability—The Microenvironment

The HVAC systems of large office buildings are designed to provide a stable and constant indoor environment throughout the building. However, postconstruction changes to either the ventilation system or interior space (190), or normal wear and tear, may result in malfunctioning of well-designed ventilation systems and substantial reduction in local ventilation effectiveness (189). In addition, there may be important differences in local indoor pollutant sources because of differences in the human occupants themselves (such as perfume use) or because of their work activities and use of equipment. Also, there may be local pollutant sources such as microbial contamination following water damage, or materials known as "sinks," which trap contaminants such as VOCs and release them slowly later (116). All these factors may result in substantial spatial variation in temperature, air velocity, and indoor pollutant levels between work sites, even on the same floor of one building (77,85,194). In addition, there may be considerable temporal variation in contaminant concentrations as a result of changes in outdoor air supply, in outdoor air pollutant levels, or in the number and activities of the workers. Spatial variability may have resulted in significant misclassification of exposure in studies where environmental measures were made at only two to seven sites and used to estimate exposure for all workers in an entire building (8,97,117,140). Temporal variability may have resulted in misclassified exposure in studies where environmental measures were not taken at the same time as measures of symptoms, or were taken only over a short period (8,85,97,140).

The unexpected finding of significant spatial variability within large office buildings has given rise to the concept of the "microenvironment" (118). When environmental parameters have been measured directly at the work sites of individual workers—so-called personal measures—associations have been detected between individual contaminants and symptoms, although even these results are not consistent. The concept of the microenvironment has provided support for the provision of personal control over the ventilation system to individual workers. This is because in the complex environment of large office buildings, it is simply not possible for a centrally controlled HVAC system to adapt rapidly and effectively to highly variable local conditions, as well as meet the demands or preferences of many workers. Sophisticated automated ventilation systems with electrochemical sensors for a number of environmental parameters are unlikely to be developed.

However, the provision of individual ventilation control offers a more practical solution because it utilizes the most sophisticated, as well as the most relevant sensor—that of the human organism itself. In a cross-sectional British survey of 4373 workers in 46 buildings, those who could regulate temperature and ventilation reported significantly higher productivity and fewer symptoms (195). Among 7043 Dutch workers in 61 office buildings, work absence related to symptoms of nonspecific BRI was 34% lower in buildings where workers could regulate the temperature (196). The provision of a personally controlled ventilation system was associated with a significant increase in objectively measured productivity in one study (197) and with persistent and prolonged improvement in symptoms, environmental ratings, and self-reported productivity in another (198).

SYNTHESIS OF EVIDENCE REGARDING NONSPECIFIC BRI

Several personal factors are associated with nonspecific BRI, which may be indicators of increased susceptibility. Symptoms are also associated with markers of individual exposure, such as use of carbonless paper, photocopiers, and VDTs or the presence of carpets and dust. Yet the specific agent(s) responsible for the associated health effects of mechanical ventilation (10,12,14,75) or humidification remains unclear (15). Cross-sectional studies to examine these factors were confounded by between-building differences among the occupants and their work, and may have been biased by occupants' awareness and attitudes. Although symptoms have consistently been associated with temperature and humidity (77,85,96), this has not been the case for measured chemical and microbial parameters, despite the indirect evidence implicating them. This may reflect the multiple agents present, their spatial and temporal variability, and that current measurement methods are expensive and not precise enough for the low levels usually present in this environment.

The failure to detect associations of nonspecific BRI with chemical and microbial contaminants may also be explained by the wide range in the threshold of response in any population (susceptibility), a spectrum of response to any given agent, and the temporal and spatial variability in exposure within large office buildings.

Health effects develop in individuals exposed to an agent or agents at concentrations above their individual threshold for response. Among healthy adults there is a wide range in the threshold for irritant effects of formaldehyde (134,137), VOCs (199), and environmental tobacco smoke (123,199). Similar between-subject variability has been demonstrated for the threshold of physiological response to (86,87) temperature; ozone, sulfates, and particulates (200); and endotoxin (51,52). Thresholds for response are lower in workers with asthma (200) or previous building-related symptoms (89), or those who are female or younger (86,88). In addition, thresholds for physiological response to allergens, VOCs, and environmental tobacco smoke have been lowered by concomitant exposure to ozone (144), higher temperature (201), and lower humidity (99), respectively.

Specific BRIs were initially identified when several workers presented with similar clinical manifestations and objective abnormalities. An important but overlooked finding in these outbreaks was the wide spectrum of clinical response to the same agents (33–35). The "tip of the iceberg" was the few seriously affected workers with specific clinical abnormalities. Among other exposed workers, some (often more than the number of initial sentinel cases) had symptoms but no objective abnormalities, whereas others were asymptomatic, yet had circulating specific antibodies (33–35). Without the sentinel cases, the cause for symptoms in these other affected workers may have been missed or the symptoms labeled nonspecific BRI.

The indoor environment of nonindustrial buildings is complex. There may be many different pollutants: from outdoor air, from humans and their activities, and from the building materials, furnishings, or even the ventilation systems themselves. The concentrations of these pollutants will vary markedly between buildings and within buildings according to local sources and local ventilation. There may be substantial temporal variation over the course of each day, from day-to-day, and between different seasons, related to differences in the indoor and outdoor pollutant sources as well as the ventilation. The relationship of health effects to this complex indoor environment is further complicated because there is a wide range in human susceptibility to individual and combinations of pollutants. For this reason, large-scale epidemiologic studies are best suited to investigate the health effects of this indoor environment.

Modern high-rise office buildings are designed to provide a stable and uniform indoor environment, but as discussed earlier, the actual environment has considerable temporal and spatial variability. This variability may create quite different microenvironments at each work station (90,92). If there was independent variation in the microenvironmental exposures and workers' susceptibility, then individuals could be symptomatic because of localized exposure to one or more agents exceeding their threshold of response. This hypothesis would be difficult to test because of the multiplicity of agents and symptoms, and the difficulties of accurately characterizing exposure. However, this could explain why past epidemiological surveys failed to identify relationships between environmental parameters measured at a limited number of work sites and symptoms of all workers within these buildings (15,97,140,202). This would provide the rationale for moving affected workers to other work stations—a simple solution that has never been evaluated formally. Another potential solution is personal control over ventilation as this would take advantage of highly sophisticated and sensitive monitors located at every workplace—the workers themselves! Individuals who sensed local adverse conditions could mitigate them by changing ventilation—even if they did not know what they were affected by.

APPROACH TO THE PATIENT

Given the complexity of the indoor environment in office buildings, and numerous contributing factors, it is difficult to envisage a simple standardized approach to an office worker with health problems that may be work related. However, certain principles can be defined.

A careful history is an essential first step. Workers may fail to recognize the office environment as the source of their symptoms, so it is important to ascertain the onset, course, and temporal relationship of symptoms with the work environment. On the other hand, if workers attribute their symptoms to the work environment, it is still important to exclude nonoccupational causes.

The physical examination is usually normal in nonspecific BRI but may be abnormal with specific illnesses. Additional investigations may be appropriate to diagnose specific entities such as a chest X ray and lung function tests for hypersensitivity pneumonitis or asthma, allergy skin tests, and serum IgE for those with allergic manifestations.

If a BRI is suspected, a work site "walk-through" is a valuable starting point in the evaluation of the work environment. A team approach including the physician, industrial hygienist, and engineer is best to identify and resolve problems in this complex indoor environment. Clinicians should familiarize themselves with public or occupational health officials at the municipal, state, or federal level who have expertise in the evaluation of these problems. An important advantage of contacting such authorities is that they may also receive reports of other affected workers in the same building. This should prompt a more thorough environmental assessment, and may enable workers to receive compensation or similar benefits. Environmental air sampling may be indicated if specific indoor contaminants are suspected, but is expensive and requires considerable expertise in measurement and interpretation.

Interventions demonstrated to mitigate nonspecific BRI, such as lowering temperature, better control of humidity, or better cleaning could be suggested, although these may not be applicable in all settings. Another possible (although untested) solution for the workers with nonspecific and unexplained symptoms would be to change microenvironments—by changing work sites—even within the same building.

Recommendations for Control—Microbial Contamination

There are two general approaches to microbial control in any indoor environment. The most effective long-term solution is elimination of all conditions allowing microbial growth (source control). The alternative, if it is impossible to eliminate all possible sources, is to eliminate airborne microbes through sterilization, filtration, or dilution.

Source control can mean prevention or remediation. Prevention means altering the conditions that influence microbial growth. Given the dependence of microbes on water, the most successful and practical method is to prevent water accumulation, condensation, or infiltration, as well as any subsequent water damage. This means installation of dehumidification systems where humidity levels are high, such as environments at or below ground level. Prevention of water infiltration means water-proofing the building shell, particularly at or below ground level. Since condensation with air-conditioning systems is inevitable, condensate should be rapidly removed before it becomes contaminated. Humidification systems should use steam, rather than ultrasonic or other forms of nebulization of cool water.

Prevention also includes careful selection of equipment, furnishings, and building materials that will not act as media for microbial growth. Carpets are an important and common source of microbial contamination, particularly in areas where food or drinks are prepared or consumed. Having no carpets, or selecting low-pile carpets, is an important preventive measure. Other furnishings and equipment should be selected with similar criteria—they should have smooth surfaces, reducing accumulation of microbial substrate (dirt) and surface area for microbial growth, and facilitating cleaning.

Remediation is the term applied to elimination of microbial sources after contamination has occurred. The most effective method is to completely remove contaminated sources such as damp-damaged carpets, furnishings, draperies, insulation, or other building materials. Cleaning can be effective, but is often a less permanent solution. In some cases, such as the cleaning of ventilation ducts or the changing of filters, the actions can result in significant release of microbial products, resulting in very high, albeit transient, microbial exposures. Therefore, these activities should be performed when the occupants are not present, and significant care must be taken to prevent an occupational hazard to those performing these tasks. Microbial reduction can also be accomplished with germicidal chemicals, but it is important to recognize that these chemicals may themselves be associated with health effects. Therefore, chemical cleaning also must be done only when the occupants are absent, and appropriate precautions must be taken to ensure that the workers doing the cleaning are not exposed. Furthermore, sufficient time should have elapsed before the occupants' return so that all traces of the chemicals have dissipated.

Reduction of airborne concentration of microbes can be achieved on sterilization by natural sunlight or ultraviolet germicidal irradiation (UVGI). Because the sterilizing ultraviolet rays of natural sunlight are largely eliminated by glass, natural sunlight is not a practical option for air sterilization within most indoor environments. UVGI has been used to sterilize air, and thereby prevent airborne transmission of certain diseases, most notably measles transmission within schools and tuberculosis transmission within hospitals and other health care facilities. UVGI is also used for sterilizing air in meat packing plants, pharmaceutical manufacturing, and operating rooms.

The efficacy of UVGI in sterilizing air is unquestioned, but direct exposure can cause eye irritation and a theoretical risk of skin cancer. Therefore, UVGI cannot be used in occupied spaces, or if used, it is only to irradiate the upper air of the room with the fixtures constructed and mounted to prevent direct irradiation of the human occupants. In other areas, such as within the HVAC system, UVGI is potentially useful within the ducts to sterilize the air, or to irradiate the air-conditioning systems to eliminate condensate-related microbial contamination. In a recent study, UVGI irradiation of air-conditioning systems in three large office buildings resulted in a significant reduction of allergic and systemic syndrome–type symptoms in 771 office workers (91). The most significant improvement was seen in the most susceptible— workers who had a history of atopy or allergy, as well as nonsmokers. UVGI appears to be underutilized at present, and may be a useful addition to the microbial control armamentarium.

A major limitation of airborne sterilization is that the killed airborne microbes, although no longer able to cause infections, may still be immunogenic and result in allergic or hypersensitivity manifestations. Filters can be effective in eliminating viable and nonviable microbes, as well as microbial particles. However, the efficiency of the filter is an important determinant of the beneficial effects. Although filters found in most HVAC systems will trap microbes that are adherent to airborne dust particles, they will not trap particles of 1 to 5 µm size. These are termed respirable particles, as they can reach the alveoli when inhaled, and may contain microbial antigens, such as proteins or cell wall parts, or viable bacteria, such as tuberculosis. These pathogenically important particles will only be trapped by the more efficient HEPA filters. HEPA filters will trap more than 99% of particles of 0.3 µm size or larger. However, these filters are much more costly, and because of their greater resistance to air flow, they require greater fan strength and energy to operate, further increasing their cost and limiting their applicability. An additional limitation of filters is that they must be changed frequently because they become contaminated.

Several reports have documented that poorly maintained filters can become a source of airborne microbial contamination. When filters are being changed there can be a substantial airborne burst of microbes released, which can pose significant hazards to those in the occupied space. Therefore, it is recommended that filters are changed when the indoor environment is not occupied and the occupational hazard for those changing the filters is prevented by suitable protection.

Recommendations for Control—Ventilation Rate

Most owners and operators of nonindustrial buildings in Canada and the United States adhere to recommendations for ventilation rate, and other parameters for this environment, established by the ASHRAE (114). These recommendations are frequently adopted in building codes promulgated by municipal, provincial, and federal agencies. The current recommendations published in 2005 (ASHRAE 62.1-2004) advocate a minimum ventilation rate of 17 cubic feet per minute (CFM) per person (or approximately 8.5 LPS) for the office environment when occupant density is unknown; when occupant density is known, the outdoor air ventilation rate is 5 CFM/person (2.5 LPS) (114).

The overall relationship between ventilation rates or indoor CO_2 concentrations and health outcomes remains somewhat unclear because of contradictory evidence. The most consistent relationships between ventilation rate and health outcomes have been found in experimental studies and in studies of infectious diseases, despite widely different techniques used to estimate ventilation rate. Studies of respiratory infections assessed objective outcomes but involved unusual populations or situations, such as an Antarctic station, prisons, nursing homes, or army barracks. Experimental studies, which are the strongest epidemiologic designs to limit sources of bias and confounding factors, measured self-reported symptoms and perceived air quality but not objective health outcomes. As shown in Figure 1, these studies consistently demonstrated that ventilation rates less than 5 LPS were associated with increased occurrence of potentially serious respiratory illnesses, poor perceived air quality, and building-related symptoms.

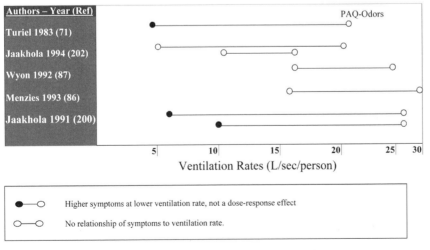

Figure 1 Experimental studies—relationship of air change rates and work-related symptoms (unless marked).

Evidence regarding the relationship between higher ventilation rates and perceived air quality and building-related symptoms, largely derived from more than a dozen large-scale cross-sectional studies, is not as consistent. The relationships between these outcomes and average CO_2 levels and/or ventilation rates are summarized in Figures 2 and 3. Some studies demonstrated a strong relationship between lower ventilation rates and symptoms, whereas others demonstrated no such relationship. Reasons for these discrepant findings include very different ventilation rates, potential selection and reporting biases, as well as confounding due to differences in personal, work, and psychosocial factors.

Interestingly, the few studies which employed objective measures, such as nasal patency, markers of nasal inflammation, and documented sickness absence were the most consistent in detecting relationships between lower outdoor air exchange rates and health outcomes.

The most consistent evidence is that adverse health effects are increased when outdoor air ventilation rates are less than 5 LPS. Evidence linking health effects to ventilation rates between 5 and 10 LPS is much more contradictory. Only a few studies have demonstrated any benefit of ventilation rates above 10 LPS; most studies demonstrated no benefit of outdoor air exchange rates greater than 10 LPS, and two actually found higher symptom prevalence at higher ventilation rates. These findings can be explained by the phenomenon that relatively small changes in ventilation strongly influence indoor pollutant levels when baseline ventilation rates are low, but have much less effect at higher ventilation levels (Fig. 4). The consistent finding that health effects were linked to ventilation rates less than 5 LPS suggests that in most buildings at least 5 LPS are needed to control indoor pollutant sources. The inconsistent results when ventilation has varied between 5 and 10 LPS suggests that this level of ventilation may be adequate in some buildings—presumably those with less indoor pollutant sources—but is not sufficient in buildings with stronger indoor

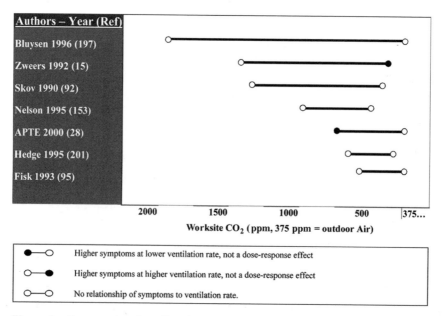

Figure 2 Cross-sectional studies. Association between average work site CO_2 concentrations and building-related symptoms.

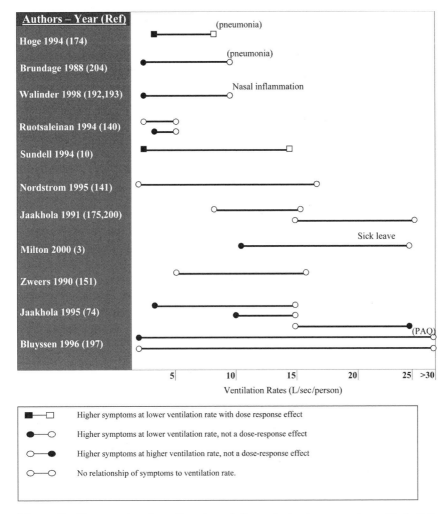

Figure 3 Cross-sectional studies. Association of air changes rates with building-related symptoms (unless marked).

pollutant sources. Therefore, the present minimum value of 10 LPS appears to provide a reasonable margin of safety for most buildings.

Present standards recommend higher but unspecified outdoor air exchange rates if smoking is allowed within the building (114). This is because cigarette smoking is associated with generation of substantial indoor air pollutants. By inference, ventilation rates should also be increased in buildings with other important identifiable pollutant sources. However, in all instances, source control is by far the best mitigation approach. In the example of cigarette smoking, the most effective approach is to ban cigarette smoking within buildings. Increased ventilation should be used only when the pollutant source cannot be identified or cannot be removed, such as when it is from building materials themselves. For example, in new or extensively renovated buildings, there may be substantial off-gassing of VOCs and formaldehyde. Such buildings may require higher ventilation levels to remove these

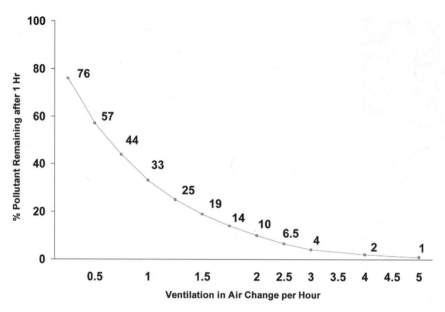

Figure 4 Air-borne pollutants remaining after one hour of ventilation at different rates.

pollutants. The only study demonstrating the potential value of increased ventilation to control greater indoor pollutants was a study of asthma among Norwegian infants. In this study, the effect of indoor pollutant sources was magnified in homes with lower outdoor air supply rate. At present, there is insufficient understanding of these sources and the magnitude of the ventilation rate required for remediation—only that increased ventilation is required.

CONCLUSIONS

Symptoms of nonspecific BRI are common. Although there is little convincing direct evidence to implicate specific causative agents, there is sufficient indirect evidence to support a number of recommendations. For example, it seems prudent to select building materials, furnishings, and equipment that are least likely to release pollutants, such as formaldehyde or VOCs; assure proper cleaning and maintenance to avoid dampness and water accumulation and infiltration; and avoid materials that may act as substrates for microbial or dust mite proliferation.

The current North American minimum of 17 CFM/person or 8.5 LPS should be considered the minimum required outdoor air exchange rate or ventilation rate for office buildings. This is roughly equivalent to a maximum CO_2 concentration of 1000 ppm. In buildings with known important indoor sources of air pollutants, the ventilation rates should be increased to account for this. In buildings where smoking is allowed, increased ventilation is recommended, and air from smoking areas should not be recirculated or transferred to no-smoking areas (114). Elimination of known sources of indoor pollutants is the most effective mitigation strategy. Therefore, smoking should be banned in all indoor environments. In circumstances of other sources of indoor pollutants where elimination is not possible (such as building materials), the increase in ventilation required is unknown and deserves further research.

In air-conditioned buildings, it is highly likely that some degree of microbial contamination will occur in the central HVAC systems. In addition, moisture barriers in air-conditioned buildings and pressure changes induced by mechanical ventilation may lead to entrainment of microbial materials from the building shell into the occupied space. Based on substantial but indirect evidence, this may account for part of the phenomenon of nonspecific BRI. If microbial contamination is heavy, then adverse health effects in building occupants may be more likely. Indoor microbial contamination may be unaffected by ventilation rate, meaning that different remediation strategies are required. The threshold of microbial contamination for causing adverse health effects and optimal methods for prevention or remediation of microbial contamination have not been established and require further research.

Workers in the indoor environment of office buildings represent more than half the entire workforce of industrialized countries. Significant proportions have symptoms at work. Given the enormous population apparently affected and our current limited understanding of the adverse health effects of this environment, further research is urgently required. Susceptibility should be assessed in experimental studies of exposures to individual and multiple pollutants at concentrations typically found in the office environment. Proposed interventions should be evaluated in properly designed trials using standardized case definitions, questionnaires, and environmental measurement methods. Such studies could help to ensure that the man-made ecosystem of modern office buildings is a healthy work environment.

RESEARCH PRIORITIES

- Exposure–response relationships in the nonindustrial indoor environment require further work.
- Variability in human susceptibility to exposures at levels commonly seen in the office-building environment.
- Human response to multiple exposures at low levels.
- Mitigation or prevention strategies for microbial contaminants such as filtration and/or ultraviolet germicidal irradiation.
- Impact on objectively measured productivity of the nonindustrial indoor environment.

ACKNOWLEDGMENTS

Dr. Menzies was supported by a Chercheur-Boursier award from the Fonds de la Recherche en Santé de Québec. Health Canada provided financial support for a review of the literature that formed part of this chapter. The authors thank Ms. Tonya Rowan and Mme. Catherine Michaud for secretarial assistance. The contents and views in this chapter are those of the authors and not of the National Institute for Occupational Safety and Health.

REFERENCES

1. Christie B. Human factors of information technology in the office. New York: John Wiley and Sons, 1985.
2. Woods JE. Cost avoidance and productivity in owning and operating buildings. Occup Med 1989; 4:753–770.
3. Milton DK, Glencross PM, Walters MD. Risk of sick leave associated with outdoor air supply rate, humidification, and occupant complaints. Indoor Air 2000; 10:212–221.
4. Mendell MJ, Fisk WJ, Kreiss K, et al. Improving the health of workers in indoor environments: priority research needs for a National Occupational Research Agenda. Am J Public Health 2002; 92(9):1430–1440.
5. Menzies D, Bourbeau J. Building-related illnesses. New Engl J Med 1997; 337: 1524–1531.
6. World Health Organization. Indoor air pollutants: exposure and health effects. Copenhagen: World Health Organization, 1983.
7. Skov P, Valbjorn O, Pedersen BV. Danish Indoor Climate Study Group. Influence of personal characteristics, job-related factors and psychosocial on the sick building syndrome. Scand J Work Environ Health 1989; 15:286–295.
8. Burge PS, Hedge A, Wilson S, Bass JH, Robertson A. Sick Building Syndrome: a study of 4373 office workers. Ann Occup Hyg 1987; 31:493–504.
9. Stenberg B, Hansson MK, Sandstrom M, Sundell J, Wall S. A prevalence study of the sick building syndrome (SBS) and facial skin symptoms in office workers. Indoor Air 1993; 3:71–81.
10. Sundell J, Stenberg B, Lindvall T. Associations between type of ventilation and air flow rates in office buildings and the risk of SBS-symptoms among occupants. Environ Int 1994; 20(2):239–251.
11. Bourbeau J, Brisson C, Allaire S. Prevalence of the sick building syndrome symptoms in office workers before and after being exposed to a building with an improved ventilation system. Occup Environ Med 1996; 53:204–210.
12. Jaakkola JJK, Miettinen P. Type of ventilation system in office buildings and sick building syndrome. Am J Epidemiol 1995; 141(8):755–765.
13. Wallace LA, Nelson CJ, Highsmith R, Dunteman G. Association of personal and workplace characteristics with health, comfort and odor: A survey of 3948 office workers in three buildings. Indoor Air 1993; 3:193–205.
14. Mendell MJ, Smith AH. Consistent pattern of elevated symptoms in air-conditioned office buildings: a re-analysis of epidemiologic studies. Am J Public Health 1990; 80:1193–1199.
15. Zweers T, Preller L, Brunekreef B, Boleij JSM. Health and indoor climate complaints of 7043 office workers in 61 buildings in The Netherlands. Indoor Air 1992; 2:127–136.
16. Menzies D, Pasztor J, Leduc J, Nunes F. The "sick building"–a misleading term that should be abandoned. In: Besch EL, ed. I.A.Q. '94 Engineering Indoor Env. Atlanta, GE: (ASHRAE) American Society of Heating Refrigiration Air Conditioning Engineer, 1994.
17. Wallace LA. Carbon monoxide in air and breath of employees in an underground office. J Air Pollut Contr Assoc 1983; 33:678–682.
18. Horvath SM, Dahms TE, O'Hanlon JF. Carbon monoxide and human vigilance. Arch Environ Health 1971; 23:343–347.
19. Heckerling PS, Leiken JB, Maturen A, Perkins JT. Predictors of occult carbon monoxide poisoning in patients with headache and dizziness. Ann Int Med 1987; 107:174–176.
20. Farkas J. Fibre glass dermatitis in employees of a project-office in a new building. Contact Dermatitis 1983; 9:79.
21. Kreiss K, Hodges MJ. Building-associated epidemics. In: Wash PJ, Dudney CS, Copenhaver ED, eds. Indoor Air Quality. Boca Raton: CRC Press Inc., 1984:87–106.

22. Tencati JR, Novey HS. Hypersensitivity angiitis caused by fumes from heat-activated photocopy paper. Ann Intern Med 1983; 98:320–322.

23. Marks JG, Trautlein JJ, Zwilich CW, Demers LM. Contact urticaria and airway obstruction from carbonless copy paper. JAMA 1984; 252(8):1038–1040.

24. LaMarte FP, Merchant JA, Casale TB. Acute systemic reactions to carbonless copy paper associated with histamine release. JAMA 1988; 260(2):242–243.

25. Morgan MS, Camp JE. Upper respiratory irritation from controlled exposure to vapor from carbonless copy forms. J Occup Med 1986; 28(6):415–419.

26. Fraser DW, Tsai TR, Orenstein W, et al. Legionnaire's disease: description of an epidemic of pneumonia. N Engl J Med 1977; 297:1189–1197.

27. Dennis PJ, Taylor JA, Fitzgerald RB, Bartlett CLR, Barnow GI. *Legionella pneumophilia* in water plumbing systems. Lancet 1982; 1:949–951.

28. Kaufman AF, McDade JE, Patton CM. Pontiac fever: isolation of the etiologic agent (*Legionella pneumophilia*) and demonstration of its mode of transmission. Am J Epidemiol 1981; 114:337–347.

29. Jaakkola JJK, Heinonen OP. Shared office space and the risk of the common cold. Eur J Epidemiol 1995; 11(2):213–216.

30. Brundage JF, Scott RMcN, Lednar WM, Smith DW, Miller RN. Building-associated risk of febrile acute respiratory diseases in army trainees. JAMA 1988; 259:2108–2112.

31. Nardell EA, Keegan J, Cheney SA, Etkind SC. Airborne infection: theoretical limits of protection achievable by building ventilation. Am Rev Resp Dis 1991; 144(2):302–306.

32. Banaszak EF, Thiede WH, Fink JN. Hypersensitivity pneumonitis due to contamination of an air conditioner. N Engl J Med 1970; 283:271–276.

33. Woodard ED, Friedlander B, Lesher RJ, Font WF, Kinsey R, Hearne FT. Outbreak of hypersensitivity pneumonitis on an industrial setting. JAMA 1988; 259:1965–1969.

34. Arnow PM, Fink JN, Schuelter DP, et al. Early detection of hypersensitivity pneumonitis in office workers. Am J Med 1978; 64:236–241.

35. Bernstein RS, Sorenson WG, Garabrant D, Reaux C, Treitman RD. Exposures to respirable, airborne penicillium from a contaminated ventilation system: clinical, environmental and epidemiologic aspects. Am Ind Hyg Assoc J 1983; 44:161–169.

36. Hoffman RE, Wood RC, Kreiss K. Building-related asthma in Denver office workers. Am J Public Health 1993; 83(1):89–93.

37. Burge PS, Finnegan MJ, Horsfield N, et al. Occupational asthma in a factory with a contaminated humidifier. Thorax 1985; 40:248–254.

38. Schneider T. Manmade mineral fibres and other fibres in the air and in settled dust. Environ Int 1986; 12:61–65.

39. Apte MG, Fisk WJ, Daisey JM. Association between indoor CO_2 concentration and sick building syndrome symptoms in U.S. office buildings: an analysis of the 1994–1996 BASE study data. Indoor Air 2000; 10:246–257.

40. Jiang Z, Haghighat F, Chen Q. Influence of air supply parameters 65 on air quality in individual workstations. ASHRAE Trans 1993.

41. Rose CS, Newman LS, Martyny JW, et al. Outbreak of hypersensitivity pneumonitis in an indoor swimming pool: clinical, pathophysiologic, radiographic, pathologic, lavage and environmental findings. Am Rev Respir Disease 1990; 141:A315.

42. Institute of Medicine (U.S.), Committee on Damp Indoor Spaces and Health. Damp Indoor Spaces and Health. Washington, D.C.: National Academic Press, 2004.

43. Bornehag CG, Blomquist G, Gyntelberg F, et al. Dampness in buildings and health. Nordic interdisciplinary review of the scientific evidence on associations between exposure to "dampness" in buildings and health effects (NORDDAMP). Indoor Air 2001; 11(2):72–86.

44. Bornehag CG, Sundell J, Sigsgaard T. Dampness in buildings and health (DBH): report from an ongoing epidemiological investigation on the association between indoor environmental factors and health effects among children in Sweden. Indoor Air 2004; 14(suppl 7):59–66.

45. Jarvis JQ, Morey PR. Allergic respiratory disease and fungal remediation in a building in a subtropical climate. Appl Occup Environ Hyg 2001; 16(3):380–388.

46. Park JH, Schleiff PL, Attfield MD, Cox-Ganser JM, Kreiss K. Building-related respiratory symptoms can be predicted with semi-quantitative indices of exposure to dampness and mold. Indoor Air 2004; 14(6):425–433.

47. Seuri M, Husman K, Kinnunen H, et al. An outbreak of respiratory diseases among workers at a water-damaged building–a case report. Indoor Air 2000; 10(3):138–145.

48. Ganier M, Lieberman P, Fink J, Lockwood DG. Humidifier lung: an outbreak in office workers. Chest 1980; 77:183–187.

49. Nordness ME, Zacharisen MC, Schlueter DP, Fink JN. Occupational lung disease related to cytophaga endotoxin exposure in a nylon plant. J Occup Environ Med 2003; 45(4):385–392.

50. Malmberg P, Rask-Anderson A, Palmgren U, Hoglund S, Kolmodin-Hedman B, Stalenheim G. Exposure to microorganisms, febrile and airway-obstructive symptoms, immune status and lung function of Swedish farmers. Scand J Work Environ Health 1985; 11:287–293.

51. Malmberg P, Rask-Andersen A, Rosenhall L. Exposure to microorganisms associated with allergic alveolitis and febrile reactions to mold dust in farmers. Chest 1993; 103:1202–1209.

52. Rylander R, Bake B, Fischer JJ, Helander IM. Pulmonary function and symptoms after inhalation of endotoxin. Am Rev Respir Dis 1989; 140:981–986.

53. Fogelmark B, Goto H, Yuasa K, Marchat B, Rylander R. Acute pulmonary toxicity of inhaled beta-1, 3-glucan and endotoxin. Agents Actions 1992; 35:50–56.

54. Smid T, Heederik D, Houba R, Quanjer PH. Dust- and endotoxin-related acute lung function changes and work-related symptoms in workers in the animal feed industry. Am J Ind Med 1994; 25:877–888.

55. Teeuw KB, Vandenbroucke-Grauls CMJE, Verhoef J. Airborne gram-negative bacteria and endotoxin in sick building syndrome. Arch Intern Med 1994; 154:2339–2345.

56. Gyntelberg F, Suadicani P, Nielsen JW, et al. Dust and the sick building syndrome. Indoor Air 1994; 4(4):223–238.

57. Reynolds SJ, Black DW, Borin SS, et al. Indoor environmental quality in six commercial office buildings in the midwest United States. Appl Occup Environ Hyg 2001; 16(11):1065–1077.

58. Park JH, Gold DR, Spiegelman DL, Burge HA, Milton DK. House dust endotoxin and wheeze in the first year of life. Am J Respir Crit Care Med 2001; 163(2):322–328.

59. Michel O, Ginanni R, Duchateau J, Vertongen F, Le Bon B, Sergysels R. Domestic endotoxin exposure and clinical severity of asthma. Clin Exp Allergy 1991; 21(4):441–448.

60. Michel O, Kips J, Duchateau J, et al. Severity of asthma is related to endotoxin in house dust. Am J Respir Crit Care Med 1996; 154(6 Pt 1):1641–1646.

61. Ohnishi H, Yokoyama A, Hamada H, et al. Humidifier lung: possible contribution of endotoxin-induced lung injury. Intern Med 2002; 41(12):1179–1182.

62. Page E, Trout D. Mycotoxins and building-related illness. JOEM 1998; 40(9):761–764.

63. Jarvis BB, Zhou Y. Toxigenic molds in water damaged buildings. J Natural Products 1996; 59(6):553–554.

64. Centers for Disease Control (CDC). Acute pulmonary hemorrhage/hemosiderosis among infants–Cleveland. Morbidity Mortality Weekly Rep 1994; 43:881–883.

65. Warshauer DW, Dick EC, Madel AD, Flynn TC, Jerde RS. Rhinovirus infections in an isolated Antarctic Station: transmission of the virus and susceptibility of the population. Am J Epidemiol 1989; 129(2):319–339.

66. Hodge CW, Reichler MR, Dominguez EA, et al. An epidemic of pneumococcal disease in overcrowded, inadequately ventilated jail. N Engl J Med 1994; 331:643–648.

67. Drinka PJ, Krause P, Schilling M, Miller BA, Shult P, Gravenstein S. Clinical investigation: reporting of an outbreak: nursing home architecture and Influenza-A attack rates. J Am Geriat Soc 1996; 44(8).
68. Menzies RI, Fanning A, Yuan L, FitzGerald JM. Hospital ventilation and risk of tuberculous infection in Canadian Health Care Workers. Ann Intern Med 2000; 133(10): 779–789.
69. Preziosi P, Czernichow S, Gehanno P, Hercberg S. Workplace air-conditioning and health services attendance among French middle-aged women: a prospective cohort study. Int J Epidemiol 2004; 33(5):1120–1123.
70. Richards AL, Hyams KC, Watts DM, Rozmajzl PJ, Woody JN, Merrell BR. Respiratory disease among military personnel in Saudi Arabia during operation desert shield. Am J Public Health 1993; 89(9):1326–1329.
71. Tuomainen A, Seuri M, Sieppi A. Indoor air quality and health problems associated with damp floor coverings. Int Arch Occup Environ Health 2004; 77(3):222–226.
72. Norback D, Wieslander G, Nordstrom K, Walinder R. Asthma symptoms in relation to measured building dampness in upper concrete floor construction, and 2-ethyl-L-hexanol in indoor air. Int J Tuberc Lung Dis 2000; 4(11):1016–1025.
73. Turiel I, Hollowell CD, Miksch RR, Rudy JV, Young RA. The effects of reduced ventilation on indoor air quality in an office building. Atmos Environ 1983; 17:51–64.
74. Vanderstraeten P, Muylle E, Verduyn G. Indoor air quality in a large hospital building 4th ed. Stockholm, Sweden: Swedish Council for Building Research, 1984.
75. Mendell MJ, Fisk WJ, Deddens JA, et al. Elevated symptom prevalence associated with ventilation type in office buildings. Epidemiology 1996; 7(6):583–589.
76. Jaakkola JJK, Miettinen P. Ventilation rate in office buildings and sick building syndrome. Occup Environ Med 1995; 52:709–714.
77. Menzies RI, Tamblyn RM, Farant JP, Hanley J, Nunes F, Tamblyn RT. The effect of varying levels of outdoor air supply on the symptoms of sick building syndrome. New Engl J Med 1993; 328:821–827.
78. Jaakkola JJK, Reinikainen LM, Heinonen OP, Majanen A, Seppanen O. Indoor air quality requirements for healthy office buildings: recommendations based on an epidemiologic study. Environ Int 1991; 17:371–378.
79. Mikatavage MA, Rose VE, Funkhouser E, Oestenstad RK, Dillon K, Reynolds KD. Beyond air quality-factors that affect prevalence estimates of sick building syndrome. Am Ind Hyg Assoc J 1995; 56:1141–1146.
80. Hill BA, Craft BF, Burkart JA. Carbon dioxide, particulates, and subjective human responses in office buildings without histories of indoor air quality problems. Appl Occup Environ Hyg 1992; 7(2):101–110.
81. Teculescu DB, Sauleau EA, Massin N, et al. Sick building symptoms in office workers in northeastern France: a pilot study. Int Arch Occup Environ Health 1998; 71:353–356.
82. Stenberg B, Eriksson N, Hoog J, Sundell J, Wall S. The sick building syndrome (SBS) in office workers. A case-referent study of personal, psychosocial and building-related risk indicators. Int J Epidemiol 1994; 23(6):1190–1197.
83. Fisk WJ, Mendell MJ, Daisey JM, et al. Phase 1 of the California healthy building study: a summary. Indoor Air 1993; 3:246–254.
84. Kleinman GD, Horstman SW. Health complaints attributed to the use of carbonless copy paper (a preliminary report). Am Ind Hyg Assoc J 1982; 43:432–435.
85. Jaakkola JJK, Heinonen OP. Sick building syndrome, sensation of dryness and thermal comfort in relation to room temperature in an office building: need for individual control of temperature. Environ Int 1989; 15:163–168.
86. Doeland HJ, Nauta JJP, Van Zandbergen JB, et al. The relationship of cold and warmth cutaneous sensation to age and gender. Muscle Nerve 1989; 12:712–715.
87. Grivel F, Candas V. Ambient temperatures preferred by young European males and females at rest. Ergonomics 1991; 34(3):365–378.

88. Ritchie IM, Lehnen RG. Formaldehyde-related health complaints of residents living in mobile and conventional homes. Am J Public Health 1987; 77(3):323–328.
89. Kjaergaard S, Molhave L, Pedersen OF. Human reactions to a mixture of indoor air volatile organic compounds. Atmos Environ 1991; 25A:1417–1426.
90. Menzies R, Tamblyn RM, Nunes F, Hanley J, Tamblyn RT. Exposure to varying levels of contaminants and symptoms among workers in two office buildings. Am J Public Health 1996; 86(11):1629–1632.
91. Menzies D, Popa J, Hanley JA, Rand T, Milton DK. Effect of ultraviolet germicidal lights installed in office ventilation systems on workers' health and wellbeing: double-blind multiple crossover trial. Lancet 2003; 362(9398):1785–1791.
92. Hodgson MJ, Collopy P. Symptoms and the micro-environment in the sick building syndrome: a pilot study. In: ASHRAE, editor. IAQ '89-The Human Equation: Health and Comfort. Atlanta, GA.: American Society of Heating Refrigeration and Air-conditioning Engineers (ASHRAE), 1989: 8–16.
93. Bauer RM, Greve KW, Besch EL, et al. The role of psychological factors in the report of building-related symptoms in sick building syndrome. J Consult Clin Psychol 1992; 60(2):213–219.
94. Karasek RA, Theorell T, Schwartz JE, Schnall PL, Pieper CF, Michela JL. Job characteristics in relation to the prevalence of myocardial infarction in the US Health Examination Survey (HES) and the Health and Nutrition Examination Survey (HANES). Am J Public Health 1988; 78(8):910–918.
95. Klitzman S, Stellman JM. The impact of the physical environment on the psychological well-being of office workers. Soc Sci Med 1989; 29(6):733–742.
96. Wyon DP. Sick buildings and the experimental approach. Environ Technol 1992; 13:313–322.
97. Skov P, Valbjorn O, Pedersen BV. Danish Indoor Climate Study Group. Influence of indoor climate on the sick building syndrome in an office building. Scand J Work Environ Health 1990; 16:363–371.
98. Reinikainen LM, Jaakola JJK, Heinonen OP. The effect of air humidification on different symptoms in office workers – an epidemiologic study. Environ Int 1991; 17:243–250.
99. Kay DL, Heavner DL, Nelson PR, et al. Effects of relative humidity on non-smoker response to environmental tobacco smoke. In: Walkinshaw DJ, ed. Proceedings of Fifth International Conference on Indoor Air Quality and Climate, Toronto, July 29–August 3, 1990. Vol 1. Canadian Mortgage and Housing, 1993:275–280.
100. Andersen I, Lundqvist GR, Jensen PL, Proctor DF. Human response to 78-hour exposure to dry air. Arch Environ Health 1974; 29:319–324.
101. Reinikainen LM, Jaakola JJK, Seppanen O. The effect of air humidification on symptoms and perception of indoor air quality. Arch Environ Health 1992; 47:8–15.
102. American Society of Heating Refrigeration and Air-conditioning Engineers. ASHRAE standard 55–1981: thermal environmental conditions for human occupancy. Atlanta: American Society of Heating Refrigeration and Air-conditioning Engineers (ASHRAE), 1981.
103. American Society of Heating Refrigeration and Air-conditioning Engineers. ASHRAE standard 62–1989: ventilation for acceptable indoor air quality. Atlanta, GA: American Society of Heating Refrigeration and Air-conditioning Engineers (ASHRAE), 1989.
104. Menzies D, Comtois P, Pasztor J, Nunes F, Hanley JA. Aeroallergens and work-related respiratory symptoms among office workers. J Allergy Clin Immunol 1998; 101:38–44.
105. Harrison J, Pickering CA, Faragher EB, Austwick PK, Little SA, Lawton L. An investigation of the relationship between microbial and particulate indoor air pollution and the sick building syndrome. Respir Med 1992; 86:225–235.
106. Hugenholtz P, Fuerst JA. Heterotrophic bacteria in an air-handling system. Appl Environ Microbiol 1992; 58(12):3914–3920.

107. Elixman J. Investigation of alleric potential induced by fungi on air filters of HVAC systems. The Seventh International Conference on Indoor Climate and Air Quality, 1996:125.

108. Smoragiewicz W, Cossette B, Boutard A, Krzystyniak K. Trichothecene mycotoxins in the dust of ventilation systems in office buildings. Int Arch Occup Environ Health 1993; 65:113–117.

109. Pasanen P, Pasanen AL, Jantunen M. Water condensation promotes fungal growth in ventilation ducts. Indoor Air 1993; 3:106–112.

110. Menzies R, Tamblyn R, Comtois P, et al. Case-control study of microenvironmental exposures to aero-allergens as a cause of respiratory symptoms–part of the sick building syndrome (SBS) symptom complex. In: Geshwiler M, ed. IAQ 1992–Environments for people. Atlanta: American Society of Heating, Refrigeration and Air-conditioning Engineers, 1992:119–128.

111. Nelson CJ, Kollander M, Clayton CA, et al. EPA's indoor air quality and work environment survey: relationships of employees' self-reported health symptoms with direct indoor air quality measurements. In: Berglund LG, ed. IAQ 1991–Healthy Buildings. Atlanta: American Society of Heating, Refrigeration and Air-conditioning Engineers, 1991:22–32.

112. Chao HJ, Schwartz J, Milton DK, Burge HA. The work environment and workers' health in four large office buildings. Environ Health Perspect 2003; 111(9):1242–1248.

113. Rylander R. Airborne $(1{\rightarrow}3)$-beta-D-glucan and airway disease in a day-care center before and after renovation. Arch Environ Health 1997; 52(4):281–285.

114. American Society of Heating RaAE. ASHRAE standard 62.1–2004: Ventilation for acceptable indoor air quality. Atlanta, GA: American Society of Heating, Refrigerating and Air-conditioning Engineers (ASHRAE), 2005.

115. American Conference of Governmental Industrial Hygienists. Guidelines for the assessment of bioaerosols in the indoor environment. Cincinnati, Ohio, 1989.

116. Brown SK, Sim MR, Abramson MJ, Gray CN. Concentrations of volatile organic compounds in indoor air: a review. Indoor Air 1994; 4:123–134.

117. Norback D, Michel I, Widstrom J. Indoor air quality and personal factors related to sick building syndrome. Scand J Work Environ Health 1990; 16:121–128.

118. Hodgson MJ, Frohliger J, Permar E, et al. Symptoms and microenvironmental measures in nonproblem buildings. J Occup Med 1991; 33(4):527–533.

119. Sundell J, Andersson B, Andersson K, Lindvall T. Volatile organic compounds in ventilating air in buildings at different sampling points in the buildings and their relationship with the prevalence of occupant symptoms. Indoor Air 1993; 3:82–93.

120. Molhave L, Bach B, Pedersen OF. Human reactions to low concentrations of volatile organic compounds. Environ Int 1986; 12:167–175.

121. Otto DA, Hudnell KH, House DE, Molhave L, Counts W. Exposure of humans to a volatile organic mixture.1 Behavioral assessment. Arch Environ Health 1992; 47(1): 23–30.

122. Otto DA, Hudnell HK, House DE, Molhave L. Exposure of humans to a volatile organic mixture. 2. Sensory. Arch Environ Health 1992; 47(1):31–38.

123. Weber A. Annoyance and irritation by passive smoking. Preventive Medicine 1984; (Symposium: Medical perspectives on passive smoking):618–625.

124. Norback D, Torgen M, Edling C. Volatile organic compounds, respirable dust, and personal factors related to prevalence and incidence of sick building syndrome in primary schools. Br Med J 1990; 47:733–741.

125. Walker JC, Nelson PR, Cain WS, et al. Perceptual and psychophysiological responses of non-smokers to a range of environmental tobacco smoke concentrations. In: Yoshizawa S, ed. IAQ 96–The Seventh International Conference on Indoor Climate and Air Quality. Nagoya: Organizing Comm. 7th Int Conf of Indoor Air Quality and Climate, 1996:1001–1006.

126. Otto D, Molhave L, Rose G, Hudnell K, House D. Neurobehavioral and sensory irritant effects of controlled exposure to a complex mixture of volatile organic compounds. Neuro Toxiocol Teratol 1990; 12:649–652.

127. Pappas GP, Herbert RJ, Henderson W, Koenig J, Stover B, Barnhart S. The respiratory effects of volatile organic compounds. Int J Occup Environ Health 2000; 6(1):1–8.

128. Gravesen S, Larsen L, Gyntelberg F, Skov P. Demonstration of microorganisms and dust in schools and offices. Allergy 1986; 41:520–525.

129. Wood RA, Eggleston PA, Lind P, et al. Antigenic analysis of household dust samples. Am Rev Resp Dis 1988; 137:358–363.

130. Wargocki P, Wyon DP, Baik YK, Clausen G, Fanger PO. Perceived air quality, sick building syndrome (SBS) symptoms and productivity in an office with two different pollution loads. Indoor Air 1999; 9(3):165–179.

131. Pejtersen J, Brohus H, Hyldgaard CE, et al. Effect of renovating an office building on occupants' comfort and health. Indoor Air 2001; 11(1):10–25.

132. Leinster P, Raw G, Thomson N, Leaman A, Whitehead C. A modular longitudinal approach to the investigation of sick building syndrome. In: Walkinshaw DJ, ed. Proceedings of the Fifth International Conference on Indoor Air Quality and Climate, Toronto, July 29–August 3, 1990. Vol 1. Toronto: Canadian Mortgage and Housing, 1990:287–293.

133. Raw GJ, Roys MS, Whitehead C. Sick building syndrome: cleanliness is next to healthiness. Indoor Air 1993; 3:237–245.

134. Horvath EP, Anderson H, Pierce WE, Hanrahan L, Wendlick JD. Effects of formaldehyde on the mucous membranes and lungs: a study of an industrial population. JAMA 1984; 259(5):701–707.

135. Main DM, Hogan TJ. Health effects of low level exposure to formaldehyde. J Occup Med 1983; 25(12):896–900.

136. De Bortoli M, Knoppel H, Peil A, Pecchio E, Schlitt H. Investigation on the contribution of volatile organic compounds to air quality complaints in office buildings of the European Parliament. In: Walkinshaw DJ, ed. Proceedings of Fifth International Conference on Indoor Air Quality and Climate, Toronto, July 29–August 3, 1990: 695–700.

137. Ahlstrom R, Berglund B, Lindvall T, Berglund V. Formaldehyde odor and its interaction with the air of a sick building. Environ Int 1986; 12:289–295.

138. Hempel-Jorgenssen A, Kjaergaard SK, Molhave L. Eye irritation in humans exposed to formaldehyde. The Seventh International Conference on Indoor Air Quality and Climate. Indoor Air 1996; 325–330.

139. Faust HS, Brilliant LB. Is the diagnosis of 'mass hysteria' an excuse for incomplete investigation of low level environmental contamination? J Occup Med 1981; 23:22–26.

140. Robertson AS, Burge PS, Hedge A, et al. Comparison of health problems related to work and environmental measurements in two office buildings with different ventilation systems. Brit Med J 1985; 291:373–376.

141. Chappell SB, Parker R. Smoking and carbon monoxide levels in enclosed public places in New Brunswick. Can J Public Health 1977; 68:159–161.

142. Dhala A, Pinsker K, Prezant DJ. Respiratory health consequences of environmental tobacco smoke. Med Clin North Am 2004; 88(6):1535–1552, xi.

143. Surgeon General. The health consequences of involuntary smoking, 1986.

144. Molfino NA, Wright SC, Katz I, et al. Effect of low concentrations of ozone on inhaled allergen responses in asthmatic subjects. Lancet 1991; 338:199–203.

145. Finnegan MJ, Pickering CAC, Burge PS. The sick building syndrome: prevalence studies. Br Med J 1984; 289:1573–1575.

146. Hedge A. Evidence of a relationship between office design and self-reports of ill health among office workers in the United Kingdom. J Arch Plan Res 1984; 1:163–174.

147. Skov P, Valjorn O. Danish Indoor Climate Study Group. The "sick" building syndrome in the office environment: the Danish Town Hall study. Environ Int 1987; 13:339–349.

148. Smedje G, Norback D, Edling C. Subjective indoor air quality in schools in relation to exposure. Indoor Air 1997; 7:143–150.

149. Vincent D, Annesi I, Festy B, Lambrozo J. Ventilation system, indoor air quality, and health outcomes in parisian modern office workers. Environ Res 1997; 75:100–112.

150. Wålinder R, Norbäck D, Wieslander G, Smedje G, Erwall C, Venge P. Nasal patency and biomarkers in nasal lavage-the significance of air exchange rate and type of ventilation in schools. Int Arch Occup Environ Health 1998; 71:479–486.

151. Wålinder R, Norbäck D, Wieslander G, Smedje G, Erwall C. Nasal congestion in relation to low air exchange rate in schools. Acta Otolaryngol (Stockh) 1997; 117:724–727.

152. Costa MFB, Brickus LSR. Effect of ventilation systems on prevalence of symptoms associated with "Sick Buildings" in Brazilian commercial establishments. Arch Environ Health 2000; 55(4):279–283.

153. Liddament MW. A review of ventilation and the quality of ventilation air. Indoor Air 2000; 10:193–199.

154. Molhave L, Thorsen M. A model for investigations of ventilation systems as sources for volatile organic compounds in indoor climate. Atmos Environ 1991; 25A(2):241–249.

155. Bluyssen PM, Fernandes EO, Groes L, et al. European Indoor Air Quality Audit Project in 56 office buildings. Indoor Air 1996; 6:221–238.

156. Morey PR, Jenkins BA. What are the typical concentrations of fungi, total volatile organic compounds, and nitrogen dioxide in an office environment? In: ASHRAE, ed. IAQ '89–The Human Equation: Health and Comfort. Atlanta, GA: American Society of Heating Refrigeration and Air-conditioning Engineers, 1989:67–71.

157. Schneider T, Nielson O, Bredsdorff P, Linde P. Dust in buildings with man-made mineral fiber ceiling boards. Scand J Work Environ Health 1990; 16:434–439.

158. Neumeister HG, Moritz M, Schleibinger H, Martiny H. Investigation of allergic potential induced by fungi on air filters of HVAC systems. In: Yoshizawa S, ed. Tokyo: Organizing Comm of 7th Int Conf of Indoor Air Quality and Climate, 1996:125–130.

159. Menzies D, Pasztor J, Rand T, Bourbeau J. Germicidal ultraviolet irradiation in air conditioning systems: effect on office worker health and wellbeing: a pilot study. Occup Environ Med 1999; 56:397–402.

160. NIOSH. Outbreaks of respiratory illness among employees in large office buildings– Tennessee, District of Columbia. J Immunol 1984; 33:506–508.

161. Baur X, Richter G, Pethran A, Czuppon AB, Schwaiblmair M. Increased prevalence of IgG-induced sensitization and hypersensitivity pneumonitis (humidifier lung) in non-smokers exposed to aerosols of a contaminated air conditioner. Respiration 1992; 59:211–214.

162. Glick TH, Gregg MB, Berman B, Mallison G, Rhodes WW, Kassanoff I. An epidemic of unknown etiology in a health department: I. Clinical and epidemiologic aspects. Am J Epidemiol 1978; 107(2):149–160.

163. Ruutu P, Valtonen V, Tiitanen L, et al. An outbreak of invasive aspergillosis in a haematologic unit. Scand J Infect Disease 1987; 19:347–351.

164. Mamolen M, Lewis DM, Blanchet MA, Satink FJ, Vogt RL. Investigation of an outbreak of "humidifier fever" in a print shop. Am J Ind Med 1993; 23:483–490.

165. Edwards HG. Microbial and immunological investigations and remedial action after an outbreak of humidifier fever. Br J Ind Med 1980; 37:55–62.

166. Kateman E, Heederik D, Pal TM, Smeets M, Smid T, Spitteler M. Relationship of airborne microorganisms with the lung function and leucocyte levels of workers with a history of humidifier fever. Scand J Work Environ Health 1990; 16:428–433.

167. Pertti P. Impurities in ventilation ducts. ASHRAE 1994:89–93.

168. Jarvis BB, Croft WA, Yatawara CS. Airborne outbreak of trichothecene toxicosis. Atmos Environ 1986; 20(3):549–552.

169. Foarde KK, VanOsdell DW, Chang CS. Evaluation of fungal growth on fiberglass duct materials for various moisture, soil, use, and temperature conditions. Indoor Air 1995; 5:1–10.

170. Zweers T, Skov P, Valbjorn O, Molhave L. The effect of ventilation and air pollution on perceived indoor air quality in five town halls. Energy Buildings 1990; 14:175–181.

171. Jaakkola JJK, Heinonen OP, Seppanen O. Mechanical ventilation in office buildings and the sick building syndrome. An experimental and epidemiological study. Indoor Air 1991; 2:111–121.

172. Ruotsalainen R, Jaakkola N, Jaakkola JJK. Ventilation rate as a determinant of symptoms and perceived odors among workers in daycare centers. Environ Int 1994; 20(6):731–737.

173. Nordstrom K, Norback D, Akselsson R. Influence of indoor air quality and personal factors on the sick building syndrome (SBS) in Swedish geriatric hospitals. Occup Environ Med 1995; 52:170–176.

174. Hedge A, Erickson WA, Rubin G. Individual and occupational correlates of the sick building syndrome. Indoor Air 1995; 5:10–21.

175. Nelson NA, Kaufman JD, Burt J, Karr C. Health symptoms and the work environment in four nonproblem United States office buildings. Scand J Work Environ Health 1995; 21:51–59.

176. Niven RMcL, Fletcher AM, Pickering CAC, et al. Building sickness syndrome in healthy and unhealthy buildings: an epidemiological and environmental assessment with cluster analysis. Occup Environ Med 2000; 57:627–634.

177. Seppanen OA, Fisk WJ, Mendell MJ. Association of ventilation rates and CO_2 concentrations with health and other responses in commercial and institutional buildings. Indoor Air 1999; 9:226–252.

178. Øie L, Nafstad P, Botten G, Magnus P, Jaakkola JJK. Ventilation in homes and bronchial obstruction in young children. Epidemiology 1999; 10(3):294–299.

179. Jaakkola JJK, Tuomaala P, Seppanen O. Air recirculation and sick building syndrome: a blinded crossover trial. Am J Public Health 1994; 84:422–428.

180. Wargocki P, Wyon DP, Sundell J, Clausen G, Fanger PO. The effects of outdoor air supply rate in an office on perceived air quality, sick building syndrome (SBS) symptoms and productivity. Indoor Air 2000; 10:222–236.

181. Scheff PA, Paulius VK, Huang SW, Conroy LM. Indoor air quality in a middle school, Part 1: use of CO_2 as a tracer for effective ventilation. Appl Occup Environ Hyg 2000; 15(11):824–834.

182. Norback D. Subjective indoor air quality in schools–the influence of high room temperature, carpeting, fleecy wall materials and volatile organic compounds (VOC). Indoor Air 1995; 5:237–246.

183. Berardi BM, Leoni E, Marchesini B, Cascella D, Raffi GB. Indoor climate and air quality in new offices: effects of a reduced air-exchange rate. Int Arch Occup Environ Health 1991; 63:233–239.

184. Jankovie JT, Ihle R, Vick DO. Occupant generated carbon dioxide as a measure of dilution ventilation efficiency. Am Ind Hyg Assoc J 1996; 57:756–759.

185. Pearson ML, Jereb JA, Frieden TR, Crawford JT. Nosocomial transmission of multidrug resistant *Mycobacterium tuberculosis*: a risk to patients and health care workers. Ann Intern Med 1992; 117(3):191–196.

186. Menzies RI, Schwartzman K, Loo V, Pasztor J. Measuring ventilation of patient care areas in hospitals: description of a new protocol. Am J Respir Crit Care Med 1995; 152:1992–1999.

187. Mudarri DH. Potential correction factors for interpreting CO_2 measurements in building. ASHRAE 1997; 106:244–255.

188. Persily AK, Axley J. Measuring airflow rates with pulse tracer techniques. Am Soc Testing Mater 2002:31–51.

189. Lindberg PR. Improving hospital ventilation systems for tuberculosis infection control. In: Tomasik KM, ed. Plant Technology and Safety Management Series. Oakbrook Terrace, Illinois: Joint Commission on Accreditation of Healthcare Organizations, 1993:19–23.

190. Tamblyn RT. Healthy building manual: systems, parameters, problems, and solutions. Ottawa: Energy, Mines, and Resources, 1988.

191. Samet JM, Marbury MC, Spengler JD. Health effects and sources of indoor air pollution. Am Rev Resp Dis 1988; 137:221–242.

192. Morey P. Mold Growth in buildings: removal and prevention. IAQ 1996; 2:27–36.

193. Johanning E, Morey P, Jarvis B. Clinical-epidemiological investigation of health effects caused by *Stachybotrys atra* building contamination. Proc Indoor Air 1993; 1:225–230.

194. Menzies RI, Tamblyn RM, Nunes F, Leduc J, Pasztor J, Tamblyn RT. Varying ventilation conditions to provide a more complete assessment of building HVAC operation and indoor air quality. In: Jaakkola JJK, Ilmarinen R, Seppanen O, eds. Indoor Air '93–Proceedings of the Sixth International Conference on Indoor Air Quality and Climate. Vol. 6. Finland: Helsinki, 1993:551–556.

195. Raw GJ, Roys MS, Leaman A. Further findings from the office environment survey: productivity? In: Walkinshaw DJ, ed. Indoor Air '90–Proceedings of the Fifth International Conference on Indoor Air Quality Climate. Toronto, Ontario, Canada. Canadian Mortgage and Housing Commission, 1990:231–236.

196. Preller L, Zweers T, Brunekreef B, Boleij JSM. Sick leave due to work-related health complaints among office workers in the Netherlands. In: Walkinshaw DJ, ed. Indoor Air '90–Proceedings of the Fifth International Conference on Indoor Air Quality and Climate. Toronto, Ontario, Canada. Toronto, Ontario, Canada: Canadian Mortgage and Housing Commission, 1990:227–230.

197. Kroner W, Stark-Martin JA, Willemain T. Rensselaer's West Bend Mutual Study: Using Advanced Office Technology to Increase Productivity. Troy, New York: Rensselaer Polytechnic Inst., 1994.

198. Menzies D, Pasztor J, Nunes F, Leduc J, Chan C. Effect of a new ventilation system on health and well-being of office workers. Arch Environ Health 1997; 52(5):360–67.

199. Cain WS, Cometto-Muniz JE. Sensory irritation potency of VOCs measured through nasal localization thresholds. In: Yoshizawa S, editor. IAQ 96 – The Seventh International Conference on Indoor Climate and Air Quality. Nagoya: Organizing Comm. 7th Int Conf of Indoor Air Quality and Climate, 1996:167–172.

200. Bascom R, Bromberg PA, Costa DA, et al. Committee of the Environmental and Occupational Health Assembly of the American Thoracic Society. Health effects of outdoor air pollution. Am J Respir Crit Care Med 1996; 153:3–50.

201. Molhave L, Liu Z, Jorgensen AH, Pedersen OF, Kjaergaard SK. Sensory and physiological effects on humans of combined exposures to air temperatures and volatile organic compounds. Indoor Air 1993; 3:155–169.

202. Burge HA. Bioaerosols: prevalence and health effects in the indoor environment. J Allergy Clin Immun 1990; 86(5):687–701.

31
Upper Airways Involvement

David C. Christiani
*Department of Environmental Health, Harvard School of Public Health, and
Department of Medicine, Massachusetts General Hospital/Harvard Medical School,
Boston, Massachusetts, U.S.A.*

Jean-Luc Malo
*Department of Chest Medicine, Université de Montréal and Sacré-Cœur Hospital,
Montreal, Quebec, Canada*

Andrea Siracusa
Department of Clinical and Experimental Medicine, University of Perugia, Perugia, Italy

INTRODUCTION—DEFINITION

In the working environment, exposures may result in inflammation of the upper airways: the nasal passages, nasopharynx, sinus, and larynx. In this chapter, the nasal passages are emphasized because of (i) the critical role of the nose in respiratory defenses; (ii) the growing body of epidemiologic and clinical data available on effects of airborne contaminants on the nose; and (iii) the recent concept of "united airways," that is, airway mucosa forms a continuum from the nose to the lower bronchi (1). Moreover, changes in the inflammatory status of the upper airways can effect asthma, and the vice-versa worsening of asthma has a deleterious effect on rhinitis (2,3). The nasal mucosa can therefore be used as a surrogate to study the inflammatory response in the airways.

The nasal passage serves several critical functions. It is the first of the respiratory mucosa to encounter inhaled particles, gases, vapors, and fumes (4). It warms and humidifies inhaled air and filters large particles, including many allergens. It is the primary absorptive surface for water-soluble gases, such as sulfur dioxide. It removes substantial quantities of even less soluble gases, such as ozone. Obstruction of the nasal passages may result in a change from nasal to oral respiration. Oral breathing bypasses the filtering functions of the nose, increasing the hazard to the lower airways and the lung.

Rhinitis is defined as inflammation of the nasal mucosa, because of a specific immune reaction or a direct irritant effect. As for occupational asthma (OA), rhinitis can occur due to a "sensitizing" mechanism or following acute exposure to high concentrations of an irritant material.

EXPOSURES

A variety of occupational exposures have been associated with rhinitis. Experimental exposures to ozone have demonstrated neutrophilia in nasal lavagate (5). This observation was confirmed in studies of children exposed to ambient ozone (6). Exposure to fuel oil ash among boilermakers resulted in a significant increase in nasal neutrophils among nonsmokers, but not smokers, although smokers had high baseline neutrophil concentrations (7). Agricultural exposures such as grain dust cause rhinitis and peripheral neutrophilia (8), and grain dust extracts and endotoxin result in upper and lower respiratory tract inflammation (9). Other agents and processes likely to cause occupational rhinitis (OR) include, but are not limited to: livestock breeding; feed manufacture and handling; wood dust; cotton, flax, and hemp processing; silicate dust; metal salts; pollens; gases (e.g., nitric oxide, ammonia, hydrogen sulfide, chlorine); insect parts; fungi and insecticides; bakers' flour; isocyanates; methacrylates; diacrylate; vegetables such as soybeans and garlic; fruit mites (citrus mite); coffee beans; pulp and paper mill exposures; wool processing; rice field harvesting; swine confinement exposure; working in the zoo and greenhouse; laboratory animal exposures; proteases; latex product (e.g., gloves) exposure; tobacco leaf processing; xerographic toner exposure; milk protein exposure; hairdressing; furniture making; and compost and waste handling.

Many agents inducing OA with a latency period, particularly those that are of high molecular weight (protein-derived), can cause rhinoconjunctivitis symptoms (10). In the latter situation, both conditions, OA and OR, are immunoglobin (Ig) E–mediated. Upper airway inflammation can occur after exposure to high concentrations of irritant materials (11).

CLINICAL FEATURES

Intermittent or persistent rhinorrhea may be caused by a variety of clinical disorders including allergic rhinitis and irritant rhinitis. Evaluation of a patient with upper airway symptoms consists of a careful study of history and physical examination. History is the single most important tool for evaluation of the upper respiratory tract. Temporal patterns of irritation, congestion, rhinorrhea, or sneezing may suggest likely causes. A symptom diary may be useful to clarify these patterns. History may also suggest concomitant symptoms of conjunctivitis and reactive airways or asthma, such as paroxysmal cough, episodic chest tightness, exertional or nocturnal wheeze or dyspnea.

Rhinitis caused by sensitization to airborne agents is characterized by rhinorrhea, sneezing, nasal obstruction, lacrimation, and occasionally, pharyngeal itching. Episodic symptoms are the hallmark of allergic rhinitis. In addition to the nasal symptoms, there may be conjunctival congestion and edema. Swelling of the nasal turbinates and mucosa with obstruction of the sinus ostia and eustachian tubes can precipitate secondary infections of the sinus and middle ear. The latter is more common in perennial (vs. seasonal) rhinitis. Washings, swabs or biopsy of the mucosa usually reveals eosinophils, but some polymorphonuclear leukocytes are also present.

There is suggestion documented in apprentices exposed to laboratory animals and who were followed prospectively that the timing of occurrence of nasoconjunctival symptoms is first characterized by an IgE-mediated type of reaction and by symptoms of sneezing, rhinorrhea, and itchy eyes followed, at a later stage in the evolution of the disease, by a more predominant congestive reaction with nasal obstruction (12).

Irritant rhinitis is often found when sensitizers are not identified or may be caused by exposure to irritants in the working environment. Nasal washings and biopsy usually reveal a predominant polymorphonuclear response. Nasal symptoms are common in bakers exposed to flour, having been documented in 16% of apprentices after one to two years of exposure to flour, but the association of symptoms with evidence of sensitization to a flour-derived allergen is ten times less common (13). There is evidence that air pollutants can initiate allergic responses among atopic individuals (14).

If the history is suggestive of a sensitized response, a referral for allergy skin tests is indicated. Another approach is to obtain a multi-allergen radioallergosorbent test (RAST), with referral for skin testing if the RAST is positive.

ASSESSMENT OF NASAL RESPONSES

Common symptoms of rhinitis and OR include rhinorrhea, nasal obstruction, and sneezing. The prevalence of OR tends to be overestimated if based only upon symptoms because of the information bias. Confirmation of OR requires response to the possible causal agent during the usual work activity or by means of an occupational nasal challenge test (ONCT). Response assessment is based on symptoms and objective methods such as assessing nasal congestion and measuring secretions as reviewed by Siracusa et al. (15) and Schumacher (16).

Assessing Congestion

Rhinomanometry and acoustic rhinometry are the best methods for assessing nasal obstruction and congestion. Rhinomanometry is widely used in clinical practice to assess anatomic variation, to quantify the effects of therapy on nasal obstruction, and to measure pathophysiological responses such as allergies. There are three major types of rhinomanometry: anterior active rhinomanometry, posterior active rhinomanometry, and passive rhinomanometry. "Active" tests are done while subjects voluntarily inhale or exhale through the manometer. In "passive" tests air is blown into the subject's nose. In anterior active rhinomanometry the tube is inserted into the nostrils, while in posterior rhinomanometry the tube is placed near the pharynx through the mouth. Rhinomanometry has also been applied to assess environmental and occupational factors causing change in nasal flow or resistance. Resistance is expressed as the pressure difference divided by flow ($R = dP/V$), which can be measured simultaneously. Increased nasal airway resistance was demonstrated by means of rhinomanometry in workers exposed to formaldehyde (17) and chlorine (18). Manometry is useful and easy, but has some limitations: the subject's degree of cooperation, collapse of nasal alae, relatively high variability, and unsatisfactory correlation with symptoms. It is sometimes not sensitive to pathology in some parts of the nasal cavity.

Acoustic rhinometry utilizes sound reflection to obtain an area–distance curve from the nostril through the nasal cavity. It is more accurate and reliable than rhinomanometry in measuring patency in terms of anatomical area, but it is based on assumptions of no turbulence, no viscous loss of acoustic energy, no influence by the contralateral cavity and wall rigidity. Although all these assumptions are not actually true, and tend to limit interpretation, acoustic rhinometry correlates well with computed tomography (CT) measurements. However, in workers exposed to soft paper or wood dusts there was no correlation between self-reported nasal obstruction and acoustic rhinometry findings (19,20). Acoustic rhinometry is also limited by its inaccuracy in the presence of severe nasal obstruction.

Nasal peak flow can be measured in forced nasal inhalation or exhalation and is of particular interest in occupational medicine because measurements can be repeated, independently by the subject, many times a day during the workdays to detect early reversible signs of nasal obstruction (21). Peak nasal expiratory flow (PNEF) has been quantified in many studies, and recently peak nasal inspiratory flow (PNIF) measurement has also been investigated, with divergent results (19,22–24). PNEF and PNIF are variably associated with nasal obstruction (19,24–27) and are less sensitive than rhinomanometry in detecting changes in nasal patency (27,28). However, measuring PNEF and PNIF is simple and inexpensive, making them useful tests for assessing nasal workplace disorders as measurements can be performed serially throughout the working day (22,23,25). PNIF has also been used in nasal challenge tests with good results (29,30).

Measuring Secretions

Nasal secretions are analyzed before and after ONCT for markers of inflammation, mediators, and cells. Secretions can also be weighed using tissue papers or plastic wrap, filter paper or disk methods, or plastic suction tips (15,31). Weighing nasal secretion is helpful in cases of abundant secretion, such as after high-dose allergen challenges. However, secretions have seldom been measured in occupational studies since the typically low exposure levels in ONCTs do not usually increase nasal secretions significantly enough for an appreciable weight difference.

BIOCHEMICAL MARKERS OF INFLAMMATORY AND IMMUNE RESPONSES

Nasal lavage has been used to collect secretions and assess the inflammatory response of the upper airways to allergens and irritants (5,14,32–37). The technique is simple, though not yet standardized. The most common method, briefly described, is, while seated, subjects tilt their heads backwards to 45°. Using a needleless syringe, 5 mL of warm (37°C) sterile phosphate buffered saline (without calcium or magnesium) is instilled into the nostril. The saline is retained for 10 seconds, and then allowed to drain passively for 30 seconds into a sterile specimen cup. The volume of lavage fluid recovered is recorded and used to adjust cell counts. Cells are counted on a hemocytometer and differential counts done on slides prepared by cytospin and stained with Wright-Giemsa. Although the method is not yet standardized, studies have indicated that intraindividual variability in polymorphonuclear neutrophils (PMN) counts is less than interindividual variability, supporting utility in epidemiological studies (38). Nasal secretions can also be analyzed for biochemical components like protein, albumin, histamine, IgE, antioxidants, and complement (38). The intra-individual variability and kinetics of these constituents in nasal fluid is as yet unknown. Although this type of challenge can be used with occupational challenges that can be diluted, it cannot be performed for occupational agents of the low-molecular-weight type, which are usually chemicals.

Table 1 Biomarkers of NAL with Potential Use in Environmental Studies

Marker	Indication
PMNs	Inflammatory response
Protein, albumin	Permeability
Eosinophils, mast cells, histamine, tryptase, kinins	Allergic response
PGD2, TAME-esterase, serotonin	Mast cell degranulation/allergic response
IgE	Allergic response
Eicosanoids, substance P, antioxidants, kallikrein, kinins, cytokines, C5a, C3a	Inflammatory/allergic

Abbreviations: NAL, nasal lavage; PGD2, prostaglandin D2; TAME, *N*-alpha-*p*-tosyl-L-arginine methyl ester; PMNs, polymorphonuclear neutrophils.
Source: From Ref. 35.

Inflammatory and immune responses of the upper airways are mostly studied to understand the pathophysiology of allergic and nonallergic rhinitis. Basic study methodology is to challenge with specific antigen or nonspecific agent such as methacholine and then collect nasal secretions to analyze the cellular and biochemical components of the secretion.

Nasal lavage has been the mainstay of collecting nasal secretion to assess inflammatory and immune responses of the upper airways to allergen or irritants in most of the recent studies. Biochemical analysis of various mediators in nasal secretions and/or morphologic analysis of cellular components are performed on the lavage fluid, after centrifugation, if needed. Measurements of molecular markers, such as cytokines, myeloperoxidase, and eosinophillic cationic protein have been measured in the nasal lavage of occupationally exposed populations (37). The brush method can be used mainly to harvest cells (39). Other techniques such as nasal blowing, smears, and imprints were also used to collect the specimen in some studies. Those methods are reviewed by Pipkorn and Karlsson (40).

Nasal secretions originate from several sources, such as transudated serum components including albumin and other proteins, locally synthesized proteins including enzymes and surface IgA, mucous glycoprotein derived from the glandular elements, and chemical mediators and other products from various cells including plasma cells, mast cells, basophils, and epithelial cells. Many studies assessed cellular or biochemical components of nasal lavage fluid before and after challenge testing using methacholine or specific allergens (41,42).

Nasal challenge of sensitive individuals with antigen or cold dry air increases the levels of histamine, *N*-alpha-*p*-tosyl-L-arginine methyl ester-esterase activity, prostaglandin D2, and kinins in nasal lavage fluid (43). These mediators originate from the influx of activated cells such as eosinophils, neutrophils, mast cells, and basophils. Neutrophils represent the greatest number of infiltrating cells in the late phase reaction.

The interpretation of the markers is well summarized by Koren and Delvin (35) and reproduced in Table 1. Nasal lavage studies in subjects exposed to agricultural dusts are limited. One study reported elevated nasal PMN counts in farmers exposed to sorghum dust (43). Another study, a controlled human-exposure experiment, reported elevated lymphocytes in subjects exposed to dusts from corn and soybean as well as for endotoxin (9). In one study, challenges were performed in 15 subjects with OA (eight due to high-molecular-weight agents—flour and guar gum—and seven due to isocyanates) on two occasions, two to four weeks apart in a random fashion (44). On one occasion, they inhaled through the nose and on the other, through the mouth. The authors showed that inhaling through the mouth and through the nose (i) yielded similar asthmatic responses, and (ii) more than doubled the peak nasal symptoms and nasal resistance when the maximum daily response was compared with the prechallenge results. This increase occurred on the days of inhalational challenges through the mouth and through the nose, and is explained by backflow of air into the upper airways on the day of challenge through the mouth. There were some significant, though low magnitude, responses assessed by nasal lavage in terms of cells and mediators, again with no differences between the days of challenges through the mouth and through the nose. Nasal challenge test has been shown by others to be useful in the diagnosis of rhinitis accompanying OA to flour (45). A study by Gorski et al. (45) included specific challenges through the nose by the nasal pool method in which a concentrated solution of flour is inserted into the nostril. In 100 subjects with OA and rhinitis caused by flour, the authors documented a significant increase in symptoms as well as in the cellular and mediator influx after the nasal challenge. As for nasal challenges performed with common inhalants, this study used concentrations that are more elevated than what occurs with natural exposure, therefore questioning the interpretation of findings. However, the authors found that 40 controls, either atopic subjects not sensitized to flour or healthy subjects, did not show significant changes after comparable challenges.

PATHOGENESIS

The pathogenesis and pathology of OR has seldom been investigated. Like OA, OR can be divided into two types:

1. The immunological, with onset after a latency period, which includes (a) IgE-mediated (allergic) OR and (b) non-IgE–mediated (nonallergic) OR; and
2. The nonimmunological, without a latency period, which includes (a) irritant-induced OR or (b) reactive upper airways dysfunction syndrome (RUDS).

The nasal mucosa is covered by a thin layer of mucus, which carries pollutants and is moved back towards the pharynx by the cilia. Most particles greater than 5 μm in size are deposited on the mucus layer and transported from the nose to the pharynx within 15 to 30 minutes. In normal subjects airway mucosa is similar in the nose and in the bronchi. Structurally, the nasal mucosa is a pseudostratified epithelium with columnar, ciliated cells, lining the basement membrane and the *lamina propria* or submucosa (46,47). Basal cells, goblet cells, and ciliated and nonciliated columnar cells are found within the epithelium, and Langerhans cells, T and B lymphocytes, macrophages, mast cells, and fibroblasts are detected in the nasal mucosa of normal subjects (46,47).

Allergic OR is caused by most high- and several low-molecular-weight sensitizers (15). The mechanism of allergic OR is the same as that of allergic rhinitis and asthma. When the IgE-mediated allergic reaction occurs, mast cell degranulation with a release of histamine and other proinflammatory mediators is followed by T lymphocyte activation, cytokine release, and adhesion molecule expression. Consequently, eosinophils and some mast cells, basophils, and CD4$^+$ T lymphocytes are recruited into the nasal epithelium and submucosa (46–49). While T lymphocytes orchestrate the allergic response through cytokine production, mast cells mediate the immediate response to the allergen, and eosinophils have an important role in the inflammatory process in allergic rhinitis (46).

Nonallergic OR is caused by several low-molecular-weight sensitizers (15). Although its mechanism is unknown and airway mucosa pathology is similar in allergic and nonallergic OA, we can presume that nasal mucosa inflammation is the same in allergic and nonallergic OR.

Irritant-induced OR or RUDS is the nonimmunological type of OR. It may occur after single or multiple episodes of exposure to irritants (11,50). Some irritants, such as formaldehyde and glutaraldehyde, may also act as sensitizers. The nasal pathology of RUDS and immunological OR are different, as the former is characterized by epithelium desquamation, glandular hyperplasia, lymphocyte infiltrates, and peripheral nerve fiber proliferation, without mast cell degranulation (18,51). Irritants have been hypothesized to damage and/or stimulate nasal epithelial cells and neurons, leading to synthesis of proinflammatory mediators and neuromediators (52).

Irritants are known to interact with allergic rhinitis. They exert a stronger effect in subjects with seasonal allergic rhinitis than in normal subjects (53), have a "priming" effect on nasal responsiveness to allergen challenge (54), and can act as adjuvants to initial sensitization (55).

OCCURRENCE AND DETERMINANTS

Occupational rhinoconjunctivitis is a frequent condition, two to three times more common than OA, especially in subjects exposed to high-molecular-weight agents (15,56). In a summary article that provides information on prevalence rates from many studies, Siracusa et al. (15) report that the ratios of rhinitis to asthma cases were most often above one and ratios up to 10 are quoted. An incidence of rhinoconjunctivitis close to 10% has been documented in 387 animal-health apprentices followed for almost four years (12). Gautrin et al. (57) report that the incidence density of occupational rhino-conjunctivitis in laboratory animal workers (defined by skin sensitization to one or the other of several animal-derived antigens and symptoms) was 5.7, whereas the comparable figure for OA was 2.7. The frequency of occupational rhinoconjunctivitis is 100% in subjects with OA due to high-molecular-weight agents and close to 50% in the case of asthma caused by low-molecular-weight agents in subjects referred for possible OA (10). As for OA due to high-molecular-weight agents, the degree of exposure and atopy are the determinants for the presence of rhinoconjunctivitis and the role of smoking is controversial (15). In the cohort previously quoted (12), determinants of the appearance of rhinoconjunctivitis were sensitization to grass pollens as well as various nasal and bronchial symptoms at the pre-exposure assessment.

NATURAL HISTORY

In the case of high-molecular-weight agents, symptoms of rhinoconjunctivitis often precede the onset of asthmatic symptoms whereas they seem to occur at the same time in the case of low-molecular-weight agents (10). However, it has been estimated that the positive predictive value of rhinoconjunctivitis for the development of OA is close to 30% only (57). Rhinoconjunctivits invariably precedes or accompanies

OA in the case of subjects exposed to laboratory animals (58). The incidence of rhinoconjunctivits is higher in the first two years after starting exposure to laboratory animals (57). Cullinan et al. (59) published figures of 12 months and 18 months for the median intervals for the onset of nasal and chest symptoms, respectively, in workers also exposed to rats. In the case of RUDS that occurs after acute inhalation of an agent at high concentration, symptoms are acute on the occasion of exposure to an irritant material (11). These are characterized by acute burning of the upper airways, followed by sneezing, secretions, and congestion. Anosmia or hyposmia may be a long-term consequence of such accidental inhalational exposures, especially if they are repeated. Symptoms of chronic rhinitis that occur in nearly 50% of subjects who suffer repeated acute inhalations of chlorine (puffs), are related to the number of accidental inhalations and are commonly associated with lower respiratory symptoms and increased bronchial responsiveness (60).

MANAGEMENT

The first line approach to managing OR is implementation of environmental measures designed to reduce or eliminate exposure to the agent causing the disease. These strategies reduce occupational exposure and successfully decrease occupational symptoms in case of exposure to latex (61) and to the proteolytic enzymes used in the manufacture of detergents (62). Steps include modifying the workplace, for example, by providing adequate ventilation and aspiration of pollutants, using less hazardous materials, and creating closed-circuit manufacturing processes. Workers should be supplied with personal protective equipment, e.g., filtering masks. Subjects affected by rhinitis symptoms due to sensitization to high-molecular-weight agents may continue to work in the same environment, provided that they have no asthma symptoms and that they take appropriate medications. These subjects should be followed up closely to ensure that they do not develop asthma or bronchial hyperresponsiveness. On the other hand, patients with OR associated with OA, anaphylaxis, etc. need to be removed from exposure to the sensitizing agent or irritants (63).

Medication for OR is similar to what is used for other types of rhinitis. Although antihistamines are helpful, their side effect—sedation—may create a workplace hazard (64) and lead to an increase in occupational injuries (65). This risk is avoided with second- and third-generation "non-sedating" antihistamines, which can be used by patients who need to be awake and alert at work (47). Corticosteroid nasal sprays effectively block the inflammatory cell influx. They should be taken regularly and will often obviate the need for antihistamines. Antihistamine nasal sprays are also effective and can be used on an as-needed basis. Nasal sprays containing anticholinergic agents, such as ipratropium bromide, might reduce anterior or posterior discharge (47,66). Intranasal decongestants are not recommended for use because they can induce rhinitis medicamentosa, which is iatrogenic nasal vasodilatation and obstruction caused by overuse of topical sympathomimetics. The role of leukotriene inhibitors, such as montelukast, in the treatment of OR remains unclear.

FUTURE RESEARCH

The development and application of new biologic markers for upper airway responses to workplace exposures will help define the prevalence, distribution, and impact of upper airway disease in the workforce. There is a pressing need for standardization of techniques such as nasal lavage and nasal airflow measurements. Molecular techniques to detect early inflammatory responses need to be developed and evaluated.

In addition to the development of techniques for evaluation of epidemiologic studies of upper airway responses, research must also focus on whether the upper airway responses to contaminants reflect or predict lower airway responses. Research should focus on whether conditions such as irritant rhinitis may be an early marker of chronic bronchitis and airflow obstruction. The methodology of nasal challenges with occupational agents, particularly low-molecular-weight agents that cannot be diluted in saline solutions, needs to be developed. Such a methodology would be very useful for diagnostic purposes in subjects with rhinitis but no asthmatic symptoms. Finally, it is known that rhinoconjunctivitis has a major influence on quality of life (67). The impact of occupational rhinoconjunctivitis on quality of life and various psychological and social outcomes needs to be examined.

REFERENCES

1. Vignola AM, Bousquet J. Rhinitis and asthma: a continuum of disease? Clin Exper Allergy 2001; 31:674–677.
2. Baraniuk JN. Mechanisms of rhinitis. Immunol Allergy Clin North Am 2000; 20: 245–264.
3. Bousquet J, Vignola AM, Demoly P. Links between rhinitis and asthma. Allergy 2003; 58:691–706.
4. Witek TJ. The nose as a target for adverse effects from the environment: applying advances in nasal physiologic measurements and mechanisms. Am J Ind Med 1993; 24:649–657.
5. Graham D, Henderson F, House D. Neutrophil influx measured in nasal lavages of humans exposed to ozone. Arch Environ Health 1988; 43:229–233.
6. Frischer TM, Kuehr J, Pulwitt A. Ambient ozone causes upper airways inflammation in children. Am Rev Respir Dis 1993; 148:961–964.
7. Hauser R, Elreedy S, Hoppin JA, Christiani DC. The upper airway response in workers exposed to fuel-oil ash: nasal lavage analysis. J Occup Env Med 1995; 52:353–358.
8. Von Essen S, OíNeill D, Robbin R. Grain sorghum dust inhalation at harvest causes nasal inflammation and peripheral blood neutrophilia. Am Rev Respir Dis 1993; 147:A528.
9. Clapp WD, Thorne PS, Frees KL, Zhang X, Lux CR, Schwartz DA. The effects of inhalation of grain dust extract and endotoxin on upper and lower airways. Chest 1993; 104:825–830.
10. Malo JL, Lemière C, Desjardins A, Cartier A. Prevalence and intensity of rhinoconjunctivitis in subjects with occupational asthma. Eur Respir J 1997; 10:1513–1515.
11. Meggs WJ. RADS and RUDS–The toxic induction of asthma and rhinitis. J Toxicol Clin Toxicol 1994; 32:487–501.
12. Rodier F, Gautrin D, Ghezzo H, Malo JL. Incidence of occupational rhinoconjunctivitis and risk factors in animal-health apprentices. J Allergy Clin Immunol 2003; 112: 1105–1111.
13. Gautrin D, Ghezzo H, Infante-Rivard C, Malo JL. Incidence and host determinants of work-related rhinoconjunctivitis in apprentice pastry-makers. Allergy 2002; 57:913–918.
14. Bascom R, Nacliero RM, Fitzgerald TK. Effect of ozone inhalation on the response to nasal challenge with antigen of allergic subjects. Am Rev Respir Dis 1990; 142:594–601.
15. Siracusa A, Desrosiers M, Marabini A. Epidemiology of occupational rhinitis: prevalence, aetiology and determinants. Clin Exp Allergy 2000; 30:1519–1534.

16. Schumacher MJ. Nasal congestion and airway obstruction: the validity of available objective and subjective measures. Curr Allergy Asthma Rep 2002; 2:245–251.
17. Giordano C, Siccardi E, Fedrighini B, et al. Nasal patency patterns observed during working hours in a group of technicians habitually exposed to formaldehyde. Acta Otorhinol Ital 1995; 15:335–344.
18. Shusterman D, Balmes J, Avila PC, Murphy MA, Matovinovic E. Chlorine inhalation produces nasal congestion in allergic rhinitis without mast cell degranulation. Eur Respir J 2003; 21:652–657.
19. Hellgren J, Eriksson C, Karlsson G, Hagberg S, Olin AC, Torén K. Nasal symptoms among workers exposed to soft paper dust. Int Arch Occup Environ Health 2001; 74:129–132.
20. Schlünssen V, Schaumburg I, Andersen NT, Sigsgaard T, Pedersen OF. Nasal patency is related to dust exposure in woodworkers. Occup Environ Med 2002; 59:23–29.
21. Cho SI, Hauser R, Christiani DC. Reproducibility of nasal peak inspiratory flow among healthy adults. Assessment of epidemiologic utility. Chest 1997; 112:1547–1553.
22. Åhman M, Söderman E. Serial nasal peak expiratory flow measurements in woodwork teachers. Int Arch Occup Environ Health 1996; 68:177–182.
23. Torén K, Hagberg S, Brisman J, Karlsson G. Nasal inflammation in pulp mill workers exposed to lime dust—Investigation before and after a reconstruction of the mill. Am J Resp Crit Care Med 1994; 149(part 2):A409.
24. Siracusa A, Pace M, Tacconi C, Sivestrelli A, Bussetti A. Prevalence of upper and lower respiratory symptoms in workers exposed to colophony and MBTS. J Allergy Clin Immunol 2004; 113(suppl 2):S61.
25. Frolund L, Madsen F, Mygind N, Nielsen NH, Svendsen UG, Weeke B. Comparison between different techniques for measuring nasal patency in a group of unselected patients. Acta Otolaryngol (Stockh) 1987; 104:175–179.
26. Fairley JW, Durham LH, Ell SR. Correlation of subjective sensation of nasal patency with nasal inspiratory peak flow rate. Clin Otolaryngol 1993; 18:19–22.
27. Clarke RW, Jones AS. The limitations of peak nasal flow measurement. Clin Otolaryngol 1994; 19:502–504.
28. Panagou P, Loukides S, Tsipra S, Syrigou K, Anastasakis C, Kalogeropoulos N. Evaluation of nasal patency: comparison of patient and clinician assessments with rhinomanometry. Acta Otolaryngol (Stockh) 1998; 118:847–851.
29. Miralles JC, Negro JM, Alonso JM, Garcia M, Sánchez-Gascón, Soriano J. Occupational rhinitis and bronchial asthma due to TBTU and HBTU sensitisation. J Invest Allergol Clin Immunol 2003; 13:133–134.
30. Miralles JC, Garcia-Sells J, Bartolome B, Negro JM. Occupational rhinitis and bronchial asthma due to artichoke (Cynara scolymus). Ann Allergy Asthma Immunol 2003; 91:92–95.
31. Pirilä T, Nuutinen J. Acoustic rhinometry, rhinomanometry and the amount of nasal secretion in the clinical monitoring of the nasal provocation test. Clin Exp Allergy 1998; 28:468–477.
32. Koren HS, Hatch GE, Graham DE. Nasal lavage as a tool in assessing acute inflammation in response to inhaled pollutants. Toxicology 1990; 60:15–25.
33. Graham DE, Koren HS. Biomarkers of inflammation in ozone-exposed humans. Am Rev Respir Dis 1990; 142:152–156.
34. Bascom R, Kulle T, Kagey-Sobotka A, Praud D. Upper respiratory-track environmental tobacco smoke sensitivity. Am Rev Respir Dis 1991; 143:1304–1311.
35. Koren HS, Devlin RB. Human upper respiratory-track responses to inhaled pollutants with emphasis on nasal lavage. Ann NY Acad Sci 1992; 641:215–224.
36. Koren HS, Graham DE, Devlin RB. Exposure of humans to a volatile organic mixture–III. Inflammatory response. Arch Env Health 1992; 47:39–44.
37. Woodin MA, Hauser R, Liu Y, et al. Molecular markers of acute upper airway inflammation in workers exposed to fuel-oil ash. Am J Respir Crit Care Med 1998; 158:182–187.

38. Hauser R, Garcia-Closas M, Kelsey K, Christiani DC. Variability of nasal lavage polymorphonuclear leukocyte counts in unexposed subjects: its potential utility for epidemiology. Arch Env Health 1994; 49:267–272.

39. Pipkorn U, Karlsson G, Enerback L. A brush method to harvest cells from the nasal mucosa for microscopic and biochemical analysis. J Immunol Meth 1988; 112:37–42.

40. Pipkorn U, Karlsson G. Methods for obtaining specimens from the nasal mucosa for morphological and biochemical analysis. Eur Respir J 1988; 1:856–862.

41. Shelhamer J, Marom Z, Michae K. The constituents of nasal secretion. Ear Nose Throat J 1984; 63:82–84.

42. Raphael GD, Druce HM, Baraniuk JN, Kaliner MA. Pathophysiology of rhinitis. 1. Assessment of the sources of protein in methacholine-induced nasal secretions. Am Rev Respir Dis 1988; 138:413–420.

43. Togias A, Naclerio RM, Proud D, et al. Studies on the allergic and nonallergic nasal inflammation. J Allergy Clin Immunol 1988; 81:782–790.

44. Desrosiers M, Nguyen B, Ghezzo H, Leblanc C, Malo JL. Nasal response in subjects undergoing challenges by inhaling occupational agents causing asthma through the nose and mouth. Allergy 1998; 53:840–848.

45. Gorski P, Krakowiak A, Pazdrak K, Palcynski C, Ruta U, Walusiak J. Nasal challenge test in the diagnosis of allergic respiratory diseases in subjects occupationally exposed to a high molecular allergen (flour). Occup Med 1998; 48:91–97.

46. Sobol SE, Christodoulopoulos P, Hamid QA. Inflammatory patterns of allergic and nonallergic rhinitis. Curr Allergy Asthma Rep 2001; 1:193–201.

47. Bousquet J, van Cauwenberge P, Khaltaev N. Organization in collaboration with the World Health. Allergic Rhinitis and Its Impact on Asthma. J Allergy Clin Immunol 2001; 108:S147–S334.

48. Kay AB. Allergy and allergic diseases. First of two parts. N Engl J Med 2001; 344:30–37.

49. Passalacqua G, Canonica GW. The asthma-rhinitis association: between the clinical hypothesis and the scientific theory. Curr Allergy Asthma Rep 2003; 3:191–193.

50. Shusterman D. Toxicology of nasal irritants. Curr Allergy Asthma Rep 2003; 3:258–265.

51. Meggs WJ. Hypothesis for induction and propagation of chemical sensitivity based on biopsy studies. Env Health Perspect 1997; 105:473–478.

52. Bachert C. Persistent rhinitis—allergic or nonallergic? Allergy 2004; 59(suppl 76):11–15.

53. Shusterman DJ, Murphy MA, Balmes JR. Subjects with seasonal allergic rhinitis and nonrhinitic subjects react differentially to nasal provocation with chlorine gas. J Allergy Clin Immunol 1998; 101:732–740.

54. Peden DB, Setzer R Woodrow, Devlin RB. Ozone exposure has both a priming effect on allergen-induced responses and an intrinsic inflammatory action in the nasal airways of perennially allergic asthmatics. J Am Respir Crit Care Med 1995; 151:1336–1345.

55. Diaz-Sanchez D, Garcia MP, Wang M, Jyrala M, Saxon A. Nasal challenge with diesel exhaust particles can induce sensitisation to a neoallergen in the human mucosa. J Allergy Clin Immunol 1999; 104:1183–1188.

56. Gautrin D, Ghezzo H, Infante-Rivard C, Malo J-L. Incidence and determinants of IgE-mediated sensitization in apprentices: a prospective study. Am J Respir Crit Care Med 2000; 162:1222–1228.

57. Gautrin D, Ghezzo H, Infante-Rivard C, Malo JL. Natural history of sensitization, symptoms and diseases in apprentices exposed to laboratory animals. Eur Respir J 2001; 17:904–908.

58. Gross NJ. Allergy to laboratory animals: epidemiologic, clinical, and physiologic aspects, and a trial of cromolyn in its management. J Allergy Clin Immunol 1980; 66:158–165.

59. Cullinan P, Cook A, Gordon S, et al. Allergen exposure, atopy and smoking as determinants of allergy to rats in a cohort of laboratory employees. Eur Respir J 1999; 13: 1139–1143.

60. Leroyer C, Malo JL, Girard D, Dufour JG, Gautrin D. Chronic rhinitis in workers at risk of RADS due to chlorine exposure. Occup Env Med 1999; 56:334–338.

61. Vandenplas O, Delwiche JP, Depelchin S, et al. Latex gloves with a lower protein content reduce bronchial reactions in subjects with occupational asthma caused by latex. Am J Respir Crit Care Med 1995; 151:887–891.

62. Pepys J, Wells ID, D'Souza MF, Greenberg M. Clinical and immunological responses to enzymes of *Bacillus subtilis* in factory workers and consumers. Clin Allergy 1973; 3: 143–160.

63. Dykewicz MS, Fineman S, Skoner DP. Diagnosis and management of rhinitis: complete guidelines of the joint task force on practice parameters in allergy, asthma and immunology. Ann Allergy Asthma Immunol 1998; 81:478–518.

64. Meltzer EO. Antihistamine- and decongestant-induced performance decrements. J Occup Med 1990; 32:327–334.

65. Hanrahan LP, Paramore LC. Aeroallergens, allergic rhinitis, and sedating antihistamines: risk factors for traumatic occupational injury and economic impact. Am J Ind Med 2003; 44:438–446.

66. Slavin RG. Occupational rhinitis. Ann Allergy Asthma Immunol 2003; 90(suppl):2–6.

67. Juniper EF. Quality of life in adults and children with asthma and rhinitis. Allergy 1997; 52:971–977.

32
Occupational Urticaria

C. G. Toby Mathias
Departments of Environmental Health and Dermatology, University of Cincinnati Medical Center and Group Health Associates, Cincinnati, Ohio, U.S.A.

Boris D. Lushniak
Office of Counterterrorism Policy and Planning, U.S. Food and Drug Administration, Rockville, Maryland, U.S.A.

INTRODUCTION

Many exposures in the workplace that can result in occupational asthma (OA) can also cause a variety of dermatological problems. These include irritant contact dermatitis, allergic contact dermatitis (type IV delayed hypersensitivity), and urticaria (type I immunologic and nonimmunologic). Urticaria will be discussed here because of its direct association with OA, in terms of both clinical coexistence and mechanistic similarities.

Urticaria is defined as the transient appearance of elevated, erythematous pruritic wheals or serpiginous exanthem, usually surrounded by an area of erythema. In addition, areas of macular erythema or erythematous papules may also be present. These skin lesions appear and peak in minutes to hours after the etiologic exposure, and individual lesions usually disappear within 24 hours. Urticarial lesions usually involve the trunk and extremities, although they can involve any epidermal or mucosal surface. Large wheal formation, where the edema extends from the dermis into the subcutaneous tissue, is referred to as angioedema. This condition is more commonly seen in the more distensible tissues, such as the eyelids, lips, ear lobes, external genitalia, and mucous membranes.

Urticarial wheals result from local subcutaneous and intradermal leakage of plasma filtrate from postcapillary venules. The erythema and surrounding swelling results from locally increased blood flow. Biopsy specimens of urticarial lesions may exhibit only subtle microscopic changes. There may be evident subcutaneous or dermal edema, an increase in the number of mast cells, and a modest perivascular lymphocytic infiltrate, perhaps intermingled with eosinophils. Electron microscopy reveals mast cell and eosinophilic degranulation (1).

797

CLASSIFICATIONS OF URTICARIA

Urticarial lesions can be classified into one or more of the following categories based on their characteristic features:

1. Duration or chronicity—acute or chronic
2. Clinical distribution of the lesions or the extra-dermal manifestations—localized, generalized, or systemic associated with rhinitis, conjunctivitis, asthma, or anaphylaxis
3. Etiology—idiopathic or cause specific
4. Route of exposure—direct contact, inhalation, or ingestion
5. Mechanisms—nonimmunologic, immunologic, or idiopathic

Acute urticaria ranges from a single episode of urticaria to recurrences lasting less than six weeks. Common causes of acute urticaria include insect bites or stings and food or drug allergies. Chronic urticaria occurs almost daily over a period longer than six weeks. Food, drugs, and infections can also be causes of chronic urticaria. However, in the chronic form, the exact causative agents may never be identified. The majority of cases of urticaria remain idiopathic.

Occupational urticaria is a general etiological classification of urticaria. It is urticaria that is presumed or proven to be caused by exposure to one or more substances or physical agents in the workplace. Beyond this definitional idiosyncrasy, occupational urticaria may fall into any of the other classifications of urticaria. It may be acute or chronic and may be localized, generalized, or associated with systemic manifestations, such as asthma. In occupational settings, direct contact with substances, and possibly inhalation, may be the more common routes of exposure inducing urticaria. The pathological mechanisms may be nonimmunologic, immunologic, or of uncertain etiology.

EPIDEMIOLOGY

Limitations of Epidemiologic Data

It can be difficult to obtain accurate epidemiologic data for occupational and nonoccupational urticaria, and all sources have their limitations. Although a case definition is a prerequisite for the gathering of epidemiologic data, there is no standard case definition in the literature to define occupational urticaria, and there is no standard approach to prove the presumed occupational-relatedness of the urticaria. Cases may be defined using a variety of criteria. These include the following: (*i*) the self-reporting of current or past episodes of urticaria in the workplace; (*ii*) histories of urticaria associated with a specific occupational exposure or work activity; (*iii*) objective signs of urticaria on clinical examination in the workplace, sometimes associated with the use of the alleged etiologic substance; and (*iv*) evidence of specific immunoglobin E (IgE) to suspect occupational antigens (e.g., radioallergosorbent test (RAST) assays or skin-prick testing). A case definition used in a study or a data source may be based on one or more of these criteria. Therefore, because the epidemiological case definition for occupational urticaria varies from one data source to another, it is difficult to compare different sources of information and different findings.

The accuracy of the diagnosis of occupational urticaria is related to the skill level, experience, and knowledge of the medical professional. The diagnosis is based on the medical and exposure history, physical findings, and in vitro or in vivo testing. The lack of a standard case definition and the difficulty of diagnosis lead to potential misclassification of occupational urticaria, which can result in either over- or under-estimation of disease frequency. In allergic contact urticarial syndromes, the lack of standardized occupational test allergens also contributes to the problem of vague case definitions.

Much of the literature on urticaria in the workplace is filled with anecdotal case reports and limited observations. This usually results in information about a single worker or a relatively small number of workers. Many of the cases in the literature are based upon clinical presentations, a determination that the urticaria is based upon a "probable" occupational exposure, and a "probable" allergic or nonallergic mechanism. Further attempts to prove etiology or mechanisms may be lacking or inadequate. Although the literature is filled with cases of occupational urticaria, tabulating these cases cannot be considered a basis for epidemiologic assessment (2).

Because of the problems with case definition and diagnosis, the limited number of subjects, and the difficulty in proving etiologies and mechanisms, the epidemiology of occupational urticaria remains obscure. The other problems in assessing the epidemiology of occupational urticaria and other occupational skin diseases are as follows (3):

1. Occupational urticaria is not a reportable disease in the United States (except in states that require reporting of all occupational diseases). This makes health department data sources useless for monitoring occupational urticaria.

2. Occupational urticaria is not a disease that commonly leads to mortality or hospitalization; thus, death certificates or hospital records are not potential data sources.

3. Occupational urticaria is a disease seen and treated (though not always specifically diagnosed) by medical professionals in multiple specialties, especially primary care practitioners, thereby making review of physician-based data sources inefficient.

4. Occupational urticaria is a disease that often goes undiagnosed and untreated; thus, many cases may never be documented in any data source.

5. Once a diagnosis of occupational urticaria is made, a case does not necessarily elicit a public health response.

6. Individuals with occupational urticaria who seek medical care may be a unique subset of those with the condition. Through this self-selection bias, the information obtained may not reflect the epidemiology of the disease in the general population.

7. Unique exposures may occur in different populations and industries, making the epidemiology of occupational urticaria in one population or workforce not necessarily generalizable to other populations.

8. The evaluation of past exposures causing occupational urticaria may be exceedingly difficult, often relying on historical information and patient recollection, which are subject to recall and information bias.

9. Cross-sectional studies of working populations, a common epidemiologic study design, are subject to survivor bias. Those with severe occupational urticaria may move out of the workforce, leaving only those who are not affected or less affected to be included in the studies.

10. An occupational urticaria case, especially if treated by a company's own occupational health personnel, may not involve lost wages or any costs to the worker. Thus, there would be no workers' compensation claim, reducing the utility of this already limited data source.

Descriptive Epidemiology of Occupational Urticaria

Accurate data on the general prevalence of urticaria are not available, although it is estimated that in a lifetime 5% to 23% of the U.S. population may have had an episode of acute urticaria (4). Of 1011 consecutive patients encountered in a dermatology practice, 26% had a history of at least one urticarial episode (5). Data from the National Ambulatory Medical Care Survey, a national probability sample survey of nonfederal office-based physicians in the United States, showed that from January 1989 to December 1990 over 25 million patient visits (4% of the total 698 million visits) were made to dermatologists. Urticaria was listed as the 17th most common principal diagnosis, accounting for 240,000 visits (1% of the total visits to dermatologists) (6). Unfortunately, similar data are not available for patient visits to allergists and immunologists.

International data are also limited. Of 4600 patients seen in a Spanish dermatology clinic from 1973 to 1977, 3.5% were given a final diagnosis of urticaria (7). A questionnaire study of 4492 respondents from a population of randomly selected Norwegians showed that 9% reported at least one episode of urticaria (8).

National occupational disease and illness data are available from the U.S. Bureau of Labor Statistics (BLS), but once again data specific for occupational urticaria are limited. The BLS conducts annual surveys of approximately 250,000 employers, selected to represent most private industries in the United States (9). The survey results are then projected to estimate the number and incidence rates of occupational injuries and illnesses in the American working population. BLS data are limited in that (*i*) they exclude several groups, including self-employed individuals, small farms, and government agencies; (*ii*) they depend on misinterpretable definitions of reportable occupational injuries and illnesses; (*iii*) they rely to a large extent on employees reporting conditions to the employer; and (*iv*) they do not provide information on the etiology of the disease.

In 1993, BLS estimated 60,200 cases of occupational skin diseases or disorders in the U.S. workforce (9). Further information is available on the 12,613 cases that involved days away from work. Of this subgroup, 142 (1.1%) were diagnosed with urticaria or hives. The median time away from work for workers with urticaria was five days. These 142 workers included 81 from the services industry, 39 from manufacturing, 9 from transportation and public utilities, and 13 not classified. It must be emphasized that because of BLS survey limitations, it has been estimated that the number of actual occupational skin diseases may be in the order of 10 to 50 times higher than reported by the BLS (10). Only limited clinically based epidemiologic information on occupational urticaria is available in the United States. Of 250 consecutive dermatology patients who had filed workers' disability compensation benefits, eight (3.2%) were found to have urticaria and/or dermatographism (11). However, in this study none were deemed to be work-related dermatoses.

In contrast, more specific occupational data are available in Finland. Between 1990 and 1994, occupational contact urticaria was responsible for 29.5% of all reported occupational dermatoses (12,13). Of the 815 cases of occupational contact urticaria, 70% were reported in women. Table 1 lists the most common causes of

Table 1 Ranking List of the Causes of Occupational Contact Urticaria and Protein Contact Dermatitis During 1990–1994 (815 Cases) According to the Finnish Register of Occupational Diseases

Ranking/cause	No. of cases	%	Men/women
Cow dander	362	44.4	132/230
Natural rubber latex	193	23.7	22/171
Flour, grains, and feed	92	11.3	ng
Handling of foodstuffs	25	3.1	9/16
Enzymes	14	1.7	ng
Cellulase	8		
Alfa-amylase	2		
Other enzymes	4		
Decorative plants	13	1.6	1/12
Roots	10	1.2	2/8
Spices	9	1.1	1/8
Pork	8	1.0	4/4
Vegetables	8	1.0	ng
Storage mites	6	0.7	5/1
Ethylhexyl acrylate	5	0.6	0/5
Onions	4	0.5	1/3
Egg	4	0.5	1/3
Fish, fish meal	3	0.4	0/3
Poultry, chicken, other birds	3	0.4	1/2
Total	815	100	248/567

Abbreviation: ng, not given.
Source: From Refs. 12, 13.

occupational contact urticaria, mostly protein allergens, which include cow dander (44%); natural rubber latex (24%); flour, grains, and feed (11%); foodstuffs (3%); industrial enzymes (2%); and decorative plants (2%). Interestingly, cow protein allergens also represented the most common cause of OA in Finland (14). Other, less common causes included roots, spices, pork, vegetables, storage mites, ethylhexyl acrylate, onions, egg, fish, fish meal, poultry, chicken, and other birds. Table 2 lists the occupations with the highest number of cases of occupational contact urticaria per 100,000 workers which included bakers (140 cases per 100,000 employed persons), processed-food preparers, dental assistants, veterinarians, animal attendants, farmers, chefs and cooks, dairy workers, horticultural supervisors, laboratory technicians, physicians, butchers, laboratory assistants, dentists, and nurses.

In general, risk factors for contact urticaria and contact anaphylaxis (e.g., natural rubber latex glove proteins) include a history of atopy, a compromise to the barrier function of intact skin (such as eczema, abrasions, ulcers, etc.), and in some cases, occupation (15).

Epidemiology of Natural Rubber Latex Allergy

Urticaria is an important manifestation of natural rubber latex allergy. Although many studies have been published on natural rubber latex allergy, the prevalence and incidence are still unknown. Still, some occupational epidemiologic details are

Table 2 Ranking List of Occupations with Occupational Contact Urticaria in Finland During 1990–1994 ($n = 815$) per 100,000 Employed Workers[a]

Ranking/occupation	No. per 100,000 workers (total no.)
Bakers	140.5
Preparers of processed food	101.8
Dental assistants	95.5
Veterinary surgeons	72.5
Domestic animal attendants	69.1
Farmers, silviculturists	57.7
Chefs, cooks, cold buffet managers	38.5
Dairy workers	37.9
Horticultural supervisors	37.8
Laboratory technicians, radiographers	35.6
Physicians	33.0
Butchers and sausage makers	28.9
Laboratory assistants	24.6
Dentists	23.4
Nurses	21.2
Waiters in cafes and snack bars, etc.	15.1
Kitchen assistants, restaurant workers, etc.	13.6
Hairdressers, beauticians, bath attendants, etc.	11.8
Housekeeping managers, snack bar managers, etc.	11.5
Packers	11.2
Horticultural workers	10.7
Assistant nurses, hospital attendants	10.2
Industrial sweepers, etc.	9.1
Cleaners, etc.	6.7
Electrical and teletechnical equipment assemblers	6.6
Homemakers, home helps (municipal)	6.2
Technical nursing assistants	4.2
Machine and engine mechanics, etc.	3.9
Shop assistants, shop cashiers	2.1
Total	3.7

[a]Occupations with at least three cases of occupational urticaria were included.
Source: From Refs. 12, 13.

available. Health care workers are the occupational group with the highest risk for developing immediate hypersensitivity reactions to natural rubber latex. A survey of hospital workers showed that 2.9% of 512 employees had positive latex skin-prick tests (16,17). Positive reactions were seen in 7.4% of the surgeons and 5.6% of the surgical nurses. Questionnaire data showed that 2% of operating as well as dental personnel reported localized contact urticaria (18) and 4% of U.S. Army dentists reported symptoms of probable latex allergy (19). Recent studies in dental students and staff revealed that 14% of 203 students and staff reported pruritus and 3% reported urticaria within minutes of exposure to latex gloves; 10% of the 131 who underwent skin-prick tests had a positive response to natural rubber latex (20). In another study of 1171 patients attending a Spanish dermatology clinic, it was found that 16.7% of health care workers were sensitized to natural rubber latex as judged by positive prick tests and specific IgE levels, compared to 2.3% in non-health care

workers. The prevalence of contact urticaria to natural rubber latex in this population was also more frequent among health care workers, who accounted for 71.4% of
all cases among this population (21).

A cross-sectional study in a large U.S. metropolitan hospital showed that
among 741 nurses, 8.9% had a positive response to anti-latex IgE antibodies (22).
The prevalence ranged from 6.4% for operating room nurses to 13.6% for labor
and delivery nurses. In this study, the factors that were most closely associated with
the presence of anti-latex IgE included non-white race, self-reported allergy to penicillin, pruritus, conjunctivitis, localized urticaria on latex exposure, history consistent
with atopy, and allergies to avocado or ragweed.

Another cross-sectional study of 1351 Canadian hospital workers showed a
prevalence of positive latex skin-prick tests of 12.1% (23). The highest prevalence
was found in laboratory workers (16.9%) and nurses and physicians (13.3%). The
latex skin-prick test–positive workers reported work-related symptoms, including
urticaria, more often than latex skin test–negative workers; 11.3% of latex skin test–
positive workers reported urticaria, compared to 2.5% of latex skin test–negative
workers (adjusted odds ratio of 6.3; confidence interval of 3.2–2.5).

Natural rubber latex allergy may be seen in other occupations as well. In a
Finnish clinic, 144 adult patients (66 health care workers and 78 from other occupations) were diagnosed with natural rubber latex allergy over a 10-year period. In
88% of the 66 health care workers, but in only 24% of the other workers, was the
sensitization determined to be work-related (24). The other affected occupations
included in the study are kitchen workers, cleaners, workers in a rubber band plant,
textile workers, farmers' wives, a paper mill worker, a gardener, a food worker, a
dairy worker, a secretary, and a private caretaker. In a survey of latex allergy in
a surgical glove manufacturing plant, 7 of 68 workers (10%) stated that they had
hives at work, and 7 of 64 workers had positive skin test reactions to latex (25).
In a study of 418 greenhouse workers who used latex gloves, 18% reported immediate symptoms associated with wearing gloves, and 5% had positive latex skin-prick
tests (26).

Epidemiology of Occupational Urticaria in Specific Occupations

The prevalence of occupational skin diseases within specific occupations is based
upon the exposures inherent within those occupations. Cross-sectional studies of
workers in a specific occupation or workplace may allow for an estimation of skin
disease within that occupation or workplace. However, there are few studies on specific occupations where occupational urticaria is a measured endpoint. In a study of
801 car mechanics, 120 (15%) reported hand eczema and five (0.6%) had a history of
contact urticaria; scratch tests were all negative (27). The overall prevalence
of allergic respiratory symptoms among exposed animal laboratory workers has
been estimated at 23%; of these, 4% to 9% develop asthma (28). In 5641 laboratory
animal handlers, 1304 (23.1%) reported one or more allergic symptoms related to the
animals (29). Of this symptomatic group 45.6% had skin symptoms and 16%
reported contact urticaria. Various combinations of symptoms were noted—19.3%
had nasal or eye and skin symptoms, and 11.6% had nasal or eye, respiratory, and
skin symptoms. A study of laboratory workers handling rats showed that of 323
workers surveyed, 31% reported at least one work-related symptom with 22% reporting eye and nose symptoms, followed by skin (15%), and chest symptoms (10%) (30).
In another study of biology laboratory workers, 27 (11.3%) of those who had

frequent exposure to animals had reactions, of whom 15 had various skin reactions, including urticaria; 21 had positive prick tests to animal dander (31). A study of 101 laboratory technicians showed that 14 cases of contact urticaria were caused by rat, seven by mouse, four by guinea pig, and two by cat exposure (32). In another study of 1064 employees exposed to a variety of proteases, lipases, cellulases, and carboxy-hydrases in an enzyme-producing plant, the frequency of asthma was 5.3%, rhinitis 3.0%, and urticaria 0.6% (33).

Case studies alone do not allow an estimation of occupational prevalence but may describe potential high-risk occupations based upon exposures to specific allergens or urticants. In one study of nine veterinary surgeons, all nine exhibited specific IgE against cow hair and dander; seven were symptomatic (34). Cow dander is the most common cause of occupational contact urticaria among veterinarians and dairy farmers in Finland (35). A study of 50 food handlers/caterers with possible immediate protein contact dermatitis showed that nine (18%) had positive prick tests, most commonly to fish (36). Another study of 33 food handlers with a similar skin condition showed that 10 had positive scratch tests to explain their dermatitis, with the major allergens being fish and shellfish (37). The prevalence of OA among workers in the fishing and seafood processing industry ranges from 7% to 36%, with protein contact dermatitis (a variant of contact urticaria) occurring in between 3% and 11% of exposed workers (38).

CONTACT URTICARIA

Contact urticaria is defined as urticaria that occurs after direct skin contact with a substance. Table 3 lists some of the many substances that can cause contact urticaria in occupational settings. Extensive lists are available in several sources, and new etiologic agents are continually being described (39–45).

There are four types of contact urticaria: (*i*) nonallergic (nonimmunologic; primary urticariogenic agents), (*ii*) allergic (immunologic), (*iii*) combined allergic and nonallergic, and (*iv*) combined allergic eczematous and urticarial (41). Some contactants affect normal skin while others require eczematized or fissured skin to produce urticaria (43,46). Small molecules may penetrate intact skin while large proteinaceous molecules may require disruption of the epidermal barrier.

There may be a variety of skin manifestations associated with contact urticaria. Because of the potential of this varied morphology, terms such as "immediate contact reactions" are also used to describe what may be different skin manifestations of urticaria (42). Contact urticaria may comprise a spectrum of manifestations "that flows continuously from wheals to erythema to pruritus" (47). Pruritus, tingling, or burning accompanied by erythema is the weakest type of immediate contact reaction. A local wheal and flare is the prototypical reaction of contact urticaria and generalized urticaria after a local contact is considered a rare phenomenon. Symptoms, such as asthma, rhinitis, conjunctivitis, orolaryngeal effects, and gastrointestinal and cardiovascular symptoms, can involve other organ systems (42). The term "contact urticaria syndrome" is used to describe both local and systemic immediate reactions caused by contact urticarial agents (48,49). The contact urticaria syndrome has been divided into the following four stages:

1. Stage 1: localized contact urticaria
2. Stage 2: contact urticaria with generalized urticaria

Table 3 Selected Causes of Occupational Contact Urticaria

Agent	Nonimmunological	Allergic

Animals and living organisms (nonplant), and their by-products	Caterpillars
	Jellyfish
	Moths
		Amniotic fluid
		Blood
		Caterpillars
		Cercariae
		Dander and hair
		Enzymes (bacterial, fungal)
		  Alpha-amylase
		  Carboxylases
		  Cellulases
		  Lipases
		  Proteases
		Grasshoppers
		Gut
		Locusts
		Mites
		Parasites
		Placenta
		Saliva
		Seminal fluid
		Silk
		Wool
		Urine (mouse)

Chemicals, miscellaneous industrial and occupational	Histamine
	Sulfur
	Turpentine
		Acrylic monomers
		Ammonium
		  persulfate
		Anhydrides
		Aziridine hardeners
		Carbonless copy paper
		Epoxy resin
		Formaldehyde resin
		Isocyanates
		Organic dyes
		  p-Phenylenediamine
		Pesticides and insecticides
		  Chlorothalonil
		  Diethyltoluamide
		   (DEET)
		  Lindane

Food substances	Spices
	Cayenne pepper
	Cinnamon
		Dairy products
		  Cheese
		  Eggs
		  Milk
		Fruits and vegetables
		  Apples
		  Bananas
		  Carrots
		  Celery

(*Continued*)

Table 3   Selected Causes of Occupational Contact Urticaria (*Continued*)

Agent	Nonimmunological	Allergic
		Kiwi
		Mango
		Peaches
		Potatoes
		Plums
		Fish and shellfish
		Grains
		Meats
		Spices
		Cinnamon
		Mustard
		Paprika
Flavorings and fragrances	Balsam of Peru	Balsam of Peru
	Cassia (cinnamon oil)	Cassia
	Cinnamic alcohol	Menthol
	Cinnamic aldehyde	Vanillin
Medications	Alcohols	Antibiotics
	Camphor	Ampicillin
	Capsaicin	Bacitracin
	Dimethyl sulfoxide	Cefotiam
	Friar's balsam	Gentamycin
	Tincture of benzoin	Idochlorhydroxyquin
		Neomycin
		Penicillin
		Piperacillin
		Rifampin
		Streptomycin
		Virginiamycin
		Benzocaine
		Pentamidine
		Phenothiazines
		Chlorpromazine
		Levomepromazine
		Promethazine
Metals		Iridium
		Nickel
		Platinum
		Rhodium
Plants and their by-products	Nettles	Algae
	Seaweed	Asparagus
		Cacti
		Christmas cactus
		Easter cactus
		Camomile
		Cornstarch
		Flowers
		Chrysanthemum

(*Continued*)

Table 3 Selected Causes of Occupational Contact Urticaria (*Continued*)

Agent	Nonimmunological	Allergic
		Alstroemeria
		Spathe
		Tulip
		Henna
		Latex (natural rubber)
		Perfumes
		Tobacco
		Weeping fig
		Woods and wood dusts
		Larch
		Mukali
		Obeche
		Teak
Preservatives and disinfectants	Benzoic acid	Benzoic acid
	Chlorocresol	Chlorhexidine
	Formaldehyde	Chlorocresol
	Sodium benzoate	Benzyl alcohol
	Sorbic acid	Formaldehyde
		Gentian violet
		Sodium hypochlorite

3. Stage 3: contact urticaria with extracutaneous symptoms (asthma, rhinitis and conjunctivitis, orolaryngeal symptoms, gastrointestinal symptoms)
4. Stage 4: contact urticaria with anaphylaxis (49)

Another variety of immediate reaction, termed "protein contact dermatitis," describes cutaneous reactions with clinical features of both immediate and delayed (eczematous) hypersensitivity and usually occurs on the palms. This condition was initially described in food handlers exposed to certain food proteins (especially fish and shellfish), who developed immediate (10–30 minutes after exposure) pruritus and erythema as well as eczematous changes including vesicle formation (37). Other causes of protein contact dermatitis include: animal proteins, enzymes, fruits, grains, plants, spices, and vegetables (50). Tests for immediate hypersensitivity (e.g., prick tests) are invariably positive, but patch tests for delayed hypersensitivity may be negative. The mechanisms for the immediate eczematous changes are unknown, but could involve an ordinary type IV allergic mechanism or a reaction mediated by IgE bound Langerhans cells (51).

Concomitant type I (urticarial) and type IV (allergic contact dermatitis) skin reactions have also been increasingly reported. Some of the contactants that can produce both an immediate and delayed reaction include acrylic acid, benzocaine, carrot, chlorhexidine, chlorocresol, chrysanthemum, cinnamic aldehyde, epoxy resin, garlic, latex, lettuce, nickel sulphate, potato, soybean, and textile dyes (43).

In terms of pathomechanisms, contact urticaria may be caused by nonimmunological, immunological, or undetermined mechanisms. In instances where the mechanism of urticaria is undetermined, both unknown nonimmunological and immunological mechanisms could be operative. Examples include urticaria owing to ammonium persulfate (used as an oxidizing hair bleach) (52,53), formaldehyde, and some physical agents (2). A recent study, however, has documented specific IgE-mediated hypersensitivity in at least some patients with persulfate hypersensitivity (54).

Nonimmunologic Contact Urticaria

Nonimmunologic (nonallergic) contact urticaria occurs in the absence of prior sensitization. The mechanisms of nonimmunologic urticaria remain unclear. It can result either from a direct influence on dermal blood vessel walls or from a nonantibody-mediated release of vasoactive substances, such as histamine, prostaglandins, leukotrienes, platelet-activating factor, and cytokines (41,55,56). Indirect provocation of mast cell degranulation by complement activation or neural reflex vasodilation can occur. Multiple stimuli can cause the nonimmunological degranulation of mast cells within the subcutaneous tissues and dermis. This causes the release of preformed mediators (e.g., histamine), which cause vasodilation and increase capillary permeability. Also, cellular regulatory factors secreted by lymphocytes, neutrophils, eosinophils, platelets, and macrophages, such as C-C chemokines (e.g., MCP-1, MCP-3) possess histamine-releasing factor (HRF) that can activate exocytosis of histamine from mast cells or basophils (57).

Nonimmunologic contact urticaria needs to be distinguished from irritant contact dermatitis reactions, although this may be difficult at times. Strong irritants, such as hydrochloric acid, formaldehyde, and phenol can cause immediate urticaria formation. However, this reaction does not disappear within 24 hours but is followed by erythema, scaling, or crusting (39). Some substances may be both primary irritants and contact urticants.

Nonimmunologic contact urticaria may be the most common form of occupational contact urticaria and is usually not associated with systemic symptoms (43). However, in one case, a severe systemic immediate reaction was reported after occupational exposure to benzoic acid–containing materials (41). A variety of agents have been shown to cause a nonimmunological contact urticaria. These include acetic acid, ethyl and butyl alcohol, balsam of Peru, benzoic acid, butyric acid, caterpillar hair, cinnamic acid, cinnamic aldehyde, cobalt chloride, diethyl fumarate, dimethyl sulfoxide, formaldehyde, insect stings, methyl nicotinate, moths, sodium benzoate, and sorbic acid (41,43). Exposures to these substances may occur in occupational settings, an example being contact urticaria owing to airborne sodium benzoate in a pharmaceutical manufacturing plant (58). Some of the physical urticarias may also be classified as nonimmunological urticarias.

Atopic and nonatopic individuals are at equal risk for developing nonimmunologic contact urticaria. Even with well-documented chemical urticants, such as benzoic acid, cinnamic acid, and methyl nicotinate, there is wide interindividual variation in response (59). In addition, there is also regional body site variation in the response to chemical urticants (60).

Immunologic Contact Urticaria

Immunologic (allergic) contact urticaria occurs in individuals previously sensitized to the offending substance. The sensitization route may be through the skin or through extracutaneous organs such as the respiratory and gastrointestinal tracts (2). Confirmation of an allergic basis for contact urticaria is achieved by demonstration of specific IgE to a causative antigen either by the presence of serum specific IgE (e.g., via a RAST assay) or by skin-prick testing. In the past, immediate hypersensitivity was demonstrated by the passive transfer of allergic serum to naive skin where wheal and flare responses could be elicited by injection of allergen (Prausnitz–Kustner reaction); at that time, the transferrable allergic factor was referred to as "reagin" which is now known to be IgE.

A variety of stimuli can cause mast cell activation and release of mediators. These include specific IgE molecules which are bound to mast cell membrane via high affinity receptors for IgE. The cross-linking of these IgE receptors by the interaction of the IgE antibody and its antigen initiates cell activation and subsequent degranulation. Other mechanisms that can effect histamine release in occupational urticaria are unproven. They include the activation of the complement cascade and generation of anaphylotoxins (C3a, C4a, C5a), which activate mast cells via specific complement receptors. A variety of peptides may activate mast cells including bradykinin and substance P. As mentioned, C-C chemokines secreted by mononuclear cells and neutrophils can induce histamine release.

Usually a low proportion of exposed individuals are affected by allergic contact urticaria, and it is likely that it is more common among atopic individuals. It is also likely that IgE mediates most cases, because nonspecific elevation of IgE is frequently reported. In many cases, specific IgE has also been documented (43). In other cases, specific IgG and perhaps immunoglobin M may be responsible by activating the classical complement system (43).

Based upon reviews of epidemiological studies, exposures, and patterns seen in case reports, several occupations may be at higher risk for the development of allergic contact urticaria. These include the following:

1. food handlers, cooks, caterers, and bakers;
2. general health care workers (61), dental professionals (62), and pharmaceutical industry workers (63);
3. animal handlers such as laboratory workers or veterinarians; and
4. gardeners, florists, woodworkers, and agricultural workers.

The following foods have been reported to produce allergic contact urticaria in food handlers, cooks, caterers, and bakers: apples, bean, beer, caraway seed, carrot, egg, endive, fish, garlic, kiwi fruit, lettuce, meat (beef, chicken, lamb, liver, pork, and turkey), milk, peach, potato, rice, shellfish, spices, and strawberries (41,43). Crab is the most common seafood allergen among seafood handlers (38). Shrimp and scallops demonstrate significant cross-reactivity among sensitized seafood handlers (64). Allergic sensitization may sometimes be caused by associated exposures, such as fish parasites (65) and live bait (66). Allergic respiratory symptoms are caused by aerosolization of proteinaceous material during processing, preparation, and cooking (38,64). Bakers can develop contact urticaria and other systemic symptoms after exposure to cereal flours, buckwheat flour, and additive flour enzymes, such as alpha-amylase (from *Aspergillus oryzae* or *Bacillus subtilis*) (43,67,68). Enzyme allergy may depend on whether the alpha-amylase is of fungal or bacterial origin (69). In the case of flour, the allergen may be the beetles contaminating it (70). A unique food-related contact urticaria in nontraditional "food handlers" has been reported in hairdressers using egg shampoos (71).

In health care, dental, and pharmaceutical environments, handling or producing a variety of medications or chemical disinfectants can put workers at risk. Exposures that can cause allergic contact urticaria include aminothiazole, bacitracin, benzocaine gel, cefotiam, cephalosporins, chloramine (a sterilizer, disinfectant, and chemical reagent), chloramphenicol, chlorhexidine (an antiseptic), chlorocresol (a disinfectant), ethylene oxide, gentamicin, neomycin, nitrogen mustard, penicillin, pentamidine isethionate, phenothiazines, piperacillin rifamycin, and streptomycin (41,43,72–75).

The initial 1979 case report of natural rubber latex allergy occurred in a woman using gloves for hand protection during housework (76). The next reported case occurred in a nurse using surgical gloves (77). Since then, natural rubber latex has been found to be an important cause of allergic contact urticaria, asthma, and anaphylaxis in health care professionals. The most frequently reported manifestation is contact urticaria, followed by rhinoconjunctivitis (78). Atopics, individuals with hand eczema, and patients with spina bifida and indwelling catheters seem to be at higher risk for developing natural rubber latex allergy (79,80). Persons sensitive to natural rubber latex may develop severe systemic urticaria by ingesting certain fruits and foods, such as banana, kiwi, and avocado, which cross-react with the latex antigen (79,80).

Allergic contact urticaria has been found to be caused by animal hair (rat and guinea pig exposure in laboratory workers), dander, insects (such as cockroaches, caterpillars, and locusts), animal placenta, saliva, seminal fluid, and serum (41,81–83). Slaughterhouse workers can develop contact urticaria by exposure to animal blood (84). Contact urticaria can be seen in veterinarians after exposure to cow's hairs and placenta, horse dander, and pig's bristles (43).

Certain woods and plants can cause allergic contact urticaria. These include the larch, limba, obeche (African maple), teak, mukali, and other exotic woods (41,85–87) and plants such as bishop's weed (*Ammi majus*), Christmas and Easter cacti, chrysanthemum, *Ficus benjamina* (weeping fig), Easter lily (*Lilium longiforum*) and Peruvian lily (*Alstroemeria*), *Limonium tataricum*, *Phoenix canariensis* (canary palm), *Spathiphyllum wallisii* (spathe flower), tulips, and fungi (shiitake mushrooms) (88–102). Those in high-risk occupations include agricultural workers, carpenters, florists, gardeners, and woodworkers. In some cases, insects associated with plants are the actual causes of allergic urticaria (e.g., caterpillars, moths, stinging insects, etc.). In an investigation of 46 farm workers with allergic symptoms, 17 had an allergic contact urticaria and respiratory complaints and 29 had respiratory complaints resulting from contact with *Tetranychus urticae* (red spider mite) (103). In another study of 24 greenhouse workers with allergic symptoms, allergy resulting from contact with red spider mite caused 15 cases of asthma, 14 cases of rhinitis, and 5 cases of urticaria (104). Agricultural workers may also be exposed to fertilizers and pesticides, some of which can cause allergic contact urticaria (105). Immediate hypersensitivity to tobacco (106) and asparagus (107) may cause urticaria, rhinitis, and asthma in field workers tending these crops.

A variety of industrial chemicals can cause allergic contact urticaria, including acrylic monomers (plastics), polyfunctional aziridine hardener (aziridine reacted with a multifunctional acrylic), aliphatic polyamines (epoxy resins), alkylphenol novolac resin (found in carbonless copy paper), ammonia, acid anhydrides, castor bean pomace (fertilizers), diethyltoluamide (DEET), formaldehyde (used in clothing, leather, fumigation, and resins), isocyanates, lindane (a parasiticide), paraphenylenediamine, phenylmercuric propionate (an antibacterial fabric softener), plastic additives (such as butylhydroxytoluene and oleylamide), reactive dyes, sodium sulfide (used in photographs, dyes, and tanning), sulfur dioxide, vinyl pyrrolidone, xylene, and other solvents (41,43,108–118). Allergic contact urticaria can occur following exposure to a variety of metal salts, including iridium, nickel, platinum, and rhodium (41,43,119,120). Also silk, wool, and nylon, which may be found in work clothing, are rare causes of allergic contact urticaria (121). Dioctylphthalate in work clothing has also caused at least one case of contact urticaria (122).

Some causes of allergic contact urticaria are well documented with in vivo and in vitro testing. An example of one of the more completely documented causes of occupational contact urticaria and asthma are the acid anhydrides, which include hexahydrophthalic anhydride, maleic anhydride, methylhexahydrophthalic anhydride, phthalic anhydride (PA), tetrahydrochlorophthalic anhydride (TCPA) and trimellitic anhydride (TMA). The anhydrides are used as cross-linking agents or hardeners in epoxy resins, which are used in paints and plastics, and for encapsulation of electronic components. Immediate allergy has been verified by an open test with undiluted PA, a scratch chamber test using 1% of PA, prick tests, specific IgE determinations, RAST inhibition studies, and chamber provocation tests (118,123). Exposure to airborne acid anhydrides has been documented as causing sensitization in some workers (112,116).

Contact urticaria, systemic urticaria, rhinitis, conjunctivitis, and asthma have been reported with increasing frequency among hairdressers and cosmetologists. The causes include exposure to persulfates (54), henna (124), glyceryl thioglycolate (125), protein hydrolysates in hair conditioners (126), and chamomile and lime flowers (127).

AIRBORNE EXPOSURE URTICARIA

Contact urticaria caused by airborne exposures is an unusual condition because most of the agents that can cause contact urticaria are not volatile and do not easily vaporize. But in some cases airborne aerosols, dusts, fumes, mists, or vapors have been shown to cause contact urticaria, usually on the exposed skin of the face and neck (128). Examples of agents that can cause airborne contact urticaria include acrylic acid, ammonia, formaldehyde, garlic, naphtha, natural rubber latex (protein alone or protein–cornstarch powder combination), PAs, sodium benzoate, soybean, 1,1,1-trichloroethane, and xylene (16,59,112,129–132).

Airborne contact urticaria is caused by direct contact of exposed skin with the causative substance. In some instances, urticaria may appear after inhalation of a substance (133). Inhaled agents, however, are considered rare causes of urticaria. Case reports have described generalized urticaria and metal fume fever–like symptoms in welders exposed to zinc oxide and polyurethane (134,135). Other occupational exposures that have been reported to induce inhalant urticaria include aminothiazide, ammonia, animal danders, castor bean dust and pomace, coffee bean dust, formaldehyde, lindane, mold spores, complex platinum salts, pollens, and sulfur dioxide (136–139). In many reports, the exact etiologies, routes of exposure, and mechanisms were circumstantial and not proven unequivocally (135). A precise distinction between an inhalational exposure and an epidermal exposure to airborne aerosols, dusts, fumes, mists, or vapors is seldom made in these reports.

PHYSICAL URTICARIAS

Urticarias that result from nonchemical exposures are commonly classified as "physical urticarias." Up to 17% of chronic urticarias may be attributable to physical causes (140). These include mechanical urticarias (caused by trauma, pressure, friction, and vibration) and urticaria resulting from local exposure to physical agents (such as cold, heat, solar radiation, and water) (141,142). The physical urticarias can also be classified mechanistically as immunological, nonimmunological, and uncertain. An allergic mechanism is supported for certain forms of the physical urticarias (e.g., dermatographism) by demonstration that the urticarial response can be passively transferred to a naive donor (i.e., the Prausnitz–Kustner reaction) (143).

Causes of trauma-induced urticaria include mechanical irritants, for example, fiberglass fragments that puncture the skin (144). Pressure urticaria, comprising less than 1% of all urticarias, occurs as deep, indurated, tender hives, usually on the buttocks, feet, or palms 3 to 12 hours following application of pressure. These lesions, which may occur after manual labor, walking, climbing stairs, and using hand tools, may persist for up to 48 hours and can be accompanied by fever, chills, and arthralgias (141). A nonimmunologic mechanism seems most likely (145). Although rare, pressure urticaria can be very disabling. This condition may be associated with chronic idiopathic urticaria and dermatographism. Dermatographism, the most common form of physical urticaria (seen in 2–5% of the population), results in a linear wheal and flare at the site of firm stroking or friction. The very rare vibratory urticaria may be acquired or familial (autosomal dominant inheritance), and can occur after occupational exposure to vibration, as in metal grinding or jackhammer operation (146,147).

Cold urticaria occurs as acquired, inherited, and secondary forms associated with serum abnormalities (cryoglobulinemia, cold agglutinins, cryofibrinogens, and cold hemolysins) (147). Urticarial lesions develop during rewarming after direct cold contact or immersion in cold water and may be associated with bronchospasm, flushing, hypotension, and syncope. A positive Prausnitz–Kustner reaction shows that acquired cold urticaria, which comprises 1% to 3% of all urticarias, may be IgE mediated (142,148). Examples of occupational exposures causing cold urticaria include contact sprays, cold lithography solutions, and cold environments (149–151).

Localized heat urticaria is a very rare entity in which pruritic lesions occur quickly after localized heat contact. These lesions can be associated with nausea, diarrhea, abdominal pain, headache, and dizziness. Urticaria caused by heat is likely to be nonimmunologic (148). Cholinergic urticaria, which may comprise 5% to 7% of all urticarias, is marked by a sensation of warmth followed by the appearance of small (1–3 mm) pruritic wheals (142). This condition, which can be accompanied by systemic symptoms, develops after increase in core body temperature and is induced by heat, exercise, or emotion (148). One report documented occupational exposures causing cholinergic urticaria in U.S. Air Force personnel (152). Cholinergic urticaria is mediated by cholinergic substances liberated from stimulated peripheral nerves (153). The rare exercise-induced anaphylactic syndrome needs to be distinguished from cholinergic urticaria. Some individuals develop symptoms only during exercise (or strenuous work) following intake of certain foods, and the condition is not related to core body temperature (142).

Solar urticaria, found in less than 1% of persons with urticaria, occurs only on exposed skin surfaces following exposure to a variety of wavelengths of light. Solar urticaria may be associated with other photosensitive disorders, such as systemic lupus erythematosus and porphyria cutanea tarda (154). Solar urticaria can be associated with systemic symptoms as well; the mechanism is uncertain.

Aquagenic urticaria is a very rare disorder associated with water contact at any temperature and is not associated with any systemic symptoms. It is typically marked by punctate, perifollicular hives. There is some evidence that a water-soluble epidermal antigen permeates the skin after contact with water and activates mast cells, although the mechanism remains uncertain (142).

DIAGNOSIS OF WORK-RELATED URTICARIA

Although a reliable diagnosis of urticaria may usually be established on the basis of clinical examination alone, reliable attribution of causation to an occupational exposure is generally difficult. In part, this difficulty is inherent to the investigation of urticaria in general. No cause can be identified in at least 70% of the cases of chronic urticaria (145). Because urticaria is common, cases will inevitably occur within the working population. In the absence of an obvious explanation, some workers and physicians will ultimately attribute the cause of the urticaria to an exposure in the workplace. While patient observation and insight may offer valuable clues to any medical investigation, the etiology of a case of urticaria may remain in question unless objective criteria can be established to support an occupational relationship.

Although no general consensus yet exists, a review of the best-documented cases of occupational urticaria cited in this review and elsewhere (155) suggests that the following seven criteria are most useful:

1. The clinical diagnosis of urticaria has been documented by medical examination. The pathognomonic lesion of urticaria is the wheal, a circumscribed, pruritic, raised, pink to erythematous, effervescent swelling of the superficial dermis without any changes (such as scaling) in the overlying epidermis. The wheal usually lasts only a few hours—rarely more than 24 hours. The appearance of new wheals, coupled with the relatively rapid disappearance of older wheals, may give rise to the patient's perception that the rash is "moving around the body." There are no particular characteristics of wheals caused by occupational exposures, which allow them to be distinguished from urticaria owing to other causes (including idiopathic).

   Urticaria may sometimes be confused with other acute erythematous cutaneous eruptions, such as morbilliform rashes caused by drugs or viruses, erythema multiforme, or even acute contact dermatitis. These latter conditions are more persistent, and individual lesions last longer than 24 hours. A skin biopsy is not usually helpful or necessary to confirm the diagnosis of urticaria, but may sometimes be useful to exclude these other dermatologic conditions (including urticarial vasculitis) in the presence of uncertainty. Objective medical documentation is essential since patients' self-reported histories of hives can be unreliable. Similarly, pruritus alone is not an objective proof of urticaria unless wheals can be observed.

2. Exposure has occurred in the workplace to an agent that has already been documented as a potential cause of urticaria, based on published medical or toxicological studies. Published studies must be critically evaluated. Upon careful scrutiny, rigorous or convincing proof is often lacking; skin tests allegedly supporting a causal relationship may not have adequate standardization or controls, and the etiologic relationship to many purported causes of occupational urticaria, such as formaldehyde, seems

to be based upon subjective historical data, such as "hives occur only when working; do not occur when not working."

3. The temporal relationship between exposure and onset of symptoms should be consistent with the diagnosis of urticaria, an immediate hypersensitivity reaction. Under ordinary circumstances, hives should develop within 30 to 60 minutes of exposure to the putative causal agent in the workplace. However, no general consensus yet exists concerning the time lag between initial exposure and first occurrence of urticaria; symptoms may not develop for weeks, months, or even years after first exposure or date of hire. One study of enzyme workers found that 50% of sensitized workers developed their allergic symptoms within 15 months of initial exposure (33).

4. Associated medical symptoms and the anatomical localization of urticaria must be consistent with the clinical route of exposure to the alleged causal agent. If the skin is the primary route of exposure, the skin should urticate first and foremost in anatomical areas (e.g., the hands and arms) where the causal substance has come in direct contact with the skin. Although hives may remain localized to the primary areas of direct contact (contact urticaria), generalized urticaria may develop if sufficient percutaneous absorption occurs. In the latter case, the appearance of hives elsewhere on the body surface should follow, not precede, the appearance of hives at the site of primary skin contact. If the primary route of exposure is airborne, urticaria is often associated with additional medical symptoms consistent with rhinitis, conjunctivitis, or asthma. These symptoms should precede, rather than follow, the onset of hives. Medical documentation of these associated symptoms is valuable, since self-reported symptoms are unreliable and difficult to distinguish from minor irritation caused by noxious vapors. In rare instances of alleged contamination of food from workplace exposures, the gastrointestinal tract will be the primary route of exposure. In this case, hives should be associated with nausea and abdominal cramping. Lip and oropharyngeal swelling may also occur as a result of direct contact with the mucous membranes of the mouth.

5. Urticaria should occur only in the workplace and should completely resolve on weekends, vacations, layoffs, or termination of employment. As urticaria is a common disorder in general, care should be taken to distinguish urticaria that may be aggravated by nonspecific workplace conditions that elevate skin temperature (such as hot environments and heavy physical exercise) from hives caused by an exposure that occurs only at work.

6. Nonoccupational causes of urticaria should be excluded. Unfortunately, since no specific cause is objectively documented in the majority of cases of chronic urticaria, a natural temptation exists to blame idiopathic cases on any temporal association (e.g., workplace exposures), although the scientific proof is seldom more than "guilt by association."

7. Medical testing should support a causal relationship between urticaria and a workplace exposure. The following tests may be employed in the investigation of contact or systemic urticaria suspected to be caused by an occupational exposure. In all cases where skin tests are performed, the patient should be off conventional antihistamine therapy for at least 72 hours and long-acting antihistamine therapy for at least two weeks. If asthma or anaphylactic symptoms have been associated with urticaria, cardiopulmonary resuscitation equipment should be readily available.

Open or closed patch test is the primary test utilized for the diagnosis of contact urticaria, and is the preferred test for the evaluation of systemic urticaria thought to be caused by skin exposure, as it most closely approximates the conditions under which exposure is actually occurring in the workplace. In the open patch test, the suspected etiologic agent is placed directly on the skin "as is" and the test site is observed up to 60 minutes for erythema or a wheal—and flare reaction. In the closed patch test, the suspected causal agent is placed on a standard commercial patch test device (e.g., Finn Chamber on Scanpor Tape) and occluded against the skin for 15 to 30 minutes. The device is then removed, and the test site is observed for a reaction for an additional 30 minutes (total of 60 minutes). The preferred test site is the ventral forearm, upper outer arm, or upper back. In cases where occupational cutaneous exposure has been occurring on eczematous skin exclusively (e.g., natural rubber latex gloves over eczematous hand dermatitis), these tests may be cautiously repeated over the eczematous skin (e.g., cutting a finger off a latex glove and placing it over an affected finger). No standardization of test concentrations exists, and ideally the interpretation of a test as "positive" should be supported by at least 20 negative controls. In some instances, published case reports supported by negative controls may serve as "literature" controls.

With prick or scratch tests, the skin is either pricked with a 26-gauge needle or blood lancet, or scratched (approximately 7- to 8-mm long scratch) with a 20-gauge needle. If the suspected causal agent is a liquid, a drop should be placed on the skin first and the skin pricked or scratched through the liquid. If the suspected causal agent is a solid, the skin should be pricked or scratched first and then the solid placed over it after moistening it with water. A variation called the scratch-chamber test has been developed and is particularly useful for solids such as food substances. With this procedure, the test substance is placed into a standard patch test device (e.g., Finn Chamber on Scanpor Tape) and then taped to the skin over a 7- or 8-mm long scratch and observed for response. These invasive tests may be necessary if the primary route of exposure is airborne, as mucous membranes are generally more permeable to absorption than the general skin surface, and false-negative patch tests (open or closed) may occur as a result of inadequate percutaneous penetration of the test substance. Unfortunately, many industrial chemicals may be nonspecifically irritating to the skin when tested in this fashion. No prick or scratch test standardization exists for most of the industrial test substances in terms of vehicle or concentration, and the onus is on the investigator to test a sufficient number of control subjects, using positive histamine and negative saline controls as well as the test substance(s), which may turn a clinical evaluation into a time-consuming research project. Ideally, controls should include other subjects with chronic urticaria unrelated to workplace chemical exposure. The mean wheal diameter (i.e., longest diameter + perpendicular diameter divided by two) should be measured for any positive reaction. Kanerva et al. (156) have recommended a test reaction grading system as follows: $1+$ = reaction diameter less than $\frac{1}{2}$ diameter of a histamine control, but at least 2 mm greater than the diameter of a saline control; $2+$ = reaction diameter greater than $\frac{1}{2}$ diameter but less than the full diameter of a histamine control; $3+$ = reaction diameter greater than or equal to, but less than twice, a histamine control; $4+$ = reaction diameter equal to or greater than twice a histamine control. A weak test reaction of $1+$ intensity can be considered significant if other aspects of the evaluation overwhelmingly support this conclusion.

Intradermal tests need not be performed ordinarily except in cases where standardized materials already exist (e.g., wheat antigen for evaluation of baker's asthma associated with hives). The lack of standardization for the majority of workplace allergens makes this test almost impossible to interpret reliably. Furthermore, the majority of workplace chemicals are likely to be highly irritating to tissue when injected intradermally, even in diluted aqueous vehicles, and some may be corrosive.

RAST materials are not commercially available for most workplace chemicals, however, with few exceptions (natural rubber latex protein, diisocyanates, and acid anhydrides). Where available, the RAST can be an extremely helpful diagnostic aid, especially in the presence of generalized urticaria. However, the test may be negative unless there is a sufficient amount of circulating specific IgE antibody to the suspected allergen. The RAST is generally considered quite specific, but not as sensitive as a properly performed and standardized skin test, for the diagnosis of immediate hypersensitivity.

Miscellaneous blood tests such as increased total serum IgE levels and peripheral blood eosinophilia are sometimes suggestive of a true allergic reaction, but none are specific for any causal agent.

Skin biopsies are seldom helpful in establishing a diagnosis of urticaria, which is usually made on clinical grounds alone, unless urticarial vasculitis is suspected. A biopsy is never helpful for establishing a specific etiologic cause.

TREATMENT

In all cases of occupational urticaria where a specific causal agent can be identified, the treatment of obvious choice is avoidance of the offending agent. In some cases, a nonallergenic substance may simply be substituted, and the affected worker kept in the same job (e.g., substitution of nitrile gloves for natural rubber latex gloves for workers allergic to latex protein). Among health care workers, the use of powder-free low–latex allergen gloves along with substitution of synthetic rubber gloves has substantially reduced the incidence of latex allergy (79). In other cases, the affected worker will have to be removed from that part of the work environment where exposure has been occurring, even if it ultimately means changing jobs. However, medical recommendations to leave employment should not be made lightly and should be supported by adequate objective medical findings, including tests that specifically identify the causal agent.

Because the overwhelming majority of cases of urticaria occurring among workers will not follow an occupational exposure, treatment may be instituted according to the same therapeutic principles used in the management of other chronic urticaria. First-generation antihistamines that block H_1 receptors (e.g., diphenhydramine and hydroxyzine) should be employed initially, but they frequently cause sedation; this may present a safety issue for certain occupations (e.g., heavy equipment operators). When sedation occurs or presents a safety concern, nonsedating second-generation antihistamines (cetirizine, loratadine, and fexofenadine) may be employed. When H_1 histamine blockers alone are not sufficient, they may be combined with H_2 blockers (e.g., cimetidine, ranitidine, and famotidine) or doxepin, a tricyclic antidepressant with potent H_1 and H_2 blocking activity. Doxepin is extremely sedating and should be used cautiously, if at all, when safety concerns arise on the job. Oral corticosteroid therapy may be employed for severe cases of chronic urticaria, especially those associated with angioedema, which are unresponsive to the above measures. Immunotherapy with a standardized latex extract has been tried in one randomized, double-blind, placebo-controlled study, which demonstrated some clinical efficacy in the treatment of contact urticaria, and some improvement in rhinitis and asthma symptoms during specific inhalation challenges (157).

REFERENCES

1. Lever WF, Schaumburg-Lever G. Histopathology of the Skin. 7th ed. Philadelphia: Lippincott, 1990:152–153.
2. Harvell J, Bason M, Maibach H. Contact urticaria and its mechanisms. Food Chem Toxicol 1994; 32:103–112.
3. Lushniak BD. The epidemiology of occupational contact dermatitis. Dermatol Clin 1995; 13:671–680.
4. Greaves MW. Chronic urticaria. N Engl J Med 1995; 332:1767–1771.
5. Elpern DJ. The syndrome of immediate reactivities (contact urticaria syndrome)–an historical study from a dermatology practice. Hawaii Med J 1985; 44:426–440.
6. Nelson C. Office visits to dermatologists: National Ambulatory Medical Care Survey, United States 1989–90. Vital and Health Statistics of the Centers for Disease Control and Prevention/National Center for Health Statistics 1994; 240:1–12.
7. Romaguera C, Grimalt F. Statistical and comparative study of 4600 patients tested in Barcelona (1973–1977). Contact Dermatitis 1980; 6:309–315.
8. Bakke P, Gulsvik A, Eide GE. Hay fever, eczema and urticaria in southwest Norway. Allergy 1990; 45:515–522.
9. Bureau of Labor Statistics (BLS). Occupational Injuries and Illnesses in the United States. US Department of Labor, BLS, published annually since 1972; data for 1993 published August 1996 in Bulletin 2478.
10. National Institute for Occupational Safety and Health (NIOSH). National Occupational Survey–pilot study for development of an occupational disease surveillance method. Rockville, MD: US Department of Health, Education, and Welfare, 1975; HEW Publications (NIOSH):75–162.
11. Plotnick H. Analysis of 250 consecutively evaluated cases of workers' disability claims for dermatitis. Arch Dermatol 1990; 160:782–786.
12. Kanerva L, Toikkanen J, Jolanki R, Estlander T. Statistical data on occupational contact urticaria. Contact Dermatitis 1996; 35:229–233.
13. Kanerva L, Jolanki R, Toikkanen J, Estlander T. Statistics on occupational contact urticaria. In: Amin S, Lahti A, Maibach HI, eds. Contact Urticaria Syndrome. Boca Raton, FL: CRC Press, 1997.
14. Kanerva L, Vaheri E. Occupational rhinitis in Finland. Int Arch Occup Environ Health 1993; 32:150–155.
15. Skinner SL, Fowler JF. Contact anaphylaxis: a review. Am J Contact Dermatitis 1995; 6:133–142.
16. Hamann CP. Natural rubber latex sensitivity in review. Am J Contact Dermatitis 1993; 4:4–21.
17. Turjanmaa K. Incidence of immediate allergy to latex gloves in hospital personnel. Contact Dermatitis 1987; 17:270–275.
18. Wrangsjo K, Osterman K, van Hage-Hamsten M. Glove-related skin symptoms among operating theatre and dental care unit personnel. Contact Dermatitis 1994; 30:102–107.
19. Berky ZT, Luciano WJ, James WD. Latex glove allergy, a survey of the US Army Dental Corps. JAMA 1992; 268:2695–2696.
20. Tarlo SM, Sussman GL, Holness DL. Latex sensitivity in dental students and staff–a cross-sectional study. J Allergy Clin Immunol 1997; 99:396–401.
21. Valkes R, Conde-Salazar L, Cuevas M. Allergic contact urticaria from natural rubber latex in healthcare and non-healthcare workers. Contact Dermatitis 2004; 50:222–224.

22. Grzybowski M, Ownby DR, Peyser PA, Johnson CC, Schork MA. The prevalence of anti-latex IgE antibodies among registered nurses. J Allergy Clin Immunol 1996; 98:535–544.

23. Liss GM, Sussman GL, Deal K, et al. Latex allergy: epidemiological study of 1351 hospital workers. Occup Environ Med 1997; 54:335–342.

24. Turjanmaa K. Update on occupational natural rubber latex allergy. Dermatol Clin 1994; 12:561–567.

25. Tarlo SM, Wong L, Roos J, Booth N. Occupational asthma caused by latex in a surgical glove manufacturing plant. J Allergy Clin Immunol 1990; 85:626–631.

26. Carillo T, Blanco C, Quiralte J, Castillo R, Cuevas M, Rodriguez de Castro F. Prevalence of latex allergy among greenhouse workers. J Allergy Clin Immunol 1995; 96:699–701.

27. Meding B, Barregard L, Marcus K. Hand eczema in car mechanics. Contact Dermatitis 1994; 30:129–134.

28. Seward JP. Occupational allergy to animals. Occup Med 1999; 14:285–304.

29. Aoyama K, Ueda A, Manda F, Matsushita T, Ueda T, Yamauchi C. Allergy to laboratory animals: an epidemiological study. Br J Ind Med 1992; 49:41–47.

30. Cullinan P, Lowson D, Nieuwenhuijsen MJ, et al. Work-related symptoms, sensitization and estimated exposure in workers not previously exposed to laboratory rats. Occup Environ Med 1994; 51:589–592.

31. Lincoln TA, Bolton NE, Garrett AS. Occupational allergy to animal dander and sera. J Occup Med 1974; 16:465–469.

32. Agrup G, Sjostedt L. Contact urticaria in laboratory technicians. Acta Derm Venereol 1985; 65:114–115.

33. Johnson CR, Sorensen TB, Ingemann Larsen A, et al. Allergy risk in an enzyme producing plant: a retrospective follow-up study. Occup Environ Med 1997; 54:671–675.

34. Prahl P, Roed-Petersen J. Type I allergy from cows in veterinary surgeons. Contact Dermatitis 1979; 5:33–38.

35. Kanerva L, Susitaival P. Cow dander: the most common cause of occupational contact urticaria in Finland. Contact Dermatitis 1996; 35:309–310.

36. Cronin E. Dermatitis of the hands in caterers. Contact Dermatitis 1987; 17:265–269.

37. Hjorth N, Roed-Petersen J. Occupational protein contact dermatitis in food handlers. Contact Dermatitis 1976; 2:28–42.

38. Jeebhay MF, Robins TG, Lehrer SB, Lopata AL. Occupational seafood allergy: a review. Occup Environ Med 2001; 58:553–562.

39. Lahti A, Maibach HI. Immediate contact reactions. Immunol Allergy Clin North Am 1989; 9:463–478.

40. Lahti A, Maibach HI. Immediate contact reactions: contact urticaria and the contact urticaria syndrome. In: Marzulli FN, Maibach HI, eds. Dermatotoxicology. New York: Hemisphere, 1991:473–495.

41. Fisher AA. Contact urticaria due to occupational exposures. In: Adams RM, ed. Occupational Skin Disease. Philadelpia: W.B. Saunders, 1990:113–126.

42. Lahti A. Immediate contact reactions. In: Rycroft RJG, Menne T, Frosch PJ, eds. Textbook of Contact Dermatitis. Berlin: Springer-Verlag, 1992:62–74.

43. Reitschel RL, Fowler JF. Contact urticaria. In: Reitschel RL, Fowler JF, eds. Fisher's Contact Dermatitis. 4th ed. Baltimore: Williams & Wilkins, 1995:778–807.

44. Hogan DJ, Tanglertsampan C. The less common occupational dermatoses. Occup Med 1992; 7:385–401.

45. Amin S, Maibach HI. Immunologic contact urticaria definition. In: Amin S, Lahti A, Maibach HI, eds. Contact Urticaria Syndrome. Boca Raton, FL: CRC Press, 1997.

46. Andersen KE, Maibach HI. Multiple application delayed onset contact urticaria: possible relation to certain unusual formalin and textile reactons. Contact Dermatitis 1984; 10:227–234.

47. Kligman AM. The spectrum of contact urticaria–wheals, erythema, and pruritus. Dermatol Clin 1990; 8:57–60.

48. Tanglertsampan C, Maibach, HI. Contact urticaria. In: Hogan DJ, ed. Occupational Skin Disorders. New York: Igaku-Shoin, 1994:81–88.

49. Maibach HI, Johnson HL. Contact urticaria syndrome. Arch Dermatol 1975; 111:726–730.

50. Janssens V, Morren M, Dooms-Goosens A, Degreef H. Protein contact dermatitis: myth or reality? Br J Dermatol 1995; 132:1–6.

51. Hannuksela M. Immediate and delayed type protein contact dermatitis. In: Amin S, Lahti A, Maibach HI, eds. Contact Urticaria Syndrome. Boca Raton, FL: CRC Press, 1997.

52. Calnan CD, Shuster S. Reactions to ammonium persulfate. Arch Dermatol 1963; 88:812–815.

53. Fisher AA, Dooms-Goosen A. Persulfate hair bleach reactions. Arch Dermatol 1976; 112:1407–1409.

54. Aalto-Korte K, Makinen-Kiljunen S. Specific immunoglobulin E in patients with immediate persulfate hypersensitivity. Contact Dermatitis 2003; 49:22–25.

55. Marks JG, DeLeo VA. Contact urticaria. In: Marks JG, DeLeo VA, eds. Contact and Occupational Dermatology. St Louis: Mosby-Year Book, 1992:309–318.

56. Beltrani VS. Urticaria and angioedema. Dermatol Clin 1996; 14:171–198.

57. Kaplan AP, Kuna P, Reddigari SR. Chemokines and the allergic response. Exp Dermatol 1995; 4:260–265.

58. Nethercott JR, Lawrence MJ, Roy AM, Gibson BL. Airborne contact urticaria due to sodium benzoate in a pharmaceutical manufacturing plant. J Occup Med 1984; 26:734–736.

59. Basketter DA, Wilhelm KP. Studies on non-immune immediate conact reactions in an unselected population. Contact Dermatitis 1996; 35:237–240.

60. Shriner DL, Maibach HI. Regional variation of nonimmunologic contact urticaria–functional map of the human face. Skin Pharmacol 1996; 9:312–321.

61. Cohen SR. Skin disease in health care workers. Occup Med 1987; 2:565–580.

62. Kanerva L, Estlander T, Jolanki R. Occupational skin allergy in the dental profession. Dermatol Clin 1994; 12:517–531.

63. Sheretz EF. Occupational skin diseases in the pharmaceutical industry. Dermatol Clin 1994; 12:533–536.

64. Goetz DW, Whisman BA. Occupational asthma in a seafood restaurant worker: cross reactivity of shrimp and scallops. Ann Allergy Asthma Immunol 2000; 85:461–466.

65. Scala E, Giani M, Pirrotta L, et al. Occupational generalized urticaria and allergic airborne asthma due to anisakis simplex. Eur J Dermatol 2001; 11:249–250.

66. Siracusa A, Marcucci F, Spinozzi F, et al. Prevalence of occupational allergy due to live fish bait. Clin Exp Allergy 2003; 33:507–510.

67. Valdivieso R, Moneo I, Pola J, et al. ccupational asthma and contact urticaria caused by buckwheat flour. Ann Allergy 1989; 63:149–152.

68. Morren MA, Janssens V, Dooms-Goosens A, et al. Alpha-amylase, a flour additive: an important cause of protein contact dermatitis in bakers. J Am Acad Dermatol 1993; 29:723–728.

69. Kanerva L, Vanhanen M, Tupasela O. Occupational allergic urticaria from fungal but not bacterial alpha-amylase. Contact Dermatitis 1997; 36:306–307.

70. Alanko K, Tuomi T, Vanhanen M, et al. Occupational IgE-mediated allergy to Tribolium confusum (confused flour beetle). Allergy 2000; 55:879–882.

71. Temesvari E, Varkonyi V. Contact urticaria provoked by egg. Contact Dermatitis 1980; 6:143–144.

72. Shimizu S, Chen KR, Miyakawa S. Cefotiam-induced contact urticaria syndrome: an occupational condition in Japanese nurses. Dermatology 1996; 192:174–176.

73. Krautheim AB, Jermann TH, Bircher AJ. Chlorhexidine anaphylaxis: case report and review of the literature. Contact Dermatitis 2004; 50:113–116.
74. Belsito DV. Contact urticaria from pentamidine isethionate. Contact Dermatitis 1993; 29:158.
75. Moscato G, Galdi E, Scibilia J, et al. Occupational asthma, rhinitis and urticaria due to piperacillin sodium in a pharmaceutical worker. Eur Respir J 1995; 8:467–469.
76. Nutter AF. Contact urticaria to rubber. Br J Dermatol 1979; 101:597–598.
77. Forstrom L. Contact urticaria from latex surgical gloves. Contact Dermatitis 1980; 6:33–34.
78. Turjanmaa K, Alenius H, Makinen-Kiljunen S, Reunala T, Palusuo T. Natural rubber latex allergy. Allergy 1996; 51:593–602.
79. Taylor JS, Erkek E. Latex allergy: diagnosis and management. Dermatol Ther 2004; 17:289–301.
80. Turjanmaa K. Contact urticaria from latex goves. In: Amin S, Lahti A, Maibach HI, eds. Contact Urticaria Syndrome. Boca Raton, FL: CRC Press, 1997.
81. Vega JM, Moneo I, Armentia A, Vega J, De la Fuente R, Fernandez A. Pine processionary caterpillar as a new cause of immunologic contact urticaria. Contact Dermatitis 2000; 42:129–132.
82. Lopata AL, Fenemore B, Jeebhey MF, Gade G, Potter PC. Occupational allergy laboratory workers cased by the African migratory grasshopper *Locusta migratoria*. Allergy 2005; 60:200–205.
83. Krakowiak A, Kowalczyk M, Palczynski C. Occupational contact urticaria and rhinoconjunctivitis in a veterinarian from bull terrier's seminal fluid. Contact Dermatitis 2004; 50:385.
84. Goransson K. Occupational contact urticaria to fresh cow and pig blood in slaughtermen. Contact Dermatitis 1981; 7:281–282.
85. Hinojosa M, Subiza J, Moneo I, Puyana J, Diez ML, Fernandez-Rivas M. Contact urticaria caused by Obeche wood (*Triplochiton scleroxylon*). Report of eight patients. Ann Allergy 1990; 64:476–479.
86. Estlander T, Jolanki R, Alanko K, Kanerva L. Occupational allergic contact dermatitis caused by wood dusts. Contact Dermatitis 2001; 44:213–217.
87. Garces Sotillos MM, Blanco Carmona JG, Juste Picon S, Rodriguez Gaston P, Perez Gimenez R, Alonso Gil L. Occupational asthma and contact urticaria caused by mukali wood dust (*Aningeria robusta*). J Investig Allergol Clin Immunol 1995; 5:113–114.
88. Kiistala R, Makinen-Kiljunen S, Heikkinen K, Rinne J, Haahtela T. Occupational allergic rhinitis and contact urticaria caused by bishop's weed (*Ammi majus*). Allergy 1999; 54:635–639.
89. Paulsen E, Skov PS, Bindslev-Jensen C, Voitenko V, Poulsen LK. Occupational type I allergy to Christmas cactus (*Schlumbergera*). Allergy 1997; 52:656–660.
90. Anderson F, Bindslev-Jensen C, Stahl Skov P, Paulsen E, Anderson KE. Immediate allergic and nonallergic reactions to Christmas and Easter cacti. Allergy 1999; 45:511–516.
91. De Greef JM, Lieutier-Colas F, Bessot JC, et al. Urticaria and rhinitis to shrubs of Ficus benjamina and breadfruit in a banana-allergic road worker: evidence for a cross-sensitization between Moracea, banana and latex. Int Arch Allergy Immunol 2001; 125:182–184.
92. Piirila P, Kanerva L, Alanko K, et al. Occupational IgE-mediated asthma, rhinoconjunctivitis, and contact urticaria caused by Easter lily (*Lilium longiflorum*) and tulip. Allergy 1999; 54:273–277.
93. Chan RY, Oppenheimer JJ. Occupational allergy caused by Peruvian lily (*Alstroemeria*). Ann Allergy Asthma Immunol 2002; 88:638–639.
94. Uter W, Nohle M, Randerath B, Schwanitz HJ. Occupational contact urticaria and late-phase bronchial asthma caused by compositae pollen in a florist. Am J Contact Dermat 2001; 12:182–184.

95. Kanerva L, Estlander T, Petman L, Makinen-Kiljunen S. Occupational allergic contact urticaria to yucca (*Yucca aloifolia*), weeping fig (*Ficus banjamina*), and spathe flower (*Spathiphyllum wallisii*). Allergy 2001; 56:1108–1111.

96. Blanco C, Carillo T, Quiralte J, Pascual C, Martin Estaban M, Castillo R. Occupational rhinoconjunctivitis and bronchial asthma due to *Phoenix canariensis* pollen allergy. Allergy 1995; 50:277–280.

97. Quirce S, Garcia-Figueroa B, Alaguibel JM, Muro MD, Tabar Al. Occupational astma and contact urticaria from dried flowers of *Limonium tartaricum*. Allergy 1993; 48:285–290.

98. Kanerva L, Makinen-Kiljunen S, Kiistala R, Granlund H. Occupational allergy caused by the spathe flower (*Spathiphyllum walisii*). Allergy 1995; 50:174–178.

99. Tanaka T, Moriwaki SI, Horio T. Occupational dermatitis with simultaneous immediate and delayed allergy to chrysanthemum. Contact Dermatitis 1987; 16:152–154.

100. Tarvainen K, Salonen JP, Kanerva L, Estlander T, Keskinen H, Rantenen T. Allergy and toxicodermia from shiitake mushrooms. J Am Acad Dermatol 1991; 24:64–66.

101. Lahti A. Contact urticaria and respiratory symptoms from tulips and lilies. Contact Dermatitis 1986; 14:317–319.

102. Axelsson IG, Johansson SG, Zetterstrom O. Occupational allergy to weeping fig in plant keepers. Allergy 1987; 42:161–167.

103. Astarita C, Di Martino P, Scala G, Franzese A, Sproviero S. Contact allergy: another occupational risk to *Tetranychus urticae*. J Allergy Clin Immunol 1996; 98:732–738.

104. Delgado J, Orta JC, Navarro AM, et al. Occupational allergy in greenhouse workers: sensitization to *Tetranychus urticae*. Clin Exp Allergy 1997; 27:640–645.

105. Dannaker CJ. Agricultural chemicals. In: Amin S, Lahti A, Maibach HI, eds. Contact Urticaria Syndrome. Boca Raton, FL: CRC Press, 1997.

106. Ortega N, Quiralte J, Blanco C, Castillo R, Alvarez MJ, Carrillo T. Tobacco allergy: demonstration of cross-reacitivity with other members of Solanaceae family and mugwort pollen. Ann Allergy Asthma Immunol 1999; 82:194–197.

107. Tabar AI, Alvarez-Puebla MJ, Gomez B, et al. Diversity of asparagus allergy: clinical immunological features. Clin Exp Allergy 2004; 34:131–136.

108. Kanerva L, Estlander T, Jolanki R, Tarvainen K. Occupational allergic contact dermatitis and contact urticaria caused by polyfunctional aziridine hardener. Contact Dermatitis 1995; 33:304–309.

109. Kanerva L, Pelttari M, Jolanki R, Alanko K, Estlander T, Suhonen R. Occupational contact urticaria from diglycidyl ether of bisphenol A epoxy resin. Allergy 2002; 57:1205–1207.

110. Sasseville D. Contact urticaria from epoxy resin and reactive diluents. Contact Dermatitis 1998; 38:57–58.

111. Valks R, Conde-Salazar L, Barrantes OL. Occupational allergic contact urticaria and asthma from diphenylmethane-4,4'-diisocyanate. Contact Dermatitis 2003; 46:166–167.

112. Kanerva L, Grenquist-Norden B, Piirila P. Occupational IgE-mediated contact urticaria from diphenylmethane-4,4-diisocyanate (MDI). Contact Dermatitis 1999; 41:50–51.

113. Tarvainen K, Jolanki R, Estlander T, Tupasela O, Pfaffli P, Kanerva L. Immunologic contact urticaria due to airborne methylhexahydrophthalic and methyltetrahydrophthalic anhydrides. Contact Dermatitis 1995; 32:204–209.

114. Kanerva L, Alanko K, Jolanki R, Estlander T. Airborne allergic contact urticaria from methylhexahydrophthalic anhydride and hexahydrophthalic anhydride. Contact Dermatitis 1999; 41:339–341.

115. Kanerva L, Alanko K. Occupational allergic contact urticaria from maleic anhydride. Contact Dermatitis 2000; 42:170–172.

116. Yokota K, Johyama Y, Miyaue H, Matsumoto N, Yamaguchi K. Occupational contact urticaria caused by airborne methylhexahydrophthalic anhydride. Ind Health 2001; 39:347–352.

117. Weiss RR, Mowad C. Contact urticaria from xylene. Am J Contact Dermat 1998; 9:125–127.
118. Jolanki R, Kanerva L, Estlander T, Tarvainen K. Skin Allergy caused by organic acid anhydrides. In: Amin S, Lahti A, Maibach HI, eds. Contact Urticaria Syndrome. Boca Raton, FL: CRC Press, 1997.
119. Bergman A, Svedberg U, Nilsson E. Contact urticaria with anaphylactic reactions caused by occupational exposure to iridium salt. Contact Dermatitis 1995; 32:14–17.
120. Nakayama H, Ichikawa T. Occupational contact urticaria syndrome due to rhodium and platinum. In: Amin S, Lahti A, Maibach HI, eds. Contact Urticaria Syndrome. Boca Raton, FL: CRC Press, 1997.
121. Dooms-Goosens A, Duron C, Loncke J, Degreef H. Contact urticaria due to nylon. Contact Dermatitis 1986; 14:63.
122. Sugiura K, Sugiura M, Hayakawa R, Shamoto M, Sasaki K. A case of contact urticaria syndrome due to di(2-ethylhexyl) phthalate (DOP) in work clothes. Contact Dermatitis 2002; 46:13–16.
123. Kanerva L, Hyry R, Jolanki R, Hytonen M, Estlander T. Delayed and immediate allergy caused by methylhexahydrophthalic anhydride. Contact Dermatitis 1997; 36:34–38.
124. Majoie IM, Bruynzeel DP. Occupational immediate-type hypersensitivity to henna in a hairdresser. Am J Contact Dermat 1996; 7:38–40.
125. Shelley WB, Shelly ED, Talanin NY. Urticaria due to occupational exposure to glyceryl monothioglycolate permanent wave solution. Acta Derm Venereol 1998; 78:471–472.
126. Niinimaki A, Niinimaki M, Makinen-Kiljunen S, Hannuksela M. Contact Urticaria from protein hydrolysates in hair conditioners. Allergy 1998; 53:1078–1082.
127. Rudzki E, Rapiejko P, Rebandel P. Occupational contact dermatitis, with asthma and rhinitis, from camomile in a cosmetician also with contact urticaria from both camomile and lime flowers. Contact Dermatitis 2003; 49:162.
128. Dooms-Goosens A, Deleu H. Airborne contact dermatitis: an update. Contact Dermatitis 1991; 25:211–217.
129. Lindskov R. Contact urticaria to formaldehyde. Contact Dermatitis 1982; 8:333–334.
130. Fowler JF. Contact urticaria to 1,1,1-Trichoroethane. Am J Contact Dermatitis 1991; 2:239.
131. Goncalo M, Chiera L, Goncalo S. Immediate and delayed hypersensitivity to garlic and soybean. Am J Contact Dermatitis 1992; 3:102–104.
132. Palmer KT, Rycroft RJG. Occupational airborne contact urticaria due to xylene. Contact Dermatitis 1993; 28:44.
133. Bjorkner BE. Industrial airborne dermatoses. Dermatol Clin 1994; 12:501–509.
134. Farrell FJ. Angioedema and urticaria as acute and late phase reactions to zinc fume exposure, with associated metal fume fever-like symptoms. Am J Ind Med 1987; 12:331–337.
135. Kanerva L, Estlander T, Jolanki R, Lahteenmaki MT, Keskinen H. Occupational urticaria from welding polyurethane. J Am Acad Dematol 1991; 24:825–826.
136. Kanerva L, Estlander T, Jolanki R. Long-lasting contact urticaria from castor bean. J Am Acad Dermatol 1990; 23:351–355.
137. Mathias CGT. Occupational dermatoses. J Am Acad Dermatol 1988; 19:1107–1114.
138. Key MM. Some unusual allergic reactions in industry. Arch Dermatol 1961; 83:3–6.
139. Morris GE. Urticaria following exposure to ammonia fumes. Arch Ind Health 1956; 13:480.
140. Champion RH, Roberts SOB, Carpenter RG, Roger JH. Urticaria and angioedema: a review of 554 patients. Br J Dermatol 1969; 81:588–595.
141. Black AK. Mechanical trauma and urticaria. Am J Int Med 1985; 8:297–303.
142. Caslae TB, Sampson HA, Hanifin J, et al. Guide to physical urticarias. J Allergy Clin Immunol 1988; 5:758–763.
143. Soter NA. Physical urticaria/angioedema. Semin Dermatol 1987; 6:302–312.

144. Farkas J. Fiberglass dermatitis in employees of a project-office in a new building. Contact Dermatitis 1983; 9:79.
145. Soter NA. Urticaria and angioedema. In: Fitzpatrick TB, Eisen AZ, Wolff K, Freedberg IM, Austen KF, eds. Dermatology in General Medicine. New York: McGraw-Hill, 1993:1483–1493.
146. Wener MH, Metzger WJ, Simon RA. Occupationally acquired vibratory angioedema with secondary carpal tunnel syndrome. Ann Intern Med 1983; 98:44–46.
147. Cohen SR, Bilinski DL, McNutt NS. Vibration syndrome: cutaneous and systemic manifestations in a jackhammer operator. Arch Dermatol 1985; 12:1544–1547.
148. Page EH, Shear NH. Temperature-deendent skin disorders. J Am Acad Dematol 1988; 18:1003–1119.
149. Bjorkner B. Occupational cold urticaria from contact spray. Contact Dermatitis 1981; 7:338–339.
150. Fitzgerald DA, Heagerty AHM, English JSC. Cold urticaria as an occupational dermatosis. Contact Dermatitis 1995; 32:238.
151. Miller SD, Pritchard D, Crowley JP. Blood histamine levels following graded cold challenge in atypical acquired cold urticaria. Ann Allergy 1992; 68:27–29.
152. Whinnery JE, Anderson GK. Environmentally induced cholinergic urticaria and anaphylaxis. Avia Space Environ Med 1983; 54:551–553.
153. Hirschmann JV, Lawlor F, English JSC, Louback JB, Winkelmann RK, Greaves MW. Cholinergic urticaria. Arch Dermatol 1987; 123:462–467.
154. Jorizzo JL, Smith EB. The physical urticarias. Arch Dermatol 1982; 118:194–201.
155. Amin A, Lahti A, Maibach HI. Contact Urticaria Syndrome. Boca Raton, FL: CRC Press, 1997.
156. Kanerva L, Estlander E, Jolanki R. Skin testing for immediate hypersensitivity in occupational allergology. In: Menne T, Maibach HI, eds. Exogenous Dermatoses: Environmental Dermatitis. Boca Raton, FL: CRC Press, 1990.
157. Sastre J, Fernandez-Nieto M, Rico P, et al. Specific immunotherapy with a standardized latex extract in allergic workers: a double-blind, placebo-controlled study. J Allergy Clin Immunol 2003; 111:985–994.

Appendix

Agents Causing Occupational Asthma with Key References

Jean-Luc Malo
Department of Chest Medicine, Université de Montréal and Sacré-Cœur Hospital, Montreal, Quebec, Canada

Moira Chan-Yeung
Occupational and Environmental Lung Disease Unit, Respiratory Division, Department of Medicine, University of British Columbia and Vancouver General Hospital, Vancouver, British Columbia, Canada

Agents Causing Occupational Asthma with Key References

Agents	Occupation	References	Subjects	Prevalence (n)	Skin (%)	Specific IgE test	Other immunologic test	Broncho-provocation test	Other evidence
High-molecular-weight agents									
Animal-derived antigens									
Laboratory animal	Laboratory workers	(1)	296	13	17%	34% of 255 +	ND	ND	
Cow dander	Agricultural workers	(2)	5	NA	100%	100 % +	– precipitin	100% +	
		(3)	49	NA	100%	ND	Immunoblotting	ND	
Monkey dander	Laboratory workers	(4)	2	NA	2	2 +	ND	ND	+
Deer dander	Farmer	(5)	1	NA	+	ND	ND	+	
Mink urine	Farmer	(6)	1	NA	+	–	ND	+	
Chicken	Poultry workers	(7,8)	NA	79% +	79% +	ND	1/1 +	+	
		(9)	4	NA	+ to feathers	ND	ND	+	
Pig	Butcher	(10)	1	NA	ND	+	ND	ND	PEF
Frog	Frog catcher	(11)	1	NA	+	+	Neg precipitin	ND	
Lactoserum	Dairy industry	(12)	1	NA	+	ND	+ basophil degranulation	+	
Bovine serum albumin	Laboratory technician	(13)	1	NA	+	ND	ND	+	
Lactalbumin	Chocolate candy	(14)	1	NA	+	+	ND	+	+ conjunctival
Casein (cow's milk)	Tanner	(15)	1	NA	ND	+	ND	+	
Egg protein	Egg producers	(16)	188	7	34% +	29% +	ND	ND	PEF, 7% +
Endocrine glands	Pharmacist	(17)	1	NA	+	ND	ND	+	
Bat guano	Various	(18)	7	NA	+	+	RAST inhibition	ND	
Ivory dust	Ivory worker	(19)	1	NA	–	ND	ND	+	FEV$_1$ at work
Nacre dust	Nacre buttons	(20)	1	NA	+	ND	Neg precipitin	+	

Sericin	Hairdresser	(21)	2	ND	1/1 +	ND	ND	ND	
Crustacea, seafoods, fish									
Crab	Snow-crab processors	(22)	303	16	22% +	ND	ND	72 % of 46 +	PEF, PC20
Prawn	Prawn processors	(23)	50	36	26% +	16% +	ND	2/2 +	
Hoya	Oyster farm	(24)	1413	29	82% of 511 with asthma	89% of ~180 + with asthma +	ND	ND	
Clam and shrimp	Food processors	(25)	2	4%	+	+	RAST inhibition	+	PC20
Lobster and shrimp	Fishmonger shop	(26)	1	NA	+	+	ND	+	
Gammarus shrimp	Fish food factory	(27)	1	NA	+	+	SDS-PAGE	+	PC20
Scallop and shrimp	Restaurant seafood handler	(28)	1	NA	+	+	SDS-PAGE	+	PEF
Cuttle-fish	Deep-sea fishermen	(29)	66	Incidence of 1%/yr	ND	ND	ND	ND	
Cuttle-fish bone	Jewelery polisher	(30)	1	NA	+	ND	ND	+	
Salmon	Processing plant	(31)	291	24 (8%)	ND	25 (9%)	Specific IgG (33%)	ND	PEF
Trout (?)	Trout processors	(32)	5	NA	ND	100% Neg	100% +	ND	
Shrimpmeal	Technician	(33)	1	NA	+	+	ND	+	
Red soft coral	Fishermen	(34)	74	9	2/2+	ND	ND	ND	
Marine sponge	Laboratory grinder	(35)	1	NA	+	ND	Precipitins	ND	Asthma attack at work
Various fishes	Fish processors	(36)	2	NA	+	+	ND	+	PEF
Arthropods									
Grain mite	Farmers	(37)	290	12	21% +	19% of 219 +	ND	ND	
	Grain-store workers	(38)	133	33	25% +	23% of 128 +	ND	1/1 +	21% of 116 with + PC 20

(*Continued*)

Agents Causing Occupational Asthma with Key References (*Continued*)

Agents	Occupation	References	Subjects	Prevalence (n)	Skin (%)	Specific IgE test	Other immunologic test	Broncho-provocation test	Other evidence
Amblyseius cucumeris	Horticulturists	(39)	472	25.7%	23%	Done in some	ND	ND	Nasal challenges
Locust	Laboratory workers	(40)	118	26	32% of 113 +	Done	Specific IgG	ND	Reduced FEV1
Screw worm fly	Flight crews	(41)	15	60	77% +	53%	RAST inhibition	ND	
	Laboratory workers	(42)	182	25	91% of 11 +	ND	ND	ND	
Cricket	Laboratory workers	(43)	2	NA	+	+	Passive transfer	+	
Insect larvae	Fish bait breeder	(44)	14	NA	+	+	RAST inhibition	+	PEF
	Fish bait farmers	(45)	76	4%	32%	19%	ND	ND	
Moth, butterfly	Entomologists	(46)	2	NA	+	ND	ND	ND	
Mexican bean weevil	Seed house	(47)	2	NA	+	ND	Passive transfer	ND	
Fruit fly	Laboratory workers	(48)	22	32	27% +	27%+	RAST inhibition	21% of 14 +	
Honeybee	Honey processors	(49)	1	NA	+	+	ND	+	
L. caesar larvae	Anglers	(50)	14	NA	13/14	13/14	RAST inhibition	7/7 +	
Lesser mealworm	Entomologists	(51)	3	NA	Neg	100% of 3 +	RAST inhibition	ND	
Mealworm larvae (*Tenibriomolitor*)	Fish bait handlers	(52)	5	NA	4/5	2/5	RAST inhibition	2/2	
Fowl mite	Poultry workers	(53)	13	NA	77% +	60%	ND	1/1 +	
Barn mite	Farmers	(54)	38	NA	100% +	~100%	ND	ND	
Mites and parasites	Flour handlers	(55)	12	NA	ND	+	ND	ND	
Various acarians									
Panonychus ulmi	Apple growers	(56)	4	NA	+	ND	Neg precipitins	ND	
Panonychus citri	Citrus farmers	(57)	16	NA	+	+	RAST inhibition	+ (one)	

Organism	Occupation	Ref	n				Method		
Tetranychus macdanieli	Vine growers	(58)	35	4/35 (11%)	100%	ND	ND	ND	
Tetranychus urticae	Farmers	(59)	16	16/46 (35%)	100%	100%	ND	ND	
Bruchus lentis	Agronomist	(60)	1	NA	+	+	Immunoblotting	+	
Daphnia	Fish food store	(61)	2	NA	+	+	ND	2/2 +	
Sheep blowfly	Technicians	(62)	53	24	ND	67% of 15 +	ND	ND	
Grasshoper	Laboratory workers	(63)	16	4 (25%)	7 (44%)	ND	ND	+ in one	
Sewer fly (*Psychoda alternata*)	Sewage plant workers	(64)	1	NA	+	+	Histamine rel.; PK +	+	
Chironimid midges	Aquarists, fish-food	(65)	225	45%	80%	34%	ND	ND	
Beetles (*Coleoptera*)	Museum curator	(66)	1	NA	+	ND	Passive transfer	ND	
Dermestidae spp. (*Coleoptera*)	Wool worker	(67)	1	NA	+	+	SDS-PAGE	+	
Confused flour beetle (*Tribolium confusum*)	Mechanics in a rye plant	(68)	1	NA	+	+	ND	ND	
Silkworm	Silk workers	(69)	53	34%	ND	ND	ND	ND	
Anisakis simplex (nematode)	Chicken breeder and fish monger	(70)	2	NA	+	+	Immunoblotting	+	
Larva of silkworm	Sericulture	(71)	5519	0.2	100% of 9(?)+	1/1(?)+	P-K reaction	100% of 9 +	
Fish-feed	Aquarium keeper	(72)	1	NA	+	+	ND	+	
(*Echinodorus larva*)	Technicians	(73)	3	23%	ND	+	ND	ND	
Arthropods Ground bugs	Bottling	(74)	1	NA	+	+	ND	ND	PEF
Molds *Dictyostelium discoideum* (mold)	Technician	(75)	1	NA	+	+	ND	Workplace +	

(Continued)

Agents Causing Occupational Asthma with Key References (*Continued*)

Agents	Occupation	References	Subjects	Prevalence (n)	Skin (%)	Specific IgE test	Other immunologic test	Broncho-provocation test	Other evidence
Aspergillus niger	Technicians	(76)	3	1%	3 +	ND	ND	ND	
Aspergillus	Beet sugar workers	(77)	1	1%	+	+	ND	ND	
Aspergillus	Baker	(78)	1	NA	+	ND	Neg precipitins	+	
Alternaria	Baker	(78)	1	NA	+	ND	Neg precipitins	+	
Trichoderma koningii	Sawmill worker	(79)	1	NA	ND	ND	Precipitins specific IgG	ND	PEF
Plasmopara viticola	Agricultural	(80)	1	NA	+	+	Various	+	
Neurospora	Plywood factory worker	(81)	1	NA	+	+	ND	+	
Chrysonilia sitophila	Logging worker	(82)	1	NA	+	+	ND	ND	PEF
Rhizopus nigricans	Coal miner	(83)	1	NA	+	+	ND	+	
Algae *Chlorella*	Pharmacist	(84)	1	NA	+	ND	ND	+	PEF
Plants Grain dust	Grain elevators	(85)	610	~40	9% +	ND	Neg precipitins	ND	Spirometry pre-postshift FEV_1, volumes
		(86,87)	502	47	~50% of 51 exposed +	ND	ND	ND	
Wheat, rye, and soya flour	Bakers, millers	(88)	22	NA	0% +	ND	Neg precipitins	27%+	50% PC 20 + FEV_1, PC20
		(89)	279	35	9% + (cereals)	ND	ND	ND	
		(90)	7	100	100% +	100%	100% Neg Western blotting, etc.	57% +	
		(91)	9	100	ND	100% +	ND	ND	
Lathyrus sativus	Flour handler	(92)	1	NA	+	ND	+ Precipitins	+	
Lathyrus odoratus	Greenhouse worker	(93)	1	NA	+	+	ND	ND	PEF

Saccharomyces cerevisiae	Baker	(94)	1	NA	+	+	ND	+	ND	+	PEF
Vicia sativa	Farmer	(95)	1	NA	+	+	+ Preciptins,	+	+	Passive transfer +	
Buckwheat	Bakers	(96)	3	NA	100% +	ND	ND	ND	ND	+	
Gluten	Bakers	(97)	1	NA	+	+	RAST inhibition	+	+	ND	
Coffee bean	Food processor	(98)	372	34	24% +	12% +	ND	ND	ND	+	Lung function
		(99)	45	9	9–40% +	ND	ND	ND	ND	ND	Spirometry
		(100)	22	NA	82% +	50% +	ND	ND	67 % of 12 +	+	PC20 + in 14
Castor bean	Oil industry	(101)	14	NA	100% +	100% +	ND	ND	ND	+	
Green bean (*Phaseolus multiflorus*)	Homemaker	(102)	1	NA	+	+	Histamine	+	+	+	
Carob bean	Jam factory	(103)	1	NA	–	+	ND	+	+	+	
Tea	Tea processors	(104)	3	NA	+	+	+ PCA with catechin	+	+	+	
Herbal tea	Herbal tea processors	(105)	1	NA	ND	Neg	ND	+	+	+	Tobacco leaf
	Tobacco manufacturers	(106)	1	NA	+	+	ND	+	+	+	
Hops	Brewery chemist	(107)	16	69	ND	ND	ND	ND	ND	ND	PEF
Baby's breath (*Gypsophila paniculata*)	Florist	(108)	1	NA	+	ND	ND	ND	ND	ND	
		(109)	1	NA	+	+	Histamine release	+	+	+	
Freesia and paprika	Horticulture	(110)	2	NA	+	+	Histamine release	+	+	ND	
Flowers (various)	Flower industry	(111)	40	7.7%	+ (21%, flowers)	ND	ND	ND	Three subjects +	+	
Bell pepper	Greenhouse workers	(39)	472	13.3%	35.4%	18.6%	ND	18.6%	ND	ND	
Bells of Ireland (*Molucella laevis*)	Grower	(112)	1	NA	+	+	ND	+	+	+	PEF
Amaryllis	Greenhouse worker	(113)	1	NA	+	+	ND	+	+	+	PEF

(Continued)

Agents Causing Occupational Asthma with Key References (*Continued*)

Agents	Occupation	References	Subjects	Prevalence (n)	Skin (%)	Specific IgE test	Other immunologic test	Broncho-provocation test	Other evidence
Camomile	Cosmetician	(114)	1	NA	+	ND	ND	+ Nasal challenge	
Cyclamen	Florists	(115)	2	NA	+ (pollen)	+	ND	ND	
Limonium tataricum	Floral worker	(116)	1	NA	+	+	ND	ND	PEF
Decorative flowers	Floral worker	(117)	4	NA	+2/4	+2/4	ND	+3/4	
Spathe flowers	Floral worker	(118)	1	NA	+	+	Immunoblotting	Neg (done 8 months later)	
Rose	Culture of roses	(119)	290	6.2%	ND	19.5%	Immunoblotting	ND	
Peach	Factory worker	(120)	1	NA	+	+	ND	+	
Chrysanthemum	Greenhouse workers	(121)	104	9%	20.2%	+ in some	ND	ND	
Solanum melongena	Greenhouse worker	(122)	1	NA	+	ND	ND	+ conjunctival	PEF
Stephanotis floribunda (Madagascar jasmine)	Greenhouse workers	(123)	4	50%	+	+	ND	+ in one	PEF
Herb material	Herbal worker	(124)	1	NA	+	+	Identification of 3 protein fractions	+	
Umbrella tree (Schefflera)	Landscape gardener	(125)	1	NA	+	+	ND	ND	
Passiflora alata and Rhamnus purshiana	Technician pharmacy	(126)	1	NA	+	+	Immunoblotting	+	
Sarsaparilla root	Herbal tea worker	(127)	1	NA	+	+	ND	+	
Soybean lecithin	Bakers	(128)	2	NA	+	+	ND	+	
Olive oilcake	Oil industry	(129)	1	NA	+	ND	ND	+	

Brazil ginseng (*Pfaffia paniculata*)	Medicinal plant processor	(130)	1	NA	+	+	Neg precipitins	+	
Voacanga africana	Chemist's spouse	(131)	1	NA	+	+	Neg precipitins	+	
Onion	Homemakers	(132)	3	NA	+	+	ND	+	
Onion seeds (*Allium cepa*, red onion)	Seed packing	(133)	1	NA	+	+	Immunoblotting	+	
Fennel seed	Sausage processing	(134)	1	NA	ND	+	Immunoblotting	ND	
Sesame seeds	Baker	(135)	1	NA	+	+	Immunoblotting	+	
Grass juice	Gardener	(136)	1	NA	+	+	Immunoblotting	+	
Potato	Housewives	(137)	2	NA	+	+	Histamine release	+	
Asparagus	Food processor	(138)	1	NA	+	+	Immunoblotting	+	
Courgette	Fruit warehouse	(139)	1	NA	+	+	ND	ND	
Swiss chard (*Beta vulgaris* L. cycla)	Housewives	(140)	1	NA	+	+	Histamine release	+	
Mushroom	Mushroom soup processors	(141)	8	NA	+	ND	ND	50% of 8 +	
	Mushroom producers	(142)	1	NA	ND	+	Immunoblotting	ND	PEF
Mushroom *Boletus edulis*	Office worker, cook, hotel manager	(143)	3	NA	+	+	ND	2+	
Cacoon seed	Decorator	(144)	1	NA	+	ND	ND	ND	
Chicory	Vegetable wholesaler	(145)	1	NA	+	+	Immunoblotting	ND	
Rose hips	Pharmaceutical	(146)	9	NA	67% +	67% +	ND	50% of 4 +	
Sunflower	Laboratory worker	(147)	1	NA	+	+	RAST inhibition	+	
Helianthus annus	Processing workers	(148)	102	16.6%	23.5%	ND	ND	ND	
Phoenix canariensis	Gardener	(149)	1	NA	+	+	ND	+	

(Continued)

Agents Causing Occupational Asthma with Key References (*Continued*)

Agents	Occupation	References	Subjects	Prevalence (n)	Skin (%)	Specific IgE test	Other immunologic test	Broncho-provocation test	Other evidence
Garlic dust	Food packaging	(150)	1	NA	+	+	ND	+	
Licuorice roots	Herbalist	(151)	1	NA	+	+	RAST inhibition	+	
Spices	Spices processing	(152)	1	NA	+	+	ND	+	
Saffron spice (*Crocus sativus*)	Saffron processors	(153)	1	NA	+	+	ND	ND	
		(154)	5	10%	6%+	26%	Immunoblotting, RAST inhibition	+ in one	
Aromatic herbs	Butcher	(155)	1	NA	+	+	ND	+	PEF
Lycopodium	Powder	(156)	30	7	ND	ND	ND	2/2 +	
Weeping fig	Plant keepers	(157)	84	7	21% +	21%	ND	100% of 6 +	PC20
Pectin	Christmas candy maker	(158)	1	NA	+	–	Specific IgG$_4$	+	
Henna (conchiolin?)	Hairdressers	(159)	2	NA	+	+	ND	1/2 +	
Fenugreek	Food industry	(160)	1	NA	+	+	ND	ND	
Aniseed	Food industry	(161)	1	NA	+	+	ND	+	
Kapok	Sewer	(162)	1	NA	–	–	ND	+	
Latex	Glove manufacturing	(163)	81	6	11%+	ND	ND	ND	Lung function PEF
	Health professionals	(164)	7	2.5%	4.7%+	ND	ND	+	
Biologic enzymes *Bacillus subtilis*	Detergent industry	(165)	1642	3.2 (over seven years)	4.5–7.5% +26% of 248 +	ND	ND	ND	Lung function
		(166)	38	NA	66% +	ND	Passive transfer 100% of 5 + precipitin (nonspecific)	90% +	Lung function
Trypsin	Plastic, pharmaceutical	(167)	14	29	+	+	ND	75% of 4+	
Papain	Pharmaceutical	(168)	29	45	34% +	34% +	ND	89% of 9 +	

Allergen	Source	Ref.	No.	%					Lung function
Pepsin	Pharmaceutical	(169)	1	NA	+	+		+	
Pancreatin	Pharmaceutical	(170)	14	NA	93% +	100% of 3 +	ND	100% of 9 +	
Flaviastase	Pharmaceutical	(171)	3	NA	+	+	+precipitin	ND	
Bromelin	Pharmaceutical	(172)	76	11	25%	ND	ND	ND	
	Pharmaceutical	(173)	2	NA	+	ND	ND	2/2 +	
Egg lysosyme	Pharmaceutical	(174)	1	NA	+	+	ND	+	PEF
Fungal amylase	Bakers	(175)	118	NA	100% of 10 +, 2% exposed, 34% occupational asthma +	ND	ND	ND	
Phytase	Technicians	(176)	1	NA	+	+	ND	+	
Fungal amyloglucosidase and hemicellulase	Bakers	(177)	53	36%	ND	+	SDS-PAGE	ND	
	Bakers	(178)	140	NA	ND	5–24%	ND	ND	
Serratial peptidase	Pharmaceutical and lysozyme	(179)	1	NA	ND	+	Immunoblotting	+	
Esperase	Detergent industry	(180)	667	NA	ND	5%	ND	ND	
Xylanase	Laboratory workers	(181)	2	NA	2	2	ND	ND	PFR
Pectinase and glucanase	Fruit processors	(182)	3	NA	ND	+	Immunoblotting	ND	PFR
Lactase	Pharmaceutical	(183)	207	4%	31% +	ND	ND	ND	
Vegetable gums									
Acacia	Printers	(184)	63	19% of 31 (selection)	ND	ND	ND	ND	
		(185)	10	NA	+	ND	Passive transfer (3 +)	ND	
Tragacanth	Gum importer	(186)	1	NA	+	ND	ND	ND	
Karaya	Hairdressers	(187)	9	4	+	ND	ND	ND	
Guar	Carpet manufacturing	(188)	162	2	8%+	ND	Passive transfer 67 of 3 +	ND	PC20

(Continued)

Agents Causing Occupational Asthma with Key References (*Continued*)

Agents	Occupation	References	Subjects	Prevalence (n)	Skin (%)	Specific IgE test	Other immunologic test	Broncho-provocation test	Other evidence
Gutta-percha	Dental hygienist	(189)	1	NA	+	ND	ND	ND	
Low-molecular-weight agents									
Diisocyanates									
Toluene diisocyanate	Polyurethane, plastics, varnish	(190)	112	12.5	3%+	0%+	0%+ PCA	45% of 11 +	
		(191)	26	NA	ND	19%+	ND	100%+	
		(192)	195	28	ND	5%+	ND	70% of 17+	
		(193)	91	NA	NA	ND	0%+ Specific IgG	ND	
		(194)	162[c]	NA	ND	ND	ND	57% +	
Diphenylmethane diisocyanate	Foundry	(195)	11	NA	ND	27%+	36%+ Specific IgG	54.5%+	
		(196)	76	13	ND	3%+	7%+ Specific IgG	ND	
		(197)	26	27	4%+	4%+	15%+ Specific IgG	ND	
1,5 Naphthylene diisocyanate	Manufacturing rubber	(198)	3	NA	ND	ND	ND	100% +	
Isophorone diisocyanate	Spray painter	(199)	1	NA	ND	ND	ND	+	
Prepolymers of TDI	Floor varnishers	(200)	2	NA	ND	0% +	Specific IgG-	+	
Prepolymers of HDI	Spray painters	(201)	9	45	ND	33%+	56% +	+	
Combination of diisocyanates									
TDI, MDI, HDI, PPI	Paint shop	(202)	51	11.8[a]	ND	ND	ND	60% of 10+ to PPI	
TDI, MDI, HDI	Various industries	(203)	24	NA	ND	ND	ND	70%+ to TDI, 33%+ to MDI, 33% of + to HDI	
		(204)	247[b]	NA	60% of 53+, 14%+	ND	ND	ND	

Substance	Source/use	Ref.	n						
TDI, MDI	Paint shop	(205)	62	NA	ND	15%+	47%+ Specific IgG	6%+ to TDI, 16%+ to MDI, 24% of + to HDI	PEF
		(206)	28	NA	ND	27% of 22+ TDI-HSA, 83% of 6+ MDI-HSA	ND	100%+	
Other hardeners									
Triglycidyl isocyanurate	Spray painter	(207)	1	NA	ND	ND	ND	+	
Polyfunctional aziridine	Hardener in paints	(208)	7	NA	33% of 7	ND	ND	+ in 7	
Anhydrides									
Phthalic anhydride	Plastics	(209)	1	NA	+	+	ND	+	
	Toolsetter, resin plant agent,	(210)	3	NA	ND	ND	ND	100%+	
		(211)	118	28	18% of 11+	ND	ND		
	Production of resins	(212)	60	14	ND	7%+	17%+ Specific IgG	ND	
Trimellitic anhydride	Epoxy resins, plastics	(213)	4	NA	100% +	75% +	100% +	100% of 1 +	
Tetrachlorophthalic anhydride	Epoxy resins, plastics	(214)	5	NA	ND	ND	ND	100% +	
Pyromellitic dianhydride	Epoxy adhesive	(215)	7	NA	100% +	100% +	ND	100% +	
		(216)	7	NA	ND	ND	ND	30% +	
Methyl tetrahydrophthalic anhydride	Curing agent	(217)	1	NA	+	+	Specific IgG−	ND	Improvement with removal
Hexahydrophthalic anhydride	Chemical worker	(218)	1	NA	ND	ND	ND	+	PEF
MTHPA + HHPA	Electrical plant	(219)	109	5.4	ND	15.4%	ND	6/17	

(Continued)

Agents Causing Occupational Asthma with Key References (*Continued*)

Agents	Occupation	References	Subjects	Prevalence (n)	Skin (%)	Specific IgE test	Other immunologic test	Broncho-provocation test	Other evidence
Himic anhydride	Manufacture of flame retardant	(220)	20	35	ND	40% of 7%	RAST inhibition	ND	
Chlorendic anhydride	Mechanics	(221)	1	NA	+	+	ND	+	PEF
Maleic anhydride	Polyester resin production	(222)	1	NA	ND	ND	ND	+	
Dioctyl-phthalate	Production of PVC	(223)	1	NA	ND	ND	ND	ND	PEF
Aliphatic amines									
Ethyleneamines									
Ethyleneamines	Shellac handlers	(224)	7	NA	100%	ND	ND	100%+	
	Photography	(225)	1	NA	ND	ND	ND	+	
Hexamethylene tetramine	Lacquer handlers	(225)	7	NA	100%	ND	ND	100%	
Aliphatic polyamines	Chemical factory	(226)	12	4/12	NA	ND	ND	ND	100% of 2 +
Triethylene tetramine	Aircraft filter	(210)	1	NA	ND	ND	ND	+	
Mixture of trimethyl-hexanediamine and isophoron-diamine	Floor covering material salesman	(227)	1	NA	−	ND	ND	+	BAL
Ethanolamines									
Monoethanolamine	Beauty culture	(225)	10	100% +	ND	ND	ND	100% +	
Triethanolamine	Metal worker	(228)	2	NA	ND	ND	ND	100% of 2	
Aminoethylethanolamine	Soldering, cable jointer	(229,230)	2	NA	ND	ND	ND	+	
Dimethylethanolamine	Spray paint	(231)	1	NA	−	ND	ND	+	

	Occupation		No.					Cross-shift change in FEV_1
Other								
3-(Dimethylamino)-propylamine (3-DMAPA)	Ski manufacture	(232)	34	11.7	ND	ND	ND	ND
Heterocyclic amines								
Piperazine hydrochloride	Chemist	(233)	2	NA	50% +	ND	ND	100%
	Pharmaceutical	(234)	131	11.4	ND	ND	ND	100% of 1+
	Chemical plant	(235)	2	50% +	100% +	ND	ND	ND
N-methyl-morpholine		(236)	48	16.6[b]	ND	ND	ND	ND
Aromatic amines								
Paraphenylene diamine	Fur dyeing	(237)	80	37.0	66%+	ND	ND	74%+
Quaternary amines (benzalkonium)	Cleaning product	(238)	1	NA	+	ND	ND	+
Mixture of amines								
EPO 60	Mould maker	(239)	1	NA	ND	ND	ND	+
Fluxes								
Colophony	Electronics workers	(240)	34	NA	ND	ND	ND	100% +
	Manufacture solder flux	(241)	68 low	4	ND	ND	ND	ND
			14 med.	21	ND	ND	ND	ND
Zinc chloride and ammonium chloride flux 95%	Metal jointing	(242)	6 high	21	ND	ND	ND	ND
			2	NA	ND	ND	ND	+ (PC20)
Alkylarul polyether alcohol +5% polypropylene glycol	Electronics assembler	(243)	1	NA	ND	ND	ND	+
Wood dust or bark								
Western red cedar (*Thuja plicata*)	Carpentry	(244)	35	NA	ND	ND	ND	ND (Improvement on removal)

(*Continued*)

Agents Causing Occupational Asthma with Key References (*Continued*)

Agents	Occupation	References	Subjects	Prevalence (n)	Skin (%)	Specific IgE test	Other immunologic test	Broncho-provocation test	Other evidence
	Furniture making	(245)	1320	3.4	1.9% +	ND	ND	ND	
	Cabinet making, carpentry	(246)	22		100% −	ND	100% −precipitin	82%	
	Sawmill	(247)	185	4.1	100%	ND	ND	100%+	Questionnaire
Eastern white cedar (*Thuja occidentalis*)	Sawmill	(248)	652	4–7%	100%	ND	ND	ND	PC20
		(249)	3		ND	ND	ND	+	
California redwood (*Sequoia sempervirens*)	Woodcarvers	(250)	2	NA	−	ND	−precipitin	+	
Cedar of Lebanon (*Cedra libani*)	Carpenter	(251)	1	NA	ND	ND	ND	+	
		(252)	6	NA	17%+	ND	100% −precipitin	ND	
Cocabolla (*Dalbergin retusa*)		(253)	3	NA	100% −	ND	ND	ND	Improvement on removal
Iroko (*Chlorophora excelsa*)		(254)	1	NA	+	ND	+ precipitin	+	
	Carpenter	(255)	1	NA	ND	ND	ND	+	
	Woodworkers	(256)	9	NA	4/9 with + intradermal test	Negative	ND	+	PEF
Oak (*Quercus robur*)		(257)	1	NA	−	ND	+ precipitin	+	
Mahogany (*Shoreal* sp.)		(258)	3	NA	ND	ND	+ precipitin	+	
		(257)	1	NA	−	ND	+ precipitin	+	
Abiruana (*Pouteria*)		(259)	2	NA	+	ND	− precipitin	+	
African maple (*Triplochiton scleroxylon*)		(260)	2	NA	+	+	Passive transfer	+	
Sauna building	Sauna building	(261)	2	NA	100% +	100% +		+	

Common name (species)	Ref.	Occupation	No.	%				
Tanganyika aningre	(262)		3	NA	100%+	100%–	100%–precipitin	100%+
Mukali (*Angineria robusta*)	(263)		1	NA	+	+	ND	+
Central American walnut (*Juglans olanchana*)	(264)		1	NA	–	–	– precipitin	+
Kejaat (*Pterocarpus angolensis*)	(265)		1	NA	+	ND	ND	ND
African zebrawood (*Microberlinia*)	(266)		1	NA	+	+	ND	+
Ramin (*Gonystylus bancanus*)	(267)	Woodworker	2	NA	+	+	ND	+
	(268)	Saponin factory	1	NA	ND	+	ND	+
Fernambouc (*Caesalpinia echinata*)	(269)	Bow making	36	33.3	100%–	ND	ND	100% of 1 +
Ash (*Fraxinus americana*)	(270)	Sawmill	1	NA	–	–	ND	+
Ash (*Fraxinus escelsior*)	(271)	Furniture	1	NA	–	+	ND	+
Pau Marfim (*Balfourodendron riedelianum*)	(272)	Woodworker	1	NA	+	+	ND	+
Capreuva (*Myyrocarpus fastigiattus* Fr. All.)	(273)	Parquet floor layer	1	NA	ND	ND	ND	+
Ebony wood (*Diospyros crassiflora*)	(274)		1	NA	–	ND	ND	+
Kotibe wood (*Nesorgordonia papverifera*)	(275)		1	NA	+	ND	Passive transfer	+
Cinnamon (*Cinnamomum zeylanicum*)	(276)		40	22.5	ND	ND	ND	100% of 1+

(*Continued*)

Agents Causing Occupational Asthma with Key References (*Continued*)

Agents	Occupation	References	Subjects	Prevalence (*n*)	Skin (%)	Specific IgE test	Other immunologic test	Broncho-provocation test	Other evidence
Imbuia (Brazilian walnut)	Furniture	(277)	1	NA	ND	ND	+ precipitin	+	Neg PEF
Blackwood (*Acacia melanoxylon*)	Furniture	(278)	3	NA	ND	ND	ND	+	+PEF
African cherry (Makore)	Cabinet worker	(279)	1	NA	–	ND	ND	+	
Antiaris	Door manufacturer	(280)	1	NA	+	+	SDS-PAGE	+	
Unidentified agent	Sawmills of Eastern Canada and United States	(281)	11	NA	ND	ND	ND	+	PEF
Metals									
Platinum	Platinum refinery	(282)	16	NA	62%+	ND	ND	62%+	
		(283)	136	29	17%+	21%+	ND	ND	
Nickel	Metal plating	(284)	1	NA	+	ND	– precipitin	+	
		(285)	1	NA	+	ND	– precipitin	+	
		(286)	1	NA	+	+	ND	+	
Cobalt	Hard metal grinders	(287)	4	NA	25%+	ND	ND	50%+	
	Diamond polisher	(288)	3	NA	ND	ND	ND	100%+	
Palladium	Assembly line	(289)	1	NA	+	ND	ND	+	
Zinc fumes	Solderers	(290)	2	NA	ND	ND	ND	+	
	Locksmith	(291)	1	NA	ND	ND	ND	+	
Tungsten carbide	Grinder	(292)	1	NA	ND	ND	ND	ND	Recovery on removal
Chromium	Printer	(293)	1	NA	+	ND	ND	ND	

Substance	Occupation/Source	Ref	No.	NA					Notes
Chromate salt	Cement floorer	(294)	1	NA	ND	ND	ND	+	
	Plater	(295)	1	NA	+	ND	ND	ND	
	Various	(296)	4	NA	+	ND	ND	+	
Chromium and nickel	Welder	(297)	5	NA	ND	ND	ND	100% of 2+	
	Tanning	(298)	1	NA	−	+	+	+	
	Electroplating	(299)	7	NA	Cr 29%+ Ni 57%+	+	ND	Cr 100% of 7	
	Cobalt and nickel	(300)	8	NA	75% cobalt / 62%+ nickel	62%+ cobalt / 50%+ nickel	62%+ cobalt / ND	100%+to both cobalt and nickel	
Aluminum	Soldering	(301)	1	NA	Nickel ND	Nickel ND	ND	+	
Drugs									
Penicillins and ampicillin	Pharmaceutical	(302)	4	NA	100% −	ND	ND	75%+	
Penicillamine	Pharmaceutical	(303)	1	NA	ND	−	ND	+	
Cephalosporins	Pharmaceutical	(304)	2	NA	+	ND	ND	+	PEF
	Pharmaceutical	(305)	91	8	71%+	ND	ND	ND	Improvement off work
Phenylglycine acid chloride	Pharmaceutical	(306)	24	29	37%+	37%+	Passive transfer	100% of 2+	
Psyllium	Laxative manufacturing	(307)	3	NA	100%+	ND	ND	60% +	
	Pharmaceutical	(308)	130	4[a]	19% of 120 +	26% of 118+	ND	27% of 18+	
	Nurses	(309)	5	NA	80%+	100% +	ND	100% +	
	Health personnel	(310)	193	4[a]	3%+	12% of 162 +	ND	26% of 15+	
Methyl dopa	Pharmaceutical	(311)	1	NA	−	ND	ND	+	
Spiramycin	Pharmaceutical	(312)	1	NA	+	ND	ND	+	
	Pharmaceutical	(313)	51	8[a]	100%−	ND	ND	25% of 12+	
	Pharmaceutical	(314)	2	NA	ND	−	ND	+	
Salbutamol intermediate	Pharmaceutical	(315)	1	NA	−	ND	ND	+	

(Continued)

Agents Causing Occupational Asthma with Key References (*Continued*)

Agents	Occupation	References	Subjects	Prevalence (n)	Skin (%)	Specific IgE test	Other immunologic test	Broncho-provocation test	Other evidence
Amprolium	Poultry feed mixer	(316)	1	NA	ND	ND	ND	+	
Tetracycline	Pharmaceutical	(317)	1	NA	ND	ND	ND	+	
Isonicotinic acid hydrazide	Hospital pharmacy	(318)	1	NA	+	+	ND	+	
Hydralazine	Pharmaceutical	(319)	1	NA	-	-	- specific IgG	+	
Tylosin tartrate	Pharmaceutical	(320)	1	NA	ND	ND	ND	+	
Ipecacuanha	Pharmaceutical	(321)	42	48	52% of 19+	66% of 18+	ND	ND	
Cimetidine	Pharmaceutical	(322)	4	NA	ND	ND	ND	25%+	
Piperacillin	Pharmaceutical	(323)	1	NA	+	ND	ND	+	
Ceftazidine	Pharmaceutical	(324)	1	NA	ND	ND	ND	+	
Opiate compounds	Pharmaceutical	(325)	39	26	+	ND	ND	ND	PEF
	Pharmaceutical	(326)	4	14	+	+	ND	+	Pre-post shift FEV_1
Amoxicillin	Pharmaceutical	(327)	1	NA	-	-	ND	+	
Mitoxantrone	Nurse	(328)	1	NA	ND	ND	ND	+	PEF Alveolar lavage
Reactive dyes									
Reactive dyes	Reactive dyes manufacture	(329)	309	25	7%+ orange 8%+ black	17%+ orange 17%+ black	ND	65% of 20+	
	Wool dye house	(330)	6	NA	ND	83%+	100%+	ND	
	Textile dye house	(331)	162	NA	NA	85% of 5 +	ND	ND	
Levafix brilliant yellow E36	Prep dye solution	(332)	1	NA	+	ND	ND	+	
Drimaren brilliant yellow K-3GL	Textile industry	(333)	1	NA	+	ND	ND	+	
Black henna	Herbal shop sales	(334)	1	NA	+	+	ND	ND	PEF monitoring

Agent	Occupation	Ref.	N						Comments
FD&C blue dye #2 Cibachrome brilliant	Food industry	(335)	1	NA	–	–	ND	+	
Scarlet 32	Textile industry	(333)	1	NA	+	ND	ND	++	
Drimaren brilliant blue K-BL	Textile industry	(333)	1	NA	+	ND	ND	++	
Lanasol yellow 4G	Dyer	(333)	1	NA	+	ND	ND	+	
Carmine	Dye manufacture	(336)	10	NA	30%+	30%+	ND	100% of 1	
Monascus ruber (food colorant)	Delicatessen plant	(337)	1	NA	+	ND	+immuno-blotting	+	PC20
Biocides									
Hexachlorophene	Hospital staff (sterilizing agent)	(338)	1	NA	ND	ND	ND	+	
Chlorhexidine	Nurse	(339)	2	NA	ND	ND	ND	+	
Glutaraldehyde	Hospital endoscopy unit	(340)	9	89	ND	ND	ND	ND	Questionnaire
Chloramine T	Endoscopy and radiology	(341)	8	NA	ND	ND	ND	7/8 +	PEF monitoring
	Chemical manufacturing	(342)	6	NA	100% +	100% +	66%+ passive transfer	ND	
	Brewery	(343)	7	NA	100% +	100% +	ND	ND	Recovery with removal
Chloramine	Janitor-cleaning	(344)	5	NA	100% of 4+	ND	ND	100% of 3+	
	Lifeguard swimming teacher	(345)	3	NA	ND	ND	ND	+	PEF
Lauryl dimethyl benzyl ammonium chloride	Pharmacist	(346)	1	NA	ND	ND	ND	+	PEF
Isothizolinone	Chemical plant	(347)	1	NA	ND	ND	ND	+	
Fungicides									
Tetracholoro-isophthalonitrile	Farmer	(348)	1	NA	ND	–	+patch test	+	FEV$_1$ recording at work

(*Continued*)

Agents Causing Occupational Asthma with Key References (*Continued*)

Agents	Occupation	References	Subjects	Prevalence (n)	Skin (%)	Specific IgE test	Other immunologic test	Broncho-provocation test	Other evidence
Tributyl tin oxide	Venipuncture technician	(349)	1	NA	–	ND	ND	+	
Captafol	Chemical manufacturing	(350)	1	NA	–	ND	ND	+	
Chemicals									
Polyvinyl chloride (fumes; powder)	Meat wrapper	(351)	96	69	ND	ND	ND	27% of 11+	
	Meat wrapper	(352)	3	NA	ND	ND	ND	ND	History only
	Manufacturing bottle caps	(353)	1	NA	ND	ND	ND	+	PEF
Organic phosphate insecticides	Chemical packaging plant	(354)	1	NA	ND	ND	ND	ND	History only PC20
Tetramethrin	Extermination	(355)	1	NA	–	ND	ND	+	
Persulfate salts and henna	Hairdressing	(356)	2	NA	+	ND	ND	+	
	Hairdressing	(357)	2	NA	+	ND	ND	100% of 4+	
	Hairdressing	(358)	23	17	4%+	ND	ND	+	
	Hairdressing	(359)	1	NA	–	ND	ND	+	
	Hairdressing	(360)	1	NA	ND	ND	ND	+	
Diazonium salt	Manufacturing of photocopy paper	(361)	1	NA	ND	ND	ND	+	
	Manufacturing of fluorine polymer precursor	(362)	45	56	ND	20%+	ND	100% of 2	
Urea formaldehyde	Resin	(363)	2	NA	–	ND	ND	+	
	Resin	(364)	3	NA	ND	ND	ND	100% of 3	

Agent	Occupation	Ref	N						
	Manufacturing of foam	(365)	1	NA	ND	ND	ND		
Freon	Refrigeration	(366)	1	NA	ND	ND	ND		
Furfuryl alcohol (furan based resin)	Foundry mold making	(367)	1	NA	ND	ND	ND	+	
Styrene	Plastics factory	(368)	2	NA	-	ND	ND	+	
Azobisformamide	Plastics, rubber	(369)	151	18.5	ND	ND	ND	ND	Removal with improvement
Iso-nonanyl oxybenzene sulfonate	Plastics	(370)	2	NA	ND	ND	ND	+	
	Plastics	(371)	4	NA	ND	ND	ND	100% of 2+	
	Laboratory technician	(372)	1	NA	ND	ND	ND	+	
Tetrazene	Detonator manufacturing	(373)	1	NA	ND	ND	ND	+	PEF
Polyethylene	Paper packer	(374)	1	NA	ND	ND	ND	+	PEF
Tall oil (pine resin)	Rubber tire manufacturer	(375)	1	NA	-	ND	- patch test	+	PEF
Sulfites	Water plant	(376)	1	NA	-	ND	oral +	oral +	
	Food processor	(377)	1	NA	ND	ND	ND	+	
	Bag manufacturer	(378)	1	NA	ND	ND	ND	+	PEF
Polyester	Painter	(379)	1	NA	ND	ND	ND	+	Alveolitis
Glacial acetic acid	Picking	(380)	1	NA	ND	+	ND	ND	
Ninhydrin	Laboratory worker	(381)	1	NA	ND	ND	ND	+	PEF
1,2-Benzisolhizolin-3-one	Chemical worker	(382)	1	NA	ND	ND	ND	+	
Metabisulfite	Agricultural producer	(377)	1	NA	ND	ND	ND	ND	
Health care									
Ethylene oxide	Nurse	(383)	1	NA	ND	+	ND	+	Changes in PC20

(Continued)

Agents Causing Occupational Asthma with Key References (*Continued*)

Agents	Occupation	References	Subjects	Prevalence (n)	Skin (%)	Specific IgE test	Other immunologic test	Broncho-provocation test	Other evidence
Enflurane	Hospital staff	(384)	1	NA	ND	ND	ND	+	
Methyl blue	Hospital staff	(385)	1	NA	ND	ND	ND	+	
Terpene	Hospital staff	(386)	1	NA	ND	ND	ND	+	
Radiographic fixative	Hospital staff	(387)	1	NA	ND	ND	ND	+	
Sulfathiazoles	Hospital staff	(388)	2	NA	−	ND	ND	+	
Formaldehyde	Hospital staff	(389)	28	29[a]	ND	ND	ND	50% of 4+	
	Different industries	(390)	15	NA	ND	ND	ND	60%+	
Methyl methacrylate and cyanoacrylates		(391)	230	5	ND	ND	ND	5%+	
	Adhesive	(392)	7	NA	ND	ND	ND	86%+	PEF 14%+
	Nurse	(393)	1	NA	ND	ND	ND	+	
	Glue	(394)	1	NA	ND	ND	ND	+	PEF monitoring
Diacrylate	Autobody shop	(395)	1	NA	ND	ND	ND	+	
Synthetic material Plexiglass	Factory	(396)	1		ND	ND	ND	+	Pre-postchange in FEV$_1$
Tooth enamel dust	Dentist	(397)	1	NA	ND	ND	ND	ND	

Agent	Occupation/industry	Ref	No. of subjects	%					Method of diagnosis
ECG ink	Laboratory nurse	(385)	1	NA	+	ND	ND	+	Questionnaire
Unidentified (?)	Respiratory therapist	(398)	194	19	ND	ND	ND	ND	Questionnaire PC20
(?)	Mineral analysis laboratory	(399)	21	24[b]	ND	ND	ND	ND	PEF recording PC20, FEV_1
(?) Oil mists	Toolsetter	(400)	1	NA	ND	ND	ND	+	PEF recording
(?) Metalworking fluid	Automobile plant	(401)	12	1.5	ND	ND	ND	ND	PC20, FEV_1
(?) Fluorine	Potroom	(402)	52	NA	ND	ND	ND	ND	History
(?) Aluminum	Potroom	(403)	227	7	ND	ND	ND	ND	Questionnaire
(?) Aluminum	Potroom	(404)	35	NA	ND	ND	ND	ND	History
(?) Aluminum	Potroom	(405)	57	NA	ND	ND	ND	ND	History
(?) Aluminum	Potroom	(406)	1	NA	ND	ND	ND	+	PEF monitoring
Aluminum chloride	Foundry worker	(407)	1	NA	ND	ND	ND	+	PEF recording
(?) Pulverized fuel ash	Power station attendant	(408)	1	NA	ND	ND	ND	+	PEF recording

Note: The number of subjects tested is not specified if it included all subjects; otherwise it is mentioned.

a Based on challenge data.

b Presence of bronchial hyperresponsiveness.† Subjects with symptoms.

c Subjects with symptoms.

PCA = Passive cutaneous analphylaxis polymethylene polyphenylisocyanate. All proportions including three or more as the denominator are expressed as %.

NA = Not assessed

ND = Not done

REFERENCES

1. Venables KM, Tee RD, Hawkins ER, et al. Laboratory animal allergy in a pharmaceutical company. Br J Ind Med 1988; 45:660–666.
2. Newman TA, Longbottom JL, Pepys J. Respiratory allergy to urine proteins of rats and mice. Lancet 1977; 2:847–849.
3. Mäntyjärvi J, Ylönen R, Taivainen A, Virtanen T. IgG and IgE antibody responses to cow dander and urine in farmers with cow-induced asthma. Clin Exp Allergy 1992; 22:83–90.
4. Petry RW, Voss MJ, Kroutil LA, Crowley W, Bush RK, Busse WW. Monkey dander asthma. J Allergy Clin Immunol 1985; 75:268–271.
5. Nahm DH, Park JW, Hong CS. Occupational asthma due to deer dander. Ann Allergy Asthma Immunol 1996; 76:423–426.
6. Gomez IJ, Anton E, Picans I, Jerez J, Obispo T. Occupational asthma caused by mink urine. Allergy 1996; 51:364–365.
7. Bar-Sela S, Teichtahl H, Lutsky I. Occupational asthma in poultry workers. J Allergy Clin Immunol 1984; 73:271–275.
8. Lutsky I, Teichtahl H, Bar-Sela S. Occupational asthma due to poultry mites. J Allergy Clin Immunol 1984; 73:56–60.
9. Perfetti L, Cartier A, Malo JL. Occupational asthma in poultry-slaughterhouse workers. Allergy 1997; 52:594–595.
10. Brennan NJ. Pig Butcher's asthma—case report and review of the literature. Irish Med J 1985; 78:321–322.
11. Armentia A, Martin-Santos J, Subiza J, et al. Occupational asthma due to frogs. Ann Allergy 1988; 60:209–210.
12. Moneret-Vautrin DA, Pupil P, Courtine D, Grilliat JP. Asthme professionnel aux protéines du lactosérum. Rev Fr Allergol 1984; 24:93–95.
13. Joliat TL, Weber RW. Occupational asthma and rhinoconjunctivitis from inhalation of crystalline bovine serum albumin powder. Ann Allergy 1991; 66:301–304.
14. Bernaola G, Echechipia S, Urrutia I, Fernandez E, Audicana M, Corres LF. Occupational asthma and rhinoconjunctivitis from inhalation of dried cow's milk caused by sensitization to alpha-lactalbumin. Allergy 1994; 49:189–191.
15. Olaguibel JM, Hernandez D, Morales P, Peris A, Basomba A. Occupational asthma caused by inhalation of casein. Allergy 1990; 45:306–308.
16. Smith AB, Bernstein DI, London MA, et al. Evaluation of occupational asthma from airborne egg protein exposure in multiple settings. Chest 1990; 98:398–404.
17. Breton JL, Leneutre F, Esculpavit G, Abourjaili M. Une nouvelle cause d'asthme professionnel chez un préparateur en pharmacie. La Presse Médicale 1989; 18:433.
18. El-Ansary EH, Gordon DJ, Tee RD, Newman-Taylor AJ. Respiratory allergy to inhaled bat guano. Lancet 1987; 1:316–318.
19. Armstrong RA, Neill P, Mossop RT. Asthma induced by ivory dust: a new occupational cause. Thorax 1988; 43:737–738.
20. Zedda S. A case of bronchial asthma from inhalation of nacre dust. Med del Lavoro 1967; 58:459–464.
21. Charpin J, Blanc M. Une cause nouvelle d'allergie professionnelle chez les coiffeuses: l'allergie à la séricine. Marseille Médical 1967; 104:169–170.
22. Cartier A, Malo JL, Forest F, et al. Occupational asthma in snow crab-processing workers. J Allergy Clin Immunol 1984; 74:261–269.
23. Gaddie J, Legge JS, Friend JAR, Reid TMS. Pulmonary hypersensitivity in prawn workers. Lancet 1980; 2:1350–1353.
24. Jyo T, Kohmoto K, Katsutani T, Otsuka T, Oka SD, Mitsui S. Hoya (Sea-squirt) asthma. In: Occupational Asthma. CA Frazier, ed. Von Nostrand Reinhold, London 1980:209–228.

25. Desjardins A, Malo JL, L'Archevêque J, Cartier A, McCants M, Lehrer SB. Occupational IgE-mediated sensitization and asthma due to clam and shrimp. J Allergy Clin Immunol 1995; 96:608–617.

26. Lemière C, Desjardins A, Lehrer S, Malo JL. Occupational asthma to lobster and shrimp. Allergy 1996; 51:272–273.

27. Baur X, Huber H, Chen Z. Asthma to Gammarus shrimp. Allergy 2000; 55:96–97.

28. Goetz DW, Whisman BA. Occupational asthma in a seafood restaurant worker: cross-reactivity of shrimp and scallops. Ann Allergy Asthma Immunol 2000; 85:461–466.

29. Tomaszunas S, Weclawik Z, Lewinski M. Allergic reactions to cuttlefish in deep-sea fishermen. Lancet 1988; 1:1116–1117.

30. Beltrami V, Innocenti A, Pieroni MG, Civai R, Nesi D, Bianco S. Occupational asthma due to cuttle-fish bone dust. Med Lav 1989; 80:425–428.

31. Douglas JDM, McSharry C, Blaikie L, Morrow T, Miles S, Franklin D. Occupational asthma caused by automated salmon processing. Lancet 1995; 346:737–740.

32. Sherson D, Hansen I, Sigsgaard T. Occupationally related respiratory symptoms in trout-processing workers. Allergy 1989; 44:336–341.

33. Carino M, Elia G, Molinini R, Nuzzaco A, Ambrosi L. Shrimpmeal asthma in the aquaculture industry. Med Lav 1985; 76:471–475.

34. Onizuka R, Inoue K, Kamiya H. Red soft coral-induced allergic symptoms observed in spiny lobster fishermen. Aerugi 1990; 39:339–347.

35. Baldo BA, Krilis S, Taylor KM. IgE-mediated acute asthma following inhalation of a powdered marine sponge. Clin Allergy 1982; 12:179–186.

36. Rodriguez J, Reano M, Vives R, et al. Occupational asthma caused by fish inhalation. Allergy 1997; 52:866–869.

37. Cuthbert OD, Jeffrey IG, McNeill HB, Wood J, Topping MD. Barn allergy among scottish farmers. Clin Allergy 1984; 14:197–206.

38. Blainey AD, Topping MD, Ollier S, Davies RJ. Allergic respiratory disease in grain workers: the role of storage mites. J Allergy Clin Immunol 1989; 84:296–303.

39. Groenewoud GCM, Jong de NW, Nes van Oorschot-van AJ, et al. Prevalence of occupational allergy to bell pepper pollen in greenhouses in the Netherlands. Clin Exper Allergy 2002; 32:434–440.

40. Burge PS, Edge G, O'Brien IM, Harries MG, Hawkins R, Pepys J. Occupational asthma in a research centre breeding locusts. Clin Allergy 1980; 10:355–363.

41. Tee RD, Gordon DJ, Hawkins ER, et al. Occupational allergy to locusts: an investigation of the sources of the allergen. J Allergy Clin Immunol 1988; 81:517–525.

42. Gibbons HL, Dille JR, Cowley RG. Inhalant allergy to the screwworm fly. Arch Environ Health 1965; 10:424–430.

43. Bagenstose AH, Mathews KP, Homburger HA, Saaveard-Delgado AP. Inhalant allergy due to crickets. J Allergy Clin Immunol 1980; 65:71–74.

44. Stevenson DD, Mathews KP. Occupational asthma following inhalation of moth particles. J Allergy 1967; 39:274–283.

45. Siracusa A, Marcucci F, Spinozzi F, et al. Prevalence of occupational allergy due to live fish bait. Clin Exp Allergy 2003; 33:507–510.

46. Randolph H. Allergic reaction to dust of insect origin. JAMA 1934; 103:560–562.

47. Wittich FW. Allergic rhinitis and asthma due to sensitization to the Mexican bean weevil (*Zabrotes subfasciatus boh*). J Allergy 1940; 12:42–45.

48. Spieksma FTM, Vooren PH, Kramps JA, Dijkman JH. Respiratory allergy to laboratory fruit flies (*Drosophila melanogaster*). J Allergy Clin Immunol 1986; 77:108–113.

49. Ostrom NK, Swanson MC, Agarwal MK, Yuninger JW. Occupational allergy to honeybee-body dust in a honey-processing plant. J Allergy Clin Immunol 1986; 77:736–740.

50. Siracusa A, Bettini P, Bacoccoli R, Severini C, Verga A, Abbritti G. Asthma caused by live fish bait. J Allergy Clin Immunol 1994; 93:424–430.

51. Schroeckenstein DC, Meier-Davis S, Graziano FM, Falomo A, Bush RK. Occupational sensitivity to *Alphitobius diaperinus* (Panzer) (lesser mealworm). J Allergy Clin Immunol 1988; 82:1081–1088.

52. Bernstein DI, Gallagher JS, Bernstein IL. Mealworm asthma: clinical and immunologic studies. J Allergy Clin Immunol 1983; 72:475–480.

53. Lutsky I, Bar-Sela S. Northern fowl mite (*Ornithonyssus sylviarum*) in occupational asthma of poultry workers. Lancet 1982; 2:874–875.

54. Cuthbert OD, Brostoff J, Wraith DG, Brighton WD. "Barn allergy": asthma and rhinitis due to storage mites. Clin Allergy 1979; 9:229–236.

55. Granel-Tena C, Cistero-Bahima A, Olive-Perez A. Allergens in asthma and baker's rhinitis. Alergia 1985; 32:69–73.

56. Michel FB, Guin JJ, Seignalet C, et al. Allergie à *Panonychus ulmi* (Koch). Rev Franç Allergol 1977; 17:93–97.

57. Kim YK, Son JW, Kim HY, et al. New occupational allergen in citrus farmers: citrus red mite (*Panonychus citri*). Ann Allergy Asthma Immunol 1999; 82:223–228.

58. Carbonnelle M, Lavaud F, Bailly R. Les acariens de la vigne sont-ils susceptibles de provoquer une allergie respiratoire? Rev Fr Allergol 1986; 26:171–178.

59. Astarita C, Franzese A, Scala G, Sproviero S, Raucci G. Farm workers occupational allergy to *Tetranychus urticae*: clinical and immunologic aspects. Allergy 1994; 49: 466–471.

60. Armentia A, Lombardero M, Barber D, et al. Occupational asthma in an agronomist caused by the lentil pest *Bruchus lentis*. Allergy 2003; 58:1200–1201.

61. Meister W. Professional asthma owing to Daphnia-allergy. Allerg Immunol (Leipz) 1978; 24:191–193.

62. Kaufman GL, Gandevia BH, Bellas TE, Tovey ER, Baldo BA. Occupational allergy in an entomological research centre. I Clinical aspects of reactions to the sheep blowfly *Lucilia cuprina*. Br J Ind Med 1989; 46:473–478.

63. Soparkar GR, Patel PC, Cockcroft DW. Inhalant atopic sensitivity to grasshoppers in research laboratories. J Allergy Clin Immunol 1993; 92:61–65.

64. Gold BL, Mathews KP, Burge HA. Occupational asthma caused by sewer flies. Am Rev Respir Dis 1985; 131:949–952.

65. Liebers V, Hoernstein M, Baur X. Humoral immune response to the insect allergen Chi t*I in aquarists and fish-food factory workers. Allergy 1993; 48:236–239.

66. Sheldon JM, Johnston JH. Hypersensitivity to beetles (Coleoptera). J Allergy 1941; 12:493–494.

67. Brito FF, Mur P, Barber D, et al. Occupational rhinoconjunctivitis and asthma in a wool worker caused by *Dermestidae spp*. Allergy 2002; 57:1191.

68. Alanko K, Tuomi T, Vanhanen M, et al. Occupational IgE-mediated allergy to *Tribolium confusum* (confused flour beetle). Allergy 2000; 55:879–882.

69. Uragoda CG, Wijekoon PMB. Asthma in silk workers. Occup Med 1991; 41:140–142.

70. Kobayashi S. Different aspects of occupational asthma in Japan. Occup Asthma. Van Nostrand Reinhold CompanyNew York1980229–244.

71. Armentia A, Lombardero M, Callejo A, et al. Occupational asthma by *Anisakis simplex*. J Allergy Clin Immunol 1998; 102:831–834.

72. Resta O, Foschino-Barbaro MP, Carnimeo N, Napoli Di PL, Pavese I, Schino P. Occupational asthma from fish-feed. Med Lav 1982; 3:234–236.

73. Lugo G, Cipolla C, Bonfiglioli R, et al. A new risk of occupational disease: allergic asthma and rhinoconjunctivitis in persons working with beneficial arthropods. Int Arch Occup Environ Health 1994; 65:291–294.

74. Lazaro MAG, Muela RA, Irigoyen JA, et al. Occupational asthma caused by hypersensitivity to ground bugs. J Allergy Clin Immunol 1997; 99:267–268.

75. Gottlieb SJ, Garibaldi E, Hutcheson PS, Slavin RG. Occupational asthma to the slime mold *Dictyostelium discoideum*. JOM 1993; 35:1231–1235.

76. Seaton A, Wales D. Clinical reactions to *Aspergillus niger* in a biotechnology plant: an eight year follow up. Occup Environ Med 1994; 51:54–56.
77. Jensen PA, Todd WF, Hart ME, Mickelsen RL, O'Brien DM. Evaluation and control of worker exposure to fungi in a beet sugar refinery. Am Ind Hyg Ass J 1993; 54:742–748.
78. Klaustermeyer WB, Bardana EJ, Hale FC. Pulmonary hypersensitivity to alternaria and aspergillus in baker's asthma. Clin Allergy 1977; 7:227–233.
79. Halpin DMG, Graneek BJ, Turner-Warwick M, Taylor AJN. Extrinsic allergic alveolitis and asthma in a sawmill worker: case report and review of the literature. Occup Environ Med 1994; 51:160–164.
80. Schaubschlager WW, Becker WM, Mazur G, Godde M. Occupational sensitization to *Plasmopara viticola*. J Allergy Clin Immunol 1994; 93:457–463.
81. Côté J, Chan H, Brochu G, Chan-Yeung M. Occupational asthma caused by exposure to neurospora in a plywood factory worker. Br J Ind Med 1991; 48:279–282.
82. Tarlo SM, Wai Y, Dolovich J, Summerbell R. Occupational asthma induced by *Chrysonilia sitophila* in the logging industry. J Allergy Clin Immunol 1996; 97: 1409–1413.
83. Gamboa PM, Jauregui I, Urrutia I, Antépara I, Gonzalez G, Mugica V. Occupational asthma in a coal miner. Thorax 1996; 51:867–868.
84. Ng TP, Tan WC, Lee YK. Occupational asthma in a pharmacist induced by *Chlorella*, a unicellular algae preparation. Respir Med 1994; 88:555–557.
85. Chan-Yeung M, Schulzer M, MacLean L, Dorken E, Grzybowski S. Epidemiologic health survey of grain elevator workers in British Columbia. Am Rev Respir Dis 1980; 121:329–338.
86. Williams N, Skoulas A, Merriman JE. Exposure to grain dust. I. A survey of the effects. JOM 1964; 6:319–329.
87. Skoulas A, Williams N, Merriman JE. Exposure to grain dust. II. A clinical study of the effects. JOM 1964; 6:359–372.
88. Chan-Yeung M, Wong R, MacLean L. Respiratory abnormalities among grain elevator workers. Chest 1979; 75:461–467.
89. Musk AW, Venables KM, Crook B, et al. Respiratory symptoms, lung function, and sensitisation to flour in a British bakery. Br J Ind Med 1989; 46:636–642.
90. Block G, Tse KS, Kijek K, Chan H, Chan-Yeung M. Baker's asthma. Clin Allergy 1983; 13:359–370.
91. Sutton R, Skerritt JH, Baldo BA, Wrigley CW. The diversity of allergens involved in bakers' asthma. Clin Allergy 1984; 14:93–107.
92. Valdivieso R, Quirce S, Sainz T. Bronchial asthma caused by *Lathyrus sativus* flour. Allergy 1988; 43:536–539.
93. Jansen A, Vermeulen A, van Toorenenbergen AW, Dieges PH. Occupational asthma in horticulture caused by *Lathyrus odoratus*. Allergy Proc 1995; 16:135–139.
94. Belchi-Hernandez J, Mora-Gonzalez A, Iniesta-Perez J. Baker's asthma caused by *Saccharomyces cerevisiae* in dry powder form. J Allergy Clin Immunol 1996; 97: 131–134.
95. Picon SJ, Carmona JGB, Sotillos MDMG. Occupational asthma caused by vetch (*Vicia sativa*). J Allergy Clin Immunol 1991; 88:135–136.
96. Ordman D. Buckwheat allergy. S Afr Med J 1947; 21:737–739.
97. Lachance P, Cartier A, Dolovich J, Malo JL. Occupational asthma from reactivity to an alkaline hydrolysis derivative of gluten. J Allergy Clin Immunol 1988; 81:385–390.
98. Jones RN, Hughes JM, Lehrer SB, et al. Lung function consequences of exposure and hypersensitivity in workers who process green coffee beans. Am Rev Respir Dis 1982; 125:199–202.
99. Zuskin E, Valic F, Kanceljak B. Immunological and respiratory changes in coffee workers. Thorax 1981; 36:9–13.
100. Osterman K, Johansson SGO, Zetterstrom O. Diagnostic tests in allergy to green coffee. Allergy 1985; 40:336–343.

101. Panzani R, Johansson SGO. Results of skin test and RAST in allergy to a clinically potent allergen (castor bean). Clin Allergy 1986; 16:259–266.

102. Igea JM, Fernandez M, Quirce S, Hoz de la B, Gomez MLD. Green bean hypersensitivity: an occupational allergy in a homomaker. J Allergy Clin Immunol 1994; 94:33–35.

103. van der Brempt X, Ledent C, Mairesse M. Rhinitis and asthma caused by occupational exposure to carob bean flour. J Allergy Clin Immunol 1992; 90:1008–1010.

104. Shirai T, Sato A, Hara Y. Epigallocatechin gallate. The major causative agent of green tea-induced asthma. Chest 1994; 106:1801–1805.

105. Blanc PD, Trainor WD, Lim DT. Herbal tea asthma. Br J Ind Med 1986; 43:137–138.

106. Gleich GJ, Welsh PW, Yunginger JW, Hyatt RE, Catlett JB. Allergy to tobacco: an occupational hazard. N Engl J Med 1980; 302:617–619.

107. Lander F, Gravesen S. Respiratory disorders among tobacco workers. Br J Ind Med 1988; 45:500–502.

108. Newmark FM. Hops allergy and terpene sensitivity: an occupational disease. Ann Allergy 1978; 41:311–312.

109. Twiggs JT, Yunginger JW, Agarwal MK, Reed CE. Occupational asthma in a florist caused by the dried plant, baby's breath. J Allergy Clin Immunol 1982; 69:474–477.

110. Toorenenbergen van AW, Dieges PH. Occupational allergy in horticulture: demonstration of immediate-type allergic reactivity to freesia and praprika plants. Int Arch Allergy Appl Immun 1984; 75:44–47.

111. Monso E, Magarolas R, Badorrey I, Radon K, Nowak D, Morera J. Occupational asthma in greenhouse flower and ornamental plant growers. Am J Respir Crit Care Med 2002; 165:954–960.

112. Miesen WM, Heide vander S, Kerstjens HA, Dubois AE, Monchy de JG. Occupational asthma due to IgE mediated allergy to the flower *Molucella laevis* (Bells of Ireland). Occup Environ Med 2003; 60:701–703.

113. Jansen APH, Visser FJ, Nierop G, et al. Occupational asthma to amaryllis. Allergy 1996; 51:847–849.

114. Rudzki E, Rapiejko P, Rebandel P. Occupational contact dermatitis, with asthma and rhinitis, from camomile in a cosmetician also with contact urticaria from both camomile and lime flowers. Contact Dermatitis 2003; 49:162.

115. Bolhaar STHP, Ginkel van CJW. Occupational allergy to cyclamen. Allergy 2000; 55:411–412.

116. Quirce S, Garcia-Figueroa B, Olaguibel JM, Muro MD, Tabar AI. Occupational asthma and contact urticaria from dried flowers of *Limonium tataricum*. Allergy 1993; 48(4):285–290.

117. Piirila P, Keskinen H, Leino T, Tupasela O, Tuppurainen M. Occupational asthma caused by decorative flowers: review and case reports. Int Arch Occup Environ Health 1994; 66:131–136.

118. Kanerva L, Makinen-Kijunen S, Kiistala R, Granlund H. Occupational allergy caused by spathe flower (*Spathiphyllum wallisii*). Allergy 1995; 50:174–178.

119. Demir AU, Karakaya G, Kalyoncu AF. Allergy symptoms and IgE immune response to rose: an occupational and an environmental disease. Allergy 2002; 57:936–939.

120. Moya CC, Hernandez AP, Calatayud MD, Baixauli EB, Salom BJM, Sastre A. Allergy to peach. Allergy 2002; 57:756–757.

121. Groenewoud GCM, Jong de NW, Burdorf A, Groot de H, Wÿk van RG. Prevalence of occupational allergy to *Chrysanthemum* pollen in greenhouses in the Netherlands. Allergy 2002; 57:835–840.

122. Gil M, Hogendjik S, Hauser C. Allergy to eggplant flower pollen. Allergy 2002; 57:652.

123. Zee vander JS, Jager de KSN, Kuipers BF, Stapel SO. Outbreak of occupational allergic asthma in a stephanotis floribunda nursery. J Allergy Clin Immunol 1999; 103:950–952.

124. Park HS, Kim MJ, Moons HB. Occupational asthma caused by two herb materials, *Dioscorea batatas* and *Pinellia ternata*. Clin Exp Allergy 1994; 24:575–581.

125. Grob M, Wuthrich B. Occupational allergy to the umbrella tree (*Schefflera*). Allergy 1998; 53:1008–1009.
126. Giavina-Bianchi PF, Castro FFM, Machado MLS, Duarte AJS. Occupational respiratory allergic disease induced by *Passiflora alata* and *Rhamnus purshiana*. Ann Asthma Allergy Immunol 1997; 79:449–454.
127. Vandenplas O, Depelchin S, Toussaint G, Delwiche JP, Weyer RV, Saint-Remy JM. Occupational asthma caused by sarsaparilla root dust. J Allergy Clin Immunol 1996; 97:1416–1418.
128. Lavaud F, Perdu D, Prévost A, Vallerand H, Cossart C, Passemard F. Baker's asthma related to soybean lecithin exposure. Allergy 1994; 49:159–162.
129. Benzarti M, Tlili MS, Klabi N, et al. Asthme aux tourteaux d'olives. Rev Fr Allergol 1986; 26:205–207.
130. Subiza J, Subiza JL, Escribano PM, et al. Occupational asthma caused by Brazil ginseng dust. J Allergy Clin Immunol 1991; 88:731–736.
131. Hinojosa M, Moneo I, Cuevas M, Diaz-Mateo P, Subiza J, Losada E. Occupational asthma caused by *Voacanga africana* seed dust. J Allergy Clin Immunol 1987; 79:574–578.
132. Valdivieso R, Subiza J, Varela-Losada S, et al. Bronchial asthma, rhinoconjunctivitis, and contact dermatitis caused by onion. J Allergy Clin Immunol 1994; 94:928–930.
133. Navarro JA, Pozo del MD, Gastaminza G, Moneo I, Audicana MT, Corres de LD. *Allium cepa* seeds: a new occupational allergen. J Allergy Clin Immunol 1995; 96:690–693.
134. Schwartz HJ, Jones RT, Rojas AR, Squillace DL, Yunginger JW. Occupational allergic rhinoconjunctivitis and asthma due to fennel seed. Ann Allergy Asthma Immunol 1997; 78:37–40.
135. Alday E, Curiel G, Lopez-Gil MJ, Carreno D. Occupational hypersensitivity to sesame seeds. Allergy 1996; 51:69–70.
136. Subiza J, Subiza JL, Hinojosa M, Varela S, Cabrera M, Marco F. Occupational asthma caused by grass juice. J Allergy Clin Immunol 1995; 96:693–695.
137. Quirce S, Gomez MLD, Hinojosa M, et al. Housewives with raw potato-induced bronchial asthma. Allergy 1989; 44:532–536.
138. Lopez-Rubio A, Rodriguez J, Crespo JF, Vives R, Daroca P, Reano M. Occupational asthma caused by exposure to asparagus: detection of allergens by immunoblotting. Allergy 1998; 53:1216–1220.
139. Miralles JC, Negro JM, Sanchez-Gascon F, Garcia M, Pascual A. Occupational rhinitis/asthma to courgette. Allergy 2000; 55:407–408.
140. Parra FM, Lazaro M, Cuevas M, et al. Bronchial asthma caused by two unrelated vegetables. Ann Allergy 1993; 70(4):324–327.
141. Symington IS, Kerr JW, McLean DA. Type I allergy in mushroom soup processors. Clin Allergy 1981; 11:43–47.
142. Michils A, Vuyst De P, Nolard N, Servais G, Duchateau J, Yernault JC. Occupational asthma to spores of *Pleurotus cornucopiae*. Eur Respir J 1991; 4:1143–1147.
143. Torricelli R, Johansson SGO, Wuthrich B. Ingestive and inhalative allergy to the mushroom *Boletus edulis*. Allergy 1997; 52:747–751.
144. Rubin JM, Duke MB. Unusual cause of bronchial asthma. Cacoon seed used for decorative purposes. NY State J Med 1974:538–539.
145. Cadot P, Kochuyt AM, Deman R, Stevens EAM. Inhalative occupational and ingestive immediate-type allergy caused by chicory (*Cichorium intybus*). Clin Exp Allergy 1996; 26:940–944.
146. Kwaselow A, Rowe M, Sears-Ewald D, Ownby D. Rose hips: a new occupational allergen. J Allergy Clin Immunol 1990; 85:704–708.
147. Bousquet OJ, Dhivert H, Clauzel AM, Hewitt B, Michel FB. Occupational allergy to sunflower pollen. J Allergy Clin Immunol 1985; 75:70–75.

148. Atis S, Tutluoglu B, Sahin K, Yaman M, Küçükusta AR, Oktay I. Sensitization to sunflower pollen and lung functions in sunflower processing workers. Allergy 2002; 57:35–39.

149. Blanco C, Carrillo T, Wuiralte J, Pascual C, Esteban MM, Castillo R. Occupational rhinoconjunctivitis and bronchial asthma due to *Phoenix canariensis* pollen allergy. Allergy 1995; 50:277–280.

150. Falleroni AE, Zeiss CR, Levitz D. Occupational asthma secondary to inhalation of garlic dust. J Allergy Clin Immunol 1981; 68:156–160.

151. Lybarger JA, Gallagher JS, Pulver DW, Litwin A, Brooks S, Bernstein IL. Occupational asthma induced by inhalation and ingestion of garlic. J Allergy Clin Immunol 1982; 69:448–454.

152. Cartier A, Malo JL, Labrecque M. Occupational asthma due to liquorice roots. Allergy 2002; 57:863.

153. van Toorenenbergen AW, Dieges PH. Immunoglobulin E antibodies against coriander and other spices. J Allergy Clin Immunol 1985; 76:477–481.

154. Feo F, Martinez J, Martinez A, et al. Occupational allergy in saffron workers. Allergy 1997; 52:633–641.

155. Lemière C, Cartier A, Lehrer SB, Malo JL. Occupational asthma caused by aromatic herbs. Allergy 1996; 51:647–649.

156. Catilina P, Chamoux A, Gabrillargues D, Catilina MJ, Royfe MH, Wahl D. Contribution à l'étude des asthmes d'origine professionnelle: l'asthme à la poudre de lycopode. Arch Mal Prof 1988; 49:143–148.

157. Axelsson IGK, Johansson SGO, Zetterstrom O. Occupational allergy to weeping fig in plant keepers. Allergy 1987; 42:161–167.

158. Kraut A, Peng Z, Becker AB, Warren CPW. Christmas candy maker's asthma. IgG4-mediated pectin allergy. Chest 1992; 102:1605–1607.

159. Starr JC, Yunginger J, Brahser GW. Immediate type I asthmatic response to henna following occupational exposure in hairdressers. Ann Allergy 1982; 48:98–99.

160. Dugue J, Bel J, Figueredo M. Le fenugrec responsable d'un nouvel asthme professionnel. La Presse Médicale 1993; 22:922.

161. Fraj J, Lezaun A, Colas C, Duce F, Dominguez MA, Alonso MD. Occupational asthma induced by aniseed. Allergy 1996; 51:337–339.

162. Kern DG, Kohn R. Occupational asthma following kapok exposure. J Asthma 1994; 31:243–250.

163. Tarlo SM, Wong L, Roos J, Booth N. Occupational asthma caused by latex in a surgical glove manufacturing plant. J Allergy Clin Immunol 1990; 85:626–631.

164. Vandenplas O, Delwiche JP, Evrard G, et al. Prevalence of occupational asthma due to latex among hospital personnel. Am J Respir Crit Care Med 1995; 151:54–60.

165. Juniper CP, How MJ, Goodwin BFJ. *Bacillus subtilis* enzymes: a 7-year clinical, epidemiological and immunological study of an industrial allergen. J Soc Occup Med 1977; 27:3–12.

166. Franz T, McMurrain KD, Brooks S, Bernstein IL. Clinical, immunologic, and physiologic observations in factory workers exposed to *B. subtilis* enzyme dust. J Allergy 1971; 47:170–179.

167. Colten HR, Polakoff PL, Weinstein SF, Strieder DJ. Immediate hypersensitivity to hog trypsin resulting from industrial exposure. N Engl J Med 1975; 292:1050–1053.

168. Baur X, Konig G, Bencze K, Fruhmann G. Clinical symptoms and results of skin test, RAST and bronchial provocation test in thirty-three papain workers: evidence for strong immunogenic potency and clinically relevant "proteolytic effects of airborne papain". Clin Allergy 1982; 12:9–17.

169. Cartier A, Malo JL, Pineau L, Dolovich J. Occupational asthma due to pepsin. J Allergy Clin Immunol 1984; 73:574–577.

170. Wiessmann KJ, Baur X. Occupational lung disease following long-term inhalation of pancreatic extracts. Eur J Respir Dis 1985; 66:13–20.

171. Pauwels R, Devos M, Callens L, Straeten Van der M. Respiratory hazards from proteolytic enzymes. Lancet 1978; 1:669.

172. Cortona G, Beretta F, Traina G, Nava C. Preliminary investigation in a pharmaceutical industry: bromelin induced pathology. Med Lav 1980; 1:70–75.

173. Galleguillos F, Rodriguez JC. Asthma caused by bromelin inhalation. Clin Allergy 1978; 8:21–24.

174. Bernstein JA, Kraut A, Warrington RJ, Bolin T, Bernstein DI. Clinical and immunologic evaluation of a worker with occupational asthma from exposure to egg lysozyme [abstr.]. J Allergy Clin Immunol 1991; 87:201.

175. Baur X, Fruhmann G, Haug B, Rasche B, Reiher W, Weiss W. Role of aspergillus amylase in baker's asthma. Lancet 1986; 1:43.

176. Birnbaum J, Latil F, Vervloet D, Senft M, Charpin J. Rôle de l'alpha-amylase dans l'asthme du boulanger. Rev Mal Respir 1988; 5:519–521.

177. Baur X, Melching-Kollmuss S, Koops F, Straßburger K, Zober A. IgE-mediated allergy to phytase—a new animal feed additive. Allergy 2002; 57:943–945.

178. Baur X, Weiss W, Sauer W, et al. Baking components as a contributory cause of baker's asthma. Dtsch Med Wschr 1988; 113:1275–1278.

179. Park HS, Nahm DH. New occupational allergen in a pharmaceutical industry: serratial peptidase and lysozyme chloride. Ann Allergy Asthma Immunol 1997; 78:225–229.

180. Zachariae H, Høegh-Thomsen J, Witmeur O, Wide L. Detergent enzymes and occupational safety. Observations on sensitization during Esperase® production. Allergy 1981; 36:513–516.

181. Tarvainen K, Kanerva L, Tupasela O, et al. Allergy from cellulase and xylanase enzymes. Clin Exp Allergy 1991; 21:609–615.

182. Sen D, Wiley K, Williams JG. Occupational asthma in fruit salad processing. Clin Exp Allergy 1998; 28:363–367.

183. Muir DCF, Verrall AB, Julian JA, Millman HM, Beaudin MA, Dolovich J. Occupational sensitization to lactase. Am J Ind Med 1997; 31:570–571.

184. Fowler PBS. Printers' asthma. Lancet 1952; 2:755–757.

185. Bohner CB, Sheldon JM, Trenis JW. Sensitivity to gum acacia, with a report of ten cases of asthma in printers. J Allergy 1941; 12:290–294.

186. Gelfand HH. The allergenic properties of vegetable gums: a case of asthma due to tragacanth. J Allergy 1943; 14:203–219.

187. Feinberg SM, Schoenkerman BB. Karaya and related gums as causes of atopy. Wiscousin Med J 1940; 39:734.

188. Malo JL, Cartier A, L'Archevêque J, et al. Prevalence of occupational asthma and immunological sensitization to guar gum among employees at a carpet-manufacturing plant. J Allergy Clin Immunol 1990; 86:562–569.

189. Boxer MB, Grammer LC, Orfan N. Gutta-percha allergy in a health care worker with latex allergy. J Allergy Clin Immunol 1994; 93:943–944.

190. Butcher BT, Salvaggio JE, Weill H, Ziskind MM. Toluene diisocyanate (TDI) pulmonary disease: immunologic and inhalation challenge studies. J Allergy Clin Immunol 1976; 58:89–100.

191. Butcher BT, O'Neil CE, Reed MA, Salvaggio JE. Radioallergosorbent testing of toluene diisocyanate-reactive individuals using p-tolyl isocyanate antigen. J Allergy Clin Immunol 1980; 66:213–216.

192. Baur X, Fruhmann G. Specific IgE antibodies in patients with isocyanate asthma. Chest 1981; 80:73S–76S.

193. Paggiaro PL, Filieri M, Loi AM, et al. Absence of IgG antibodies to TDI-HSA in a radioimmunological study. Clin Allergy 1983; 13:75–79.

194. Mapp CE, Boschetto P, Vecchio DL, Maestrelli P, Fabbri LM. Occupational asthma due to isocyanates. Eur Respir J 1988; 1:273–279.

195. Zammit-Tabona M, Sherkin M, Kijek K, Chan H, Chan-Yeung M. Asthma caused by diphenylmethane diisocyanate in foundry workers. Clinical, bronchial provocation, and immunologic studies. Am Rev Respir Dis 1983; 128:226–230.
196. Tse KS, Johnson A, Chan H, Chan-Yeung M. A study of serum antibody activity in workers with occupational exposure to diphenylmethane diisocyanate. Allergy 1985; 40:314–320.
197. Liss GM, Bernstein DI, Moller DR, Gallagher JS, Stephenson RL, Bernstein IL. Pulmonary and immunologic evaluation of foundry workers exposed to methylene diphenyldiisocyanate (MDI). J Allergy Clin Immunol 1988; 82:55–61.
198. Harris MG, Burge PS, Samson M, Taylor AJ, Pepys J. Isocyanate asthma: respiratory symptoms due to 1,5 naphthylene diisocyanate. Thorax 1979; 34:762–766.
199. Clarke CW, Aldons PM. Isophorone diisocyanate induced respiratory disease (IPDI). Aust NZ J Med 1981; 11:290–292.
200. Vandenplas O, Cartier A, Lesage J, Perrault G, Grammer LC, Malo JL. Occupational asthma caused by a prepolymer but not the monomer of toluene diisocyanate (TDI). J Allergy Clin Immunol 1992; 89:1183–1188.
201. Vandenplas O, Cartier A, Lesage J, et al. Prepolymers of hexamethylene diisocyanate (HDI) as a cause of occupational asthma. J Allergy Clin Immunol 1993; 91:850–861.
202. Séguin P, Allard A, Cartier A, Malo JL. Prevalence of occupational asthma in spray painters exposed to several types of isocyanates, including polymethylene polyphenyli-socyanates. JOM 1987; 29:340–344.
203. O'Brien IM, Harries MG, Burge PS, Pepys J. Toluene di-isocyanate-induced asthma. I. Reactions to TDI, MDI, HDI and histamine. Clin Allergy 1979; 9:1–6.
204. Baur X, Dewair M, Fruhmann G. Detection of immunologically sensitized isocyanate workers by RAST and intracutaneous skin tests. J Allergy Clin Immunol 1984; 73:610–618.
205. Cartier A, Grammer L, Malo JL, et al. Specific serum antibodies against isocyanates: association with occupational asthma. J Allergy Clin Immunol 1989; 84:507–514.
206. Pezzini A, Riviera A, Paggiaro P, et al. Specific IgE antibodies in twenty-eight workers with diisocyanate-induced bronchial asthma. Clin Allergy 1984; 14:453–461.
207. Piirila P, Estlander T, Keskinen H, et al. Occupational asthma caused by triglycidyl isocyanurate (TGIC). Clin Exp Allergy 1997; 27:510–514.
208. Kanerva L, Keskinen H, Autio P, Estlander T, Tuppurainen M, Jolanki R. Occupational respiratory and skin sensitization caused by polyfunctional aziridine hardener. Clin Exp Allergy 1995; 25:432–439.
209. Maccia CA, Bernstein IL, Emmett EA, Brooks SM. In vitro demonstration of specific IgE in phthalic anhydride hypersensitiviy. Am Rev Respir Dis 1976; 113:701–704.
210. Fawcett IW, Newman-Taylor AJ, Pepys J. Asthma due to inhaled chemical agents-epoxy resin systems containing phthalic acid anhydride, trimellitic acid anhydride and triethylene tetramine. Clin Allergy 1977; 7:1–14.
211. Wernfors M, Nielsen J, Schutz A, Skerfving S. Phthalic anhydride-induced occupational asthma. Int Arch Allergy Appl Immunol 1986; 79:77–82.
212. Nielsen J, Welinder H, Schütz A, Skerfving S. Specific serum antibodies against phthalic anhydride in occupationally exposed subjects. J Allergy Clin Immunol 1988; 82:126–133.
213. Zeiss CR, Patterson R, Pruzansky JJ, Miller MM, Rosenberg M, Levitz D. Trimellitic anhydride-induced airway syndromes: clinical and immunologic studies. J Allergy Clin Immunol 1977; 60:96–103.
214. Schlueter DP, Banaszak EF, Fink JN, Barboriak J. Occupational asthma due to tetra-chlorophthalic anhydride. JOM 1978; 20:183–187.
215. Howe W, Venables KM, Topping MD, et al. Tetrachlorophthalic anhydride asthma: evidence for specific IgE antibody. J Allergy Clin Immunol 1983; 71:5–11.
216. Meadway J. Asthma and atopy in workers with an epoxy adhesive. Br J Dis Chest 1980; 74:149–154.

217. Nielsen J, Welinder H, Skerfving S. Allergic airway disease caused by methyl tetrahydrophthalic anhydride in epoxy resin. Scand J Work Environ Health 1989; 15:154–155.

218. Chee CBE, Lee HS, Cheong TH, Wang YT. Occupational asthma due to hexahydrophthalic anhydride: a case report. Br J Ind Med 1991; 48:643–645.

219. Drexler H, Weber A, Letzel S, Kraus G, Schaller KH, Lehnert G. Detection and clinical relevance of a type I allergy with occupational exposure to hexahydrophthalic anhydride and methyltetrahydrophthalic anhydride. Int Arch Occup Envir Health 1994; 65:279–283.

220. Rosenman KD, Bernstein DI, O'Leary K, Gallagher JS, D'Souza L, Bernstein IL. Occupational asthma caused by himic anhydride. Scand J Work Environ Health 1987; 13:150–154.

221. Keskinen H, Pfaffli P, Lelttari P, et al. Chlorendic anhydride allergy. Allergy 2000; 55:98–99.

222. Lee HS, Lang YT, Cheong TH, Tan KT, Chee BE, Narendran K. Occupational asthma due to maleic anhydride. A case report diagnosed by inhalation challenge test. Br J Ind Med 1991; 48:283–285.

223. Cipolla C, Belisario A, Sassi C, Auletti G, Nobile M, Raffi GB. Occupational asthma due to dioctyl-phthalate in a bottle stopper production worker. Med Lav 1999; 90: 513–518.

224. Lam S, Chan-Yeung M. Ethylenediamine-induced asthma. Am Rev Respir Dis 1980; 121:151–155.

225. Gelfand HH. Respiratory allergy due to chemical compounds encountered in the rubber, lacquer, shellac, and beauty culture industries. J Allergy 1963; 34:374–381.

226. Ng TP, Lee HS, Malik MA, Chee CBE, Cheong TH, Wang YT. Asthma in chemical workers exposed to aliphatic polyamines. Occup Med 1995; 45:45–48.

227. Aleva RM, Aalbers R, Koëter GH, Monchy de JGR. Occupational asthma caused by a hardener containing an aliphatic and cycloliphatic diamine. Am Rev Respir Dis 1992; 145:1217–1218.

228. Savonius B, Keskinen H, Tuppurainen M, Kanerva L. Occupational asthma caused by ethanolamines. Allergy 1994; 49:877–881.

229. Pepys J, Pickering CAC. Asthma due to inhaled chemical fumes—amino-ethil ethanolamine in aluminium soldering flux. Clin Allergy 1972; 2:197–204.

230. Sterling GM. Asthma due to aluminium soldering flux. Thorax 1967; 22:533–537.

231. Vallières M, Cockcroft DW, Taylor DM, Dolovich J, Hargreave FE. Dimethyl ethanolamine-induced asthma. Am Rev Respir Dis 1977; 115:867–871.

232. Sargent EV, Mitchell CA, Brubaker RE. Respiratory effects of occupational exposure to an epoxy resin system. Arch Env Health 1976; 31:236–240.

233. Pepys J, Pickering CAC, Loudon HWG. Asthma due to inhaled chemical agents-piperazine dihydrochloride. Clin Allergy 1972; 2:189–196.

234. Hagmar L, Bellander T, Bergöö B, Simonsson BG. Piperazine-induced occupational asthma. JOM 1982; 24:193–197.

235. Welinder H, Hagmar L, Gustavsson C. IgE antibodies against piperazine and N-methyl-piperazine in two asthmatic subjects. Int Arch Allergy Appl Immunol 1986; 79:259–262.

236. Belin L, Wass U, Audunsson G, Mathiasson L. Amines: possible causative agents in the development of bronchial hyperreactivity in workers manufacturing polyurethanes from isocyanates. Br J Ind Med 1983; 40:251–257.

237. Silberman DE, Sorrell AH. Allergy in fur workers with special reference to paraphenylenediamine. J Allergy 1959; 30:11–18.

238. Bernstein JA, Stauder T, Bernstein DI, Bernstein IL. A combined respiratory and cutaneous hypersensitivity syndrome induced by work exposure to quaternary amines. J Allergy Clin Immunol 1994; 94:257–259.

239. Lambourn EM, Hayes JP, McAllister WA, Taylor NAJ. Occupational asthma due to EPO 60. Br J Ind Med 1992; 49:294–295.

240. Burge PS, Harries MG, O'Brien I, Pepys J. Bronchial provocation studies in workers exposed to the fumes of electronic soldering fluxes. Clin Allergy 1980; 10:137–149.
241. Burge PS, Edge G, Hawkins R, White V, Taylor AN. Occupational asthma in a factory making flux-cored solder containing colophony. Thorax 1981; 36:828–834.
242. Weir DC, Robertson AS, Jones S, Burge PS. Occupational asthma due to soft corrosive soldering fluxes containing zinc chloride and ammonium chloride. Thorax 1989; 44: 220–223.
243. Stevens JJ. Asthma due to soldering flux: a polyether alcohol-polypropylene glycol mixture. Ann Allergy 1976; 36:419–422.
244. Milne J, Gandevia B. Occupational asthma and rhinitis due to western (Canadian) red cedar. Med J Aust 1969; 2:741–744.
245. Ishizaki T, Sluda T, Miyamoto T, Matsumara Y, Mizuno K, Tomaru M. Occupational asthma from Western red cedar dust (*Thuja plicata*) in furniture factory workers. JOM 1973; 15:580–585.
246. Chan-Yeung M, Barton GM, MacLean L, Grzybowski S. Occupational asthma and rhinitis due to western red cedar (*Thuja plicata*). Am Rev Respir Dis 1973; 108: 1094–1102.
247. Chan-Yeung M, Lam S, Koerner S. Clinical features and natural history of occupational asthma due to western red cedar (*Thuja plicata*). Am J Med 1982; 72:411–415.
248. Chan-Yeung M, Vedal S, Kus J, Maclean L, Enarson D, Tse KS. Symptoms, pulmonary function, and bronchial hyperreactivity in Western Red Cedar workers compared with those in office workers. Am Rev Respir Dis 1984; 130:1038–1041.
249. Malo JL, Cartier A, L'Archevêque J, Trudeau C, Courteau JP, Bhérer L. Prevalence of occupational asthma among workers exposed to eastern white cedar. Am J Respir Crit Care Med 1994; 150:1697–1701.
250. Chan-Yeung M, Abboud R. Occupational asthma due to California redwood (*Sequoia sempervirens*) dusts. Am Rev Respir Dis 1976; 114:1027–1031.
251. doPico GA. Asthma due to dust from redwood (*Sequoia sempervirens*). Chest 1978; 73:424–425.
252. Greenberg M. Respiratory symptoms following brief exposure to cedar of Lebanon (*Cedra libani*) dust. Clin Allergy 1972; 2:219–224.
253. Eaton KK. Respiratory allergy to exotic wood dust. Clin Allergy 1973; 3:307–310.
254. Pickering CAC, Batten JC, Pepys J. Asthma due to inhaled wood dusts—western red cedar and iroko. Clin Allergy 1972; 2:213–218.
255. Azofra J, Olaguibel JM. Occupational asthma caused by iroko wood. Allergy 1989; 44:156–158.
256. Ricciardi L, Fedele R, Saitta S, et al. Occupational asthma due to exposure to iroko wood dust. Ann Allergy Asthma Immunol 2003; 91:393–397.
257. Sosman AJ, Schlueter DP, Fink JN, Barboriak JJ. Hypersensitivity to wood dust. New Engl J Med 1969; 281:977–980.
258. Malo JL, Cartier A, Desjardins A, Weyer RV, Vandenplas O. Occupational asthma caused by oak wood dust. Chest 1995; 108:856–858.
259. Booth BH, Lefoldt RH, Moffitt EM. Hypersensitivity to wood dust. J Allergy Clin Immunol 1976; 57:352–357.
260. Hinojosa M, Moneo I, Dominguez J, Delgado E, Losada E, Alcover R. Asthma caused by African maple (*Triplochiton scleroxylon*) wood dust. J Allergy Clin Immunol 1984; 74:782–786.
261. Reijula K, Kujala V, Latvala J. Sauna builder's asthma caused by obeche (*Triplochiton scleroxylon*) dust. Thorax 1994; 49:622–623.
262. Paggiaro PL, Cantalupi R, Filieri M, et al. Bronchial asthma due to inhaled wood dust: tanganyika aningre. Clin Allergy 1981; 11:605–610.
263. Sotillos MMG, Carmona JGB, Picon SJ, Gaston PR, Gimenez RP, Gil LA. Occupational asthma and contact urticaria caused by mukali wood dust (*Aningeria robusta*). J Invest Allergol Clin Immunol 1995; 5:113–114.

264. Bush RK, Clayton D. Asthma due to central American walnut (*Juglans olanchana*) dust. Clin Allergy 1983; 13:389–394.

265. Ordman D. Wood dust as an inhalant allergen. Bronchial asthma caused by kejaat wood (*Pterocarpus angolensis*). S Afr Med 1949; 23:973–975.

266. Bush RK, Yunginger JW, Reed CE. Asthma due to African zebrawood (*Microberlinia*) dust. Am Rev Respir Dis 1978; 117:601–603.

267. Hinojosa M, Losada E, Moneo I, Dominguez J, Carrillo T, Sanchez-Cano M. Occupational asthma caused by African maple (Obeche) and Ramin: evidence of cross reactivity between these two woods. Clin Allergy 1986; 16:145–153.

268. Raghuprasad PK, Brooks SM, Litwin A, Edwards JJ, Bernstein IL, Gallagher J. Quillaja bark (soapbark)-induced asthma. J Allergy Clin Immunol 1980; 65:285–287.

269. Hausen BM, Herrmann B. Bow-makers disease: an occupational disease in the manufacture of wooden bows for string instruments. Dtsch Med Wochenschr 1990; 115: 169–173.

270. Malo JL, Cartier A. Occupational asthma caused by exposure to ash wood dust (*Fraxinus americana*). Eur Respir J 1989; 2:385–387.

271. Fernandez-Rivas M, Pérez-Carral C, Senent CJ. Occupational asthma and rhinitis caused by ash (*Fraxinus excelsior*) wood dust. Allergy 1997; 52:196–199.

272. Basomba A, Burches E, Almodovar A, Rojas D, de Hernandez F. Occupational rhinitis and asthma caused by inhalation of *Balfourodendron riedelianum* (Pau Marfim) wood dust. Allergy 1991; 46:316–318.

273. Innocenti A, Romeo R, Mariano A. Asthma and systemic toxic reaction due to cabreuva (*Myrocarpus fastigiatus Fr. All.*) wood dust. Med del Lavoro 1991; 82:446–450.

274. Maestrelli P, Marcer G, Dal Vecchio L. Occupational asthma due to ebony wood (*Diospyros crassiflora*) dust. Ann Allergy 1987; 59:347–349.

275. Reques FG, Fernandez RP. Asthme professionnel à un bois exotique. *Nesorgordonia papaverifera* (danta ou kotibe). Rev Mal Respir 1988; 5:71–73.

276. Uragoda CG. Asthma and other symptoms in cinnamon workers. Br J Ind Med 1984; 41:224–227.

277. Jeebhay MF, Prescott R, Potter PC, Ehrlich RI. Occupational asthma caused by imbuia wood dust. J Allergy Clin Immunol 1996; 97:1025–1027.

278. Wood-Baker R. Occupational asthma due to Blackwood (*Acacia melanoxylon*). Aust NZ J Med 1997; 27:452–453.

279. Obata H, Dittrick M, Chan H, Chan-Yeung M. Occupational asthma due to exposure to African Cherry (Makore) wood dust. Intern Med 2000; 39:947–949.

280. Higuero NC, Zabala BB, Villamuza YG, et al. Occupational asthma caused by IgE-mediated reactivity to Antiaris wood dust. J Allergy Clin Immunol 2001; 107:554–555.

281. Malo JL, Cartier A, Boulet LP. Occupational asthma in sawmills of eastern Canada and United States. J Allergy Clin Immunol 1986; 78:392–398.

282. Pepys J, Pickering CAC, Hughes EG. Asthma due to inhaled chemical agents-complex salts of platinum. Clin Allergy 1972; 2:391–396.

283. Brooks SM, Baker DB, Gann PH, et al. Cold air challenge and platinum skin reactivity in platinum refinery workers. Chest 1990; 97:1401–1407.

284. McConnell LH, Fink JN, Schlueter DP, Schmidt MG. Asthma caused by nickel sensitivity. Ann Int Med 1973; 78:888–890.

285. Block GT, Yeung M. Asthma induced by nickel. JAMA 1982; 247:1600–1602.

286. Malo JL, Cartier A, Doepner M, Nieboer E, Evans S, Dolovich J. Occupational asthma caused by nickel sulfate. J Allergy Clin Immunol 1982; 69:55–59.

287. Hartmann AL, Walter H, Wuthrich B. Allergisches berufsasthma auf pektinase, ein pektolytisches enzym. Schweiz Med Wschr 1983; 113:265–267.

288. Gheysens B, Auxwerx J, Van Den Eeckhout A, Demedts M. Cobalt-induced bronchial asthma in diamond polishers. Chest 1985; 88:740–744.

289. Daenen M, Rogiers Ph, Van de Walle C, Rochette F, Demedts M, Nemery B. Occupational asthma caused by palladium. Eur Respir J 1999; 13:213–216.

290. Malo JL, Cartier A. Occupational asthma due to fumes of galvanized metal. Chest 1987; 92:375–377.
291. Vogelmeier C, König G, Bencze K, Fruhmann G. Pulmonary involvement in zinc fume fever. Chest 1987; 92:946–949.
292. Bruckner HC. Extrinsic asthma in a tungsten carbide worker. J Occup Med 1967; 9: 518–519.
293. Smith AR. Chrome poisoning with manifestations of sensitization. JAMA 1931; 94: 95–98.
294. deRaeve H, Vandecasteele C, Demedts M, Nemery B. Dermal and respiratory sensitization to chromate in a cement floorer. Am J Ind Med 1998; 34:169–176.
295. Joules H. Asthma from sensitization to chromium. Lancet 1932; 2:182–183.
296. Park HS, Yu HJ, Jung KS. Occupational asthma caused by chromium. Clin Exp Allergy 1994; 24:676–681.
297. Keskinen G, Kalliomaki PL, Alanko K. Occupational asthma due to stainless steel welding fumes. Clin Allergy 1980; 10:151–159.
298. Novey HS, Habib M, Wells ID. Asthma and IgE antibodies induced by chromium and nickel salts. J Allergy Clin Immunol 1983; 72:407–412.
299. Bright P, Burge PS, O'hickey SP, Gannon PFG, Robertson AS, Boran A. Occupational asthma due to chrome and nickel electroplating. Thorax 1997; 52:28–32.
300. Shirakawa T, Kusaka Y, Fujimura N, Kato M, Heki S, Morimoto K. Hard metal asthma: cross immunological and respiratory reactivity between cobalt and nickel. Thorax 1990; 45:267–271.
301. Vandenplas O, Delwiche JP, Vanbilsen ML, Roosels J, Joly D. Occupational asthma caused by aluminium welding. Eur Respir J 1998; 11:1182–1184.
302. Davies RJ, Hendrick DJ, Pepys J. Asthma due to inhaled chemical agents: ampicillin, benzyl penicillin, 6 amino penicillanic acid and related substances. Clin Allergy 1974; 4:227–247.
303. Lagier F, Cartier A, Dolovich J, Malo JL. Occupational asthma in a pharmaceutical worker exposed to penicillamine. Thorax 1989; 44:157–158.
304. Coutts II, Dally MB, Taylor AJN, Pickering CAC, Horsfield N. Asthma in workers manufacturing cephalosporins. Br Med J 1981; 283:950.
305. Briatico-Vangosa G, Beretta F, Bianchi S, et al. Bronchial asthma due to 7-aminocephalosporanic acid (7-ACA) in workers employed in cephalosporine production. Med Lav 1981; 72:488–493.
306. Kammermeyer JK, Mathews KP. Hypersensitivity to phenylglycine acid chloride. J Allergy Clin Immunol 1973; 52:73–84.
307. Busse WW, Schoenwetter WF. Asthma from psyllium in laxative manufacture. Ann Inter Med 1975; 83:361–362.
308. Bardy JD, Malo JL, Séguin P, et al. Occupational asthma and IgE sensitization in a pharmaceutical company processing psyllium. Am Rev Respir Dis 1987; 135:1033–1038.
309. Cartier A, Malo JL, Dolovich J. Occupational asthma in nurses handling psyllium. Clin Allergy 1987; 17:1–6.
310. Malo JL, Cartier A, L'Archevêque J, et al. Prevalence of occupational asthma and immunologic sensitization to psyllium among health personnel in chronic care hospitals. Am Rev Respir Dis 1990; 142:1359–1366.
311. Harries MG, Newman TA, Wooden J, MacAuslan A. Bronchial asthma due to alpha-methyldopa. Br Med J 1979:1461.
312. Davies RJ, Pepys J. Asthma due to inhaled chemical agents—the macrolide antibiotic Spiramycin. Clin Allergy 1975; 1:99–107.
313. Malo JL, Cartier A. Occupational asthma in workers of a pharmaceutical company processing spiramycin. Thorax 1988; 43:371–377.
314. Moscato G, Naldi L, Candura F. Bronchial asthma due to spiramycin and adipic acid. Clin Allergy 1984; 14:355–361.

315. Fawcett IW, Pepys J, Erooga MA. Asthma due to "glycyl compound" powder—an intermediate in production of salbutamol. Clin Allergy 1976; 6:405–409.

316. Greene SA, Freedman S. Asthma due to inhaled chemical agents—amprolium hydrochloride. Clin Allergy 1976; 6:105–108.

317. Menon MPS, Das AK. Tetracycline asthma—a case report. Clin Allergy 1977; 7:285–290.

318. Asai S, Shimoda T, Hara K, Fujiwara K. Occupational asthma caused by isonicotinic acid hydrazide (INH) inhalation. J Allergy Clin Immunol 1987; 80:578–582.

319. Perrin B, Malo JL, Cartier A, Evans S, Dolovich J. Occupational asthma in a pharmaceutical worker exposed to hydralazine. Thorax 1990; 45:980–981.

320. Lee HS, Wang YT, Yeo CT, Tan KT, Ratnam KV. Occupational asthma due to tylosin tartrate. Br J Ind Med 1989; 46:498–499.

321. Luczynska CM, Marshall PE, Scarisbrick DA, Topping MD. Occupational allergy due to inhalation of ipecacuanha dust. Clin Allergy 1984; 14:169–175.

322. Coutts II, Lozewicz S, Dally MB, et al. Respiratory symptoms related to work in a factory manufacturing cimetidine tablets. Br Med J 1984; 288:1418.

323. Moscato G, Galdi E, Scibilia J, et al. Occupational asthma, rhinitis and urticaria due to piperacillin sodium in a pharmaceutical worker. Eur Respir J 1995; 8:467–469.

324. Stenton SC, Dennis JH, Hendrick DJ. Occupational asthma due to ceftazidime. Eur Respir J 1995; 8:1421–1423.

325. Moneo I, Alday E, Ramos C, Curiel G. Occupational asthma caused by *Papaver somniferum*. Allergol Immunopathol 1993; 21:145–148.

326. Biagini RE, Bernstein DM, Klincewicz SL, Mittman R, Bernstein IL, Henningsen GM. Evaluation of cutaneous responses and lung function from exposure to opiate compounds among ethical narcotics-manufacturing workers. J Allergy Clin Immunol 1992; 89:108–117.

327. Jiminez I, Anton E, Picans I, Sanchez I, Quinones MD, Jerez J. Occupational asthma specific to amoxicillin. Allergy 1998; 53:104–105.

328. Walusiak J, Wittczak T, Ruta U, Palczynski C. Occupational asthma due to mitoxantrone. Allergy 2002; 57:461.

329. Alanko K, Keskinen H, Byorksten F, Ojanen S. Immediate-type hypersensitivity to reactive dyes. Clin Allergy 1978; 8:25–31.

330. Romano C, Sulotto F, Pavan I, Chiesa A, Scansetti G. A new case of occupational asthma from reactive dyes with severe anaphylactic response to the specific challenge. Am J Ind Med 1992; 21:209–216.

331. Nilsson R, Nordlinder R, Wass U, Meding B, Belin L. Asthma, rhinitis, and dermatitis in workers exposed to reactive dyes. Br J Ind Med 1993; 50:65–70.

332. Park HS, Lee MK, Kim BO, et al. Clinical and immunologic evaluations of reactive dye-exposed workers. J Allergy Clin Immunol 1991; 87:639–649.

333. Topping MD, Forster HW, Ide CW, Kennedy FM, Leach AM, Sorkin S. Respiratory allergy and specific immunoglobin E and immunoglobin G antibodies to reactive dyes used in the wool industry. J Occup Med 1989; 31:857–862.

334. Scibilia J, Galdi E, Biscaldi G, Moscato G. Occupational asthma caused by black henna. Allergy 1997; 52:231–232.

335. Miller ME, Lummus ZL, Bernstein DI. Occupational asthma caused by FD&C blue dye no.2. Allergy Asthma Proc 1996; 17:31–34.

336. Quirce S, Cuevas M, Olaguibel JM, Tabar AI. Occupational asthma and immunologic responses induced by inhaled carmine among employees at a factory making natural dyes. J Allergy Clin Immunol 1994; 93:44–52.

337. Vandenplas O, Caroyer JM, Cangh F Binard-van, Delwiche JP, Symoens F, Nolard N. Occupational asthma caused by a natural food colorant derived from *Monascus ruber*. J Allergy Clin Immunol 2000; 105:1241–1242.

338. Nagy L, Orosz M. Occupational asthma due to hexachlorophene. Thorax 1984; 39:630–631.

339. Waclawski ER, McAlpine LG, Thomson NC. Occupational asthma in nurses caused by chlorhexidine and alcohol aerosols. Br Med J 1989; 298:929–930.

340. Jachuck SJ, Bound CL, Steel J, Blain PG. Occupational hazard in hospital staff exposed to 2 per cent glutaraldehyde in an endoscopy unit. J Soc Occup Med 1989; 39:69–71.

341. Gannon PFG, Bright P, Campbell M, O'Hickey SP, Burge PS. Occupational asthma due to glutaraldehyde and formaldehyde in endoscopy and x ray departments. Thorax 1995; 50:156–159.

342. Feinberg SM, Watrous RM. Atopy to simple chemical compounds-sulfonechloramides. J Allergy 1945; 16:209–220.

343. Bourne MS, Flindt MLH, Walker JM. Asthma due to industrial use of chloramine. Br Med J 1979; 2:10–12.

344. Dijkman JG, Vooren PH, Kramps JA. Occupational asthma due to inhalation of chloramine-T. 1. Clinical observations and inhalation-provocation studies. Int Archs Allergy Appl Immunol 1981; 64:422–427.

345. Thickett KM, McCoach JS, Gerber JM, Sadhra S, Burge PS. Occupational asthma caused by chloramines in indoor swimming-pool air. Eur Respir J 2002; 19:827–832.

346. Burge PS, Richardson MN. Occupational asthma due to indirect exposure to lauryl dimethyl benzyl ammonium chloride used in a floor cleaner. Thorax 1994; 49:842–843.

347. Bourke SJ, Convery RP, Stenton SC, Malcolm RM, Hendrick DJ. Occupational asthma in an isothiazolinone manufacturing plant. Thorax 1997; 52:746–748.

348. Honda I, Kohrogi H, Ando M, et al. Occupational asthma induced by the fungicide tetrachloroisophthalonitrile. Thorax 1992; 47:760–761.

349. Shelton D, Urch B, Tarlo SM. Occupational asthma induced by a carpet fungicide—tributyl tin oxide. J Allergy Clin Immunol 1992; 90:274–275.

350. Royce S, Wald P, Sheppard D, Balmes J. Occupational asthma in a pesticides manufacturing worker. Chest 1993; 103:295–296.

351. Andrasch RH, Bardana EJ, Koster F, Pirofsky B. Clinical and bronchial provocation studies in patients with meatwrapper's asthma. J Allergy Clin Immunol 1976; 58:291–298.

352. Sokol WN, Aelony Y, Beall GN. Meat-wrapper's asthma. A new syndrome? JAMA 1973; 226:639–641.

353. Lee HS, Yap J, Wang YT, Lee CS, Tan KT, Poh SC. Occupational asthma due to unheated polyvinylchloride resin dust. Br J Ind Med 1989; 46:820–822.

354. Weiner A. Bronchial asthma due to the organic phosphate insecticides. Ann Allergy 1961; 19:397–401.

355. Vandenplas O, Delwiche JP, Auverdin J, Caroyer JM, Cangh Binard-Van F. Asthma to tetramethrin. Allergy 2000; 55:417–418.

356. Pepys J, Hutchcroft BJ, Breslin ABX. Asthma due to inhaled chemical agents-persulphate salts and henna in hairdressers. Clin Allergy 1976; 6:399–404.

357. Baur X, Fruhmann G, Liebe VV. Occupational asthma and dermatitis after exposure to dusts of persulfate salts in two industrial workers. Respiration 1979; 38:144–150.

358. Blainey AD, Ollier S, Cundell D, Smith RE, Davies RJ. Occupational asthma in a hairdressing salon. Thorax 1986; 41:42–50.

359. Pankow W, Hein H, Bittner K, Wichert P. Asthma in hairdressers induced by persulphate. Pneumologie 1989; 43:173–175.

360. Gamboa PM, de la Cuesta CG, García BE, Castillo JG, Oehling A. Late asthmatic reaction in a hairdresser, due to the inhalation of ammonium persulphate salts. Allergol Immunopathol 1989; 17:109–111.

361. Graham V, Coe MJS, Davies RJ. Occupational asthma after exposure to a diazonium salt. Thorax 1981; 36:950–951.

362. Luczynska CM, Hutchcroft BJ, Harrison MA, Dornan JD, Topping MD. Occupational asthma and specific IgE to diazonium salt intermediate used in the polymer industry. J Allergy Clin Immunol 1990; 85:1076–1082.

363. Cockcroft DW, Hoeppner VH, Dolovich J. Occupational asthma caused by cedar urea formaldehyde particle board. Chest 1982; 82:49–53.

364. Lemière C, Desjardins A, Cloutier Y, et al. Occupational asthma due to formaldehyde resin dust with and without reaction to formaldehyde gas. Eur Respir J 1995; 8:861–865.

365. Frigas E, Filley WV, Reed CE. Asthma induced by dust from urea-formaldehyde foam insulating material. Chest 1981; 79:706–707.

366. Malo JL, Gagnon G, Cartier A. Occupational asthma due to heated freon. Thorax 1984; 39:628–629.

367. Cockcroft DW, Cartier A, Jones G, Tarlo SM, Dolovich J, Hargreave FE. Asthma caused by occupational exposure to a furan-based binder system. J Allergy Clin Immunol 1980; 66:458–463.

368. Moscato G, Biscaldi G, Cottica D, Pugliese F, Candura S, Candura F. Occupational asthma due to styrene: two case reports. J Occup Med 1987; 29:957–960.

369. Slovak AJM. Occupational asthma caused by a plastics blowing agent, azodicarbona-mide. Thorax 1981; 36:906–909.

370. Normand J-C, Grange F, Hernandez C, et al. Occupational asthma after exposure to azodicarbonamide: report of four cases. Br J Ind Med 1989; 46:60–62.

371. Malo JL, Pineau L, Cartier A. Occupational asthma due to azobisformamide. Clin Allergy 1985; 15:261–264.

372. Hendrick DJ, Connolly MJ, Stenton SC, Bird AG, Winterton IS, Walters EH. Occupational asthma due to sodium iso-nonanoyl oxybenzene sulphonate, a newly developed detergent ingredient. Thorax 1988; 43:501–502.

373. Burge PS, Hendy M, Hodgson ES. Occupational asthma, rhinitis, and dermatitis due to tetrazene in a detonator manufacturer. Thorax 1984; 39:470–471.

374. Gannon PFG, Burge PS, Benfield CFA. Occupational asthma due to polyethylene shrink wrapping (paper wrapper's asthma). Thorax 1992; 47:759.

375. Tarlo SM. Occupational asthma induced by tall oil in the rubber tyre industry. Clin Exper Allergy 1991; 22:99–102.

376. Valero AL, Bescos M, Amat P, Mallet A. Asma bronquial por exposicion laboral a sulfitos. Bronchial asthma caused by occupational sulfite exposure. Allergol Immuno-pathol 1993; 21:221–224.

377. Malo JL, Cartier A, Desjardins A. Occupational asthma caused by dry metabisulphite. Thorax 1995; 50:585–586.

378. Malo JL, Cartier A, Pineault L, Dugas M, Desjardins A. Occupational asthma due to heated polypropylene. Eur Respir J 1994; 7:415–417.

379. Cartier A, Vandenplas O, Grammer LC, Shaughnessy MA, Malo JL. Respiratory and systemic reaction following exposure to heated electrostatic polyester paint. Eur Respir J 1994; 7:608–611.

380. Kivity S, Fireman E, Lerman Y. Late asthmatic response to inhaled glacial acetic acid. Thorax 1994; 49:727–728.

381. Piirila P, Estlander T, Hyrtonen M, Keskinen H, Tupasela O, Tuppurainen M. Rhinitis caused by nihydrin develops into occupational asthma. Eur Respir J 1997; 10:1918–1921.

382. Moscato G, Omodeo P, Dellabianca A, et al. Occupational asthma and rhinitis caused by 1,2-benzisothiasolin-3-one in a chemical worker. Occup Med 1997; 47:249–251.

383. Dugue P, Faraut C, Figueredo M, Bettendorf A, Salvadori JM. Asthme professionnel à l'oxyde d'éthylène chez une infirmière. Presse Méd 1991; 20:1455.

384. Schwettmann RS, Casterline CL. Delayed asthmatic response following occupational exposure to enflurane. Anesthesiology 1976; 44:166–169.

385. Rodenstein D, Stanescu DC. Bronchial asthma following exposure to ECG ink. Ann Allergy 1982; 48:351–352.

386. Seaton A, Cherrie B, Turnbull J. Rubber glove asthma. Br Med J 1988; 296:531–532.

387. Cullinan P, Hayes J, Cannon J, Madan L, Heap D, Taylor AN. Occupational asthma in radiographers. Lancet 1992; 340:1477.

388. Rosberg M. Asthma bronchiale caused by sulphathiazole. Acta Med Scand 1946; 126:185–190.

389. Hendrick DJ, Lane DJ. Formalin asthma in hospital staff. Br Med J 1975; 1:607–608.

390. Burge PS, Harries MG, Lam WK, O'Brien IM, Patchett PA. Occupational asthma due to formaldehyde. Thorax 1985; 40:255–260.

391. Nordman H, Keskinen H, Tuppurainen M. Formaldehyde asthma—rare or overlooked? J Allergy Clin Immunol 1985; 75:91–99.

392. Lozewicz S, Davison AG, Hopkirk A, et al. Occupational asthma due to methyl methacrylate and cyanoacrylates. Thorax 1985; 40:836–839.

393. Pickering CAC, Bainbridge D, Birtwistle IH, Griffiths DL. Occupational asthma due to methyl methacrylate in an orthopaedic theatre sister. Br Med J 1986; 292:1362–1363.

394. Chan CC, Cheong TH, Lee HS, Wang YT, Poh SC. Case of occupational asthma due to glue containing cyanoacrylate. Ann Acad Med 1994; 23:731–733.

395. Weytjens K, Cartier A, Lemière C, Malo JL. Occupational asthma to diacrylate. Allergy 1999; 54:289.

396. Kennes B, Garcia-Herreros P, Sierckx P. Asthma from plexiglas powders. Clin Allergy 1981; 11:49–54.

397. Housholder GT, Chan JT. Tooth enamel dust as an asthma stimulus. Oral Surg Oral Med Oral Pathol 1993; 75:599–601.

398. Kern DG, Frumkin H. Asthma in respiratory therapists. Ann Int Med 1989; 110:767–773.

399. Musk AW, Peach S, Ryan G. Occupational asthma in a mineral analysis laboratory. Br J Ind Med 1988; 45:381–386.

400. Hendy MS, Beattie BE, Burge PS. Occupational asthma due to an emulsified oil mist. Br J Ind Med 1985; 42:51–54.

401. Zacharisen MC, Kadambi AR, Schlueter DP, et al. The spectrum of respiratory disease associated with exposure to metal working fluids. J Occup Environ Med 1998; 40:640–647.

402. Midttun O. Bronchial asthma in the aluminium industry. Acta Allerg 1960; 15:208–221.

403. Saric M, Godnic-Cvar J, Gonzi M, Stilinovic L. The role of atopy in potroom workers' asthma. Am J Ind Med 1986; 9:239–242.

404. Wergeland E, Lund E, Waage JE. Respiratory dysfunction after potroom asthma. Am J Ind Med 1987; 11:627–636.

405. O'Donnell TV, Welford B, Coleman ED. Potroom asthma: New Zealand experience and follow-up. Am J Ind Med 1989; 14:43–49.

406. Desjardins A, Bergeron JP, Ghezzo H, Cartier A, Malo JL. Aluminium potroom asthma confirmed by monitoring of forced expiratory volume in one second. Am J Respir Crit Care Med 1994; 150:1714–1717.

407. Burge PS, Scott JA, McCoach J. Occupational asthma caused by aluminium. Allergy 2000; 55:779–780.

408. Davison AG, Durham S, Taylor AJN. Asthma caused by pulverised fuel ash. Br Med J 1986; 292:1561.

Index

Acid anhydride, 96–97, 100, 141, 150, 309–310
  effect of exposure to, 148
  respiratory symptoms, 267
Acoustic rhinometry, 787–788
Active sampling, 256–257, 299
Adenosine 5′-monophosphate (AMP), 112
Adult-onset asthma, 115. *See also* Asthma.
Aeroallergens, 55
Air pollution, 737
Airborne exposure, 694
  to natural rubber latex, 449
  urticaria from, 811
Airborne particulates, effects of, 257
Airborne sterilization, 768
Air-conditioning systems, 754, 767–768
Airflow limitations, 694
Airflow obstruction
  acute, 109–110
  chronic, 109, 111, 685, 692, 695
  in grain handlers, 657
  nonallergen-induced, 656
Airway disease, 663–665
  chronic, 683, 691
Airway hyper-reactivity, 581
Airway hyperresponsiveness (AHR), 109, 111, 142, 583–584, 589–591, 651, 657–658, 666
Airway inflammation, 121–122
  cellular components of, 123
  changes in, 188
  chronic, 71
  noninvasive assessment of, 124–125, 187–188
  phases of, 123
Airway microvascular leakage, 128
Airway narrowing, 110–111
Airway reactivity, heightened, 642
Airway remodeling, 71, 142, 150
Alastat microtiter plate assay, 446

Alcalase1®, 377, 380, 384, 388
Allergen dispersion, 276–277, 292
Allergens, 164
  animal, 420–421
  fish and shellfish, 428
  high-molecular weight protein, 151–153, 163
  insect, 426–427
  low-molecular weight, 163
  soybean hull, 266
Allergen-specific IgE, measurement of, 183–186
Allergy,
  enzyme-induced, 265
  laboratory animal allergy (LAA), 415–417, 425
  latex, 152
  symptoms, 744
Alpha-amylase, 54
Aluminum, 544–546
Alveolar macrophages, 668
Alveolitis, 125, 245–246
American Medical Association (AMA) Guidelines for Evaluation of Permanent Impairment, 340
American National Standards Institute, disease coding, 322
American Thoracic Society, 50, 169, 700
  guidelines, 338, 344
Americans with Disabilities Act, 341
Amines, 311
Analyte-specific reagents (ASR), 185
Animal allergens, 419–421
Antibody-mediated immunity, in occupational asthma, 118
Antigen-presenting cells, 113
Arachidonic acid, 123, 128
Arterial blood gas analysis, 339
Asbestosis, 69
Aspergillus, and *Alternaria*, 465, 469, 655